EMERGENCY PEDIATRICS
A Guide to Ambulatory Care

Editor

ROGER M. BARKIN, M.D., M.P.H., F.A.A.P., F.A.C.E.P.

Vice-President for Pediatric and Newborn Programs
HealthONE;
Professor of Surgery, Division of Emergency Medicine
University of Colorado Health Sciences Center
Denver, Colorado

Associate Editor

PETER ROSEN, M.D., F.A.C.E.P.

Director of Education, Department of Emergency Medicine;
Director, Emergency Medicine Residency Program;
Clinical Professor of Medicine and Surgery;
Assistant Director, Department of Emergency Medicine
University of California San Diego Medical Center
San Diego, California

FIFTH EDITION

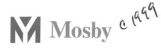 Mosby ©1999

St. Louis Baltimore Boston Carlsbad Chicago Minneapolis New York Philadelphia Portland
London Milan Sydney Tokyo Toronto

Mosby
Dedicated to Publishing Excellence

A Times Mirror Company

Publisher: Susie Baxter
Managing Editor: Kathryn H. Falk
Acquisitions Editor: Liz Fathman
Developmental Editor: Ellen Baker Geisel
Project Manager: Patricia Tannian
Senior Production Editor: Melissa Mraz Lastarria
Book Design Manager: Gail Morey Hudson
Manufacturing Supervisor: Linda Ierardi
Cover Designer: Teresa Breckwoldt

FIFTH EDITION
Copyright © 1999 by Mosby, Inc.

Previous editions copyrighted 1984, 1986, 1990, and 1994

Composition by Graphic World Inc.
Printing/binding by R.R. Donnelley & Sons Company
Jacket/Cover by Pinnacle Press, Inc.

Mosby, Inc.
11830 Westline Industrial Drive
St. Louis, Missouri 63146

Library of Congress Cataloging in Publication Data
Emergency pediatrics: a guide to ambulatory care / editor, Roger M.
   Barkin ; associate editor, Peter Rosen. — 5th ed.
       p.   cm.
    Includes bibliographical references and index.
    ISBN 0-323-00326-5
    1. Pediatric emergencies. I. Barkin, Roger M. II. Rosen, Peter.
    [DNLM: 1. Emergencies—in infancy & childhood. 2. Ambulatory
Care—in infancy & childhood.   WS 200E53   1999]
RJ370.E44   1999
618.92′0025—dc21
DNLM/DLC
for Library of Congress   98-26889
                                                                          CIP

99   00   01   02   03 / 9 8 7 6 5 4 3 2 1

CONTRIBUTORS

ADAM Z. BARKIN, B.A.
Vanderbilt University School of Medicine
Nashville, Tennessee

SUZANNE Z. BARKIN, M.D.
Director, Pediatric Imaging
Denver Health Medical Center;
Associate Professor of Radiology
University of Colorado Health Sciences Center
Denver, Colorado

GARY K. BELANGER, D.D.S.
Associate Professor and Chairman
Department of Pediatric Dentistry
University of Colorado School of Dentistry
Denver, Colorado

DIANE M. BOURLIER, D.O.
Pediatric Emergency Physician
CarePoint
Denver, Colorado

MICHELE CHETHAM, M.D.
Medical Director of Pediatric Emergency Services
CarePoint
Denver, Colorado

JOSEPH T. FLYNN, M.D.
Assistant Professor, Division of Pediatric
  Nephrology
University of Michigan Medical Center
Ann Arbor, Michigan

ROGER H. GILLER, M.D.
Associate Professor of Pediatrics
University of Colorado Health Sciences Center
Denver, Colorado

BENJAMIN HONIGMAN, M.D.
Director, Emergency Department
University Hospital;
Associate Professor of Surgery
Interim Head, Division of Emergency Medicine
Department of Surgery
University of Colorado Health Sciences Center
Denver, Colorado

ROBERT C. JORDEN, M.D.
Department of Emergency Medicine
Maricopa Medical Center
Phoenix, Arizona;
Clinical Professor of Emergency Medicine
University of Arizona
Tucson, Arizona

SUSAN B. KIRELIK, M.D.
Medical Director of Pediatric Urgent Care Services
CarePoint
Denver, Colorado

PAUL A. KOZAK, M.D.
Department of Emergency Medicine
Maricopa Medical Center
Phoenix, Arizona

KENNETH W. KULIG, M.D.
Toxicology Associates;
Associate Clinical Professor, Department of Surgery
Division of Emergency Medicine and Trauma
University of Colorado Health Sciences Center
Denver, Colorado

RONALD D. LINDZON, M.D.
Coordinator, Post-Graduate Residency Program
Emergency Medicine;
Assistant Professor, Department of Medicine
University of Toronto;
Staff Attending Physician, Emergency Department
Toronto General Hospital
Toronto, Ontario, Canada

VINCENT J. MARKOVCHICK, M.D.
Director, Emergency Medical Services
Denver Health Medical Center;
Associate Professor, Division of Emergency
   Medicine
Department of Surgery
University of Colorado Health Sciences Center
Denver, Colorado

JOHN A. MARX, M.D.
Chairman, Department of Emergency Medicine
Carolinas Medical Center
Charlotte, North Carolina;
Clinical Professor, Division of Emergency Medicine
University of North Carolina
Charlotte, North Carolina

DOUGLAS V. MAYEDA, M.D.
Associate Staff Physician, Department of Emergency
   Medicine
Penrose and St. Francis Health Services Hospital
Colorado Springs, Colorado

JAMES C. MITCHINER, M.D.
Associate Director, Department of Emergency
   Medicine
Hospital Emergency Medicine Residency Program
University of Michigan;
St. Joseph Mercy Hospital
Ann Arbor, Michigan

SANDY MOON, M.D.
Regional Medical Director, Pediatric Division
CarePoint
Denver, Colorado

ANTHONY F. PHILIPPS, M.D.
Professor of Pediatrics
Chief, Section of Neonatology and Developmental
   Biology
Department of Pediatrics
University of Arizona Health Sciences Center
Tucson, Arizona

PETER T. PONS, M.D.
Associate Director, Department of Emergency
   Medicine
Denver Health Medical Center;
Assistant Professor of Surgery
Division of Emergency Medicine
Department of Surgery
University of Colorado Health Sciences Center
Denver, Colorado

JEFFREY RICHKER, M.D.
Pediatric Emergency Physician
CarePoint
Denver, Colorado

THOMAS J. SMITH, M.D.
Childhood Hematology-Oncology Associates
Denver, Colorado

JAMES B. SPRAGUE, M.D.
Associate Clinical Professor, Department of
   Ophthalmology
Georgetown University School of Medicine and
   Health Sciences
Washington, D.C.

REGINALD L. WASHINGTON, M.D.
Rocky Mountain Pediatric Cardiology;
Associate Professor, Department of Pediatrics
University of Colorado Health Sciences Center
Denver, Colorado

ROCHELLE A. YANOFSKY, M.D.
Associate Professor, Section of Pediatric
   Hematology/Oncology
Department of Pediatrics
University of Manitoba
Winnipeg, Manitoba, Canada

FOREWORD

Over the past 36 years, a great number of medical students and some residents have told me something like the following: "I am afraid I cannot handle medicine as a career. Last night I worked in the emergency department, and a desperately ill accident victim was brought in for treatment. My only thought was to flee out the back door, and I was in a panic." I have always replied that I was so pleased to hear that because only people devoid of conscience will run toward such acute disasters with joy; to be scared is to be honest as well as intelligent.

The unprepared student soon acquires experience by working alongside senior role models, nurses, paramedics, and other physicians— learning that team care is essential. All emergencies require more than one set of hands. Practitioners must be well trained and intellectually as well as emotionally prepared to deal with anything that comes through the door. I always urge practicing physicians, residents, and students to "play" at situations where a mother rushes her child to the office or to the emergency department or where an urgent call comes from a ward and the immediate needs for survival must be practiced: an airway established, breathing ensured, and the vascular bed brought back to a capacity to carry oxygen to all organs. The entire team must maintain its competency to maximize each patient's chances. The ability to tell a four-star from a one-star emergency is learned with time.

Often the patient's history is obtained while urgent care for life support is given. It isn't easy to do both at the same time, yet both are required. This is no moment for textbooks or lengthy dissertations; ready access to a broad range of diagnostic and therapeutic information is needed. The basics are crucial and must be learned by heart. Where are vital medications? Where is a working laryngoscope? Who will assist the primary members of the team? What are the most important drug dosages, fluids, and electrolytes? Practice, expertise, organizations, and cooperation make the components flow smoothly.

Emergency care is always a bit scary, and it should be! It needs the best kind of quick and broadly based diagnostic thought and action. Yet, regardless of where the emergency is treated—even in the best-equipped and trained units—some patients will die. This is always a very bad time for all who have worked so hard to pull a youngster through. Recriminations between parents and relatives abound.

Among the members of the health care team,

there are similar frustrations, anger, and sorrow, and the temptation to scapegoat somebody must be avoided at all costs. It is best to lock the door, pick up, clean the dead child, and have the provisional rites of baptism administered to a Catholic child.* Important too is taking a few minutes to calm down before talking to the parents in a quiet place and with plenty of time. The response to "I am sorry we lost your baby" is often disbelief. Properly run emergency departments will already have seen that a supportive relative or a minister is in the waiting room. Relatives usually want to see the child, and they will remember these next moments forever.

Then follows the time of questioning. It is simply bad medicine to blame anyone, tempting though it may be. It is useless to tell a mother that she should have brought in the child 2 hours earlier or that the child's regular doctor should have diagnosed the problem better and sooner, even though that may be true. A devastated family needs compassion and support, wherever it can be found. In my experience, when families have been treated with respect and kindness, permission for diagnostic autopsies is routinely given.

---

*Note that any person of any faith can administer provisional baptism: "I baptize you in the name of the Father, the Son, and the Holy Spirit. Amen."

The field of emergency care is continuing to expand rapidly and well. Recent technical advances have made for better survival rates, and greater understanding of physiology has led to new and better medications. Thus emergency medicine has become a new and highly sophisticated specialty. Yet all physicians are expected to perform basic life-support procedures in any setting and, sometimes, without any help or tools.

This book addresses the field of pediatric emergencies in a comprehensive and readily accessible format, focusing on information that is immediately required. It contains these priority items, as well as those many conditions that permit more thought and time. It prepares the conscientious physician, resident, student, and other members of the team to overcome and thus lessen the anxiety that signifies a good conscience while capably performing all that is needed in an outwardly calm manner. In this field, experience allows rapid growth in building the confidence that management will be proficient.

I shall always trust and admire the competent, yet honestly frightened, practitioner.

The late C. Henry Kempe, M.D. (1922-1984)
Former Professor of Pediatrics and Microbiology,
University of Colorado Health Sciences Center,
Denver, Colorado

PREFACE

The fifth edition of *Emergency Pediatrics: A Guide to Ambulatory Care* reflects the dedication of clinicians, scientists, and teachers to the ongoing growth of an evolving specialty. Pediatric emergency medicine represents a redefined biology: pathophysiologic principles and research applied to the pediatric patients. This rapid evolution of knowledge necessarily generates controversy; concurrently, it stimulates searching, discussion, and analysis.

Children present a unique challenge and rare opportunity to the health care professional. Although medical and traumatic illnesses progress rapidly, the vast majority are expected to leave the child without sequelae and with a full life ahead.

The child is often frightened, and the history may be obtained only from parents. The data may initially be nonspecific, and frustration may be encountered in gaining cooperation and performing examinations, procedures, and tests.

A child's dependency on a familiar environment necessitates sensitivity to the concerns, fears, anxieties, and grief of families whose youngsters are experiencing major illness. Children are constantly looking for support from parents, who simultaneously are seeking small reassurances from a child, such as an infrequent smile or nod. This dependency is exaggerated during illness.

Understanding the time frame during which clinical decisions are based is the fundamental philosophy of managing the emergently ill child. Emergency physicians are unique in their need to solve problems within the time constraints of an acute illness, frequently modified by field considerations as well as the logistical demands of concurrent priorities and patients. Perhaps more than any other area of medicine, when the database conflicts with the clinical assessment, the clinician must often go with judgment and "gestalt"; it is often too easy to endow laboratory numbers with infallibility and ignore pertinent clinical findings.

This book brings together in an accessible format, that which is immediately required for the care of the acutely ill child by the health care provider, whether that individual is a pediatrician, emergency medicine physician, nurse practitioner, emergency medicine technician, or student of medicine. *Emergency Pediatrics* is a resource for the clinician to consult, analyze, alter, and add to as experience dictates but certainly not to leave on the bookshelf for leisure reading.

For those practitioners desiring greater clinical or pathophysiologic background in the management of pediatric patients in the emergency setting, *Pediatric Emergency Medicine: Concepts and Clinical Practice,* 2nd edition (St. Louis, 1997, Mosby) has recently been published.

This fifth edition incorporates many suggestions of readers for which we are most appreciative. It reflects the rapid expansion of available pharmacologic agents, changing recommendations for advanced life support, greater understanding of analgesia and sedation, evolving clinical entities, and broadened scientific and clinical literature. Emergency departments have increasingly become community clinics for children without routine sources of primary care; this is reflected in the scope of this book.

The initial sections of this book emphasize nontraumatic and traumatic conditions that may be life threatening, presenting strategies and diagnostic considerations crucial to stabilization. Resuscitation of the newborn and child reflects the latest in our knowledge base.

Throughout this book, diagnostic categories are organized alphabetically. Differentials are encompassed within the mnemonic *INDICATIVE:*

*i*nfection/*i*nflammation
*n*eoplasm
*d*egenerative/*d*eficiency
*i*ntoxication
*c*ongenital
*a*utoimmune/*a*llergy
*t*rauma
*i*ntrapsychic
*v*ascular
*e*ndocrine

Tables are used extensively to facilitate access to material; commonly encountered conditions are set in **boldface type** for ease of identification.

Diagnostic entities are the focus of a major section. The systems approach provides a resource for the vast majority of children's problems seen at any ambulatory facility. Specific attention is given to parental education, follow-up, and prevention. Appendixes are intended to provide a database for the practitioner.

We hope that this text will serve the clinician, stimulating future changes and advancement in the management of ambulatory patients whom we will encounter and to educate trainees who are committed to becoming clinicians. Clinical judgment is based on the combination of experience, reason, and an appropriate database. This synthesis must form the basis for our care of children.

Roger M. Barkin
Peter Rosen

ACKNOWLEDGMENTS

This book is a tribute to the outstanding medical and nursing staffs with whom it has been our pleasure to work with during the last three decades. It is a synthesis of many individuals' knowledge, experience, concerns, and sensitivities toward patient care in general, and children in particular.

We are grateful to HealthONE, the Department of Surgery at the University of Colorado Health Sciences Center, and the Department of Emergency Medicine of the University of California San Diego Medical Center for their ongoing support.

Beyond the numerous contributors who have generously written chapters, we are also appreciative of the expertise provided by the authors of *Pediatric Emergency Medicine: Concepts and Clinical Practice,* 2nd edition, that has been incorporated in this revision.

A host of dedicated professionals have produced this book through encouragement, cajoling, and compulsive attention to detail. The authors and editors have made it happen and kept it on schedule. Kathi Thompson facilitated and watched over the many administrative and organizational aspects of producing this book. We especially want to thank Kathy Falk, Robin Sutter, Patricia Tannian, Melissa Lastarria, and Ellen Baker Geisel of Mosby, Inc., and Suzanne Copple of Graphic World who have been there throughout the process of revising this book.

We would also like to thank our readers, who we hope will take this book with them to the front lines and use it with expertise and confidence in caring for pediatric patients to whom all of our efforts are dedicated.

Note: The indications for and dosages of medications recommended conform to practices at present; clinician judgment may alter management of a specific patient. References to specific products are incorporated to serve only as guidelines; they are not meant to exclude a practitioner's choice of other, comparable drugs. Many oral medications may be given with more scheduling flexibility than implied by the specific time intervals noted. Individual drug sensitivity and allergies must be considered in drug selection. Adult dosages are provided as a gauge of the maximum dosage commonly used.

Every attempt has been made to ensure accuracy and appropriateness. New investigations and broader experience may alter present dosage schedules, and it is recommended that the package insert of each drug be consulted before administration. Often there is limited experience with established drugs for neonates and young children. Furthermore, new drugs may be introduced, and indications for use may change. This rapid evolution is particularly noticeable in the use of antibiotics and cardiopulmonary resuscitation. The clinician is encouraged to maintain expertise concerning appropriate medications for specific conditions.

Contents

I

PEDIATRIC CARE IN THE EMERGENCY DEPARTMENT

1 APPROACHING THE PEDIATRIC PATIENT

Each encounter is an opportunity to observe a child and speak with parents. Unless the condition is life threatening, the initial focus should be on reducing anxiety by being friendly and interacting before threatening or painful aspects of the evaluation are undertaken. In approaching children, it is useful to assess their growth and development and provide counsel and assistance as appropriate and needed. Gleaning information about prior behavior, family and environmental issues, and unusual stress and pressures may point toward a functional rather than organic basis for a sign or symptom.

Understanding behavior may make the visit go more smoothly and allow the clinician to influence many aspects of care. Parental presence and participation during the encounter usually ease the process. Occasionally it is necessary to redirect a child's activity and redefine appropriate limits; consistency must be the basis for all such efforts. Expectations and limits should be appropriate for the child's development. Two-year-old children should not be asked to sit still and be "angels" while their parents speak to the physician. Anxiety is probably tremendous for everyone involved and may escalate "acting out behaviors."

THE DEVELOPING CHILD

Understanding the growth and development of children during their early years provides tremendous insight into pediatric care. Babies are unique, and during the first 2 years of life gain skills with a rapidity that is astounding. Each day new things are learned, new behaviors are evident, and new sounds and responses are present. Part of the excitement is that all children develop on somewhat different timetables. Although the pattern and general framework are consistent, the variability makes child development fun and full of surprises (see "Denver Development Screening Test," Appendix B-6).

Normal development provides insights into behavior and disease mechanisms and allows for a more thoughtful, age-specific evaluation of the child in the emergency department (ED). Children adopt behaviors that may occasionally be frustrating but are usually a part of normal development. Independence, separation anxiety, and jealousy are recurrent themes that form the basis for many developmental changes that have an impact on behavior. Most behaviors that pose problems are actually exaggerations of normal development and may be a reflection of the variability that exists among children in acquiring new skills. It is essential to recognize this in encouraging children to take age-appropriate risks and challenges that allow them to explore and experiment. Supporting and encouraging growth and the expansion of horizons lead to self-confidence.

Newborn

Babies arrive to anticipation and fanfare but create unexpected stress and time demands. Although babies have little control of muscles and can barely (if at all) hold their heads up, they have an amazing ability to look at their environment and respond to people, sounds, colors, and shapes. Babies' eyes follow to the midline, and infants enjoy looking at faces and occasionally interact with bright, shiny moving objects. They should be talked to, played with, and entertained.

The early weeks are ones of bonding with mother, father, and siblings. Time demands are intense: feedings to give, diapers to change, and laundry to do. These tasks fill the time between enjoying the baby and ensuring that other children are included and that spouses are not forgotten. Everyone must be part of the excitement and get pleasure from the new arrival while some semblance of family functioning is maintained.

The stress and sibling rivalry may lead to somatization in older children.

Six Weeks

Children by 6 weeks are increasingly able to do things and respond in a more positive and animated way to sounds, faces, actions, and so on. Even as newborns, babies are taking everything in; they are just not responding. By 6 weeks some children are making some sounds and smile in response to faces. They now follow past the midline.

Interactive playing is essential. Babies follow brightly colored objects better than dull objects and even make early attempts at grabbing things. However, they will not hold them or play with them in a consistent manner.

Babies sleep continuously but now there is greater responsiveness, and more noises are made; part of this becomes a response to the actions of others. They feed with somewhat more purpose and are less passive in terms of position and demands.

Four Months

By age 4 months, the infant is sociable and responds with an exciting array of facial expressions, sounds, and motions to every word. The baby constantly makes sounds, such as squeals, coos, and babbles, because he or she either gets pleasure from the noise or provokes a response from someone. Now babies will respond to most people who are willing to play, crawl, squeal, or make funny faces. Smiling becomes more common.

Muscle control improves, and physical interaction with the environment is more frequent. Children look at their hands and grab for things and are able to grasp an object with a wide swing of the arms and hands. They slowly develop the ability to self-support while in someone's arms or in an infant seat. One of the most exciting events is when a child finally turns over. Often the baby will not understand what has just happened and begin to cry after this tremendous feat. Some evidence also exists that babies enjoy being held in a standing position. All of this increased control allows children to entertain themselves and keep track of what is going on in a more active fashion. Their interest is still primarily in people.

Six Months

Children at 6 months are constantly exploring. Eyes, fingers, hands, and mouth become essential parts of this process. Everything is new and needs to be held, looked at, tasted, and chewed. Things can now be grabbed with more skill and even transferred from one hand to another. Cubes are common play toys. All of a sudden children become social beings, making sounds for themselves or anyone who will respond. Sitting becomes an important landmark at this age, and it may happen suddenly. Children are in constant motion, but crawling is limited by the inability to keep the stomach off the floor.

Nine Months

Increasingly, interaction with the world becomes more sophisticated. Body movements become more purposeful, usually in moving toward something that appears attractive. Standing is accomplished while they hold on to something. Babies reach out to learn about things, places, and people. Picking up objects and touching everything become common. The index finger and thumb can now work together in an efficient pincer action, and the baby's world is thereby expanded immeasurably.

For the baby, being included in everything is essential; games such as peek-a-boo are fun. At least the tone of "no" is understood. Sounds are made in a meaningful fashion, and "Dada" and "Mama," as well as imitation sounds, become incorporated into the language pattern. Children listen to readings of books with pictures for longer periods. Stranger anxiety becomes a dominant force. Parents are clearly preferred to everyone else, and children who a month earlier loved for anyone to hold them and pay attention now cry whenever someone else picks them up. There is tremendous variability in this stage and it will pass. It is part of the development toward being a healthy, independent person.

Sitting is now perfected; children also scoot or crawl, permitting mobility that is astounding. Many children never crawl much if they can scoot efficiently. Remember that the object is to get from one place to another, not necessarily to acquire skills that are not needed. Children enjoy standing up while holding on to some object.

Twelve Months

The first birthday is a landmark, and walking is the big achievement; children may not become efficient walkers for a few more months. The pincer grasp has improved, and playing with cubes and other objects is more sophisticated.

Communication skills have escalated and single words, especially "Mama" and "Dada," are clearly understood. Simple directions are understood and limit setting becomes a reality. Children are much more responsive, waving good-bye and wanting to do things by themselves. They now have the ability to ambulate and find things; feeding requires compromise because the child wants to hold the spoon while combining, smearing, and spilling foods. Dependency is still paramount. Although they like to do things by themselves, separation is still difficult. The security of the favorite blanket is essential, and often parents need to stay by the crib for a few minutes until the child goes to sleep.

Mobility is essential and becomes a part of the child's desire to explore and be independent, but the child still always wants the security of a loved one around. Providing an area that is safe to explore is helpful in assisting in this growth.

Eighteen Months

The 18-month-old child is an explorer whose world has expanded over the last few months. Walking has opened a whole new world and when combined with crawling leaves no place safe from the curiosity and initiative of the youngster. There is a tremendous sense of independence and a much greater focus on what he or she really wants. Separation from parents is now more acceptable, but frequent checks for eye contact are reassuring.

Behavior becomes somewhat inconsistent; children may develop fears of certain things, such as baths or loud noises. "No" becomes an important part of an expanded vocabulary, particularly when the child's desires are not met. Often children demonstrate their temper and displeasure with these limits. Diverting attention to more acceptable activities is usually easy at this age. At this time consistency is important to internalizing appropriate behavior patterns for children.

Vocabulary has increased to several single words, and there is constant babbling. Words are imitated, and usually one or more body parts are incorporated into normal play. Playing with friends is now more fun, although it is often done in parallel, with minimal interaction with peers. Often children become frustrated when they cannot do something; diverting their attention may be useful. Children can turn pages by themselves and they like to draw and scribble. They can partially undress themselves at this time.

Two Years

Independence is the hallmark of the 2-year-old child, who is trying to build new skills and competencies. Two-year-old children want to do everything themselves and have everything exactly their way. They want choices, and these should be given when appropriate (e.g., a choice of what clothes to wear but not a choice about when to go to bed or eat). The 2-year-old child has emblazoned the word "No" on all communications. Periodically, these intense feelings of independence do give way to a need to be held, praised, and supported; enjoy these moments while they last.

Obviously, children can now move around with tremendous skill, even using tricycles. Balls can be kicked, steps climbed, and objects jumped. Vocabulary becomes increasingly sophisticated, and sentences can be understood and words combined. Pictures can often be named and body parts identified. Cooperative play and sharing remain limited. Listening to stories is a favorite activity, as is helping with housework.

Three Years

Three-year-old children can pedal the tricycle and go up stairs using alternate steps. They enjoy playing with blocks and can even stack them. Balls can usually be thrown overhand a small distance. Copying drawings is tremendous fun. Speech is more understandable, and children can describe pictures by combining different objects and describing the action within the story. Play is more interactive. Masturbation may occur.

Four Years

Hopping is a favorite activity, and sense of balance greatly improves at age 4 years. People increasingly become the subject of their drawings, and they still love to copy and imitate pictures. Speech is totally understandable and naming opposites is a favorite game. "Why," "how," and "when" are constantly included in all questions and should be recognized as important parts of the learning process.

Children can usually dress themselves with help, and many are toilet trained. Separation from parents is easier, and play groups work cooperatively.

Five to Eight Years

Balancing is possible at 5 to 8 years, and the child plays with a bouncing ball with improved eye-hand coordination and speed. Drawings of people are more complicated, including multiple body parts. Exploring is constant. More control of their environment is expected and self-reliance is observed. Increasingly group activities, sports, and diversions are requested by the child.

Language is tremendously important and children know body parts; vocabulary is expanded and counting improves.

They can dress themselves.

Older Children

With more years, children develop enhanced and increasing independence. The ED encounter can be less frightening if particular attention is directed to communicating with and relieving anxiety in the child and parents. Parents increasingly become allies in this process. With this growth also comes greater experimentation, which on occasion may lead to "acting out" and other patterns that increase the risk of injury. The rationality of this age group should be considered but not overestimated. Children's fears, anxiety, and concern over body image must be respected.

Children and adolescents are developing and responding to their environment. A responsiveness to behavioral, physical, familial, and environmental stresses and problems will provide a more optimal focus in the care of the pediatric patient in the ED.

The ED clinician must understand the growth and development of children. An awareness of these unique patterns provides unique challenges and delights for all those involved in patient care and allows greater sensitivity in approaching children and their families during times of stress.

II

ADVANCED CARDIAC LIFE SUPPORT

2 EMERGENCY DEPARTMENT ENVIRONMENT

The expansion of emergency services is a response to a growing demand for accessible, efficient, and superior health care facilities. The pediatric patient is seen in a variety of emergency department (ED) settings. Often the patient is integrated into a general ED with a specific environment and staff for children: Equipment, supplies, and expertise must be available. More and more EDs are developing separate physical areas for children, providing personnel, equipment, and space conducive to caring for youngsters, but integrating major resuscitation activities with the expertise and responsiveness of the entire staff. Children's hospitals with EDs have provided for the needs of children through triage, evaluation, and treatment systems. The growth of pediatric emergency medicine fellowships has broadened the cadre of physicians with a specific pediatric focus.

Approximately 25% to 35% of patients in the general ED are pediatric, presenting problems ranging from benign, self-limited conditions to those that are life threatening. Fewer than 5% require admission, a statistic that emphasizes the noncritical nature of most encounters. Parents take children to the ED for a variety of reasons. Many who have private health care providers have been frustrated in their attempts to schedule an appointment with their regular physician and feel that their children require immediate attention to relieve discomfort. Others prefer the anonymity of the emergency facility and use it as their primary source of health care. A significant number of patients have been directed to the emergency facility by health care professionals.

The ED is a major focus of pediatric health care in the United States and a central component of the emergency medical services system. In balancing the medical, nursing, and related needs of pediatric patients, it is essential to ensure that EDs reflect the unique medical and nursing care requirements of this age group. Whether the child is seen in an area that treats only children or one that treats all ages, certain aspects need to be addressed prospectively to ensure family-oriented, high-quality, effective care.

CLINICAL ASPECTS

Traditional components of triage, history, physical, laboratory assessment, and management are essential. Children who require emergent care should be treated, irrespective of formal consent. Adults cannot generally make decisions that significantly jeopardize the health of a child by the refusal of care. Emancipated minors are those who live apart from their parents, are self-supporting, and are not subject to parental control as well as those individuals who are married, pregnant, or members of the armed forces. Many states have special provisions related to venereal disease, pregnancy, and drug related problems.

Federal regulations (EMTALA and COBRA) require a screening examination for all patients presenting to an ED.

Beyond the traditional clinical components of

Box 2-1

INITIAL NURSING ASSESSMENT OF PEDIATRIC PATIENTS

1. Age
2. Chief complaint: history of present illness (brief), recent interventions, and contacts with health professionals/facilities
3. Previous medical history
4. Weight
5. Medications
6. Allergies
7. Immunizations: identify any deficiencies, and encourage parent to make health maintenance appointment at usual health care facility
8. Source of routine care
   NOTE:
   a. Vital signs and laboratory tests must be individualized for each patient. Oximetry is generally done in all patients with altered mental status/behavior, abnormal vital signs, or respiratory signs/symptoms.
   b. If abnormalities in pulse, respiration, oximetry, or blood pressure are recorded, notify MD immediately.
   c. Antipyretic should be initiated in children with temperatures about 39° C if none has been given in the past 2-4 hr (e.g., acetaminophen 15 mg/kg/dose PO).
   d. Any patient seen at a health care facility earlier in the day and brought back within a few hours is a source of concern. Notify MD.
   e. Document concerns about parenting and home environment, if any.

---

the evaluation, it is essential to respond to the relatively transient nature of the interface between patients and health professionals. This requires some specific attention to routine health maintenance in children, including identifying a primary care provider (PCP) and immunization status. Although controversial, many believe that ED immunization is ineffective because of the inability to ascertain status and parental refusal to accept immunizations in the ED. Follow-up is increased when the PCP is notified in a timely manner of the ED visit. Noncompliance is associated with a parental belief that the child was not seriously ill as well as ED visits without laboratory tests.

Ongoing quality improvement programs should be initiated specific to diagnostic categories and evaluations of children.

DESIGN

Physical constraints are often produced by waiting areas, room design, and layout. Pediatric patients should be cared for in well-defined areas, ideally providing some physical separation. Space should be provided to facilitate parental presence during procedures; parental presence has not been documented to impact the ability to do a procedure. Observation and monitoring capacity should be incorporated into the structure. A variety of observation unit structures within either the ED area or the inpatient unit have been established. It is estimated that approximately 150 patients per 10,000 pediatric ED visits could benefit from an observation unit whereby patients are discharged within 24 hours of admission. Play areas, toys, and other mechanisms for distracting anxious children should be provided. Waiting times should be monitored because perception of parents is often inaccurate and is a central issue in achieving patient satisfaction.

EQUIPMENT

Special age-specific equipment must be available in an organized fashion as outlined in Appendix C-3. Oximetry, overhead warmers, and other relevant supplies should be present.

PERSONNEL

Staff must be trained and competent in the care of pediatric patients. Pediatric advanced life support training has provided a mechanism

TABLE 2-1   Major Pediatric Triage Categories*

Emergent				Urgent†
ABNORMAL VITAL SIGNS				**Abuse, child**
Age	Systolic BP (mm Hg)	Pulse (beats/min)	Respirations (breaths/min)	**Abuse, sexual**
0-2 yr	<60	<80	<15 or >40	**Acute symptoms in child <2-3 mo**
2-5 yr	<70	<60	<10 or >30	**Behavioral alteration**
>5 yr	<90	<50	<5 or >25	**Bite, poisonous snake**
				Bleeding, moderate
RESPIRATIONS				**Dehydration**
Irregular				**Drowning (near)**
Labored				**Eye: alkali, acid, or chemical burn**
				Fever >40° C
PULSE				**GI hemorrhage**
Irregular				**Headache: acute and severe**
Dysrhythmia				**History of apnea**
				Hypertension
COMA				**Hyperthermia**
				Hypothermia
CYANOSIS				**Neck pain or stiffness**
				Pain: acute and severe
STATUS EPILEPTICUS				**Poisoning**
				Rash (isolate patient)
MULTIPLE OR MAJOR TRAUMA				**SIDS (near) or ALTE**
Head				
Loss of consciousness				
Altered mental status				
Changing or asymmetric neurologic findings				
Cerebrospinal fluid leak				
Depressed fracture				
Neck or spinal injury				
Chest				
Abdomen				
Orthopedic				
Two or more long bone fractures				
Pelvic fracture				
Potential neurovascular compromise				
Amputation				
MAJOR BURN				
BLEEDING: ACUTE AND SIGNIFICANT				

SIDS, Sudden infant death syndrome; *ALTE,* apparent life-threatening event.

*If none of these emergent or urgent problems is present, the patient should be appropriately screened and treated according to normal facility flow patterns unless there is a complicating condition.

†May be emergent, depending on patient's condition. Repeat visits or very anxious parents may require that the visit be categorized as urgent.

TABLE 2-2 Initial Nursing Assessment: Pediatric Patients

Condition	Temp	Resp	Pulse	BP	CBC	UA	Other	Parent instruction (in text)	Comments
									Procedures
Abdominal pain	+		±	±0	±	+	± β-hCG		
Anemia			±	±0	+			Yes	Do reticulocyte count, assess diet
Asthma	+	+	+	+				Yes	Assess medications; nebulizer
Behavioral alteration	+	+	+	+	±	+	Glucose,* electrolytes, ± LP		Exhaustive work-up required, monitor, oximetry
Burn	+	+	+	+	±	+	± Electrolytes	Yes	Notify MD if >5%
Child abuse		+	+	+			Growth parameters		Reassure, observe
Communicable disease	+	+	+	+					Isolate patient
Cough	+	+						Yes	Oximetry
Croup	+	+	+					Yes	Notify MD, oximetry
Diabetic ketoacidosis	+	+	+	±0		+	Glucose,* acetone		± IV, electrolytes, pH
Diarrhea	+	+	+	±0	±	+	± Electrolytes	Yes	Assess hydration; also hematuria or proteinuria
Dysuria (painful urination)	+			+		+ and urine culture		Yes	
Earache	+							Yes	
Eye infection	+	+						Yes	

Condition						Laboratory	Procedure	Nursing assessment/intervention
Eye injury	+	+						Screen vision
Fever <2 mo old	+	+	+				Yes	Notify MD
>2-3 mo old	+	+	+		+		Yes	+ Antipyretics
Head injury	+		+	+			Yes	Do brief neurologic examination
Headache	+	+	+					Do brief neurologic examination; ± vision screen
Ingestion	+	+	+	+		± Toxicology screen		Obtain history, do neurologic examination, ± ipecac/lavage, ± charcoal/cathartic, prevention talk
Laceration	+	+	±⊖				Yes	Clean; ± apply pressure
Nosebleed	+	+	⊖				Yes	Apply pressure
Rash	+							± Isolate patient
Seizure	+	+	+	+	±	Glucose*		Give O₂, maintain airway, monitor, ± IV, ± antipyretics, do neurologic examination
Sore throat	+	+	+			± Throat culture	Yes	± Rapid strep screen
Sprain/fracture		±	±⊖			X-ray study	Yes	± Ultrasound
Vaginal bleeding	+	+	+	+		β-hCG		
Vomiting	+	+	±⊖	+		± Electrolytes	Yes	Assess hydration

The initial assessment steps noted for a specific condition are the minimal required database. The patient's presentation, history, and level of toxicity may suggest the need for additional initial nursing evaluation.

+, Perform procedure; ±, perform if indicated by patient's condition; ⊖, obtain orthostatic BP if appropriate; *BP*, blood pressure; *CBC*, complete blood count; *UA*, urinalysis.

*May be performed initially by bedside techniques (Dextrostix or Chemstrip).

for preparing health professionals to care for children.

Physicians must ensure that the patient with a life-threatening problem who expresses only nonspecific complaints is readily identified. The nurse often complements the physician's unique clinical skills with a broad psychosocial base that facilitates early evaluation.

Emergency physicians and pediatric emergency physicians should staff the ED with appropriate pediatric and surgical expertise readily available. The certification of pediatric emergency medicine physicians and the expanded pediatric training based on emergency medicine residencies provide greater expertise in the stabilization of children.

Support staff from radiology, laboratory, respiratory therapy, and other departments should be oriented to the care of the pediatric patient.

Personnel must function independently and interdependently. Communication is vital for all members of the health care team. It provides the basis for team functioning and ensures a coordinated effort.

PROTOCOLS

Protocols specific for the pediatric patient should be developed or a book such as this one readily available for reference. A triage system needs to be established. Decisions must be made on the basis of a short history, vital signs, and brief physical assessment. Tables 2-1 and 2-2 provide a foundation for triage and effective screening that may serve as a basis for formalizing this process. Obviously, many of the management approaches outlined in *Emergency Pediatrics,* 5th edition, need to be individualized for a specific institution. Referral, transport, and follow-up protocols should be established.

Emergency medical services for children (EMS-C) should be organized within the emergency medical services system to ensure appropriate ED preparation. Prevention, access, prehospital care, ED care, inpatient services, and rehabilitation are all central components that must be considered as protocols and systems are developed. The growth of special needs and technologically dependent children adds an additional challenge to the entire EMS-C. Transport considerations for all children are discussed in Chapter 3. A coordinated approach for children will improve care and ensure access to an efficient and high-quality level of emergency care during times of stress and tremendous need. Within this environment, sharing, communication, and trust can ensure optimal patient care.

REFERENCES

Baker DW, Stevens CD, Brook RH: Determinants of emergency department use by ambulatory patients at an urban public hospital, *Ann Emerg Med* 25:311, 1995.

Baucher H, Vinci R, Bak S, et al: Parents and procedures: a randomized controlled trial, *Pediatrics* 98:861, 1996.

Bond GR, Wiegand CB: Estimated use of a pediatric emergency department observation unit, *Ann Emerg Med* 29:739, 1997.

Emergency Medical Services for Children: Recommendations for coordinating care for children with special health care needs, *Ann Emerg Med* 30:274, 1997.

Foltin GL, Tunik MG: Emergency medical services for children: organizational and operational principles. In Barkin RM, editor: *Pediatric emergency medicine: concepts and clinical practice,* ed 2, St Louis, 1997, Mosby.

Gausche M, Rutherford M, Lewis RL: Emergency department quality assurance/improvement practices for the pediatric patient, *Ann Emerg Med* 25:804, 1995.

Goodman DC, Fisher ES, Gittelsohn A, et al: When are children hospitalized? The role of non clinical factors in pediatric hospitalization, *Pediatrics* 93:896, 1994.

King C, Nilsen GJ, Henretig FM, et al: Proposed fellowship training program in pediatric emergency medicine for emergency medicine graduates, *Ann Emerg Med* 22: 542, 1993.

Leffler S, Hayes M: Analysis of parental estimates of children's weights in the ED, *Ann Emerg Med* 30:167, 1997.

Mellick LB, Asch SM: Pediatric emergency department environment. In Barkin RM, editor: *Pediatric emergency medicine: concepts and clinical practice,* ed 2, St Louis, 1997, Mosby.

Mower WR, Sachs C, Nickline EL, et al: Pulse oximetry as a fifth pediatric vital sign, *Pediatrics* 99:681, 1997.

Robinson PE, Gausche M, Gerardi MJ, et al: Immunization of the pediatric patients in the emergency department, *Ann Emerg Med* 28:334, 1996.

Rodewald LE, Szilagyi PG, Humiston SG, et al: Effect of emergency department immunization rates and subsequent primary care visits, *Arch Pediatr Adolesc Med* 150:1271, 1996.

Sacchetti A, Lichenstein R, Carracaio CA, et al: Family member presence during pediatric emergency department procedures, *Pediatr Emerg Care* 12:2688, 1996.

Scarfone RJ, Jaffe MD, Wiley JF, et al: Noncompliance with scheduled revisits to a pediatric emergency department, *Arch Pediatr Adolesc Med* 150:948, 1996.

Storgion SA: Care of the technology-dependent child, *Pediatr Ann* 25:677, 1996.

Weinberg JA, Medearis DN: Emergency medical services for children: the report of the Institute of Medicine, *Pediatrics* 93:821, 1994.

Thompson DA, Yarnold PR, Adams SL, et al: How accurate are waiting time perceptions of patients in the emergency department, *Ann Emerg Med* 28:652, 1996.

Zimmerman DR, McCarten-Gibbs KA, DeNoble DH, et al: Repeat pediatric visits to a general emergency department, *Ann Emerg Med* 28:467, 1996.

3 TRANSPORT OF THE PEDIATRIC PATIENT

Systems for pediatric care in the emergency department (ED) must be established to provide for prehospital stabilization and transport of patients, as well as interhospital transport to ensure appropriate care within the emergency medical services system. Children account for 5% to 10% of all ambulance runs; 0.3% to 0.5% of transported children require tertiary care, and 5% of cases involve potentially life-threatening problems. Younger children often have medical problems, whereas those older than 2 years of age have predominantly traumatic conditions.

Pediatric patients in the prehospital setting are often a source of inordinate anxiety, primarily because of the inexperience of prehospital care providers with this age group. However, the principles of resuscitation and management that are used every day for older patients parallel those used for the younger patient. Judgment forms the basis for management of emergency situations.

The prehospital care provider enters the patient's environment. Paramedics and emergency medical technicians (EMTs) develop "street sense," an ability to create order out of chaos: to "read" the scene, the people, and the emotions, and then to intervene. Personnel, education and training, and equipment must be provided. Management strategies and protocols must be established. The concept of "pick up and run" is not uniformly appropriate, given the current sophistication of prehospital care. Each action must be individualized to the particular circumstances, patient's stability, anticipated length of transport, and so on, and close coordination with the base station and receiving hospital is essential. The expansion of technology such as ventilators that facilitate home care enhances the complexity of patients encountered in the prehospital setting. A warm and safe environment must be provided. Aggressive management should be maintained throughout the transport.

Field triage, using specific criteria, has been developed and may be useful in communication with the base station and in assessment of outcome. Trauma scores such as the Champion and Pediatric Trauma Scores are discussed in Chapter 56 and the Glasgow Coma Scale in Chapter 57.

The prehospital setting presents additional unique difficulties when the death of a child is involved. Controversy abounds regarding the best approach when death seems apparent, but many believe that the standard should be to initiate all-out resuscitative efforts and to expedite transport to an ED. This resuscitation obviously can be modified by the base station in circumstances involving major trauma, nonaccidental injuries, sudden infant death syndrome (SIDS), the family's acceptance of the outcome, or an obviously nonviable child.

INTERHOSPITAL TRANSPORT

Patients' conditions may be stabilized at an institution that does not have adequate staff and equipment to deal with the acute or long-term medical problems of a child. Transfer becomes a priority.

Before transport can be considered, resuscitation must be initiated and immediate therapy instituted. The airway requires stabilization and adequate ventilation must be ensured, often through administration of oxygen and active airway management. An intravenous line (or lines) should be started to permit fluid resuscitation and administration of lifesaving medications.

An urgent evaluation is appropriate. The physical examination should be completed, baseline laboratory values obtained, and x-ray tests performed as indicated by the apparent medical or traumatic condition. Early pharmacologic therapy, including administration of antibiotics, anticonvulsants, β-adrenergic agents, and bronchodilators, should be initiated as necessary. Traumatic injuries may require surgical, neurosurgical, or orthopedic intervention before transport.

Once stabilization has been achieved, the physician must carefully analyze facilities that can adequately care for the child in terms of personnel, equipment, and distance. Special needs such as dialysis, intensive care, or cardiac catheterization programs should be considered. The institution selected should be contacted and transport discussed and arranged. It is imperative that communication at this time be adequate between the physicians and nursing staffs at the two hospitals to ensure a smooth transfer.

The mechanism of transfer should be a joint decision of the referring and receiving institutions, focusing on equipment, speed, distance, weather, traffic patterns, and level of expertise of medical personnel required to care for the child. Many communities have access to formal ground (ambulance) or air (helicopter or airplane) transport systems that are particularly useful for critically ill patients who will be admitted to an intensive care unit (ICU) on arrival at the receiving hospital or who experience respiratory, cardiovascular, or neurologic deterioration during the transport. Clinicians should know how to arrange for transport through these systems.

Active management of the patient must continue until transfer of care to the receiving hospital or transport team. Concurrently, charts, x-ray films, laboratory results, and past records should be duplicated and readied for transport with the patient. Intravenous lines and tubes should be secured and fractures stabilized to prevent disruption.

Parents and patients should be involved throughout the resuscitation and stabilization processes to help them feel comfortable with the transfer and understand its benefits.

REFERENCES

Baker MD, Ludwig S: Pediatric emergency transport and the private practitioner, *Pediatrics* 88:691, 1991.

Day S, McCloskey K, Orr R, et al: Pediatric interhospital critical care transport: consensus of a national leadership conference, *Pediatrics* 88:696, 1991.

Dernocoeur K: *Streetsense*, Bowie, Md, 1985, Brady Communication.

McCloskey KA, Orr RA: Interhospital transport. In Barkin RM, editor: *Pediatric emergency medicine: concepts and clinical practice*, ed 2, St Louis, 1997, Mosby.

4 CARDIOPULMONARY ARREST

ALERT: Cardiopulmonary arrest in children is commonly respiratory in origin, emphasizing the importance of stabilization of the airway, breathing, and then circulation (the ABCs). The coordinated effort of a team of professionals is required for optimal care.

The outcome of cardiopulmonary arrests in children is poor, reaching a 90% mortality rate in some studies. Most of the patients (87%) have an underlying disease. In contrast, respiratory arrest has been associated with a mortality rate of 33%; most affected children are less than 1 year of age. Mortality is affected by whether the arrest occurs in the prehospital or hospital setting. Survival is better in the ED than in the prehospital setting but worse than in an inpatient arrest. Out-of-hospital cardiac arrests in children less than 18 years old are commonly a result of sudden infant death syndrome (SIDS), drowning, and respiratory arrest, and they occur most commonly in children less than 1 year of age.

ANTICIPATING CARDIOPULMONARY ARREST

Progressive deterioration of respiratory and ultimately circulatory function may lead to cardiopulmonary arrest in infants and children. The underlying condition is usually *respiratory* in origin, stemming from obstruction and hypoxia, secondarily leading to cardiac arrest. Hypoxia may be acute or chronic, resulting from either an acquired or underlying disease. Respiratory arrest and hypoxia almost always precede cardiac standstill; with careful observation, they can be recognized and prevented.

Respiratory failure is recognizable in the compensated state. Prevention can be facilitated by noting abnormal respirations characterized by tachypnea, bradypnea, apnea, or increased work of breathing.

Decompensation of *cardiac* function leads to a shock state associated with impaired cardiac output. Excessive output from stool or vomitus or inadequate intake is often contributory. Tachycardia, hypotension (note orthostatic changes), and poor peripheral circulation are present. Ultimately, impaired perfusion causes delayed capillary refill time (>2 seconds), mottling, cyanosis, cool skin, an altered level of consciousness, poor muscle tone, and finally, decreased urine output.

Recognizing this typical pattern may prevent dysfunction from progressing to failure and arrest. Intervention can then be initiated in a timely and effective manner.

Etiology

The precipitating causes of a catastrophic event often can be identified and prevented:

1. Respiratory disease (see Chapters 20 and 84)
   a. Upper airway obstruction: croup, epiglottitis, foreign body, suffocation, strangulation, and trauma
   b. Lower airway disease: pneumonia,

asthma, bronchiolitis, foreign body aspiration, near-drowning, smoke inhalation, and pulmonary edema
2. Infection: sepsis and meningitis (Infection may be the underlying process leading to respiratory or circulatory compromise.)
3. Intoxication: narcotic depressants, sedatives, and antidysrhythmics (see Chapter 54)
4. Cardiac disorders: congenital heart disease, myocarditis, pericarditis, and dysrhythmias, often associated with congestive heart failure (CHF) and pulmonary edema
5. Shock: cardiogenic, hypovolemic, or distributive (see Chapter 5)
6. Central nervous system (CNS): meningitis, encephalitis, head trauma, anoxia, and other causes of hypoventilation (see Chapter 81)
7. Trauma/environment: multiple organ failure, child abuse, hypothermia or hyperthermia, and near-drowning
8. Metabolic: hypoglycemia, hypocalcemia, and hyperkalemia
9. Near-SIDS or apparent life-threatening event (ALTE) (see Chapter 22)

The cause of cardiopulmonary arrest in children may also be divided by age group. *Newborn* causes primarily include prematurity, uteroplacental insufficiency, congenital malformations, sepsis, and nuchal cord. Problems in *infancy* include SIDS, child abuse, pulmonary or congenital heart disease, ingestions, congenital malformations, and sepsis. The *adolescent* experiences cardiopulmonary arrest primarily from trauma, drug overdose, dysrhythmias, and congenital heart disease.

TEAM APPROACH

The management of cardiorespiratory arrest in children requires the combined efforts of several professionals working as a team. The team captain must be immediately identifiable and provide direction, expertise, and coordination in a precise way. This individual must be responsible for ensuring that everything gets done; he or she should delegate responsibilities rather than assuming them single-handedly. Beyond dealing with the immediate logistics of procedures and medication and monitoring their effects, the leader must also be able to delineate issues that are crucial to the outcome and that may alter management.

1. Etiology
   a. What condition preceded the arrest?
   b. What process caused the arrest (i.e., hypoxia, hypovolemia)?
   c. Why is the patient in shock (hypovolemic, distributive, or cardiogenic)?
   d. Why are we having difficulty oxygenating or ventilating the patient?
   e. Why are we not making progress (e.g., cardiac tamponade, pneumothorax, electromechanical dissociation [EMD] or pulseless electrical activity [PEA], electrolyte or acid-base disturbance, inadequate ventilation, or coagulopathy)?
2. Time
   a. How long have we been treating the patient?
   b. How much time (including time before arrival in the emergency department) has elapsed since initiating cardiopulmonary resuscitation (CPR), and how long was the patient in arrest before CPR was begun?
3. End point. When do we stop, and what criteria do we have for stopping?
4. Evaluation
   a. Can we learn about our performance from this resuscitation?
   b. How can we improve techniques, equipment, personnel training, and team functioning?

BASIC LIFE SUPPORT (Table 4-1)

Basic life support of the child provides immediate intervention until additional capabilities are

TABLE 4-1   Basic Life Support Procedures

	Infant (<1 yr)	Child (1-8 yr)	Adult*
AIRWAY	Head tilt-chin lift (if trauma present, use jaw thrust)		
BREATHING	Initially, 2-5 breaths at 1.5 sec (adult 1.5 sec)/breath, then		
	20 breath/min	20 breath/min	10-12 breath/min
CIRCULATION			
Pulse check	Brachial/femoral	Carotid	Carotid
Site of compression over sternum	Lower third	Lower third	Lower third
Mechanism	2-3 fingers	Heel of hand	Two hands
Depth	Approx. $\frac{1}{3}$ of chest	Approx. $\frac{1}{3}$ of chest	Approx. $\frac{1}{3}$ of chest
Rate/min	At least 100	100	100
COMPRESSION:VENTILATION RATIO†	5:1	5:1	5:1 (2 rescuers)
			15:2 (1 rescuer)
FOREIGN BODY OBSTRUCTION	Back blow-chest thrust	Abdominal thrust	Abdominal thrust

*Two rescuers.
†Pause for ventilation.

available. The basic principles parallel those evolved for adults. The importance of the elements known as the ABCs cannot be overemphasized. These elements are stabilizing the *airway,* establishing adequate *breathing,* and facilitating *circulation.* Basic CPR using the ABCs should be interrupted only for defibrillation or intubation. Following is a list of the skills and procedures of the ABCs. They require practice and repetition.

1. Establish unresponsiveness or respiratory difficulty. Gently shake the patient; if conscious, he or she should display motor activity.
2. Call for help.
3. Position the patient supine, on a firm, flat surface. Do not subject the patient to further injury.
4. Open the *airway* using the head tilt–chin lift method (place hand closest to child's head on forehead and gently tilt head back into a "sniffing" position).
5. Assess *breathing* to ensure air move-

ment by demonstrating movement of the chest or abdomen with ventilation, by feeling air moving through the mouth, or by hearing noise during expiration. Look, feel, and listen. Assess use of accessory muscles.

6. If the patient is an infant who is not breathing, cover both the mouth and the nose (mouth to nose and mouth) and establish a seal. If the child is too large, cover the child's mouth (mouth to mouth) while pinching the nose.
7. Give two slow breaths, using enough volume to cause the chest to rise. If air enters freely, the airway is clear. If air does not enter, the airway is obstructed (see item number 12).
8. Begin rescue breathing if breathing is not noted.
9. Assess pulse for *cardiac function.* In infants less than 1 year old, use the brachial or femoral arteries. The carotid artery should be used in older children.

10. Begin chest compressions if no pulse is present.
    a. In the infant less than 1 year old, compress one finger width below the imaginary line between the nipples on the sternum.
    b. In older children, compress over the lower third of the sternum.
    c. Some clinicians have suggested that the compression rate be increased to more than 100/min to improve coronary perfusion pressure.
11. Coordinate compressions and breathing. In the infant and child, a 5:1 compression/ventilation ratio is maintained.
12. ***Upper airway foreign body*** may be present and requires urgent intervention (p. 791).
    a. In the infant (<1 year), do five back blows with the child straddled over the rescuer's arm. Then do five chest thrusts at the location described for chest compressions. Repeat until relieved.
    b. If the conscious child is more than 1 year of age, perform a Heimlich maneuver or abdominal thrust. Repeat until obstruction is relieved.
    In the unconscious child, visible obstructing objects should be removed. If ventilation is unsuccessful, reposition the head and resume efforts.

ADVANCED LIFE SUPPORT

Basic life support must be initiated immediately and followed by advanced life support and more sophisticated intervention on the basis of stabilization of the airway, breathing, and circulation.

Specific components of the resuscitation that must be emphasized and are unique to children include the following:

1. Children usually respond to initial airway, ventilation, and fluid therapy.
2. All drugs, medications, invasive catheters, and tubes must be age and weight specific. Children should be monitored aggressively as appropriate.
3. Fluid resuscitation must reflect the child's size and volume. Intravascular fluid is about 80 ml/kg. Laboratory studies requiring extensive blood samples should be minimized.
4. Children are developing physically and psychologically, and the team must be responsive to the needs of the child and family.
5. Iatrogenic injuries may occur in as many as 3% of patients undergoing CPR, including retroperitoneal hemorrhage, pneumothorax, and so on.

Airway

Anatomic differences in children compared with adults may be considered in approaching stabilization of the child's airway.

1. The child's head and occiput are proportionately larger, causing neck flexion and airway obstruction when the child is supine. Moderate extension is necessary.
2. The tongue is relatively larger with less muscle tone.
3. The epiglottis is shorter, narrower, more horizontal and softer.
4. The larynx is more anterior and higher, at the C2 level in children while it is at the C6 level in adults.
5. The trachea is shorter, increasing the risk of a right main stem intubation.
6. The airway is narrower, increasing airway resistance. The cricoid is the narrowest portion.

Patency should be established by one of the techniques outlined. The options are restricted if there is a question of neck trauma.

An airway should be established to ensure patency, facilitate suctioning, prevent aspiration, or administer drugs. In contrast to an adult, the child has a relatively large head and a forward-placed larynx. In addition, there is greater redundancy of mucosal tissues, a relatively large adenoidal tissue, and anterior placement of C1, C3, and C4. Also, the smaller pediatric airway is subject to a variety of conditions that increase airway resistance.

The following adjuncts to airway management may be used in conjunction with appropriate barrier devices and universal precautions:

1. *Oxygen:* administered by hood, mask, or cannula: 3-6 L/min by mask or cannula produces a forced inspiratory oxygen (Fio_2) of 40% to 50%. To get higher oxygen (O_2) concentrations, a mask with reservoir is required (100% or non-rebreathing bag).

2. *Oropharyngeal airway:* a semicircular-shaped apparatus of plastic curved to fit over the back of the tongue and inserted into the lower posterior pharynx. It is introduced into the mouth backward and rotated as it approaches the posterior wall of the pharynx near the back of the tongue (poorly tolerated in conscious patients).

3. *Nasopharyngeal airway:* a soft rubber or plastic tube inserted into the nose close to the midline along the floor of the nostril and into the posterior pharynx behind the tongue (tolerated fairly well in conscious patients).

4. *Self-inflating bag-valve ventilation* is usually effective (see p. 26).
   a. Neonatal size (250 ml) for premature infants. May be inadequate for full-term neonates and infants, who may require a minimum value of 450 ml.
   b. Infant size (450 ml) for full-term neonates, infants, and children.
   c. Adult size (1600 ml). When large bags are used, care must be taken to use only that force and tidal volume necessary to produce effective chest expansion.
   d. If a pop-off valve is present, it should usually be bypassed because pressures required for adequate ventilation during CPR may exceed the pop-off limit. This is especially true in patients with poor lung compliance.
   e. Self-inflating bag delivers 21% unless supplemental oxygen is provided. A reservoir permits delivery of concentrations of 60% to 95% at a flow of 10% to 15% oxygen.
   f. Two hands are needed: one to create a tight seal between the mask and face and the other to compress the bag.

5. *Laryngeal mask airway:* Potentially fills the gap between self-inflating bag valve mask and endotracheal intubation. Available in six sizes, it is passed without visualization into the hypopharynx. It is not useful when there is high airway resistance, pharyngeal disease, low pulmonary compliance, or a small mouth. The role in the ED is unclear, given the potential risk of aspiration and damage to facial or pharyngeal structures. Experience is predominantly in the controlled environment of the operating room.

6. *Endotracheal (ET) intubation:* provides and protects a stable airway for more efficient ventilation. The size of the ET tube varies with the age and size of the child but may be estimated by selecting a tube that approximates the diameter of the patient's little (fifth) finger. An estimate also may be made by adding 16 to the child's age (up to 16 years) and dividing this total by 4. Below the age of 7 or 8 years, uncuffed tubes are used because the airway is narrowest at the cricoid in this age group; cuffed tubes are used in older children. Cuffed tubes must be treated as if they were 0.5 mm larger in size (e.g., 6.0 mm cuffed = 6.5 mm uncuffed tube). Although patient-to-patient variability exists, the following guidelines may be useful in

estimating the correct tube size (see Appendix B-2):

Age	Tube size (mm)	Suction catheter (FR)
Newborn	3.0	6
1 mo	3.5	8
6 mo	3.5	8
1 yr	4.0	8
2-3 yr	4.5	8
4-5 yr	5.0	10
6-8 yr	6.0	10
10-12 yr	6.5	12
16 yr	7.0	12
Adult female	7.0-8.0	12
Adult male	7.5-8.5	14

a. Prepare by checking the laryngoscope to ensure adequate functioning and light source. Be certain that suction is available. In the newborn, a DeLee trap suction may be helpful. If a stylet is used, it should not protrude beyond the tip of the ET tube. Lighted stylets and endoscopic laryngoscopes are available.

b. Oxygenate patient and attach heart monitor. Position patient in sniffing position.

c. Visualize the esophagus, epiglottis, and cords. Laryngeal pressure may be helpful.

d. Whether orally or nasotracheally intubating the patient, watch the tube pass through the cords, and pass it 1 to 2 cm beyond.

e. If the patient becomes bradycardic or cyanotic, abort the procedure, administer oxygen, and ventilate. Start again once signs have stabilized.

f. Gastric inflation can be reduced by cricoid pressure (Sellick maneuver).

g. Check the position of the tube by listening on both sides of upper chest and stomach. Make sure the tube is not in the right stem bronchus or esophagus. Confirm by x-ray film. The tip should be at T2-T3 vertebral level or at the level of the lower edge of the medial aspect of the clavicle. Further confirmation can be achieved by using end-tidal CO_2 detectors. Colorimetric, semiquantitative monitors are available.

h. Stabilize the tube with adhesive tape or other device. The skin to which adhesive tape is to be affixed should be cleansed and dried, followed by an application of tincture of benzoin.

i. Blind nasotracheal intubation is relatively safe in the hypoventilating patient. The tube may also be introduced under direct visualization.

7. Cricothyroidotomy is indicated as a temporizing measure in children more than 3 years old when acute upper airway obstruction cannot otherwise be relieved. It is, however, rarely needed.

8. If unable to ventilate on an emergent basis with intubation, bag and mask, or cricothyroidotomy (not readily available as alternative), a 14-gauge catheter over the needle may be inserted into the cricothyroid membrane. The adapter from a 3-mm nasotracheal or ET tube may be inserted into the Luer adapter of the catheter for application of oxygen and positive pressure for a limited time.

9. Patients with pure respiratory arrest not associated with trauma often respond rapidly to bag and mask or mouth-to-mouth (or mouth-to-mouth and nose) ventilation. However, if no response is seen within 60 seconds, intubation should be considered. Respiratory arrests complicated by such findings as cyanosis and hypotension usually require intubation.

10. Prophylactic intubation of nontraumatized patients in the ED setting is rarely indicated because of a concern about depression of respirations resulting from pharmacologic management of such diseases as seizures with diazepam (Valium), lorazepam (Ativan), or phe-

nobarbital and agitation with sedatives. Flumazenil (Mazicon) may be a useful agent to reduce benzodiazepine overdose effects. Intubate when necessary.

11. Although judgment ultimately becomes the prime determinant of a patient's need for intubation, each situation must be individualized to consider the patient's condition, the progression of disease, potential therapeutic maneuvers, and personnel and equipment availability.

Muscle Relaxants

Muscle relaxants may be required to achieve intubation; this is sometimes the case in patients with excessive muscle tone, as seen with seizures, tetanus, or neurologic disease. Obviously, the problems inherent in using such agents relate to the inability to further evaluate the patient neurologically and the potential inability to intubate the patient after relaxation, aspiration, and dysrhythmias.

Neuromuscular blocking agents may either cause or prevent depolarizing of the end-plate (if a nondepolarizing or competitive agent is used).

Succinylcholine is the classic depolarizing agent and is contraindicated in patients with hyperkalemia, burns, glaucoma, penetrating ocular injury, and increased intracranial pressure.

The patient's anatomy is initially evaluated, looking for oral or dental abnormalities, trauma to the neck or face, and systemic abnormalities. Equipment is checked.

One suggested protocol is as follows:

1. The patient is preoxygenated. If the patient is hypoventilating, hyperventilate while the Sellick maneuver is performed. Position the head of adolescents and adults with a towel under it to elevate it about 10 cm off the bed.

2. Administer vecuronium (Norcuron), 0.01 mg/kg IV (adults: 1 mg IV), to reduce fasciculations. It is a nondepolarizing agent. Allow 3 to 5 minutes before proceeding with succinylcholine. This step is unnecessary in children less than 5 years old.

3. Atropine, 0.01-0.02 mg/kg IV (minimum 0.10 mg/dose), may be given to children less than 7 years old to reduce bradycardia or if ketamine is used. In the presence of significant head injury, administer lidocaine, 1.0-1.5 mg/kg IV, and allow 2 minutes before giving succinylcholine.

4. Sedate patient with thiopental, 3-5 mg/kg IV, if he or she is not hypotensive or in status asthmaticus. Alternatives include midazolam up to 0.1 mg/kg IV (maximum 4 mg) or ketamine, 1 mg/kg IV, if no head injury.

5. Give succinylcholine, 1.0-1.5 mg/kg IV, to adults and 2 mg/kg IV to children less than 10 kg. Allow 45 to 60 seconds for muscle relaxation. Cricoid pressure should be maintained.

6. Orally intubate the patient, verify position, and release cricoid pressure. When paralysis wears off, pancuronium up to 0.1 mg/kg IV may be used if needed.

Obviously, this procedure should be performed with tremendous caution if any concern about being unable to intubate the patient is present.

Breathing

Breathing is demonstrated by detecting movement of the chest or abdomen with ventilation, by feeling air moving through the mouth, or by hearing noise during expiration.

1. Limit ventilation to the amount of air needed to cause the chest to rise (excessive volumes exacerbate gastric distension and increase the risk of pneumothorax).

2. Use a self-inflating bag-valve ventilation system whenever possible, optimally with a pop-off valve or in-line manometer to override the pop-off valve. An oxygen reservoir is useful in increasing the oxygen concentration. Bags are available for neonates (stroke volume of 250 to 300 ml), infants and children (stroke volume of 550 to 600 ml), and adults (stroke volume of

1.0 to 1.5 L). Neonatal bags are usually inadequate for full-term neonates and infants; infant size should be used in these children. Tidal volume should be about 10 ml/kg. An oxygen reservoir should be used to enhance the oxygen concentration achieved:

Flow rate (L/min)	Adult bag Fio_2	Pediatrics bag Fio_2	Infant bag Fio_2
5	—	59%	75%
10	67%	85%	94%
15	78%	95%	95%

Masks are available in infant, child, and adult sizes.

Circulation

Circulation must be assessed by checking brachial, femoral, or carotid pulses, blood pressure, heart rate, and capillary refilling (normally <2 seconds).

All patients should be monitored if possible.

1. Initiate external chest compressions if there is no effective pulse as described previously. Monitor pulse and blood pressure during compression. Children older than 1 year of age require a hard surface.

2. Intravenous cannulation for fluid and drug administration is achieved by a variety of peripheral modalities; most common is the catheter over the needle. The butterfly or scalp vein-type needle is useful but less commonly used in the resuscitation setting. The size and type of catheter depend on the clinician's level of comfort and the availability of sites. If access is difficult, rapid consideration of a cutdown or central line may be appropriate (Box 4-1).

3. Intraosseous infusion of crystalloid solution can be used as an alternative route for establishment of venous access in children 6 years of age or younger. However, it is indicated only in life-threatening or potentially life-threatening situations in which intravenous cannulation is not achieved.

Insert a bone marrow needle or special

Box 4-1
PRIORITIES FOR VASCULAR ACCESS

Attempt peripheral venous access. If not successful in timely fashion, consider alternative route.

FOR DRUGS

If ET tube present, may give atropine, epinephrine, lidocaine, or naloxone.

If no ET tube, consider intraosseous on central lines.

FOR CRYSTALLOID AND OTHER FLUIDS

If ≤6 years, consider intraosseous infusion.

If >6 years, consider central or surgical access.

---

intraosseous needle (less desirable alternatives include a spinal needle or other similar device with a stylet) into the anterior tibia (midline flat surface of the tibia) 2 to 3 cm below the tibial tuberosity. Under aseptic conditions, insert the needle perpendicular to the skin or directed inferiorly, away from the epiphysis.

The needle is in the marrow when a lack of resistance is felt and the needle stands up by itself, bone marrow can be aspirated, and fluid runs in safely. The procedure appears to be safe for infusion of crystalloid and a number of drugs (see Appendix A-3).

4. *Atropine, epinephrine, lidocaine,* and *naloxone* also can be administered by ET tube. Although the exact dosing by this route has not been established, it is suggested that the dose of epinephrine be greater than the initial IV dose. Instill the dose as deeply as possible into the tracheobronchial tree by using a catheter or feeding tube inserted beyond the distal tip of the ET tube. Dilution of the drug in

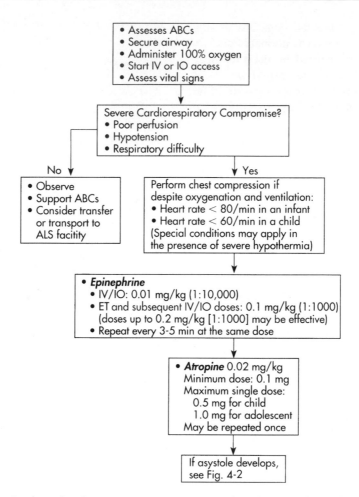

Fig. 4-1   Bradycardia decision tree. *ABC,* Airway, breathing, and circulation; *ALS,* advanced life support; *ET,* endotracheal; *IO,* intraosseous; *IV,* intravenous. (From *JAMA* 268:2171, 1992.)

1 to 2 ml of saline solution may assist delivery.

5. Central venous catheters, preferably inserted into the internal jugular or femoral veins, may be used by the experienced practitioner. Because most children have normal renal and cardiac function and respond rapidly to resuscitation, such monitoring is rarely required.

   If CVP monitoring is appropriate, the middle approach to the internal jugular cannulation is preferred but still carries a risk of lung puncture. Insert a guide wire,

then insert a larger catheter (see Appendix A-3).

6. If there is any question of hypovolemia, give a rapid infusion of normal saline or lactated Ringer's solution at 20 ml/kg over 10 to 20 minutes. This may be repeated. If no response is seen, initiate further evaluation of fluid status on the basis of underlying conditions, the nature of the acute insult, and hemodynamic parameters such as central venous pressure, heart rate, blood pressure, and capillary refill. If the patient is considered

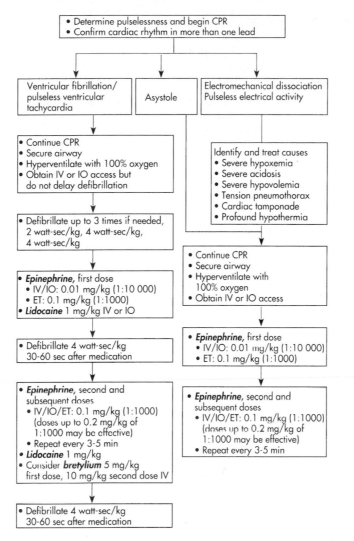

- Determine pulselessness and begin CPR
- Confirm cardiac rhythm in more than one lead

| Ventricular fibrillation/ pulseless ventricular tachycardia | Asystole | Electromechanical dissociation Pulseless electrical activity |

Ventricular fibrillation / pulseless ventricular tachycardia branch:

- Continue CPR
- Secure airway
- Hyperventilate with 100% oxygen
- Obtain IV or IO access but do not delay defibrillation

- Defibrillate up to 3 times if needed, 2 watt-sec/kg, 4 watt-sec/kg, 4 watt-sec/kg

- *Epinephrine,* first dose
  - IV/IO: 0.01 mg/kg (1:10 000)
  - ET: 0.1 mg/kg (1:1000)
- *Lidocaine* 1 mg/kg IV or IO

- Defibrillate 4 watt-sec/kg 30-60 sec after medication

- *Epinephrine,* second and subsequent doses
  - IV/IO/ET: 0.1 mg/kg (1:1000) (doses up to 0.2 mg/kg of 1:1000 may be effective)
  - Repeat every 3-5 min
- *Lidocaine* 1 mg/kg
- Consider *bretylium* 5 mg/kg first dose, 10 mg/kg second dose IV

- Defibrillate 4 watt-sec/kg 30-60 sec after medication

Electromechanical dissociation / Pulseless electrical activity branch:

Identify and treat causes
- Severe hypoxemia
- Severe acidosis
- Severe hypovolemia
- Tension pneumothorax
- Cardiac tamponade
- Profound hypothermia

- Continue CPR
- Secure airway
- Hyperventilate with 100% oxygen
- Obtain IV or IO access

- *Epinephrine,* first dose
  - IV/IO: 0.01 mg/kg (1:10 000)
  - ET: 0.1 mg/kg (1:1000)

- *Epinephrine,* second and subsequent doses
  - IV/IO/ET: 0.1 mg/kg (1:1000) (doses up to 0.2 mg/kg of 1:1000 may be effective)
  - Repeat every 3-5 min

Fig. 4-2 Asystole and pulseless arrest decision tree. *CPR,* Cardiopulmonary resuscitation; *ET,* endotracheal; *IO,* intraosseous; *IV,* intravenous.
(From *JAMA* 268:2171, 1992.)

normovolemic and shock persists, give dopamine, 5-20 µg/kg/min IV, and begin a rapid evaluation for shock (see Chapter 5).

Essential Medications and Measures

First-line drugs are given to virtually all patients who have a cardiopulmonary arrest and who do not respond to initial airway and ventilatory intervention and support (Figs. 4-1 and 4-2). The recommendation of the International Liaison Committee on Resuscitation (ILCR) varies slightly in suggesting that 2-4 watt-sec/kg be used for the second and third shock. Furthermore, lidocaine was not used with epinephrine and up to three shocks were recommended. Although the guidelines outlined in these figures are standard protocols, working groups continue to develop consensus on these and other issues.

The patient is given the following:
1. Oxygen.
2. Epinephrine. The recommended initial dose for asystolic and pulseless arrest is 0.01 mg/kg (0.1 ml/kg of 1:10,000 solution) given IV or intraosseous (IO). If it is given endotracheally (ET), the initial dose is 0.1 mg/kg (0.1 ml/kg of 1:1000 solution [10 times the initial IV dose]).

Because the outcome is poor and high-dose epinephrine has been suggested to be more effective, second and subsequent doses have been recommended to be 0.1 mg/kg (0.1 ml/kg of 1:1000 solution). This larger dose should be administered within 3 to 5 minutes of the initial dose and repeated every 3 to 5 minutes. Further doses as high as 0.2 mg/kg (0.2 ml/kg of 1:1000 solution) have also been suggested. This approach has not been documented to be beneficial; timing and other factors may influence efficacy.

If asystolic or pulseless arrest continues, a continuous infusion of epinephrine at 20 µg/kg/min may be used until effective pulses are noted, at which time an infusion may be used. Low-dose infusions (<0.3 µg/kg/min) produce β-adrenergic effects; larger doses result in α-adrenergic vasoconstriction.

The measures and medications for resuscitation are outlined in Table 4-2.

Blood pressure, pulse, and heart rhythm must be monitored constantly throughout the resuscitation to ensure that therapeutic measures are appropriate and effective. Additional steps may include treatment of the following:
1. Acidosis. Acidosis is undesirable pathophysiologically because it depresses myocardial contractility, decreases the threshold for ventricular fibrillation, impairs normal cardiac automaticity, and blocks the cardioaccelerator and vasopressor action of catecholamines. Acidosis in children is primarily a problem of ventilation and oxygenation.

   The benefits of bicarbonate therapy in the arrest situation are unclear; furthermore, this type of therapy does not improve the ability to defibrillate. It causes oxygen to bind more tightly to oxyhemoglobin, and it may lead to hyperosmolality and hypernatremia. Bicarbonate therapy also worsens the mixed venous acidosis and inactivates simultaneously administered catecholamines.

   Bicarbonate administration may be initiated after resuscitation efforts have been tried for some time (usually 10 minutes) and ventilation is effective. Further doses ideally are administered in response to arterial blood gas (ABG) determinations.
2. EMD or PEA. The role of calcium blockers in cerebral resuscitation is under investigation. Calcium salts may not be beneficial in EMD/PEA, and their use should be restricted to circumstances in which a benefit is documented (hyperkalemia, hypocalcemia, calcium channel blocker overdose, fluoride poisoning, and hypermagnesemia). Reversible causes of EMD/PEA should be sought, including hypovolemia, tension pneumothorax, pericardial tamponade, and severe acidosis.
3. Dysrhythmias (see Chapter 6 and Figs. 4-1 and 4-2).
4. Congestive heart failure (see Chapter 16).
5. Seizure (see Chapter 21).
6. Malignant hypertension (see Chapter 18).
7. Increased intracranial pressure (see Chapter 57).
8. Cortical blindness after cardiac arrest usually has a good recovery if the neurologic status returns.

Ancillary Data and Measures

Laboratory tests and other procedures beyond those required for evaluation of the patient's underlying disease must be performed:
1. Complete blood count with hematocrit done in ED
2. Chemical evaluations: electrolytes, blood

Text continued on p. 37

TABLE 4-2 Common Primary and Secondary Measures in Resuscitation

Drug availability	Dose/route	Indications	Adverse reactions	Comments
Adenosine (Adenocard) Vial: 3 mg/ml	0.1 mg/kg IV (rapid) and repeat in 2 min; adult: 6 mg IV, if no response in 2 min, give 12 mg IV	Supraventricular tachycardia	Flushing, shortness of breath	Rapid half-life (10 sec); do not use for 2nd or 3rd degree AV block (unless pacemaker present) or sick sinus syndrome
Albuterol (Proventil, Ventolin) soln (inhalation) (0.5%–5 mg/ml)	Inhalation 0.03 ml/kg/dose (maximum: 1.0 ml/dose) diluted in 2 ml saline; repeat as necessary	Bronchoconstriction	Tachycardia, nausea	β_2 agonist; also available as MDI (90 µg/dose)
Atropine (0.1, 0.4, 1.0 mg/ml)	0.02 mg/kg/dose (minimum: 0.1 mg/dose) (adult: 0.6–1.0 mg/dose; maximum 2 mg) q5min prn IV, ET, IO	Bradycardia, asystole, ↑ vagal tone Heart block (temporary); increases AV node conduction	Tachycardia, dysrhythmias, anticholinergic	Parasympatholytic (Table 6-4); use 2-3 times dose for ET
Bicarbonate, sodium ($NaHCO_3$) (8.4%–50 mEq/50 ml) (7.5%–44.5 mEq/50 ml)	1 mEq/kg/dose q10min prn IV	Metabolic acidosis Hyperkalemia	Metabolic alkalosis, hyperosmolality, hypernatremia	Incompatible with calcium, catecholamine infusion; monitor ABG
Bretylium (50 mg/ml)	5 mg/kg/dose IV followed prn by 10 mg/kg/dose q15min IV up to 30 mg/kg	Ventricular dysrhythmias refractory to lidocaine	Hypotension (orthostatic), bradyrhythmias	Inhibits release of catecholamines (i.e., norepinephrine) from sympathetic nerves; blocks adrenergic nerve endings; do not give ET; use if defibrillation and lidocaine fail (Table 6-4)
Calcium chloride (10%–100 mg/ml) (1.36 mEq Ca^{++}/ml)	20-30 mg (0.2–0.3 ml)/kg/dose (maximum: 500 mg/dose) q10min prn IV slowly	Hyperkalemia Calcium channel blocker OD	Rapid infusion causes bradycardia, hypotension Extravasation-necrosis	Inotropic; monitor; use caution with digitalized patient; probably no benefit in asystole or electromechanical dissociation

Continued

IV drugs may generally be given intraosseously (IO). *TDD,* Total digitalizing dose.

TABLE 4-2 Common Primary and Secondary Measures in Resuscitation—cont'd

Drug availability	Dose/route	Indications	Adverse reactions	Comments
Crystalloid 0.9% NS, LR, D5W 0.9% NS, D5WLR	20 ml/kg over 20-30 min IV; repeat as necessary	Hypovolemia	Fluid overdose and pulmonary edema	Monitor volume status; see Chapter 5
Defibrillation	2 watt-sec/kg (adult: 200 watt-sec)	Ventricular fibrillation Ventricular tachycardia		Use correct paddle size and paste; if initial dose is unsuccessful, use 2-4 watt-sec/kg, which may be repeated once; if still unresponsive, give 4 watt-sec/kg after lidocaine; synchronized cardioversion (0.5-1.0 watt-sec/kg)
Dexamethasone (Decadron) (4,24 mg/ml)	0.15-0.60 mg/kg/dose IM, IV	Croup, asthma, meningitis	Hypoglycemia	Delayed onset
Diazepam (Valium) (5 mg/ml)	0.2-0.3 mg/kg/dose (maximum: 10 mg/dose) IV	Status epilepticus	Respiratory depression	Also begin maintenance medication (Table 81-6); may give higher dose rectally (0.5 mg/kg PR)
Diazoxide (Hyperstat) (15 mg/ml)	1-3 mg/kg q4-24hr IV	Hypertension	Hypotension, hyperglycemia	Monitor (very prompt onset) (Table 18-2)
Digoxin (0.1, 0.25 mg/ml)	Preemie: 0.01-0.02 mg/kg TDD IV 2 wk-2 yr: 0.03-0.05 mg/kg TDD IV Newborn and >2 yr: 0.04 mg/kg TDD IV ½ TDD initially, then ¼ q4-8hr IV × 2	Congestive heart failure Supraventricular tachycardia	Dysrhythmia, heart block, vomiting	Monitor ECG; may also load PO in stable, nonurgent situation; if mild CHF, may give PO without loading (Table 16-2)

Drug	Dosage	Indications	Side Effects	Comments
Dobutamine (Dobutrex) (vial: 250 mg)	2-20 µg/kg/min IV	Cardiogenic shock	Tachycardia, dysrhythmia, hypotension or hypertension	β Adrenergic; positive inotropic; may be synergistic with dopamine or isoproterenol (Table 5-2)
Dopamine (200 mg/5 ml)	Low: 2-5 µg/kg/min IV Mod: 5-20 µg/kg/min IV High: >20 µg/kg/min IV	Cardiogenic shock (moderate dose) Maintain renal perfusion Septic shock	Tachycardia, bradycardia, vasoconstriction (increases with higher doses)	β Adrenergic; avoid in hypovolemic shock; may use in combination with isoproterenol or levarterenol (norepinephrine) (Table 5-2)
Epinephrine (1:10,000) (0.1 mg/ml)	0.01 mg/kg (or 0.1 ml/kg of 1:10,000 solution) IV or IO followed by 0.1 mg/kg (0.1 ml/kg of 1:1000 solution) q3-5min prn; subsequent doses may be as high as 0.2 mg/kg (0.2 ml/kg of 1:1000 solution)	Ventricular standstill Ventricular fibrillation (fine) Anaphylaxis Hemodynamically significant bradycardia	Tachycardia, dysrhythmia, hypertension, decreased renal and splanchnic blood flow	α and β Adrenergic; inotropic; not effective if acidotic (Table 5-2); endotracheal dose is 0.1 mg/kg (1:1000 solution) initially
Epinephrine (1:1000) (1 mg/ml)	0.01 ml/kg/dose SC (max: 0.35 ml/dose) q10-20min SC × 3 prn	Reactive airway disease	Tachycardia, headache, nausea	See above for high-dose epinephrine or ET administration
Epinephrine racemic (Vaponefrin) (2.25% solution)	0.25-0.75 ml/dose in 2.5 ml saline by inhalation	Croup	Tachycardia, rebound stridor	Observe, concurrent steroids
Fentanyl (Sublimaze, Innovar) 50 µg/ml	1-5 µg/kg/dose IV, IM	Analgesia	Respiratory depression, muscle rigidity	Monitor
Furosemide (Lasix) (10 mg/ml)	1 mg/kg/dose q6-12hr IV up to 6 mg/kg/dose; may repeat q2hr prn	Fluid overload, pulmonary edema, cerebral edema	Hypokalemia, hyponatremia, prerenal azotemia	Reduce dosage in newborn to q12hr; if no response in urine output in 30 min, repeat; do not use if hypovolemic (Table 16-3)

Continued

TABLE 4-2 Common Primary and Secondary Measures in Resuscitation—cont'd

Drug availability	Dose/route	Indications	Adverse reactions	Comments
Glucagon 1 mg (1 unit)/ml	0.03-0.1 mg/kg/dose q20min prn IV, SC, IM	β-Blocker overdose, Hypoglycemia		Not adequate as only glucose support in neonate, inotropic
Glucose (D50W-0.5 gm/ml)	0.5-1.0 g (2-4 ml D25W or 1-2 ml D50W)/kg/dose IV	Hypoglycemia, with coma or seizure	Hyperglycemia	Draw glucose; if possible use D25W
Hydralazine (Apresoline) (20 mg/ml)	0.1-0.4 mg/kg/dose q4-6hr IV/IM	Hypertension	Tachycardia, tachyphylaxis	Prompt onset (Table 18-2); may also be given as 1.5 µg/kg/min IV infusion; limited availability
Hydrocortisone (Solu-Cortef) (100, 250, 500 mg)	Asthma: 4-5 mg/kg/dose q6hr IV	Adrenal failure, Asthma		May be detrimental in shock (controversial) (Table 74-2)
Isoproterenol (1 mg/5 ml)	0.05-1.5 µg/kg/min Begin at 0.1 µg/kg/min and increase q5-10min prn	Bradycardia or heart block (S/P atropine)	Tachyrhythmias	β Adrenergic; avoid in hypovolemic shock; do not use with digoxin (Table 5-2)
Lidocaine (1%-10 mg/ml) (2%-20 mg/ml)	1 mg/kg/dose q5-10min IV, ET up to 5 mg/kg, then 20-50 µg/kg/min	Ventricular dysrhythmias, Cardiac arrest caused by ventricular fibrillation	Hypotension, bradycardia with block, seizures	↓ Automaticity and ectopic pacemaker (Table 6-4); for ET administration give 1:1 dilution, with 2-3 times IV dose
Lorazepam (Ativan) (2,4 mg/ml)	0.05-0.10 mg/kg/dose (maximum: 4 mg/dose) IV; may repeat	Status epilepticus	Respiratory depression	Longer acting than diazepam
Methylprednisolone (Solu-Medrol) (40, 125, 500, 1000 mg)	Asthma: 1-2 mg/kg/dose q6hr IV; usual maximum is 12.5-25 mg/dose	Adrenal failure, Asthma	Hypoglycemia	May be detrimental in shock (controversial) (Table 74-2)
Midazolam (Versed) (1, 5 mg/ml;	0.05-0.1 mg/kg/dose (maximum: 5 mg/dose IV)	Sedation	Respiratory depression, hypotension	Monitor, must be prepared to manage airway

Drug	Dosage	Indications	Side Effects	Comments
Morphine (8, 10, 15 mg/ml)	0.1-0.2 mg/kg/dose (maximum: 15 mg/dose) q2-4hr IV	Pulmonary edema, Tetralogy spell, Reduce preload and afterload	Hypotension, respiratory depression	Antidote: naloxone (Narcan)
Naloxone (Narcan) (0.4, 1 mg/ml)	0.1 mg/kg/dose (minimum: 0.4 mg/dose; maximum: 2.0 mg/dose) IV, ET	Narcotic overdose; ? septic shock		Give empirically in suspected opiate overdose; may be given ET; higher dosage may be used for unresponsive overdose
Nitroglycerin (Nitrostat, Nitro-Bid) (0.5, 0.8, 5, 10 mg/ml)	IV 0.5-10 µg/kg/min	Pulmonary edema, angina pectoris, perioperative hypertension	Hypotension, headache, nausea, vomiting, palpitations	Contraindicated with hypotension, increased ICP, hypovolemia, cardiac tamponade, pericarditis, inadequate cerebral circulation
Nitroprusside (50 mg/vial)	0.5-10 µg (average: 3 µg)/kg/min IV	Hypertensive emergency, Afterload reduction	Hypotension, cyanide poisoning	Monitor closely; light sensitive (Table 18-2); thiocyanate toxicity in patient with impaired renal function
Oxygen	100% mask, ET	Hypoxia, Major injury	Toxicity not a problem with acute short-term use	Use high flow (3-6 L/min); monitor ABG, oximetry
Pancuronium (Pavulon) (1, 2 mg/ml)	0.04-0.1 mg/kg/dose IV; may repeat 0.01-0.02 mg/kg/dose q20-40min IV prn	Muscle relaxation	Tachycardia	Rapid onset; support respirations; lower dose in newborn
Phenobarbital (65 mg/ml)	15-20 mg/kg load IV/IM (adult: 100 mg/dose q20min prn × 3), then 5 mg/kg/24 hr PO, IV, IM	Seizures	Sedation	If not controlled after load, repeat 10 mg/kg/dose IV; administer <1 mg/kg/min IV; IM erratically absorbed (Table 81-6)

Continued

TABLE 4-2   Common Primary and Secondary Measures in Resuscitation—cont'd

Drug availability	Dose/route	Indications	Adverse reactions	Comments
Phenytoin (Dilantin) (50 mg/ml)	10-20 mg/kg load IV slowly, then 5-10 mg/kg/24 hr q12-24hr PO, IV	Seizures	Hypotension, bradycardia when given too fast; cerebral disturbance	Do not give faster than 0.5 mg/kg/min; dilute in normal saline (Table 81-6); fosphenytoin (Cerebyx) (50 mg/ml) is available for IV or IM administration with less toxicity and local reaction
	5 mg/kg/dose IV q5-20min × 2 prn	Dysrhythmia		
Succinylcholine (20 mg/ml)	1-2 mg/kg/dose IV (larger dose in children <20 kg)	Muscle relaxation	Dysrhythmia Hypotension	Must be able to control ventilation
Vecuronium (Norcuron) (10 mg/ml)	0.08-0.1 mg/kg/dose IV	Nondepolarizing muscle blockade	Profound skeletal muscle weakness; respiratory arrest	Monitor; to be used only by persons with advanced airway skills
Verapamil (Calan, Isoptin) (2.5 mg/ml)	0.1-0.2 mg/kg/dose (maximum: 5 mg/dose) IV; may repeat in 30 min	Supraventricular tachycardia	Dizziness, hypotension, bradycardia, AV block	Monitor; contraindicated in patients <1 yr or with ventricular dysfunction, sick sinus syndrome, heart block, atrial fibrillation or flutter

urea nitrogen (BUN), creatinine, sugar, calcium, phosphorus levels

3. ABG levels and oximetry

4. X-ray film: chest x-ray study for underlying disease, placement of ET and nasogastric (NG) tubes, and monitoring of potential complications.

5. Ultrasound: assess cardiac function and exclude pneumothorax and tamponade

6. Electrocardiogram (ECG) and ongoing cardiac monitoring

7. Type and cross match, if appropriate

8. NG tube insertion: determine nature of aspirate and output monitoring

9. Urinary catheter: urinalysis and output monitoring

Disposition/Termination

If resuscitation is successful, ongoing support and monitoring is mandatory. Patients seen in the ED in arrest despite prehospital intervention usually have a poor outcome.

Efforts should be terminated if obvious brain death has not occurred, remembering that the brain of the infant and child is relatively resistant to hypoxic damage. Clinical evidence that is useful includes the oculocephalic reflex (doll's eyes reflex), oculovestibular reflex (calorics), absent corneal reflex, and fixed, dilated pupils. Resuscitation should be continued if evidence of drug depression or hypothermia is present. Underlying disease may modify the aggressiveness of resuscitation.

Psychologic Support

Support of the child and the entire family is essential throughout the resuscitation period. The child is separated from the parents and is in a strange environment, surrounded by unfamiliar nurses and physicians. If the resuscitation is successful and vital signs and consciousness are restored, time should be taken to reassure and calm the child.

1. A member of the health care team should be assigned to provide the family with information, explanations, and emotional support. Health professionals must recognize their own personal feelings while being available and allowing parents to verbalize their feelings and emotions.

2. The decision regarding whether to allow parents to stay with the child must be individualized, on the basis of the child's medical condition and level of consciousness and the emotional state of the family. Family members often find it reassuring to be in the resuscitation room, even if the outcome is poor. There may be specific individuals such as relatives or clergy who can be supportive and should be called.

3. If the child dies, support and compassion are needed while attempting to relieve the family of feelings of guilt and facilitating the normal grieving process. Most parents will want to touch and hold their child after the youngster has been made as presentable as possible (see Foreword). Some parents have found it useful to have a lock of the child's hair or a footprint (using nursery's print pad identification system) taken at this time. Arrangements should be made for support during the next days and weeks to ensure that appropriate resources have been mobilized to assist the family.

When faced with the sudden death of a child, all concerned experience grief at the loss. It is essential that support be provided not only for the family but also for the entire health care team.

REFERENCES

Ahrens W, Hart R, Maruyama N: Pediatric death: the aftermath in the emergency department, *J Emerg Med* 15:601, 1997.

American Academy of Pediatrics and American College of Physicians: *APLS-the pediatric emergency medicine course*, ed 2, Dallas, 1993, The College.

American Academy of Pediatrics and American Heart Association: *Textbook of pediatric advanced life support*, Elk Grove, Ill, 1994, The Academy and The Association.

American Heart Association: Guidelines for cardiopulmonary resuscitation (CPR) and emergency cardiac care (ECO), *JAMA* 268:2171, 1992.

Barton C, Callaham M: High-dose epinephrine improves the return of spontaneous circulation rates in human victims of cardiac arrest, *Ann Emerg Med* 20:722, 1991.

Benumof JL: Laryngeal mask airway, *J Anesthesiology* 77: 843, 1992.

Bhendi MS, Thompson AE: Evaluation of an end-tidal CO_2 detector during pediatric cardiopulmonary resuscitation, *Pediatrics* 95:395, 1995.

Bush CM, Jones JS, Cohle SD, et al: Pediatric injuries from cardiopulmonary resuscitation, *Ann Emerg Med* 28:40, 1996.

Chameides L: CPR challenges in pediatrics, *Ann Emerg Med* 22:388, 1993.

Cook RT, Moglia BB, Consevage MW, et al: The use of Beck Airway Airflow Monitor for verifying intratracheal endotracheal tube placement in patients in the pediatric emergency department and intensive care unit, *Pediatr Emerg Care* 12:331, 1996.

Fiser D: Intraosseous infusion, *N Engl J Med* 322:1579, 1990.

Cerardi MJ, Sacchetti AD, Cantor RM, et al: Rapid sequence intubation of the pediatric patient, *Ann Emerg Med* 28:55, 1996.

Halperin HR, Chandra NC, Levin HR, et al: Newer methods of improving blood flow during CPR, *Ann Emerg Med* 27:553, 1996.

Hebert P, Weitzman BN, Stiell IC, et al: Epinephrine in cardiopulmonary resuscitation, *J Emerg Med* 9:481, 1991.

Hickey RW, Cohen DM, Strausbaugh S, et al: Pediatric patients requiring CPR in the prehospital setting, *Ann Emerg Med* 25:495, 1995.

Hooker EA, Danzl DF, Brueggmeyer M, et al: Respiratory rate in pediatric emergency patients, *J Emerg Med* 10:407, 1992.

Internation Liason Committee on Resuscitation: Pediatric resuscitation, *Circulation* 95:2185, 1997.

Johnston C: Endotracheal drug delivery, *Pediatr Emerg Care* 8:94, 1992.

King BR, Baker MD, Braitman LE, et al: Endotracheal tube selection in children: a comparison of four methods, *Ann Emerg Med* 22:530, 1993.

Luten RC, Wears RL, Broselow J, et al: Length-based endotracheal tube and emergency equipment selection in pediatrics, *Ann Emerg Med* 21:900, 1992.

Quan L, Craves JR, Kinder DR, et al: Transcutaneous cardiac pacing in the treatment of out-of-hospital pediatric cardiac arrest, *Ann Emerg Med* 21:905, 1993.

Schindler MB, Bohn D, Cox PN, et al: Out of hospital cardiac arrest, *N Engl J Med* 335:1473, 1995.

Schlessel JS, Rappa HA, Lesser M, et al: CPR knowledge, self-efficacy and anticipated anxiety as functions of infant/child CPR training, *Ann Emerg Med* 25:618, 1995.

Seidel JS, Henderson DP, Spencer PE: Education in pediatric basic and advanced life support, *Ann Emerg Med* 22:489, 1993.

Staudinger T, Brugger S, Watchinger B, et al: Emergency intubation with the Combitube: with endotracheal airway, *Ann Emerg Med* 22:1573, 1993.

Teach SJ, Moore PE, Fleisher CR: Death and resuscitation in the pediatric emergency department, *Ann Emerg Med* 25:799, 1995.

Tobias JD: The laryngeal mask airway: a review for emergency physicians, *Pediatr Emerg Care* 12:370, 1996.

Todres ID: Pediatric airway control and ventilation, *Ann Emerg Med* 22:400, 1993.

Zaritsky A, Nadharni V, Hazinshi MR, et al: Recommended guidelines for uniform reporting of pediatric advanced life support: pediatric resuscitation pharmacology, *Ann Emerg Med* 26:487, 1993.

5 SHOCK

Shock occurs when acute circulatory dysfunction is marked by progressive impairment of blood flow to the skin, muscles, kidneys, mesentery, lungs, heart, and brain. Patients in shock have diminished perfusion manifested by decreased blood pressure, tachycardia, poor capillary refill, decreased skin temperature, altered mental status, diminished urinary output, and multiple system failure. In children, hypovolemia is the most common cause. Compensatory mechanisms initially prevent functional deterioration, but with progression, cellular metabolic changes are marked by anaerobic metabolism, leading to further injury and eventually cell death and release of proteolytic enzymes and cellular by-products.

Blood pressure depends on cardiac output (rate and volume) and peripheral resistance. Although normal blood pressure and pulse values are summarized in Appendix B-2, it is useful to remember that the maximum effective heart rate in infants is 200 beats/min; in preschool children, 150 beats/min; and in older individuals, 120 beats/min. Normal systolic blood pressures in individuals 1 to 20 years of age can be estimated by adding twice the age in years to 80. Diastolic blood pressure is usually two thirds of systolic blood pressure.

Normal blood volume is averaged as 80 ml/kg; age-specific volumes are as follows:

Preterm infant	90-105 ml/kg
Term newborn	85 ml/kg
>1 mo	75 ml/kg
>1 yr	67-75 ml/kg
Adult	55-75 ml/kg

STAGES OF SHOCK AND DIAGNOSTIC FINDINGS
Compensated Shock

Vital organ functions are maintained by intrinsic compensatory mechanisms that stabilize vital signs. As fluid loss progresses, compensation causes venous capacitance to decrease by 10% to 25%, fluid to shift from the interstitial to intravascular compartments, and arteriolar constriction to increase. With compensation the central venous pressure (CVP) is decreased, as are stroke volume and urine output; heart rate and systemic vascular resistance increase. Perfusion to the periphery (skin and muscles) and to the kidneys and intestine may be compromised, even without major alterations in blood pressure. Decreased skin perfusion may produce decreased skin temperature, impaired capillary refill (>2 seconds), and a pale, blue, or mottled appearance. Poor central nervous system (CNS) perfusion ultimately produces impaired mentation and poor responsiveness.

Capillary refill is measured in the fingernail bed after applying just the amount of pressure necessary to blanch the nailbed. In children 2 to 24 months of age, a turgor time less than 1.5 seconds is consistent with less than 5% deficit, 1.5 to 3 seconds occurs with a 5% to 10% deficit, and more than 3 seconds time with more than a 10% deficit. Other factors that prolong the capillary refill are hyponatremia, hypothermia, and congestive heart failure. It is less reliable in patients with edema or malnutrition.

Ultimately, the efficacy of compensatory mechanisms depends on the patient's preexisting cardiac and pulmonary status and the rate and volume of blood loss.

Diagnostic Findings

Orthostatic changes (systolic blood pressure decreases >15 mm Hg or pulse increases >20 beats/min from supine to seated or erect position) reflect primarily intravascular volume but are difficult to delineate in the child under less than 5 years of age.

1. An acute volume deficit of 10% may be marked by an increase in pulse rate of 20 beats/min, and a 20% deficit has an associated heart rate increase of 30 beats/min, with a variable decrease in blood pressure. Larger volume deficits have a consistent blood pressure decrease (>15 mm Hg) and pulse increase (>30 beats/min).

2. A 10% to 15% gradual volume loss produces minimal physiologic change. On the other hand, a 20% to 30% gradual volume deficit is marked by compensation, but no related hypotension is present. Progressive hypotension is noted with 30% to 50% gradual volume loss.

In acute blood loss, *supine* blood pressure may remain normal with a 20% or greater deficit. Orthostatic changes *must* be measured. Acidosis, which may be the most sensitive indicator of inadequate perfusion, must also be monitored closely.

Uncompensated Shock

Cardiovascular dysfunction and impairment of microvascular perfusion lead to lowered perfusion pressures, increased precapillary arteriolar resistance, and further contraction of venous capacitance; with progressive blood stagnation, anaerobic metabolism and release of proteolytic enzymes and vasoactive substances occur. This exacerbates myocardial depression. Platelet aggregation and release of tissue thromboplastin produce hypercoagulability and disseminated intravascular coagulation (DIC).

Diagnostic Findings

Hypotension, tachycardia, decreased cardiac output, and variable central venous pressures are observed. Multiple organ system failure occurs with adult respiratory distress syndrome (ARDS), liver and pancreatic failure, coagulopathies with DIC, oliguria and renal failure, gastrointestinal (GI) bleeding, impaired mental status, acidosis, abnormal calcium and phosphorus homeostasis, and ongoing cellular damage. Although variability does exist, the following observation may be useful:

Type of shock	Appearance of skin	Neck veins
Hypovolemic	Cold, clammy, pale	Flat
Cardiogenic	Cold, clammy, pale	Bulging
Distributive	Warm, dry, flushed; then cold, clammy	Variable

Terminal Shock

Irreversible damage to the heart and brain as a result of altered perfusion and metabolism ultimately leads to death.

ETIOLOGY AND DIAGNOSTIC FINDINGS

The clinical presentation and progression of findings partially reflect the underlying condi-

---

Box 5-1
ETIOLOGIC CLASSIFICATION OF SHOCK

HYPOVOLEMIC

1. Hemorrhage
   a. External: laceration
   b. Internal: ruptured spleen or liver, vascular injury, fracture (neonate: intracerebral/intraventricular hemorrhage)
   c. Gastrointestinal: bleeding ulcer, ruptured viscus, mesenteric hemorrhage
2. Plasma loss
   a. Burn
   b. Inflammation or sepsis; leaky capillary syndrome
   c. Nephrotic syndrome
   d. Third spacing: intestinal obstruction, pancreatitis, peritonitis
3. Fluid and electrolyte loss
   a. Acute gastroenteritis
   b. Excessive sweating (cystic fibrosis)
   c. Renal disorder
4. Endocrine
   a. Adrenal insufficiency, adrenal-genital syndrome
   b. Diabetes mellitus
   c. Diabetes insipidus
   d. Hypothyroidism (myxedema coma)

CARDIOGENIC

1. Myocardial insufficiency
   a. Dysrhythmia: bradycardia, atrioventricular (AV) block, ventricular tachycardia, supraventricular tachycardia
   b. Cardiomyopathy: myocarditis, ischemia, hypoxia, hypoglycemia, acidosis
   c. Drug intoxication
   d. Hypothermia
   e. Myocardial depressant effects of shock
   f. Status after cardiac surgery
2. Filling or outflow obstruction
   a. Pericardial tamponade
   b. Pneumopericardium
   c. Tension pneumothorax
   d. Pulmonary embolism
   e. Congenital heart disease, including patent ductus arteriosus (PDA)—dependent lesion such as coarctation of the aorta or critical pulmonary stenosis

DISTRIBUTIVE (VASOGENIC)

1. High or normal resistance (increased venous capacitance)
   a. Septic shock
   b. Anaphylaxis
   c. Barbiturate intoxication
2. Low resistance, vasodilation: CNS injury (i.e., spinal cord transection)

---

tion and the stage and classification of shock (Box 5-1). Patients demonstrate altered vital signs associated with tachycardia; poor capillary refill (abnormal if >2 seconds); cool, mottled, and pale skin; and altered mental status. They may have evidence of impaired cardiac function. Blood pressure changes may develop, often preceded by earlier orthostatic changes. Respiratory alkalosis and metabolic acidosis are common.

Specific focus must be directed toward defining the underlying disease and its specific sequelae and complications, as well as understanding the pathophysiology of the disease process.

Hypovolemic Shock

Reduction in circulating blood volume produces progressive dysfunction:

1. Decreased preload through capillary pooling and leakage accompanied by extrinsic and intrinsic loss of intravascular volume and decreased cardiac output

2. Increased afterload secondary to arteriolar constriction
3. Myocardial ischemia resulting from impairment of subendocardial blood flow and decreased supply of oxygen to myocardium; concurrently, an increased myocardial oxygen requirement is associated with tachycardia, increased afterload, and cardiac distension
4. Excessive aldosterone secretion with sodium and water retention, leading to pulmonary edema and further hypoxia

Compensatory homeostasis is achieved at the expense of regional blood flow initially to the skin and muscles and then to the kidneys, mesentery, lungs, heart, and brain. Because children have highly reactive vascular beds, an adequate blood pressure can be maintained, even in the presence of significant intravascular volume depletion; when hypotension does develop, it is profound and rapid.

Cardiogenic Shock

Dysfunction of the heart with depressed cardiac output may result from myocardial insufficiency or mechanical obstruction of the flow of blood into and out of the heart. Inadequate preload, with accompanying hypovolemia, capillary injury, vascular instability, decreased cardiac output, and tissue perfusion, produces a rapid downhill spiral of microcirculatory failure. Children rarely go through a prolonged compensated phase before decompensation.

Hemodynamically, patients have decreased cardiac output and elevated central venous pressure, pulmonary wedge pressure, and systemic vascular resistance. These may be the terminal events associated with primary shock of other origin (Fig. 5-1).

Distributive or Vasogenic Shock

Distributive or vasogenic shock is associated with an abnormality in the distribution of blood flow, initially resulting from acute arteriolar dilation and increased venous capacitance accompanied by decreased intravascular volume secondary to leaky capillaries. This early hyperdynamic phase is associated with decreased afterload; it is less common in children than adults. The early phase is followed by rapid decompensation with decreased cardiac output and increased systemic vascular resistance secondary to hypoxemia and acidosis and increased venous capacitance. Clinically, warm, dry, flushed skin may be noted initially. This occurrence is followed by rapid progression to a vasoconstrictive phase.

In septic shock the endotoxin inhibits platelet function while injuring the endothelium and activating intrinsic clotting factors with subsequent DIC.

Although the initial hyperdynamic phase is rare in children, when present it may respond to volume therapy. With progression, volume administration must be rapidly combined with agents that decrease peripheral resistance (alpha effect), whereas cardiac function is improved with positive inotropic agents (β_1).

Complications

Complications are common, reflecting the stage of shock, rapidity of response, underlying disease process, and problems secondary to therapy.

1. ARDS (p. 44)
2. Acute tubular necrosis (ATN) with renal failure (p. 809)
3. Myocardial dysfunction with failure (p. 145)
4. Stress ulcers, GI bleeding, ileus

Ancillary Data

1. Chest radiographic studies on all patients to evaluate for cardiac size, pneumothorax, pneumonia, and pulmonary edema.
2. Arterial blood gas (ABG) level to monitor progression of acidosis and diffusion and

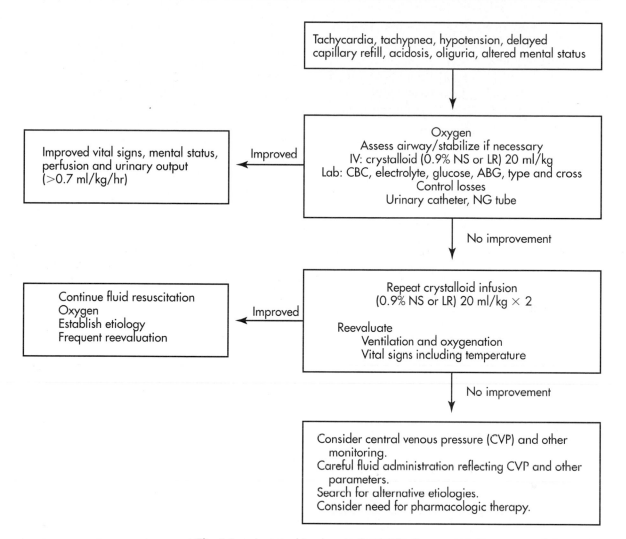

Fig. 5-1   Approaching hypovolemic shock.

ventilation problems associated with respiratory distress syndrome.

3. Electrocardiography (ECG) and echocardiography to evaluate cardiac function, exclude dysrhythmias, monitor preload, and exclude effusion.

4. Chemical studies: electrolytes, blood urea nitrogen (BUN), creatinine, glucose, liver functions, calcium, phosphorus, cardiac enzymes, as indicated.

5. Hematologic evaluation: complete blood count (CBC), platelets, coagulation (prothrombin time [PT], partial thromboplastin time [PTT]), and DIC (fibrinogen, fibrin split products) screening (p. 683). Hemoglobin (Hb) and hematocrit (Hct) may be artificially normal in the face of markedly decreased intravascular volume and must be measured on a continuing basis.

6. Type and cross match because of the potential for hemorrhage, DIC, or intravascular hemolysis, which are common.

7. Urinalysis to exclude hematuria, proteinuria, and infection. Output must be continuously monitored.
8. Cultures of blood and urine. Spinal fluid as indicated. Counterimmunoelectrophoresis (CIE) may be useful with negative culture results.

MANAGEMENT

Initial resuscitation must be followed by a systematic approach to fluid therapy, pharmacologic support, and diagnostic evaluation. It is imperative to monitor perfusion constantly through hemodynamic parameters, including blood pressure, heart rate and capillary refill, urine output, acid-base status, and mental alertness. If one approach is not effective, the fluid and pharmacologic approach must be adjusted on an empiric basis.

After stabilization of the airway and ventilation and initiation of resuscitation of the cardiovascular system, the underlying disease process requires urgent attention.

Airway and Ventilation

1. Administer oxygen at 3-6 L/min by cannula, mask, etc. (see Chapter 4).
2. Determine need for intubation and mechanical ventilation. The indications for intubation include the following:
   a. Arterial oxygen tension (Pao_2) less than 50 mm Hg (sea level) when oxygen is administered with Fio_2 of 50%
   b. Arterial carbon dioxide tension ($Paco_2$) greater than 50 mm Hg (unless caused by compensation from prolonged condition such as bronchopulmonary dysplasia or cystic fibrosis)
   c. Decreasing vital capacity, increasing respiratory rate, or rapidly progressive disease
   d. Severe metabolic acidosis
   e. Inability to protect airway
   f. Severe pulmonary edema or marked respiratory distress after drowning or a similar accident requiring positive end-expiratory pressure (PEEP)

ARDS may develop with increased extravascular pulmonary water, thereby increasing both the work of breathing and permeability secondary to damage of the alveolar epithelium and the pulmonary capillary endothelium (alveolar-capillary membrane). This syndrome is not a single disease but a group of disorders with similar clinical, pathologic, and pathophysiologic findings. No one mediator can explain every case, and for a given insult, more than one pathogenic process can occur simultaneously.

As a result of the cellular injury, the pulmonary capillaries become permeable, and proteinaceous fluid leaks into the interstitial space and alveoli. This is characterized by progressive hypoxemia, hypercapnia, respiratory alkalosis, increased shunting, and decreased compliance.

Ventilation with early introduction of PEEP is essential if Pao_2 does not respond to PEEP alone or if other indications for intubation are present. A PEEP of 3 to 6 cm H_2O should be started with and titrated upward using an adequate Pao_2 as the end-point, without decreasing cardiac output. Chest radiographic films and ABGs should be monitored.

NOTE: PEEP may increase intrapulmonary shunting, with a potential decrease in cardiac output and decreased delivery of oxygen to the tissues. This usually does not occur until PEEP reaches above 15 cm H_2O.

Intravenous Fluids

Fluids should be initiated after insertion of one or two large-bore intravenous (IV) lines (see p. 400 and Appendix A-3). In administering IV fluids, it is essential to remember the relationship between preload and stroke volume described by the Frank-Starling curve; excessive fluid administration actually may impair cardiac function, emphasizing the importance of monitoring the central venous pressure or pulmonary capillary wedge pressure (PCWP).

Hypovolemic Shock (see Fig. 5-1)

1. Administer 0.9% normal saline solution (NS) at a rate of 20 ml/kg over 20 minutes. D5W 0.9% NS may be used if the cause is gastroenteritis and low glucose levels are anticipated. Monitor urine output, pulse, perfusion, and blood pressure.

2. If no response, repeat the infusion of 0.9% NS with ongoing evaluation of ventilatory status, temperature, electrolytes, glucose, ABG, and ECG.

3. Place a CVP line if no response after two infusions. Observe CVP or PCWP for 10 minutes after fluid challenge.

   a. If elevated (>10 mm Hg CVP* or >12 mm Hg PCWP), consider other causes, including tension pneumothorax, pericardial tamponade, myocardial insufficiency, congestive heart failure, PDA-dependent lesion with closing of PDA (coarctation of aorta in newborn), or myocarditis.

   b. If decreased (<10 mm Hg CVP or <12 mm Hg PCWP), administer crystalloid (0.9% NS) in increments of 5-10 ml/kg over 20 to 30 minutes while monitoring CVP response. Observe response for at least 10 minutes after infusion. If CVP returns to within 3 mm Hg of the preinfusion value, continue infusion and repeat until either hemodynamic parameters are corrected or the CVP persistently exceeds the initial value by 3 mm Hg.

   c. CVP may not reflect left ventricular function. PCWP may be needed, particularly if positive pressure ventilation is used, if pulmonary disease or mitral stenosis is present, or if there is evidence of failure of either the left or right side of the heart.

4. If hemorrhage is the cause of hypovolemia, type-specific or cross-matched blood should be administered after an initial crystalloid resuscitation. Once 40-50 ml/kg of crystalloid has been infused, it is increasingly important to administer blood. Whole blood is particularly useful for massive ongoing acute bleeding; however, packed red blood cells may be appropriate after the infusion of large amounts of crystalloid in an acute situation or in a more chronic process (Table 5-1).

   a. If completely cross-matched blood is not available, administer type-specific blood. It is usually available within 10 to 15 minutes after delivery of a clot to the blood bank. O-negative blood should be reserved for those patients in profound shock secondary to hypovolemia who have no response to crystalloid or who are in cardiac arrest after trauma.

   b. Fresh-frozen plasma and platelets are often indicated to correct coagulation defects rapidly. Coagulation status should be monitored.

   c. Massive blood transfusions (equivalent to one blood volume of 80 ml/kg) require the use of blood warmers and micropore filters.

5. If hypovolemia exists concurrently with hypoproteinemia, use 5% *albumin* in 0.9% NS (Plasmanate) or fresh-frozen plasma at 5-10 ml/kg over 30 minutes with careful monitoring. This infusion may be repeated until the patient is hemodynamically stable or the CVP increases.

6. The role of *colloid* in severe shock or capillary leak syndromes is controversial. There may be a role for 5% albumin or products like 6% hetastarch combined with crystalloid to improve intravascular blood flow, but this has not been consistently demonstrated to be superior to crystalloid. Colloid is not used for initial burn therapy.

---

*0.75 mm Hg = 1 cm H_2O.

TABLE 5-1   Pediatric Blood Component Therapy

Problem	"Classic" coagulation panel abnormalities	Blood component	Quantity
Acute blood loss	Hematocrit <40 (infants) <30 (children)	Whole blood* P-RBCs	To replace loss or 10-20 ml/kg 10 ml/kg should raise Hct 10 points
Chronic anemia	Hematocrit <15% to 20% Hemoglobin <5-7 gm/dl Patient symptomatic	P-RBCs If frequent or multiple transfusions are required, or history of febrile reactions, consider leukocyte-poor RBCs (buffy coat removed to prevent reactions with WBCs)	Administer *slowly:* 3 ml/kg/hr (consider diuretics)
Anemia in child with T-cell immune deficiency	Hematocrit <40 (infants) <30 (children) (consider patient baseline)	If time and patient stability allows, consider irradiated blood cells	As above (see acute blood loss)
Thrombocytopenia	↓ platelets (isolated) ↑ template bleeding time Clot formation but lack of clot retraction	Platelets	1 U/5 kg (maximum: 10 U)
Thrombocytopathia	Normal or only slightly decreased platelet count, template bleeding time	Platelets	1 U/5 kg (maximum: 10 U)
Disseminated intravascular coagulation (DIC)	↓ fibrinogen and platelets (lower than expected) ↑ PT, PTT ↑ fibrin split products	Treat cause If fibrinogen <50, cryoprecipitate plus fresh-frozen plasma (FFP) should be given; if fibrinogen >50 FFP alone may be effective	FFP: 10 ml/kg Cryoprecipitate: 1 bag/5 kg Titrate to achieve improvement in fibrinogen and platelet count
DIC with purpura fulminans	As above with evidence of peripheral embolic phenomena	Administer FFP to restore levels of antithrombin III, then heparin	FFP: 10 ml/kg Heparin: Load: 50 U/kg IV: 10-25 U/kg/hr Titrate to achieve rise in fibrinogen and platelet count and fall in PTT

From Hazinski MF: Cardiovascular disorders. In Hazinski MF, editor: *Nursing care of the critically ill child,* ed 2, St Louis, 1992, Mosby.
*Generally unavailable; largely replaced by P-RBC (packed red blood cells).

TABLE 5-1 Pediatric Blood Component Therapy—cont'd

Problem	"Classic" coagulation panel abnormalities	Blood component	Quantity
Hemophilia A (Table 79-2)	Bleeding ↓ factor VIII activity	Purified factor VIII	Severe life-threatening bleeding or major surgery: up to 50 U/kg or continuous infusion of 2 U/kg/hr to maintain factor VIII activity at 100% Minor bleeding: up to 25 U/kg
Lack of coagulation factors in general†	↑ PT, PTT, thrombin time ↓ fibrinogen Slow clot formation	Fresh-frozen plasma	10 ml/kg
Heparin excess‡	↑↑ PTT, thrombin time, and template bleeding time PT may be slightly ↑ Platelet count normal (initially) Slow clot formation	Protamine sulfate (titrated to correct thrombin time)	1 mg/kg (slowly): 1 mg IV each 100 U Heparin given concurrently; 0.5 mg IV each 100 U Heparin given in previous 30 min, and so on; maximum: 50 mg/dose (slowly)
Protamine sulfate excess‡	↑↑ PTT, thrombin time, and template bleeding time PT may be slightly ↑ Platelet count normal (initially) Slow clot formation	When protamine is titrated and thrombin time does not improve, heparin may be administered	Heparin IV: 50 U/kg Infusion: 10-15 U/kg/hr
Effects of aspirin (ASA)	↑ template bleeding time	Platelets	1 U/5 kg (maximum: 10 U)

†Usually, this condition results from a complex function of dilution and lack of replacement during surgery, inability of the liver to compensate, and occasionally from excessive loss of plasma protein (large proteins) via chest tubes.
‡The only way to distinguish between these two problems is through protamine sulfate titration.

Cardiogenic Shock

1. A fluid push may improve cardiac output by increasing filling pressure in accordance with the Frank-Starling curve, particularly if the CVP is less than 15 mm Hg. The PCWP is a more reliable measure of the response to fluid challenge in cardiogenic shock and should be measured if possible, but insertion of a Swan-Ganz catheter should not delay aggressive stabilization. At 5 ml/kg over 30 minutes, 0.9% NS may be administered with careful monitoring of response.

2. Pressor agents (Table 5-2) are usually necessary with an inadequate response to IV fluid challenge. Ultimately, inotropic and vasodilating drugs may be needed to normalize blood pressure.

TABLE 5-2   Commonly Used Drugs for Shock*

| Drug | Mechanism | | | Dose (IV) | Comments |
	Alpha	β₁	β₂		
Isoproterenol (Isuprel)	±	+++	+++	0.05-1.5 µg/kg/min	Positive inotropic and chronotropic effect; peripheral vasodilation; increased cardiac oxygen requirement; relatively large increase in cardiac output; decreased coronary blood flow Use: decreased cardiac contractility; bradycardia and third-degree atrioventricular (AV) block
Dopamine (Inotropin)	At high dosage	++ to +++	±	Low: 2-5 µg/kg/min Mod: 5-20 µg/kg/min High: >20 µg/kg/min	Low: increased renal and mesenteric blood flow, little effect on heart (dopaminergic effect) Mod: increased renal blood flow, heart rate, cardiac contractility, and cardiac output High: systemic vasoconstriction May be used synergistically with isoproterenol or dobutamine
Dobutamine (Dobutrex)	±	++ to +++	±	2-20 µg/kg/min (usually 10-15 µg/kg/min)	Positive inotropic effect with minimal chronotropic; minimal β₂; useful in cardiogenic shock; may use with low-dose dopamine
Norepinephrine (Levophed)	+++	+++	±	0.1-1.0 µg/kg/min	Positive inotropic; intense alpha vasoconstrictor, with compromised peripheral tissue and organ perfusion Useful in cardiogenic shock caused by myocardial insufficiency; seldom used without an α blocker

Drug				Dose	Comments
Epinephrine (Adrenalin)	+++	+++	+++	0.1-1.0 µg/kg/min	Use only when isoproterenol and dopamine are ineffective; positive inotropic and chronotropic effects; renal and mesenteric ischemia; tachyrhythmia; increased cardiac oxygen requirements; intense alpha effect if >0.3 µg/kg/min
Sodium nitroprusside (Nipride)				0.5-10 µg/kg/min (average: 3 µg/kg/min)	Arterial and venous dilator; afterload reduction; rapid response, short duration
Phentolamine (Regitine)	Antagonist			0.05-0.1 mg/kg/dose q1-4hr IV prn	Counteracts vasoconstriction; useful for high CVP or in combination with vasoconstrictive drug; rapid onset, short activity; may also be given by continuous infusion
Naloxone (Narcan)				0.1 mg/kg/dose (0.8-2.0 mg/dose) IV q3-5min × 2 prn	May have unproven role in septic shock; endorphin antagonist; alternative regimen: bolus of 0.03 mg/kg, then 0.03 mg/kg/hr IV infusion
Calcium chloride				0.2 ml/kg/dose q10min prn IV slowly (20 mg/kg/dose) (maximum: 0.5 gm)	Positive inotropic and chronotropic effects; may cause bradycardia; controversial and unproven role

+, ++, +++, Relative degree present; ±, variable.
*Inotropic agents are not useful in hypovolemic shock: volume replacement is required.

3. Evaluation of the adequacy of preload (by CVP or PCWP measurements) and afterload is essential in monitoring the efficacy of therapy. Monitoring by echocardiography in consultation with a cardiologist is extremely important.

Distributive (Vasogenic) Shock

1. Septic shock. Intravenous fluids do not usually improve vital signs because cardiac output actually decreases when preload is increased. Pressor agents commonly are required after adequate preload has been established and documented. Filling pressure should be kept at the lowest level consistent with adequate tissue perfusion.
2. Anaphylaxis (see Chapter 12).
3. Head and spinal cord trauma (see Chapters 57 and 61). Pressor agents are usually required after adequate preload has been established and documented.

Cardiac Function

1. Treatment of dysrhythmias (see Chapters 4 and 6). Bradycardia, AV block, and tachyrhythmias are particularly detrimental to cardiac output. Predisposing conditions include electrolyte abnormalities, acidosis, alkalosis, drugs, fever, and pericardial disease, as well as ischemic or hypoxic damage.
2. Inotropic agents (see Table 5-2). Although an evaluation of the adequacy of preload by echocardiography, CVP, or PCWP optimally should be done before initiating pharmacologic support, it must not delay aggressive stabilization. The efficacy of the agent can then be measured. Inotropic agents have no role in hypovolemic shock, but they are fundamental components of therapy for cardiogenic and distributive shock.

a. Classification

Effector organ	Mechanism/effect		
	Alphas	β_1	β_2
Heart			
Rate		Increase	Increase
Contractility		Increase	
Conduction velocity		Increase	
Arterioles	Constrict		Dilate
Veins	Constrict		Dilate
Lung-bronchiolar smooth muscles	Constrict		Dilate

b. If local infiltration of an agent with significant alpha effects (vasoconstriction) occurs during infusion, a significant risk of skin necrosis and ulceration exists. To minimize this when infiltration occurs, phentolamine (α antagonist), 1 to 5 mg diluted in 1 to 5 ml of 0.9% NS, depending on the size of the child, is infiltrated locally.

c. Often a combination of pressor agents is required to maximize the clinical effect. A typical combination includes dopamine in low dosages (0.5-3 µg/kg/min) as one drug to maintain renal perfusion by dilating the splanchnic and renal vascular beds and a second drug such as dobutamine (5-15 µg/kg/min). Continuous infusions of isoproterenol and epinephrine may be used in severe, unresponsive situations.

3. Vasodilators

a. An evaluation of the adequacy of preload and cardiac function by echocardiography and CVP or PCWP measurement should be done if possible before pharmacologic therapy is initiated, carefully monitoring improvement of function with intervention.

b. In cardiogenic shock, vasodilators such as nitroprusside (0.5-10 µg/kg/min IV) (p. 49) may be helpful for pulmonary congestion. Vasodilators are useful when peripheral hypoperfusion is present and when the patient is hypervolemic or a major outflow obstruction secondary to arteriolar vasoconstriction exists. Vasodilators are usually used in combination with an inotropic drug. These agents may simultaneously reduce the preload, and therefore volume repletion may be required.

Hypovolemic Shock

Inotropic agents are not indicated for hypovolemic shock.

Cardiogenic Shock

1. Inotropic agents (e.g., dopamine, dobutamine) should be initiated if there is poor peripheral perfusion after an initial infusion of fluids to improve cardiac function. Periodically during inotropic therapy, a fluid challenge should be administered to reassess intravascular volume status.
2. If pulmonary congestion exists or there is peripheral hypoperfusion in hypervolemic patients, vasodilators (e.g., nitroprusside) may be useful adjunctive therapy.

Distributive Shock

Primary therapy is to initiate positive inotropic agents while maintaining intravascular volume. In the early hyperdynamic phase (rare in children), there is a decreased afterload requiring volume administration. Later, with the decreased cardiac output and increased systemic vascular resistance secondary to hypoxemia and acidosis, isoproterenol (0.05-1.5 μg/kg/min) is particularly useful because it decreases peripheral resistance and has a positive inotropic effect.

Ancillary Procedures

These procedures require appropriate priority in the initial evaluation and stabilization.

1. Elevate legs unless respiratory distress or pulmonary edema is present.
2. Place urinary catheter to monitor renal output and evaluate renal injury.
3. Insert nasogastric tube to initiate decompression and provide information of GI bleeding.
4. Normalize temperature (see Chapters 50 and 51).
5. Consider and perform peritoneal lavage to exclude peritoneal blood loss (see Chapter 63) or peritonitis after trauma or, if appropriate, in the patient with ascites.
6. Insert CVP catheter. This is particularly important in hypovolemic shock if positive pressure ventilation is required or there is significant pulmonary, renal, or cardiac disease. A Swan-Ganz catheter permits measurement of the PCWP, which is particularly useful in cardiogenic or distributive shock.
7. Perform pericardiocentesis (see Appendix A-5) to exclude pericardial tamponade, or do thoracentesis (see Appendix A-8) to treat tension pneumothorax if specific indications are present.
8. If available, in unresponsive hypovolemic patients with no evidence of pulmonary edema or cardiogenic shock, consideration may be given to pneumatic military antishock trousers (MAST). The trousers provide an autotransfusion into the upper circulation by compression of the venous beds in the legs and abdomen, but there is no evidence of a beneficial impact on patient outcome. Complications include acidosis, ventilatory and renal compromise, and reduced visibility of the patient. This device rarely has been used on children.

Other Considerations

1. *Electrolyte* and *acid-base* abnormalities must be corrected because they impair ventilation, depress the myocardium, predispose to dysrhythmias, and alter response to catecholamines. All corrections require frequent monitoring of response.
   a. *Acidosis* is a consistent finding, which

must be at least partially corrected if the pH is less than 7.15. Early treatment of a pattern of deteriorating acid-base status may prevent complications. If acidosis is a result of hypoventilation, consider active airway management. If the cause is metabolic, give 1-2 mEq/kg sodium bicarbonate ($NaHCO_3$) over 5 minutes IV. Repeat according to ABG levels. Correct only to 7.25 to 7.30, but monitor closely. Calculation: deficit mEq HCO_3^- = weight (kg) × base excess × 0.3.

b. *Hypocalcemia* develops with decreased serum ionized calcium level; it is associated with impaired tissue perfusion. Hypocalcemia depresses myocardial function, as does hypophosphatemia. Give $CaCl_2$ 10% 10-20 mg/kg (0.1-0.2 ml/kg) IV slowly, optimally through a central venous line, while monitoring vital signs. Simultaneously check phosphorus level; a deficit being treated with potassium phosphate 5-10 mg/kg slowly if K^+ is normal. If phosphorus level is high, care must be exercised in administering calcium.

2. *Urine output* is optimally maintained at 1-2 ml/kg/hr. Pharmacologic agents may be required to supplement volume repletion in maintaining urine flow. The choice of regimen must be individualized, reflecting the experience of the clinician and the response to one or more of the agents. Oliguria is a common finding secondary to prerenal failure and acute tubular necrosis (p. 809). It is essential to know the intravascular volume before initiating pharmacologic therapy. Treatment options in addition to fluid therapy include the following:

a. Furosemide (Lasix), 1 mg/kg/dose up to 6 mg/kg/dose q2-6hr IV as needed

b. Mannitol, 0.25-1.0 gm/kg/dose q4-6hr IV

c. Low-dose dopamine (0.5-3 µg/kg/min IV continuous infusion)

d. Monitoring input and output meticulously and replacing urine output milliliter by milliliter

e. Dialysis, which is required in unresponsive hyperkalemia, acidosis, or hypervolemia

3. *Antibiotics* are appropriate because of the nonspecific nature of the clinical presentation. The critically ill child with shock from unknown cause is thus treated empirically. Ideally antibiotics are initiated after obtaining at least one blood culture result and optimally all other relevant culture findings. Broad-spectrum antibiotics should be used initially to cover all potential pathogens and then modified to reflect the results of culture and sensitivity data.

a. Cefotaxime, 50-150 mg/kg/24 hr q6-8hr IV (or ceftriaxone, 50-100 mg/kg/24 hr q12hr IV; or cefuroxime, 100-200 mg/kg/24 hr q6-8hr IV). In the newborn, ampicillin should be added and the dose altered.

These antibiotics should be modified if there are specific clinical indications such as a perforated abdominal organ or toxic shock syndrome.

4. *Corticosteroid* use continues to be debated. The use of steroids in the treatment of gram-negative sepsis is probably detrimental. Administration may be lifesaving if a patient has adrenal cortical insufficiency. Routine use is recommended in patients with bacterial meningitis. The exact role in patients in whom shock develops remains unclarified.

5. *Coagulopathy* may occur after shock of any cause. DIC is common (p. 683). With many coagulopathies associated with shock, fresh-frozen plasma is a rapid approach to correcting abnormalities and additionally provides volume expansion.

6. Mediator-specific therapy, including anti-

endotoxin and anti–tumor necrosis factor (TNF) agents and LI-1 receptor antagonists, has been found to be effective in selected models. The role in pediatric septic shock remains experimental.

7. Naloxone (Narcan) use is controversial; it serves as an endorphin antagonist and has some questionable efficacy in the treatment of septic shock by improving hemodynamic parameters when initiated early. High dosages are recommended initially with a continuous drip thereafter. Empirically, one suggested regimen provides an IV bolus of 0.03 mg/kg followed by a continuous IV infusion of 0.03 mg/kg/hr (adult: 0.4 mg/hr).

8. Anaphylactic shock is discussed in Chapter 12.

9. Patients who fail to respond to resuscitation efforts must be rapidly reevaluated to ascertain whether other causes may concurrently exist. Consultation is mandatory. Factors that must be considered include the following:

   a. Multiple organ failure
   b. Myocardial injury, ischemia, or other damage, as well as coronary artery disease
   c. Outflow or filling obstruction, such as tension pneumothorax or pericardial tamponade
   d. Coagulopathy and DIC

   e. Renal failure
   f. Respiratory failure
   g. Uncontrolled sepsis
   h. Ongoing blood loss

DISPOSITION

All patients require immediate admission to an ICU. Cardiac, pulmonary, and infectious disease consultations should be requested immediately.

REFERENCES

American Academy of Pediatrics Committee on Drugs: Emergency drug doses for infants and children, *Pediatrics* 81:462, 1988.

Bone RC: Sepsis and its complications: the clinical problem, *Crit Care Med* 22:88, 1994.

Bone RC, Fisher CJ, Clemmer TP, et al: A controlled clinical trial of high dose methylprednisolone in the treatment of severe sepsis and septic shock, *N Engl J Med* 317:653, 1987.

Hazinski MF, Barkin RM: Shock. In Barkin RM, editor: *Pediatric emergency medicine: concepts and clinical practice*, ed 2, St Louis, 1997, Mosby.

Hinshaw L, Veterans Administration Systemic Sepsis Cooperative Study Group: Effect of high-dose glucocorticoid therapy on mortality in patients with clinical signs of systemic sepsis, *N Engl J Med* 324:659, 1987.

Royall JA, Levin DL: Adult respiratory distress syndrome in pediatric patients, *J Pediatr* 112:169, 335, 1988.

Saavedra JM, Harris GD, Li S, et al: Capillary refilling (skin turgor) in the assessment of dehydration, *Am J Dis Child* 145:296, 1991.

Seffredini AF: Current prospects for the treatment of clinical sepsis, *Crit Care Med* 22:821, 1994.

6 DYSRHYTHMIAS

Dysrhythmias are uncommon in pediatric patients. Because of the differences in causes, particularly in infants and children, and the absence of ischemic heart disease, only a few types of disturbances are seen with any frequency.

Cardiac stimuli arise in specialized neuromuscular tissues within the heart, consisting of the sinus (sinoatrial [SA]) node, AV (atrioventricular) junction, bundle of His, right and left branches, and Purkinje fibers. The primary pacemaker is the sinus node. When this node is suppressed or fails to propagate impulses, a secondary pacemaker sets the cardiac rate. The stimuli become progressively slower as the site becomes more distal. The sympathetic and vagal fibers modify stimuli through the sinus node and AV junction. The sympathetic nervous system stimulates the heart, and the vagal or parasympathetic system has a suppressive effect, mostly on the sinus node and AV junction. Increased heart rate may result from increased sympathetic activity or decreased vagal tone; bradycardia is commonly caused by increased vagal tone, often secondary to myocardial hypoxia.

Dysrhythmias are caused by abnormal impulse formation or conduction or by a combined mechanism. *Automaticity* occurs when myocardial tissue independently depolarizes, reaches threshold, and fires. Automaticity is increased by hypokalemia, hypercalcemia, catecholamines, drugs (e.g., digitalis), and ischemia.

Reentry dysrhythmias occur when some areas of the heart are repolarized while other areas are not. Reentry can occur only when two pathways are connected proximally and distally.

Triggered automaticity occurs as a result of instability of the resting membrane potential after myocardial ischemia, fibrosis, or drug (e.g., calcium, digitalis) administration.

Tachyrhythmias in children result from increased sympathetic activity, decreased vagal tone, ectopic pacemakers, or reentrant pathways that often involve abnormal or accessory connections. Accessory pathways produce preexcitation syndromes such as Wolff-Parkinson-White (WPW), which predisposes to paroxysmal atrial tachycardia (PAT), or supraventricular tachycardia (SVT).

Therapy is focused on interruption of the reentry or prevention of premature beats that trigger the cycle. Ectopic pacemakers are treated by suppression of the focus. Adenoside, an endogenous nucleoside, causes a temporary block through the AV node and interrupts the reentry circuit in stable patients with SVT; the dosage is 0.1 mg/kg IV (rapid). The adult dose is 6 mg initially, which may be doubled up to 12 mg if there is no effect. Lidocaine is indicated in hemodynamically stable patients with ventricular dysrhythmias.

Bradyrhythmias usually are caused by slowing of the intrinsic pacemaker, often caused by increased vagal tone or a conduction abnormality. The block in conduction may be complete, in which circumstance a more distal, slower pacemaker controls the rate, or it may be incomplete, allowing only a few impulses to pass (Tables 6-1 and 6-2).

Children at risk of dysrhythmias may have congenital or acquired heart disease, systemic disease, intoxication, or acute hemodynamic alterations.

Text continued on p. 59

TABLE 6-1   Characteristics of Common Dysrhythmias

Dysrhythmia	Rate/min (>6 yr old)	Rhythm	P wave (atrial)	QRS complex	AV conduction	Response to vagotonic maneuver	Comments
BRADYRHYTHMIAS							
Sinus bradycardia	<60	Regular	Upright I, II, aVF	WNL	WNL	None	Found in athletes, hypothyroidism, increased intracranial pressure, with drugs (propranolol or digitalis); if no symptoms, no treatment; if serious, use atropine, pacemaker; rate is age specific
Sinus dysrhythmia	60-120	Irregular	Upright I, II, aVF	WNL	WNL	Transient slowing	Normal variation with respiration and varying vagal tone; reassurance needed
SUPRAVENTRICULAR TACHYRHYTHMIAS							
Sinus tachycardia	120-200	Regular	Upright I, II, aVF	WNL	WNL	Transient slowing	Secondary to fever, exercise, anemia, shock, hyperthyroidism; treat condition
Premature atrial complex (PAC)	60-120	Irregular	Variable	WNL	WNL, may be first-degree block	Slows	Stimulants (caffeine, smoking, alcohol), digitalis toxicity; early congestive heart failure (CHF), hypoxia; if infrequent, no treatment; avoid stimulants; if frequent, treat condition; rarely need propranolol or quinidine

Continued

WNL, Within normal limits; *NA,* not applicable.

TABLE 6-1   Characteristics of Common Dysrhythmias—cont'd

Dysrhythmia	Rate/min (>6 yr old)	Rhythm	P wave (atrial)	QRS complex	AV conduction	Response to vagotonic maneuver	Comments
SUPRAVENTRICULAR TACHYRHYTHMIAS—cont'd							
Paroxysmal supraventricular (atrial) tachycardia (PAT or SVT)	150-250	Regular	Buried; nonsinus, variably retrograde	WNL	WNL	None or converts	Most common significant dysrhythmia in children (reentry); children <5 yr: infection, fever, congenital heart disease; older children: WPW (short PR segment, ± prolonged QRS complex, delta wave); may cause cardiac decompensation secondary to inadequate filling time; occurs with digitalis toxicity, particularly with block
Junctional premature contraction	NA	Irregular	Retrograde, often obscured	WNL or aberrant	Variable	None	Same as PAC
Atrial flutter	100-300 (atrial: 200-300)	Regular	Flutter (saw toothed) waves II, III, aVF	WNL	Variable block	None	Heart disease, thyrotoxicosis, pulmonary embolism, myocarditis, chest trauma

	Rate	Rhythm	P waves	QRS			
Atrial fibrillation	60-190 (atrial: 400-700)	Irregularly irregular	No P waves; fibrillation waves	WNL	Variable block	Transient slowing	As above (atrial flutter); severe valvular disease (mitral stenosis, tricuspid insufficiency, aortic stenosis), WPW and without heart disease
VENTRICULAR TACHYRHYTHMIAS							
Premature ventricular complex (PVC)	NA	Irregular	Usually obscured	≥0.12 sec, premature, bizarre	Compensatory pause, variable retrograde	None	ST segment and T wave opposite in polarity to QRS complex; variably significant if >6/min, multifocal, occurs near T wave, increases with exercise, or occurs in bigeminy or trigeminy; associated with cardiac ischemia, digitalis toxicity, ↓ K⁺, hypoxia, alkalosis
Ventricular tachycardia	150-220	Regular or slightly irregular	Usually not recognizable	≥0.12 sec, bizarre	None	None	ST segment and T wave opposite in polarity to QRS complex; may cause hemodynamic compromise requiring immediate treatment
Ventricular fibrillation	Indeterminate	None	Not recognizable	Irregular undulation	None	None	Disorganized, ineffective cardiac activity without pulse or blood pressure; medical emergency: defibrillate

TABLE 6-2 Characteristics of Conduction Disturbances*

Type	Atrial rate	Ventricle rate	PR interval	Ventricular rhythm	P-QRS relation	QRS complex	Comment
First degree	Unaffected	Same as atrial	Prolonged for age	Same as atrial	Consistent 1:1	Unaffected	Delay anywhere from AV node to bundle branches; may be caused by digitalis; no therapy necessary
Second degree (Wenckebach Mobitz I)	Unaffected	Slower than atrial	Progressive increase until P wave is dropped	Irregular	Variable† (recurring)	Narrow; constant; irregular	Delay at AV node; may be caused by digitalis or quinidine; therapy rarely needed; do not give potassium
Second degree (Mobitz II)	Unaffected	Slower than atrial	Normal or prolonged; constant	Irregular or regular	Fixed†	Usually wide; constant	Delay at bundle of His or below; may be precursor to complete block; pacemaker needed; temporize with atropine or isoproterenol
Third degree	Unaffected	Slower than atrial	Variable	Regular	None†	Constant; regular	Delay is anywhere from AV node to bundle branches; life threatening; pacemaker; temporize with atropine or isoproterenol

*May be idiopathic, acquired (nonsurgical), postoperative, or congenital.
†More Ps than QRSs.

Assessment requires a careful history and physical examination, focusing on the vital signs, cardiac evaluation, and evidence of systemic disease. Prompt analysis of the ECG and hemodynamic parameters is imperative.

Symptomatic patients may show evidence of congestive heart failure (see Chapter 16), including pallor, irritability, poor eating, dyspnea, decreased cerebral blood flow associated with syncope and altered behavior, decreased coronary blood flow and anginal pain, or a perception of a rhythm disturbance marked by palpitations or missed beats.

Newborns and infants with SVT commonly have tachypnea, lethargy, decreased feeding, and respiratory distress that may progress to hypotension and shock. Older children have chest discomfort/pain, palpitations, faintness, and may have syncope or cardiac arrest.

ANALYSIS OF ELECTROCARDIOGRAM
(see Appendix B-3)

1. Rate
   a. Rate is age dependent (newborn: 100 to 160, infant: 120 to 160, toddler: 80 to 150, child older than 6 years: 60 to 120).
   b. Each small box is 0.04 seconds, and time between vertical lines at top of strip is 3 seconds. Determine rate by multiplying number of complexes between vertical lines by 20.
2. Axis: Axis is age specific, also reflecting hypertrophy or conduction defects.
3. Rhythm
   a. Regular or irregular.
   b. Voltage (low with myocarditis or effusion)
4. P wave
   a. Presence implies atrial activity, although it may be buried in QRS interval, ST segment, or T wave. Seen best in leads II, III, and aVF.
   b. Enlarged or biphasic (V1) (atrial hypertrophy); normal: 0.08 to 0.10 second.
   c. Configuration (normal vs. ectopic foci).
5. PR interval
   a. A fixed relationship between the P wave and QRS interval implies that the rhythm is supraventricular in origin.
   b. Interval is age and rate dependent, ranging from 0.10 to 0.20 second.
   c. Prolongation occurs with first-degree block, hyperkalemia, digitalis, propranolol, verapamil, adenosine, quinidine, and carditis (acute rheumatic fever).
   d. Short in WPW syndrome, it also has delta wave.
6. QRS complex
   a. Duration is normally less than 0.10 second.
   b. Prolongation occurs with conduction defect, ventricular focus, severe hyperkalemia, and quinidine.
   c. Abnormal configuration demonstrates that the focus is ventricular in origin or that there is a conduction defect.
   d. High voltage implies hypertrophy or overload pattern.
7. ST segment
   a. Elevated with transmural injury, pericarditis, ventricular aneurysm
   b. Depressed with subendocardial injury, digitalis, systolic overload, and strain
8. T wave
   a. Peaks in hyperkalemia (if severe, also has widened QRS interval); flat with hypokalemia
   b. Inverted with conduction defect or ischemia
9. QT segment
   a. Duration is rate dependent, but correction (QTc) should be less than 0.42 second.
   b. Prolonged with quinidine, procainamide, cyclic antidepressant overdose, hypokalemia, hypocalcemia, hypomagnesemia, and hypothermia.

ANCILLARY DATA

1. The patient's response to *vagotonic maneuvers* should be evaluated. Vagotonic maneuvers include massage of the carotid (unilateral), Valsalva's maneuver, cold water applied to face briskly, deep inspiration, coughing, drinking cold water, and gagging. The resulting increased vagal tone should result in at least a transient slowing of the heart rate if the rhythm is supraventricular. Do not perform eyeball compression or simultaneous, bilateral carotid massage.

Continuous monitoring is essential. In the hospital setting this should be done in a monitored unit. After discharge, transtelephonic electrocardiography has been useful in defining dysrhythmias and monitoring the efficacy of drug and pacemaker therapy.

Electrophysiologic studies may be indicated.

   a. Tachyrhythmias. Supraventricular (preexcitation WPW) with syncope and frequent episodes of SVT unresponsive to vagotonic maneuvers or medication. Ventricular dysrhythmias requiring study include patients with associated heart disease and those with cardiac tumors, myocarditis, or metabolic disorders.

   b. Bradyrhythmias requiring investigation include sick sinus syndrome and AV conduction defects.

MANAGEMENT (Tables 6-3, 6-4, and 6-5)

Once a dysrhythmia apparently has been identified, it is imperative to determine whether there is any compromise in cardiac output or hemodynamic parameters or if the rhythm is potentially life threatening. Six questions must be addressed:

1. Does the patient truly have a dysrhythmia?
2. Is the heart rate fast or slow?

TABLE 6-3   Overview of Dysrhythmia Management*

Heart rate/QRS	Hemodynamic stability	
	Unstable	Stable
SLOW	Atropine Isoproterenol Pacing (see Fig. 4-2)	Oxygen Ventilation Atropine
FAST		
Narrow QRS	Synchronized cardioversion	Adenosine Verapamil† Digitalis
Wide QRS	Defibrillation	Lidocaine Defibrillation Bretylium
ABSENT		

Ventricular
   fibrillation
	Defibrillation
	   (see Fig. 4-3)	

Asystole	See Fig. 4-3	
EMD/PEA	See Fig. 4-3	

*Assumes resuscitation efforts are ongoing.
†Do not use if child <1 year old.

3. If the heart rate is fast, is the QRS wide (>0.08 second) or narrow?
4. Does the patient require therapy (i.e., how stable is the patient)?
5. How soon is therapy required?
6. What is the most effective and safest therapy?

Management must focus on prevention, control of the underlying condition, and specific therapy for the dysrhythmia.

1. Administer oxygen during stabilization of the airway, ventilation, and circulation. Treatment of the underlying condition, which often causes hypoxia, may adequately resolve the dysrhythmia.
2. Usually, *one medication* is initiated until the therapeutic effect is achieved or toxicity is noted (see Figs. 4-1 and 4-2). If the agent fails, additional medications should be used (see Tables 6-3, 6-4, and 6-5).

Text continued on p. 65

TABLE 6-4 Common Antidysrhythmic Drugs

Drug	ECG effect	Half-life	Blood level		Dosage		Adverse reactions
			Therapeutic	Toxic	Initial	Maintenance	
Digoxin (Table 16-2)	Prolongs PR	24 hr	1-3.5 µg/ml	>3.5 µg/ml (variable)	TDD premature infant: 0.01-0.02 mg/kg IV; TDD 2 wk-2 yr: 0.03-0.05 mg/kg IV; TDD newborn and >2 yr: 0.04 mg/kg IV; ½ TDD initially, then ¼ q4-8hr IV × 2	¼-⅓ TDD q12-24hr PO, or IV	Ventricular ectopy, tachycardia, fibrillation, atrial tachycardia, AV block, vomiting; slow onset
Lidocaine	Shortens QT	5 hr	1-5 µg/ml	>10 µg/ml	1 mg/kg/dose IV (may repeat in 10 min) to max 5 mg/kg	20-50 µg/kg/min IV (adult: 2-4 mg/min)	Seizure, drowsiness, euphoria, muscle twitching; may give ET (dilute 1:1)
Quinidine	Prolongs QRS, QT, ± PR	6 hr	2-6 µg/ml	>9 µg/ml	15-60 mg/kg/24 hr q6hr PO (adult: 300-400 mg q6hr PO)	Same	GI symptoms, PVC, syncope, hypotension, anemia
Procainamide	Prolongs QRS, QT, ± PR	3-4 hr	4-10 µg/ml	>10 µg/ml	2-6 mg/kg/dose IV slowly (adult: 100 mg/dose IV q10min prn or 25-50 mg/min, and titrate up to total dose of 1 gm)	20-80 µg/kg/min IV (adult: 1-3 mg/min IV) 15-50 mg/kg/24 hr q4-6hr PO (adult: 250-500 mg/dose q4-6hr PO up to 4 gm/24 hr)	Hypotension, lupuslike syndrome, urticaria, GI symptoms

Continued

±, Variable effect; *TDD*, total digitalizing dose.

TABLE 6-4   Common Antidysrhythmic Drugs—cont'd

Drug	ECG effect	Half-life	Blood level		Dosage		Adverse reactions
			Therapeutic	Toxic	Initial	Maintenance	
Propranolol	Prolongs PR, shortens QT	2-4 hr	20-150 μg/ml	NA	0.01-0.1 mg/kg/dose IV over 10 min (adult: 1 mg/dose IV q5min up to 5 mg)	0.5-1.0 mg/kg/24 hr q6hr PO (adult: 10-80 mg/dose q6-8hr PO)	Bradycardia, hypotension, cardiac failure, asthma, hypoglycemia; do not give to patient with asthma; overdose treated with glucagon 0.1 mg/kg/dose IV
Bretylium	No change	6-10 hr	0.5-1.5 μg/ml	NA	5 mg/kg/dose IV over 10 min; may be increased to 10 mg/kg	5 mg/kg/dose q6-8hr IV	Hypotension, initial increase of dysrhythmias, nausea; little experience in children
Verapamil	Shortens QT, prolongs PR	3-7 hr (variable)			0.1 mg/kg/dose IV over 1-2 min repeated in 10-30 min prn (adult: 5-10 mg/dose IV)	NA	Bradycardia, hypotension, apnea, AV block, negative inotropic agent; do not use in children <1 yr or if patient is taking β blocker; adenosine usually preferred

Drug	Action	Half-life	Therapeutic level	Toxic level	Dose (IV)	Dose (PO)	Side effects
Adenosine	Slows AV nodal conduction	10 sec	NA	NA	0.1 mg/kg IV (rapid); may repeat in 2 min; adult: 6 mg IV (rapid) and if no response in 2 min give 12 mg IV (rapid)	NA	Transient AV block; half-life is 10 sec
Phenytoin (Dilantin)	Shortens QT	20-26 hr	10-20 µg/ml	>20 µg/ml	5 mg/kg/dose IV over 5 min (<0.5 mg/kg/min) (adult: 100 mg/dose IV q5min up to 1 gm)	6 mg/kg/24 hr q12hr PO (adult: 300 mg/24 hr PO)	Ataxia, nystagmus, hypotension; new formulation available to reduce adverse reaction
Atropine	Increases rate	<5 min	NA	NA	0.02 mg/kg/dose IV; repeat q2-5min × 2 prn	NA	Tachycardia, mydriasis, dry mouth
Isoproterenol	Increases rate	<5 min	NA	NA	0.05-1.5 µg/kg/min IV; begin 0.1 µg/kg/min and increase q5-10min (adult: 2-20 µg/min/IV)	NA	Tachycardia, PVC

NA, Not applicable.

TABLE 6-5   Acute Treatment of Common Dysrhythmias*

Dysrhythmia	Treatment	Comments
SUPRAVENTRICULAR TACHYRHYTHMIA (FAST HEART RATE; NARROW QRS)		
Supraventricular (atrial) tachycardia (PAT, VT)	Vagotonic maneuvers	Attempt in all patients first: carotid sinus massage, Valsalva's maneuver
With critical hemodynamic compromise	DC-synchronized cardioversion (0.5-1.0 watt-sec/kg) Adenosine Verapamil	Do not use verapamil if child <1 yr
Without critical hemodynamic compromise	Adenosine Verapamil Digoxin Edrophonium	Do not use digoxin if any question of WPW; adenosine may be used with WPW
Atrial flutter	Digoxin DC-synchronized cardioversion (0.5-1.0 watt-sec/kg) Propranolol	Do not use digoxin with WPW; verapamil slows ventricular response; cardioversion if hemodynamic compromise occurs; potentially unstable
Atrial fibrillation	Same as atrial flutter	Same as atrial flutter; considered anticoagulation with prolonged atrial fibrillation
VENTRICULAR TACHYRHYTHMIA (FAST HEART RATE; WIDE QRS)		
Premature ventricular contractions (PVC)	Lidocaine Procainamide	Quinidine, procainamide, propranolol, or phenytoin for long-term suppression
Ventricular tachycardia		
With critical hemodynamic compromise	DC-synchronized cardioversion (0.5-1.0 watt-sec/kg) Lidocaine Bretylium	Administer lidocaine bolus and infusion simultaneously with cardioversion; maintenance therapy includes quinidine or procainamide
Without critical hemodynamic compromise	Lidocaine Procainamide Bretylium DC-synchronized cardioversion (0.5-1.0 watt-sec/kg)	Same as above
Ventricular fibrillation	DC defibrillation (2-4 watt-sec/kg) Lidocaine Bretylium	Initiate lidocaine infusion simultaneously with defibrillation
BRADYRHYTHMIA (SLOW HEART RATE)		
Sinus bradycardia	Ventilation, oxygen, atropine	Hypoxia is most common cause; therapy if unstable

*Oxygen, CPR, and other supportive treatment may be required. Cardiology consultation should be requested. (See also Figs. 4-1 and 4-2.)

TABLE 6-5   Acute Treatment of Common Dysrhythmias—cont'd

Dysrhythmia	Treatment	Comments
BRADYRHYTHMIA (SLOW HEART RATE)—cont'd		
Atrioventricular block	Atropine Isoproterenol (temporize) Pacemaker	Therapy if unstable; be certain not digoxin induced
DIGITALIS-INDUCED		
Paroxysmal atrial tachycardia (PAT) with block	Potassium chloride (40 mEq/L peripheral IV or 0.5-1.0 mEq/kg/hr central IV) Phenytoin	Stop drug, self-limited; avoid cardioversion, propranolol; worsened by $\downarrow K^+$ $\downarrow Mg^{++}$, $\uparrow Ca^{++}$
PVC or ventricular tachycardia	Potassium chloride Phenytoin Lidocaine	Avoid cardioversion, bretylium; see above

New agents may be useful once the clinician has acquired greater experience in treating children. Adenosine in an initial dose of 0.1 mg/kg IV (rapid) is generally preferred in children with SVT. Amiodarone is good for life-threatening refractory atrial flutter, ventricular tachyrhythmias, and SVTs. An initial dosage of 10 mg/kg/24 hr PO is suggested; maintenance should be reduced slowly to 6 mg/kg/24 hr PO.

Other drugs include mexiletene, propaferone, encainide, and ethmozine, all of which require greater clinical experience in treating children.

3. *Electrical conversion* is used to treat ventricular fibrillation and symptomatic tachyrhythmias that are unresponsive to pharmacologic therapy or for hemodynamic compromise. Sedation is often advantageous before this procedure. Children can usually tolerate tachyrhythmias for long periods before cardiac decompensation occurs.
   a. Defibrillation is the untimed depolarization used to convert ventricular fibrillation. Cardioversion is a timed depolarization that prevents stimulation of the heart during the vulnerable part of the cardiac cycle, thereby preventing the initiation of lethal ventricular dysrhythmias. Cardioversion is useful in conversion of ventricular tachyrhythmias.
   b. Direct current (DC) defibrillators are used; it is crucial that the low watt-second range be appropriately calibrated. Paddle size should ensure full contact with the chest. Many models have a "quick-look" feature, allowing immediate assessment of the rhythm.
   Transthoracic impedance can be minimized with an adult-sized paddle (8 to 10 cm in diameter) as soon as the chest is large enough to permit electrode-to-chest contact over the entire paddle surface, usually by 1 year or 10 kg. Smaller pediatric paddles should be used for infants less than 10 kg.
   c. The paddles are placed on the anterior chest, one to the right of the sternum at the second intercostal space and the other to the left of the midclavicular line at the level of the xiphoid. Electrode cream or paste is applied to the paddles before they are placed on the chest.

d. Defibrillation uses 2 watt-sec/kg initially. This may be repeated if the first attempt is unsuccessful and repeated with double the dose. If still unsuccessful, repeat at 4 watt-sec/kg. The International Liaison Committee on Resuscitation has suggested that 2-4 watt-sec/kg be used for the second and third shock. If the third administration still is unsuccessful, lidocaine is administered with oxygen and correction of the acid-base status and temperature abnormalities. Epinephrine should also be considered. Defibrillation is then repeated, if necessary at 4 watt-sec/kg.

e. Cardioversion is useful for tachyrhythmias. Commonly, 0.5 watt-sec/kg is administered with the synchronizer circuit and, if unsuccessful, doubled. Hypoxia, acidosis, hypoglycemia, and hyperthermia should be corrected.

4. Pacemakers are the definitive therapeutic modality in the treatment of bradyrhythmias and AV conduction abnormalities associated with hemodynamic compromise. External, transcutaneous, temporary transvenous, and permanent pacemakers are available. Transesophageal pacing may be effective for cardioversion of atrial flutter and SVTs, but experience in children is limited.

5. Radiofrequency ablation may emerge as a primary therapy in the future.

DISPOSITION

Cardiology consultation is usually indicated in recurrent or unresponsive dysrhythmias, as well as in those causing hemodynamic compromise. These parameters should also determine the need for hospitalization and the urgency of initiating therapy. It is imperative not only to treat the dysrhythmia but also to institute a program to prevent recurrence. Caffeine and other stimulants should be avoided.

REFERENCES

American Heart Association: Guidelines for cardiopulmonary resuscitation (CPR) and emergency cardiac care, *JAMA* 268:2171, 1992.

Atkins DL, Sirna S, Kieso R: Pediatric defibrillation: importance of paddle size in determining transthoracic impedance, *Pediatrics* 82:914, 1988.

Binder LS, Boeche R, Atkinson D: Evaluation and management of supraventricular tachycardia in children, *Ann Emerg Med* 20:51, 1991.

Cairns CB, Niemann JT: Intravenous adenosine with emergency department management of paroxysmal supraventricular tachycardia, *Ann Emerg Med* 20:717, 1991.

Chameides L: Dysrhythmias. In Barkin RM, editor: *Pediatric emergency medicine: concepts and clinical practice*, ed 2, St Louis, 1997, Mosby.

Dubin D: *Rapid interpretation of EKG's*, Tampa, Fla, 1981, Cover Publishing.

Harken AH, Honigman B, VanWay CW: Cardiac dysrhythmias in the acute setting: recognition and treatment or anyone can treat cardiac dysrhythmias, *J Emerg Med* 5:129, 1987.

Klitzner TS, Wetzel GT, Saxon LA, et al: Radiofrequency ablation: a new era in the treatment of pediatric arrhythmias, *Am J Dis Child* 147:769, 1993.

Magayzel C, Quan Land, Graves JC, et al: Out-of-hospital ventricular fibrillation in children and adolescents: causes and outcomes, *Ann Emerg Med* 25:484, 1995.

Ralston MA, Knilans TK, Hannon DW, et al: Use of adenosine for diagnosis and treatment of tachyarrhythmias in pediatric patients, *J Pediatr* 124:139, 1994.

Reyes G, Stanton R, Galvis AG: Adenosine in the treatment of paroxysmal supraventricular tachycardia in children, *Ann Emerg Med* 21:1499, 1992.

Ros SP, Fisher EA, Bell TJ: Adenosine in the emergency management of supraventricular tachycardia, *Pediatr Emerg Care* 7:222, 1991.

Truong JH, Rosen P: Current concepts in electrical defibrillation, *J Emerg Med* 15:331, 1997.

III

FLUID AND ELECTROLYTE BALANCE

Management of the pediatric patient with fluid and electrolyte disturbance requires an understanding of maintenance requirements and sources of abnormal losses. It is imperative to correlate history, physical, and laboratory data in patient management.

7 DEHYDRATION

DIAGNOSTIC FINDINGS

Clinical assessment with ancillary laboratory data determines the urgency and type of therapy required.

Degree of Dehydration

	Mild (<5%)	Moderate (10%)	Severe (15%)
Signs and symptoms			
Dry mucous membrane	+	+	‖
Reduced skin turgor (pinch retraction)	−	±	+
Depressed anterior fontanel	−	+	−
Mental status	Alert	Irritable	Lethargic
Sunken eyeballs	−	+	+
Hyperpnea	−	±	+
Hypotension (orthostatic)	−	±	+
Increased pulse	−	+	+
Capillary refill	≤2 sec	>2 sec	>2 sec
Laboratory			
Urine			
Volume	Small	Oliguria	Oliguria/anuria
Specific gravity*	≤1.020†	>1.030	>1.035
Blood			
BUN	WNL†	Elevated	Very high
pH (arterial)	7.40-7.30	7.30-7.00	<7.10

+, Present; −, absent; ±, variable.
*Specific gravity can provide evidence that confirms the physical assessment.
†Not usually indicated in mild or moderate dehydration.

In the child with only very mild dehydration (2% to 3%), a slight decrease in mucosal membrane moisture and the relative dryness and prominence of the papillae of the tongue may be all that is noted on physical examination. In the younger child it is important, as a guide to hydration status, to determine specifically the number of diapers changed and their dampness in the preceding 6 to 8 hours.

Beyond those parameters indicated above, the percentage of dehydration may be estimated by calculating:

$$\% \text{ Dehydration} = 1 - \left(\frac{\text{Present weight}}{\text{Recent known weight}} \right) \times 100\%$$

Orthostatic vital signs should be obtained in older children. When the patient rises from a lying to a standing (or sitting) position, a decrease in blood pressure of 15 to 20 mm Hg or an increase in pulse of 20 beats/min after 2 or 3 minutes is significant. These changes may be seen in children without hypovolemia.

Children can often compensate for fluid losses because of their ability to constrict peripheral blood vessels and redistribute blood flow centrally. With uncompensated shock, vital organ functions are maintained. Perfusion to the peripheral (skin and muscles) blood vessels may be compromised, causing prolonged capillary refill (>2 seconds) and a pale, blue, or mottled appearance. Poor central nervous system perfusion may impair mental activity. An acute volume deficit of 10% may produce a minimal pulse increase, but progressive changes occur with further fluid deficit. Gradual volume losses are better tolerated.

The amount of fluid deficit can be calculated by multiplying the percentage of dehydration (e.g., 3%, 5%, 10%) by the weight of the child (e.g., a 10-kg child who is 10% dehydrated has a total deficit of 1000 ml or 100 ml/kg). Clinical assessment when combined with an HCO_3^- less than 17 mEq/L is useful in predicting dehydration more than 5%. The electrolyte composition of this fluid deficit depends on the rapidity of progression of dehydration (normally 60% extracellular fluid [ECF] and 40% intracellular fluid [ICF]). In general, the percentage of loss from ECF increases with a more acute progression and decreases with more chronic loss. The electrolyte composition of these compartments may be simplified as ECF: 140 mEq Na^+/L and ICF: 150 mEq K^+/L.

Types of Dehydration

The types of dehydration are based on serum sodium concentration, reflecting osmolality in the moderately and severely dehydrated patient. Clinical assessment of the patient with hypernatremia tends to underestimate the degree of dehydration because perfusion is preserved longer.

	Isotonic	Hypotonic	Hypertonic
Serum sodium level			
(mEq/L)	130-150	<130	>150
Physical signs			
Skin			
Color	Gray	Gray	Gray
Temperature	Cold	Cold	Cold
Turgor	Poor	Very poor	Fair
Feel	Dry	Clammy	Thick, doughy
Mucous membrane	Dry	Dry	Parched
Sunken eyeballs	+	+	+
Depressed anterior fontanel	+	+	+
Mental status	Lethargic	Coma/seizure	Irritable/seizure
Increased pulse	++	++	+
Decreased blood pressure	++	+++	+

+, ++, +++, Relative prominence of finding.

Complications

Complications of dehydration are shock (see Chapter 5) and acute tubular necrosis (p. 809).

Ancillary Data

The following laboratory findings to assess hydration status are indicated for all moderately and severely dehydrated children but rarely for mildly dehydrated youngsters.
   1. Serum electrolyte and glucose levels.

2. Blood urea nitrogen (BUN) level: often elevated; with appropriate rehydration will decrease by 50% over first 24 hours. If fall does not occur, consider hemolytic-uremic syndrome as an etiologic consideration (p. 801). If intake is poor or the child is malnourished, BUN level may be low because of low protein.
3. Specific gravity of urine to confirm physical findings.
4. Complete blood count (CBC) to assess risk of infection.
5. Other studies as indicated by underlying condition.

MANAGEMENT OF SEVERE AND MODERATE DEHYDRATION
Restoration of Vascular Volume: Phase I

Patients require immediate infusion of fluids, particularly patients with abnormal vital signs. If possible, orthostatic blood pressure and pulse should be obtained in the recumbent position on older patients with normal vital signs. While the patient goes from a lying to a standing (or sitting) position, a decrease of 15 mm Hg in blood pressure or an increase of 20 beats/min in pulse after 2 to 3 minutes is considered significant. These changes may be seen in the absence of hypovolemia and therefore require clinical correlations.

Fluid Therapy

1. In the moderately or severely dehydrated child, 0.9% NS (normal saline) solution or lactated Ringer's (LR) solution should be given at 20 ml/kg (adult = 1 to 2 L) over 20 minutes.
2. If a poor therapeutic response is noted, the initial infusion should be followed by 10 to 20 ml/kg (adult: 0.5 to 1.0 L) over 20 to 30 minutes, assuming normal renal and cardiac function.
3. The initial phase I bolus of 20 to 40 ml/kg to restore vascular volume is not routinely computed into phase II and III water deficit and maintenance corrections.
4. Glucose infusion with crystalloid as D5W 0.9% NS or D5WLR may be used for the initial bolus in children who have experienced prolonged vomiting, diarrhea, or inadequate intake, and a low glucose is anticipated. Blood glucose levels should be checked and monitored.
5. If a poor therapeutic response is noted in the severely dehydrated child after two fluid pushes (i.e., no urine, continued abnormal vital signs, poor perfusion) with ongoing losses or with suspected cardiac or renal disease, central venous pressure or pulmonary capillary wedge pressure may need to be monitored (see Chapter 5).

Specific Therapeutic Plans

Case examples of the three major categories of dehydration (isotonic, hypotonic, and hypertonic) provide a basis for fluid management. Maintenance requirements are summarized in Chapter 8. Ongoing abnormal losses need additional replacement therapy either on the basis of approximations (see Chapter 8) or by direct determination of the electrolyte composition of fluid losses. Vital signs, intake and output, and ancillary data (electrolyte, BUN, and glucose levels) must be monitored constantly. These patients require hospital observation and often admission.

Isotonic Dehydration

1. Initial findings
   a. Preillness weight: 10.0 kg (a 1-year-old child)

  b. Degree of dehydration: moderate (10%)
  c. Body weight on admission: 9.0 kg
  d. Electrolytes:

$$Na^+ \; 135 \; mEq/L \quad K^+ \; 5 \; mEq/L \quad Cl^- \; 115 \; mEq/L \quad HCO_3^- \quad 12 \; mEq/L$$

2. Summary of fluid requirements

	H_2O	Na^+ (mEq)	K^+ (mEq)
Maintenance	1000	30	20
	(100 ml/kg)	(3 mEq/kg)	(2 mEq/kg)
Deficit (100 ml/kg)			
ECF (60%)	600	84 (140 mEq/L × 0.6)	
ICF (40%)	400	—	30 (150 mEq/L × 0.4 × 50% correction)
TOTAL	1000	84	30

3. Fluid schedule

		Fluids
Phase	Calculation	Administered
I. 0-½ hr	20 ml/kg	200 ml 0.9% NS or LR over 20 min
II. ½-9 hr	½ deficit: 500 ml D5W with 42 Eq NaCl and 15 mEq KCl	833 ml (~100 ml/hr) of D5W 0.45% NS with 22 mEq KCl (~27 mEq KCl) (this approximation facilitates care)
	⅓ maintenance: 333 D5W with 10 mEq NaCl and 7 mEq KCl	
	Total: 833 ml with 52 mEq NaCl and 22 mEq KCl	
III. 9-25 hr	½ deficit	1167 ml (~75 ml/hr) of D5W
	⅔ maintenance	0.45% NS with 28 mEq KCl (~24 mEq/L) (this approximation facilitates care)

NOTE: If the patient is acidotic with HCO_3^- less than 11 mEq/L or pH less than 7.1 (on the basis of metabolic acidosis), one third of the sodium is administered during phase II (½ to 9 hours) as $NaHCO_3$. Glucose should be checked initially.

In general, after a bolus of normal solution, D5W 0.45% NS with 20 mEq KCl/L is the appropriate fluid, infused at a rate reflecting both deficit and maintenance requirements.

Oral rehydration has been recommended in specific circumstances for children who can tolerate oral fluids and who have no contraindications, including shock, intractable vomiting, voluminous diarrhea that cannot be matched with oral intake, intestinal obstruction, or short bowel syndrome.

Oral glucose facilitates the absorption of sodium and water across the mucosal cells of the small intestine, an osmolality in the range of 250 mOsm/L being preferable to a higher osmolality. Current recommendations in young children distinguish between fluids used for initial oral rehydration under close supervision and careful monitoring followed by maintenance solutions:

Composition	Rehydration solution (treatment of acute dehydration)	Maintenance solution
Sodium	70-90 mEq/L	40-60 mEq/L
Potassium	20-30 mEq/L	20 mEq/L
Glucose	2-2.5 gm/dl	2-2.5 gm/dl

In infants, Rehydralyte is an excellent rehydration solution, whereas Pedialyte or Infalyte are excellent liquids for maintenance.

Management using oral hydration may be approached as follows:
a. 100 ml/kg over 4 hours; *or*
b. Twice the deficit volume over 6 to 12 hours; *or*
c. Deficit plus 12 hours of maintenance fluids over 12 hours; *or*
d. Ad lib feedings to a maximum of 200 ml/kg/24 hr.

If vomiting occurs, increase the feeding aliquots in 5- to 10-ml increments. Small amounts of vomiting are not a contraindication to enteral therapy. For each diarrhea stool seen in the emergency department (ED), 10 ml/kg should be added.

If the child refuses to feed actively, passive enteral therapy can be instituted with a nasogastric (NG) tube or repeated 2 to 5 ml syringe boluses to the back of the mouth. Obviously, if these are unsuccessful, parenteral therapy should be considered.

Hypotonic Dehydration

In children the most common form of hyponatremia also is associated with hypovolemia (decreased total body water [TBW]) (p. 79) caused by abnormal gastrointestinal (GI) losses. Glucose should be monitored.

1. Initial findings
   a. Preillness weight: 10.0 kg (a 1-year-old child)
   b. Degree of dehydration: moderate (10%)
   c. Body weight on admission: 9.0 kg
   d. Electrolytes:

$$Na^+ \text{ 110 mEq/L} \quad K^+ \text{ 5 mEq/L} \quad Cl^- \text{ 90 mEq/L} \quad HCO_3^- \text{ 12 mEq/L}$$

2. Summary of fluid requirements

	H_2O (ml)	Na^+ (mEq)	K^+ (mEq)
Maintenance	1000 (100 ml/kg)	30 (3 mEq/kg)	20 (2 mEq/kg)
Deficit (100 ml/kg)			
ECF (60%)	600	84 (140 mEq/L × 0.6)	
ICF (40%)	400		30 (150 mEq/L × 0.4 × 50% correction)
Sodium*	_____	125	_____
TOTAL	1000	209	30

*Sodium deficit calculation
A. Na^+ required to correct to 135 mEq/L = 135 mEq/L − 110 mEq/L (observed Na^+) = 25 mEq.
B. TBW (L/kg) = 0.6 L/kg (preillness TBW) − 0.1 L/kg (water loss) = 0.5 L/kg.
C. Preillness weight = 10 kg.
Sodium deficit = A × B × C = 25 mEq/L × 0.5 L/kg × 10 kg = 125 mEq.

3. Fluid schedule

Phase	Calculation	Fluids Administered
I. 0-½ hr	20 ml/kg	200 ml 0.9% NS or LR over 20 min
II. ½-9 hr	½ deficit: 500 ml D5W with 105 mEq NaCl and 15 mEq KCl	833 ml (~100 ml/hr) of D5W 0.9% NS with 22 mEq KCl (~27 mEq KCl) (this approximation facilitates care)
	⅓ maintenance: 333 ml D5W with 10 ml NaCl and 7 mEq KCl	
	Total: 833 ml with 115 mEq NaCl and 22 mEq KCl	
III. 9-25 hr	½ deficit	1167 ml (~75 ml/hr) of D5W 0.9% NS with 28 mEq KCl (~24 mEq/L) (this approximation facilitates care)
	⅔ maintenance	

NOTE: If the patient is acidotic with an HCO_3^- less than 11 mEq/L or pH less than 7.1 (on the basis of metabolic acidosis), one third of the sodium is administered as $NaHCO_3$. Glucose levels should be checked initially and monitored.

In general, after an initial bolus of normal saline solution, D5W 0.9% NS with 20 mEq KCl/L is the appropriate fluid, infused at a rate reflecting both deficit and maintenance requirements. In the presence of severe hyponatremia with decreased TBW in symptomatic patients, hypertonic 3% saline solution may be given to raise the serum sodium level to 125 mEq/L. A 3% saline solution contains approximately 0.5 mEq Na^+/ml. Patients may be given 3% saline solution 4 ml/kg IV over 10 minutes and the response monitored. Once seizures have stopped, one half of the deficit may be corrected over the next 8 hours as outlined in the fluid schedule.

In patients with increased TBW, whether associated with normal or slightly increased total body sodium level, fluid restriction is usually necessary. Excess water may be calculated as follows:

$$\text{Present TBW (L)} = \text{Weight (kg)} \times 0.6$$
$$\text{Desired TBW (L)} = \frac{\text{Weight (kg)} \times 0.6 \times \text{Measured Na}^+ \text{ (mEq/L)}}{\text{Desired Na}^+ \text{ (mEq/L)}}$$
$$\text{Water excess (L)} = \text{Present TBW} - \text{Desired TBW}$$

NOTE: Sodium is usually corrected to 125 mEq/L.

In addition, in the moderately symptomatic patient, furosemide (Lasix), 1 mg/kg/dose IV, should be administered. During the subsequent diuresis, urinary sodium, potassium, and chloride levels should be measured and replaced milliequivalent for milliequivalent with 3% saline solution and supplemental potassium chloride (beginning with 20 mEq KCl/L). Demeclocycline may be useful in patients more than 8 years old with chronic severe syndrome of inappropriate antidiuretic hormone (SIADH) in whom water restriction is inadequate to correct the abnormality.

Hypernatremic Dehydration

Most patients have a deficit of free water, but rapid rehydration often results in serious neurologic complications, including seizures. The degree of hydration is difficult to assess.

If hypotension exists, phase I stabilization is used to expand the intravascular volume—initiating 20 ml/kg of 0.9% NS or LR over the first hour. Glucose should be checked and monitored.

The underlying emphasis of therapy must be a slow and deliberate schedule designed to correct deficits over 48 hours. Guidelines are as follows:

1. If the serum sodium concentration is 175 mEq/L or greater, the deficit therapy should decrease serum sodium concentration by 15 mEq/L/24 hr.
2. If the serum sodium concentration is less than 175 mEq/L, the deficit therapy should decrease the serum sodium half the way to normal in the first day of therapy.
3. If the loss is primarily water, some suggest that the water deficit is 50 ml/kg if the Na^+ is 150 mEq/L, 90 ml/kg if 160 mEq/L, and 140 ml/kg if 170 mEq/L.

Other recommendations:

1. Fluids to be used should be D5W 0.2% NS. With altered mental status or seizures, higher sodium concentration may be needed.
2. The volume of free water needed to lower a serum sodium concentration above 145 mEq/L is about 4 ml/kg of free water for each 1 mEq/L evenly over 48 hours.
3. Maintenance fluids should be continued.

Ongoing Management: Phases IV and V

1. After parenteral hydration, oral fluids should be initiated slowly—initially with Lytren or Pedialyte—advancing the diet slowly in both volume and composition.
2. If the dehydration has followed an episode of acute gastroenteritis, a lactase deficiency is commonly present, and a lactose-free formula may be used.
3. After severe, prolonged diarrhea, an elemental formula such as Pregestimil or Alimentum may be necessary. Such patients require a deliberate, conservative approach, which may necessitate continuous NG feeding of dilute formula (one-fourth to one-half strength) and slow advancement to bolus feeding, with subsequent increase in volume and finally osmolality (p. 78).

Phases of Response

Phase	Therapeutic plan	Pattern of response
I. Up to ½ hr Restoration of vascular volume	20 ml/kg 0.9% NS or LR over 20-30 min; may repeat 10-20ml/kg	Improved vital signs Increased urine flow Improved state of consciousness
II. ½-9 hr Partial restoration of ECF deficit and acid-base status	⅓ maintenance daily fluids ½ deficit fluids	Gain in body weight Stabilization of vital signs Improved urine flow Partial restoration of normal acid-base status
III. 9-25 hr Restoration of ECF, ICF, and acid-base status	⅔ maintenance daily fluids ½ deficit fluids	Sustained gain in body weight Fall in BUN level (50% in 24 hr) Sustained urine flow Improved electrolytes
IV. 25-48 hr Total correction of acid-base and K^+ status	Ongoing parenteral ± oral hydration Maintenance fluids and replacement of ongoing losses	Sustained gain in body weight Normal electrolytes
V. 2-14 days Restoration of caloric and protein deficits	Ongoing oral support	Steady gain in weight Plasma constituents normal

MANAGEMENT OF MILD DEHYDRATION (<5%)

1. Oral hydration is usually adequate in the child who is less than 5% dehydrated *if that patient can tolerate oral intake.* An approach to oral rehydration is outlined on p. 72. If the patient cannot tolerate oral fluid, another approach is to administer fluids by NG tube usually beginning as 10-20 ml/kg/hr by continuous NG infusion.
2. If oral fluids are not retained, parenteral fluids should be given. Many children can tolerate fluids after the initial phase I flush of 20 ml/kg of 0.9% NS or LR over 30 to 45 minutes. However, if fluids continue to be vomited, the patient requires admission and calculation of fluids as outlined.
3. Patients require careful monitoring of intake, output, and weight. Laboratory data are rarely necessary.
4. Clear fluids (Table 7-1) should be pushed, although slowly in the child who is vomiting. Do not use rice water, tea, or boiled milk. Many fruit juices (especially apple juice) are hyperosmolar and may draw water into the intestinal lumen, worsening diarrhea. Kaolectrolyte, a powder packet, is an alternative.

TABLE 7-1   Common Oral Hydrating Solutions

Solution	Na$^+$ (mEq/L)	K$^+$ (mEq/L)	Cl$^-$ (mEq/L)	HCO$_3^-$/citrate (mEq/L)	Glucose* (gm/dl)	mOsm/L
REHYDRATION						
Rehydralyte	75	20	65	30	2.5	270
WHO Solution	90	20	80	10	2.0	310
MAINTENANCE						
Lytren	50	25	45	30	2.0	
Pedialyte	45	20	35	30	2.5	270
Infalyte	50	25	45	34	1.9	200
CLEAR LIQUIDS						
Gatorade	20	3			2.1	
Cola	3	0.1-0.9		7-13	10.0	
Ginger ale	4	0.2			9.0	

*May be long-chain oligosaccharide subject to hydrolysis.

5. In infants it is particularly important to provide adequate electrolytes while minimizing potential errors in formulation of solutions. Therefore fluids such as Rehydralyte are recommended during initial rehydration, followed by Lytren or Pedialyte.
6. Once ongoing losses have stopped, the diet may be advanced. No clear evidence exists that clinicians need to prescribe elaborate dietary manipulations after an episode of diarrhea in previously healthy children. In children who have had prolonged (>7 days) gastroenteritis, many suggest a lactose-free product initially, although this is controversial.
7. Applesauce, strained carrots, dry toast, and bananas have been found useful in advancing to solids. Attention should be given to caloric intake to facilitate mucosal healing.

Disposition

If fluids are tolerated, patients with mild dehydration may be discharged when close follow-up observation and good compliance are ensured and no underlying medical conditions necessitate early intervention (e.g., diabetes and sickle cell disease).

Parental Education

1. Give only clear liquids; give as much as your child wants. The following may be used during the first 24 hours:
   a. Rehydralyte, during initial rehydration followed by Pedialyte or Lytren is ideal.
   b. Give defizzed, room-temperature soda or Gatorade to older children (>2 years) if diarrhea is only mild.
2. If your child is vomiting, give clear liquids slowly. In younger children, start with 1 teaspoonful and slowly increase the amount. If vomiting occurs, let your child rest for a while and then try again. About 8 hours after vomiting has stopped, your child can gradually return to a normal diet.
3. After 24 hours, your child's diet may be advanced if the diarrhea has improved. If your child is

taking only formula, mix the formula with twice as much water to make up half-strength formula, which should be given over the next 24 hours. Applesauce, bananas, and strained carrots may be given if your child is eating solids.

If this is tolerated, your child may advance to a regular diet over the next 2 to 3 days.

4. If your child has had a prolonged course of diarrhea, it may be helpful in the younger child to advance from clear liquids to a soy formula (Isomil, ProSobee, or Soyalac) for 1 to 2 weeks. Children more than 1 year old should not have cow's milk products (milk, cheese, ice cream, or butter) for several days.

5. Do not use boiled milk. Kool-Aid and soda are not ideal liquids, particularly for younger infants, because they contain few electrolytes.

6. Call your physician if:
   a. The diarrhea or vomiting is increasing in frequency or amount.
   b. The diarrhea does not improve after 24 hours of clear liquids or does not resolve entirely after 3 to 4 days.
   c. Vomiting continues for more than 24 hours.
   d. The stool has blood or the vomited material contains blood or turns green.
   e. Signs of dehydration, including decreased urination, less moisture in diapers, dry mouth, no tears, weight loss, lethargy, or irritability, develop.

8 MAINTENANCE REQUIREMENTS AND ABNORMALITIES

MAINTENANCE FLUIDS AND ELECTROLYTES

Fluids

Fluid balance is closely regulated. Intake of water is controlled by the hypothalamic regulation of thirst, whereas absorption is largely a reflection of the gastrointestinal (GI) tract. Excretion occurs via the lungs, skin, GI tract, and kidneys. An antidiuretic hormone (ADH) regulates urinary volume and concentration.

Normal maintenance fluids reflect the necessity to replace daily water and electrolyte losses from the skin and the respiratory, urinary, and GI tracts. These may be divided into insensible, urinary, and fecal components; they amount to 100 ml/kg/24 hr up to age 1 year and decrease thereafter.

Insensible losses (30 ml/kg/24 hr) occur through the skin and respiratory tract. Water loss is affected by humidity, body temperature, respiratory rate, and ambient temperature. Fever increases insensible water loss by 7 ml/kg/24 hr for each degree rise in temperature above 37.2° C (99° F).

Urinary losses (60 ml/kg/24 hr) reflect the solute load and obligate excretion and urine concentration. Normal fecal water losses (10 ml/kg/24 hr) are small and, in older children, insignificant.

Water requirements

Children <10 kg	100 ml/kg/24 hr
Children 11-20 kg	1000 ml plus 50 ml/kg/24 hr for each kilogram over 10 kg
Children >20 kg	1500 ml plus 20 ml/kg 24 hr for each kilogram over 20 kg
Adult	2000-2400 ml/24 hr

Beyond the newborn period, total body water makes up about 60% of body weight; 40% is intracellular fluid (ICF) and the remaining 20% is extracellular fluid (ECF). The intravascular volume represents 5% of the ECF in adults and is as much as 8% (80 ml/kg) in younger children.

Electrolytes

Cation	Daily requirement			Compartment
	0-10 kg	**10-20 kg**	**>20 kg**	
Na$^+$	3 mEq/kg	30 mEq + 1.5 mEq for each kilogram over 10 kg	45 mEq + 0.6 mEq/kg for each kilogram over 20 kg	ECF (includes intravascular)
K$^+$	2 mEq/kg	20 mEq + 1 mEq/kg for each kilogram over 10 kg	30 mEq + 0.4 mEq/kg for each kilogram over 20 kg	ICF

Osmolality

Osmolality is regulated by osmoreceptors in the hypothalamus. When a receptor detects increased ECF osmolality, ADH release is stimulated. Because cell membranes are permeable to water and osmotic equilibrium is homeostatically maintained, the volume of ICF is determined by the tonicity of ECF. The osmolality of plasma and therefore ICF can be approximated as follows:

$$\text{Plasma osmolality} = 2 \times (\text{Na}^+) + \frac{(\text{Glucose})}{18} + \frac{\text{BUN}}{2.8}$$

Plasma osmolality normally ranges between 280 and 295 mOsm/kg water.

If the measured osmolality is normal but the calculated osmolality is low, the difference most likely is caused by a decrease in serum water content. This can occur in hyperglobulinemia, triglyceridemia, and hyperglycemia.

Acid-Base Balance

Compensatory Mechanisms

The relationship between pH and bicarbonate-carbonic acid concentration is best expressed by the Henderson-Hasselbalch equation:

$$pH = pK + \log \frac{(\text{HCO}_3^-)^{\text{Renal}}}{(\text{H}_2\text{CO}_3)_{\text{Respiratory}}}$$
$$\text{H}_2\text{CO}_3 = \text{H}_2\text{O} + \text{Dissolved (CO}_2)$$

The renal and respiratory compensatory systems determine acid-base balance.

1. *Respiratory* systems can provide a *rapid* alteration in pH by changing the respiratory rate and tidal volume. The classic example is Kussmaul's pattern breathing in diabetic ketoacidosis. Respiratory alkalosis may be due to central nervous system (CNS) (increased intracranial pressure [ICP], anxiety, encephalitis/meningitis), hypotension, sepsis, or liver toxic (salicylates) conditions.

2. *Kidneys* provide a *slow* response, balancing the excretion of HCO_3^- and the secretion of H^+, primarily by the distal nephron.

Anion Gap

In addition to determining pH, $P\text{co}_2$, and HCO_3^- as determinants of acid-base balance, the anion gap should be determined in considering potential causes:

$$\text{Anion gap} = \text{Na}^+ + \text{K}^+ - (\text{Cl}^- + \text{HCO}_3^-)$$

The normal anion gap is 8-12 mEq/L, comprised primarily of phosphates, sulfates, and organic acids. The gap is usually normal in metabolic acidosis resulting from diarrhea in which there is a loss of bicarbonate ion through the GI tract and kidneys. It is increased with excessive production of organic acids (ketones), lactic acid (shock, sepsis, congestive heart failure [CHF]), toxins (salicylates), or renal failure. A useful mnemonic for remembering entities that produce a metabolic acidosis with a large anion gap is MUDPILES: *m*ethanol, *u*remia, *d*iabetic ketoacidosis, *p*araldehyde overdose, *i*soniazid or iron overdose, *l*actic acidosis, *e*thanol or ethylene glycol, and *s*alicylate overdose or starvation.

ELECTROLYTE AND ACID-BASE ABNORMALITIES

The two major cations, sodium and potassium, are the primary determinants of the distribution of water between the ECF and ICF spaces. These compartments depend on active transport of potassium into the cells and sodium out of the cells by an energy-requiring process.

Sodium

Sodium regulation is a balance of intake, total body water, and excretion through urine, sweat, and feces. Disorders can result in hyponatremia or hypernatremia, both significantly affecting plasma osmolality.

1. *Hyponatremia.* Clinical presentation is variable, reflecting the rapidity of progres-

sion and severity of hyponatremia. Early signs may include apathy, difficulty in concentrating, and agitation, progressing to confusion, irritability, coma, and seizures. Nausea, vomiting, muscle weakness and cramps, myoclonus, and decreased deep tendon reflexes may be noted. Several mechanisms may produce hyponatremia, reflecting the balance between total body water and sodium:

a. Decreased total body water (hypovolemia) and decreased total body sodium. Examples: renal salt loss (diuretics, adrenal insufficiency, renal tubular acidosis), extrarenal salt loss (severe sweating, cystic fibrosis, GI losses, vomiting, diarrhea), and third spacing (burns, peritonitis, pancreatitis). Sodium is usually less than 20 mEq/L in urine.

b. Increased total body water and normal total body sodium. Examples: syndrome of inappropriate antidiuretic hormone (SIADH) (pulmonary disease, CNS trauma, drugs such as hypoglycemic agents, antineoplastic drugs, tricyclics, and thiazide diuretics), hypothyroidism, severe potassium depletion, and psychogenic water drinking. Urine sodium is usually more than 20 mEq/L.

c. Increased total body water (hypervolemia) relatively greater than increased total body sodium. Examples: CHF, renal or hepatic failure, nephrosis, and hypoproteinemia.

d. Pseudohyponatremia. Examples: hyperglycemia, hyperproteinemia, and hyperlipidemia. NOTE: Serum sodium level decreases 1.6 mEq/L for each increment of 100 mg/dl in serum glucose level.

2. *Hypernatremia.* Symptoms of altered mental status, irritability, seizures, and coma may develop, with associated skeletal muscle rigidity and hyperactive reflexes. This may result from one of two mechanisms:

a. Decreased total body water and normal total body sodium (dehydration). Examples: increased insensible or renal water loss, excessive solute loss (mannitol, urea), abnormal water loss (diarrhea), and diabetes insipidus.

b. Normal total body water and increased total body sodium. Examples: salt poisoning, rehydration with boiled milk, and CNS disease affecting hypothalamus. Urine sodium is more than 20 mEq/L.

Potassium

Potassium is of central importance in the maintenance of ICF osmolality. Only 1.5% to 2.0% of the total body potassium is ECF, as reflected by serum measurements.

During metabolic acidosis, renal secretion of hydrogen ions is increased while that of potassium is decreased. For every 0.1 decrease in pH, serum potassium increases by about 0.5 mEq/L, with a similar reverse relationship.

To alkalinize the urine as required in treatment of barbiturate or aspirin ingestions, adequate amounts of potassium must be administered to facilitate renal excretion of sodium bicarbonate.

1. *Hypokalemia.* Patients may have muscle weakness, abdominal distension, and decreased bowel sounds (ileus), impaired renal concentrating ability, and hypochloremic alkalosis. Delayed ventricular depolarization is noted, with a relatively flat T wave on electrocardiogram (ECG). Decreased potassium commonly results from excessive loss of potassium from the GI tract (diarrhea, vomiting, or nasogastric [NG] suction), kidneys (diuretic, renal tubular acidosis), drug ingestion, and insulin or glucose therapy.

Significant hypokalemia (3.0 mEq/L), especially in patients taking digoxin or in those with myocarditis, should be treated cautiously. Such patients may receive 0.1-0.2 mEq/kg infusions of KCl every 4 to 6 hours while their serum levels are monitored. Larger boluses (0.2-0.3 mEq K^+/kg/hr) ideally should be given through a central line.

2. *Hyperkalemia.* The primary toxicity of cardiac conduction is common. A peaked T wave progresses to a widened QRS and ventricular dysrhythmias, and muscle weakness often is noted. Renal or metabolic disease may be present, as well as acidosis or excessive intake. Hemolysis of red blood cells during heelsticks or venipuncture may artificially elevate the measured serum potassium level. Management is discussed on p. 814.

Calcium

Ninety percent of calcium is in the skeletal system. About 40% is protein bound, primarily to albumin.

1. *Hypocalcemia.* Patients may be symptomatic, with neuromuscular findings of tetany, positive Chvostek's and Trousseau signs, laryngospasm, and seizures. Vitamin D and nutritional deficiency, malabsorption or abnormal metabolism of vitamin D, parathyroid disease, magnesium deficiency, and pancreatitis may be causative.

   Treatment of symptomatic patients begins with a dose of 0.5-1.0 ml/kg of 10% calcium gluconate IV over 5 minutes. Ongoing management includes a combination of parenteral (5-8 ml/kg/24 hr 10% calcium gluconate given in four to six doses IV) and oral calcium gluconate (200-500 mg/kg/dose q6hr PO) as needed. Magnesium level should be monitored and supplemented as needed. Cardiac monitoring is essential.

2. *Hypercalcemia.* Calcium level may be more than 11 mg/dl. Headache, irritability, lethargy, weakness, seizures, or coma may develop. Anorexia, dehydration, polydipsia, and polyuria may be noted. Hyperparathyroidism, vitamin D toxicity,

immobilization, and malignancies may be contributory. Management focuses on hydration and intermittent furosemide (1 mg/kg/dose q6hr IV). Malignancies require mithramycin therapy.

Acid-Base

Alterations in acid-base status, which represent a balance of compensatory mechanisms (p. 79), may be summarized as follows:

	pH	P_{CO_2}	HCO_3^-
Metabolic acidosis	↓	↓	↓*
Metabolic alkalosis	↑	↑	↑*
Respiratory acidosis	↓	↑*	↑
Respiratory alkalosis	↑	↓*	↓

*Indicates primary abnormality.

NOTE: Mixed metabolic and respiratory disorders are common. In a simple disturbance without compensatory reaction, both the $Paco_2$ and HCO_3^- level abnormalities are in the same direction.

Metabolic acidosis is initially accompanied by compensatory tachypnea and may be associated with cardiac dysrhythmias and cellular dysfunction. Initially, the $Paco_2$ level decreases, with a fall 1 to 1.5 times the reduction in the HCO_3 level. Specific correction of the underlying condition requires treatment (often correction of intravascular volume); in addition, it may require supplemental HCO_3^- therapy. If the HCO_3^- level is less than 10 mEq/L in acute conditions, it should be corrected to at least 12 to 15 mEq/L. The initial correction should replace a maximum of *half* of the deficit:

$$\text{Deficit mEq } HCO_3^- = \text{Weight (kg)} \times \text{Base deficit}$$
$$\text{(mEq/L desired} - \text{mEq/L observed)} \times 0.6 \times 0.5$$

Metabolic alkalosis may be accompanied by muscle cramps, weakness, paresthesias, seizures, hyperreflexia, tetany, and dysrhythmias. The $Paco_2$ level increases 0.5 to 1.0 mm Hg for each mEq/L increase in HCO_3^-. Primary treatment of the causative condition often requires restoration of intravascular volume or discontinuation of diuretics as appropriate. If alkalosis is severe, with a pH of 7.7 (lower if symptomatic), treatment options include the following:

1. Acetazolamide (Diamox), 5 mg/kg/24 hr q6-24hr (adult: 250-375 mg/24 hr) PO, IV. Use only if K^+ level is normal; or
2. Ammonium chloride (NH_4Cl), 150-300 mg/kg/24 hr q6hr (adult: 8-12 gm/24 hr) PO.

ELECTROLYTE COMPOSITION OF BODY FLUIDS

Knowing the electrolyte composition of body fluids may be useful in delineating potential abnormalities associated with fluid loss.

ELECTROLYTE COMPOSITION OF BODY FLUIDS

	Electrolyte Composition of Body Fluids				
Fluid	Na^+ (mEq/ L)	K^+ (mEq/ L)	Cl^- (mEq/ L)	H^+ (mEq/ L)	HCO_3^- (mEq/ L)
Sweat	10-30	3-10	10-35		
Gastric	20-80	5-20	100-150	90	
Pancreas	120-140	5-40	50-120		90
Small intestine	100-140	15-40	90-130		25
Diarrhea	10-90	10-80	10-110		45

REFERENCES

Avery ME, Snyder JD: Oral therapy for acute diarrhea, *N Engl J Med* 323:891, 1990.

Brown KH, Peerson JM, Fontaine O: Use of non-human milks in the dietary management of young children with acute diarrhea: a meta-analysis of clinical trials, *Pediatrics* 93:17, 1994.

Cohen MB, Mezoff AC, Laney DW, et al: Use of a single solution or oral rehydration and maintenance therapy of infants with diarrhea and mild to moderate dehydration, *Pediatrics* 95:639, 1995.

Finberg L, Kravath RE, Fleischman AR: *Water and electrolytes in pediatrics: physiology, pathophysiology, and treatment*, Philadelphia, 1982, WB Saunders.

Margolis PA, Litteer T, Hare N, et al: Effects of unrestricted diet on mild infantile diarrhea: a practice based study, *Am J Dis Child* 144:162, 1990.

MacKenzie A, Barnes G, Shann F: Clinical signs of dehydration in children, *Lancet* 2:605, 1989.

Pizarro D, Castillo B, Posada G, et al: Efficacy comparison of oral rehydration solutions containing either 90 or 75 millimoles of sodium per liter, *Pediatrics* 79:190, 1987.

Pizzaro D, Posada G, Sandi L, et al: Rice based oral electrolyte solutions for the management of infantile diarrhea, *N Engl J Med* 324:517, 1991.

Santosham M, Fayad I, Zikri MA, et al: A double blind clinical trial comparing World Health Organization oral rehydration solution with a reduced osmolality solution containing equal amounts of sodium and glucose, *J Pediatr* 128:45, 1996.

Vega RM, Avner JR: A prospective study of the usefulness of clinical and laboratory parameters for predicting the percentage of dehydration in children, *Pediatr Emerg Care* 13:179, 1997.

IV
NEWBORN EMERGENCIES

ANTHONY F. PHILIPPS

Care providers faced with a distressed newborn in the delivery room or emergency department may be forced to make rapid therapeutic decisions without an adequate patient database. Under such conditions, standardized guidelines for resuscitation, diagnosis, and management provide a basis for intervention.

ANTICIPATION

A number of *maternal "high-risk" factors* have been associated with poor outcome for the newborn. Notification prenatally of any of the factors listed below will help alert the neonatal care provider of specific diseases processes to be aware of and, therefore, of specific treatment strategies to be made available.

Maternal factors commonly associated with poor outcome are the following:
1. Previous obstetric history: premature delivery or miscarriage, perinatal loss, previous baby with fetal growth retardation or malformation
2. Third-trimester or intrapartum disorders: toxemia of pregnancy, gestational diabetes, prolonged rupture of membranes, clinical chorioamnionitis, prolonged labor, breech or face presentation, abruptio placentae, or placenta previa
3. "Chronic" factors: type 1 diabetes, chronic hypertension, Rh sensitization, multifetal gestation, history of oligohydramnios or polyhydramnios, or history of drug or ethanol exposure/abuse

Fetal factors associated with poor outcome are as follows:
1. Lack of fetal well-being: history of decreased fetal movement, heart rate abnormalities (particularly late or severe variable decelerations), meconium-stained amniotic fluid, or history of abnormal nonstress or stress test result
2. Fetal immaturity: prematurity as estimated by dates, ultrasound, uterine size, or amniocentesis (lecithin/sphingomyelin [L/S] ratio <2.0 or absent phosphatidylglycerol suggests inadequate lung maturation)
3. Fetal growth: history of poor intrauterine growth or postdate delivery
4. Specific fetal malformations (detected by ultrasound) such as diaphragmatic hernia or omphalocele or other abnormalities such as fetal edema or ascites

Equipment

Adequate preparation is essential.
1. Temperature: radiant warmer present and preheated. Special wraps (e.g., Thinsulate [3M]) are specifically designed to function as an effective insulating head wrap and bunting.
2. Airway and ventilation (see Chapter 4 and Table 9-1): bulb syringe, suction trap (adapters are available for use with low wall suction), face masks (newborn and premature sizes), endotracheal (ET) tubes (2.5-, 3.0-, and 3.5-mm ET tube; malleable stylet [sterile]), suction catheters (one 5 Fr and two 8 Fr), laryngoscope, laryngoscope blades (straight 0 and 1), extra batteries and bulbs, and a resuscitation bag (non–self-inflating, able to deliver 90% to 100% oxygen; adaptable with a manometer and positive end-expiratory pressure [PEEP] valve). Although less optimal, standard self-inflating (750-ml) resuscitation bags may also be used. Several types of disposable infant resuscitation bags that include an adjustable PEEP valve and adapter for a manometer are now

TABLE 9-1   Intubation Equipment

Weight (kg)	ET tube (mm)	Suction catheter	Laryngoscope blade
1	2.5	5 Fr	0
2	3.0	6 Fr	0
3	3.5	8 Fr	0-1
4	3.5-4.0	8 Fr	1

available. A sterile, disposable end-tidal CO_2 device is now commercially available for use in conjunction with neonatal or infant intubation to test whether the ET tube has been properly placed within the airway.

3. Medications (Table 9-2): epinephrine (1:10,000), sodium bicarbonate (dilute 1:1 to 4.2%), volume expander (e.g., 5% albumin or normal saline), and naloxone.
4. Equipment to initiate administration of parenteral fluids: normal equipment plus umbilical catheterization supplies, including catheter (3.5 and 5.0 Fr), three-way stopcock, and sterile umbilical vessel catheterization tray containing towels, gauze pads, scissors, hemostats, curved iris forceps, scalpels, and umbilical tape.
5. Warm, dry towels to dry infant.
6. Obstetric (OB) kit/cord-cutting material.
7. Gloves and other protective devices.

Personnel

A team approach is absolutely necessary for re-suscitation of the depressed neonate. This approach calls for close cooperation among physicians, nurses, nurse practitioners, and other health care providers in the delivery room setting, as well as a team leader previously designated to direct efforts of the resuscitation. Periodic practice drills are strongly recommended.

Optimally, this team should be very familiar with the principles of resuscitation and management of neonatal asphyxia, including the practical uses of bag and mask ventilation, ET intubation, chest massage, and umbilical vein and artery catheterization. In addition, completion of the Neonatal Resuscitation Program (NRP) curriculum (available through the American Heart Association and American Academy of Pediatrics, 141 Northwest Point Blvd., P.O. Box 927, Elk Grove Village, IL, 60009-0927) with certification should be essential for personnel involved in delivery room care of the neonate.

MANAGEMENT

Immediately after delivery in high-risk situations, if poor color or flaccidity is evident or if there is no cry:

1. Maintain temperature. Minimize heat loss by towel drying and placing infant under radiant warmer (avoid overheating) or in warm blankets.
2. Assess respiratory pattern and rate visually. Heart rate may be determined rapidly by either auscultation or palpation of the umbilical cord (pulsations). Perfusion is best assessed by determining capillary refill time after gentle pressure over the midsternum (<2 to 3 seconds refill time after the release is the norm). Visually inspect the patient quickly to determine the presence of any major external anomalies (e.g., myelomeningocele, omphalocele).
3. Calculate Apgar score (Table 9-3) at 1 and 5 minutes, evaluating *a*ppearance (color), *p*ulse, *g*rimace (reflex irritability), *a*ctivity (muscle tone), and *r*espirations. The score is a useful indicator of neonatal depression and may also be used to evaluate the response to resuscitation during asphyxia (i.e., at 10 minutes, 15 minutes, etc.). It is recommended that observation be continued at intervals until a score of 7 or higher is achieved. Optimally, the score should be assigned by someone not directly involved in resuscitation efforts.

TABLE 9-2   Drugs Used in Resuscitation of Newborns

Drug	Availability	Indications	Dosage
Epinephrine	1:10,000	Bradycardia	0.1-0.3 ml/kg IV, ET
Calcium gluconate	10% (100 mg/ml) 0.45 mEq Ca^{++}/ml	Decreased cardiac output (controversial)	100 mg (1 ml)/kg IV
Calcium chloride	10% (100 mg/ml) 1.36 mEq Ca^{++}/ml	Decreased cardiac output (controversial)	33 mg (0.3 ml)/kg IV
Sodium bicarbonate	4.2% (0.5 mEq/ml)	Metabolic acidosis	1-2 mEq/kg (give slowly over at least 2 min)
Dextrose (glucose)	10%	Hypoglycemia	2-4 ml (10%)/kg for term or preterm, given slowly over 10 min IV
Albumin	5%	Hypovolemic shock	10 ml/kg IV; may repeat
Naloxone (Narcan)	0.4, 1 mg/ml	Narcotic-induced respiratory depression	0.1 mg/kg IV, ET

TABLE 9-3   Apgar Score

Sign	Score		
	0	1	2
Muscle tone (activity)	Limp	Some flexion	Active, good flexion
Pulse	Absent	<100/min	>100/min
Reflex irritability* (grimace)	No response	Some grimace or avoidance	Cough, cry, or sneeze
Color (appearance)	Blue, pale	Pink body, blue hands/feet	Pink
Respirations	Absent	Slow, irregular, ineffective	Crying, rhythmic, effective

*Nasal or oral suction catheter stimulus.

After stabilization and during transfer to the nursery, several routine steps are carried out:

1. Routine prophylaxis against ophthalmia neonatorum is performed with silver nitrate (1%) drops or erythromycin (0.5%) or tetracycline (1%) ophthalmic ointments.
2. Vitamin K (0.5 to 1.0 mg phytonadione) is administered IM to prevent vitamin K–dependent hemorrhagic disease of the newborn. (Note that oral administration of vitamin K preparations to the newborn, in lieu of parenteral injection, has not been found to be as efficacious. In addition, no available oral preparation is approved for use currently.)
3. Cord blood is obtained for later studies as deemed appropriate (e.g., hemoglobin, blood gas, bilirubin). Note that most institutions accept cord blood only for testing of infant blood type, not for cross-matching.

GENERAL RESUSCITATION MEASURES
(See Chapters 4 and 5 and Fig. 9-1)

Although depression of the newborn at delivery may be the result of a variety of different insults, the most typical symptoms of neonatal depression are significant hypotonia and respiratory compromise. The latter is usually evidenced by apnea or moderate to severe hypoventilation with concomitant cyanosis and bradycardia. Unless cord blood gases reveal a condition of metabolic acidosis, a diagnosis of intrapartum

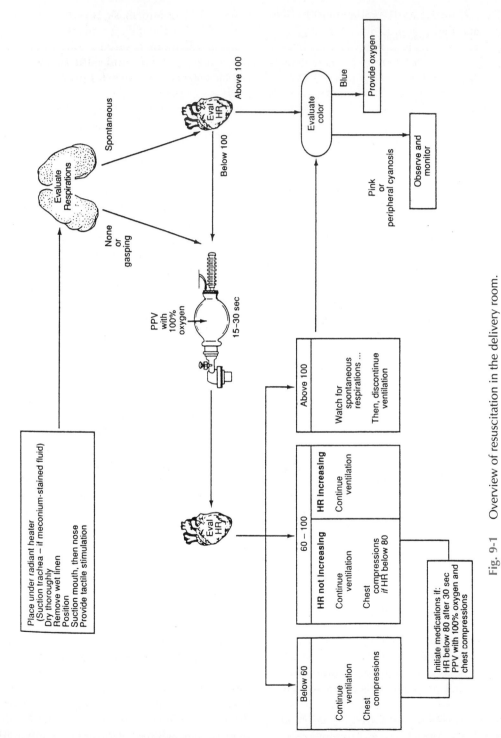

Fig. 9-1 Overview of resuscitation in the delivery room.
(From *Textbook of neonatal resuscitation*, Dallas, 1992, American Heart Association.)

asphyxia cannot be made with certainty. However, if perinatal depression is not addressed in an appropriate and timely manner, tissue hypoxia, acidosis, and resultant organ damage (particularly to the central nervous system [CNS], heart, kidneys, and lungs) can occur. Delivery of a premature infant, particularly less than 32 weeks' gestation, is often accompanied by signs of respiratory distress, temperature instability, and hypotonia.

Resuscitation of the newborn rarely requires advanced life support techniques; adequate resuscitation is usually achieved with relatively simple measures, such as the following:

1. Use *tactile stimulation* by drying and suctioning the oropharynx and nares to remove amniotic fluid. Flicking the soles of the feet or gently rubbing the infant's back may be useful.
2. Place the infant in Trendelenburg position in a *radiant warmer.*
3. If thick or particulate meconium has been noted in the amniotic fluid before or at delivery, do *not* initiate positive pressure ventilation immediately (see below).
4. If labor was not complicated by fetal meconium passage:
   a. Use deep airway suction if the infant is apneic and has no response to stimulation. This procedure is *not* done routinely on all delivered newborns because of the risk of severe reflex bradycardia when performed within 5 minutes of delivery.
   b. Assess the airway. If evidence of nasal obstruction or mandibular hypoplasia is present, insert oral airway. Administer free flowing oxygen. If normal airway, proceed to (c).
   c. If the infant is apneic and does not respond to stimulation, administer oxygen and begin *bag and mask inflation* at 40 to 60/min. Insufflation bags should have an oxygen reservoir to deliver close to 100% oxygen. Positive pressure ventilation administered with

a bag and mask is optimally achieved with the infant's head in the sniffing position. It often is helpful to place a small towel under the infant's neck to prevent hyperextension.
   d. If the response is poor (no increase in heart rate or improvement in color), *intubate* and continue with bag to ET tube ventilation.
   e. Assess the heart rate and, if less than 80 beats/min and not readily responsive to ventilation, initiate *closed chest massage* at midsternum. This is best achieved in the term newborn by either (1) encircling the chest with both hands, placing the thumbs over the midsternum and the tips of fingers over the spine or (2) touching the midsternum region with the tips of the middle finger and either ring or index finger of one hand. The sternum is then compressed approximately one third of the depth of the chest in a ratio of three compressions/breath at a compression rate of approximately 120/min until spontaneous heart rate is greater than 80/min.

Medications are usually unnecessary for the neonate with perinatal depression unless there is advanced vascular collapse or decreased cardiac output that has not responded to previous resuscitative measures. The most common drug used as a cardiac stimulant in the delivery room is epinephrine, which can be given through the ET tube before obtaining vascular access. Such access can be achieved easily in the emergency setting, however, via the umbilical vein (see p. 90). Specific drugs and volume expanders can also be administered.

Volume resuscitation is rarely indicated because many depressed babies have normal blood volume. Volume expanders may be appropriate, however, if there are signs of inadequate blood volume (poor perfusion or severe metabolic acidosis). Hypovolemia most commonly is associated with placenta previa or abruptio placentae but can also be noted after twin-to-twin or fetomaternal transfusion. Rupture of membranes with relative oligohydramnios may produce umbilical cord compression during labor, probably a common, as well as occult, cause of fetal blood loss (fetal-placental transfusion). Volume expansion with solutions such as 5% albumin or fresh-frozen plasma are optimal (10 ml/kg over 15 to 60 minutes), but normal saline solution infusion (at the same volume and interval) is acceptable and often more readily available.

Factors that should be considered when resuscitation efforts are unsuccessful include equipment failure, ET tube malposition, pneumothorax, and congenital anomalies such as diaphragmatic hernia or pulmonary hypoplasia.

Umbilical Catheterization

In an emergency, the umbilical cord provides easy access for administration of intravascular drugs and fluid.

1. Restrain extremities, prepare abdomen and cord with antiseptic solution (surgical scrub), and drape lower abdomen and legs with sterile towels.
2. After placing loosely knotted umbilical tape around the base of the cord, trim the umbilical cord to 1 to 2 cm above the skin surface (vertical traction with hemostats will control venous bleeding).
3. Identify the umbilical vein (single, thin wall, large-diameter lumen) and umbilical artery (paired, thick wall, small-diameter lumen).

Umbilical Venous Catheterization

The umbilical venous catheterization technique is easier and more practical in the delivery room. This vessel can often be catheterized in the first 4 to 5 days after birth as well.

1. With caudal countertraction on the umbilical cord, insert a 5-Fr end-hole catheter (previously filled with saline solution and attached to a three-way stopcock and syringe) into the lumen. Gently pass the catheter cephalad in the direction of the liver 5 to 8 cm or until blood return is noted. If resistance to passage is encountered once the catheter has gone beyond the peritoneal fascia, the tip is probably in a portal vein radical, and the catheter should be pulled back until blood can be withdrawn smoothly. Occasionally (e.g., in severe congenital heart disease, hydrops, septic shock), it may be helpful to have a central vein catheterized. If no resistance is encountered, it may be possible (roughly 50% chance) to pass this catheter above the ductus venosus to a position near the right atrium 8 to 10 cm in the term newborn (Fig. 9-2). However, for most simple resuscitations, the more shallow position is adequate. In both situations, great care should be taken to prevent injection of air intravenously and to prevent injury of vessels within the liver caused by advancing the catheter tip too forcefully. If a central catheter is deemed necessary, radiographic confirmation of catheter tip location should be obtained.
2. Remove the catheter only when resuscitation is completed and patient is stable. If it is deemed necessary to continue IV fluid or drug therapy, the central catheter should be removed only when stable peripheral venous access has been achieved. Prolonged maintenance of indwelling umbilical venous catheters may be associated with neonatal bacteremia and portal vein thrombosis.

Umbilical Arterial Catheterization

Umbilical arterial catheterization requires more time than umbilical venous catheterization and may not be appropriate for achieving vascular access in an emergency.

1. Gently dilate vessel with an iris forceps. Avoid trauma to the vessel wall.
2. Insert a 3.5- or 5.0-Fr end-hole catheter (previously filled with saline solution and attached to a three-way stopcock and sy-

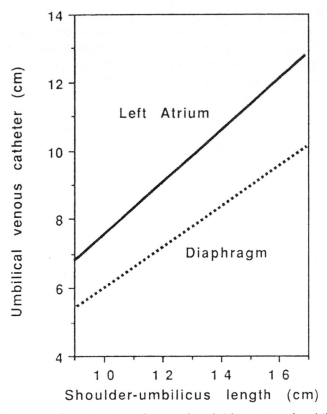

Fig. 9-2   Nomogram for estimation of proper length of insertion of umbilical venous catheter (distance from lateral end of clavicle to umbilicus versus length of catheter to reach designated level).

(From Dunn PM: *Arch Dis Child* 41:69, 1966.)

ringe) into the lumen until blood return is noted, then advance so catheter is at diaphragm or aorta bifurcation. The catheter should be angled slightly caudad to conform with the direction of the umbilical arteries. Estimate the length of catheter required for proper insertion, using markings on the catheter and Fig. 9-3.

3. Resistance to passage is caused by vasoconstriction and usually can be overcome by gentle, steady pressure. Reposition or replace the catheter if resistance persists. Observe the extremities and buttocks for evidence of arterial obstruction.

4. If the catheter is to be left in place after the resuscitation, check the position of the tip with abdominal roentgenography. The optimal position above the diaphragm is at T6-T9 and below the diaphragm at the aortic bifurcation (L4-L5). A catheter tip facing caudad is in the external iliac artery and must be removed. Secure the catheter with a 3-0 silk purse-string suture through the cord.

5. Infuse parenteral solutions at a rate of at least 2 to 3 ml/hr IV. Heparinized saline solution (1 U/ml) may be used but is usually unnecessary. Hyperosmolar solutions infused through the catheter may cause significant ischemic reactions.

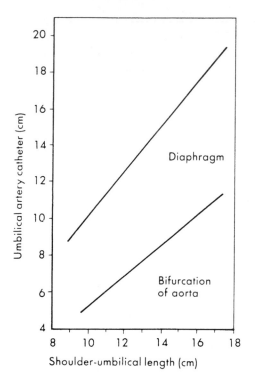

Fig. 9-3 Nomogram for estimation of proper length of umbilical artery catheter (distance from lateral end of clavicle to umbilicus versus length of catheter to reach designated level).

(From Dunn PM: *Arch Dis Child* 41:69, 1966.)

MECONIUM-STAINED AMNIOTIC FLUID

1. Meconium staining of the amniotic fluid, which complicates 10% to 15% of all pregnancies, predominantly in the term or postterm gestation, is usually benign, particularly when the meconium is noted to be thin and nonparticulate. However, in some cases, meconium passage into the amniotic fluid may be associated with intrapartum asphyxia. Under these circumstances, fetal distress may promote gasping, allowing meconium passage below the vocal cords. Fetal distress or depression at birth is more likely if the meconium is thick or particulate. Meconium as-

piration syndrome (MAS) (see Chapter 11) may result, with significant morbidity and mortality rates. Management at delivery depends on the character of the meconium and the presence or absence of significant neonatal depression.

2. Diagnostic findings: Meconium staining of cord and skin and perinatal depression may or may not be present.

3. Management: In all babies who have passed meconium in utero, clear mouth and pharynx of meconium with a suction device before delivery of the thorax from the perineum or hysterotomy site.

   If thick or particulate meconium was present in amniotic fluid:

   a. After moving the patient to a warmer, remove any remaining meconium from hypopharynx with laryngoscopy and suctioning. If meconium is present at the level of the vocal cords or if the newborn is depressed, initiate ET intubation to suction out remaining meconium from the trachea. While applying continuous suction, withdraw the ET tube slowly. Adapters are now available to be used to attach a suction apparatus to the ET hub. An alternate method (less efficient, but faster) is to pass a suction catheter through the ET tube for suctioning of the airway. In the former situation, intubation may be required twice (maximum). In the latter case, particulate meconium may not be easily removed.

   b. Begin other measures of resuscitation involving support of ventilation and circulation after (a) has been performed.

   c. Clearly, considerable judgment must be used. Although debatable from the point of view of trauma related to intubation of vigorous neonates, symptomatic meconium aspiration has occurred in nondepressed term infants. Thus rapid and efficient intubation of these babies seems indicated. Reintubation to remove residual meconium probably should be limited to two to three times maximum before beginning positive pressure ventilation if required.

If only thin, watery (green-tinged) amniotic fluid has been noted:

(1) Most would advocate suctioning the mouth and nose alone, particularly for the vigorous neonate, without laryngoscopy or intubation.

(2) This subject remains controversial. However, for the depressed neonate with thinly stained fluid, laryngoscopy is an acceptable alternative approach. If meconium is noted at the cords, intubation with suction before resuscitation is indicated.

10 DISTRESS AT BIRTH

*S*everal diagnostic entities may be associated with distress or depression of the newborn immediately after birth.

INTRAPARTUM ASPHYXIA

1. Etiology: decreased transplacental gas exchange with resultant fetal hypoxemia, acidosis, and ischemia
2. Diagnostic findings: pallor or cyanosis, bradycardia, apnea, and flaccidity
3. Management: resuscitation as outlined in Chapter 9

MECONIUM ASPIRATION
(see Chapters 9 and 11)

MATERNAL DRUGS

Narcotics, sedatives, and magnesium sulfate may cause depression of the newborn.
1. Etiology: transplacental passage of agent with subsequent central or neuromuscular depression
2. Diagnostic findings: apnea, decreased muscle tone
3. Management
   a. If depression is believed to be the result of narcotics, administer naloxone (Narcan), 0.1 mg/kg/dose (0.4 mg/ml or 1.0 mg/ml solution) q3-5min prn IM or IV, and support. Larger doses may be required. Note that use of naloxone is *contraindicated* in babies exposed in utero to opiates, including methadone, because it may induce convulsions.
   b. If magnesium sulfate is suspected as cause, give calcium gluconate, 100 mg/kg/dose IV, slowly with cardiac monitoring. Note that resultant improvement in clinical status may be temporary and patients must be monitored closely. In addition, the potential risk of calcium extravasation may make repetitive doses impractical and potentially dangerous. In premature infants, temporary artificial ventilation may be required.

CONGENITAL ANOMALIES (see Chapter 20)

Upper Airway Disorders

1. Etiology: choanal atresia, micrognathia, and macroglossia are most common. Less common causes include laryngeal atresia, cyst, or web; vascular ring; goiter; cystic hygroma; vocal cord paralysis; and tracheal anomalies.
2. Diagnostic findings: substernal and intercostal retractions, cyanosis, apnea, and inspiratory stridor. May note neck mass, hypoplastic mandible, etc. Passage of feeding tube or suction catheter through the nasopharynx is impossible in choanal atresia.
3. Management
   a. Oxygen and oral airway. Prone position, with micrognathia.

b. Intubation if obstruction is unrelieved or apnea develops. Laryngoscopy may reveal cause of obstruction.

c. Surgical consultation as needed.

Lower Airway and Pulmonary Disorders

1. Etiology: diaphragmatic hernia, tracheo-esophageal fistula (TEF), or Potter's syndrome (oligohydramnios, lung hypoplasia, and characteristic facies). Less commonly observed are neonatal chylothorax, congenital pneumonia, cystic adenomatoid malformation of the lung, and lobar emphysema. Some of these abnormalities may be identified prenatally.

2. Diagnostic findings

  a. Severe respiratory distress with poor air entry and cyanosis

    (1) Scaphoid abdomen is occasionally prominent in diaphragmatic hernia.

    (2) TEF is suggested by excessive mucus production, crowing respirations, hoarse cry, and inability to place nasogastric (NG) tube in stomach. Usually associated with esophageal atresia.

    (3) Potter's syndrome suggested by resistance to lung inflation, early pneumothorax, flattened facies, redundant skin folds, renal dysgenesis, and history of oligohydramnios.

  b. X-ray studies. Characteristic presentation in diaphragmatic hernia (unilateral lung hypoplasia with multiple bowel loops in chest, tip of stomach tube in chest if left-sided hernia), TEF (NG tube coiled in air-filled esophageal pouch), and Potter's syndrome (lung hypoplasia often with pneumothorax).

3. Management: strong suspicion is important, particularly if oligohydramnios or scaphoid abdomen is present or significant early respiratory distress in a term infant.

  a. Oxygen, intubation, and ventilatory support as indicated. Bag and mask ventilation in diaphragmatic hernia is contraindicated because it will inflate intrathoracic stomach and bowel and compromise ventilation further.

  b. Early insertion of large (e.g., 8 to 10 Fr) NG tube and suction for decompression.

  c. Portable ultrasound to identify kidneys, cystic tumors, or pleural fluid (chylothorax or hydrops presentation).

  d. Appropriate surgical consultation.

NEUROMUSCULAR DISORDERS

1. Etiology: although individually these are rare entities, they have a common presentation. Neonatal myotonic dystrophy, congenital fiber-type disproportion, muscular dystrophy, and a number of other relatively rare entities should be considered.

2. Diagnostic findings: flaccidity, little to absent spontaneous respiration, and poor to absent spontaneous movement and swallowing efforts. Breech presentation and polyhydramnios are also intrauterine clues to diagnosis. Family history may be useful, but these disorders often occur as sporadic events. Muscle and nerve biopsies may be indicated with neurologic consultation.

3. Management: for the most part supportive, once initial resuscitative efforts have been carried out. These infants often pose difficult diagnostic dilemmas because postpartum hypoxia may obscure the clinical picture.

OTHER

More common abnormalities such as sepsis, respiratory distress syndrome, and shock, may present with symptoms while the patient is still in the delivery room setting. These disorders are discussed in Chapter 11.

11 POSTNATAL EMERGENCIES

CARDIOVASCULAR DISORDERS

DYSRHYTHMIAS (see Chapter 6)

In the premature infant, the most common dysrhythmias are premature atrial and ventricular beats. These are usually benign.

Paroxysmal atrial tachycardia (PAT, supraventricular tachycardia, SVT) may require therapy if it persists more than 1 hour or if there is associated hemodynamic compromise (e.g., respiratory distress, oxygen requirement, shock, poor feeding). Treatment should be undertaken in consultation with a pediatric cardiologist, if practical. Cardiac monitoring with chart recorder should be available. Management includes the following:

1. Adenosine is an effective therapeutic and diagnostic tool. Give 100 µg/kg IV. Must be given rapidly. Follow immediately with 2 to 3 ml normal saline (NS) at same IV site using a three-way stopcock apparatus to flush this small amount of adenosine into the circulation. May repeat one time with 100-200 µg/kg in 10 to 15 minutes if no response. Note that brief but significant bradycardia may ensue.

    Other therapies include:
2. Give propranolol, 0.05-0.15 mg/kg/dose IV over 10 minutes. Maintenance is 0.2-0.5 mg/kg/24 hr q6hr PO.
3. Use of digoxin (see Table 16-3).
4. In general, avoid vagal stimulation. However, application of ice (small bag with ½ ice, ½ water) centered over the bridge of the nose for 15 to 20 seconds) can be

effective in some circumstances. May be repeated two to three times, maximum. Do *not* perform ocular maneuvers in the newborn.
5. If condition deteriorates, synchronized cardioversion at 2 watt-sec/kg.
6. Consult with pediatric cardiologist.

CONGENITAL HEART BLOCK

The uncommon dysrhythmia of congenital heart block may be due to either major congenital heart malformations or an underlying maternal collagen vascular disease. It is often recognized prenatally and, in some cases, has resulted in emergency delivery because of the mistaken interpretation of fetal distress. If associated with a malformation, the electrophysiologic and anatomic combination is often fatal. In situations without associated congestive heart failure (CHF) (ascites, pleural effusions, anasarca), no emergent therapy may be necessary. Management includes the following:

1. Make diagnosis with electrocardiogram (ECG): usually shows evidence of normal atrial rate (120 to 150/min) and dissociated ventricular rate (50 to 60/min).
2. Establish venous access (see Chapter 9).
3. Evaluate for respiratory and circulatory insufficiency.
4. Consult with pediatric cardiologist and consider possible pacemaker placement.
5. In the presence of CHF or evidence of tissue hypoxia (significant metabolic acidosis), infusion of isoproterenol, 0.05-0.5 µg/kg/min, or epinephrine, 0.1-1.0

μg/kg/min IV in 5% dextrose solution, may be necessary.

CYANOTIC CONGENITAL HEART DISEASE (see Table 16-1)

Cyanotic congenital heart disease results from fixed right-to-left shunts at any level. It is more common in infants of insulin-dependent diabetic mothers, in those with chromosomal disorders (e.g., trisomy 13 or 18), or after the use of specific drugs in the first trimester of pregnancy (e.g., lithium). The most prevalent lesions in the neonate include transposition of the great vessels, tetralogy of Fallot, and pulmonary atresia. Characteristically, cyanosis (or desaturation noted on pulse oximeter) remains in trials of 100% O_2. Evaluation is outlined in Chapters 16 and 17, and consultation with a pediatric cardiologist is advised. Chest x-ray films and Doppler echocardiography are indicated for preliminary diagnosis. Cardiac catheterization and, in some cases, magnetic resonance imaging (MRI) may be indicated.

NONCYANOTIC CONGENITAL HEART DISEASE

Obstruction to or absence of aortic flow in the neonate is often unrecognized in the first days of life because of patency of the ductus arteriosus. With closure of the ductus in the presence of either coarctation of the aorta, interruption of the aortic arch, or hypoplastic left heart syndrome, femoral pulses are lost and perfusion to the trunk deteriorates. Massive shock and metabolic acidosis result, mimicking the appearance of septic shock or inborn errors of metabolism. Suspicion is necessary for diagnosis, with prompt involvement of a pediatric cardiologist and ultrasound assessment of cardiac anatomy. Catheterization and, in some cases, MRI may also be indicated.

Positive pressure ventilation and IV fluid and bicarbonate support are often necessary. Prostaglandin E_1 infusion IV (0.05-0.1 μg/kg/min)

can be instituted if appropriate (or if the diagnosis is suspected but cannot be immediately confirmed). Note that infusion of prostaglandin E_1 may lead to respiratory depression or apnea, particularly in premature infants.

PERSISTENT PULMONARY HYPERTENSION OF THE NEWBORN (OR PERSISTENCE OF THE FETAL CIRCULATION)

Persistent pulmonary hypertension of the newborn (PPHN) is more common than "fixed shunt" disorders, which it may mimic. PPHN is commonly seen in term or near-term neonates, in those with significant intrapartum asphyxia, and in infants delivered postdate. PPHN is occasionally associated with polycythemia or diaphragmatic hernias. It also may complicate pulmonary disease, such as respiratory distress syndrome (RDS), meconium aspiration syndrome (MAS), or bacterial pneumonia. PPHN is presumed to be caused in many instances by failure of the pulmonary arteriolar bed to vasodilate, as well as by a hyperreactive pulmonary arteriolar medial muscle mass, with resultant continued pulmonary hypertension and right-to-left shunting through fetal channels (ductus arteriosus and foramen ovale).

Diagnostic Findings

Cyanosis with quiet but persistent tachypnea occurs in the first 12 hours of life. If associated with pulmonary disease (e.g., MAS or diaphragmatic hernias), there may be significant dyspnea with retractions.

Ancillary Data

1. X-ray films: results often normal or may show nonspecific pattern much milder than the clinical presentation would indicate. May suggest decreased pulmonary vascularity. In PPHN with associated pulmonary disease, there may be associated typical findings (e.g., aspiration pattern in MAS).

2. ECG: finding of nonspecific right ventricular hypertrophy.
3. Pulse oximeter saturation: usually below 85% and often below 75% in room air. Right upper extremity saturation is often 5% to 10% above lower extremity saturation, suggesting right-to-left ductal shunting.
4. Arterial blood gas (ABG): determination of Pao_2 less than 50 mm Hg in room air without significant response to 100% oxygen. Radial artery Pao_2 is often 15 mm Hg above umbilical artery Pao_2, suggesting ductal shunting. Acidosis secondary to hypoxemia may be present. $Paco_2$ is usually normal or decreased initially.

Management

1. Consultation with a tertiary care facility and with pediatric cardiologists should be obtained. A "fixed shunt" disorder cannot be excluded without further evaluation.
2. A minority of patients respond to increased ambient oxygen alone. Inducement of metabolic alkalosis by use of bicarbonate infusion or respiratory alkalosis achieved by ventilator-assisted hyperventilation may be useful. Both conventional and high-frequency ventilation strategies are now commonly applied to babies with severe PPHN.
3. Other drugs in the management of PPHN may be useful. For example, cardiotonic agents such as dopamine and dobutamine may improve cardiac output and enhance pulmonary blood flow significantly. However, these should not be administered with an uncertain diagnosis and without the support of a tertiary care center because of the lability of these patients and the systemic side effects encountered with drug therapy. This is particularly true of vasodilators such as tolazoline, which may increase pulmonary blood flow but also induce severe systemic hypotension. Similarly, surfactant administered by endotracheal (ET) tube may also be of benefit in selected patients but should be given only by qualified individuals with significant experience in use of surfactants and in managing ventilated newborns.
4. Extracorporeal membrane oxygenation (ECMO) is a heroic but occasionally lifesaving modality now available for affected term or near-term neonates in a number of specialized centers.
5. Other therapies, such as liquid ventilation and inhaled nitric oxide, show promise and are currently undergoing clinical research trials but have not been approved for general use in the newborn.

CONGESTIVE HEART FAILURE
(see Chapter 16)

CHF occurs most commonly as a result of a patent ductus arteriosus (PDA) in the premature neonate, often during recovery from hyaline membrane disease (HMD). Other causes of CHF include coarctation of the aorta, aortic stenosis or atresia, hypoplastic left ventricle, tachydysrhythmias, heart block, viral myocarditis, arteriovenous fistula (central nervous system [CNS] or liver), and structural cardiac lesions, with either a single large shunt or shunts at multiple levels. "Acyanotic" structural lesions (septal defects) rarely cause CHF in the first weeks.

Fetal echocardiography has made intrauterine diagnosis possible. CHF in the fetus may be demonstrated by scalp edema, pericardial effusion, ascites, and decreased fetal movement.

Shock may develop rapidly with closing of the PDA if there is a PDA-dependent lesion such as coarctation or critical pulmonary stenosis.

Patients should be transferred to a tertiary care facility after appropriate consultation and initial stabilization.

HYPERTENSION (see Chapter 18)

In the term newborn, a consistent systolic blood pressure (BP) measurement above 100 mm Hg is considered elevated. The most common conditions associated with neonatal hypertension are RDS and asphyxia. Often the cause is never determined. However, renovascular disease (anomalies, injury, renal vein thrombosis), coarctation of the aorta, and intracranial hemorrhage have been noted as proven causes of hypertension often enough to warrant investigation.

ENDOCRINE/METABOLIC DISORDERS

HYPOGLYCEMIA (see Chapter 38)

Hypoglycemia is a blood sugar concentration below 30 mg/dl (1.7 mmol/L) in the neonate, although consistent values below 40 mg/dl in the first days after birth warrant further observation.

Etiology

1. Most commonly caused by decreased availability of mobilizable substrates, as in intrauterine growth retardation (IUGR), postdate birth, asphyxia, cold stress, sepsis, polycythemia, or prematurity.
2. Less commonly caused by hypermetabolic states, usually a result of erythroblastosis or hyperinsulinism in infants of diabetic mothers. Rare causes also include congenital hyperthyroidism and genetic inborn errors, predominantly disorders of glycogen storage or release, amino acid metabolism, or mitrochondrial enzymopathies. These latter disorders are often associated with severe lactic acidosis.

Diagnostic Findings

1. Adrenergic: pallor, cool extremities, irritability
2. Central: jitteriness, poor feeding, seizures, apnea
   NOTE: Hypoglycemia may not be accompanied by identifiable symptoms, particularly in the premature or asphyxiated newborn.

Management

Anticipatory management is important, particularly in premature and other high-risk infants.

1. In initial management, maintain high suspicion when a history of maternal diabetes (discussed later), asphyxia, sepsis, and other risk factors are present.
2. If stable condition and more than 34 weeks, begin enteral feedings with 15 to 30 ml of D5W or D10W or formula or breast milk and advance, as tolerated, with feedings every 2 to 3 hours. Perform serial tests (Dextrostix or Chemstrip) until three normal determinations are recorded. At least one confirmatory serum glucose level determination is indicated.
3. If unstable or premature less than 34 weeks, begin D10W at 100-150 ml/kg/24 hr IV. Enteral feeding when stable.
4. If symptomatic or serum glucose less than 20 mg/dl, administer D10W 2-4 ml/kg IV over 5 minutes. Stable venous access is required. Follow by a constant infusion of D10W 100-150 ml/kg/24 hr. Avoid higher concentrations of glucose in hyperinsulinemic or premature neonates because of the risks of rebound hypoglycemia and hypertonicity.
5. If neither IV glucose solution nor infusion site is available, glucagon, 0.1-0.2 mg/kg IM, may be given in an emergency. Glucagon is ineffective in states of limited substrate availability, as in prematurity or growth retardation. The umbilical vein may be patent for several days after birth (see Chapter 9).

INFANT OF DIABETIC MOTHER

Births of infants of diabetic mothers (IDMs) are common as the mortality and fetal morbidity rates attributable to this disorder have fallen dramatically over the last 20 to 30 years. Common findings in infants of gestational and insulin-dependent mothers include macrosomatia and postnatal metabolic disorders such as hypoglycemia, hypocalcemia, polycythemia, and hyperbilirubinemia. The incidence of RDS (when corrected for gestational age) may be slightly increased. Infants born to insulin-dependent diabetic mothers have an increased risk of heart (ventricular septal defect [VSD], transposition of great vessels, coarctation), CNS (holoprosencephaly, myelocele), skeletal (sacral dysgenesis), gastrointestinal (GI) (anal atresia, small left colon), and renal anomalies. Cardiac septal hypertrophy is seen occasionally. In general, IUGR is the more common growth disturbance observed in fetuses of women with long-standing or severe insulin-dependent diabetes.

Diagnostic Findings

Excessive weight and length for gestational age and cushingoid or "cherubic" facies are common. Other findings relate to a particular anomaly, metabolic disorder, or concurrent problem. In addition, because of excessive fetal weight, birth trauma (clavicular fracture, axillary nerve injury) during vaginal delivery may be noted. Cardiac septal hypertrophy is evidenced by cardiomegaly, heart failure, and occasionally shock.

Management

1. A comprehensive history of mother's diabetes and complications is essential, as is a thorough newborn physical examination.
2. Close observation for early hypoglycemia and hypocalcemia. Treat each disorder as above (p. 99). Hypomagnesemia may coexist with hypocalcemia. May treat hypomagnesemia with magnesium sulfate, 25-50 mg/kg dose q4-6hr for three to four doses.
3. Watch closely for development of hyperbilirubinemia, particularly on days 3 to 5. May require office visits after nursery discharge to assess severity of jaundice.

4. Even near-term and term IDMs may be hypotonic for several days postnatally. Poor feeding is also a transient problem.
5. If symptomatic cardiac septal hypertrophy is suspected, pediatric cardiologist consultation is necessary. In an emergency, propranolol, 0.01-0.10 mg/kg/dose, slow IV push q6-8hr, is the drug of choice. AVOID α and β agonists, such as dopamine and epinephrine.

HYPOCALCEMIA

Hypocalcemia is serum calcium level below 7 mg/dl or ionized calcium level below 1.0 mmol/L. It is usually transient and in the nconate may be associated with maternal diabetes or perinatal asphyxia. After the first week of postnatal life, it may also be noted in infants with poor renal function. Rare disorders include isolated parathyroid hormone deficiency and DiGeorge syndrome (typical facial appearance, conotruncal cardiac anomalies, thymic and parathyroid dysfunction).

Diagnostic Findings

Findings may include jitteriness and irritability, occasional seizures in infants, low serum calcium level, and ECG with prolonged QT interval.

Management
1. Calcium gluconate, 100 mg (1 ml)/kg IV slowly. Watch for extravasation and bradycardia. Do not administer intraarterially.
2. Begin maintenance calcium gluconate, 200-300 mg/kg/24 hr q6-8hr IV or PO, until full feedings are tolerated. Adjust diet. (Occasionally, dosages as high as 600 mg/kg/24 hr are required.)
3. If little response, obtain serum magnesium level. If magnesium is less than 1.5 mEq/L, treat with magnesium sulfate, 20 mg/kg/dose q12hr IV.

HYPERKALEMIA (p. 814)

Hyperkalemia is defined as a serum potassium concentration above 6.5 mEq/L. Sampling site should be taken into account, particularly in the newborn, because of the effects of hemolysis from sampling bruised heels (capillary blood samples). It is common in babies with renal failure or severe renal anomalies, severely depressed babies, or those of very low birth weight (<1.0 kg). Although rare, congenital adrenal hyperplasia (CAH) should be considered, particularly if ambiguous genitalia are present. Note, however, that males with CAH have normal genitalia at birth.

Diagnostic Findings

Often asymptomatic until well advanced. Dysrhythmias or bradycardia is common. Earlier ECG findings include peaked T waves and widened QRS complex.

Management (see Chapter 85)

1. If the condition is stable, but potassium is 7.5-8.0 mEq/L or greater, give sodium polystyrene sulfonate (Kayexalate), 1 gm/kg/dose (25% sorbitol solution) q6hr rectally. Insulin and glucose have a more rapid onset of action. Infusion of human insulin in 5% albumin solution, 0.05-0.1 U insulin/kg/hr (1 unit of insulin per 10 ml of 5% albumin is given); piggyback into existing IV fluid such as D7.5W to D10W at 100-150 ml/kg/24 hr. Follow serum glucose and dipstick glucose level closely.
2. If dysrhythmia, treat immediately with sodium bicarbonate, 1-3 mEq/kg IV over 5 to 15 minutes, *or* calcium gluconate, 100-200 mg/kg IV over 5 to 15 minutes.
3. Determine and treat (if possible) the cause of hyperkalemia.

Other Disorders

1. Hyponatremia (see Chapter 8)
2. Hypernatremia (see Chapter 8)

GASTROINTESTINAL DISORDERS

Most significant GI diseases in neonates are caused by obstruction, usually evident shortly after birth or in the first few weeks of life (see Chapter 44).

ESOPHAGEAL ATRESIA AND TRACHEOESOPHAGEAL FISTULA

Tracheoesophageal fistula (TEF) symptoms may or may not be present at birth. The incidence of premature delivery increases with TEF and polyhydramnios. Esophageal atresia is associated with fistula between the trachea and distal esophagus in 85% of cases.

Diagnostic Findings

Early respiratory distress in "mucousy" infant with hoarse cry or stridor. Vomiting and aspiration occur when infant is fed. Nasogastric (NG) tube will not pass. Small fistula causes coughing with feeding. Associated anomalies such as imperforate anus, limb defects, and vertebral or renal anomalies may be present.

Complications
Aspiration pneumonia.

Ancillary Data
1. X-ray studies. Anteroposterior (AP) chest film shows tip of NG tube in air-filled upper esophageal pouch.
2. Contrast study should not be attempted without surgical consultation and is often unnecessary.

Management

1. Administer oxygen, maintain NPO status, and replace fluid deficits (see Chapter 7) as required.
2. Elevate patient's head 15 to 20 degrees (may raise end of incubator or crib).
3. Perform intermittent low suction with double-lumen nasoesophageal tube or equivalent (e.g., 8- to 10-Fr catheter).

4. Arrange immediate surgical consultation.

OBSTRUCTIVE LESIONS

Obstructive lesions are most commonly congenital in origin, with an overall rate of 1:2700 live births.

Etiology

1. Pyloric stenosis (p. 658).
2. Intestinal atresia: Proximal jejunum and distal ileum are the most common sites. Duodenal atresia is common with Down syndrome.
3. Meconium ileus: Ileal obstruction is most commonly associated with cystic fibrosis.
4. Volvulus (p. 659).
5. Imperforate anus: If associated with intestinal obstruction, perineal fistula is either absent or inadequate to permit elimination, particularly in males. Incidence of associated malformations (vertebral, cardiovascular, and tracheoesophageal) is as high as 50%.
6. Hirschsprung's disease (p. 652).

Diagnostic Findings

1. High obstructions (midjejunum and above) are associated with less abdominal distension but persistent vomiting, which may be bilious if distal to the ampulla of Vater. Patients are hungry after emesis. They may have a history of polyhydramnios.
2. Low obstructions are associated with more distension, less vomiting, and only occasionally a history of polyhydramnios. Palpable and visible bowel loops may be prominent. Respiratory distress or apnea as a result of elevated intraabdominal pressure and limited diaphragmatic excursion may be noted. High-pitched bowel sounds are often present.

3. Palpable mass, if present, is caused by volvulus or meconium ileus. Perforation may be accompanied by hypotension and sepsis.

Ancillary Data

1. X-ray studies. Supine and upright abdominal films are often helpful, demonstrating air-fluid levels, distended bowel, and mass effects. Free air may be noted in the presence of a perforation.
2. Electrolytes and complete blood count (CBC).

Management

1. Oxygen and fluid deficit replacement as required (see Chapter 7); NPO.
2. Large-bore NG tube (e.g., 8 to 10 Fr) for drainage at atmospheric pressure or intermittent low suction.
3. Immediate surgical and radiologic consultation as indicated by specific process.

ABDOMINAL WALL DEFECTS

Abdominal wall defects occur in 1:2500 live births.

1. Gastroschisis: abdominal wall defect lateral to umbilicus with herniation of abdominal viscera. Associated anomalies are rare, but atretic bowel may be an associated finding.
2. Omphalocele: herniation of abdominal viscera through omphalomesenteric duct into umbilical cord. Sac may rupture. Associated congenital anomalies are common (e.g., trisomy 13, trisomy 18, Beckwith syndrome).

Diagnostic Findings

A mass is noted at birth either in the cord itself (omphalocele) or paraumbilically (gastroschisis). The physician may visualize bowel loops, stomach, and occasionally, the liver within the herniated mass. With the advent of intrauterine ultrasound, prenatal diagnosis is relatively common. Green-tinged amniotic fluid may be mistaken for meconium but, when nonparticulate, probably represents in utero bilious reflux.

Management

1. Promptly prevent fluid loss. Cover herniated viscera loosely with saline-solution-moistened gauze, and enclose mass and lower portion of patient in a plastic wrap or aluminum foil. Support mass in midline position if possible.
2. Prevent hypothermia by heated incubator or radiant warmer.
3. Promptly administer IV fluids: D5W 0.2% NS solution at 20-40 ml/kg over 2 to 6 hours. Maintain NPO status.
4. Insert large-bore (e.g., 8 to 10 Fr) NG tube for drainage.
5. Monitor BP, urine output, and serum electrolyte levels.
6. Arrange immediate surgical consultation.

NECROTIZING ENTEROCOLITIS

Intestinal ischemia with secondary bacterial invasion is thought to be the most likely cause of necrotizing enterocolitis (NEC). Pneumatosis intestinalis and portal venous "air" are probably the results of bacterial production of hydrogen gas. This condition may quickly progress to intestinal necrosis and, occasionally, perforation and may also be accompanied by symptoms of gram-negative septicemia and shock. NEC is commonly found in the middle of distal ileum, but involvement of the stomach, as well as other portions of the small and large intestines, has been reported. Prematurity, high tonicity of feedings, umbilical catheterization, hypoxic stress, polycythemia, and *Klebsiella* nosocomial infection have been implicated as risk factors. NEC occurs predominantly in preterm infants after the onset of feedings. However, a somewhat more benign entity has been observed in near-term or term newborns with only colonic involvement.

Diagnostic Findings

Insidious or rapid onset of abdominal distension, with significant gastric residual (or emesis) of feedings, which are commonly bile stained. Nonspecific but early signs may also include lethargy, tachycardia, and temperature instability. These may progress rapidly to more worrisome findings of hypotension, pallor, tachypnea (or apnea), bloody stools, and tenderness to palpation indicated by abdominal examination.

Ancillary Data

1. X-ray studies. Early findings may include intestinal dilation with or without evidence of bowel-wall edema. The presence of pneumatosis intestinalis, with bubbly or linear air shadows in the bowel wall, confirms the diagnosis. Portal venous gas, which is occasionally seen, is a poor prognostic sign. Free air suggests intestinal perforation.
2. White blood cell (WBC) count is markedly elevated or depressed, with a shift to the left and presence of toxic granulations. Thrombocytopenia (platelet count $<50,000/mm^3$) is present in 50% of patients.
3. Serum electrolyte and glucose concentrations may demonstrate hyperglycemia and hyponatremia.
4. ABG results often show a significant metabolic acidosis.
5. Blood culture should be obtained before antibiotic therapy.
6. Disseminated intravascular coagulation (DIC) may be demonstrated by coagulation studies.

Management

1. IV hydration, with an initial bolus of D5W 0.2% NS or D5W 0.45% NS at 20-40 ml/kg over 2 to 3 hours if fluid deficit is present.

In addition, colloid or blood may be required when peripheral perfusion is diminished. Maintain NPO status.

2. Large-bore NG (e.g., 8 to 10 Fr) tube placed for drainage. Suction is unnecessary, but tube should be irrigated every 2 to 3 hours with 1 to 2 ml 0.9% NS.

3. Antibiotics initiated after culture results are obtained:
   a. Ampicillin, 100-150 mg/kg/24 hr q12hr IV; and
   b. Gentamicin, 5.0 mg/kg/24 hr q12hr IM or IV (if <7 days old); 7.5 mg/kg/24 hr q8hr IM or IV (if 7 to 28 days old), **or** cefotaxime, 100 mg/kg/24 hr q12hr IV or IM (if ≤7 days old); 150 mg/kg/24 hr q8hr IV or IM (if >7 days old).
   c. If rapid development of symptoms and signs occurs, *Clostridium* species must be considered as an etiologic agent. Initiation of clindamycin, 15 mg/kg/24 hr q8hr IV (or if full-term >7 days, 20 mg/kg/24 hr q6hr IV), is warranted. Clindamycin is also commonly administered if intestinal perforation occurred or is deemed likely.
   d. Antibiotic therapy should not be delayed if technical problems ensue in obtaining blood culture.

4. Surgical consultation, preferably as soon as concerns regarding NEC as a potential diagnosis are raised.

HEMATOLOGIC DISORDERS

ANEMIA (see Chapter 26)

Normal hematocrit at birth is 45% to 65%.

Etiology

1. Hemorrhage
   a. Prenatal or intrapartum hemorrhage or transfusion (e.g., abruptio placentae or fetomaternal transfusion)
   b. Internal hemorrhage caused by trauma or bleeding dyscrasia

2. Hemolysis
   a. Immune: erythroblastosis fetalis (EBF) caused by Rh, ABO, or minor blood incompatibilities
   b. Nonimmune: relatively uncommon; caused by red blood cell (RBC) membrane defect (e.g., glucose-6-phosphate dehydrogenase [G6PD] deficiency, spherocytosis) or intravascular coagulation

Diagnostic Findings

1. Pallor, tachypnea, weak pulse, hypotension (BP <30 to 40 mm Hg), and tachycardia if hemorrhage is recent and significant (10% blood volume)

2. Hemolysis, usually chronic, often associated with jaundice, hepatosplenomegaly, edema, and other signs of CHF

Ancillary Data

Hematocrit (Hct) and hemoglobin (Hb) concentration low (normal term newborn Hct 45 to 65; Hb, 14 to 21 gm/dl) if chronic blood loss but may still be in normal range if acute. RBC structure may show a significant hemolytic picture. Chronic blood loss or hemolysis is usually accompanied by reticulocytosis. Blood and cerebrospinal fluid (CSF) cultures if symptoms are vague and any suspicion of sepsis is present.

Management

1. Hemorrhagic, hypovolemic shock (see Chapter 5).

2. Without shock but with Hct less than 30%; 10 ml/kg of packed RBC over 1 to 2 hours.

3. If caused by EBF (Rh incompatibility), see p. 108.

4. If immune hemolysis is a result of ABO or minor group incompatibility, follow serial serum bilirubin levels and hematocrits, and maintain adequate hydration. Use phototherapy. Patient may require exchange transfusion.

POLYCYTHEMIA

A venous Hct above 65% may be associated with increased blood viscosity and vascular resistance. An increased incidence is noted in infants with IUGR, in those with Down syndrome or diabetic mothers, or in the recipient of monozygotic twins with twin-to-twin transfusion syndrome. Polycythemia caused by intercurrent dehydration is less common and can be dealt with simply by rehydration.

Etiology

There is an absolute increase in fetal RBC mass with normal blood volume (chronic in utero hypoxemia) or an actual increase in blood volume (cord "milking" or transfusion syndrome).

Diagnostic Findings

Most commonly, symptoms are absent. If pronounced hyperviscosity is present, the infant may have plethora, tachypnea, respiratory distress, hypoglycemia, irritability, jitteriness, or seizures. Less common findings include frank CHF, oliguria, cyanosis, gangrene, or NEC.

Ancillary Data

Peripheral venous Hct above 65%. Capillary Hct is usually 4% to 7% above that in a peripheral or central vein.

Management

Guidelines are controversial because later neurologic outcome appears not to be affected by a decision to perform partial exchange transfusion for neonatal polycythemia. One protocol that has been found useful follows:

1. With Hct 65% to 70%, observation is warranted if the patient is asymptomatic (usually). However, if significant CNS, cardiopulmonary, or renal signs develop, partial exchange transfusion via umbilical vein may be indicated. Because this procedure is less commonly performed than in previous decades, risk of the procedure versus risk of the disease (e.g., minor

symptoms such as mild respiratory distress or irritability) must be considered. Exchange transfusion should use the umbilical venous approach with 0.9% NS solution. Albumin solution (5%) or fresh frozen plasma is an acceptable alternative. The volume (milliliters) to be exchanged is as follows:

$$\frac{\text{Weight (kg)} \times 90 \times (\text{Initial Hct} - \text{Hct desired})}{\text{Initial Hct}}$$

2. With peripheral venous Hct above 70%, partial exchange is often indicated; symptoms (particularly oliguria, respiratory distress, CNS symptoms, hypoglycemia) are more common.
3. Monitor for hypoglycemia and treat if present.
4. NPO status for 6 to 12 hours after exchange transfusion is conservative but reasonable.
5. Watch for hyperbilirubinemia.

THROMBOCYTOPENIA (p. 694)

Thrombocytopenia may be a nonspecific sign of sepsis, anoxia, prematurity, or DIC. Maternal factors include toxemia of pregnancy, collagen vascular disease, idiopathic thrombocytopenic purpura (ITP), and platelet group incompatibilities.

Diagnostic Findings

Findings reflect the underlying cause and potential sequelae of bleeding.

Management

1. Treat the underlying process, including sepsis, hypoxemia, and DIC if present.
2. Administer platelet transfusion: 10 ml/kg/dose over 1 to 2 hours. Half-life of random donor platelets should be 2 to 4 days in peripheral blood.
3. In isoimmune thrombocytopenia, half-life of platelets is greatly reduced if random

donors are used. Treat with maternal platelet concentrates 10 ml/kg over 1 to 2 hours. Consider infusion of IV gamma globulin, 0.4-0.5 gm/kg/24 hr given over 4 to 6 hours IV.

4. Avoid intramuscular injections and other trauma.

DISSEMINATED INTRAVASCULAR COAGULATION (p. 683)

Etiology

Common initiating events (triggers) in the neonate include the following:

1. Maternal factors of acute hemorrhage, amniotic fluid embolism, or dead fetal twin
2. Neonatal factors such as hypoxemia, bacterial or viral sepsis, erythroblastosis, NEC, and severe HMD

Diagnostic Findings

Findings include petechiae, purpura, and evidence of underlying disease. This disorder in the neonate can range from severe to extremely mild in presentation. Results of clotting studies, fibrin degradation products, and hemolysis noted on RBC smear are diagnostic.

Management

1. Treatment of trigger with oxygen, ventilation, antibiotics, etc.
2. Transfusion of fresh frozen plasma, 10 ml/kg over 1 to 2 hours.
3. Blood platelet concentrate infusion if count is less than 30,000/mm^3.
4. Vitamin K, 1 mg IV slowly.
5. If DIC continues, further therapy may be indicated:
   a. If fibrinogen concentration is low (<100 mg/dl) and partial thromboplastin time (PTT) remains very prolonged (>75 to 80 seconds), give cryoprecipitate, 1 bag/3 kg IV.
   b. Two-volume (neonatal blood volume 80 to 90 ml/kg) exchange transfusion with fresh heparinized blood or citrate-phosphate-dextrose (CPD) blood less than 72 hours old via umbilical vein in 5- to 10-ml increments. Alternatively, packed RBCs reconstituted in fresh frozen plasma to an Hct of 50% to 55% is acceptable. For exchange transfusion in neonates, particularly premature neonates, use of cytomegalovirus (CMV) negative, irradiated product is warranted because of risk of graft versus host syndrome.
   c. Consideration of heparin infusion of 100 U/kg/dose every 4 hours IV, although it is rarely required.

UNCONJUGATED HYPERBILIRUBINEMIA (NEWBORN JAUNDICE)

Physiologic jaundice in the term newborn is common, self-limited, and generally without sequelae. However, more severe jaundice in the first week of life may be caused by an occult disease process and may require intervention. "Physiologic" unconjugated hyperbilirubinemia with peak bilirubin concentration below 12 mg/dl occurs by day 3 to 4 in the term neonate (mean concentration = 6-7 mg/dl on day 3). In preterm infants, peak bilirubin concentrations occur later and are more severe if untreated. Severe unconjugated hyperbilirubinemia in babies with erythroblastosis fetalis has been related to kernicterus with irreversible deafness, choreoathetosis, and mental retardation. However, risk factors for kernicterus appear to include not only elevation of bilirubin concentration (probably above 25 mg/dl in the term neonate) but also degree of maturity, intactness of blood-brain barrier (influenced by recent neurologic insult or prematurity), acidosis, hypoxia, hypoalbuminemia, and perinatal depression. However, significant uncertainty remains regarding a direct cause and effect relationship between those factors listed above and the development of kernicterus.

Etiology

The most common disorders associated with nonphysiologic unconjugated (indirect) hyperbilirubinemia in the first week of life are Rh or ABO incompatibility, prematurity, polycythemia, intestinal obstruction, sepsis, and asphyxia. Infants of diabetic mothers are also at high risk. Hypothyroidism must also be considered but is a relatively rare cause of early hyperbilirubinemia. Breast milk jaundice rarely occurs before 10 days of life and usually does not peak above 15 mg/dl. Conjugated (direct) hyperbilirubinemia must be excluded. Beyond the first week of life, consideration must include sepsis, biliary atresia, hepatitis, rubella, galactosemia, and hypothyroidism.

Diagnostic Findings

1. Serial bilirubin determination. Clinically apparent jaundice usually indicates a serum bilirubin concentration below 6 mg/dl.
2. Conjugated bilirubin is usually less than 10% of total bilirubin (maximum normal concentration 2.0-2.5 mg/dl).
3. Blood type and Coombs' test, CBC, and RBC morphology.
4. Hepatomegaly may indicate extramedullary hematopoiesis in response to chronic hemolysis (unconjugated hyperbilirubinemia) or hepatitis (conjugated hyperbilirubinemia).

Management
1. Adequate hydration. Treat sepsis, asphyxia, intestinal obstruction, or erythroblastosis as indicated. In cases of hyperbilirubinemia related to dehydration and inadequate milk intake in the first several days after birth, hydration (oral and IV) plus phototherapy often produces a marked fall in serum bilirubin

concentration within 4 to 6 hours. No current evidence exists that excessive fluid administration in an otherwise normally hydrated infant will alter serum bilirubin concentrations.
2. Treat acidosis because bilirubin precipitates in acid media (CNS).
3. Phototherapy is indicated at given indirect bilirubin levels. See Table 11-1: recommendations for phototherapy:
   a. Term neonate more than 15-18 mg/dl.
   b. Premature neonate more than 7-15 mg/dl, depending on degree of immaturity and associated illness.
   c. In either group, if hemolytic disease is evident and cord blood bilirubin concentration is above 5 mg/dl.
   d. In-home phototherapy, on the basis of preestablished guidelines related to specific risk factors, is now possible but, in general, requires strict criteria for recommendation and follow-up.
4. Exchange transfusion may be indicated on the basis of unconjugated bilirubin levels:
   a. Term neonate above 25 mg/dl. Clinical judgment must still play a major role here, particularly in vigorous babies. Lethargy, hypotonia, poor feeding, etc. are all worrisome findings, even in patients with lower serum bilirubin values.
   b. Premature neonate above 10-15 mg/dl (see Table 11-1).
   c. In either group if significant hemolysis is associated with bilirubin concentration more than 10-12 mg/dl in first 24 hours of life and/or falling Hct.
   d. At present, risk of kernicterus from hyperbilirubinemia in a specific neonate cannot be assessed with accuracy. The guidelines provided should be tempered by risk factors such as prematurity and acidosis. The risk of intervention (specifically, exchange transfusion) must also be considered.

TABLE 11-1   Suggested Phototherapy Guidelines: Premature (<37 wk) and Sick Term Infants

	Serum bilirubin level (mg/dl)						
	Days of age						
Birth weight (gm)	1	2	3	4	5	6	7
<1000	3	3	3	5	5	7	7
1000-1249	5	5	5	7	8	10	12
1250-1499	8	8	8	10	12	12	12
1500-1749	10	10	10	12	12	13	13
1750-1999	10	10	12	13	13	13	13
2000-2499	10	12	12	15	15	15	15
>2500	10	12	13	15	17	17	17

Suggested Treatment Guidelines Term, Well* Newborns (Term ≥37 wk and/or ≥2500 gm)

	Total serum bilirubin level (TSB) (mg/dl)			
Age (hr)	Consider phototherapy	Institute phototherapy	Exchange transfusion if phototherapy fails	Exchange transfusion and phototherapy
≤24	Require further evaluation and treatment			
25-48	≥12	≥15	≥20	≥25
49-72	≥15	≥18	≥25	≥30
≥72	≥17	≥20	≥25	≥30

Modified from AAP Practice Parameter, Provisional Committee on Quality Improvement, October 1994.
*No hemolysis, sepsis, or shock.

5. Late anemia (4 to 6 weeks) is common sequelae of neonatal ABO or Rh incompatibility.

ERYTHROBLASTOSIS FETALIS

Erythroblastosis fetalis (EBF) produced by Rh disease is now relatively unusual because of maternal prophylaxis with Rh immunoglobulin (Rhogam). However, minor blood group incompatibility and Rh disease itself continue to occur with high enough frequency to warrant some discussion.

Etiology

Maternal-fetal antibody passage after maternal sensitization to fetal RBC antigens.

Diagnostic Findings

1. As in unconjugated hyperbilirubinemia, evidence of hemolysis may be indicated by RBC morphology, anemia, or a positive Coombs' test result.
2. Hepatomegaly caused by a long-standing hematopoietic response to anemia.
3. In severe disease, pronounced anemia (cord Hct <30%), edema (hydrops), CHF, pleural effusions, and ascites.

Management

The severely affected neonate who has EBF should be transferred to a tertiary care center as soon as possible. However, certain emergency measures may be required before or during transportation. Much depends on the degree of hemolysis apparent at birth.

Nonhydropic State

1. If cord blood bilirubin is below 5 mg/dl and/or Hct is above 30%, may observe in nursery for increasing serum bilirubin concentration. High reticulocyte count

(>10% to 15%) and hepatomegaly are useful indicators of severe prenatal hemolytic disease. Phototherapy may be justified and probably will not obscure severity of hemolysis (e.g., need for early exchange transfusion). Note that many sensitized fetuses (particularly if several in utero transfusions were received) have clinically insignificant hemolysis.

2. If cord blood bilirubin is above 5 mg/dl and/or Hct is below 30%, administer immediate partial exchange transfusion via umbilical venous catheter. Exchange 20-25 ml/kg of patient's blood with O-negative packed RBCs with an Hct of 70% to 80%. This should be done in the first hour of life, without waiting for type-specific blood, in 5- to 10-ml increments. Follow serial serum bilirubin determinations and Hct. Give phototherapy. Neonatology consultation is indicated because subsequent double-volume exchange transfusion is often performed once the patient is deemed stable to remove sensitized RBCs and to treat severe hyperbilirubinemia.

3. Subsequent exchange transfusions for hyperbilirubinemia may be performed, following the guidelines in the unconjugated hyperbilirubinemia discussion. For exchange transfusions in neonates, particularly premature neonates, use of CMV negative, irradiated product is warranted because of risk of graft versus host reaction. In emergent situations, however, this may not be practical, such as for the immediate partial exchange transfusion procedure recommended above.

4. Late anemia (4 to 6 weeks) is common. Follow-up observation and serial Hct determinations are indicated.

Hydropic State

The hydropic state signifies advanced anemia and CHF.

1. Support airway; patients often require mechanical ventilation.

2. Take chest x-ray film to diagnose pleural effusions (although these may be present,

they are rarely large enough to cause major pulmonary dysfunction).

3. Obtain umbilical venous access and begin partial exchange transfusion, using the guidelines for nonhydropic states for immediate treatment of anemia in those children as noted above.

4. Metabolic acidosis as evidenced by serum bicarbonate concentration of 18-20 mEq/L or less is worrisome and may indicate tissue hypoxia caused by anemia.

5. Neonatology and cardiology consultation is indicated.

INFECTIOUS DISORDERS

CONGENITAL AND PERINATALLY ACQUIRED INFECTIONS

Congenital infectious disorders are commonly associated with TORCHS agents (*Toxoplasma gondii,* other viruses, *r*ubella, *c*ytomegalovirus [CMV], *h*erpes, *s*yphilis). "Other" viruses of increasing importance include human immunodeficiency virus (HIV) and hepatitis B. Overall, such infections may be associated with growth retardation, lethargy, thrombocytopenia, anemia, rash, hepatosplenomegaly, and seizures. Several "classical" congenital infections such as those caused by toxoplasmosis or rubella are now relatively rare (for rubella, in part because of enhanced efforts to screen for antibody during pregnancy). However, the incidences of sexually transmitted diseases that affect the newborn, such as HIV, hepatitis B, and herpes simplex virus (HSV), are on the rise. Acquired immunodeficiency syndrome (AIDS) is of major concern as an agent transmissible to the fetus or newborn. Current evidence suggests that HIV infection can cause both embryopathy and postnatal infection, often of a fatal nature. Predominant modes of transmission include sexual contact (heterosexual and homosexual), skin breakage (e.g., needles), and perinatal transmission. The increase in infection rate in women of childbearing age has been alarming, with concern raised regarding subsequent increases in the rate of maternal to infant transmission. Cord blood and postnatal HIV antibody screening may be helpful, but the legal status of maternal consent for performing such studies is still in question. Routine testing with consent of pregnant women for HIV has been strongly recommended. Diagnosis of neonatal infection may be difficult in the neonatal period because of transplacental passage of maternal antibodies as long as 18 months after birth. Preferred testing of the newborn includes sampling blood for polymerase chain reaction (PCR) evidence of HIV RNA or direct culture for the HIV virus itself.

Because of the proven risk of maternal-infant transmission of hepatitis B virus (HBV) and the current data indicating a link between chronic hepatitis and liver carcinoma, stronger efforts to diagnose this disorder during pregnancy and to eradicate passage to the newborn have been undertaken. Immunization against HBV in infancy is now recommended. Perinatal acquisition of HSV-2 by the neonate is an increasing concern because of rising rates of apparent and unapparent maternal genital infection, as well as high neonatal mortality and morbidity rates associated with neonatal infection. Infection caused by HSV-1 (10% to 15% of neonatal HSV infections) also may occur and is related to contact with infected oral lesions and/or secretions. It is important to identify those children at risk early in life by obtaining an adequate history. The risk of acquisition of neonatal HSV-2 infection is far greater if the mother has primary genital infection and baby is delivered vaginally. Although neonatal HSV infection has occurred after recurrent or inapparent HSV genital infection, the risk is much lower.

Diagnostic Findings

The signs and symptoms indicating a risk of infection warrant a physical and laboratory investigation to detect the etiologic agent. Adjunct examinations may include radiographic (syphilis: periostitis, epiphyseal bands, and/or osteochondritis in long bones; CMV: osteitis in long bones, intracerebral calcifications; rubella:

osteitis in long bones) and ophthalmologic (rubella: cataract; toxoplasmosis, CMV, or rubella: chorioretinitis) findings.

Ancillary Data

1. Toxoplasmosis: Specific IgM and IgG antibody tests are available.
2. Other viruses:
   a. HIV antibody using enzyme immunoassay antigen detection is the most common; PCR or culture also available.
   b. Hepatitis B surface antigen (HBsAg) in serum detects acute or chronic infection; antibody-to-surface antigen (Anti-HBs) detects past infection or response to vaccine.
3. Rubella: Culture (nasopharynx) is diagnostic; rubella-specific IgM or IgG antibody may be helpful.
4. CMV: Urine cultures for CMV is diagnostic. Maternal and newborn convalescent titers (CMV-specific IgM) may also be helpful but should be reserved for situations in which a high likelihood of congenital infection is present.
5. HSV: Direct culture for HSV (e.g., mouth, nasopharynx, vesicle scraping, blood, stool) remains the easiest technique for diagnosis. Other techniques such as direct immunofluorescence antibody staining or PCR are available.
6. Syphilis: The Venereal Disease Research Laboratory (VDRL) and rapid plasmin reagin (RPR) tests remain the "gold standards."

Isolation for most agents listed above appears no longer indicated as long as "universal precautions" are taken. Pregnant hospital staff, however, should be particularly fastidious. Isolation for proven or suspected HSV infection (see below) is recommended, however.

Management

Treatment is usually supportive, supplemented by specific therapy:

1. Congenital toxoplasmosis: pyrimethamine

combined with sulfadiazine has been recommended for symptomatic newborns with proven disease after the risk of neonatal jaundice has passed. Optimal dosage and duration of treatment have not been determined. Treated patients should be given folinic acid supplementation.

2. Other viruses:

   a. HIV: Zidovudine (ZDV) is now routinely given to pregnant HIV-positive women and their newborns. Prenatal ZDV treatment has been shown to decrease the transmission of HIV by 68%. The protocol for neonates born to HIV-positive women recommended by the Centers for Disease Control and Prevention consists of:

   ZDV syrup, 2 mg/kg/dose q6hr PO for 6 weeks, starting 8 to 12 hours after birth. This therapy is also recommended for babies of HIV-positive women who did not receive prenatal ZDV.

   Last, if practical, HIV-positive women should be counseled against breast feeding because of the known risk of transmission of HIV through infected milk.

   b. Hepatitis B: Immunization against HBV in infancy is now recommended. Additional treatment with hepatitis B immunoglobulin (HBIG) is indicated if the mother proves to be antigen positive (see p. 639, Gastrointestinal Disorders). Immune globulins, in general, have no preventive effects for hepatitis C virus (a major cause of non-A, non-B hepatitis).

3. HSV: Although treatment is controversial, the following guidelines may be helpful:

   a. With active maternal genital infection, infant isolation should be used in most instances. Isolation is also recommended for neonates with active HSV disease or with positive cultures in the absence of disease.

   b. A patient in labor with active primary genital lesions of HSV-2 and either intact membranes or those ruptured less than 4 to 6 hours should be delivered by cesarean section. Under these circumstances, most physicians would advocate performing surface cultures on the baby at delivery and observing the infant in the hospital without specific chemotherapy until culture results are available. Some, however, have recommended delay of 24 hours in obtaining cultures if the neonate is asymptomatic. Fetal scalp monitors in patients at risk of acquiring neonatal herpes in labor should be avoided.

   c. If active maternal lesions are present at the time of vaginal delivery in a patient with primary genital herpes (or if the primary-recurrent status is unclear) and the membranes were ruptured for more than 4 to 6 hours before delivery, most would begin acyclovir, 30 mg/kg/24 hr q8hr IV for 10 to 14 days. However, some are now recommending higher dosages between 45 and 60 mg/kg/24 hr, but neither optimum dosage or length of therapy have been established.

   d. Infants born to women with recurrent herpes genital lesions of HSV-2 have a low risk of contracting herpes if the mother is asymptomatic at the time of delivery. Because of the low attack rate for babies whose mothers have recurrent active disease, treatment of the newborn under these circumstances is controversial. Many would advocate observation alone for these neonates after appropriate cultures have been obtained pending the results of the topical cultures.

   e. In the absence of active genital lesions but a positive maternal or paternal history, negative peripartum maternal cervical cultures would allow the guideline described in (b) to be used.

4. Syphilis: Proven or probable congenital syphilis ([a] physical or x-ray evidence of syphilis, [b] serum VDRL or RPR titer more than four times the mother's, [c] positive CSF VDRL or abnormal CSF protein or cell count, [d] positive IgM test, or [e] histologic evidence of treponemes in placenta or cord) should be treated with either (1) aqueous penicillin G, 50,000 U/kg/dose IV, IM q12hr (<7 days of age) or 50,000 U/kg/dose IM, IV q8hr (7 to 28 days of age), in both cases for a course of 10 to 14 days, or (2) aqueous procaine penicillin G, 50,000 U/kg IM QD for 10 to 14 days. Adequate CSF levels are not always achieved with this latter regimen, however. Because accelerated progression to early neurosyphilis has been reported in babies with coexistent HIV infection, HIV testing in patients with congenital syphilis is strongly recommended.

NOTE: Lumbar puncture may be performed to rule out early neurosyphilis (increased CSF protein, pleocytosis, positive CSF VDRL). These findings will not affect the treatment regimen but will necessitate more extensive follow-up observation.

ACQUIRED NEONATAL BACTERIAL SEPSIS

Acquired neonatal bacterial sepsis occurs in 3 to 5 newborns per 1000 live births. Its incidence increases with prematurity, prolonged rupture of membranes (>24 hours), maternal history of recent fever, chorioamnionitis, urinary tract infection (UTI), foul lochia, intrapartum asphyxia, and intravascular catheters in the neonate.

Etiology

Acquired neonatal bacterial sepsis is commonly caused by organisms present in maternal perineal flora, including *Escherichia coli,* group B or D hemolytic streptococci, *Listeria monocytogenes, Haemophilus* sp., and *Staphylococcus aureus.* Nosocomial infection with *Staphylococcus epidermidis* is of increasing concern in premature infants, particularly those given IV fluids via indwelling venous catheters.

Diagnostic Findings

1. Often subtle, they include irritability, vomiting, poor feeding, temperature instability (usually hypothermia), and lethargy. They may progress to more overt (but nonspecific) symptoms, including respiratory distress, apnea, poor peripheral perfusion, abdominal distension, jaundice, and excessive bleeding or bruising.
2. Group B streptococci and *L. monocytogenes* commonly have an early (up to 3 days) form, with sepsis predominating and a late (4 to 14 days) form; the primary presentation is meningitis.

Ancillary Data
1. Severe neutropenia (<2000 PMN/mm^3) or neutrophilia (>16,000 PMN/mm^3), immature band forms, toxic granulations, thrombocytopenia, and coagulopathy may be present. Erythrocyte sedimentation rate (ESR) and C-reactive protein concentrations may be elevated.
2. Cultures of blood, CSF, stool, and urine should be obtained once the diagnosis is suspected.
3. Chest x-ray films should be taken to exclude pneumonia.

Management

1. Treat under the following circumstances:
   a. If there are any of the overt signs discussed previously unless other obvious causes (e.g., jaundice caused by incompatibility) exist.
   b. In the presence of any symptoms noted previously and with an abnormal WBC count, particularly neutropenia.
   c. If the delivery is premature, with any overt symptoms or if risk factors (maternal fever, asphyxia, amnionitis, or foul smell) are present.

d. For babies who are at increased risk of invasive group B streptococcal (GBS) disease, see below.

2. Obtain cultures, particularly of blood and CSF.

  a. Obtain before initiating antibiotics. If venipuncture is unsuccessful, heelstick blood culture (0.2 ml) is acceptable if the skin is properly cleansed with antiseptic (Betadine) and alcohol.

  b. If conditions of hemodynamic instability warrant, lumbar puncture may be delayed 6 to 12 hours; blood cultures should be obtained. However, treatment should not be delayed, nor should prolonged attempts be allowed to compromise the patient's clinical status.

3. Administer antibiotics.

  a. Ampicillin, 100 mg/kg/24 hr q12hr IV or IM; and

  b. Gentamicin, 5 mg/kg/24 hr q12hr IV or IM (if <7 days of age), 7.5 mg/kg/24 hr q8hr IV or IM (if 7 to 28 days of age).

  c. Clindamycin should not be used for neonatal sepsis unless specifically indicated by culture and sensitivity data and then only if serum concentrations can be assessed. The dosage is 15 mg/kg/24 hr q8hr IV.

  d. Specific therapy for resistant organisms should await full culture reports. However, if conditions or suspicions warrant or the patient's condition continues to deteriorate, oxacillin (or equivalent) may be added: 75 mg/kg/24 hr q12hr IV or IM. For penicillin-resistant *Staphylococcus epidermidis* septicemia, give vancomycin, 15 mg/kg/dose q12hr IV. If the infant is older than 7 days, give dose every 8 hours IV.

  e. The decision regarding continuation of antibiotics should be made only after the cultures are 72 hours old. Treat for 7 to 10 days if the blood culture findings are positive or if the patient is clinically precarious or greatly improved on initiating antibiotics, making sepsis likely. The last two situations may be associated with negative blood culture results.

  f. To prevent the potential toxicity of aminoglycosides, cefotaxime may be substituted for gentamicin (b) at a dosage of 100 mg/kg/24 hr q12hr IM or IV. If the infant is older than 7 days, give 150 mg/kg/24 hr q8hr.

  g. Colloid or blood (10 ml/kg over 2 to 3 hours) for shock or decreased peripheral perfusion.

  h. IV gamma globulin (0.75 gm/kg) has been advocated by some, but its efficacy remains clinically in question.

  i. Granulocyte transfusions (irradiated) for sepsis-induced severe neutropenia (particularly group B β-hemolytic streptococcus) with prolonged absolute neutrophil counts below 1500/mm^3 may be efficacious if available. They are most often indicated if no clinical improvement or resolution of neutropenia has occurred after 4 to 6 hours of therapy.

Group B Streptococcal (GBS) Disease Strategies

GBS invasive disease in the newborn remains a significant cause of morbidity and mortality. The organism is relatively ubiquitous and the colonization rate in pregnant women may be as high as 10% to 30%. Specific strategies (ACOG and AAP) have been suggested to deal with treatment of this deadly disease and are summarized below.

For the mother:

It is recommended that women at risk receive intrapartum penicillin prophylaxis (1) if they have had a previous baby with invasive GBS disease, (2) if they have had GBS bacteriuria with the current pregnancy, or (3) if delivery of a baby less than 37 weeks' gestation is likely. Without these three criteria, one recommendation is to screen all pregnant women at 35 to 37 weeks' gestation (rectal or vaginal culture) and offer intrapartum penicillin prophylaxis if positive.

If culture results are unavailable or have not been obtained, it is recommended to give intrapartum penicillin prophylaxis if (1) mother is febrile, (2) likely to deliver a baby less than 37 weeks' gestational age, or (2) rupture of membranes occurred 18 hours or more before delivery.

For the delivered newborn:

If the mother received intrapartum penicillin prophylaxis for GBS, a joint recommendation of ACOG and AAP has been the following:

1. For asymptomatic newborns less than 35 weeks' gestation, a limited diagnostic evaluation consisting of CBC and blood culture is indicated. Such infants should then be observed for at least 48 hours, but no specific antibiotic treatment is necessary.
2. For asymptomatic newborns 35 weeks' gestation or more, the duration of maternal prophylaxis determines the course of action.
   a. If two or more doses of antibiotics given before delivery, observation for at least 48 hours is recommended, but no specific antibiotic treatment is necessary.
   b. If a single dose of antibiotics given before delivery, a limited diagnostic evaluation consisting of CBC and blood culture is indicated. Observation as in (1) is then indicated.
   c. Symptomatic newborns should be treated as in the guidelines listed above for newborn sepsis in general.

BACTERIAL MENINGITIS (p. 725)

The most common organism is the group B streptococcus *(S. agalactiae).* Less commonly, *E. coli,* group D streptococcus, *Haemophilus* sp., and *Klebsiella* organisms are noted. A high rate of significant neurologic sequelae and mortality (20% to 40%) makes early diagnosis of paramount importance.

INTOXICATION

NEONATAL NARCOTIC ABSTINENCE

The neonatal narcotic abstinence symptom complex is caused by withdrawal from passive addiction to maternal use of narcotics such as heroin, morphine, codeine, or methadone.

Diagnostic Findings

Symptoms are voracious appetite, vomiting, sneezing, hypertonicity, diarrhea, jitteriness, and irritability. Seizures are uncommon. Symptoms usually begin within 48 hours of delivery. Later manifestations (2 to 3 weeks) may occur in some patients, particularly with methadone withdrawal.

Cocaine use in pregnancy appears to be associated with an increased incidence of fetal loss and neonatal depression but not with classic symptoms of withdrawal, although irritability and tremulousness may be prominent.

Management

1. Oral morphine is now commonly used to treat symptomatic opiate withdrawal in the newborn. In general, opiates are preferred over other agents (see below) if irritability is accompanied by GI symptoms such as diarrhea or vomiting. Morphine dosage is 0.08 mg/kg/dose PO q3-4hr. May increase by 0.02 mg/kg/dose with maximum of 0.2 mg/kg/dose. Tincture of opium has been used previously, but the solution is not well standardized and may no longer be available in many hospital pharmacies. (Dose: tincture of opium = 2 mg/5 ml or 0.4 mg morphine/ml. Give 0.2-0.3 ml/dose q3-4hr PO. Maximum dosage 1 to 2 ml/kg/24 hr.)
2. Other agents occasionally used include chlorpromazine (Thorazine), 0.5 mg/kg/

dose q6-8hr IV, IM, or PO; or phenobarbital, 5 mg/kg/24 hr q8-12hr IV, IM, or PO.

3. Treat for 1 to 3 weeks while gradually tapering dosage.

4. Monitor for apnea and bradycardia until the patient's condition is stable.

5. Testing for VDRL, hepatitis B antigen, and HIV may be warranted.

6. As noted in Chapter 10, use of naloxone is contraindicated in babies exposed in utero to opiates because it may induce convulsions.

NEUROLOGIC DISORDERS

SEIZURES (p. 738)

Etiology

1. Seizures result from widely divergent CNS insults. Time of appearance after birth and history of pregnancy, delivery, drugs, and nutrition may be helpful in determining cause.

2. Intrapartum complications: symptoms apparent at less than 24 hours of age.
   a. Hypoxia and cerebral ischemia during labor. Increased incidence in IUGR, large-for-gestational-age infants, multifetal gestations, and premature infants and after prolonged labor.
   b. Hemorrhage. Subarachnoid and subdural hemorrhages are more common in term infants with breech extraction, forceps, or asphyxia. Intraventricular or intracerebral bleeding occurs in premature infants less than 34 weeks' gestation, with increased risk if asphyxia or respiratory distress is present. In term infants with intracerebral or intraventricular hemorrhage, arteriovenous malformation should be considered.

3. Infection
   a. Bacterial meningitis (group B streptococci [S. agalactiae] and E. coli are most common), accounting for two thirds of cases. Increased incidence with prolonged rupture of membranes (PROM), chorioamnionitis, and maternal UTI.
   b. Viral and other infections: seizures caused by congenital herpes, CMV, and toxoplasmosis infection usually appear shortly after birth. Echovirus and coxsackievirus B are seasonal and rarely seen in the first few days of life.

4. Metabolic
   a. Hypoglycemia (see Chapter 38). Blood glucose concentration less than 30 mg/dl. Increased risk in first postnatal day associated with growth retardation, prematurity, postdate delivery, infant of diabetic mother, and polycythemia.
   b. Hypocalcemia (<7 mg/dl). Peak incidence at less than 3 days related to prematurity or neonatal asphyxia or from 4 to 10 days because of elevated intake of phosphorus, dehydration, or renal failure.
   c. Hyponatremia or hypernatremia, amino or organic acid abnormalities, severe hyperbilirubinemia, and pyridoxine dependency are all rare causes of neonatal seizures.

5. Drug abuse in the mother, including cocaine and amphetamines.

Diagnostic Findings

1. Subtle evidence of seizures, including eye deviation, drooling, repetitive movements of mouth, and writhing movements of hips and shoulders, are more common than classic tonic-clonic seizures seen in older patients.

2. Focal seizures are most commonly found during infections such as herpes; generalized disturbances are caused by asphyxia and metabolic problems.

3. Color change (flushing, cyanosis), bradycardia, and apnea or hypoventilation may

accompany motor manifestations but are rarely found alone.

4. There may be associated asphyxia, hemorrhage, or infection, with bulging fontanelle, lethargy, pallor, or apnea.

Ancillary Data

1. Serum glucose and calcium concentrations and lumbar puncture (cell count, protein and glucose concentrations, culture, and Gram stain). Urine toxicology screen may be indicated.

2. Ultrasound (if <34 weeks or if unstable) to rule out intracerebral/intraventricular hemorrhage or midline shift. If more than 34 weeks and stable, computed tomographic (CT) scanning is preferred. MRI (with or without flow studies) may better help identify arteriovenous malformation but is usually not indicated as an initial step in seizure evaluation.

3. Electroencephalogram (EEG) may be useful if appropriate staff is available to interpret newborn study results.

Management (see Chapter 21 and p. 743)

1. Anticonvulsant alternatives
   a. Phenobarbital is the drug of choice. Loading dose: 15 mg/kg IV; maintenance: 5 mg/kg/24 hr q12hr PO or IV. Follow blood levels; 10-25 µg/ml is adequate.
   b. Phenytoin (Dilantin) is a useful adjunct to phenobarbital in the asphyxiated newborn who continues to have seizures. Poorly absorbed enterally by the newborn. Loading dose: 15 mg/kg IV; maintenance: 5 mg/kg/24 hr q12hr IV. Follow blood levels; maintain at 10-20 µg/ml.
   c. Lorazepam (Ativan), 0.01-0.04 mg/kg/dose q6-8hr IV, for acute control.

2. Supportive care, including maintenance of IV fluids, oxygen, incubator, and monitoring of electrolyte, glucose, and calcium levels

3. Metabolic abnormalities (hypoglycemia, hypocalcemia) require immediate correction

4. Consultation with neurologist for ongoing seizures

5. Serial head circumferences and ultrasound to exclude posthemorrhagic or postinfectious hydrocephalus

6. Long-term follow-up observation essential; many children require maintenance anticonvulsants and supervision to monitor for potential developmental delays

MYELOMENINGOCELE

Myelomeningocele occurs in 1:500 live births. The posterior neuropore fails to close, leaving a spinal defect containing both neural and meningeal components. Distal limb and sphincter disturbances reflect the level of defect. Associated disorders include hydrocephalus, Arnold-Chiari malformation, and talipes equinovarus.

Diagnostic Findings

A posterior midline deficit (with or without dural or epidermal covering) reflects the level of the vertebral defect. May have enlarged head circumference or full fontanelle. Sacral dimple alone (unless draining or infected) is usually benign.

Management

1. Keep patient prone.
2. Cover defect with sterile saline-solution-soaked gauze pads, and wrap lower trunk in plastic to prevent drying.
3. Consult neurosurgeon. Although some controversy still clouds the issues of survival and quality of life (if associated hydrocephalus or other major malformations exist), supportive care and early closure of defects are recommended in most cases.
4. Other manifestations of neurologic defi-

cit (e.g., neurogenic bladder or vocal cord paralysis) should be watched for closely.

PULMONARY DISORDERS

APNEA (see Chapter 13)

Apnea is cessation of respiratory activity for more than 15 to 20 seconds. It is often associated with cyanosis and bradycardia (<100/min).

Etiology

1. Central: apnea of prematurity, particularly less than 34 weeks or with a history of maternal narcotic or magnesium ingestion before delivery.
2. Metabolic: hypoglycemia, hypothermia.
3. Infection: sepsis, pneumonia, meningitis.
4. CNS damage: hemorrhage, hypoxic injury, seizures.
5. Pulmonary: respiratory distress caused by hyaline membrane disease, pneumonia, airway obstruction.
6. Obstructive: usually related to occult gastroesophageal reflux. More commonly seen in larger preterm or term infants, in those with preexisting CNS damage, or in those with chronic lung disease.

Diagnostic Findings

Examination is indicated for rales, rhonchi, stridor, quality of air exchange, neurologic status, anterior fontanelle tension, temperature, and gestational age.
Ancillary Data
Included may be chest x-ray films, pulse oximeter saturation, ABG measurements, blood glucose concentration, WBC count with differential, and as indicated, lumbar puncture and blood culture. Barium swallow or esophageal pH probe may be necessary to diagnose occult reflux as the cause if symptoms are severe and no other cause is identified.

Management

1. Resuscitation, support, treatment for underlying disease, and ongoing cardiac and apnea monitoring.
2. Apnea of prematurity: a diagnosis based on exclusion of other causes. All patients with this disorder, if significant, require inpatient cardiac and apnea monitoring.
   a. Mild spells: require gentle stimulation and 22% to 23% oxygen. Rocking water beds are recommended by some clinicians but are of indeterminate value.
   b. Frequent or severe spells: may require ventilation or continuous positive airway pressure (CPAP) applied using a nasal CPAP device, without ET tube placement. Pharmacologic approaches include theophylline (loading dosage of 5 mg/kg/dose IV followed by 1-2 mg/kg/dose q8hr IV or PO for 2 to 3 weeks, maintaining a plasma drug level of 5-10 µg/ml) or caffeine sodium citrate (10 mg/kg IM initially followed by maintenance of 2.5 mg/kg/24 hr q24hr PO, achieving plasma level of 8-16 µg/ml).
3. Neonatal and pulmonary consultation.
4. Proven or suspected reflux may be dealt with as follows:
   a. Thickening feedings with rice cereal
   b. Smaller, more frequent feeding schedule
   c. Bed or crib elevation, prone positioning, upright positioning ("Danny" sling)
   d. Metoclopramide, 0.1 mg/kg/dose QID IV or PO (maximum dosage: 0.5 mg/kg/24 hr)

RESPIRATORY DISTRESS SYNDROME (OR HYALINE MEMBRANE DISEASE)

Risk of respiratory distress syndrome (RDS, HMD) increases in premature infants (<36 weeks' gestation), particularly males, infants of diabetic mothers, and infants with intrapartum asphyxia.

Etiology

This respiratory disorder is caused by developmental deficiency of surfactant (surface active lecithins) with subsequent generalized microatelectasis and pulmonary edema.

Diagnostic Findings

Tachypnea (respiratory rate >50 to 60/min), cyanosis in room air, dyspnea with xiphisternal and intercostal retractions, expiratory grunting, and flaring of alae nasi. Auscultation may reveal decreased air entry and fine rales within 2 to 4 hours after delivery. Peak of disease occurs at 36 to 48 hours of age.

Ancillary Data

1. Chest x-ray films: diffuse fine reticulogranular infiltrates, often with significant air bronchogram findings; may have loss of volume bilaterally
2. CBC, blood cultures to exclude sepsis; serial ABG

Management

1. Administer oxygen by hood with ongoing monitoring of arterial pulse oximetry, ABG. Umbilical artery catheter is recommended if Pao_2 is less than 50 mm Hg in 40% to 50% O_2. CPAP may be administered by nasal prongs or by nasal or ET tubes. Normally, CPAP is begun at 4 to 6 cm H_2O. Ventilator support may be needed if unable to maintain Pao_2 above 50 mm Hg (oximeter saturation 90% to 95%) or if $Paco_2$ is more than 55 to 60 mm Hg. Ventilator support (or ventilation using a resuscitation bag attached to ET tube if mechanical ventilator unavailable) should also be considered on purely clinical grounds if severe respiratory distress and cyanosis are present and blood gas analyses either cannot be obtained or are unavailable.
2. Increase ambient temperature (incubator or other device) to achieve core temperature of 37° C.
3. With significant distress, keep patient NPO, and begin D10W at 80-90 ml/kg/24 hr IV. Salt usually is not needed during the first 24 hours because of a postnatal physiologic contraction of the extracellular fluid compartment. Withhold potassium supplementation until urine output is well established and patient more than 24 hours old.
4. Consult neonatal specialists, with consideration of transfer to tertiary care nursery.
5. Studies have demonstrated the efficacy of surfactant administration via ET tube in the first 24 to 48 hours of postnatal life. Both an artificial surfactant and calf lung extract are approved for use (FDA). Great caution should be used during administration of surfactant because of rapid changes that occur in neonatal lung compliance. In general, surfactant should be administered in an intensive care setting by professionals experienced in its use. Dose: 4-5 ml/kg by ET tube.

MECONIUM ASPIRATION SYNDROME
(see Chapter 10)

Prenatal aspiration of meconium-stained amniotic fluid below the glottis causes meconium aspiration syndrome (MAS). After delivery, meconium progresses into bronchi and distally, with postnatal respiratory activity. Meconium causes intense tissue reaction and chemical pneumonitis, as well as mechanical obstruction.

Diagnostic Findings

Early asphyxial syndrome (low Apgar score, apnea, flaccidity), meconium staining of the skin, umbilicus, and nails, with presence of meconium at level of vocal cords. Respiratory distress is often present within 1 to 2 hours of birth, with peak of severity at 24 to 48 hours. Dyspnea is present with retractions, tachypnea, and cyanosis in room air. Coarse rales and rhonchi, with alternating areas of decreased air entry, are auscultated.

Complications

Pneumothorax and pneumomediastinum occur in 15% to 30% of cases.

Ancillary Data

1. X-ray films: patchy asymmetric infiltrates, often perihilar in nature, with greater involvement of right middle and lower lobes. Hyperinflation evident on lateral views.
2. CBC and glucose and electrolyte concentrations: usually normal. Blood cultures to exclude sepsis.

Management

1. For delivery room management of the newborn with meconium-stained amniotic fluid, see Chapter 10.
2. After delivery room resuscitation, if respiratory symptoms develop, treat as with RDS. Give humidified oxygen by hood, keeping pulse oximeter saturations above 95%. Affected infants are usually near or at term, so risk of hyperoxemic retinal damage (retinopathy of prematurity) is nil. Because serial blood gas determinations are useful, umbilical artery catheterization or transcutaneous Po_2/Pco_2 monitors are helpful adjuncts in management. As in RDS, patients with significant respiratory distress should be kept NPO and placed on D10W at 80-90 ml/kg/24 hr. Monitor glucose concentration.
3. Neonatology consultation is advisable, with probable transfer to the tertiary center if a patient has any of the following characteristics:
   a. More than 40% O_2 required to maintain Pao_2 above 50 mm Hg.

   b. Severe respiratory distress in the first 24 hours of life.
   c. $Paco_2$ above 50 mm Hg (exclude pneumothorax). Intubation may be required.
   d. Recurrent apnea.
   e. Evidence of pneumothorax or pneumomediastinum.
4. Patients with meconium aspiration pneumonia often have pulmonary hypertension (PPHN, see above). Pulmonary vasodilation may be achieved through hyperoxia, alkalinization (sodium bicarbonate 2-4 mEq/kg IV over 2 to 4 hours), and sedation. Pressor support may also be of assistance (dopamine and/or dobutamine).
5. Surfactant administration via ET tube has been found efficacious in selected patients. As noted for RDS, surfactant should be administered in an intensive care setting by professionals experienced in its use.

BACTERIAL PNEUMONIA (p. 794)

Bacterial pneumonia is generally associated with prematurity and in infants with prolonged rupture of membranes (>24 hours) or other signs of chorioamnionitis.

Etiology

Infection is caused most commonly by β-hemolytic streptococci (particularly group B), *S. aureus* or *E. coli,* and other gram-negative organisms.

Diagnostic Findings

Comparable to HMD, tachypnea, expiratory grunting, and sternal retractions. Fine rales and asymmetrically decreased breath sounds often are noted. Peripheral vasoconstriction with decreased pulses and hypothermia may suggest vascular collapse and sepsis. Cyanosis and vascular instability are often disproportionately great in relationship to the degree of respiratory distress.

Ancillary Data

1. X-ray films: asymmetric patchy infiltrates often unilateral; a minority of patients will show pleural effusion. X-ray studies of infants with group B β-hemolytic streptococcal pneumonia may mimic findings noted with HMD.
2. WBC may be increased or greatly decreased with a shift to the left and decreased platelets. Serial ABG determinations may show hypoxemia and metabolic acidosis. Polymorphonuclear leukocytes and bacteria may be noted in tracheal effluent and gastric aspirate if obtained within 6 hours of delivery. Cultures of blood, spinal fluid, and urine should be obtained.
3. Gram stain of tracheal secretions in the newborn may demonstrate bacteria that are associated with congenital pneumonia.

Management

1. Oxygen, support of ventilation, and serial ABG as outlined for HMD. Umbilical artery catheter may be useful.
2. Antibiotics. Administer after appropriate specimens (blood, CSF, and urine) are obtained for culture:
   a. Ampicillin, 100 mg/kg/24 hr q12hr IV, *and* if culture is positive for group B streptococcus, may change to penicillin G, 100,000 U/kg/24 hr q12hr IV.
   b. Gentamicin, 5.0-7.5 mg/kg/24 hr q12hr IM or IV. Cefotaxime may be substituted for gentamicin at a dosage of 100 mg/kg/24 hr q12hr IM or IV. If the infant is older than 7 days, give cefotaxime, 150 mg/kg/24 hr q8hr.
   c. If *S. aureus* is a concern, add oxacillin, 75 mg/kg/24 hr q12hr IV.
3. Neonatology consultation, particularly in presence of severe respiratory distress or vascular instability, is suggested. Treatment with exchange transfusion or granulocyte transfusion is advocated by some physicians.

TRANSIENT TACHYPNEA OF THE NEWBORN

Transient tachypnea of the newborn (TTN) is also called amniotic fluid aspiration syndrome, "drowned newborn syndrome," neonatal wet lung, and a variety of other terms that reflect the lack of knowledge of the causes. The symptoms of TTN likely are due to excessive pulmonary fluid, both intravascular and extravascular. TTN is usually a self-limited disorder of term or near-term infants and is often evident 2 to 4 hours postnatally. It is somewhat more common after cesarean section or heavy maternal narcotic administration. A severe variant with associated pulmonary hypertension is seen in less than 10% of cases.

Diagnostic Findings

Tachypnea with a respiratory rate often at 80 to 100/min. Dyspnea is common but less prominent than in MAS or RDS. There are mild to moderate sternal retractions with coarse rales and rhonchi; increased AP diameter of the chest is possible. Maximum severity of distress occurs within 24 to 48 hours with gradual resolution thereafter.

Ancillary Data

1. X-ray films: nonspecific increase in perihilar markings with fluid in the right minor fissure. Mild to moderate hyperinflation on lateral views.
2. CBC, gastric aspirate, and blood cultures to exclude sepsis. Serial pulse oximeter saturation and ABG determinations to adjust oxygen delivery. Umbilical arterial catheterization is usually unnecessary.

Management

1. Administer oxygen by hood with Fio_2 adjustment based on serial blood gas

determinations. Rarely requires more than 40% O_2 to maintain oximeter saturation 90% to 95%.

2. If respiratory rate is above 60/min, keep NPO and give D10W, 80-90 ml/kg/24 hr IV.

3. Consider consultation if:
   a. There is respiratory distress with Pao_2 less than 50 mm Hg in 40% O_2 or $Paco_2$ more than 50 mm Hg.
   b. Apnea or increasing distress develops.

PNEUMOTHORAX

Pneumothorax usually is associated with sudden deterioration of the patient with preexisting respiratory distress, particularly MAS or RDS. "Spontaneous" pneumothorax may be present at birth.

Diagnostic Findings

Severe respiratory distress with deterioration and cyanosis. Tamponade and vascular collapse if under tension. Decreased breath sounds on the affected side. If on the left, the heart sounds may be heard in the right side of the chest.

Ancillary Data

1. X-ray films: AP and lateral decubitus views are best for diagnosis. Clear shadow lateral to lung field with no lung markings present. Shift in carina from midline or depression of ipsilateral hemidiaphragm suggests tension pneumothorax. In pneumomediastinum (not life threatening and rarely requiring therapy), the air is noted lateral to the heart borders, with lung markings seen peripherally.

2. Asymmetric fiberoptic transillumination.

Management

1. If distress is not severe and there is no evidence of tension pneumothorax, increase ambient oxygen to 40% to 70% and monitor x-ray films and ABG. This may be effective if the pneumothorax is small (<10% to 20%) and little underlying lung disease is present.

2. If large or tension pneumothorax is present, temporize by inserting a 14- or 16-gauge intravenous cannula (over-the-needle type) at the anterior axillary line, at the fourth to fifth interspace, with the tip angled anteromedially. Take care to introduce the needle only far enough to enter the pleural space. Remove needle and advance the cannula 1 cm. Attach the cannula to IV extension tubing; connect to three-way stopcock and a 30-ml syringe. Tape in place and evacuate as needed until the chest tube is inserted, preferably by a person experienced in newborn care. Attach the chest tube, once in place, to a neonatal water seal and suction device (see Appendix A-9).

3. Transilluminate and repeat chest x-ray film to ensure adequate air evacuation.

4. Obtain neonatal or surgical consultation.

RENAL AND GENITOURINARY DISORDERS

ACUTE RENAL FAILURE (p. 809)

Most neonates (95%) void before 36 hours of age. Failure to void should initiate a diagnostic evaluation, particularly if certain risk factors are present, including hypotension, sepsis, polycythemia, dehydration, or intrapartum asphyxia.

OBSTRUCTIVE UROPATHY

Obstructive uropathy must be considered if there is an early history of oliguria with maternal history of oligohydramnios or abnormal in utero ultrasound and the presence of abdominal mass or spontaneous pneumothorax.

Etiology

1. Ureteropelvic or ureterovesicle obstruction, megaloureter (Hirschsprung's disease, prune belly syndrome), or urethral

obstruction. In males, consider posterior urethral valves.

2. Neurogenic bladder resulting from my-elomeningocele or severe CNS insult.

Diagnostic Findings

1. Unilateral or bilateral flank mass, often cystic in nature. Palpable bladder may indicate urethral obstruction or neurogenic bladder. Poor feeding and emesis are common.
2. Ultrasonography may be diagnostic.

Management

1. Gentle bladder catheterization with 3.5- to 5-Fr feeding tube
2. Urologic consultation

AMBIGUOUS GENITALIA ("INTERSEX")

Many of these patients are identified at birth. More minor degrees such as hypospadias would not generally qualify as a disorder requiring emergency management. However, more serious anomalies of the genital area should be addressed by qualified professionals, such as urologists, pediatric surgeons, geneticists, pediatricians, and neonatologists, often working in a team approach to care. Virilization of a genotypic female (congenital adrenal hyperplasia, maternal androgens) or incomplete virilization of a genotypic male (partial or complete hypopituitarism, septooptic dysplasia) are examples of ambiguous genitalia disorders that carry a high risk of early metabolic consequences, such as adrenal failure. These disorders should be considered in any patient with a potential intersex anomaly. Qualified medical professionals, as listed above, should be consulted immediately. In addition, although difficult because of parental concerns and anxiety,

the assignment of male or female sex should be deferred until definitive diagnostic testing can be accomplished.

REFERENCES

AIDS Clinical Trials Group Protocol (Centers for Disease Control and Prevention): Recommendations for the use of zidovudine to reduce perinatal transmission of human immunodeficiency virus, *MMWR* 43(RR-11):1-11, 1994.

American Academy of Pediatric Committee on Infectious Diseases and Committee on Fetus and Newborn: Revised guidelines for prevention of early-onset group B streptococcal infection, *Pediatrics* 99:489, 1997.

American Academy of Pediatrics Provisional Committee for Quality Improvement, Subcommittee on Hyperbilirubinemia: Practice parameter: management of hyperbilirubinemia in the healthy term newborn, *Pediatrics* 94:558-565, 1994.

American Heart Association: Guidelines for cardiopulmonary resuscitation and emergency cardiac care, *JAMA* 268:2276, 1992.

American Heart Association and American Academy of Pediatrics: *Textbook of neonatal resuscitation,* Dallas, 1994, American Heart Association.

Bratlid D: Criteria for treatment of neonatal jaundice, *J Perinatol* 16:S83-S88, 1996.

Burton BK: Inborn errors of metabolism: the clinical diagnosis in early infancy, *Pediatrics* 79:359, 1987.

Committee on Infectious Diseases, American Academy of Pediatrics: *Report on the Committee on Infectious Diseases,* ed 24, Elk Grove, Ill, 1997, The Academy.

Committee on Infectious Diseases: Universal hepatitis B immunization, *Pediatrics* 89:795, 1992.

Guidelines for perinatal care, ed 4, Evanston, Ill, 1997, American Academy of Pediatrics and American College of Obstetrics and Gynecology.

Manroe BL, Weinberg AG, Rosenfeld CR, et al: The neonatal blood count in health and disease. I. Reference values for neutrophilic cells, *J Pediatr* 95:89, 1979.

Meropol SB, Lubert A, DeJong AR, et al: Home phototherapy: use and attitudes among community pediatricians, *Pediatrics* 91:97, 1993.

Prevention of perinatal Group B streptococcal disease: a public health perspective, *MMWR* 45(RR-7):1-24, 1996.

Wisnell TE, Baumgart S, Gannon CM, et al: No lumbar puncture in the evaluation for early neonatal sepsis: will meningitis be missed? *Pediatrics* 95:803, 1995.

Wisnell TE, Tuggle JM, Turner BS: Meconium aspiration syndrome: have we made a difference? *Pediatrics* 85:715, 1990.

V
EMERGENT COMPLAINTS

12 ANAPHYLAXIS

ALERT: Acute respiratory distress caused by upper airway obstruction or lower airway bronchospasm requires prompt intervention.

Anaphylaxis is a multisystem allergic reaction elicited in a hypersensitive subject on reexposure to a sensitizing antigen. The syndrome is caused by antibodies, usually immunoglobulin E (IgE), which release chemical mediators, including histamine, leukotrienes, and other vasoactive substances.

ETIOLOGY

Antigens that produce a systemic reaction may be ingested, inhaled, or administered by injection. Although parenteral exposures have the highest risk, anaphylaxis may occur with oral ingestion.

Common agents responsible for anaphylaxis include the following:

1. Antigen extracts used for desensitization of skin testing
2. Antibiotics, particularly penicillin
3. Insect stings, including Hymenoptera order (bee, wasp, yellow jacket, hornet, certain ants) (p. 306)
4. Foods, ranging from shellfish to nuts, eggs, milk, and legumes
5. Insulin and adrenocorticotropic hormone (ACTH)
6. Biologic agents, including foreign serum (usually horse), gamma globulin, and vaccines
7. Latex, especially in health care workers and children with spina bifida or urogenital anomalies
8. Inhaled allergens such as dust, animal danders, and pollens
9. Diagnostic agents (e.g., radiologic contrast media); low osmolarity contrast media reduce the risk
10. Local anesthetics
11. Aspirin
12. Narcotics such as morphine or codeine

NOTE: Agents 9 to 12 are not IgE mediated and are called *anaphylactoid*.

DIAGNOSTIC FINDINGS

A wide range of reaction to antigenic exposures, from mild distress, with a sense of anxiety, to true anaphylaxis, with respiratory distress and cardiovascular collapse exists. Patients often note a sense of "impending doom."

There may be upper and lower airway involvement of the respiratory tract. Patients may have rhinorrhea and initial sneezing that does not progress. Patients with significant distress have dyspnea, tachypnea with retractions, respiratory compromise, and cyanosis.

1. Upper airway problems may cause stridor, laryngeal and epiglottic edema, and obstruction.
2. Lower airway bronchospasm may cause coughing, wheezing, and marked distress.

Circulatory collapse may develop. Patients have mild hypotension or true vascular collapse and shock.

1. Initially, chest pain may be noted, sometimes secondary to myocardial ischemia.
2. Dysrhythmias and syncope are common.

Other Diagnostic Features

1. Urticaria, pruritus, and erythema are observed.
2. Nausea, vomiting, abdominal cramping, and diarrhea may occur.

Complications

The major life-threatening complications include the following:
1. Upper airway obstruction
2. Bronchospasm
3. Dysrhythmias and cardiac ischemia
4. Circulatory collapse and shock

Ancillary Data

1. Arterial blood gas (ABG) determinations for all patients with moderate or severe respiratory distress. Oximetry on all patients.

Severity of airway obstruction	Pao_2	$Paco_2$	pH
Mild	WNL	↑↑	↓
Moderate	↓↓	WNL/↓	WNL/↑
Severe	↑↑↑	↑	↓↓

2. Electrocardiogram (ECG) to assess for dysrhythmias, conduction abnormalities, and ischemic changes

DIFFERENTIAL DIAGNOSIS

The differential diagnosis is usually distinctly established by the clear temporal relationship of exposure to an antigenic agent. Special diagnostic considerations include the following:
1. Asthma
2. Infection—septic shock (see Chapter 5)
3. Vasovagal reaction
4. Procaine reaction from inadvertent intravascular injection of penicillin (may cause confusion, syncope, or seizures)

MANAGEMENT

The management of the patient must reflect the severity of the illness and focus on stabilization.
1. Those with *mild* disease and no evidence of respiratory distress or cardiovascular compromise may be easily treated with antihistamines (diphenhydramine [Benadryl], 5 mg/kg/24 hr q4-6hr PO), and epinephrine subcutaneously if indicated.
2. Patients with *moderate* or *severe* distress present a potentially life-threatening emergency and require immediate stabilization and intervention (see Chapter 4).
3. Attention must be directed to the airway and ventilation (assisted ventilation is rarely needed):
   a. Oxygen administered at 3-6 L/min by mask or cannula
   b. Intubation if there is airway obstruction or respiratory failure
   c. With significant bronchospasm, administration of bronchodilators:
      (1) *Epinephrine.* Administer 0.01 ml/kg subcutaneously (maximum 0.35 ml) of 1:1000 dilution. With absent or partial response, repeat twice at 20-minute intervals. Do not give until heart rate is 180 beats/min or less.
         (a) If the patient is in shock, epinephrine should be administered IV. With severe disease, many prefer administration by continuous infusion: start in child with 0.1 µg/kg/min, titrating response with increasing dosage up to 1.5 µg/kg/min to maintain pressure (prepare by adding 1.0 mg or 1.0 ml of 1:1000 solution to 250 ml D5W to make concentration

of 4 μg/ml). In an adult, administer bolus with 0.1 mg (0.1 ml of 1:1000 solution mixed in 10 ml D5W to make dilution of 1:100,000), followed by infusion of 1 μg/min increased to 4 μg/min if needed (prepared by adding 1 mg or 1 ml of 1:1000 epinephrine to 250 ml D5W to make a solution of 4 μg/ml). The risk of dysrhythmias increases when infused at a rate greater than 5 μg/kg/min.

NOTE: 0.1 ml of 1:1000 solution contains 100 μg, whereas 0.1 ml of 1:10,000 solution contains 10 μg.

(b) Epinephrine may also be injected directly into the site of administration of the offending agent, if appropriate, in cases of insect or allergen injections. After a tourniquet is applied (in case of parenteral drugs), inject 0.05 to 0.2 ml of 1:1000 solution.

(2) Albuterol can be given by inhalation (p. 769) as a supplement to epinephrine.

4. Antihistamines may be helpful. Administer diphenhydramine (Benadryl) at a dosage of 2 mg/kg/dose IV, IM, or PO followed by repeat administration every 4 to 6 hours to treat urticaria, itching, and angioedema.

5. Histamine (H_2) blockers have been found useful in cases of refractory anaphylaxis
   a. Mild: give Cimetidine, 5-10 mg/kg/dose PO (adult: 300 mg/dose), or ranitidine, 1-2 mg/kg/dose PO (adult: 150 mg/dose).
   b. Moderate (angioedema, decreased blood pressure): give Cimetidine, 5-10 mg/kg/dose IM or IV q6hr (adult: 300

mg/dose), or ranitidine, 0.5-1.0 mg/kg/dose q8hr IV (adult: 50 mg).

6. Steroids are usually indicated, although their benefit is delayed: hydrocortisone (SoluCortef), 4-5 mg/kg/dose q6hr IV.

7. For hypotension, several maneuvers are indicated.
   a. Keep the patient with legs raised in Trendelenburg position.
   b. Initiate appropriate fluids, initially infusing 20 ml/kg IV of 0.9% normal saline (NS) or lactated Ringer's (LR) solution over 10 to 20 minutes. May repeat infusion.
   c. If hypotension continues, initiate dopamine, to be administered as a continuous IV infusion at a rate of 5-20 μg/kg/min.

8. A tourniquet proximal to the site of injection of antibiotics, insulin, antigen extract, or insect sting may be useful.

DISPOSITION

1. Patients with only mild reactions may be observed for 4 to 6 hours and discharged to continue antihistamine therapy at home.

2. All patients with moderate or severe disease require admission to an ICU.

3. Prevention is an important aspect of management.
   a. Patients should be aware of allergies and avoid exposure. A Medic-Alert bracelet should be worn.
   b. Parenteral medications should be used only when appropriate. Patients should be observed at least 20 to 30 minutes after administration of such medications.

   NOTE: Prophylaxis with steroids and antihistamines may be indicated before exposure to radiocontrast media for patients with previous reactions.
   c. In settings where parenteral medica-

tions are administered, personnel should have access to emergency supplies, including epinephrine, oxygen and airway support, diphenhydramine (Benadryl), and aminophylline.

    d. Patients with a history of anaphylaxis, particularly to insect bites, should carry an emergency kit, including syringes, epinephrine, and diphenhydramine. Epinephrine is available as autoinjectable premeasured kits:

      EpiPen delivers 0.3 ml (1 : 1000)
      EpiPen Jr. delivers 0.3 ml (1 : 2000)
      Ana-Kit delivers 0.6 ml (1 : 1000)
        (0.3 ml at one time)

Such patients should be considered for desensitization.

REFERENCES

Abramowicz M: Penicillin allergy, *Med Lett Drugs Ther* 30:79, 1988.

Atkinson TP, Kaliner MA: Anaphylaxis, *Med Clin North Am* 76:841, 1992.

Bochner BS, Lichtenstein LM: Anaphylaxis, *N Engl J Med* 324:1785, 1991.

Edwards KH, Johnston C: Allergic and immunologic anaphylaxis. In Barkin RM, editor: *Pediatric emergency medicine: concepts and clinical practice*, ed 2, St Louis, 1997, Mosby.

Reisman RE: Staging insect, *Med Clin North Am* 76: 889, 1992.

13 APNEA

Apnea occurs with the cessation of airflow for more than 20 seconds, or less than 20 seconds if accompanied by bradycardia, cyanosis, pallor, or limpness. It must be distinguished from normal periodic breathing irregularities during sleep, which may consist of alternating periods of regular breathing and respiratory pauses of 10 seconds without color change in up to 3% of sleep time. If this latter pattern occurs in a premature infant, it is considered apnea of prematurity and generally resolves by 37 weeks of age. Those older than 37 weeks of age who experience an apneic episode have apnea of infancy.

An episode characterized by a combination of apnea, color change (usually cyanosis but occasionally erythema or plethora), marked change in muscle tone (usually limpness), and choking or gagging is referred to as an *apparent life-threatening event* (ALTE), previously termed near-miss SIDS (see Chapter 22).

DIAGNOSTIC FINDINGS AND ETIOLOGY

Central apnea is marked by an absence of respiratory efforts caused by a lack of activation of the musculature that produces flow. This is particularly common in newborn infants. The incidence in the preterm infant is inversely proportional to the gestational age and decreases with maturation. Other conditions that exacerbate the condition include infection, metabolic derangements, anemia, and hypoxic or vascular cerebral damage. Some premature infants have periodic breathing, and rarely, some fail to maintain central ventilation during sleep (*Ondine's* curse) (see Chapter 11).

Obstructive apnea occurs when airflow ceases even though chest and abdominal breathing movement continues; that is, respiratory efforts continue. Airway patency is a reflection of airway constricting and dilating forces and the size of the upper airway lumen. Mixed mechanisms also may exist.

Infants may experience apnea from a wide variety of clinical conditions, often reflecting a mixed pathophysiologic mechanism involving components of central and obstructive mechanisms. Although ALTE is the most common and widely recognized, also encountered are seizures, trauma, breath holding, and problems with gastroesophageal reflux or feeding.

Children may experience obstructive apnea, often related to sleep. They demonstrate restless sleep patterns and apnea. Tonsillar and adenoidal hypertrophy is most common, resulting in a relative upper airway obstruction. Pulmonary hypertension may be a secondary complication.

DIAGNOSTIC FINDINGS

A history is essential in evaluating the child with apnea. Ultimately, the issue is to determine the significance of the episode.

1. Nature of the episode, including appear-

TABLE 13-1   Apnea: Diagnostic Considerations

	Apnea in infancy	Obstructive apnea
HISTORY	Intercurrent illness Relationship to sleep, feeding, position (reflux) Prenatal, neonatal history Appearance (color, tone) Duration, sequelae Response to stimuli History of seizures	Sleeping: snoring, fitful, restless, hypersomnolence Irritability Obesity Mouth breathing Pattern of progression Response to stimuli
ETIOLOGY		
Infection	Viral: respiratory syncytial virus (RSV), enterovirus, parainfluenza Bacterial: pertussis (p. 716)	**Tonsillitis, pharyngitis** (p. 604)
CNS	**Seizure** (p. 738) **Trauma** (p. 397) **Meningitis/encephalitis** (p. 725) Encephalopathy	Muscular dystrophy Cerebral hypotonia
Endocrine/metabolic	Hyponatremia Hypoglycemia Hypocalcemia	Hypothryoidism (p. 624) Cushing's disease Obese: Prader Willi, pickwickian syndromes Mucopolysaccharides
Congenital		Pierre Robin syndrome
Vascular	Vascular ring Congenital heart disease: atrial septal defect (ASD), patent ductus arteriosus (PDA), ventricular septal defect (VSD) Dysrhythmia (Chapter 6)	
Miscellaneous	**Near-SIDS or ALTE** (Chapter 22) Anemia (Chapter 26) **Gastroesophageal reflux** **Feeding problems** **Breath holding** (p. 724) **Overdose or ingestion** (Chapter 54)	**Tonsillar/adenoidal hypertrophy** **Laryngomalacia** Anemia (Chapter 26) Tumors

ance of the child with respect to color, tone (increased with seizures, choking, and aspiration; decreased with prolonged seizures or hypoxia), activity, respirations, precipitating events, duration, sequelae, response to intervention, and pattern of progression.

2. Nature of sleep, feeding reflux, and chalasia. Sleep pattern should be defined with respect to snoring, fitfulness, restlessness, and hypersomnolence.

3. Intercurrent illnesses, including viral or bacterial disease. Recurrent episodes of tonsillitis.
4. Medical history, including prenatal and neonatal history, seizures, and metabolic or congenital abnormalities.
5. Family history of apnea, SIDS, ALTE, and respiratory or cardiac problems.

The physical examination findings are commonly normal, revealing no specific entity to account for the episode. Assurance should

TABLE 13-1   Apnea: Diagnostic Considerations—cont'd

	Apnea in infancy	Obstructive apnea
ANCILLARY DATA (selectively indicated)	CBC, electrolytes, glucose, Ca^{++}, ABG Chest x-ray films Cerebrospinal fluid (CSF) Cultures: bacterial, viral ECG (consider Holter monitoring) EEG CT scan Barium swallow, manometry, nuclear scanning or esophageal pH studies as appropriate Oximetry monitoring and pneumogram (sleep study)	Lateral neck x-ray film ECG Chest x-ray film Laryngoscopy Formal sleep study
MANAGEMENT	Admit if episode is within 2 days of contact, is life threatening, or if follow-up is difficult Treat underlying cause Reflux precautions Consider continuous positive airway pressure (CPAP) or pharmacologic approach (p. 117) Close home monitoring	Admit as indicated Treat underlying problem Consider supplemental O_2, CPAP by nasal prongs Consider nasopharyngeal tube Consider tonsillectomy and adenoidectomy (nasal beclomethasone may provide temporary aid) Tracheostomy only as last resort

be obtained that the child is stable without evidence of cardiac, neurologic, or respiratory disease. Search for underlying conditions.

MANAGEMENT

Evaluation, as outlined in Table 13-1, must focus on the suspected pathophysiologic mechanism and the underlying condition. Treatment after stabilization must account for contributing abnormality while being supportive. Patients normally require admission for observation and evaluation if the episode occurred within 2 days of contact, if it was clinically significant, if it was potentially fatal, or if follow-up observation and evaluation will be difficult.

Consultation, monitoring, support, or pharmacologic (p. 117) intervention may be appropriate. Evaluation should be specific for the individual child, often including a barium swallow to exclude reflux, oximetry, and electrolytes.

REFERENCES

Demain JG, Goetz DW: Pediatric adenoidal hypertrophy and nasal airway obstruction, reduction with aqueous nasal beclomethasone, *Pediatrics* 95:355, 1995.

Kattwinkel J, Brooks J, Myerberg D: Positioning and SIDS: AAP Task Force on Infant Positioning and SIDS, *Pediatrics* 89:1120, 1992.

Mathew OP: Maintenance of upper airway patency, *J Pediatr* 106:863, 1985.

National Institutes of Health: Consensus development conference on infantile apnea and home monitoring—1986, *Pediatrics* 79:292, 1987.

Stradling JR, Thomas G, Warley ARH, et al: Effect of adenotonsillectomy on nocturnal hypoxemia, sleep disturbance and symptoms in snoring children, *Lancet* 335:249, 1990.

Weese-Mayer DE, Morrow AS, Conway LP, et al: Assessing clinical significance of apnea exceeding fifteen seconds with event reading, *J Pediatr* 117:568, 1990.

14 CHEST PAIN

ALERT: Potentially life-threatening conditions must be excluded by history, physical examination, and ancillary data.

Chest pain in children is usually not an ominous symptom and rarely suggests a serious underlying condition. Of those patients who have the problem for less than 6 months, 65% have a definable cause (Table 14-1). More than one fifth of children who experience chest pain have no defined cause, 15% have a musculoskeletal origin, 10% a cough, 9% costochondritis, 9% a psychogenic basis, and 7% asthma. Up to 15% of children who receive medical attention have cardiac disease. In 47% of the children ill enough to require admission, the chest pain was secondary to heart disease (dysrhythmia, pericarditis, cardiomyopathy, myocarditis, and coronary ischemia [Kawasaki syndrome]) (see Box 14-1 and Table 14-1).

Box 14-1

CAUSES OF MYOCARDIAL INFARCTION IN CHILDREN

CATEGORY	SPECIFIC CONDITIONS
Congenital cardiac disease	Stenosis or atresia of any of the valves, supravalvular aortic stenosis, atrioventricular canal, truncus arteriosus, patent ductus arteriosus, transposition of the great vessels, tetralogy of Fallot, coarctation of the aorta
Coronary artery anomalies	Anomalous origin of coronary arteries, single right or left coronary artery, aneurysm of the coronary arteries (Kawasaki syndrome)
Primary endocardial or myocardial disease	Endocardial fibroelastosis, cardiomyopathy
Collagen disorders	Rheumatic fever, systemic lupus erythematosus, mucocutaneous lymph node syndrome, rheumatoid arthritis
Hematologic/oncologic	Polycythemia, hemoglobinopathy (S-C, SS, H types), anemia, leukemia
Neuromuscular disease	Friedrich ataxia, muscular dystrophy
Primary cardiac tumors	Myxoma, rhabdomyosarcoma, teratoma, fibroma, lipoma, hamartoma
Miscellaneous	Cocaine use

Adapted from Perry LW: *Contemp Pediatr* 27:Nov-Dec, 1985.

TABLE 14-1   Chest Pain: Diagnostic Considerations

Condition	Diagnostic findings
TRAUMA (Chapter 62)	
Muscle strain	Point tenderness; pain reproducible with pressure or activity; often associated with new activity, particularly weightlifting; also may be secondary to prolonged coughing
Direct trauma to chest wall	
Fractured rib Contusion	History of trauma or hard, paroxysmal coughing; localized, point tenderness; may be associated with pneumothorax
Costochondritis (Tietze syndrome)	Firm, painful, tender swelling over one or more costochondral or chondral-sternal junctions; localized, superficial, nonexertional; may be painful with deep inspiration or direct palpation
Pneumothorax	Acute onset of pain, often associated with shortness of breath, respiratory distress, and cyanosis; decreased breath sounds with hyperresonance; often no history of trauma
Abdominal trauma (Chapter 63) Splenic or liver laceration/ bleeding Diaphragmatic injury	Acute onset of abdominal or referred chest pain (often shoulder pain as well); abdominal examination and vital signs variable; possible anemia
INFECTION/INFLAMMATION	
Pneumonia (p. 794)	Cough, fever, tachypnea, variable respiratory distress, systemic illness; abnormal lung examination; possible shoulder pain
Pleurisy	Superficial, localized, sharp pain, and tenderness; accentuated with deep breathing, cough, and movement of arms
Pleurodynia	Sharp pain, tenderness; unilateral or bilateral; accentuated by movement, breathing, cough; may have fever and abdominal pain; cause: coxsackievirus B
Pericarditis/myocarditis (p. 564) Viral Bacterial Tuberculosis Rheumatic fever Uremic	Sudden onset, sharp pain, substernal over precordium, epigastrium, or entire thorax; friction rub; pulsus paradoxus; accentuated by deep breathing, cough, swallowing, twisting; may have associated myocarditis (p. 563)
Herpes zoster (Chapter 42)	May be prodrome before developing vesicles

Continued

Somatic and visceral structures share sensory pathways. Visceral abnormalities may have somatic manifestations at the level of T1-T6. Abdominal disorders may cause chest pain because the posterior and lateral portions of the diaphragm are innervated by intercostal nerves and may be referred to the lower thorax and abdomen. The central and anterior portions are referred to the shoulder and neck regions.

In the history the focus is on past medical problems of the heart and lungs, family history of heart disease, presence of trauma, medications (particularly cocaine or oral birth control pills), coagulopathies, sickle cell disease, and other predisposing factors. The pain should be characterized with respect to onset and progression, character, intensity, location, radiation, relationship to position, breathing, activity, repro-

TABLE 14-1   Chest Pain: Diagnostic Considerations—cont'd

Condition	Diagnostic findings
Abdomen (Chapter 24) Esophagitis/gastritis Peritonitis Appendicitis Hepatitis Pancreatitis Cholecystitis	Referred pain; symptoms specific for disorder; empiric trial of antacids may be useful
VASCULAR	
Angina, ischemia, and infarct (see Box 14-1) Sickle cell disease (p. 698) Pulmonary stenosis Aortic stenosis and left ventricular outflow obstruction Dysrhythmia (Chapter 6) Anomalous coronary artery	Crushing, sharp pain over left chest with radiation to left arm, neck, or jaw; associated shortness of breath, anxiety, and other signs of cardiac decompensation, including tachycardia, tachypnea, gallop, rales, edema, associated signs and symptoms; ECG indicated
Pulmonary embolism and infarct (p. 568)	Acute onset of dyspnea, tachypnea, tachycardia, hemoptysis, and chest pain; $\dot{V}/\dot{Q}$ scan indicated; exclude hyperventilation, rare without predisposing condition
Dissecting aortic aneurysm	Acute onset of sharp pain in chest, abdomen, or back; pulsating mass; asymmetric lower extremity blood pressures; murmur or bruit; rare in children; Marfan's syndrome predisposes
Mitral valve prolapse	Usually asymptomatic but may have chest pain, palpitations, syncope; midsystolic click with late systolic murmur; most likely seen in young adults
INTRAPSYCHIC	
Functional (p. 758)	Acute stress, attention getting; story inconsistent; no effect on sleep or desired activity
Hyperventilation	Rapid and deep respirations; weakness, tingling; dyspnea; response to rebreathing; may mimic pulmonary embolism
CONGENITAL	
Hiatal hernia/esophagitis/reflux (Chapter 44)	Acute or chronic substernal pain and discomfort, vomiting, fullness after eating, and evidence of reflux; influenced by position and food; response to antacids
NEOPLASM	
Thoracic Mediastinal Spinal	May have organ involvement, pressure, or cord compression
MISCELLANEOUS	
Idiopathic	Most common category
Pneumothorax/pneumomediastinum (Chapters 20 and 62)	Acute onset of pain, often associated with tachypnea, respiratory distress, and cyanosis; may be spontaneous, traumatic, or associated with pulmonary disease (asthma, pneumonia, cystic fibrosis) or with forced inspiration (marijuana)
Asthma	Exercise-induced asthma; usually midsternal sharp pain

ducibility, ameliorating factors, and associated signs and symptoms. Other somatic complaints, sleep disturbances, syncope, shortness of breath, and exercise intolerance need specific questioning.

During the physical examination, attention to vital signs is crucial, as are careful auscultation, percussion, and palpation of the lungs, heart, and abdomen. Trauma should be excluded.

A minimal evaluation should include a chest x-ray film. Other ancillary data, such as electrocardiography (ECG), arterial blood gas (ABG) determination, echocardiography, cardiac enzyme evaluation, ventilation-perfusion ($\dot{V}/\dot{Q}$) scanning, or abdominal evaluation, rarely are needed unless there are specific indications from the history or physical examination of underlying cardiac or systemic disease. An exercise stress test or Holter monitoring may be helpful in unique circumstances.

If the patient appears symptomatic on arrival or if the pain is not obviously functional or musculoskeletal, oxygen and cardiac monitoring are appropriate until the diagnosis is clarified and no significant disease is defined. Treatment of the underlying abnormality and reassurance are indicated. An empiric trial of nonsteroidal antiinflammatory agents may be useful after trauma once significant abnormality is excluded.

REFERENCES

Asnes RS, Santulli R, Bemporad JR: Psychogenic chest pain in children, *Clin Pediatr* 20:788, 1981.

Brenner JI, Ringel RE, Berman MA: Cardiologic perspective of chest pain in childhood: a referral problem? to whom? *Pediatr Clin North Am* 31:1241, 1984.

Brown RT: Costochondritis in adolescents, *J Adolesc Health Care* 1:198, 1981.

Hirsch P, Landt Y, Porter S, et al: Cardiac troponin I in pediatrics: normal values and potential use in the assessment of cardiac injury, *J Pediatr* 130:872, 1997.

Pantell RH, Goodman BW: Adolescent chest pain: a prospective study, *Pediatrics* 71:881, 1983.

Reynolds JL: Precordial catch syndrome in children, *South Med J* 82:1228, 1989.

Rowe BH, Dulberg CS, Peterson RG, et al: Characteristics of children presenting with chest pain to a pediatric emergency department, *Can Med Assoc J* 143:388, 1990.

Selbst SM, Ruddy RM, Clark BJ, et al: Pediatric chest pain: a prospective study, *Pediatrics* 82:319, 1988.

Wiens L, Sabath R, Ewing L, et al: Chest pain in otherwise healthy children and adolescents is frequently caused by exercise-induced asthma, *Pediatrics* 90:350, 1992.

Zavaras-Angelidou KA, Weinhouse E, Nelson DB: Review of 180 episodes of chest pain in 134 children, *Pediatr Emerg Care* 8:189, 1992.

15 Coma

ETIOLOGY

Coma in children is caused by a wide variety of pathologic processes. Physiologically, hypoxia, hypoglycemia, or direct tissue injury are usually present. Most patients have meningitis, encephalitis, head trauma, or poisoning. Metabolic and endocrine abnormalities, prolonged seizures, and vascular accidents also must be considered. Tables 15-1 and 15-2 outline the common entities causing coma, primarily focusing on signs and symptoms noted with the deterioration of mental status from lethargy to stupor to coma. Common treatable causes of coma include infection (meningitis, empyema, abscess, encephalitis), trauma (subdural or epidural hematoma), intoxications (alcohol, barbiturates, opiates, carbon monoxide, lead), endocrine/metabolic disorders (hypoglycemia, uremia), vascular disorders (shock, hypertension), and epilepsy. Intussusception does not cause coma but does produce lethargy, with decreased response to environmental stimuli (p. 654).

A useful mnemonic is I SPOUT A VEIN: *i*nsulin (too much, too little), *s*hock, *p*sychogenic, *o*piates and other drugs, *u*remia and other metabolic abnormalities, *t*rauma, *a*lcohol, *v*ascular, *e*ncephalopathy, *i*nfection, and *n*eoplasm. Another mnemonic is AEIOU TIPS: *a*lcohol, *e*ncephalopathy/endocrinopathy/electrolytes, *i*nsulin/intussusception, *o*piates, *u*remia, *t*rauma, *i*nfection, *p*sychiatric, and *s*eizure.

DIAGNOSTIC FINDINGS

A thorough history should be obtained from friends or relatives and should focus on the progression of changes in mental status, medical history, associated signs and symptoms, and localized findings. A history of head trauma, medications, or possible ingestions (see Table 54-3) is imperative in the assessment.

Physical examination is crucial, not only in determining the patient's status, but also in providing diagnostic information to ascertain the level of injury. A complete neurologic examination is imperative. Useful diagnostic clues are outlined in Box 15-1. The Glasgow Coma Scale (p. 414) provides a means of serially monitoring patient responsiveness.

The location of the lesion may be further delineated by findings:

Supratentorial lesions have findings suggestive of focal hemispheric disease that progress from a rostral to a caudal direction. Pupillary reflexes are usually depressed, and motor signs are asymmetric.

Infratentorial lesions demonstrate brainstem findings and are not rostral to caudal in evolution. Respiratory patterns may be abnormal, and cranial nerve palsies are common.

Toxic or metabolic lesions are associated with changes in mental status that occur before changes in motor signs develop; the latter are symmetric. Pupillary reactions are preserved,

TABLE 15-1   Coma: Diagnostic Considerations

Condition	Diagnostic findings	Ancillary data	Comments
INFECTION (p. 725)			
Meningitis	Fever, headache, nuchal rigidity, seizures, lethargy, irritability, usually no focal findings; may have otitis media or other infection	CSF: ↑ WBC, ↑ protein, ↓ glucose, ↑ pressure, culture result positive	Viral or bacterial; consider in febrile patient with mental status change; antibiotics
Encephalitis	Fever, headache, variable nuchal rigidity, tremor, ataxia, hemiplegia, cranial nerve VI palsy, irritability, lethargy, or focal findings; may have only minimal symptoms	CSF: ↑ WBC (mononuclear), ↑ protein, ↑ pressure, culture result negative	Viral: measles, mumps, rubella, chickenpox, Epstein-Barr virus (infectious mononucleosis); bacterial: pertussis; immunization: pertussis, mumps
Intracranial abscess	Fever, headache, focal neurologic signs, increased intracranial pressure	CT scan; CSF: ↑ WBC, ↑ protein, culture result negative	Extension otitis media, mastoiditis; risks: congenital heart disease and polycythemia
Subdural empyema	Toxic, fever, focal neurologic signs, increased intracranial pressure	CT scan; subdural tap; CSF: ↑ WBC, ↑ protein, ↑ pressure, culture finding negative	Follows trauma or complication of meningitis
TRAUMA (Chapter 57)			
Cerebral concussion	Dizziness, nausea, vomiting, headache, lethargy, amnesia, ataxia, transient blindness, no focal findings	Variable CT scan, depending on course	Rule out mass lesions
Subdural hematoma	After trauma, immediate onset of altered mentation, headache, focal neurologic findings, increased intracranial pressure	CT scan immediately	Symptoms usually progress immediately after injury; rarely may be delayed days to weeks
Epidural hematoma	Patient often awakens from concussion and, after a brief period of lucidity, lapses into coma; focal findings, headache, increased intracranial pressure	CT scan immediately	Delayed onset unless injury is very severe

CSF, Cerebrospinal fluid; *WBC,* white blood cell; *CT,* computed tomography.   *Continued*

TABLE 15-1 Coma: Diagnostic Considerations—cont'd

Condition	Diagnostic findings	Ancillary data	Comments
TRAUMA (Chapter 57)—cont'd			
Drowning (Chapter 47)	No focal findings, variable increased intracranial pressure	CSF normal, CT WNL or edema	Injury reflects hypoxia
Heat stroke (Chapter 50)	Febrile (>40° C), headache, anorexia, confusion, posturing, acidosis	CSF WNL; ABG, electrolytes variable	Complications can be life threatening
INTOXICATION (Chapters 54 and 55; Table 54-2)			
Sedatives/hypnotics	Lethargy, stupor, possibly dilated pupils, no focal findings	Toxicology screen	Support; forced alkaline diuresis
Narcotics	Miotic, pinpoint pupils, depressed respiratory, GI, and GU activity, hypotensive; no focal findings	Narcotic screen	Support; Narcan 0.1 mg/kg/dose (0.4-2.0 mg/dose) IV, repeated prn
Ethanol	Lethargy, ataxia, slurred speech, visual hallucinations, poor coordination, seizures; no focal findings	Levels >100 mg/dl (depending on chronicity)	Support; metabolized at about 30 mg/dl/hr; glucose, K$^+$
Salicylates	Tachypnea, hyperthermia, vomiting, tinnitus, excitability; lethargy, seizures; no focal findings	Level >90 mg/dl at 6 hr, ABG, electrolytes, ↓ glucose	Chronic ingestion—levels not helpful; metabolic acidosis with anion gap
Carbon monoxide	Throbbing headache, dizziness, nausea, vomiting, collapse, progressing with diminished brainstem function; no focal findings	Carboxyhemoglobin level	Emergency oxygen therapy; hyperbaric chamber
Lead	Weakness, irritability, weight loss, vomiting, personality change, ataxia, increased intracranial pressure, seizures; no focal findings	Urine lead levels; glycosuria, proteinuria, acidosis; LP: ↑ WBC, ↑ pressure	Dimercaprol, EDTA
EPILEPSY (p. 738)	Following prolonged seizures, postictal period; may have focal findings (Todd paralysis)	Anticonvulsant levels; evaluation of cause	Support, oxygen; need to evaluate cause of seizures

WNL, Within normal limits; *ABG,* arterial blood gas; *GI,* gastrointestinal; *GU,* genitourinary; *LP,* lumbar puncture.

TABLE 15-1   Coma: Diagnostic Considerations—cont'd

Condition	Diagnostic findings	Ancillary data	Comments
ENDOCRINE/METABOLIC			
Hypoglycemia (Chapter 38)	Sweating, weakness, tachycardia, tachypnea, tremor, anxiety; no focal findings; seizures	Hypoglycemia; LP WNL	Administer 0.5-1.0 gm/kg/dose IV of D25W—rapid improvement; maintain glucose
Diabetic ketoacidosis (p. 615)	Kussmaul breathing, orthostatic BP changes, polydipsia, polyphagia, weight loss; no focal findings	Hyperglycemia, ketonemia, acidosis; LP WNL	Fluids, insulin; variable bicarbonate therapy
Hyponatremia/ hypernatremia (Chapter 8)	Dehydration, edema, seizures, intracranial bleeding; no focal findings	Electrolytes abnormal; LP WNL	Treat multiple causes in addition to sodium imbalance
Renal failure (p. 809)	Decreased urine output, edema, lethargy, dysrhythmia (secondary to $\uparrow K^+$), CHF, tachypnea, hypertension; no focal findings	Electrolytes, BUN, creatinine levels abnormal; LP WNL	Support; multiple causes; dialysis may be needed
Reye syndrome (p. 646)	URI with vomiting followed by lethargy, stupor, hepatic dysfunction, delirium, increased intracranial pressure; no focal findings	Liver function test results abnormal, LP WNL, elevated ammonia, bilirubin WNL	Multiple causes; support; intracranial monitor
Addison disease (p. 614)	Muscle weakness, pigmentation of skin, lethargy, anorexia, hypotension, weight loss; no focal findings	Electrolytes: $\downarrow Na^+$, $\uparrow K^+$, $\downarrow$ glucose; LP WNL	May follow stress (trauma, infection); IV glucose, hydrocortisone (Solu-Cortef) 5 mg/kg/dose IV q6hr IV
Amino/organic acid abnormality	Deteriorating growth and development; mental status change; no new focal findings	Acidosis, LP WNL	Evaluation of inborn errors; infection often precipitates problem
VASCULAR			
Subarachnoid hemorrhage	Acute onset of severe headache, nuchal rigidity, listlessness; usually no focal findings	CT scan; LP bloody	May be caused by trauma, AV malformation
Hypertensive encephalopathy (Chapter 18)	Rapid rise in BP, headache, vomiting, seizures, hemiparesis, lethargy	LP WNL; evaluate potential causes	Responds rapidly to reducing diastolic BP to 100 mm Hg

Continued

TABLE 15-1   Coma: Diagnostic Considerations—cont'd

Condition	Diagnostic findings	Ancillary data	Comments
VASCULAR—cont'd			
Cerebral vascular accident	Usually focal findings; seizures, hemiplegia after dehydration (cerebral vein or sagittal sinus thrombosis); papilledema, proptosis, conjunctival hemorrhage, ophthalmoplegia (cavernous sinus thrombosis)	CT scan, LP variable	Support, anticoagulation; causes include cyanotic heart disease, endocarditis, sickle cell disease, thrombocytopenia, hemophilia, trauma, birth control pills, and anticoagulants
INTRAPSYCHIC (Chapter 83)			
Hysterical	Inconsistent findings, often focal; if arm is held up, when dropped it does not hit patient; history of depression, anxiety	LP WNL	Usually history of mental illness
NEOPLASM			
Multiple cell types	Variable presentation	CT scan	Neurosurgical consultation

TABLE 15-2   Differential Diagnosis of Coma

No focal signs: normal CSF*	No focal signs: abnormal CSF*	Focal signs: normal CSF*	Focal signs: abnormal CSF*
Postictal	Infection	Subdural hematoma	Subdural hematoma
Intoxication	Meningitis	Epidural hematoma	Epidural hematoma
Concussion	Encephalitis	Todd paralysis	Infection
Metabolic/endocrine disorder	Subdural hematoma	Hypertensive encephalopathy	Brain abscess
Hypertensive encephalopathy	Epidural hematoma		Subdural empyema
	Subarachnoid hemorrhage		Encephalitis
Hysteria	Cerebral vein thrombosis		AV malformation
Hydrocephalus	Lead poisoning		Neoplasm
	Midline tumor		

*Check for cells, protein, glucose, Gram stain, culture, and pressure, if lumbar puncture is done. Perform lumbar puncture after consultation if clinical suspicion of elevated pressure exists.

seizures are common, and abnormal motor movement is seen.

Acid-base imbalance may suggest the underlying cause. A *metabolic acidosis* with increased anion gap may be due to lactic acidosis (hypoxia or inadequate perfusion), diabetic ketoacidosis, renal failure, or ingestion (methanol, ethylene glycol, salicylates [late]). *Respiratory acidosis* associated with apnea/hypoventilation may be secondary to supratentorial or infratentorial lesions, ingestion (sedative, narcotics), respiratory muscle fatigue, neuromuscular disease, metabolic encephalopathy, and generalized seizures. *Respiratory alkalosis* caused by an

Box 15-1

DIAGNOSTIC SIGNS IN COMA

RESPIRATORY PATTERN

Cheyne-Stokes (alternating apnea and hypernoia)
1. Bilateral cerebral or diencephalic lesion
2. Metabolic abnormality
3. Incipient temporal lobe herniation

Hyperventilation
1. Lesion between low midbrain and midpons
2. Metabolic acidosis
   a. Diabetic ketoacidosis
   b. Uremia
   c. Intoxication — ethanol, salicylates
   d. Fluid or electrolyte abnormalities
3. Hypoxia

Ataxic breathing (irregular rate and depth): lesion of medulla

POSITION

Decorticate (arms flexed and abducted, legs extended): corticospinal tract lesion within or near the cerebral hemisphere

Decerebrate (arms extended and internally rotated against the chest, legs extended)
1. Midbrain — midpons lesion
2. Metabolic abnormality (hypoxia, hypoglycemia)
3. Bilateral hemispheric lesion

PUPILS

Pinpoint (1-2 mm), fixed
1. Pontine lesions
2. Metabolic abnormality
3. Intoxication—opiates, barbiturates (not fixed)

Small (2-3 mm), reactive
1. Medullary lesion
2. Metabolic abnormality

Midsize (4-5 mm), fixed: midbrain lesion
Dilated, fixed
1. Bilateral
   a. Irreversible brain damage (shock, massive hemorrhage, encephalitis)
   b. Anticholinergic (atropine-like) drugs
   c. Barbiturates (late, secondary to hypoxia)
   d. Hypothermia
   e. Seizures

Continued

Box 15-1

DIAGNOSTIC SIGNS IN COMA—cont'd

2. Unilateral
   a. Rapidly expanding lesion on ipsilateral side (subdural hemorrhage, tumor)
   b. Tentorial herniation
   c. Lesion of III nerve nucleus
   d. Anticholinergic eyedrops
   e. Seizures

Dilated, reactive
   1. Postictal
   2. Anticholinergic drugs

BLOOD PRESSURE

Hypertension
   1. Increased intracranial pressure
   2. Subarachnoid hemorrhage
   3. Intoxication

Hypotension
   1. Associated injury with hypovolemia, spinal shock, or hypoxemia
   2. Adrenal failure

NUCHAL RIGIDITY

   1. Meningitis/encephalitis
   2. Subarachnoid hemorrhage
   3. Posterior fossa tumor

EYE MOVEMENT

Oculocephalic reflex (doll's eye): with the eyes held open, the head is turned quickly from side to side. Clear cervical spine first.
   1. Comatose patient with an intact brainstem responds by eye movement in the direction opposite to that which the head is turned, as if still gazing ahead in initial position.
   2. Comatose patient with midbrain or pons lesions has random eye movement.

Oculovestibular reflex with caloric stimulation: with head elevated 30 degrees, ice water is injected through a small catheter lying in the ear canal (up to 200 ml is used in an adult)
   1. Comatose patient with an intact brainstem responds by conjugate deviation of the eyes toward the irrigated ear.
   2. Comatose patient with brainstem lesions demonstrates no response.

Conjugate deviation
   1. Cerebral lesion
      a. Toward destructive lesion
      b. Away from irritative lesion
   2. Brainstem lesion: away from destructive lesion

Box 15-1

DIAGNOSTIC SIGNS IN COMA—cont'd

VI nerve palsy — eye(s) cannot move laterally
1. Increased intracranial pressure
2. Meningeal infection
3. Pontine lesion
4. Injury (e.g., trauma, neoplasm)

III nerve palsy — eyes point down and out
1. Tentorial herniation
2. III nerve entrapment (skull fracture)
3. Intrinsic III nerve lesion (e.g., diabetes)
4. Compression (aneurysm, tumor)

increased respiratory rate is associated with intracranial hypertension, septic shock, hepatic failure, salicylate ingestion, Reye syndrome, and brainstem dysfunction.

Laboratory evaluation should focus on potential causes. Chemical evaluations should always include glucose and electrolyte concentrations, liver function tests, ammonia and blood urea nitrogen (BUN) levels, and specific tests should be done as indicated. Complete blood count (CBC) and cultures are appropriate for evaluation of an infectious origin. Oximetry should be continuous. A lumbar puncture is particularly helpful once increased intracranial pressure is excluded (see Table 15-2). Urine and blood toxicologic screens may be done. Radiologically, computed tomography (CT) scanning, often with contrast medium if a nontraumatic condition is suspected, should take place early in the assessment.

In examining the child and assessing responsiveness, a number of concurrent conditions may interfere with this assessment, potentially leading to an incorrect diagnosis of brain death. Other possible causes of findings that may be associated with brain death include the following:

1. Pupils fixed: anticholinergic drugs (systemic or topical), neuromuscular blockade, and preexisting eye disease
2. No oculovestibular reflex: ototoxic agent, vestibular suppressant, and preexisting disease
3. No respirations: posthyperventilation apnea and neuromuscular blockade
4. No motor activity: neuromuscular blockade and sedative drugs
5. Isoelectric electroencephalogram (EEG): sedative drugs, hypoxia, trauma, hypothermia, and encephalitis

MANAGEMENT

Management must initially focus on administering fluids and stabilizing the airway and providing oxygen to support cardiac and respiratory status. Active intervention may be required. Thereafter all patients should receive oxygen, glucose (0.5-1.0 gm/kg/dose IV), and naloxone (Narcan), 0.1 mg/kg/dose IV initially, up to 2.0 mg/dose IV. A urinary catheter should be inserted and urine evaluation for toxic substances as well as output done. Blood is sent for glucose, electrolytes, BUN, arterial blood gas

(ABG), toxicology screening, and other specific studies, as indicated. After stabilization, a rapid approach to delineating etiologic conditions is imperative to initiating specific therapy. Obviously, a parallel approach is indicated in patients with altered mental status.

REFERENCES

American Academy of Pediatrics: Guidelines for the determination of brain death in children, *Pediatrics* 80:298, 1987.

Fields AI, Cable DH, Pollack NH, et al: Outcomes of children in a persistent vegetative state, *Crit Care Med* 21:18901, 1993.

Kraus J, Fife D, Conroy C: Pediatric brain injuries: the nature, clinical course and early outcomes in a defined United States population, *Pediatrics* 79:501, 1987.

Plum F, Posner JB: *The diagnosis of stupor and coma*, ed 3, Philadelphia, 1980, FA Davis.

Seshia S, Johnston B, Kasia G: Non-traumatic coma in childhood: clinical variables in prediction of outcome, *Dev Med Child Neurol* 25:493, 1983.

Yager JY, Johnston B, Seshia SS: Coma scales in pediatric practice, *Am J Dis Child* 144:1088, 1990.

16 Congestive Heart Failure

ALERT: Infants may have feeding difficulty, poor weight gain, irritability, and labored respirations without rales. Older children often have fatigue and anorexia accompanied by tachycardia, cardiomegaly, tachypnea with rales, rhonchi and wheezing, cyanosis, and evidence of venous congestion.

Congestive heart failure (CHF) is caused by the inability of the heart to pump adequate blood volume to meet circulatory and metabolic needs. Heart failure may result from volume overload (increased preload), pressure overload (increased afterload), myocardial dysfunction, and dysrhythmias.

Of those children in whom CHF develops, 90% experience it the first year of life because of congenital heart disease. The younger the infant with initial signs and symptoms of heart failure, generally the worse the prognosis if the condition remains untreated. Although older children may have CHF caused by congenital heart disease, they more commonly have acquired disease from cardiomyopathy, bacterial endocarditis, or rheumatic carditis. About 25% of children with congenital heart disease have associated extracardiac anomalies.

ETIOLOGY

See Box 16-1 and Table 16-1.

DIAGNOSTIC FINDINGS

Symptoms reflect cardiac decompensation and the underlying disorder. The acuteness of the process and the nature of any anatomic lesions determine the pattern of progression. Patients may have right, left, or combined heart failure, and the clinical findings will reflect the chamber(s) involved.

A careful history is essential, focusing on preexisting cardiac disease or surgery, hematologic conditions (sickle cell anemia or thalassemia), pulmonary problems, decreased exercise tolerance or associated orthopnea, altered behavior, and weight loss and eating habits.

The cardiac examination demonstrates evidence of dysfunction, reflecting a physiologic response to the inadequate cardiac output and underlying abnormality:

1. Tachycardia secondary to increased adrenergic tone and catecholamine release.
2. Cardiomegaly by examination and x-ray study. The point of maximal impulse is usually lateral to the midclavicular line in the fifth or sixth intercostal space. Hypertrophy occurs first with pressure overload, but dilation is initially more common with volume overload.
3. Gallop rhythm with prominent third sound reflecting impaired ventricular compliance and increased resistance to filling.
4. Tachypnea, often with rales, rhonchi, wheezing, retractions, and symptoms

> **Box 16-1**
> ## CAUSES OF CONGESTIVE HEART FAILURE
>
> **VOLUME OVERLOAD** (increased preload)
>
> 1. Vascular-congenital heart disease (Table 16-1)
>   Left-to-right shunt: ventricular septal defect (VSD)
>   Anomalous pulmonary venous return
>   Valvular regurgitation (aortic insufficiency)
>   Patent ductus arteriosus (PDA)
>   Arteriovenous fistula
> 2. Anemia
> 3. Hypervolemia (malnutrition, iatrogenic)
>
> **PRESSURE OVERLOAD** (increased afterload)
>
> 1. Vascular-congenital heart disease (Table 16-1)
>   Ventricular outflow obstruction (aortic stenosis, coarctation)
>   Left ventricular inflow obstruction (cor triatriatum)
> 2. Hypertension (Chapter 18)
>
> **DYSRHYTHMIA** (Chapter 6)
>
> 1. Vascular
>   Atrial or ventricular: ectopic pacemaker or reentry pathway
>   Conduction defect
> 2. Metabolic: electrolyte, Ca^{++}, Mg^{++} abnormalities
> 3. Intoxication: digitalis, cyclic antidepressants, etc.
>
> **MYOCARDIAL DYSFUNCTION**
>
> 1. Vascular
>   Pulmonary embolism (p. 568)
>   Endocardial fibroelastosis (endocardial fibrosis)
>   Anomalous coronary artery
>   Pulmonary hypertension (obesity, pickwickian)
>
> 2. Infection/inflammation
>   Cardiomyopathy
>   Viral: coxsackie, influenza
>   Bacterial: diphtheria, meningococcemia, sepsis, toxic shock syndrome
>   Miscellaneous: toxoplasmosis, spirochetes, parasites
>   Bacterial endocarditis (p. 569)
>   Pericarditis: viral, bacterial, mycobacterial
>   Pulmonary disease: chronic infection, aspiration, cystic fibrosis
> 3. Endocrine/metabolic
>   Newborn: infant of diabetic mother, hypocalcemia, hypomagnesemia
>   Hypothyroidism or hyperthyroidism
>   Hypoglycemia: glycogen storage disease, etc.
>   Pheochromocytoma
> α_1-Antitrypsin deficiency
> 4. Trauma/environment (Chapter 62)
>   Cardiac tamponade, contusion or rupture secondary to blunt or penetrating trauma (p. 472)
>   Hyperthermia (Chapter 50)
> 5. Autoimmune/allergy
>   Asthma
>   Acute rheumatic fever (ARF) (p. 566)
>   Systemic lupus erythematosus (SLE)
> 6. Deficiency/degeneration
>   Anemia
>   CNS disease: progressive or degenerative
>   Malnutrition: kwashiorkor, beri beri (thiamine), etc.
> 7. Intoxication: alcohol abuse, heavy metals, cardiac toxins (digitalis, β blockers)
> 8. Neoplasm: metastatic or infiltration, atrial myxoma
> 9. Postsurgical condition

of orthopnea and dyspnea. Pulmonary edema (see Chapter 19) commonly is present.

5. Venous congestion associated with hepatomegaly, jugular venous distension, and peripheral edema, especially with right-sided failure.

6. Peripheral pulses often are weak with impaired perfusion. Extremities are cool. Peripheral edema may develop on the

TABLE 16-1   Congenital Heart Disease: Differentiation by Chest X-Ray Film and ECG

Cyanotic				
Decreased pulmonary blood flow **(right-to-left shunt)**			**Increased pulmonary blood flow** **(right-to-left or left-to-right shunt)**	
RVH	**LVH**	**LVH, RVH, CVH**	**RVH**	**LVH, RVH, CVH**
Pulmonary stenosis with variable VSD: CHF	Tricuspid atresia Pulmonary atresia with hypoplastic right ventricle: CHF	Transposition of great vessels with pulmonary stenosis: CHF	Total anomalous pulmonary venous return: CHF	Transposition and VSD: CHF Single ventricle Truncus arteriosus:
Tetralogy of Fallot: CHF Pulmonary atresia with variable VSD Ebstein: CHF		Truncus arteriosus with hypoplastic pulmonary artery: CHF	Hypoplastic left heart: CHF	CHF Tricuspid atresia with transposition: CHF

Acyanotic			
Normal pulmonary blood flow (no shunts)		**Increased pulmonary blood flow (left-to-right shunt)**	
RVH	**LVH**	**RVH**	**LVH or CVH**
Pulmonary stenosis (severe): CHF Mitral stenosis: CHF	Coarctation: CHF Mitral regurgitation Aortic stenosis Anomalous left coronary artery: CHF	Atrial septal defect: CHF Left-to-right shunt (increased pulmonary pressure) (PDA, VSD, ASD): CHF	Patent ductus arteriosus: CHF Ventricular septal defect: CHF Arteriovenous fistula: CHF

RVH, Right ventricular hypertrophy; *LVH,* left ventricular hypertrophy; *CVH,* combined ventricular hypertrophy; *VSD,* ventricular septal defect; *PDA,* patent ductus arteriosus; *ASD,* atrial septal defect; *CHF* indicates lesion is often associated with congestive heart disease.

dorsum of the hands and feet, over the sacrum, and in the periorbital region if right-sided failure is present.

7. Cyanosis resulting from pulmonary or cardiac causes. Primary cardiac cyanosis because of significant shunting (see Table 16-1) will not respond to 100% oxygen administration, in contrast to pulmonary disease (see Chapter 17), which shows no significant improvement of the cyanosis with administration of oxygen.

8. Growth failure, undernutrition, and feeding difficulties are common in infants. Older children may experience fatigue and anorexia.

9. Altered mental status may result from decreased cerebral perfusion. Infants are typically irritable.

10. Pulsus paradoxus may accompany pericardial tamponade, pneumothorax, or severe asthma. Its presence is determined by having the patient breathe quietly and by lowering the blood pressure cuff toward the systolic level. The pressure when the first sound is heard is noted. The pressure is further dropped until sounds can be heard throughout the respiratory cycle. A difference of 15 mm Hg or more indicates the presence of a paradoxic pulse.

11. Pulses alternans is evidence of left-sided failure. When it is present, the systolic

pressure rhythmically alternates between high and low pressures.

Complications

1. Pulmonary edema (see Chapter 19)
2. Dysrhythmias (see Chapter 6)
3. Shock (see Chapter 5)
4. Superimposed pulmonary infection (p. 794)
5. Renal failure secondary to decreased renal perfusion (p. 809)
6. Cardiac arrest and death (see Chapter 4)

Ancillary Data

Specific studies clarify cardiac and pulmonary status. Additional studies may be indicated to further evaluate the underlying cause of CHF.

1. Chest x-ray films: posteroanterior (PA) and lateral. Anteroposterior (AP) view may be sufficient for initial evaluation of the critically ill patient.
   a. Cardiac silhouette will demonstrate cardiomegaly. Other findings reflect the nature of any anatomic or functional lesion and may be diagnostic of a specific congenital defect.
   b. Pulmonary edema causes fluffy infiltrates with perihilar haziness, Kerley B lines, and periodically, pleural effusion. Pneumonia, if present, must be distinguished from pulmonary edema.
   c. Noncardiac causes may be partially excluded: aortic aneurysm (widened mediastinum on PA film), signs of trauma (e.g., broken ribs), and chronic pulmonary disease.
2. Electrocardiogram (ECG), which is useful in the evaluation of a number of entities:
   a. Congenital heart disease (ventricular enlargement; axis deviation; abnormalities of P, QRS, or T waves) (see Table 16-1)
   b. Cardiac ischemia, infarction, or contusion
   c. Cardiomyopathy or pericardial disease
   d. Metabolic abnormalities (e.g., hypokalemia, hypocalcemia) (see Chapter 8)
   e. Dysrhythmias (see Chapter 6)
3. Arterial blood gas (ABG) to determine acid-base abnormalities on the basis of respiratory, circulatory (perfusion), or metabolic inadequacies. The response to oxygen may assist in distinguishing primary cardiac from pulmonary disease. Ongoing monitoring is essential.
4. Chemical evaluation: electrolytes, glucose, blood urea nitrogen (BUN), creatinine, calcium, and magnesium levels. This is particularly important for patients with dysrhythmias and for those receiving diuretic therapy and to evaluate renal status and exclude prerenal azotemia.
5. Hematologic evaluation: complete blood count (CBC) to evaluate for anemia or infection. Erythrocyte sedimentation rate (ESR) is often decreased in active CHF.
6. Measuring pulmonary artery end diastolic pressure or mean pulmonary capillary wedge pressure (PCWP) with a Swan-Ganz catheter often is essential in monitoring the patient. Patients with moderate or severe disease require careful measurement of these parameters to assess cardiac function and fluid balance. Because central venous pressure (CVP) is usually inadequate, this becomes particularly important in trying to balance inotropic agents with volume administration. Consultation should be sought.
7. Cardiac enzymes: creatine phosphokinase (CPK-MB), serum glutamic-oxaloacetic transaminase (SGOT), and lactate dehydrogenase (LDH) if perfusion abnormality, ischemia, or inflammatory response is suspected.
8. Thoracentesis (see Appendix A-8).
9. Pericardiocentesis (see Appendix A-5).
10. Ultrasonography: Echocardiography is a

safe, noninvasive technique that may be performed at the bedside with portable equipment. It is particularly useful in assessing cardiac function, pericardial thickening or effusion, cardiac valve vegetations, and atrial myxoma. It is essential in monitoring the response of the failing heart to inotropic drugs. In the fetus, heart disease may be associated with scalp edema, ascites, and pericardial effusion.

11. Nuclear scanning: useful in the assessment of ventricular contractility, myocardial perfusion, and cellular viability. The ejection fraction as a measure of function represents the percentage of end-diastolic volume that is ejected per stroke using ^{99m}Tc radioisotope. Experience with small infants is still limited.

DIFFERENTIAL DIAGNOSIS

1. Vascular
   a. Noncardiogenic pulmonary edema. Evaluation of heart will determine level of dysfunction, if any. History may be helpful in focusing on other causes (see Chapter 19).
   b. Intrapulmonary hemorrhage.
   c. Pulmonary embolism (p. 568).
   d. Infection: pneumonia (p. 794)
   e. Allergy: asthma (p. 765)

MANAGEMENT

Initial cardiac and respiratory stabilization must be achieved while evaluating and treating the underlying condition. General management focuses on improving cardiac contractility and reducing the work load. It is important to distinguish between pump and muscle function because it is possible that abnormal loads imposed on the heart may result in failure of the heart as a pump in the absence of depression of intrinsic myocardial contractility. Myocardial contractility may be depressed, but favorable

loading conditions may reduce the impact of this impairment on the contractile quality of the myocardial fibers as reflected in the Frank-Starling curve. Often this interaction requires careful titration in the management of inotropic and unloading agents with volume status.

Therapeutic goals must be to improve cardiac performance, augment peripheral perfusion, and decrease systemic and pulmonary venous congestion.

The airway, breathing, and circulation need immediate attention. Oxygen should be administered. When the condition is stabilized, the patient should be kept in a semirecumbent position with ongoing cardiac monitoring and oxygen administration. Temperature should be normalized.

Inotropic Agents: Digoxin (Table 16-2)

Digoxin is the drug of choice in improving the inotropic action of the heart. The inotropic response is determined by pharmacokinetic variables, including bioavailability, absorption, volume of distribution, metabolism, and plasma protein binding. End-organ response is affected by the sensitivity of the myocardium and by myocardial uptake. Infants often require a larger dose than adults because of the infant's

TABLE 16-2   Digoxin: Total Digitizing Dose (TDD)

Age	IV	PO
Premature	0.01-0.02 mg/kg	0.02-0.03 mg/kg
Newborn-2 wk	0.03-0.04 mg/kg	0.03-0.05 mg/kg
2 wk-2 yr	0.03-0.05 mg/kg	0.04-0.06 mg/kg
>2 yr	0.04 mg/kg	0.05 mg/kg
Adult	0.5-1.0 mg	1.0-1.5 mg

1000 µg = 1 mg. IV dose is generally 75% of PO dose.
NOTE: Oral maintenance daily dose is usually one fourth to one third of TDD.

higher body clearance and larger volume of distribution; children require similar or lower doses than adults. Digoxin is contraindicated in idiopathic hypertropic subaortic stenosis (IHSS) and tetralogy of Fallot and should be used with caution in patients with myocarditis or electrolyte abnormalities.

Characteristics

1. Onset of action: 5 to 30 minutes when administered IV (IM absorption is erratic)
2. IV dose: usually about 75% of oral dose
3. Renal excretion: 48 to 72 hours
4. Oral absorption: 66% to 75%
5. Preparations:
   a. Vial: 0.1 mg (100 μg)/ml; 0.25 mg (250 μg)/ml
   b. Elixir: 0.05 mg/ml
   c. Tablet: 0.125, 0.25, and 0.50 mg

Dosage

1. Give half of total digitalizing dose (TDD) initially, then one fourth of TDD in 6 to 8 hours, then one fourth of TDD 6 to 12 hours later, depending on severity of CHF.
2. The condition of relatively stable patients may be digitalized slowly by beginning the maintenance dose of digoxin. Therapeutic levels are reached in 5 to 7 days.
3. Maintenance daily dose is one fourth to one third of TDD divided into a morning and evening dose (mg/kg/24 hr in one or two daily doses): premature (0.005 mg/kg/24 hr), newborn (0.005-0.010 mg/kg/24 hr), infants less than 2 years (0.010-0.012 mg/kg/24 hr), children older than 2 years (0.008-0.010 mg/kg/24 hr), and adults (0.125-0.375 mg/24 hr).
4. Therapeutic level: 1-2.0 ng/ml
   a. Infants and children may not show toxicity until levels of 4 ng/ml are reached; some require this level for therapeutic effect.
   b. Obtain levels 4 hours after IV dose and 8 hours after PO dose.
   c. Variability exists among laboratories and the individual toxic level in a specific patient.

Other Considerations

1. The dose of digoxin should be reduced in the presence of myocarditis, pulmonary hypertension, decreased renal function, electrolyte abnormalities, hypoxia, and acidosis. Digoxin is contraindicated in IHSS and tetralogy of Fallot.
2. Pulse and rhythm strips should be obtained before each parenteral dose until therapeutic levels are achieved. Normal ECG findings associated with therapeutic digoxin include T wave depression, ST segment depression (scooped), and prolongation of PR interval.

Toxicity

The range between the optimal therapeutic dose and toxicity is relatively narrow. Factors that predispose to toxicity caused by *high serum digoxin levels* include decreased renal excretion (premature infant, renal disease), hypothyroidism, high dosage, and drug interaction (quinidine, verapamil). *Increased sensitivity of the myocardium* results from an altered myocardium (ischemia, myocarditis), hypokalemia, hypercalcemia, hypoxemia, alkalosis, sympathomimetic drugs, and a postoperative state.

The *signs of toxicity* are diverse:

1. Dysrhythmias (see Chapter 6)
   a. Bradycardia (infant <80 to 90/min, child <60 to 70/min, and older child and adult <50 to 60/min)
   b. Atrioventricular (AV) dissociation with second- and third-degree block
   c. Premature ventricular complex (PVC)
   d. Ventricular bigeminy
   e. Paroxysmal atrial tachycardia (PAT) with block
2. Vomiting, nausea, and decreased intake
3. Blurring of vision (rare in children)

Treatment of toxicity is as follows:

1. Discontinue the drug, which has a half-life of 24 to 36 hours.
2. Give an infusion of D5W with 40 to 80 mEq KCl/L at a rate of 0.3 mEq KCl/kg/hr IV with close monitoring. Do not use if second- or third-degree block is present.

3. Give atropine, 0.01-0.02 mg/kg/dose (minimum: 0.1 mg/dose; maximum: 0.6 mg/dose) IV, for severe bradycardia.
4. Dysrhythmias (see Chapter 6).
   a. Give phenytoin, 1 mg/kg/dose IV over 1 to 2 minutes, which may be repeated every 5 minutes up to a total dose of 5 mg/kg. Hypocontractility may develop.
   b. Lidocaine and propranolol are sometimes helpful.
      NOTE: These drugs depress the myocardium and aggravate failure and must be used carefully.
   c. Digoxin-specific Fab antibody fragments are useful in life threatening situations. There is little experience with children, and cardiology consultation is advised.

Inotropic Agents: Shock (see Chapter 5)

CHF is often accompanied by cardiogenic shock and low output states requiring aggressive management. Evaluation of fluid status is mandatory before initiating therapy.

1. A *fluid* push may improve cardiac output by increasing filling pressure, particularly if the PCWP is 15 to 20 mm Hg or less; 0.9% NS (normal saline) solution at 5 ml/kg over 30 minutes may be administered with careful monitoring of response.
2. *Pressor* agents are usually necessary with an inadequate response to fluid challenge. The agents of choice (see Table 5-2) are the following:
   a. Dopamine administered by continuous IV infusion at a rate of 5-20 µg/kg/min up to 40 µg/kg/min (the higher infusion), the latter only if an α-blocking agent is used simultaneously; or
   b. Dobutamine by continuous IV infusion at a rate of 2-20 µg/kg/min (usually 10-15 µg/kg/min). Patients may respond to a low dosage of 0.5 µg/kg/min, but others require 40 µg/kg/min.

Dobutamine is more effective in children older than 12 months of age.
   c. Low dosage of dopamine (2-5 µg/kg/min) to maintain renal flow combined with inotropic dosage of dobutamine.

Pulmonary Edema (see Chapter 19)

1. Airway and ventilation require immediate attention.
   a. Administer oxygen at 3-6 L/min by mask or nasal cannula.
   b. Determine the need for intubation and mechanical ventilation. Intubation is indicated for the patient receiving supplemental oxygen with Fio_2 of 50% if Pao_2 is below 50 mm Hg (sea level) and known cyanotic heart disease is not present. Other indications for intubation with ventilation include a $Paco_2$ above 50 mm Hg (without preexisting disease), decreasing vital capacity, severe acidosis, and progressive disease or fatigue.
   c. If intubation is indicated, initiate positive end-expiratory pressure (PEEP) at 4 to 6 cm H_2O if severe pulmonary edema is present. Titrate upward as necessary, monitoring ABGs to maximize Pao_2 without decreasing cardiac output.
2. *Fluid* resuscitation. Fluids (D5W) should be used to maintain urine output, administered at 0.5 ml/kg/hr after stabilization of intravascular volume. Although fluids usually can be maintained at about 60% of normal maintenance, this must be individualized for each patient. Observe for renal failure (p. 809) and fluid overload.
3. *Diuretics* (Table 16-3). In the acute situation, use furosemide (Lasix), 1 mg/kg/dose up to 6 mg/kg/dose q8-12hr IV. May be repeated q2hr if indicated. Do not use if anuria is present.
4. *Morphine* sulfate lowers the PCWP and relieves anxiety.

TABLE 16-3 Diuretics

Drug	Availability	Route	Frequency	Dosage Initial	Maximum	Onset of action	Comments/site of action
Chlorothiazide (Diuril)	Solution: 50 mg/ml Tablet: 250, 500 mg	PO	q8-12hr	10 mg/kg/24 hr	20 mg/kg/24 hr (2 gm/24 hr)	1-2 hr	↓ K⁺, ↓ Na⁺, alkalosis, hyperglycemia; distal tubule
Hydrochlo-rothiazide (HydroDiuril)	Tablet: 25, 50, 100 mg	PO	q8-12hr	1 mg/kg/24 hr	2 mg/kg/24 hr (200 mg/24 hr)	1-2 hr	↓ K⁺, ↓ Na⁺, alkalosis, hyperglycemia; distal tubule
Furosemide (Lasix)	Ampule: 10 mg/ml Solution: 10 mg/ml Tablet: 20, 40 mg	IV, IM / PO	q6-12hr / q6-12hr	1 mg/kg/dose / 1-3 mg/kg/dose	6 mg/kg/dose / 6 mg/kg/dose	5-15 min / 30-60 min	↓ K⁺, ↓ Na⁺, alkalosis, deafness; may give more often; ascending loop of Henle
Spironolactone (Aldactone)	Tablet: 25 mg	PO	q8-12hr	1 mg/kg/24 hr	3 mg/kg/24 hr (200 mg/24 hr)	3-5 days	↑ K⁺, ↓ Na⁺; useful as adjunct, not alone; aldosterone antago-nist; collecting tubule
Mannitol	Vial: (250 mg/ml) 25%	IV (slow)		0.5 gm/kg/dose	2.0 gm/kg/dose	10-30 min	Reduced intracranial pressure
Acetazolamide (Diamox)	Vial: 500 mg Tablet: 125, 250 mg	IV / PO	q6-24hr	5 mg/kg/24 hr	8 mg/kg/24 hr	1-6 hr	Carbonic anhydrase inhibitor; hyper-chloremic acidosis
Metolazone (Zaroxolyn)	Tablet: 2.5, 5, 10 mg	PO	q24hr	0.2 mg/kg/24 hr	0.4 mg/kg/24 hr (adult: 10 mg/24 hr)	1-2 hr	Useful when marked ↓ glomerular filtration rate; no experience in children; renal tubule
Bumetanide (Bumex)	Tablet: 0.5, 1, 2 mg	PO	q12-24hr	0.015-0.1 mg/kg/dose	0.5-2 mg/dose (max: 10 mg/24 hr)		Limited experience in children; side effects: cramps, dizziness, ↓ K⁺, ↓ Ca⁺⁺, ↓ Na⁺, encephalopathy; 40 mg furosemide comparable to 1 mg bumetanide; cross-allergenicity to sulfonamides
	Vial: 0.25 mg/kg	IV	q8-12hr	0.1 mg/kg dose	0.5-1 mg/dose over 1-2 min (max: 10 mg/24 hr)		

a. In severe pulmonary edema with CHF, 0.1-0.2 mg/kg IV should be administered slowly.

b. Respirations may be depressed. Do not give if there is evidence of unstable vital signs, intracranial hemorrhage, chronic pulmonary disease, asthma, or narcotic withdrawal.

c. *Bronchodilators* are indicated if there is wheezing or evidence of broncho-constriction (p. 769).

VOLUME OVERLOAD

Reducing the volume and cardiac preload may be beneficial if the PCWP and CVP can be maintained. Fluids and diuretics, as outlined in the previous section, must be cautiously monitored to provide the best balance between volume status and cardiac function. In patients with volume overload and renal failure, peritoneal dialysis has been used successfully.

PRESSURE OVERLOAD (see Table 18-2)

Afterload reduction may be useful if there is an inadequate response to digoxin, diuretics, pressors, and fluid management. Agents that diminish afterload by decreasing peripheral resistance may improve cardiac output. Pharmacologic reduction of afterload should be used only with indwelling arterial monitoring and a Swan-Ganz catheter in place; it usually is deferred until admission to the ICU.

1. Sodium nitroprusside (Nipride) dilates systemic veins.
   a. Dosage: 0.5-10 µg/kg/min IV by infusion. Begin with an infusion rate of 0.1 µg/kg/min and increase until the desired response is achieved. The average therapeutic dosage is about 3 µg/kg/min.
   b. The clinical response is noted in 1 to 2 minutes and lasts 5 to 10 minutes after stopping the infusion. Do not use in presence of renal failure.

2. Nitroglycerine dilates the systemic veins and is occasionally useful for patients taking digoxin and diuretics who have severe CHF and pulmonary edema, particularly if these are secondary to aortic or mitral regurgitation.
   a. Dosage for sublingual administration has not been established for children (nor is there adequate experience); administration must be titrated against clinical response. The adult dosage is 0.15 to 0.6 mg q5min sublingually up to a maximum of three doses in a 15-minute period. May be routinely repeated in 1 to 2 hours. Onset of action is 1 to 2 minutes, lasting 30 minutes.
   b. IV nitroglycerine (Nitrostat) has been used effectively in adults. In adults the infusion is usually begun at 5 µg/min with increments of 5 µg/min q3-5min until a therapeutic response is noted. Suggested pediatric dosage is not defined.
   c. Other pharmacologic options include captopril (Capoten), hydralazine (Apresoline), and prazosin (Minipress) (see Table 18-2).

DYSRHYTHMIAS (see Chapter 6)

Dysrhythmias require urgent attention. Brady-rhythmias are primarily secondary to slowing of the intrinsic pacemaker or a conduction defect; tachyrhythmias result from ectopic pacemakers or reentrant pathways.

Other Considerations

1. *Sedation* may be essential in the anxious patient. If morphine sulfate is not used because of concern for depression of respiration, chloral hydrate, 20 mg/kg/dose PO up to 50 mg/kg/24 hr, or phenobarbital, 2-3 mg/kg/dose PO, IV, or IM up to q8hr, may be used.

2. *Anemia* should be treated if significant (hematocrit [Hct] <20%) to improve oxygenation. Give 5-10 ml/kg of packed red blood cells (RBCs) over 4 to 8 hours with careful monitoring. An exchange transfusion may need to be considered.

3. *Premature* infants with CHF secondary to large patent ductus arteriosus (PDA) may respond to indomethacin, 0.1-0.2 mg/kg administered q12hr up to a maximum dose of 0.6 mg/kg IV, after consultation with a cardiologist to exclude a ductal-dependent lesion.

   Closure of the PDA in coarctation of the aorta or other ductal-dependent lesion may produce severe CHF, requiring immediate intervention. Dilation of the PDA to maintain patency may be achieved by prostaglandin E_1 0.05-0.1 µg/kg/min IV infusion in consultation with a cardiologist.

4. *Surgery* may occasionally be required on an emergent basis where the lesion is amenable to surgical correction and medical management is unsuccessful, such as PDA, total anomalous pulmonary venous return, transposition of the great vessels, pulmonic stenosis, aortic stenosis, ventricular septal defect, atrioventricular canal, and coarctation of the aorta.

5. Unresponsive patients should have immediate cardiology and cardiac surgery (if appropriate) consultations. Other entities that require consideration include the following:

   a. Reactivation of rheumatic heart disease or concurrent infection (endocarditis, pericarditis, pneumonia, urinary tract infection)

   b. Electrolyte abnormality: hypochloremic alkalosis, hypokalemia, hyponatremia

   c. Digitalis toxicity (pp. 150 and 375)

   d. Dysrhythmias (see Chapter 6)

   e. Pulmonary embolism (p. 568)

DISPOSITION

Patients with CHF should be admitted to the hospital for immediate therapy. Those with moderate or severe disease require monitoring in an ICU with appropriate expertise and equipment. Rarely, patients with mild, slowly progressive or chronic CHF and pulmonary edema of known cause may be relatively asymptomatic and respond to an oral digitalizing regimen over 5 to 7 days as outpatients, if compliance and appropriate follow-up observation can be arranged.

A cardiologist should be involved with all patients to ensure follow-up attention. Most patients require digoxin and diuretic therapy on a long-term basis.

REFERENCES

Park MK: Use of digoxin in infants and children with specific emphasis on dosage, *J Pediatr* 108:871, 1986.

Rheuban KS, Carpenter MA, Ayers CA, et al: Audi hemodynamic effects of converting enzyme inhibition in infants with congestive heart failure, *J Pediatr* 117:668, 1990.

Smith TW: Digitalis: mechanisms of action and clinical use, *N Engl J Med* 318:358, 1988.

Smith TW, Butler VP, Haber E, et al: Treatment of life-threatening digitalis intoxication with digoxin-specific Fab antibody fragments, *N Engl J Med* 307:1357, 1982.

Talner NS: Heart failure. In Emmanouilides AC, Riemenschneider TA, Allen HD, et al, editors: *Heart disease in infants, children, and adolescents,* ed 5, Baltimore, 1995, Williams & Wilkins.

17 CYANOSIS

ALERT: Impaired ventilation or perfusion on the basis of cardiac or pulmonary abnormality is very common. Pending evaluation, oxygen should be administered and airway and ventilation stabilized.

Cyanosis results from decreased oxygenation of the blood. For it to be clinically apparent, there must be at least 5 gm of reduced hemoglobin per deciliter (Hb/dl). Because of the increased affinity of fetal hemoglobin for oxygen, the infant may have hypoxia without cyanosis. Cyanosis is most evident where the epidermis is relatively thin, pigmentation minimal, and capillaries abundant (tips of finger and toes, under the nail beds, and buccal mucosa).

Central cyanosis involves cyanosis of the tongue, mucosal membranes, and peripheral skin. It may be caused by the following:

1. Decreased pulmonary and alveolar ventilation with impaired oxygen intake
2. Decreased pulmonary perfusion
3. An abnormal hemoglobin (Methemoglobin produces cyanosis when it represents more than 15% of the total hemoglobin. It should be considered when there is a history of exposure or of central cyanosis that does not respond to oxygen and congenital heart disease is not suspected.)

The history should focus on potential contributing conditions. Congenital heart, lung, or gastrointestinal (GI) disease should be excluded in the patient and family. The pattern of onset of cyanosis and respiratory distress may be distinct, as may those factors that exacerbate the finding. Recent fever, infection, shortness of breath, trauma, foreign body ingestion, and neurologic changes should be sought.

The physical examination must assess cardiovascular stability, as well as seeking clues to the etiology.

Evaluation for central cyanosis should include oximetry, arterial blood gas (ABG) analysis, chest x-ray film, complete blood count (CBC), and electrocardiogram (ECG), as well as other studies related to the differential possibilities (see Chapter 13). In addition, the response to

Text continued on p. 160

	Pulmonary disease (ventilation)		Heart disease (perfusion)	
	Room air	**100% O$_2$**	**Room air**	**100% O$_2$**
Color	Blue	Pinker	Blue	Blue
Pao$_2$ (mm Hg)	35	120 (range: 60-250)	35 or less	Little change
Saturation	60%	99%	60%	62%

TABLE 17-1 Central Cyanosis: Diagnostic Considerations

Condition	Mechanism	Respiratory pattern	Response to 100% O₂	Ancillary data	Comments
VASCULAR: CARDIAC (Chapter 16)					
Congenital heart disease*					
↓ *Pulmonary blood flow (PBF)*	↓ perfusion	RR 20-50/min	Little	ABG: ↓ Pao_2, ↓↑ pH CXR: ↓ PBF, ↑ heart ECG: Variable Hypoglycemia	R → L shunt; prostaglandin E may be helpful
Pulmonary vascular obstruction					
Pulmonary atresia					
Pulmonary stenosis					
Tetralogy of Fallot					
Tricuspid atresia					
Transposition with pulmonary stenosis					
↑ *Pulmonary blood flow*		RR 30-60/min	Little	ABG: ↓ Pao_2, ↑↓ pH CXR: ↑ PBF, ↑ heart ECG: Variable Hypoglycemia	R → L shunt
Transposition of great vessels					
Total anomalous venous return					
Truncus arteriosus					
Hypoplastic L heart					
Congestive heart failure	↓ alveolar ventilation, perfusion	RR 40-120/min	Moderate	ABG: ↓ Pao_2, ↓ pH, ↓↑ $Paco_2$ CXR: ↑ PBF, variable pulmonary edema, ↑ heart ECG: Variable	
Pulmonary edema (Chapter 19)	↓ alveolar ventilation	RR 40-120/min	Moderate	ABG: ↓ Pao_2, ↓↑ pH, ↑ $Paco_2$ CXR: Interstitial infiltrate ECG: Variable	Variable associated CHF
Shock (Chapter 5)	↓ perfusion	RR 20-80/min	Good	ABG: ↓ Pao_2, ↓ pH, ↑↓ $Paco_2$ CXR: Variable	Associated conditions

VASCULAR: PULMONARY

Condition	Mechanism	Clinical	Distress	Diagnosis	Comments
Pulmonary hemorrhage	↓ alveolar perfusion	RR 30-60/min	Moderate	ABG: ↓ Pao_2, ↑↓ pH, ↑↓ $Paco_2$; CXR: Abnormal; ECG: WNL or RVH	May shunt
Pulmonary embolism (p. 568) Persistent fetal circulation (newborn) (Chapter 11)	↓ perfusion	RR 30-60/min	None	ABG: ↓ Pao_2, ↑↓ pH, ↑ $Paco_2$; CXR: Variable; ECG: Variable	R → L shunt
Pulmonary AV fistula Pulmonary hypertension Vascular ring	↓ ventilation	Stridor, retraction	Good	ABG: ↓ Pao_2, ↑ $Paco_2$; CXR: Hyperexpansion; ECG: WNL or RVH	Barium swallow or bronchoscopy may be useful Catheterization

VASCULAR: CNS HEMORRHAGE (Chapters 18 and 57)

Condition	Mechanism	Clinical	Distress	Diagnosis	Comments
Subdural Intracranial	↓ ventilation	RR <20/min, apnea, seizures	Moderate	ABG: ↓ Pao_2, ↑ $Paco_2$; CXR, ECG: WNL	Associated CNS findings

INTOXICATION (Chapter 54)

Condition	Mechanism	Clinical	Distress	Diagnosis	Comments
Nitrates Nitrites } Well water, vegetables Aniline dyes Sulfonamides	Methemoglobinemia	Little distress unless >50%	None	ABG, CXR, ECG: WNL Methemoglobin high in blood; chocolate color when exposed to air	Rx: Methylene blue 1-2 mg (0.1-0.2 ml)/kg/dose IV over 5-15 min
Carbon monoxide (p. 371)	Displacement of O_2 by CO	RR 30-60/min	Good	Carboxyhemoglobin level	May have CNS symptoms, pulmonary edema Rx: 100% O_2

CXR, Chest x-ray; RVH, right ventricular hypertrophy.
*Complex heart lesions may have variable pulmonary blood flow.

Continued

TABLE 17-1 Central Cyanosis: Diagnostic Considerations—cont'd

Condition	Mechanism	Respiratory pattern	Response to 100% O_2	Ancillary data	Comments
INFECTION/INFLAMMATION					
Lower airway disease (Chapter 20)	↓ alveolar ventilation, perfusion	RR 30-120/min, flaring, grunting, wheezing	Moderate	ABG: ↓ Pao_2, ↓ pH, ↓ $Paco_2$ CXR: Abnormal ECG: WNL or RVH	Some shunting; also see asthma below
Pneumonia (p. 794)					
Bronchiolitis					
Emphysema					
Hyaline membrane disease (Chapter 11)					
Bronchopulmonary dysplasia (Chapter 11)					
Atelectasis					
Aspiration					
Cystic fibrosis					
Upper airway disease (Chapter 20)	↓ ventilation	Stridor, retraction	Good	ABG: ↓ Pao_2, ↑↓ pH, ↓ $Paco_2$	
Croup (p. 784)					
Epiglottitis					
Retropharyngeal abscess (p. 608)					
Meningitis (p. 725)	↓ perfusion ↓ ventilation	RR 10-80/min	Good	ABG: ↓ Pao_2, ↓ pH, ↑↓ $Paco_2$	
DEGENERATIVE					
CNS: Seizures Progressive disease	↓ ventilation	RR 10-30/min, apnea, seizures	Good	ABG: ↓ Pao_2, ↓ pH, ↑ $Paco_2$	Associated CNS findings
ALLERGIC					
Asthma (p. 765) Anaphylaxis (Chapter 12)	↓ ventilation ↓ alveolar ventilation	RR 40-80/min, flaring, wheezing, coughing	Good	ABG: ↓ Pao_2, ↑↓ pH, ↑↓ $Paco_2$ CXR: Variable	Also see infection/inflammation, lower airway disease, above

Condition	Mechanism	Clinical	Compensation	Diagnosis	Treatment
TRAUMA (Chapter 62)					
Upper airway foreign body (p. 791)	↓ ventilation	Stridor, retraction	Good	ABG: ↓ Pao_2, ↑↓ pH, ↑ $Paco_2$; CXR: Lateral neck positive result	
Lower airway Pneumothorax Drowning (Chapter 47) Contusion	↓ ventilation ↓ alveolar ventilation	RR 30-120/min, flaring	Good	ABG: ↓ Pao_2, ↑ $Paco_2$; CXR: Abnormal	
Cardiac	↓ perfusion	RR 20-80/min	Good	ABG: ↓ Pao_2, ↓ pH; CXR: Variable; ECG: Variable	
INTRAPSYCHIC					
Breath holding (p. 724)	↓ ventilation	RR 0-10/min	Moderate	ABG: ↓ Pao_2, ↑ $Paco_2$	Self-limited
CONGENITAL (Chapters 11 and 20)					
Hereditary hemoglobinemia	Methemoglobinemia	Little distress unless >50%	None	ABG, CXR, ECG: WNL Methemoglobin high in blood; chocolate color when exposed to air	Rx: Methylene blue 1-2 mg (0.1-0.2 ml)/kg/dose IV over 5-15 min
Diaphragmatic hernia Atresia nasal choanal Macroglossia Hypoplastic mandible Tracheolaryngomalacia	↓ ventilation	RR 30-80/min	Good	ABG: ↓ Pao_2, ↑↓ pH, ↑ $Paco_2$; CXR: Abnormal; ECG: WNL or RVH	Requires surgery

100% oxygen should be measured by comparing ABG in room air and during the administration of high-flow oxygen (see p. 155). This assists in differentiating primarily cardiac disease resulting from major shunting and decreased perfusion from pulmonary disease, which has primarily ventilation deficits (Table 17-1).

Tetralogy of Fallot hypoxemic spells may cause sudden onset or deepening of cyanosis, dyspnea, alterations in consciousness, and decreased intensity of the systolic murmur. These episodes usually begin in the neonatal period. Treatment consists of providing oxygen, attending to the ABCs (airway, breathing, and circulation), and placing the child in the knee-chest position. Acidosis should be corrected. Sedation with morphine sulfate, 0.1 mg/kg/dose IV, is helpful, as well as providing hemodynamic changes. Pharmacologic agents that should be considered include the following:

1. Propranolol: 0.05-0.1 mg/kg/dose IV (maximum: 0.1 mg/kg/dose not to exceed 1 mg/dose).
2. Esmolol (ultrashort β blocker): initial bolus 0.5-1.0 mg/kg IV followed by infusion of 100-300 μg/kg/min.
3. Phenylephrine: initial bolus 10-50 μg/kg/min. May repeat and double bolus to a maximum total bolus of 50 μg/kg/min. Follow by continuous infusion of 1-10 μg/kg/min. Avoid digitalis preparations.

Peripheral cyanosis is accompanied by a bluish discoloration of the skin caused by increased arterial-venous oxygen differences, with normal arterial saturation. It has a vascular origin:

1. Vasomotor instability
   a. Common in newborns, particularly with temperature changes, sepsis, or metabolic abnormalities
   b. May be related to sepsis in older children
2. Capillary stasis or venous pooling
3. Raynaud phenomenon
4. Hematologic
   a. Polycythemia
      (1) Congenital heart disease or chronic hypoxia
      (2) Maternal-fetal transfusion or twin-twin transfusion
   b. Hyperviscosity
5. Harlequin color changes (Half of body becomes pale or acutely reddened. This lasts only a few minutes and is not physiologically significant.)

REFERENCES

Driscoll DJ: Evaluation of the cyanotic newborn, *Pediatr Clin North Am* 37:1, 1990.

Kulick RM: Pulse oximetry, *Pediatr Emerg Care* 3:127, 1987.

Martin L, Khalil H: How much reduced hemoglobin is necessary to generate central cyanosis? *Chest* 97(1):182, 1990.

18   HYPERTENSION

The definition of high blood pressure in children is relative to the age and size of the patient. In adults, diastolic blood pressures of 90 to 104 mm Hg are considered mild elevations, 105 to 114 mm Hg as moderate, above 114 mg mm Hg as severe, and diastolic pressure of 129 mm Hg malignant. Children are considered hypertensive if they are at or above the 95th percentile for their age, unless they have excessive height or lean body mass for that age. Two classes of hypertension are further defined: significant, between the 95th and 99th percentiles, and severe, at or above the 99th percentile. These measurements should be obtained on at least three occasions.

Hypertensive crisis occurs with a severe sudden increase in blood pressure without end-organ damage. The diastolic blood pressure may rise to 140 mm Hg or more, with a corresponding rise in systolic pressure to 250 mm Hg or more (values for an adolescent or adult). These potentially life-threatening episodes may result from acute glomerulonephritis, head injury, drug reaction, pheochromocytoma, toxemia, or pregnancy. Commonly the result is an accelerated phase of poorly controlled chronic hypertension.

Hypertensive emergencies have associated symptoms affecting the central nervous system (CNS) (confusion, visual problems, seizures), heart (congestive heart failure [CHF]), or kidneys. *Malignant and accelerated hypertension* implies severe hypertension with progressive end-organ damage.

Assessment of a child's blood pressure requires the use of an appropriately sized cuff, based on the size of the inner inflatable bladder. The cuff should be long enough to encircle the arm completely (with or without overlap) and wide enough to cover about 75% of the upper arm between the top of the shoulder and the olecranon. A cuff that is too narrow will show a false elevation of blood pressure; a cuff that is too wide will give a low reading. Commonly available blood pressure cuffs include the following:

Cuff name	Age	Bladder width (cm)	Bladder length (cm)
Newborn	Newborn	2.5-4.0	5.0-9.0
Infant	6 mo	4.0-9.0	11.5-18.0
Child	1-10 yr	7.5-9.0	17.0-19.0
Adult	>10 yr	11.5-13.0	22.0-26.0

Measurement by auscultation, palpation, flush, and Doppler methods is useful, the last being particularly important for the young infant. Normal values for diastolic and systolic blood pressures vary with age (see Appendix B-2).

ETIOLOGY

Hypertension in children less than 12 years old usually is associated with anatomic abnormality; older children more commonly have essential hypertension. Conditions suggesting an increased risk for hypertension in infants include abdominal bruit or mass, coarctation of the aorta, congenital adrenal hyperplasia, neurofibromatosis, failure to thrive, history of indwelling umbilical artery catheter, unexplained heart failure or seizure, or renal disease.

Hypertension in *neonates* most commonly is caused by coarctation of the aorta, renal artery

Box 18-1
COMMON CAUSES OF HYPERTENSION IN CHILDREN

RENAL PARENCHYMAL DISEASE

1. Glomerulonephritis
2. Pyelonephritis
3. Henoch-Schönlein purpura (nephritis)
4. Hemolytic-uremic syndrome
5. Polycystic kidney disease
6. Dysplastic kidney
7. Obstructive uropathy
8. Autoimmune process: systemic lupus erythematosus, other vasculitides

RENAL VASCULAR DISEASE

1. Arterial anomalies or thrombosis, especially in newborns
2. Venous anomalies or thrombosis

VASCULAR DISEASE

1. Coarctation of the aorta
2. Renal artery stenosis
3. Vasculitis
4. Aortic or mitral insufficiency

NEUROLOGIC DISEASE

1. Encephalitis
2. Brain tumor
3. Dysautonomia
4. Guillain-Barré syndrome
5. Stress, including major burns

ENDOCRINE DISEASE

1. Pheochromocytoma
2. Steroid therapy—Cushing disease, congenital adrenal hyperplasia, birth control pills
3. Hyperthyroidism
4. Neuroblastoma

INTOXICATION—lead, mercury, amphetamine, cocaine, LSD, licorice, steroids

ESSENTIAL HYPERTENSION

thrombosis, renal artery stenosis, congenital renal malformations, bronchopulmonary dysplasia, and intracranial hemorrhage. Underlying conditions causing hypertension in children *less than 6 years* of age include renal parenchymal disease (cystic, hydronephrosis, pyelonephritis, and Wilms' tumor), renal artery stenosis, or coarctation of the aorta. Those *6 to 10 years* may have renal artery stenosis, renal parenchymal disease (cystic, pyelonephritis), and primary hypertension. *Older* children may have renal parenchymal disease (cystic, pyelonephritis, glomerulonephritis, and collagen) or essential, primary hypertension.

A systematic approach is required to determine the cause and achieve control. Many entities that cause mild hypertension on a chronic or transient basis are outlined in Box 18-1.

DIAGNOSTIC FINDINGS

It often is difficult to define juvenile hypertension and to distinguish children with this disorder from normotensive children. When a blood pressure measurement is stipulated, the average of at least two measurements should be used. Appendix B-2 may be used as a guide in approaching children with hypertension.

In the medical history, it is essential to focus on any family history of hypertension, preeclampsia, toxemia, renal disease, tumor, complicated neonatal history, headaches, dizziness, epistaxis, joint pain, edema, weight loss, weakness, abnormal menses, or drug ingestion.

The physical examination may indicate underlying renal, endocrine, or genetic disease, as well as cardiovascular, abdominal, retinal, or neurologic abnormalities (Box 18-2).

Box 18-2

SIGNS AND SYMPTOMS OF HYPERTENSIVE PATIENT

CAUSE	SIGNS AND SYMPTOMS
Pheochromocytoma	Flushing, palpitations, diarrhea, tachycardia
Renal	Poor growth, fever, UTI, edema, hematuria, proteinuria, trauma, family history
Congenital adrenal hyperplasia	Virilization
Cushing syndrome	Striae, moon facies, truncal obesity
Coarctation of the aorta	Heart murmur, decreased femoral pulse or leg BP, abdominal bruit
Chronic hypertension	Funduscopic changes, Bell's palsy, stroke, CHF, cardiomegaly

Ancillary Data

1. Hematologic: complete blood count (CBC) (hemolytic anemia, thrombocytopenia), elevated erythrocyte sedimentation rate (ESR)
2. Chemical evaluation: elevated blood urea nitrogen (BUN) and creatinine levels; electrolytes and PO_4^{--} consistent with renal function; uric acid; fasting cholesterol, triglycerides, high-density lipoprotein cholesterol, and calculated low-density lipoprotein cholesterol
3. Urinalysis: microscopic hematuria, proteinuria, and red blood cell (RBC) casts (see Chapter 85)
4. Chest x-ray film: cardiomegaly and left ventricular hypertrophy; possibly pulmonary edema
5. Electrocardiogram (ECG): left ventricular hypertrophy
6. Studies indicated to evaluate specific diagnostic considerations, including radiologic and radioisotope (intravenous pyelography, ultrasonography, angiography, computed tomography) and hormonal studies (e.g., quantitation of urine or plasma catecholamines and metabolites, urinary aldosterone, and electrolytes)

Malignant Hypertension

Malignant or accelerated hypertension is a subacute, accelerated phase of blood pressure elevation accompanied by retinopathy. Common underlying disorders include acute glomerulonephritis, hemolytic-uremic syndrome, obstructive uropathy, pyelonephritis, and other causes of hypertension.

Blood pressure should be brought under control in hours to days to prevent complications, including encephalopathy, intracranial hemorrhage, acute left ventricular failure, or renal failure.

Diagnostic Findings

Headaches are common, classically described as constant, occipital, and most severe in the morning. Blurred vision, dizziness, anorexia, nausea, vomiting, and weight loss are common. Retinal hemorrhages, exudate, and papilledema often are present. Cardiomegaly is common. Neurologically, patients are normal but persistent focal deficits may develop.

Ancillary data as indicated may be useful.

Hypertensive Cerebrovascular Syndromes

Hypertension associated with mental status changes may be caused by a number of cerebrovascular events that have a pathognomonic presentation and require rapid control of blood pressure. The decision to lower blood pressure must be individualized and may be accomplished by a variety of modalities.

1. Hypertensive encephalopathy
   a. Associated with rapid increase of blood pressure
   b. Gradual onset over 24 to 48 hours
   c. Variable neurologic findings: confusion, apprehension, and lethargy, progressing to stupor and coma, seizures, and hemiparesis
   d. Headache, nausea, vomiting, and anorexia concomitantly with progression of mental status deterioration; visual blurring with transient blindness may be accompanied by retinal hemorrhages, exudates, and papilledema
   NOTE: Patients respond dramatically to a decrease in diastolic blood pressure less than 100 mm Hg (adolescent or adult values).
2. Intracerebral hemorrhage
   a. Rapid onset with loss of consciousness, hemiplegia, and sensory loss
   b. Often accompanied by headache, nausea, and vomiting
   c. Focal neurologic findings usually fixed
3. Subarachnoid hemorrhage
   a. Rapid onset of a violent headache, with initial pain localized. Most patients have a stiff neck and progress to loss of consciousness; often have unequal pupils and variable, transient focal neurologic findings.
   b. Spinal fluid is usually bloody.
4. Trauma: head or neck (see Chapter 57)
5. Neoplasm

Other Presentations

1. Left ventricular failure with pulmonary edema (see Chapters 16 and 19).
2. Dissection of leaking aortic aneurysm.
3. Pheochromocytoma.

4. Monoamine oxidase (MAO) inhibitors. Patients taking MAO inhibitors should not use alcohol and ripened cheeses (Brie, cheddar, Camembert, and Stilton) because these contain tyramine, which might produce an acute catecholamine release.
5. Emergency surgery on individuals with uncontrolled hypertension may exacerbate hypertension. Anesthesia and postoperative care must be individualized for these patients.
6. Intoxication (see Table 54-1): sympathomimetics (amphetamine), hallucinogens (PCP, LSD), heavy metals.
7. Toxemia of pregnancy with maternal convulsions, left ventricular failure, or fetal distress.

MANAGEMENT

All patients must be evaluated rapidly to consider the acuteness of the rise in blood pressure, preexisting medical problems, potential etiologic factors, clinical factors related to the blood pressure, and compliance with medications.

The patient's hemodynamic status must be evaluated by measuring orthostatic blood pressure changes and the potential impact on cardiac, cerebral, and renal perfusion.

Mild Hypertension

For the patient with only mild hypertension without evidence of crisis, a slow, sequential, *stepped-care* approach is appropriate.

1. *Nonpharmacologic therapy*
   a. Weight reduction, if patient is obese
   b. Exercise and conditioning
   c. Dietary modification (sodium intake 1.5-2.0 mEq/kg/24 hr)
2. *Pharmacologic therapy* is indicated when the blood pressure is between the 90th and 95th percentiles for age and sex, when there is evidence of target organ injury, or when symptoms or signs related

to elevated blood pressure are present. The goals of the stepped-care approach to therapy are as follows:

a. Lower diastolic BP below the 90th percentile

b. Minimize side effects

c. Minimize drugs used to maximize patient compliance

Ultimately, the choice of agents depends on urgency of treatment, knowledge of agents, availability of monitoring equipment, and source of long-term follow-up.

Step 1: Initiate a thiazide-type diuretic at a low dosage, which may be increased to full dosage. In adolescents and young adults with hyperkinetic hypertension (rapid pulse), a β blocker may be preferable if the patient is neither diabetic nor asthmatic. Loop diuretics (furosemide) should be reserved for patients with impaired renal function (<50%).

a. Hydrochlorothiazide (HydroDiuril), 1 mg/kg/24 hr q12hr PO; or

b. Chlorothiazide (Diuril), 10 mg/kg/24 hr q12hr PO

c. Spironolactone (Aldactone), 1-3 mg/kg/24 hr q6-12hr PO, if potassium losses are not compensated by supplements and diet and if additional diuresis is needed

Step 2: If the BP is still not controlled, add an β-adrenergic inhibitor at small dose and slowly increase to maximal dose. Do not use if CHF or asthma is present.

a. Propranolol (Inderal), 0.5-3 mg/kg/dose q6hr PO. Another increasingly used alternative is labetalol, 0.4-1.0 mg/kg IV slow push, which may be repeated up to three times (up to 3 mg/kg) in the first hour of management. Nifedipine, 0.25-0.5 mg/kg, may also be used, often given sublingually or by biting into a capsule (see p. 166).

b. Another β blocker that is used extensively in *adults* and more recently in children is

TABLE 18-1   Agent of Choice in Hypertensive Crisis

Hypertensive crisis	Agent of choice	Contraindicated agents
Malignant (accelerated) hypertension	Nitroprusside, diazoxide	Reserpine (causes sedation)
Primary renal disease	Nitroprusside, labetalol, diazoxide	Trimethaphan (decreases renal flow), β agonists
Encephalopathy	Nitroprusside, labetalol, diazoxide	Trimethaphan (dilates pupils), β agonist Reserpine/methyldopa (causes sedation)
Head injury	Nitroprusside	Reserpine/methyldopa (causes sedation) Trimethaphan (dilates pupils) Diazoxide (causes hypotension), β agonists
Acute left ventricular failure with pulmonary edema	Nitroprusside, labetalol, nitroglycerin	Diazoxide/hydralazine (increases cardiac output), minoxidil
Aortic dissection	Propranolol and nitroprusside*	Diazoxide/hydralazine (increases cardiac output), minoxidil
Pheochromocytoma/MAO inhibitor	Phentolamine, nitroprusside	All others
Eclampsia	Hydralazine, nitroprusside, labetalol, diazoxide, magnesium sulfate	Trimethaphan (decreases uterine flow), diuretics, β agonists

*Initiate propranolol first.

TABLE 18-2   Useful Drugs in Management of Hypertensive Emergencies

Drug	Availability	Action		Dose
		Onset	Duration	
DIURETICS		See Table 16-3		
PERIPHERAL VASODILATOR				
Sodium nitroprusside (Nipride) (arterioles and veins)	50 mg/vial for reconstitution	1-2 min	1-5 min	0.5-10 µg/kg/min IV; average: 3 µg/kg/min; initial 0.25 µg/kg/min for eclampsia and renal insufficiency
Diazoxide (Hyperstat) (arterioles)	15 mg/ml (20 ml)	3-5 min	½-12 hr	1-3 mg/kg/dose rapid push
Hydralazine (Apresoline) (arterioles)	20 mg/ml (1 ml)	10-30 min (IV)	3-6 hr	0.1-0.4 mg/kg/dose q6hr (1.7-3.5 mg/kg/24 hr) (use with propranolol)
	10, 25, 50, 100 mg			0.5-7.0 mg/kg/24 hr
Minoxidil (Loniten)	2.5, 10 mg	1 hr	4-8 hr	0.1-1.0 mg/kg/24 hr
CALCIUM CHANNEL BLOCKER				
Nifedipine (Procardia)	10, 20, 30, 60, 90 mg	5-15 min	3-5 hr	0.25-0.5 mg/kg
GANGLIONIC BLOCKERS				
Trimethaphan (Arfonad)	50 mg/ml (10 ml)	5-10 min	5-10 min	50-150 µg/kg/min
CENTRALLY ACTING				
Clonidine (Catapres)	0.1, 0.2, 0.3 mg	½-2 hr	6-8 hr	5-10 µg/kg/24 hr initial dose up to 5-25 µg/kg/24 hr q6hr PO (maximum: 0.9 mg/24 hr)
Methyldopa (Aldomet)	50 mg/ml (5 ml)	2-3 hr	4-8 hr	2.5-5 mg/kg/dose (maximum: 20-40 mg/kg/24 hr)
	125, 250, 500 mg			10 mg/kg/24 hr (maximum: 40 mg/kg/24 hr)

Frequency/route	Adult dose (>12 yr)	Advantages	Disadvantages
Continuous light-shielded IV infusion	0.5-10 µg/kg/min	Precise control; protects myocardial perfusion	Constant monitoring; light sensitive; cyanide poisoning; fatigue, nausea, disorientation
q4-24hr IV (if first dose ineffective, repeat in 30 min)	75-150 mg/dose	Prompt; no reduction of renal or coronary perfusion	$\uparrow$ HR, $\uparrow$ cardiac output, variable hypotension, hyperglycemia, sodium retention; requires close monitoring
q4-6hr IV	10-20 mg/dose (maximum: 300 mg/24 hr)	Prompt; maintains cerebral, renal, coronary perfusion	$\uparrow$ HR, $\uparrow$ cardiac output; tachyphylaxis, systemic lupus erythematosus (SLE) reactions; if sole agent, need higher dose; limited availability
q6-12hr PO	10-75 mg (maximum: 300 mg/24 hr)		
q12hr PO	10-40 mg/24 hr	Gradual decrease	Limited experience in children; fluid retention, tachycardia; often used in conjunction with propranolol and furosemide
Titrate q15-30min PO, sublingual, buccal	10-20 mg	Rapid onset	Negative inotropic effect; contraindicated in intracranial hemorrhage; variable response
Continuous IV infusion	0.5-1 mg/min	Precise control	Constant monitoring; use with dissecting aortic aneurysm; tachyphylaxis; autonomic blockage—paralysis, pupils, bladder, bowel
q12hr PO	Initial: 0.1-0.2 mg/dose Maint: 0.2-0.8 mg/24 hr	Rapid onset; oral	Little experience in children; sedation; central sympatholytic agent
q6-8hr IV	500-1000 mg/dose	Gradual decrease	Variably effective; somnolence; ulcerogenic; orthostatic hypotension; bradycardia
q6-12hr PO	250-750 mg/dose		

Continued

TABLE 18-2 Useful Drugs in Management of Hypertensive Emergencies—cont'd

| Drug | Availability | Action | | Dose |
		Onset	Duration	
CENTRALLY ACTING—cont'd				
Reserpine	0.1, 0.25 mg	2-4 hr	4-8 hr	0.01-0.02 mg/kg/dose
α-β-ADRENERGIC BLOCKER				
Propranolol (Inderal)	10, 20, 40, 80 mg	1-2 min	12 hr	0.5-3 mg/kg/dose and increase (maximum: 320 mg/24 hr)
Labetalol	5 mg/ml	5-10 min	3-6 hr	0.4-1.0 mg/kg IV slow push; repeat up to 3 mg/kg in 1 hour
Esmolol (Brevibloc)	250 mg/10 ml	2-10 min	10-30 min	0.5-0.6 mg/kg/dose IV over 1-2 min; then 0.3-1.0 mg/kg/min beginning at 0.2 mg/kg/min and titrate by 0.05 µg/kg/min q5min
Atenolol (Tenormin)	25, 50, 100 mg	2-4 hr	4-6 hr	1 mg/kg/24 hr PO
Prazosin (Minipress)	1, 2, 5 mg	3 hr	8 hr	First dose 5 µg/kg PO up to 25 µg/kg/dose
Phentolamine (Regitine)	5 mg/ml (1 ml)	1-2 min	5-20 min	0.05-0.1 mg/kg/dose (repeat q5min until control)
ANGIOTENSIN-CONVERTING ENZYME INHIBITOR				
Captopril (Capoten)	25, 50, 100 mg	15 min	4-6 hr	0.5-6 mg/kg/24 hr (newborn; 0.1-0.4 mg/kg/dose q6-12hr PO)

atenolol (Tenormin), 1 mg/kg/24 hr PO q12-24hr (adult: 50-100 mg/24 hr).

Step 3: If BP is still uncontrolled, add a third agent, such as a vasodilator, after consultation. Hydralazine (Apresoline), 0.75-3.0 mg/kg/24 hr q6-12hr PO, is the common dose. Hydralazine may have limited availability because it is being reformulated.

When several drugs are required, consultation is appropriate for immediate management and follow-up.

Hypertensive Crisis

Hypertensive crisis requires more rapid control, reflecting the clinical presentation and the ur-

Frequency/route	Adult dose (>12 yr)	Advantages	Disadvantages
q12hr PO	0.1-.025 mg/24 hr	Gradual decrease	Somnolence, depression, ulcerogenic; rarely used, often combined with other agents
Titrate IV	2 mg/min or 20 mg/dose initially; then 20-80 mg q10min	Can be followed by some drug orally	Hypotension; first dose evaluates effect
q6-12hr IV	10-40 mg/dose (maximum: 320 mg/24 hr)		Dysrhythmia (monitor); fatigue; hypoglycemia; β blocker; contraindicated: CHF, asthma
Titrate IV	0.5 mg/kg/min over 1 min; then 0.1-0.3 mg/kg/min beginning at 0.05 mg/kg/min and titrate q5min		Hypotension, dysrhythmia
q12-24hr	50-100 mg/24 hr	β selective	Limited experience in children; headache, nausea, hypotension, bradycardia, exacerbates CHF
q6hr PO	0.5-7 mg/dose		
q1-4hr IV	2.5-5 mg/dose	Rapid onset; specific for pheochromocytoma and MAO inhibitor	Hypotension, dysrhythmia
q6-12hr PO	25-150 mg/dose	Rapid onset; oral; useful when other drug combinations fail, esp. if high plasma renin level	Variable response, hypotension; proteinuria, neutropenia, azotemia; absorption falls if taken with food

gency of signs and symptoms. The level of control must reflect the hemodynamic status of the patient. *Usually only a moderate reduction in pressure is needed in the acute situation, often to the range of 100 mm Hg diastolic pressure:*

1. Furosemide (Lasix), 1-3 mg/kg/dose q6-12hr IV. May be repeated every 2 hours.

In most cases, the physician cannot wait for significant diuretic effect but must use specific antihypertensive drugs.

2. Antihypertensive drugs
   a. Agents are summarized in Tables 18-1 and 18-2.
   b. *Parenteral therapy* (usually vasodilators such as nitroprusside, diazoxide,

or hydralazine) is indicated with severe acute hypertension (greater than the 95th percentile) associated with acute glomerulonephritis, hemolytic-uremic syndrome, or head injuries.

c. In general, nitroprusside is an excellent agent for initial control in most conditions causing a hypertensive crisis.

d. *Oral antihypertensive therapy* lowers blood pressure less rapidly than parenteral medications and has been used extensively in hypertensive emergencies without encephalopathy or cardiac decompensation. Many prefer this approach. Medications for this purpose include the following:

(1) Clonidine (Catapres): Adult dose is 0.2 mg PO initially, then 0.1 mg/hr PO up to a maximum dose of 0.8 mg/24 hr. Onset: 2 hours; duration: 6 to 8 hours. Disadvantages: sedation, hypertension. Mechanism: central sympatholytic.

(2) Nifedipine (Procardia): 0.25-0.5 mg/kg/dose PO or sublingual. May repeat in 30 minutes but usually q6-8hr (average: 0.33 mg/kg total dose [adult: 10 to 20 mg/dose PO or sublingual]). Onset: 5 to 15 minutes; duration: 3 to 5 hours. To give sublingually, draw contents of 10-mg capsule (0.34 ml) in 1-ml syringe.

Disadvantages: may cause tachycardia (β blocker may be given concurrently); variable response. Mechanism: calcium channel blocker.

DISPOSITION

A patient with only *mild* hypertension may be followed closely as an outpatient if compliance can be ensured.

A *hypertensive crisis* requires immediate hospitalization in an ICU.

REFERENCES

Beronson GS: Combined low-dose medication and primary intervention over a 30-month period for sustained high blood pressure in childhood, *Am J Med Sci* 299:79, 1990.

Bunchman TE, Lynch RE, Wood EG: Intravenously administered labetalol for treatment of hypertension in children, *J Pediatr* 120:140, 1992.

Calhoun DA, Oparil S: Treatment of hypertension crisis, *N Engl J Med* 323:1177, 1990.

Farine M, Arbus GS: Management of hypertensive emergencies in children, *Pediatr Emerg Care* 5:51, 1989.

Harshfield GA, Alpert BS, Pulliam DA, et al: Ambulatory blood pressure recordings in children and adolescents, *Pediatrics* 94:180, 1994.

Hulman S, Edwards R, Chen YQ, et al: Blood pressure patterns in the first three days of life, *J Perinatol* 11:231, 1991.

Ingelfinger JR: Pediatric hypertension, *Curr Opin Pediatr* 6:198, 1994.

Lauer RM, Burns TL, Clarke WR: Assessing children's blood pressure—considerations of age and body size: the Muscatine study, *Pediatrics* 75:1981, 1985.

Mirkin BL, Newman TJ: Efficacy and safety of captopril in the treatment of severe childhood hypertension: report of the international collaborative study group, *Pediatrics* 75:1091, 1985.

National Institute of Health: Update on the task force report on high blood pressure in children and adolescents: NIH Publication No. 96.3790, 1996.

Siegler RL, Brewer ED: Effect of sublingual or oral nifedipine in the treatment of hypertension, *J Pediatr* 112:811, 1988.

Sinaiko AR: Treatment of hypertension in children, *Pediatr Nephrol* 8:603, 1994.

Skalina ME, Kleigman RM, Fanaroff AA: Epidemiology and management of severe symptomatic neonatal hypertension, *Am J Perinatol* 3:235, 1986.

19 PULMONARY EDEMA

ALERT: Cardiac causes of pulmonary edema often are accompanied by congestive heart failure; noncardiogenic causes result from a wide variety of clinical entities. The chest x-ray film is particularly helpful in making this differentiation. All patients require oxygen and respiratory support.

Pulmonary edema may occur secondary to diverse mechanisms, including increased pulmonary capillary pressure (cardiac or noncardiac), decreased colloid osmotic pressure (renal or hepatic dysfunction, malnutrition), altered membrane permeability (pneumonia, drowning, adult respiratory distress syndrome [ARDS], drugs, toxins), changes in transpulmonary pressure (upper airway obstruction and relief), decreased lymphatic drainage, and mixed mechanisms (high-altitude pulmonary edema [HAPE], head trauma, seizures).

Most patients have cardiogenic pulmonary edema resulting from an elevated left atrial pressure with increased pulmonary hydrostatic pressure.

ETIOLOGY

1. Vascular
   a. Congestive heart failure (see Chapter 16)
   b. Pulmonary embolism (p. 568)
   c. Cerebrovascular accident
   d. Fat embolism
2. Trauma/physical agent
   a. Central nervous system (CNS): cerebral anoxia, embolism, head trauma (see Chapter 57)
   b. Near-drowning (see Chapter 47)
   c. HAPE (see Chapter 49)
   d. Radiation exposure
   e. Upper airway foreign body or after removal of obstruction
3. Intoxication
   a. Inhaled toxins: smoke, CO, phosgene, ozone, etc.
   b. Circulating toxins: snake venom, endotoxin
   c. Drugs: sulfonamides, narcotics (methadone, heroin), naloxone, propoxyphene, salicylates, hydrocarbon, phenytoin, organophosphates, amphetamines, thiazides
4. Infection/inflammation
   a. Pneumonia and other pulmonary infections (p. 794)
   b. Pulmonary aspiration
   c. Pancreatitis (p. 644) or peritonitis
   d. Upper airway obstruction (croup, epiglottitis, markedly enlarged tonsils and adenoids) or after relief of obstruction
   e. Disseminated intravascular coagulation (DIC): infection, eclampsia (p. 683)
5. Iatrogenic
   a. Fluid overload
   b. Decompression of pneumothorax
6. Metabolic: decreased oncotic pressure from hypoalbuminemia, as in liver failure

7. Seizures
8. Allergy/autoimmune
   a. Asthma (p. 765)
   b. Systemic lupus erythematosus
9. Neoplasm: CNS, pulmonary

DIAGNOSTIC FINDINGS

Although there are specific findings with pulmonary edema, most presenting signs and symptoms are related to the underlying cause and must be evaluated systematically. Historically, patients report progressive dyspnea with orthopnea, cough, and pink, frothy sputum.

Vital signs are variable. Blood pressure often is elevated with cardiac decompensation. It may be increased in noncardiogenic pulmonary edema secondary to anxiety and catecholamine release. Tachycardia is present. Patients have pale, clammy skin.

Tachypnea is uniformly apparent (unless decreased by narcotics). Cyanosis results from ventilation-perfusion abnormalities. Patients demonstrate rales, wheezing, and occasionally, pleural effusions. Unilateral effusions, when present, are usually on the right.

Cardiac findings reflect the underlying disorder associated with congestive heart failure, demonstrating gallop rhythm, increased heart sounds, and elevated jugular venous pressure (see Chapter 16).

Mental status may be decreased, with associated anorexia, listlessness, and headache, and occasionally, the patient may progress to coma, Cheynes-Stokes respirations, or apnea, which occurs with cerebral hypoxia.

Complications

1. Cardiac failure with left or right ventricular failure (see Chapter 16)
2. Superimposed pulmonary infection (p. 794)
3. Acute respiratory failure with Pao_2 less than 50 mm Hg and $Paco_2$ greater than 50 mm Hg at room air, sea level, progressive

disease or fatigue, and respiratory acidosis
4. DIC (p. 683)
5. Cardiopulmonary arrest and death

Ancillary Data

Studies must reflect the primary cause, in addition to those directly related to pulmonary status:

1. Chest x-ray studies
   a. Fluffy alveolar infiltrates, with diffuse perihilar haziness, Kerley B lines, cardiomegaly, and possibly pleural effusions.
   b. If cardiac in origin, findings usually are associated with underlying cardiac lesion(s). Cardiomegaly is usually present.
2. Arterial blood gases (ABGs): hypoxia with respiratory acidosis or alkalosis; continuous oximetry
3. Electrocardiogram (ECG): reflects underlying heart disease, strain, or ischemia
4. Electrolytes: particularly with diuretics (hypokalemia, blood urea nitrogen [BUN], creatinine)
5. Thoracentesis: if patient has pleural fluid leading to respiratory decompensation (see Appendix A-8)
   NOTE: Analysis should include protein, glucose, cell count, lactic dehydrogenase (LDH), culture, and Gram stain.
6. Other studies, as indicated
   a. Swan-Ganz catheter to measure pulmonary wedge pressure when cardiac failure is severe. It is usually inserted in the ICU.
   b. Echocardiogram to evaluate pulmonary hypertension and cardiac function and to determine whether effusion is present.

DIFFERENTIAL DIAGNOSIS

1. Infection: pneumonia (p. 794)
2. Vascular

a. Intrapulmonary hemorrhage, accompanied by hemoptysis, chest pain, and infiltrate on chest x-ray film

b. Pulmonary embolism (p. 568) with hemoptysis, pleuritic chest pain, and dyspnea

3. Allergy: asthma (p. 765)

MANAGEMENT

The pulmonary status initially may be stabilized during the treatment of the underlying condition. For treatment of specific entities, see appropriate chapter.

The patient should be kept in a semirecumbent position with cardiac monitor.

1. Airway and breathing.

   a. Oxygenation is a necessity. Administer humidified oxygen at 3-6 L/min by mask or nasal cannula (or 50%).

   b. Intubate and initiate positive end-expiratory pressure if the Pao_2 less than 50 mm Hg at an Fio_2 of 50%, beginning at 5 cm H_2O and increasing with close monitoring in ICU.

   c. Perform mechanical ventilation after intubation for respiratory failure (Pao_2 <50 mm Hg and $Paco_2$ >50 mm Hg at room air, sea level) to protect airway, to avoid rapid progression of disease or fatigue, or to treat unresponsive metabolic acidosis.

   d. Bronchodilator therapy including albuterol may be useful (p. 769).

2. *Fluid* resuscitation.

   a. Fluid therapy must be a balance between expanding the intravascular volume necessary to improve cardiac output and controlling the subsequent increased pulmonary flow and edema. This may require the insertion of a Swan-Ganz catheter and observation of patient for renal failure.

   b. Crystalloid solution is used to maintain urine output at 0.5 ml/kg/hr in cardiogenic pulmonary edema but must be

individualized in noncardiogenic pulmonary edema. Patients in general are maintained with fluids at a rate well below maintenance, while urine output is monitored.

   c. Albumin (25% salt poor administered 1 gm/kg/dose over 2 to 4 hours) is indicated if pulmonary edema is secondary to hypoalbuminemia.

   d. Fluid management for patients with cardiac tamponade requires pushing fluids and pericardiocentesis (see Appendix A-5).

3. Diuretics to reduce volume overload (see Table 16-3).

   a. Administer diuretics for pulmonary edema that is cardiogenic in origin. If noncardiogenic, use diuretics only if the underlying pathophysiologic condition is associated with fluid overload.

   b. Furosemide (Lasix): 1 mg/kg/dose up to 6 mg/kg/dose q6hr. May be repeated every 2 hours, if indicated. Not to be used if patient is anuric.

4. Morphine sulfate: lowers pulmonary wedge pressure and relieves anxiety.

   a. In severe pulmonary edema, slowly administer 0.1-0.2 mg/kg IV.

   b. Do not give morphine if there is evidence of unstable vital signs, intracranial hemorrhage, chronic pulmonary disease, asthma, or narcotic withdrawal.

   c. Use with caution in patients with respiratory depression or progressive disease. Close monitoring is essential.

   d. Nalbuphine (Nubain) is a useful substitute for morphine. The experience with children is still limited.

5. Shock. Cardiogenic shock or low output state may accompany pulmonary edema and must be treated aggressively. The adrenergic agents of choice (see Chapter 5) are as follows:

   a. Dopamine administered by continuous

IV infusion at a rate of 5-20 µg/kg/min. May be used at a higher dosage if α-blocking agents are used. There is extensive experience with children.

b. An alternative is dobutamine administered by continuous IV infusion at a rate of 2-20 µg/kg/min. Some patients may respond to a low dosage of 0.5 µg/kg/min; others may require 40 µg/kg/min. It may be used with low-dose dopamine (0.5-3 µg/kg/min).

6. Afterload reduction to diminish pressure overload. If an inadequate response to these measures is present, agents that diminish afterload by decreasing peripheral resistance may improve cardiac output. These drugs should be used only with indwelling arterial monitoring and a Swan-Ganz catheter in place (see Appendix A-3).

  a. Sodium nitroprusside (Nipride). Dosage: 0.5-8 µg/kg/min IV by infusion. Begin with rate of infusion of 0.1 µg/kg/min, and increase until the desired response is achieved. Average therapeutic dose is about 3 µg/kg/min. The clinical response is noted in 1 to 2 minutes and lasts for 5 to 10 minutes after stopping the infusion. Do not use if renal failure is present.

  b. Nitroglycerin has no established dosage in children. Sublingual administration in adults (0.15-0.6 mg q5min up to a maximum of three doses in a 15-minute period) may be useful for acute treatment, particularly in the prehospital setting in the patient with obvious cardiac decompensation. IV nitroglycerin (Nitrostat) similarly has been used in adults (5 µg/min with increments of 5 µg/min q3-5min titrated to response) in the hospital environment.

7. Other considerations:
  a. Dysrhythmias require urgent treatment (see Chapter 6).
  b. Steroids are not useful unless they have efficacy for the underlying condition.
  c. Bronchodilators are indicated if there is wheezing and evidence of bronchoconstriction (p. 769).

DISPOSITION

Patients require admission to an ICU for appropriate intervention, immediate treatment and monitoring of the pulmonary edema, and management of the underlying condition.

The rare patient with mild, slowly progressive pulmonary edema of known cause may be managed on an ambulatory basis, if compliance and follow-up care can be ensured.

A cardiologist should be involved immediately.

REFERENCES

Feinberg AN, Shabino CL: Acute pulmonary edema complicating tonsillectomy and adenoidectomy, *Pediatrics* 75: 112, 1985.

Kanter RK, Watchko JF: Pulmonary edema associated with upper airway obstruction, *Am J Dis Child* 138:356, 1984.

Mulroy JJ, Mitchell JJ, Tonk TK, et al: Postictal pulmonary edema in children, *Neurology* 35:403, 1985.

20 RESPIRATORY DISTRESS (DYSPNEA)

Dyspnea or labored, rapid respirations usually reflect an impairment in ventilation, perfusion, or a metabolic or central nervous system (CNS) drive. Upper airway problems produce primarily ventilatory abnormalities associated with stridor; lower airway disease may impair both ventilation and perfusion.

Respiratory failure is commonly associated with altered consciousness, increased work of breathing and respiratory rate, poor color, sweating, grunting and flaring, decreased air movement, and abnormal arterial blood gas (ABG) or oximetry results.

ETIOLOGY

Stridor is the major complaint with significant upper airway disease. A variety of entities may commonly produce stridor (Table 20-1).
- Infection—croup, epiglottitis, tracheitis
- Allergic—anaphylaxis, angioneurotic edema
- Congenital/anatomic—laryngeal edema, web
- Neurologic
- Psychogenic

Inspiratory stridor is usually supraglottic, whereas expiratory stridor emanates from the trachea. Patients with inspiratory and expiratory stridor or expiratory stridor alone usually have more significant obstructions, demanding urgent intervention.

Supraglottic stridor is usually quiet and wet, and it is associated with a muffled voice, dysphagia, and a preference to sit; a patient with subglottic lesions producing a loud stridor often has a hoarse voice, barky cough, and possibly, facial edema.

Lower airway disease consists of a more diverse group of entities that inhibit the ability of oxygen to diffuse into the capillaries. The most common are pneumonia and asthma. Pulmonary pathology often is associated with exertional dyspnea; cardiac disease, on the other hand, causes orthopnea and paroxysmal nocturnal dyspnea.

Most upper and lower airway disease result from one of several entities:

Upper airway disease	Lower airway disease
Stridor Present	**Stridor Absent**
Croup	Pneumonia
Epiglottitis	Asthma
Foreign body	Bronchiolitis
Tracheitis	Foreign body

Text continued on p. 180

See also Chapter 84: Pulmonary Disorders.

175

TABLE 20-1 Respiratory Distress: Diagnostic Considerations

Disease	Etiology	Signs and symptoms	Ancillary data	Comments/management
		UPPER AIRWAY OBSTRUCTION		
INFECTION				
Epiglottitis (p. 784)	*Haemophilus influenzae*	Toxic, febrile, inspiratory stridor, cyanosis, muffled voice, drooling, labored respirations, cherry-red epiglottis	↑WBC (shift left), positive lateral neck x-ray	Visualization and intubation, optimally in operating room; antibiotics; incidence down with routine immunization
Croup (laryngotracheal bronchitis) (p. 784)	Virus: parainfluenza, respiratory syncytial virus	Inspiratory stridor, hoarse voice, croupy cough, variably labored respirations, epiglottis WNL	Variable WBC, negative lateral neck x-ray	Cool mist; nebulized racemic epinephrine if needed; steroids
Peritonsillar abscess (p. 603)	Group A streptococci	Fever, severe throat pain, late inspiratory stridor, drooling, dysphagia, tonsil displaced, posterior pharyngeal mass	↑WBC	Nafcillin (or equivalent), surgical incision and drainage; usually child <3 yr old
Retropharyngeal/ esophageal abscess (p. 608)	*S. aureus*, group A streptococci		↑WBC, positive lateral neck x-ray	
Bacterial tracheitis	*S. aureus*	High temperature, toxic, inspiratory stridor, brassy cough, fails to respond to croup therapy	↑WBC (shift to left)	Nafcillin (or equivalent); may require intubation to remove thick secretions
Diphtheria (p. 708)	*Corynebacterium diphtheriae*	Toxic, slight fever, membrane, hoarse	Culture	History of exposure, no immunization; antitoxin and penicillin
TRAUMA				
Foreign body (p. 791) Pharynx, larynx, trachea, esophagus	Aspiration of vegetable or inanimate matter	History reflects level of obstruction, inspiratory or expiratory stridor, cyanosis, labored respirations, wheezing, variable respiratory arrest	Chest (inspiratory and expiratory) and lateral neck x-ray; foreign body, wide mediastinum; findings vary with location	Back blow, chest/abdominal thrust, mechanical removal, surgical airway
Neck injury (Chapter 61)		History and findings of trauma, instability or disruption of neck, larynx, variable stridor	Clear cervical spine, look for signs of laryngeal injury	Stabilization of airway and neck

Condition	Etiology	Clinical Features	Diagnosis	Treatment
Cord paralysis	Congenital, traumatic, iatrogenic	Acute or chronic, voice change, inspiratory stridor, respiratory distress	Direct laryngoscopy	If acute, intubation or surgical airway
Subglottic stenosis	Trauma to glottis such as intubation; rarely congenital	Respiratory distress, usually insidious; may be exacerbated by respiratory infection	Direct laryngoscopy	Surgical airway may be needed
CONGENITAL (Chapters 10 and 11)				
Vascular ring, Laryngeal web or polyp, Small mandible (Pierre Robin), Large tongue (hypothyroid)	Congenital or acquired	Chronic inspiratory or expiratory stridor, variable respiratory distress (or both), wheezing	Laryngoscopy/bronchoscopy	Surgical or medical approach to underlying problem
Choanal atresia	Congenital	Nasal obstruction, discharge; variable respiratory distress	Catheter passage, visualization	Oral airway; surgical correction may be required if significant
Tracheomalacia	Abnormal collapse of supraglottic area	Expiratory stridor		Need oxygen until stable; usually resolves spontaneously; may have feeding problem
Laryngomalacia	Floppiness of trachea	Inspiratory stridor		
ALLERGIC				
Spasmodic croup (p. 791)	Exposure to irritant or sensitizing agent	Rapid onset inspiratory stridor, croupy cough, variable labored respirations		Cool mist; nebulized racemic epinephrine
Anaphylaxis (Chapter 12)	Allergic response	Rapid onset stridor, respiratory distress, wheezing		Removal of sensitizing agent; β agonists, antihistamines, steroids
Angioneurotic edema	Allergic response, hereditary	Rapid onset after eating, bee sting, environmental exposure		Airway support, epinephrine, etc. (Chapter 12)
NEOPLASM				
Tracheal, laryngeal, esophageal, neck	Carcinoma, teratoma, hemangioma, polyp	Insidious progression of stridor, dysphagia, labored respirations		Radiologic and surgical evaluation

Continued

TABLE 20-1   Respiratory Distress: Diagnostic Considerations—cont'd

Disease	Etiology	Signs and symptoms	Ancillary data	Comments/management
UPPER AIRWAY OBSTRUCTION—cont'd				
INFECTION				
Pneumonia (p. 794)	Viral Bacterial: *S. pneumoniae, H. influenzae* Other	Febrile, recent onset tachypnea, cough, unequal breath sounds or rhonchi, variable chest pain	Variable WBC count; chest x-ray: infiltrate; blood culture (if toxic)	Antibiotics as indicated
Bronchiolitis (p. 781)	Viral: parainfluenza, respiratory syncytial virus	Variable fever, very tachypneic, nontoxic, wheezing, variable cyanosis	Chest x-ray: hyperexpanded, infiltrate variable; oximetry	Support: hydration, oxygen; nebulized β agonists (albuterol); ribavirin in selected children
Pleural effusion	Infections (viral or bacterial), CHF, nephrosis, liver failure	No fever, tachypneic with unequal breath sounds, variable chest pain	Chest x-ray (include lateral decubitus)	May need to aspirate; exudate (LDH >200 U, LDH fluid/blood ratio >0.6, or protein fluid/blood ratio >0.5)
Empyema	*S. aureus*	Fever, toxic, tachypneic, cough, variable pain, unequal breath sounds	Chest x-ray, fluid culture, blood culture	Thoracentesis for diagnosis, then closed chest tube drainage and antibiotics
LOWER AIRWAY DISEASE				
VASCULAR				
Congestive heart failure (Chapter 16)	Congenital or acquired heart disease	Fatigue, anorexia, cough, orthopnea, basilar rales, edema	Chest x-ray, ECG, ABG	Diuretics, oxygen, digitalis, morphine, nitrates
Congenital heart disease	R → L shunt, pulmonary edema	Cyanosis	Chest x-ray, ECG, ABG	Cardiology consult
Pulmonary edema (Chapter 19)	Heart, liver, renal vascular disease	Tachypnea, basilar rales, fatigue, cough, orthopnea, wheezing	Chest x-ray, serum protein, BUN, SGOT, electrolytes, UA	Evaluate systems involved; diuretics
Pulmonary embolism (p. 568)	Abnormal clotting, trauma, birth control pills	Tachypnea, hemoptysis, chest pain, variable fever	Chest x-ray, ABG, ventilation-perfusion scan	Immediate anticoagulation

Polycythemia	Heart, pulmonary, renal disease, abnormal Hb	Plethoric	CBC with indexes	Hematology consultation; may require partial exchange
Anemia (Chapter 26)	$\downarrow$ production or $\uparrow$ loss; high output failure	Pale, fatigue, poor exercise tolerance	CBC with indexes, reticulocyte count	Hematology consultation; transfusion
ALLERGIC				
Asthma (p. 765)	Exposure to irritant or sensitizing agent; infection; emotional stress	Insidious or rapid onset of tachypnea, wheezing, cough		Oxygen, nebulized β agonists, bronchodilators, and steroids
Anaphylaxis (Chapter 12)	Exposure to sensitizing agent	Rapid onset wheezing, tachypnea	Chest x-ray, ABG	
TRAUMA				
Foreign body Bronchial (p. 791)	Vegetable or inanimate material	History, cough, wheezing, asymmetric breath sounds	Chest x-ray; inspiratory and expiratory fluoroscopy	Bronchoscopy
Pneumothorax (Chapter 62)	Chest wound, spontaneous	Tachypnea, chest pain, asymmetric breath sounds	Chest x-ray	Needle aspiration, chest tube
CONGENITAL				
Cystic fibrosis	Autosomal recessive, Caucasians	Progressive pulmonary disease (hemoptysis, atelectasis, pneumothorax, obstructive pulmonary disease, concurrent infection); poor growth; GI (steatorrhea, pancreatitis, rectal prolapse); hyponatremia	Chest x-ray, sweat test	Pulmonary consultation
NEOPLASM		Progressive pulmonary disease	Chest x-ray	Oncology consultation
DEGENERATIVE				
Kyphoscoliosis Progressive CNS disease	Multiple	Progressive pulmonary disease, secondary hypoventilation	Chest x-ray, ABG, pulmonary function	Neurology, pulmonary, orthopedic consultation

Common causes of respiratory distress in children less than 2 years old include pneumonia, asthma, croup, congenital heart disease, foreign body inhalation, congenital anomalies of the airway (tracheal web, cysts, lobar emphysema), and nasopharyngeal obstruction (large tonsils and adenoids). The underlying disorder in older children more often is asthma, pneumonia, foreign bodies, poisoning, drowning, trauma, cystic fibrosis, peripheral neuritis, or encephalitis.

In addition to those conditions listed in Table 20-1, oxygen demand may be increased (increased activity, fever, hyperthyroidism), oxygen transport may be deficient (anemia, methemoglobinemia, or shock), the respiratory system may be stimulated as a compensatory mechanism in metabolic acidosis (diabetes mellitus, uremia, drug ingestions), the ambient oxygen may be low, or there may be a central neurogenic stimulation.

Adult respiratory distress syndrome (ARDS) may result from a variety of conditions that cause pulmonary damage (p. 44).

DIAGNOSTIC FINDINGS (Fig. 20-1)

The initial focus must be on the assessment of the airway and ventilatory status with intervention on an emergent basis as required. This often must occur before definitive diagnostic evaluation has been completed. Oximetry is a more reliable indicator of hypoxemia than solely a clinical evaluation.

Airway integrity and ventilatory status can be rapidly assessed initially by evaluating for the presence of stridor and auscultating to determine the adequacy of air movement and the presence of wheezing, rales, or rhonchi.

The history must focus on the presenting problems. The characterization of the current episode should include the nature of progression, associated signs and symptoms, cough (productive versus unproductive), fever, chest pain, trauma, and foreign body ingestion. Evidence of retractions, tachypnea, wheezing, stridor, and relationship to eating should be defined. Past medical problems related to respiratory distress; recurrent problems with shortness of breath, cough, pneumonia, retractions, fever; and exposure to chemical or environmental irritants should be noted. Pulmonary or cardiac disease, infectious exposures, tuberculosis, and early death in other family members may be important.

On physical examination, after stability has been ensured, respiratory status, including air entry, type of breathing, color (and oximetric findings), retractions, and breath sounds, should be evaluated. Stridor, adequacy of air movement, wheezing, rales, or rhonchi must be excluded.

Respiratory rates suggestive of pneumonia are less than 6 months (>59/min), 6 to 11 months (>52/min), and 1 to 2 years (>42/min).

Ancillary Data

1. *Upper airway obstruction.* Laboratory evaluation is usually ancillary to direct visualization, particularly in patients with respiratory distress. This must be done with great caution and anticipation. Specific measures are indicated for patients with potential foreign bodies (p. 791).
2. *Lower airway disease.* Chest x-ray films and ABG (or oximetry) provide initial data. Specific tests for the suspected causes must be obtained (see Table 20-1).

MANAGEMENT

Stabilization of the airway is central to any management plan and must not be delayed by obtaining excessive confirmatory data before instituting definitive therapy. All patients with respiratory distress require evaluation of the airway and ventilatory status and intervention as needed, often empirically. Oxygen and cardiac monitoring should be initiated on arrival.

It is important to remember that upsetting the child should be prevented when possible.

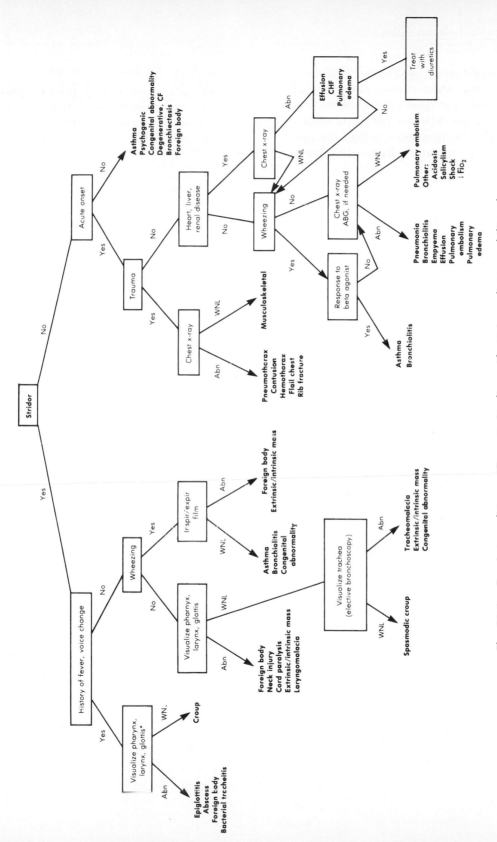

Fig. 20-1   Respiratory distress. ×Do not visualize without immediate capability of airway intervention. If epiglottitis is suspected, procedure should be performed under controlled conditions, often in the operating room.

The degree of distress should never be underestimated, and the child should never be left unattended in the emergency department, x-ray department, or any other area of the hospital.

Specific intervention must reflect the patient's degree of respiratory distress and potential causative conditions.

REFERENCES

MacPherson RL, Leithiser RE: Upper airway obstruction in children: an update, *RadioGraphics* 5:339, 1985.

Meneker AJ, Petrack EM, Krug SE: Contribution of routine pulse oximetry to evaluation and management of patients with respiratory illness in a pediatric emergency department, *Ann Emerg Med* 25:36, 1995.

Ruddy RM: Respiratory distress in a child in the office, *Pediatr Emerg Care* 6:314, 1990.

Santamacria JD, Schafermeyer R: Stridor: a review, *Pediatr Emerg Care* 8:229, 1992.

Taylor J, DelBeccaro M, Done S, et al: Establishing clinically relevant standards for tachypnea in febrile children younger than 2 years, *Arch Pediatr Adolesc Med* 149: 283, 1995.

21 STATUS EPILEPTICUS

ALERT: Maintain airway; administer oxygen, dextrose, and naloxone (Narcan) (if appropriate) and then anticonvulsants. Consider diagnostic entities.

Patients are considered to be in status epilepticus when they experience continuous seizures for 20 to 30 minutes or have two or more seizures without a lucid period.

Poor compliance is the most common explanation, although some patients may have lowered thresholds caused by fever and infection, head trauma, hypoglycemia and metabolic abnormalities, ingestions, drug interactions, hypertension, or an exacerbation of the underlying condition. It may be the first seizure in a child who goes on to have epilepsy (p. 738). Animal studies have shown that cellular ischemic changes begin within 10 to 15 minutes of onset of continuous seizures.

The morbidity rate of aggressively treated status epilepticus in the absence of an acute neurologic result or progressive neurologic disorder is low. Status epilepticus is the initial seizure in most children with epilepsy. In children less than 1 year old, 75% of episodes are associated with an acute cause; in children less than 3 years old, 47% have an acute etiology.

DIAGNOSTIC FINDINGS

Grand mal seizures are most common, although other seizure categories may occur. Several patterns may be as follows:

1. Recurrent generalized seizures with persistent cortical depression between seizures
2. Nonconvulsive seizures producing continuous or fluctuating altered mental status

3. Recurrent partial seizure producing focal motor convulsions, focal sensory symptoms, or focal impairment of function (i.e., aphasia) not associated with altered consciousness

Patients experience seizure activity, loss of consciousness, and cyanosis. Temperature may be increased before the seizures because of meningitis or other infection or secondary to the increased muscle activity. Tachycardia and increased blood pressure are common.

Mydriasis and upward deviation of the eyes are present. The corneal reflex is decreased, and a positive Babinski reflex is present. Fecal and urinary incontinence occur.

Complications

1. Death caused by anoxia, aspiration, or trauma associated with the loss of consciousness
2. Encephalopathy from hypoxia
3. Acute renal failure associated with myoglobinuria and rhabdomyolysis
4. Respiratory arrest caused by medications

Ancillary Data

Appropriate studies should be done:

1. A sample for blood glucose determination before infusion of D25W; also rapid glucose approximation (Dextrostix/ Chemstrip)

183

2. Arterial blood gas (ABG) assessment of acidosis and hypoxia
3. Anticonvulsant levels, if patient has been taking medications
4. If the cause is unknown: electrolytes, Ca^{++}, Mg^{++}, PO_4^{--}, complete blood count (CBC), and toxicologic screen (Consider lumbar puncture and computed tomographic [CT] scanning as appropriate.)

MANAGEMENT

Initial attention must be supportive, particularly to the airway, and ventilation with administration of supplemental oxygen.

1. Intubation may be required to oxygenate the patient and minimize the risk of aspiration. Prophylactic intubation is rarely indicated unless seizures are unresponsive or the patient has compromised airway or ventilation.
2. Traumatic injuries should be prevented by protecting the patient against self-injury. Trauma to the tongue rarely causes significant problems. Putting a soft cloth in the mouth to prevent the teeth from closing may prevent dental damage. Attempting to force an airway into the mouth can cause obstruction.

Glucose has an immediate metabolic effect and should be considered. A glucose level should be drawn before administration of glucose for later confirmation, if possible.

- Glucose D25W, 0.5-1.0 gm (2-4 ml)/kg/dose IV slowly; for preterm infant, D10W. For children more than 3 years old, D50W may be used.

The following should be considered:

1. Naloxone (Narcan), 0.1 mg/kg/dose up to 2.0 mg IV. With no response and suspicion of opiates, give 2 mg IV. Available in vials of 0.4 mg/ml and 1.0 mg/ml. Very large doses may be required for propoxyphene (Darvon) and pentazocine (Talwin) overdoses.

2. Consider Thiamine, 100 mg/dose IV or IM initially and then BID PO for maintenance. Administer if alcoholism or malnutrition is suspected.
3. All *metabolic* abnormalities must be corrected. Rarely will anticonvulsants be totally effective in the presence of a significant metabolic abnormality.
   a. Hypoglycemia: D25W, 0.5-1.0 gm (2-4 ml)/kg/dose IV; then use extra glucose in maintenance fluids (at least D10W) (p. 268).
   b. Hyponatremia: 3% saline solution (0.5 mEq Na^+/ml) given at rate of 4 ml/kg IV over 10 minutes; then correct deficit over 16 hours.
   c. Hypernatremia: correct over 48 hours.
   d. Hypocalcemia: 0.5 ml/kg of 10% calcium gluconate solution over 5 minutes. Ongoing management combines 5-8 ml/kg/24 hr IV of 10% calcium gluconate solution given in four to six doses and oral calcium gluconate (200-500 mg/kg/dose q6hr PO).
   e. Hypomagnesemia: $MgSO_4$ 25-50 mg/kg/dose q4-6hr for three to four doses IM or IV slowly (adult: 1 gm 10% solution IV slowly).

Anticonvulsants (see Table 81-6) should be considered, although the appropriate drug and the order of administration are controversial. Diazepam (Valium), lorazepam (Ativan), phenobarbital, or phenytoin (Dilantin) may be used. Diazepam or lorazepam is usually preferred for acute termination; both require initiation of a second drug for long-term management. The risk of respiratory depression is thereby increased.

1. Diazepam (Valium)
   a. Dosage: 0.2-0.3 mg/kg/dose IV over 2 to 3 minutes at a rate of 1 mg/min. May have to repeat in 5 to 10 minutes if seizures continue. Maximum total dose: child, 10 mg; adult, 30 mg.
   b. Although it is not preferred, rectal

administration has been successfully used. Undiluted commercial IV preparation is administered directly into the rectum using a plastic tube or angiocath.

- An initial dosage of 0.5 mg/kg/dose PR is recommended.

c. Intramuscular administration is unreliable, largely dependent on site and method of administration. In adults there have been good results when it is administered intramuscularly into the deltoid. Endotracheal administration may cause pneumonitis.

d. Peak effect: 1 to 2 minutes, with an anticonvulsant effect for 20 to 30 minutes.

e. Toxicity: respiratory depression synergistic with barbiturates. Flumazenil (Mazicon) (0.1 mg/ml) may be used to reverse suspected benzodiazepine overdose. Pediatric dosage is 10 µg/kg/dose IV, which may be repeated. Adult dosage is 0.2 to 0.3 mg IV, repeating doses up to 3 mg. May increase to total dose of 5 mg if only partial responses.

NOTE: Intramuscular (and possibly intranasal) midazolam (Versed), 0.2 mg/kg, may be an alternate if venous access is unavailable. Further studies are necessary.

2. Lorazepam (Ativan)

a. Dosage: 0.05-0.15 mg/kg/dose IV over 1 to 3 minutes at a rate of 2 mg/min. Repeat doses have decreasing effectiveness but may be considered. Maximum total dose in child, 0.15 mg/kg up to a total dose of 4 mg; adult, 2.5 to 10 mg.

b. Intramuscular injection is somewhat erratic in absorption. Sublingual (0.05 mg/kg) administration has been used.

c. Onset: 5 minutes (peak level: 45 to 60 minutes).

d. Half-life: 16 hours.

e. Toxicity: respiratory depression synergistic with barbiturates. See Flumazenil above.

3. Phenobarbital

a. Loading dosage: 15-20 mg/kg/dose IV; infusion not to exceed 1 mg/kg/min. Adult: 100 mg/dose IV q20min prn at a rate of 30 mg/min but not to exceed three doses. If more is given as load, be prepared to support blood pressure and ventilation. Although not preferred, it may be given deep IM, but there is a somewhat erratic absorption. If no response in status epilepticus, may give additional dose.

b. Maintenance dosage: 3-5 mg/kg/24 hr IV, IM, or PO.

c. Therapeutic level: 10-25 µg/ml.

d. Toxicity: respiratory depression synergistic with diazepam or lorazepam.

4. Phenytoin (Dilantin)

a. Loading dosage: 10-20 mg/kg/dose IV infusion (concentration of 6.7 mg/ml or less in saline solution, not water; not to exceed 40 mg/min or 0.5 mg/kg/min). Maximum: 1250 mg total dose. Fosphenytoin (Cerebyx), 50 mg/ml, is available for IV or IM administration with less toxicity and local reaction.

b. Maintenance dose: 5 mg/kg/24 hr IV or PO.

c. Peak effect in 15 to 20 minutes.

d. Therapeutic level: 10-20 µg/ml.

e. Toxicity: cardiac conduction block.

5. Paraldehyde

a. Dosage: 0.3 ml/kg (maximum: <10 years—5 ml; adult—10 ml) mixed 1:2 in mineral or vegetable oil (1:3 in neonate) and given per rectum (PR).

b. Useful in intractable situations. Contraindicated in presence of hepatic, pulmonary, or renal disease.

If seizure control is difficult, a neurologist should be involved in the pharmacologic management of the patient. A common practice is to use drugs in a sequential fashion until control is achieved. Although there is no agreement, many clinicians start with diazepam (Valium) or lorazepam (Ativan) and concurrently administer phenytoin (Dilantin) or phenobarbital. Another option is to omit diazepam or lorazepam and proceed directly to phenytoin or phenobarbital to avoid the marked respiratory depression noted in young children from diazepam or lorazepam, particularly when used in combination with phenobarbital. In children who have received diazepam or lorazepam, phenytoin has the advantage as the second drug because there is no synergistic respiratory depression.

Patients who continue to be resistant after loading with phenobarbital and phenytoin should receive paraldehyde. Another modality for resistant seizures after administration of appropriate drugs is general anesthesia (e.g., pentobarbital, 5 mg/kg IV slowly, followed by 1-3 mg/kg/hr infusion). Respiratory support is required while monitoring blood pressure continuously in conjunction with neurologic consultation. The barbiturate coma is followed with electroencephalogram (EEG), titrating to a burst suppression pattern.

If the patient previously had taken an anticonvulsant and the levels are subtherapeutic, the maintenance dosage should be increased. If poor compliance is the basis for low levels, the patient should be reloaded (in full or part, depending on the level) and educated about the importance of taking the medication. Close follow-up observation with measurements of drug levels is necessary.

Concurrently, a therapeutic and diagnostic evaluation must be done to determine the potential cause, while attempting to treat seizure activity with anticonvulsants. Metabolic causes require correction of the underlying abnormalities rather than additional anticonvulsants. Mass lesions and cerebral edema, for example, require specific therapeutic intervention. Infections should be treated expeditiously.

DISPOSITION

All patients should be admitted to the hospital to ensure ongoing control of seizure activity. When poor compliance was the causative factor, a period of observation (4 hours) after reloading may substitute for admission if intervention is possible in the home environment. Careful follow-up observation is required.

If seizures are refractory to normal medications, a neurologist should immediately be involved and the patient admitted to an ICU.

REFERENCES

Abromowicz M, editor: *Drugs for epilepsy*, New Rochelle, NY, 1995, Medical Letter.

Brickman KB, Rega P, Guinness M: A comparative study of intraosseous versus peripheral intravenous infusion of diazepam and phenobarbital in dogs, *Ann Emerg Med* 16:1141, 1987.

Chamberlain J, Altieri M, Futterman C, et al: A prospective, randomized study comparing intramuscular midazolam with intravenous diazepam for the treatment of seizures in children, *Pediatr Emerg Care* 13:92, 1997.

Crawford TO, Mitchell WG, Snodgrass ST: Lorazepam in childhood status epilepticus and serial seizures: effectiveness and tachyphylaxis, *Neurology* 37:190, 1987.

Dieckman RA: Rectal diazepam for prehospital pediatric status epilepticus, *Ann Emerg Med* 23:216, 1994.

Dooley JM, Tibbles JAR, Rumney DG, et al: Rectal lorazepam in the treatment of acute seizures in childhood, *Ann Neurol* 18:412, 1985.

Epilepsy Foundation of America Working Group on Status Epilepticus: Treatment of convulsive status epilepticus, *JAMA* 270:854, 1993.

Leppick IE, Derivan AT, Homan RN, et al: Double-blind study of lorazepam and diazepam in status epilepticus, *JAMA* 249:1452, 1983.

Maytel J, Shinnar S, Moshe SL, et al: Low morbidity and mortality of status epilepticus in children, *Pediatrics* 83:323, 1989.

Phillips SA, Shanahan RJ: Etiology and mortality of status epilepticus in children, *Arch Neurol* 48:74, 1989.

Selbst SM: Office management of status epilepticus, *Pediatr Emerg Care* 7:106, 1991.

Yager JY, Seshia SS: Sublingual lorazepam in childhood serial seizures, *Am J Dis Child* 142:931, 1988.

22 SUDDEN INFANT DEATH SYNDROME

ALERT: The child who suffers near–sudden infant death syndrome (SIDS) or an apparently life-threatening event (ALTE) requires aggressive resuscitation and support. Families who have lost a child through SIDS or ALTE should receive immediate and ongoing support.

Sudden infant death syndrome (SIDS) is the sudden death of a young child between 1 month and 1 year of age that is not predicted by history and in which a thorough postmortem examination fails to define an adequate cause of death. The peak incidence of SIDS is in infants 2 to 4 months of age; 88% of deaths occur in those less than 5.5 months. It commonly occurs in the fall and winter months; many children had experienced a recent respiratory infection. The overall incidence of SIDS in the United States has decreased with the onset of the "Back to Sleep" campaign, which has emphasized the benefits of infants sleeping on their back rather than on the side or prone.

As discussed in Chapter 13, near-SIDS is commonly referred to as an apparently life-threatening event (ALTE) characterized by a combination of apnea, color change (usually cyanosis but occasionally erythema or plethora), marked change in muscle tone (usually limpness), and choking or gagging.

ETIOLOGY

There are multiple contributing factors (e.g., infection, sleep, poor growth, aspiration, maternal smoking or multiparity, absent prenatal care, low birth weight, genetics) leading to respiratory obstruction and central apnea with associated hypoxia and death. Siblings of prior SIDS/ALTE victims are at increased risk. Although infantile apnea (see Chapter 13) may precede SIDS, no evidence suggests that this occurs in most cases of SIDS.

Recent evidence has suggested that well infants who are born at term and have no medical complications should be placed down for sleep on either the side or back to reduce the incidence of SIDS.

DIAGNOSTIC FINDINGS

The child who has had a SIDS death experiences irreversible cardiac and respiratory arrest. The child who has experienced near-SIDS or ALTE will have variable vital signs, depending on the duration of cardiac and respiratory arrest before intervention.

Complications of Near-SIDS or ALTE

1. Pulmonary edema (see Chapter 19)
2. Aspiration pneumonia
3. Neurologic sequelae secondary to hypoxia, including seizures

Ancillary Data

1. An autopsy should be performed on all SIDS deaths by a competent and experienced pathologist.

187

2. Supportive data should be obtained in accordance with procedures for resuscitation (see Chapter 4).

3. In the child with near-SIDS or ALTE, an evaluation for causes of apnea (see Chapter 13) must be conducted, including oximetry, electrolyte and calcium levels, complete blood count (CBC), chest x-ray, and electrocardiogram (ECG). Infection and other metabolic abnormalities should be excluded. Evaluations may also include pneumography, polycomnography, continuous ECG recording, electroencephalography (EEG), and computed tomographic (CT) scanning of the head. Because gastroesophageal reflux is a common associated finding, a barium swallow is usually indicated.

DIFFERENTIAL DIAGNOSIS

1. Trauma. Head trauma or child abuse may be difficult to distinguish in the absence of a reliable history.

2. Infection.
   a. Overwhelming and acute infection may occur; preceding signs and symptoms should be consistent with an infectious process.
   b. Central nervous system (CNS) infection (encephalopathy or meningitis) may have a similar presentation.

3. Congenital. Metabolic derangements, particularly those producing hypoglycemia (e.g., glycogen storage disease or severe acidosis) may result in apnea and seizures. Hypoadrenalism.

4. Gastroesophageal reflux or aspiration may contribute to ALTE.

5. Vascular.
   a. Subarachnoid bleeding may occur, with acute loss of consciousness and cardiac arrest.
   b. Cardiac dysrhythmias rarely occur in children.

6. Intoxication. Accidental or intentional poisoning can produce coma, with subsequent hypoventilation, arrest, hypoxia, and death.

7. Infantile apnea (see Chapter 13).

MANAGEMENT

The child with near-SIDS or ALTE requires rapid evaluation and resuscitation efforts (as outlined in Chapter 4). Admission to the hospital for ongoing management is indicated, usually in the ICU. Eventually a pneumogram will be required.

Intense psychologic support for families and friends, both immediately and on a long-term basis, is required. Parents of children who die of SIDS normally demonstrate denial, anger, and then self-reproach and guilt. Verbalization of feelings, with reunion and ultimate separation from the child, are important. Assistance in arranging the funeral may be helpful.

Ongoing support must be ensured. Many communities have parents' groups. Where they are not available, the National Center for the Prevention of Sudden Infant Death Syndrome, 441314 Bedford Avenue, Suite 210, Baltimore, MD 21208 (800-638-7437) may be helpful.

DISPOSITION

After stabilization in the hospital, the child with near-SIDS (ALTE) may be discharged. Counseling must be provided. Many of these patients should be placed on chalasia regimens with slow, careful feedings in an upright position for 30 to 60 minutes after meals.

When appropriate, apnea monitors are available for home use. Although no evidence documents its effectiveness, sleeping on the back is also beneficial. When awake, encourage "tummy time" for development and to prevent flat spots on the occiput. Children with gastroesophageal reflux or upper airway problems are managed individually. Long-term follow-up care provided by supportive health personnel is mandatory.

REFERENCES

AAP Task Force on Infant Positioning and SIDS: Positioning and SIDS, *Pediatrics* 89:1120, 1992.

Brooks JG: Apnea of infancy and sudden infant death syndrome, *Am J Dis Child* 136:1012, 1982.

Haglund B, Cnattingius S: Cigarette smoking as a risk factor for sudden infant death syndrome: a population based study, *Am J Public Health* 80:29, 1990.

Hunt CE: Sudden infant death syndrome, *Pediatrics* 95:431, 1995.

Hunt CE, Brouillette RT: Sudden infant death syndrome, *J Pediatr* 110:669, 1987.

Merritt TA, Bauer WI, Hasselmeyer EG: Sudden infant death syndrome: the role of the emergency room physician, *Clin Pediatr* 14:1095, 1975.

National Institutes of Health: Consensus development conference on infantile apnea and home monitoring, *Pediatrics* 79:292, 1987.

Peterson DR, Sabotta EE, Daling JR: Infant mortality among subsequent siblings of infants who died of sudden infant death syndrome, *J Pediatr* 108:911, 1986.

Willinger M, Hoffman HJ, Hartford RB: Infant sleep position and risk of sudden infant death syndrome, *Pediatrics* 93:814, 1994.

23 Syncope (Fainting)

ALERT: Unless syncope is obviously self-limited, patients should be placed on a monitor and be given glucose and oxygen. The history is essential to determining potential cause.

Syncope is a transient, acute loss of consciousness. It is caused by relative cerebral hypoxia or hypoglycemia. Although it most commonly results from benign conditions, cardiac, vascular, and infectious causes should be excluded.

The history must focus on recent medications, past medical problems, intercurrent illness, metabolic abnormalities, social interactions, and family history. The episodes of syncope must be carefully described in regard to the precipitating factors and accompanying signs and symptoms (Table 23-1). A history of syncope during exercise points toward cardiac disease such as aortic stenosis. Syncope should be characterized with regard to suddenness of onset and progression, duration, sequelae, and accompanying problems, such as seizures.

The physician should focus on cardiac and pulmonary status, as well as performing a careful neurologic examination. A head-up tilt test may be useful in reproducing syncope if associated with vasovagal reactions, neurocardiogenic syncope, or hyperventilation. Vital signs should include orthostatic measurements.

The patient with positional syncope has venous pooling with decreased venous return, stroke volume, and cardiac output. This produces baroreceptor inhibition, increased adrenergic tone, myocardial contraction, and parasympathetic tone. Syncope may be blocked acutely in older children with metoprolol, 0.2 mg/kg IV. If there is a response, the patient may be treated with 1-2 mg/kg/24 hr PO given in two doses (morning and early afternoon). The dosage should be rounded to the nearest 25 mg/24 hr.

Ancillary data may include a chest x-ray study, electrocardiogram (ECG) (Holter monitoring as indicated), two-dimensional (2D) or Doppler echocardiogram; electrolyte, Ca^{++}, Ma^{++}, and glucose concentrations; complete blood count (CBC); and drug screening. An arterial blood gas (ABG) (or oximetry) determination is sometimes helpful, but procedures such as electroencephalogram (EEG) and computed tomographic (CT) scanning are not routinely needed unless indicated by the history or physical examination. Consultations may be useful in specific patients.

Distinguishing syncope from seizures is sometimes difficult. Seizures are usually prolonged (≥ 5 minutes) and accompanied by tonic-clonic movements and incontinence, followed by a period of confusion and sleepiness. In contrast, syncope usually lasts only seconds, and there are no abnormal movements or incontinence. On awakening from an episode of

TABLE 23-1   Syncope: Diagnostic Considerations

Condition	Diagnostic findings	Comments
INTRAPSYCHIC (Chapter 83)		
Hyperventilation	Rapid and deep respirations; secondary weakness, tingling, numbness of hands; feeling of dyspnea	Response to anxiety; common in adolescents; responds to rebreathing
Breath holding (p. 724)	Cyanosis and frequent unconsciousness after vigorous crying	Usually self-limited; triggers usually easily defined (e.g., crying, anger)
Hysteria	No preceding nausea, vomiting, or somatic symptoms; no anxiety; avoids injury (falls while sitting)	Responds to environmental stimulus, unconscious; adolescents (females)
VASCULAR (decreased cardiac output)		
Vasomotor (vasovagal)	Rapid drop in blood pressure (BP), bradycardia; accompanying nausea, vomiting, sweating, pallor, numbness, blurred vision, weakness	Precipitated by fear, pain, anxiety, noxious stimuli; usually in hot, humid, closed space; common in adolescents; vasodilation and decreased vascular resistance
Postural hypotension (orthostatic)	Episode follows prolonged standing or upon rising from a recumbent position; orthostatic changes variably present on examination	Poor cerebral perfusion initially; avoid rapid position changes; check hematocrit (Hct), BP standing and supine
Neurocardiogenic	Episode follows standing	Overlap with vasomotor and postural hypotension
Congenital or acquired heart disease (Chapter 16) Pulmonary stenosis Aortic stenosis Tetralogy of Fallot	Cardiac murmur, low output with poor perfusion, pallor, variable large pulse pressure	Poor cerebral perfusion
Congestive heart failure (Chapter 16)	Tachypnea, dyspnea, rales, wheezing, tachycardia, cardiomegaly, diaphoresis, cyanosis	Poor cerebral perfusion
Dysrhythmia (Chapter 6) Heart block Others	Bradycardia, irregular rhythm	Stokes-Adams attack: ECG required; if finding normal, Holter monitor and exercise evaluation; Ca^{++}, Mg^{++}, echocardiogram; antidysrhythmics
Supraventricular tachycardia Ventricular tachycardia WPW	Abnormal rhythm, rate, poor perfusion; vital signs variable	
Hypertension, malignant (Chapter 18)	Headache, dizziness, visual change, nausea, vomiting; variable change in mental status and focal neurologic signs	May require treatment for encephalopathy
Posttussive cough	Episode after coughing	Caused by decreased venous return; may require cough suppressant

Continued

TABLE 23-1   Syncope: Diagnostic Considerations—cont'd

Condition	Diagnostic findings	Comments
INFECTION		
Upper airway obstruction (p. 784) Croup Epiglottitis	Inspiratory stridor, cyanosis, labored respirations, variably toxic, febrile	
Lower airway disease Pneumonia (p. 794) Empyema	Fever, toxicity, tachypnea, rhonchi, rare chest pain	Secondary to cerebral hypoxia
TRAUMA		
Upper airway: foreign body (p. 791)	History, inspiratory or expiratory stridor, cyanosis, respiratory distress, wheezing, rare respiratory arrest	Secondary to cerebral hypoxia
ALLERGY		
Asthma (p. 765)	Wheezing, tachypnea, cough	Secondary to cerebral hypoxia
METABOLIC		
Hypoglycemia (Chapter 38)	Pallor, sweating, nausea, vomiting, tachycardia, tachypnea	Secondary to cerebral hypoglycemia
INTOXICATION		
(Chapter 54)	Hypotension, poor peripheral perfusion, dysrhythmia	Any drug that causes hypotension or hypoventilation (e.g., narcotics, sedatives, alcohol, CO, antihypertensives, phenothiazines, diuretics) or dysrhythmias (digitalis)
MISCELLANEOUS		
Epilepsy (p. 738)	May be tonic-clonic (grand mal), transient lapse of consciousness (petit mal) or psychomotor	EEG required; may be difficult to differentiate
Anemia (Chapter 26)	Pale, tachycardia, light-headed	Decreased oxygen-carrying capacity and cerebral hypoxia
Dehydration (Chapter 7)	Hypotensive (orthostatic), poor perfusion, dry membrane	Secondary to poor cerebral perfusion
Micturition	Syncope during voiding	
Cough	Associated with paroxysms of coughing	Increased intrathoracic pressure and decreased venous return

syncope, patients usually are normal or only very mildly confused.

Because the episode is ordinarily self-limited, management involves a brief but appropriate evaluation and follow-up. Patients who have altered consciousness when they arrive at the emergency department should be administered dextrose, naloxone (Narcan), and oxygen and should be placed on a cardiac monitor pending evaluation.

REFERENCES

Gordon RA, Moodie DS, Passalacqua M, et al: A retrospective analysis of the cost-effective work-up of syncope in children, *Cleve Clin Q* 54:931, 1987.

Lerman-Sagie T, Rechavia E, Strasberg B, et al: Head-up tilt for the evaluation of syncope of unknown origin in children, *J Pediatr* 118:676, 1991.

Pratt JL, Fleischer GR: Syncope in children and adolescents, *Pediatr Emerg Care* 5:80, 1989.

Samoil D, Grubb BP, Kip K, et al: Head-upright tilt table testing in children with unexplained syncope, *Pediatrics* 92:426, 1993.

VI
URGENT COMPLAINTS

24 ACUTE ABDOMINAL PAIN

ALERT: Severe abdominal pain lasting more than 6 hours in a previously well patient usually requires surgery; evaluation and support are always indicated.

Acute abdominal pain in the child presents a diagnostic dilemma. The most common medical problem is acute gastroenteritis, although more serious causes must be excluded. Beyond this, the clinician must synthesize historical and physical data with anatomic and physiologic considerations.

ETIOLOGY

Diffuse abdominal pain results from one of several processes. A ruptured viscus produces peritonitis with rebound, guarding, and tenderness, commonly accompanied by sepsis and shock. Abdominal distension with high-pitched sounds and minimal rebound results from intestinal obstruction. Systemic disease may produce a diffuse pattern.

Pain that is sudden in onset may be related to a perforation, intussusception, ectopic pregnancy, or torsion, whereas a more insidious pattern is associated with appendicitis, pancreatitis, or cholecystitis. Colicky pain is usually related to intestinal abnormality, as well as the biliary tree, pancreatic duct, uterus, or fallopian tube.

Pain is commonly referred. Diaphragmatic involvement from such entities as basilar pneumonia, subphrenic abscess, pleurisy, pancreatitis, peritonitis, or disease of the spleen, gallbladder, or liver may produce shoulder pain, which may be bilateral if the median segment of the diaphragm is irritated. Testicular pain may represent renal or appendiceal abnormality. Complaints of back pain may be referred from a retroperitoneal hematoma, pancreatitis, or uterine or rectal disease. Pelvic abscesses may not produce diffuse peritonitis because of the relative absence of sensory innervation in that region.

Common diagnostic considerations vary with the age of the child. In the *infant* acute gastroenteritis is most common, but it is essential to exclude intussusception, volvulus, perforated viscus, incarcerated hernia, colic, and Hirschsprung disease. In *preschool* children the most common underlying causes of acute abdominal pain are acute gastroenteritis, urinary tract infections, trauma, appendicitis, pneumonia, viral syndromes, and constipation. The *school-age* child often has acute gastroenteritis, urinary tract infection, trauma, appendicitis, gynecologic entities such as pelvic inflammatory disease (PID) or ectopic pregnancy, inflammatory bowel disease, functional pain, constipation, or a viral syndrome associated with the pain.

DIAGNOSTIC FINDINGS

The history must define the acuteness and progression of the pain and its timing, quality, location, radiation, severity, and effect on activity.

197

TABLE 24-1   Acute Abdominal Pain: Diagnostic Considerations

	Infection/inflammation	Congenital	Trauma	Endocrine/metabolic	Other
Systemic	**Influenza** Acute rheumatic fever	Sickle cell disease	Black widow spider bite	Diabetic ketoacidosis Porphyria Uremia Hyperparathyroidism Hypothyroidism	**Constipation, functional** Henoch-Schönlein purpura Neoplasm: leukemia, lymphoma, neuroblastoma Lead, heavy metal poisoning
Skin	Herpes zoster Cellulitis		Contusion		
Abdominal wall		Hernia—inguinal, umbilical	Retroperitoneal hematoma		
Pulmonary	Pneumonia Pleurodynia				
Gastro-intestinal	**Acute gastroenteritis** (virus, bacteria, parasite) **Mesenteric adenitis** **Appendicitis** Gastritis Hepatitis Cholecystitis, cholelithiasis Pancreatitis Esophagitis Diverticulitis Peptic ulcer Peritonitis	Meckel's diverticulum Volvulus Intussusception Hiatal hernia Hirschsprung's disease	Laceration: spleen, liver Perforation Intramural hematoma Pancreatic pseudocyst		**Colic** Mesenteric infarct Ulcerative colitis Regional enteritis Neoplasm
Urinary	**Pyelonephritis** **Cystitis**	Hydronephrosis	Renal contusion	Renal stone	Wilms' tumor
Genital	**Pelvic inflammatory disease** Salpingitis Tuboovarian abscess Epididymitis/oophoritis	Testicular torsion		**Mittelschmerz** **Dysmenorrhea** Hematocolpos Ovarian cyst Threatened abortion Ectopic pregnancy	
Other	Osteomyelitis Pelvic abscess		Pelvic or vertebral fracture Herniated disk		Lactose intolerance Dissecting aortic aneurysm Abdominal epilepsy

Factors that worsen or lessen the pain may provide clues. The potential for referred pain must be considered. If the pain is recurrent, events surrounding the initial episode and the nature of the subsequent pain should be defined. The response to therapeutic trials such as antacids often focuses on specific disease processes.

Associated vomiting, diarrhea, nausea, dysuria, frequency, vaginal discharge, and other systemic signs and symptoms must be carefully delineated. Menstrual history should be defined. Concurrent events such as toilet training, stress at home or school, and trauma may be contributory. Secondary gain from the abdominal pain may require attention.

Physical examination must include vital signs (including orthostatics), temperature, and an overall assessment of the appearance and hydration status of the patient. The chest must be examined. The abdomen should be auscultated to assess bowel sounds and then palpated for masses and evidence of rebound, guarding, tenderness, and psoas or obturator signs. Hyperesthesia indicates parietal peritoneum inflammation. Rectal examination, with specimen testing for occult blood and polymorphonuclear leukocytes, is indicated in most patients. A pelvic examination should be done in all pubescent females with lower abdominal pain or any signs of pelvic disease.

Laboratory evaluation should include a urinalysis on all patients and, in those with severe pain, a complete blood count (CBC) and electrolytes and blood sugar analysis. Gonorrhea cultures and a Pap smear should be done if a pelvic examination is performed. Abdominal (supine and upright) and posteroanterior and lateral chest x-ray films may be helpful. Abdominal radiographs are particularly helpful in patients with prior abdominal surgery, foreign body ingestion, abdominal distension, peritoneal signs, or abnormal bowel sounds. If there is a significant abnormality and further diagnostic evaluation is indicated, other useful studies that may be considered include erythrocyte sedimentation rate (ESR), amylase concentra-

tion, liver function tests (LFTs), pregnancy test, peritoneal lavage, ultrasound, computed tomographic (CT) scanning, esophagoscopy, and contrast studies, including intravenous pyelogram (IVP), upper gastrointestinal (GI) series, barium enema, and cholecystogram. See Table 24-1 for diagnostic considerations.

MANAGEMENT

The management of the patient with abdominal pain must reflect the severity, acuteness, and likely causes. Patients who must be seen immediately include those with prolonged, severe pain, high temperatures (>39° C), crying and doubling over with pain, associated trauma, potential dehydration, tachypnea or grunting; patients with more prolonged fever (>2 days) with progression of pain made more comfortable by lying down should be seen on an urgent basis. Observation may be an important option.

Many patients with prolonged pain, particularly those with nausea, vomiting, or diarrhea, have fluid deficits and benefit from intravenous hydration during the evaluation process (see Chapter 7). Gastric decompression (nasogastric tube) also may be useful. Surgical consultation should be sought for all patients with severe pain and a significant abdominal examination finding. Pain relief may be administered after consultation.

A therapeutic trial of antacids may be useful if gastritis/esophagitis is suspected.

REFERENCES

Attard AR, Corlett MJ, Kidner NJ, et al: Safety of early pain relief for acute abdominal pain, *BMJ* 305:554, 1997.

Hatch EI Jr: The acute abdomen in children, *Pediatr Clin North Am* 32:1151, 1985.

Reef S, Sloven DG, Lebenthal E: Gallstones in children, *Am J Dis Child* 145:105, 1991.

Rothrock SG, Green SM, Hummel CB: Plain abdominal radiography in the detection of major disease in children: a prospective analysis, *Ann Emerg Med* 21:1423, 1992.

Silen W: *Cope's early diagnosis of the acute abdomen*, ed 17, New York, 1987, McGraw-Hill.

25 ABUSE

ALERT: Suspicion is the key to recognition. All cases must be reported.

CHILD ABUSE: NONACCIDENTAL TRAUMA

Children less than 18 years of age who have a nonaccidental trauma (NAT) or physical injury that threatens their health or welfare are abused. This may take any one of several forms, including physical or emotional abuse, neglect (physical, emotional, medical, or educational), or sexual assault. Consideration of abuse is mandatory in evaluating children who have suspicious injuries, particularly in settings that treat patients who are transient and whose care lacks continuity.

DIAGNOSTIC FINDINGS

Unique interpersonal dynamics form the basis for potential abuse and identify children who are at greatest risk.
1. The abused child
   a. Usually less than 4 years of age
   b. Often handicapped, retarded, hyperactive, or temperamental
   c. Premature birth or neonatal separation
   d. Multiple birth
2. The abusive parent
   a. Low self-esteem, depressed, a substance abuser
   b. Often abused as a child
   c. History of mental illness or criminal activity
   d. Violent temper outbursts toward child
   e. Rigid and unrealistic expectations of child
   f. Young maternal age
3. Family
   a. Monetary problems, often with unemployment
   b. Isolated and highly mobile
   c. Marital problems
   d. Pattern of husband/wife abuse
   e. Poor parent-child relationships
   f. Unwanted pregnancies, illegitimate children, youthful marriage

The introduction of one of the following triggers exacerbates the individual and family stresses, possibly resulting in child abuse: a family argument, discipline problem, substance abuse, loss of job, eviction, illness, or other environmental stresses. The child is often brought for care with a complaint other than the one associated with abuse or neglect ("somatic complaint").

Characteristics of History

1. Injury inconsistent with the history
2. Parents reluctant to give information or deny knowledge of how trauma might have occurred
3. Child developmentally incapable of specified self-injury (e.g., 9-month-old falling off tricycle)
4. Inappropriate response to severity of injury
5. Delay in seeking health care

TABLE 25-1   Differential Diagnosis of Child Abuse

Diagnostic findings		
Physical examination	**Ancillary data**	**Differential diagnosis**
CUTANEOUS LESIONS		
Bruising (rope, tie, bite, cigarette burns)	History	Trauma, accidental
	Bleeding screen	Hemophilia, von Willebrand
	Sepsis workup	Henoch-Schönlein purpura
	Sepsis workup	Purpura fulminans/ meningococcemia
	CBC, bone marrow	Malignancy—leukemia
	History	Mongolian spot
Local erythema or bullae	History	Burn, accidental
(abrasion or burns)	Culture, Gram stain	Impetigo, cellulitis
(shape delineated)	History, sensitizing agent	Contact or photo dermatitis
SKELETAL DISORDER		
(Chapters 66-70)	History	Trauma, accidental
Fractures (multiple, unexplained,	Radiograph, blue sclera	Osteogenesis imperfecta
various stages of healing,	Nutritional history, levels	Nutritional deficiency, copper, rickets, scurvy
metaphyseal or epiphyseal,		
subperiosteal ossification)	History	Birth trauma
	CBC, bone marrow	Malignancy—leukemia, neuroblastoma
	History	Neurogenic sensory deficit
	Serology	Syphilis
	History	Drugs—prostaglandin, methotrexate, vitamin A toxicity
OCCULAR FINDINGS		
(Chapter 59 and p. 626)		
Retinal hemorrhage	History	Trauma, accidental or resuscitation
	Bleeding screen	Bleeding disorder
Conjunctival hemorrhage	History	Trauma, accidental or coughing
	History	Conjunctivitis
Hyphema	History	Trauma, accidental

Continued

Physical Examination (Table 25-1)

Bruises on the skin go through a typical evolutionary pattern that is useful in relating the objective findings to the history. The age of the bruise should be only one criterion in a child's evaluation because the accuracy of timing is limited. Factors to consider include the following:

1. Bruise with any yellow is older than 18 hours.
2. Red, blue and purple, or black may occur from 1 hour after injury to resolution.
3. Red may be present in any bruise, irrespective of age.
4. Bruises of identical age and cause on the same person may appear to be different.

The mechanism of a burn may be distinguished by physical findings. Accidental burns have an irregular pattern, often a splash configu-

TABLE 25-1   Differential Diagnosis of Child Abuse—cont'd

Diagnostic findings		
Physical examination	**Ancillary data**	**Differential diagnosis**
ACUTE ABDOMEN		
(Chapters 24 and 63)	History	Trauma, accidental
Lacerated/contused liver, spleen, kidney, intramural hematoma, retroperitoneal hematoma	Radiographs, stool tests, etc.	GI disease (obstruction, peritonitis, inflammatory bowel disease)
	Urinalysis, culture	Urinary tract infection, anomaly
	Ultrasound, IVP	Other (e.g., genital problem, mesenteric adenitis, hernia)
	Specific studies	
MENTAL STATUS CHANGE		
(Chapters 15, 54, and 57)	CT scan	Trauma, accidental (subdural, epidural, intracranial)
	Drug screen	Intoxication
	Lumbar puncture	Meningitis
	Specific studies	Hypoglycemia, methylmalonic acidemia
SUDDEN INFANT DEATH		
(Chapter 22)	Sepsis work-up	Infection
	History	Trauma, accidental

ration, and varying degrees of damage. Inflicted burns often have a clear line of demarcation without splash marks and a uniform degree of burn throughout. Palm and sole burns suggest prolonged immersion.

Specific patterns include the dunking burn in which the buttocks and genitalia are involved. Stocking or glove burns or doughnut-shaped burns may be noted after immersion injuries. Cigarette burns are usually second degree.

Retinal hemorrhage, although commonly associated with child abuse, has also been reported secondary to cardiopulmonary resuscitation usually in children less than 2 years (because of elevated intrathoracic pressures), accidental trauma, blood dyscrasias (leukemia, sickle cell disease), infections (Rocky Mountain spotted fever, tick fever), general anesthesia, intraocular surgery, and intracranial disease (aneurysm, subarachnoid hemorrhage, subdural hemorrhage).

Behavioral signs that may either provoke or result from abuse or neglect include the following:

1. Anger, social isolation, or destructive patterns, with evidence of negativism
2. Difficulty in developing relationships
3. Evidence of developmental delays
4. Depression or suicidal signals
5. Repeated ingestions
6. Poor school attendance and poor performance
7. Poor self-esteem
8. Regressive behavior

Ancillary Data (see Table 25-1)

1. X-ray studies are indicated for all children less than 5 years of age to rule out unsuspected injuries in cases of physical abuse. For those older than 5 years of age, x-ray

films are taken of areas of tenderness, deformity, etc. Skeletal or trauma series, including skull (posteroanterior [PA] and lateral), chest (PA), pelvis (anteroposterior [AP]), spine, and long bones (AP) should be obtained.

2. Bleeding screen (see Chapter 29) is appropriate if there is a history of recurrent bruising and bruising is the predominant manifestation of abuse. May usually be done electively.

3. Specific studies as indicated. Methylmalonic acidemia is a genetic disorder leading to an accumulation of propionic acid. The condition may be seen with lethargy caused by central nervous system (CNS) hemorrhage.

DIFFERENTIAL DIAGNOSIS

See Table 25-1 for differential diagnosis.

MANAGEMENT (Fig. 25-1)

The key to management is early recognition of actual and potential abuse situations. Of course, the immediate medical problems must receive attention.

1. Evaluate the family and the child's environment in a nonjudgmental and supportive fashion. A social worker should be involved in this phase.

2. Determine the extent of ongoing risk to the child.

3. Contact the appropriate protective services worker immediately. *In most states there is a legal obligation to report suspected abuse.* A representative of the agency will discuss the case and arrange for involvement of a staff member. A full written report is required within 24 to 48 hours (depending on the state). Each hospital should have its own routine for expediting this process. Usually a special form is completed and forwarded with the encounter form.

DISPOSITION

Hospitalization is indicated when it is medically appropriate, in the absence of an alternative placement facility, or if the child cannot return home because of ongoing danger. The child should not be discharged until the medical problems are receiving appropriate treatment, social and protective services have agreed on a temporary disposition, and the case is fully evaluated.

Optimally, a temporary crisis center is desirable if the patient is medically stable. If there is no ongoing risk, the patient may be discharged and sent home, with close monitoring and continuing evaluation. Attention should also be focused on the potential of ongoing domestic violence. Follow-up observation for medical problems should be arranged before the patient is discharged.

Social services and protective services must arrange for continuing evaluation and management of psychosocial problems.

REFERENCES

American Medical Association: AMA diagnostic and treatment guidelines concerning child abuse and neglect, *JAMA* 254:796, 1985.

Ellerstein NS, Norris KJ: Value of radiologic skeletal survey in assessment of abused children, *Pediatrics* 74:1075, 1984.

Gayle MO, Kissoon N, Hered RW, et al: Retinal hemorrhage in the young child: a review of etiology, predisposed conditions and clinical implications, *J Emerg Med* 13:233, 1995.

Hymel KP, Abshire TC, Luckey DW, et al: Coagulopathy in pediatric abusive head trauma, *Pediatrics* 99:371, 1977.

Johnson DC, Braum D, Friendly D: Accidental head trauma and retinal hemorrhage, *Neurosurgery* 33:231, 1993.

Marshall WN, Puls T, Davidson C: New child abuse spectrum in an era of increased awareness, *Am J Dis Child* 142:664, 1988.

Schwartz AJ, Ricci LR: How accurately can bruises be aged in abused children? Literature review and synthesis, *Pediatrics* 97:254, 1996.

Stewart GM, Rosenberg NM: Conditions mistaken for child abuse. Parts I and II, *Pediatr Emerg Care* 12:116, 217, 1996.

Wright RJ, Wright RO, Isaac NE: Response to battered mothers in the pediatric emergency department: a call for an interdisciplinary approach to family violence, *Pediatrics* 99:186, 1997.

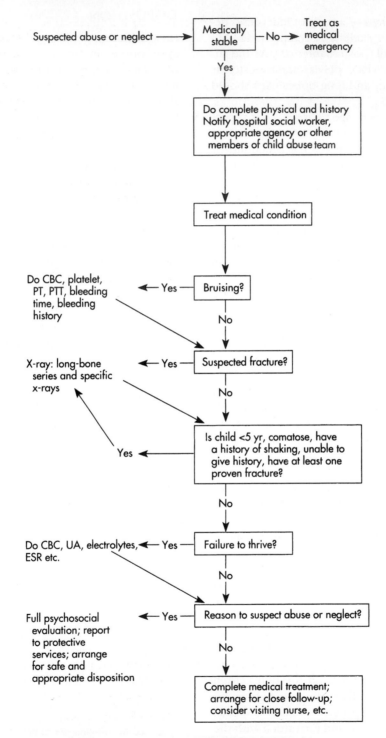

Fig. 25-1   Management of suspected child abuse.

SEXUAL ABUSE

Sexual assault—rape, molestation, or incest—may occur at any age. Evaluation and management require considerable suspicion and sensitivity. Appropriate authorities should be notified, and the assessment must reflect local guidelines.

DIAGNOSTIC FINDINGS

Initially, confidence and rapport must be established. When younger children are involved, it is often the parent who is most upset. A detailed history of the incident must be documented. In addition, information about the medical history, menstrual and pregnancy history, contraceptive status, recent intercourse, and bathing or douching since the assault should be obtained.

The examination should be individualized, and with younger children, the mother usually should be present. Time, patience, and gentleness are needed. Severely assaulted patients may be angry and withdrawn.

The child's general appearance must be assessed and signs of external trauma, abrasions, lacerations, contusions, bites, and child abuse noted. An internal examination is often not required in infants and young children. Younger children often can be examined in the froglike position; older children may require the lithotomy position (p. 666).

The patient with acute trauma will demonstrate perineal contusions or lacerations and hymenal tears with bleeding, fissures, erythema, and discharge. The uterus and adnexa may be tender. Signs of chronic molestation are residual findings of hymenal remnants, healed lacerations, a large introitus, and discharge (p. 671). A hymenal diameter of 4 mm may be associated with sexual abuse, although there is tremendous natural variation in the shape and location of the opening of hymens, and the assessment should be used as only one component of the evaluation.

Beyond the neonatal period, nonsexual transmission of sexually transmitted diseases is uncommon in prepubescent females. In general, sexual abuse should be considered in infants and prepubertal children with any of the following:

1. Genital or rectal *Chlamydia trachomatis* or herpes simplex virus
2. Genital or pharyngeal *Neisseria gonorrhoeae*
3. Anogenital warts in children more than 2 years of age
4. Human immunodeficiency virus (HIV) infection or syphilis in infant or child where mother is seronegative
5. Vaginal *Trichomonas vaginalis*
6. *Phthirus pubis* (crab louse) infestations of eyelashes

Complications

Emotional trauma varies with the age of the victim and the circumstances of the assault.

Ancillary Data

1. Specimens and data are used to assist in documenting the circumstances and appropriately treating the patient. Many centers have kits for collecting specimens. Their use should be individualized. However, their value is minimal if more than 48 hours have elapsed or if the patient has bathed.
2. Cultures are taken of the cervix for *N. gonorrhoeae* and *C. trachomatis,* as well as of the rectum and pharynx, if appropriate, and repeated 2 weeks after the assault. Wet preparation for trichomonas.
3. A wet mount of vaginal discharge for *Gardnerella vaginalis* and *T. vaginalis.*
4. The Venereal Disease Research Laboratory (VDRL) (syphilis) test taken at the visit is repeated in 2 weeks.
5. A pregnancy test (if appropriate) is used to determine status at the time of assault.
6. Vaginal fluid to test for spermatozoa (wet

preparation and dried) and prostatic acid phosphatase concentration is studied.

7. Saliva for ABO-antigen typing determines whether the victim is secretor.

8. A hair specimen is obtained by combing pubic area of the victim.

9. Clothing and other items are submitted for forensic examination when appropriate.

NOTE: To maintain the chain of custody, all specimens must be handled carefully and remain in the physician's possession at all times until sealed. To ensure that the specimens are not altered before the introduction of the data in the courtroom, the "chain of evidence" must not be violated.

MANAGEMENT

The initial management of the patient must be supportive and understanding. The examination should proceed only after appropriate support services have assisted the patient and parents in dealing with the episode. Many institutions have specially trained individuals (often volunteers) to participate in this process. The examination must be individualized, reflecting the age of the child and the circumstances of the assault. If more than 48 hours have elapsed, specimens will be of little value. The episode must be reported to the appropriate child protective services agency.

Pregnancy may be prevented, and a number of options exist:

1. Diethylstilbestrol (DES): 25 mg two times/day for 5 days within 48 hours of the incident. It is associated with considerable nausea and vomiting. An antiemetic may be needed.

2. Ovral (norgestrel 0.5 mg and ethinyl estradiol 0.05 mg): two tablets taken within 72 hours of abuse and two more tablets 12 hours later.

3. Do nothing, and await next menses.

4. Recheck monoclonal antibody agglutination test to beta subunit of human chorionic gonadotropin (hCG) in urine or radioimmunoassay against beta subunit of hCG in blood 7 days after incident. If the result is negative, likelihood of pregnancy is low, but if positive, consider therapeutic abortion.

Prophylactic antibiotic regimens for sexual abuse include the following:

1. Tetracycline, 500 mg QID PO for 7 days, or doxycycline, 100 mg BID for 7 days (*N. gonorrhoeae, C. trachomatis,* incubating syphilis). Tetracycline-resistant *N. gonorrhoeae* may be present. Do not use in children 9 years old or younger.

2. For pregnant women, amoxicillin, 3 gm plus 1 gm probenecid, as single dose (*N. gonorrhoeae,* syphilis).

3. Erythromycin base, 500 mg QID PO for 7 days (*C. trachomatis*).

4. Ceftriaxone, 125 to 250 mg IM (*N. gonorrhoeae,* syphilis).

Follow-up observation with appropriate support groups and health care professionals is crucial. The patient should be seen in 2 weeks to assess the reaction and repeat the cervical culture and VDRL test. If follow-up care will be difficult, treatment for gonorrhea at the initial encounter should be considered (p. 672).

Presumptive antibiotic treatment of prepubertal children is not widely recommended because of the lower risk of ascending infection.

Ongoing support may be necessary because of persistent problems.

REFERENCES

American Academy of Pediatrics: Guidelines for the evaluation of sexual abuse in children, *Pediatrics* 87:254, 1991.

Bays J, Jenny C: Genital and anal conditions confused with child sexual abuse trauma, *Am J Dis Child* 144:1319, 1990.

Dubowiitz H, Black M, Starrington D: The diagnosis of child sexual abuse, *Am J Dis Child* 146:688, 1992.

Gardner JJ: Descriptive study of genital variation in healthy, nonabused premenarchal girls, *J Pediatr* 120:251, 1992.

Hermann-Giddens ME, Frothingham TE: Prepubertal female genitalia: examination for evidence of sexual abuse, *Pediatrics* 80:203, 1987.

McCann J, Voris J, Simon M: General injuries resulting from sexual abuse: a longitudinal study, *Pediatrics* 89:307, 1992.

Neinstein LS, Goldenring J, Carpenter S: Non-sexual transmission of sexually transmitted disease: an infrequent occurrence, *Pediatrics* 74:67, 1984.

Ricci LR: Photographing the physically abused child, *Am J Dis Child* 145:275, 1991.

Swanson HY, Tebbutt JS, O'Toole BI, et al: Sexually abused children 5 years after presentation: a case-controlled study, *Pediatrics* 100:600, 1997.

26 ANEMIA

THOMAS J. SMITH and ROGER H. GILLER

ALERT: Anemia, which most commonly is caused by iron-deficiency, requires a systematic evaluation of hematologic parameters.

Anemia is a manifestation of a primary disease or nutritional deficiency. Because the hemoglobin and hematocrit vary with age, anemia in children and adolescents is defined as that hemoglobin concentration that falls below the third percentile for a patient's age group (Fig. 26-1).

ETIOLOGY (Fig. 26-2)

Nutritional iron-deficiency is the most common cause of anemia in children between 6 months and 2 years of age. It typically results from excessive cow's milk intake (>24 to 30 ounces/day) and inadequate consumption of iron-rich foods as the child outgrows inborn iron stores. Iron-deficiency anemia in those older than 2 years of age should prompt an investigation for causes of chronic blood loss. Iron-deficiency anemia may adversely influence performance on developmental testing; that effect may persist beyond correction of the anemia.

Anemias unrelated to iron-deficiency can be divided into two major categories:

1. Anemias caused by impaired red cell production, maturation, or release from the bone marrow

Disease	Mechanism
Malignancy: storage disease	Marrow infiltration
Fanconi anemia, drugs, Blackfan-Diamond anemia, transient erythroblastopenia of childhood (TEC), aplastic anemia	Marrow aplasia/hypoplasia

Disease	Mechanism
Infection	Marrow hypoplasia or hemolysis
Folate, B_{12}, B_6, copper deficiency	Impaired maturation of red cell precursors in bone marrow
Thalassemia syndrome, iron-deficiency, lead poisoning, sideroblastic anemia, pyridoxine deficiency	Impaired hemoglobin production, intramedullary hemolysis (thalassemias)
Chronic disease, inflammation, renal disease, hypothyroidism	Impaired erythropoiesis

2. Destruction, sequestration, or acute loss of circulating red cells

Disease	Mechanism
Sickle cell disease and other hemoglobinopathies, ABO or Rh incompatibility (in newborn), vitamin E deficiency, autoimmune hemolytic anemia, RBC enzyme deficiency, RBC membrane defect, hemolytic-uremic syndrome (HUS), disseminated intravascular coagulation (DIC), hemangioma, cardiac defect, prosthetic heart valve	Hemolysis
Portal hypertension, sickle cell disease	Splenic sequestration
Trauma, surgery, bleeding disorder, peptic ulcer disease	Hemorrhage

The physiologic nadir occurs at 6 to 12 weeks of age. In normal term infants the hemoglobin can drop to 9 gm/dl, in normal preterm infants to 75 gm/dl (see Chapter 11).

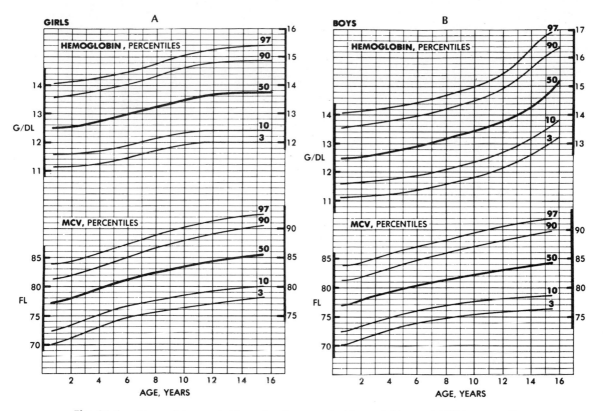

Fig. 26-1   Normal hemoglobin value by age. **A,** Hemoglobin and MCV percentile curves for girls. **B,** Hemoglobin and MCV percentile curves for boys. *MCV,* Mean corpuscular volume.

(From Dallman PR, Siimes MA: *J Pediatr* 94:26, 1979.)

DIAGNOSTIC FINDINGS

Historically, it is important to consider age, sex, ethnic background, blood type (in infants), and dietary history (especially intake of cow's milk); to determine the duration of symptoms; and to inquire about chronic illness or infection, bleeding, and pica. Family history must be reviewed in regard to history of anemia, jaundice, gallbladder disease, splenomegaly, or splenectomy.

The presenting signs and symptoms reflect the severity of the anemia, rapidity of onset, and underlying cause.

1. With rapid onset of anemia (e.g., blood loss, sudden hemolysis), headache, dizziness, postural hypotension, tachycardia, hypovolemia, or high-output cardiac failure may be present (see Chapters 5 and 16).

2. Insidious onset (e.g., nutritional deficiency, leukemia) is typically associated with pallor and decreased exercise tolerance.

3. Children with iron-deficiency anemia may display behavioral disturbances, learning problems, and delayed motor development. Severe iron-deficiency disrupts the integrity of the gastrointestinal (GI) mucosa and may lead to a protein-losing enteropathy with blood in

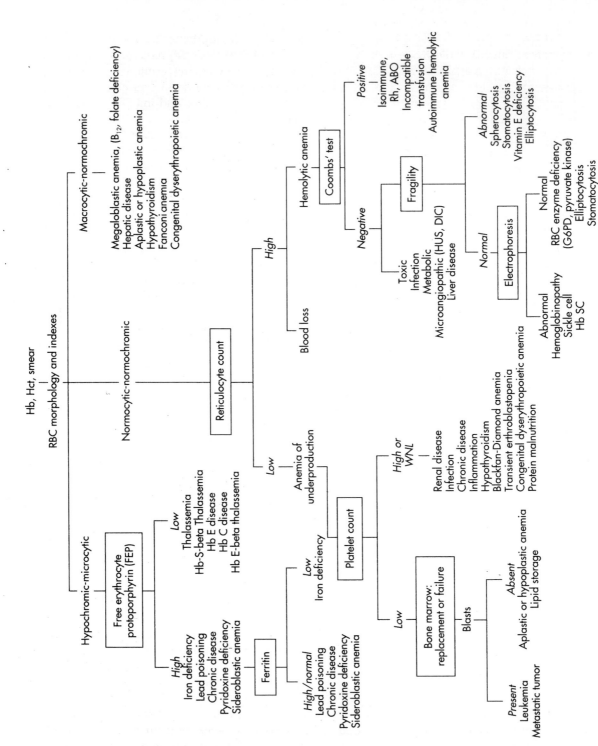

Fig. 26-2   Evaluation of anemia.

the stools, along with decreased iron absorption.

4. Hemolytic anemia typically causes jaundice and splenomegaly. If it is chronic, symptomatic cholelithiasis may develop during the teenage years. Underlying autoimmune disease (e.g., systemic lupus erythematosus) may be present.

Complications

Diminished oxygen-carrying capacity is generally well compensated for by an increased cardiac output. However, severe tissue hypoxia can occur if onset of the anemia is rapid or there is concomitant high-output cardiac failure.

Ancillary Data

1. Initial laboratory includes complete blood count (CBC) with hemoglobin (Hb), hematocrit (Hct), RBC indexes, white blood cell (WBC) count, platelet count, peripheral smear, and reticulocyte count.
2. Anemia in association with microcytosis strongly suggests iron-deficiency. For further confirmation, determine the free-erythrocyte protoporphyrin (FEP) or serum ferritin. An FEP level greater than 3 μg/gm of Hb and a serum ferritin level of less than 12 ng/ml are typical of iron-deficiency. Fasting iron saturation (serum iron/total iron-binding capacity × 100) of less than 20% also is indicative of iron-deficiency but is subject to greater error because of diurnal and acute diet-related fluctuations in serum iron level. An FEP of greater than 18 μg/gm of Hb strongly suggests lead poisoning.
3. Check stool for occult blood.
4. Perform other studies, as indicated in Fig. 26-2.

Samples for diagnostic studies to determine the cause of anemia are best drawn before transfusion therapy, if such therapy is required.

MANAGEMENT

In children 6 months to 2 years of age with no history of blood loss or prematurity, a hypochromic, microcytic anemia is most likely caused by dietary iron-deficiency anemia. It is appropriate to forgo iron studies and initiate a therapeutic trial with careful follow-up observation. Many recommend that iron supplementation be started in breast-fed children at 9 months of age. However, in children older than 2 years of age, among whom nutritional deficiency is less common, a more extensive evaluation to confirm iron-deficiency and exclude chronic blood loss is indicated.

For initial treatment of suspected iron-deficiency anemia:

1. Prescribe elemental iron 5-6 mg/kg/24 hr q8hr PO. Ferrous sulfate (Fer-in-Sol), 75 mg (15 mg elemental iron)/0.6 ml dropper, is a useful formulation. The iron supplement should be continued for 2 months after anemia is corrected to replenish iron stores.

   NOTE: With good compliance, normal absorption, and no ongoing iron losses, the reticulocyte count should increase in 3 to 5 days, and the hemoglobin should begin to rise during the first week of treatment.
2. Encourage iron-rich foods.
3. Limit cow's milk intake to 24 oz/day or less.
4. Blood transfusions should be reserved for those with evidence of cardiovascular compromise.

A profound degree of anemia may produce life-threatening cardiovascular instability, requiring emergency intervention with blood products and fluids (see Chapters 5 and 16). Other forms of anemia requiring specialized evaluation and treatment should be handled on an individual basis in consultation with a hematologist.

DISPOSITION

Most children may be followed as outpatients. Admission is indicated if the Hct is below 20% (Hb <7 mg/dl) or if there is evidence of cardiac decompensation, hypoxia, rapid ongoing blood loss, or hemolysis.

Parental education for iron-deficiency anemia:

1. Give an iron supplement three times a day, preferably between meals to enhance absorption.

   If there is any nausea, the iron may be given with foods. Keep the medication in a safe place because accidental ingestion of a large amount can be dangerous.

2. Increase your child's intake of iron-rich foods such as meat, eggs, green vegetables, and enriched cereals and breads. Limit milk intake to 24 oz/day.

3. Take your child back for a recheck of blood counts in 1 to 2 weeks and at 1 and 2 months to be certain the youngster is no longer anemic.

REFERENCES

Beutler E: The common anemias, *JAMA* 259:2433, 1988.

Eden AN, Mir MA: Iron deficiency in 1- to 3-year-old children, *Arch Pediatr Adolesc Med* 151:986, 1997.

Lozoff B, Jimenez E, Wolf AW: Long-term developmental outcome of infants with iron deficiency, *N Engl J Med* 325:687, 1991.

Walter T, De Andraea I, Chadud P, et al: Iron deficiency anemia: adverse effects on infant psychomotor development, *Pediatrics* 84:7, 1989.

27 ARTHRALGIA AND JOINT PAIN

ALERT: Septic arthritis must be excluded in all patients.

Pain, swelling, and joint discomfort accompany arthralgia. If the joint is inflamed with accompanying redness, warmth, swelling, and pain, the patient has arthritis.

The patient must be questioned regarding the nature of the joint discomfort or pain with specific reference to the progression of signs and symptoms: severity, duration, type of pain, ameliorating factors, and family history. Any relationship to trauma and infection or systemic, vascular, or degenerative disease must be defined. Associated signs and symptoms, especially gastrointestinal, renal, and neurologic, should be sought. Knowledge of previous medical problems and exposures and consideration of the patient's age may be helpful.

The patient must have a careful examination of the joint, with particular attention to the severity of involvement—defining objective parameters, including warmth, tenderness, pain, presence of fluid, and limitation of motion. Hip pain may be referred to the knee.

Ancillary data often are essential. If a fever or an elevated erythrocyte sedimentation rate (ESR) (>30 mm/hr) is present, an infectious or autoimmune process is eight times more likely than if both are absent. If both are present, only

See also Chapters 40 and 82.

7% of these patients lack a condition in either of these categories. Radiographs should be obtained. Follow-up plain films are often useful, given that callus or periosteal reaction may not be present for 7 to 10 days in patients with hairline fractures or osteomyelitis. Complete blood count (CBC), blood culture, bone scan, antinuclear antibody (ANA) tests, and rheumatoid factor and immunoglobulin levels may be selectively obtained.

If there is any question of the diagnosis and joint fluid is present, a joint aspirate should be obtained, usually after consultation with an orthopedist (see Appendix A-2). The procedure usually is contraindicated if there is any overlying infection of the joint or if only small joints are involved. Typical findings are outlined in Tables 27-1 and 82-1.

A therapeutic trial of nonsteroidal antiinflammatory agents or aspirin may be useful in inflammatory-induced disease.

REFERENCES

Kunnamo I, Kallio P, Pelkonen P, et al: Clinical signs and laboratory tests in the differential diagnosis of arthritis in children, *Am J Dis Child* 141:34, 1987.

McCarthy PL, Wasserman D, Spiesel SZ, et al: Evaluation of arthritis and arthralgia in the pediatric patient, *Clin Pediatr* 19:183, 1980.

Schallee JG: Arthritis in children, *Pediatr Clin North Am* 33:1565, 1986.

TABLE 27-1   Arthralgia and Joint Pain: Diagnostic Considerations and Management

Condition	Diagnostic findings	Joints	Ancillary data	Comments/management
TRAUMA (Chapter 66)				
Sprain **Fracture**	History of trauma; joint tenderness, swelling; fracture may be occult	Usually monoarticular	X-ray study findings variable	Orthopedic consult; consider child abuse (NAT)
"Little League elbow"	Swelling, tenderness; pitcher's elbow	Elbow on dominant arm	X-ray study findings WNL	Restrict pitching
INFECTION				
Toxic synovitis of the hip (Chapter 69)	Preceding viral illness; non-toxic; often accompanied by limp; rarely warm, tender, limited range of motion	Hip	CBC, ESR: WNL; x-ray study findings—variable effusion; aspirate if question of septic arthritis	Self-limited; common in 1½ to 7 year olds
Arthritis, septic (p. 751)	Acute onset, febrile; local swelling, warmth, tenderness	Monoarticular, large weight-bearing: knee, hip, wrist, elbow, shoulder; rarely polyarticular (gonococcal)	↑WBC, ↑ESR; x-ray study findings; joint aspirate; may need bone scan	Requires urgent drainage and antibiotics
Arthritis, viral Rubella Rubella vaccine Hepatitis Epstein-Barr virus Chickenpox	Local swelling, warmth, tenderness; associated symptoms	Polyarticular; often large joints (knee)	CBC, viral titers, liver functions; x-ray study findings—effusion; joint aspirate	Usually self-limited
Arthritis, uncommon Mycobacteria Fungi Syphilis	Often indolent with subacute progression; joint swelling, tenderness	Usually monoarticular, large joints	Joint aspirate; CBC, syphilis serologic test, PPD, as indicated	
Osteomyelitis	Fever, variable systemic toxicity, local swelling, tenderness, warmth	Monoarticular long bones (femur, tibia)	↑CBC, ↑ESR; x-ray study; bone scan; joint and bone aspirate	May have arthritis and osteomyelitis concurrently; antibiotics

AUTOIMMUNE

Juvenile rheumatoid arthritis (JRA)

Disease	General signs	Joint involvement	Laboratory	Notes/Treatment
Acute febrile systemic (Still's) disease (30% JRA patients)	Irritable, listless, anorexic; hyperpyrexia (may precede arthritis); 90% have maculopapular rash; lymphadenopathy	Minimal or widespread; often only arthralgia; 25% severe arthritis	↑CBC, ↑ESR (70%); negative ANA, negative rheumatoid factor	Peak onset: 1-3 yr; ASA trial (100 mg/kg/24 hr q4hr PO) helpful; if fails: steroids; average age: 7½ yr
Polyarticular (25% JRA patients)	Listless, anorexic; low-grade fevers, daily spike; rare maculopapular rash; rare iridocyclitis	≥4 joints (knee, ankle, wrist, elbow, hand); abrupt or insidious onset; swollen, red, tender; morning stiffness	↑CBC, ↑ESR (70%); positive ANA (25%); positive rheumatoid factor (10%-15%)	ASA trial; if fails: steroids
Monoarticular, pauciarticular (45% JRA patients)	Low-grade to no fever; rare rash; iridocyclitis (25%)	One or few joints—knee most common (others: ankle, elbow, wrist, fingers, sacroiliac); swollen, red, tender; morning stiffness	CBC, ESR: WNL; positive ANA result (25%), positive rheumatoid factor result rare; bone x-ray study finding: acclimated maturation, periosteal proliferation; synovial fluid aspiration	Average age: 7½ yr; ASA trial; if fails: steroids
Rheumatic fever (p. 566)	Carditis, chorea, rheumatoid nodule, erythema marginatum, fever	Migratory, polyarticular, involving knee, ankle, wrist, elbow, shoulder; joints swollen, red, tender, hot, and painful	Variable CBC, ↑ESR; ↑streptozyme; throat culture result variably positive	ASA trial; consider steroids; penicillin
Henoch-Schönlein purpura (anaphylactoid purpura) (p. 805)	Purpuric rash on ankles, buttock, elbow, beginning on lower extremity on extensor surface; abdominal pain, diarrhea, bleeding, intussusception; nephritis	Migratory polyarthritis of large joints	CBC, platelet: WNL; hematest stool, urine; ↑streptozyme, throat culture	Monitor for renal failure
Kawasaki syndrome (p. 710)	Persistent fever (<5 days), conjunctivitis, rash, mucosal membrane changes, migratory polyarthritis, erythema and induration of hand and feet		CBC, platelets: elevated; ↑ESR, ↑CRP	Specific diagnostic criteria; IV gamma globulin, aspirin

Continued

TABLE 27-1 Arthralgia and Joint Pain: Diagnostic Considerations and Management—cont'd

Condition	Diagnostic findings	Joints	Ancillary data	Comments/management
AUTOIMMUNE—cont'd				
Systemic lupus erythematosus	Multisystem disease: weakness, fever, butterfly cheek eruption, hepatosplenomegaly, lymphadenopathy, nephritis; CNS: seizures, psychosis	Migratory; transient with arthralgia or redness, swelling, stiffness	↓ WBC, ↑ Hct; ↑ platelets; positive ANA result; variable hematuria and proteinuria	Prednisone 1 mg/kg/24 hr PO; involve nephrologist
Serum sickness	Fever, rash, lymphadenopathy	Polyarthritis with redness, swelling, pain, stiffness, and large-joint effusion	↑↓ WBC; variable hematuria and proteinuria; reduced complement	Prevent exposure; antihistamine; consider nonsteroidal antiinflammatory agents or steroids
Inflammatory bowel disease Ulcerative colitis Regional ileitis	Diarrhea, variable rectal bleeding, abdominal pain	Polyarthritis, large joints	Sigmoidoscopy, barium swallow	Antiinflammatory agents, possibly surgery
Reiter syndrome	Insidious onset; conjunctivitis, urethritis	Polyarticular, small joints	CBC, ESR: WNL, UA: WNL	Rare in children
CONGENITAL				
Hemophilia (p. 685)	Healthy male, variable history of trauma; history of hemophilia	Monoarticular; joint swollen, tender with hemarthrosis	X-ray study result; abnormal bleeding screen	Factor replacement
Sickle cell disease (p. 698)	Systemic disease	Usually polyarticular; often insidious onset joint and bone pain	X-ray study finding: Hct; positive Sickledex; bone scan variable	May have concurrent infection; may be crisis or infarct
Developmental hip dislocation	Normal newborn except for instability of joint; positive Ortolani sign (abduction)	Abnormal placement and range of motion of hip	X-ray study result abnormal	Orthopedic consultation; splint hip in flexion and abduction

VASCULAR

Legg-Calvé-Perthes (avascular necrosis of proximal femoral head)		Insidious onset; pain of hip with limp or limitation of movement; pain may be referred to knee	X-ray study result: bulging capsule, widening joint space, decreased bone density around joint	Peak: males, 4-10 yr; orthopedic consultation; treat hip in abduction and internal rotation

DEGENERATIVE

Slipped capital femoral epiphysis	Usually obese child or tall, thin child with rapid growth	Unilateral or bilateral; knee pain (referred) on medial aspect thigh above knee; hip or knee pain made worse by activity; limp; limitation abduction and internal rotation	X-ray study result: widening of epiphyseal growth plate	Peak: 12-15 yr; orthopedic consult, surgical immobilization

OSTEOCHONDROSIS

Osteochondritis dissecans	No systemic signs	Knee is painful, stiff with effusion	X-ray, tunnel view shows demineralization of medial femoral condyle	Teenagers; decreased activity; muscle stengthening

NEOPLASM

Ewing's sarcoma Osteogenic sarcoma Leukemia Neuroblastoma	Systemic signs often present	Local pain, effusion, with warmth and tenderness	CBC; x-ray study; biopsy	Orthopedic consultation

28 ATAXIA

ALERT: Children with ataxia require attention to the diagnostic alternatives that permit early initiation of therapy when appropriate.

Ataxia is a disorder that causes impaired balance and incoordination of intentional movement. Infectious and inflammatory processes and intoxication cause most incidents of acute ataxia in children. Hysteria, trauma, ear problems, sinusitis, migraines, and cerebellar and spinal cord tumors may also be causative (Table 28-1). A host of congenital (Friedreich's ataxia, ataxia telangiectasia) and metabolic conditions (Hartnup disease, maple syrup urine disease) have insidious onset of ataxia as a component of their presentations.

Neurologic findings should be defined historically. Progression, acuteness, and recurrence of ataxia and other neurologic finding should be assessed. Preceding events such as

trauma, ingestion of drugs, infection, and respiratory symptoms should be delineated. A family history may be useful.

Cerebellar ataxia is associated with a wide-based, unsteady, and staggering gait, with difficulty in turning. The patient cannot stand with the feet together whether the eyes are open or closed (Romberg sign). *Sensory* ataxia from injury of the peripheral nerve or posterior column of the spinal cord also appears as a wide-based gait. However, the patient can stand with the feet together when the eyes are open but not when closed (positive Romberg sign). This often is associated with lethargy, stupor, and altered mental functioning, although ataxia may be the predominant finding.

TABLE 28-1   Acute Ataxia: Diagnostic Considerations

Condition	Diagnostic findings	Ancillary data	Comments
INFECTION/INFLAMMATION			
Acute cerebellar ataxia	Prodrome of fever, respiratory or GI illness; abrupt onset; cerebellar ataxia; no evidence of intracranial pressure increase; normal mental function	CSF: WNL or slight lymphocytosis	2- to 6-year-olds; resolves in 2-3 mo; usually viral (consider varicella)
Postinfectious encephalitis	Preceding headache, exanthem, stiff neck, fever; changed mental status; cerebellar ataxia	CSF: ↑ protein, lymphocytosis	Usually viral; usually resolves

TABLE 28-1   Acute Ataxia: Diagnostic Considerations—cont'd

Condition	Diagnostic findings	Ancillary data	Comments
INFECTION/INFLAMMATION—cont'd			
Bacterial: meningitis/ encephalitis (p. 725)	Fever, toxic, stiff neck, changed mental status; cerebellar ataxia may be early symptom or postinfectious sequela	CSF: ↑ protein, ↑ WBC, ↓ glucose	Usually resolves after treatment
Cerebellar abscess	Fever, headache, cerebellar ataxia; may be signs of increased intracranial pressure	CT scan	Neurosurgical consultation
Acute labyrinthitis/ sinusitis	Cerebellar ataxia, vertigo, nystagmus, tinnitus, hearing loss, headache, nausea, vomiting; may accompany otitis media		May also be traumatic
Multiple sclerosis	Cerebellar ataxia; spastic weakness; optic neuritis, diplopia; multiple neurologic deficits; relapsing	CSF: ↑ cells, ↑ protein, ↑ gamma globulin	Steroids (ACTH); physiotherapy
INTOXICATION (Chapter 54)			
Phenytoin	Cerebellar ataxia, nystagmus	Level >30 µg/ml	
Phenobarbital	Cerebellar ataxia, lethargy	Level >50 µg/ml	Tranquilizers also
Alcohol	Cerebellar ataxia, slurred speech, visual impairment, progressing to stupor and coma	Level depends on whether acute or chronic use	
Carbon monoxide	Headache, confusion, cerebellar ataxia, seizures, stupor to coma	CO elevated	Oxygen therapy, hyperbaric oxygen
Lead (also mercury and thallium)	Anorexia, vomiting, lethargy, cerebellar ataxia, increased intracranial pressure, papilledema, anemia; history of pica		Dimercaprol, EDTA
TRAUMA			
Head injury (Chapter 57)	Head trauma; headache; concussion; cerebellar ataxia	CT scan	Close monitoring
Heat stroke/exhaustion (Chapter 50)	Fatigue, weakness, headache, cerebellar ataxia, seizures, psychosis, coma	Electrolytes; variable ABG and ECG	Treatment varies with condition
INTRAPSYCHIC (Chapter 83)			
Hysteria	Anxious; inconsistent findings		Psychiatric consultation

Examination of the younger child must rely heavily on observation and cerebellar function demonstrated through play activities.

Ancillary data should usually include a spinal tap and drug levels, if indicated. A computed tomography (CT) or magnetic resonance imaging (MRI) scan may exclude mass lesions or increased intracranial pressure. Other tests must focus on potential causes.

REFERENCES

Chutorian AM, Pavlaxis SG: Acute ataxia. In Pellock JM, Meyer EC, editors: *Neurologic emergencies in infancy and childhood,* ed 2, Boston, 1993, Butterworth-Heinemann.

Peters ACB, Versteeg J, Lindeman J, et al: Varicella and acute cerebellar ataxia, *Arch Neurol* 35:769, 1978.

Stumpf DA: Acute ataxia, *Pediatr Rev* 8:303, 1987.

29 BLEEDING

ALERT: Patients with abnormal bleeding should be evaluated by an initial assessment that includes CBC, platelet count, PT, PTT, and bleeding time. Hemorrhage should be controlled when significant, usually by application of direct pressure. Resuscitation may be required with severe hemorrhage.

The evaluation of the patient with bleeding requires careful attention to the pattern of bleeding, its location, and whether it is spontaneous or a response to minor or major trauma. A history of bleeding problems should be pursued by asking about prior experience with procedures, such as circumcision; lacerations; tooth extraction; or menstruation, which typically cause transient bleeding. A family history may indicate a hereditary basis for the bleeding disorder.

The physical examination should classify the nature of the bleeding and ascertain its severity and any potential hemodynamic complications. Orthostatic vital signs may be helpful. If bruises or bleeding is unexplained or inconsistent with the history, additional evaluation for child abuse should be considered (Table 29-1).

Ancillary data that should be obtained on all patients with excessive or abnormal bleeding include the following:

1. Complete blood count (CBC), peripheral blood smear, and platelet count
2. Bleeding time (BT)
3. Partial thromboplastin time (PTT)
4. Prothrombin time (PT)

TABLE 29-1 Patterns of Bleeding

Diagnostic findings	Small-vessel hemostasis defect (platelet or capillary)	Intravascular defect (coagulation)
Preceding injury		
None (spontaneous)	Small, superficial, diffuse bleeding involving mucous membranes (epistaxis, gastrointestinal, menorrhagia)	Major bleeding (musculoskeletal, central nervous system)
Superficial cut or abrasion	Profuse, prolonged	Minimal
Deep cut or tooth extraction	Immediate; good response to pressure	Delayed; poor response to pressure
Joint trauma	Hemarthrosis uncommon	Hemarthrosis common
Petechiae	Common	Rare
Ancillary data	Prolonged bleeding time Abnormal platelets	Prolonged partial thromboplastin time, prothrombin time

TABLE 29-2   Screening of the Bleeding Patient

Condition	Screening tests					Comments
	Platelet count	BT	PTT	PT	TT	
NORMAL (WNL) (varies with lab)	150,000-400,000/ml	4-9 min	25-35 sec	12-13 sec	8-10 sec	Fibrinogen level 190-400 mg/dl
HEREDITARY DISORDERS						
Hemophilia						
Factor VIII (Classic: A)	WNL	WNL	↑	WNL	WNL	Factor assay
Factor IX (Christmas: B)	WNL	WNL	↑	WNL	WNL	Factor assay
Factor XI	WNL	WNL	↑	WNL	WNL	Factor assay
Factor XII	WNL	WNL	↑	WNL	WNL	Factor assay
Factor II, V, X	WNL	WNL	↑	↑	WNL	Factor assay
Factor VII	WNL	WNL	WNL	↑	WNL	Factor assay
von Willebrand (many variants)	WNL	↑	↑	WNL	WNL	vWF antigen, vWF activity, ristocetin cofactor
Platelet dysfunction	WNL/↓	↑	WNL	WNL	WNL	Platelet aggregation studies
ACQUIRED DISORDERS						
Disseminated intravascular coagulation (p. 683)	↓	↑	↑	↑	↑	↓ fibrinogen level, ↑ fibrin split products, ↑ D-dimer, microangiopathy
Idiopathic thrombocytopenic purpura (p. 694)	↓	↑	WNL	WNL	WNL	Increased destruction of platelets—immune
Henoch-Schönlein purpura (p. 805)	WNL	WNL	WNL	WNL	WNL	
Liver failure (severe)	WNL/↓	WNL/↑	↑	↑	WNL/↑	↓ fibrinogen level, ↑ fibrin split products
Uremia (p. 809)	WNL/↓	↑	WNL	WNL	WNL/↑	Secondary to hepatic dysfunction or protein loss
Anticoagulants						
Heparin	WNL	WNL	↑	WNL/↑	↑↑	Also lupuslike and inactivating anticoagulant
Coumadin	WNL	WNL	WNL/↑	↑	WNL	
Aspirin, other NSAID	WNL	↑	WNL	WNL	WNL	
Hemolytic-uremic syndrome (p. 801), thrombotic thrombocytopenic purpura	↓	Varies with platelet count	WNL	WNL	WNL	Platelet activation, microangiopathic hemolytic anemia, renal failure

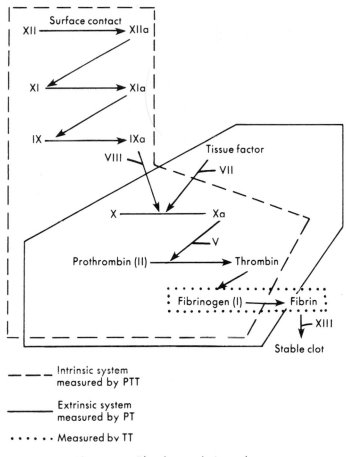

Fig. 29-1 Blood coagulation scheme.

5. Thrombin time (TT)

6. Fibrinogen

These tests assess various components of hemostasis (Fig. 29-1) and, in combination with factor assays and platelet-function studies, define most common bleeding abnormalities (Table 29-2). Once classified, specific management can be initiated in consultation with a hematologist.

REFERENCES

Bennett JS: Blood coagulation and coagulation tests, *Med Clin North Am* 68:557, 1985.

Clouse LH, Comp PC: The regulation of hemostasis: the protein C system, *N Engl J Med* 314:1298, 1986.

Montgomery RR, Hathaway WE: Acute bleeding emergencies, *Pediatr Clin North Am* 27:327, 1980.

30 CONSTIPATION

ALERT: Constipation is commonly functional, although organic conditions must be excluded.

Constipation is present when children have difficulty with bowel movements because of an abnormality in the character of the stool rather than frequency. With persistent pain and discomfort, frequency decreases. Elimination patterns reflect familial, cultural, and social factors. It is essential to determine whether the stool pattern being described is actually normal. Constipation in the newborn often is associated with an anatomic problem, but in older children it is usually functional or dietary in origin.

ETIOLOGY

1. Dietary.
   a. Lack of fecal bulk, causing an inadequate peristaltic stimulus; inadequate intake of roughage
   b. Excessive cow's milk intake and early introduction of solids such as cereals and yellow vegetables
2. Intrapsychic.
   a. Abnormal or difficult toilet training, voluntary retention, or habit; possible history of prolonged, difficult toilet training, or constipation may begin with an anal fissure and be perpetuated
   b. Psychogenic; associated with parent-child and environmental problems and stresses; commonly fecal impaction, with secondary liquid stools soiling around the fecal mass (encopresis)
3. Trauma. Anal fissures appear as small tears at the anus, often accompanied by blood streaking of the stools and pain.
4. Intoxication.
   a. Excessive use of suppositories and enemas, causing the bowel to be insensitive to normal physiologic peristalsis
   b. Excessive use of antihistamines, diuretics, calcium channel blockers, diphenoxylate (Lomotil), or codeine-containing substances
5. Congenital (see Chapter 11).
   a. Atresia of the colon or rectum
   b. Meconium plug syndrome in newborns, associated with cystic fibrosis and Hirschsprung's disease
   c. Hirschsprung's disease (p. 652)
   d. Myelomeningocele and other neurologic problems
6. Ileus secondary to infection or inflammatory bowel disease.
7. Degenerative central nervous system (CNS) diseases.
8. Metabolic/endocrine.
   a. Hypothyroidism
   b. Hypercalcemia
   c. Hypokalemia

DIAGNOSTIC FINDINGS

It is imperative to determine whether the stool pattern is abnormal and the constipation is an isolated finding or associated with systemic signs and symptoms. The characteristics of the stool must be assessed with respect to frequency, consistency, color, odor, and previous patterns. Common complaints include anorexia, tenesmus, and abdominal pain. The pain may be crampy or constant and is usually recurrent. Occasionally, it may be severe enough to mimic a surgical abdomen. Patients may develop urinary incontinence and recurrent urinary tract infections that generally resolve with relief of constipation. Personal and family stresses and maternal/paternal interactions should be evaluated.

Previous dietary manipulation and therapeutic trials should be determined.

Physical examination may demonstrate a palpable, cylindric abdominal mass. Bowel sounds are variable. Distension and minimal diffuse tenderness are often present. The rectum is usually full of stool.

Ancillary Data

If the diagnosis is in doubt, abdominal x-ray films may demonstrate retained stool that is granular or rocklike in appearance. Stool should be assessed for blood. Ultimately, rectal manometry is diagnostic of aganglionic megacolon. Rectal biopsy or barium enema may be useful.

MANAGEMENT
Simple Constipation

Usually, the elimination pattern is normal, and reassurance is all that is necessary after determining that there is no organic cause. Generally, dietary manipulation is sufficient given the patient's age, severity of symptoms, and degree of parental anxiety. If constipation develops during bowel training, the pressure on training must be reduced.

1. For babies, add 1 to 2 tsp of syrup (Karo) to each bottle. If the child is older than 4 months of age, strained apricots, peaches, pears, and other fruits may be introduced. Avoid rectal stimulation with suppositories.

2. Older children should be encouraged to increase their intake of fruits and vegetables. These include prunes, figs, raisins, beans, celery, and lettuce. Prune juice is excellent and may be diluted with soda to improve the taste. Bran should be given in cereals, muffins, crackers, and other sources. Milk products may be constipating in some children. Push other fluids temporarily.

3. Maltsupex to 2 Tbsp/day BID PO may be helpful. Docusate (Colace), 5-10 mg/kg/24 hr q6-12hr PO, may be initiated for 5 to 7 days.

4. Stool softeners may also be helpful in the child without impaction. Mineral oil (1-2 ml/kg/dose BID PO; adolescent: 60 ml/dose) may be used; emulsified forms have a better taste. This may occasionally be supplemented by laxatives to stimulate the bowel. Such agents include milk of magnesia (1 ml/kg/dose BID PO), Senokot (<5 years: 1 to 2 tsp syrup; >5 years: 2 to 3 tsp syrup), or Castoria (<5 years: 1 to 2 tsp; >5 years: 2 to 3 tsp).

5. Enemas and suppositories should not be given routinely.

Anal fissures usually disappear once the bowel movement pattern has improved. Very rarely, chronic fissures require surgical excision.

Long-Standing Constipation

Severe constipation in the older child, often with fecal impaction, requires a more aggressive approach after excluding organic considerations. Cleanout may be accomplished "from above and below."

1. Perform fecal disimpaction by manual removal or by administering hypertonic phosphate enema (Fleet pediatric: 30-60 ml/10 kg/dose; adolescent: 120 ml/dose) after overnight mineral oil. Add 100 mg docusate (Colace) to each enema.

Enemas usually have to be repeated once or twice.

2. Begin mineral oil at 1-2 ml/kg/dose up to 120 ml/dose BID PO for 2 to 7 days until the rectal effluent contains no fecal material. The dose may gradually be increased to 300 ml BID PO as a maximum. Senokot may be used as an alternative.

3. Referral for complete psychologic evaluation, support, and follow-up observation may be indicated.

REFERENCES

Dohil R, Roberts E, Verries Jones K, et al: Constipation and reversible urinary tract abnormalities, *Arch Dis Child* 70:56, 1994.

Gleghorn EE, Heyman MB, Rudolph CD: No-enema therapy for idiopathic constipation and encopresis, *Clin Pediatr* 30:669, 1990.

Leoning-Baucke V: Urinary incontinence and urinary tract infection and their resolution with treatment of chronic constipation of childhood, *Pediatrics* 100:228, 1997.

Leoning-Baucke V, Cruickshank B, Savage C: Defecation dynamics and behavioral profiles in encopretic children, *Pediatrics* 80:672, 1987.

31 COUGH

ALERT: Upper and lower airway disease may produce coughing. Patients should be evaluated for respiratory distress (see Chapter 20).

Coughing follows forceful expiration and opening of a closed glottis. An initial inspiration is followed by closure of the glottis. The intrathoracic pressure increases with sudden opening of the glottis and release of intrathoracic air and contraction of the diaphragm, chest, abdominal wall, and pelvic floor musculature. The cough reflex, which is controlled in the medulla, receives vagal stimuli from the pharynx, larynx, trachea, and other large airways, as well as the ear. A number of different stimuli trigger the reflex, including mechanical, chemical, thermal, and psychogenic factors.

ETIOLOGY AND DIAGNOSTIC FINDINGS

The predominant cause of coughing is upper respiratory tract infection (Table 31-1). Other significant causes vary by age group. In *infants,* structural abnormalities of the airway, gastroesophageal reflux, tracheoesophageal fistula, vascular rings, and physiologic mechanisms must be considered. *Toddlers* may have a foreign body, irritation of the airway (especially passive smoking), or asthma; *school-age* children often have asthma, sinusitis, or chronic rhinitis. *Adolescents* commonly have a cough caused by smoking or psychogenic factors. A chronic cough may be the only clinical presentation of reactive airway disease, but other entities to be considered with a prolonged cough include a foreign body, an unusual infection, or a congenital anomaly.

The type of cough may be useful in considering specific differential entities. Staccato, paroxysmal coughs accompany pertussis or chlamydia infections, but productive coughs imply a lower airway or parenchymal infection. Purulent sputum is associated with bacterial pneumonia, lung abscess, bronchiectasis, and cystic fibrosis. Coughs that worsen at night usually are caused by posterior nasal drips from allergy or infection, and those coughs that improve during sleep often are psychogenic in origin.

Historically, it is imperative to determine the duration, frequency, quality, timing, and productivity of the cough. Inciting and ameliorating conditions should be defined, as well as associated signs and symptoms such as fever, shortness of breath, wheezing, allergies, and growth pattern. A family history should be obtained, focusing particularly on asthma, cystic fibrosis, tuberculosis, or any chronic pulmonary disease.

The physical examination must assess the patient's clinical condition, primarily in terms of a careful evaluation of the airway, lungs, and heart. Color, oximetry, respiratory rate, pattern, effort, retractions, and flaring should be noted. The level of respiratory tract involvement may be defined by the presence of stridor, wheezing, rhonchi, rales, altered breath sounds, and symmetry. Evidence of acute infection may be supported by the presence of fever, adenopathy, productive cough,

TABLE 31-1 Cough: Diagnostic Considerations

Condition	Diagnostic findings	Ancillary data	Comments
INFECTION/INFLAMMATION			
Upper respiratory infection (p. 609)	Acute onset, prolonged course; rhinorrhea, congestion, fever, pharyngitis, laryngitis, nonproductive cough	Throat cultures, if indicated	Self-limited; vagal stimulation; also croup (p. 784)
Pneumonia (p. 794)	Variable onset; fever, tachypnea, anorexia, irritability, productive cough, pleuritic pain; hemoptysis (group A streptococcus, TB)	Chest x-ray study; CBC; oximetry, ABC as needed	Viral, bacterial, mycoplasma, tuberculosis, chlamydial, pneumocystis; antibiotics, if needed
Bronchiolitis (p. 781)	Wheezing, tachypnea, nonproductive cough, fever, relatively little respiratory distress early but may develop with cyanosis	Chest x-ray study; oximetry, ABG, if needed	Viral; children <1 yr; support, hydrate, bronchodilator (albuterol)
Aspiration pneumonia	History of incident or patient with reduced level of consciousness; fever, productive cough; respiratory distress may be delayed 12-24 hr	Chest x-ray study; serial ABG	May follow aspiration of gastric contents, bacteria, hydrocarbons; may be recurrent
Pulmonary abscess	Insidious; fever, malaise, anorexia, hemoptysis, productive cough; chest pain	Chest x-ray study; culture of abscessed material	Aspiration of infected material or complication of pneumonia; drainage, antibiotics
Pertussis (whooping cough) (p. 716)	Catarrhal phase followed by paroxysmal cough with cyanosis and vomiting; prolonged cough	Chest x-ray study; ↑ CBC (lymphocytes); fluorescent antibody	Hospitalize, support; erythromycin with catarrhal phase
Measles (Chapter 42)	Coryza, conjunctivitis, and productive cough, with generalized morbilliform rash, fever	Chest x-ray study if significant and prolonged	Self-limited; complications of secondary infection
Pleurisy	Sharp, intense pain, worsens with inspiration; irritative, dry cough	Chest x-ray study to exclude pneumonia, effusion	Self-limited; analgesia
Retropharyngeal abscess (p. 608)	Fever, difficulty swallowing, drooling, sore throat; irritative, dry cough	Lateral neck x-ray study, CBC, culture material	Incision and drainage, antibiotics, analgesia
ALLERGIC			
Asthma (p. 765)	Wheezing, tachypnea, mild to moderate respiratory distress; nonproductive cough may be only symptom, unaccompanied by wheezing (may be induced by exercise); may be worse at night	Chest x-ray study; oximetry, ABG, pulmonary functions, as indicated	Responds to bronchodilator, steroids, oxygen

Condition	Signs and symptoms	Diagnostic studies	Treatment
Posterior nasal drip (p. 609)	Prolonged, productive cough, often after respiratory infection; worse when lying down; rhinorrhea, bronchorrhea, congestion		Empiric treatment with decongestant before bedtime
TRAUMA			
Foreign body (p. 791)	If tracheal: partial or total obstruction of airway; bronchial: nonproductive cough, without accompanying illness; asymmetric wheezing	Chest x-ray study; inspiration and expiration; direct visualization	Remove by bronchoscopy; bronchial and <24 hr, consider postural drainage
Atelectasis	Fever, productive cough, hemoptysis; may have splinting; may be caused by trauma	Chest x-ray study	Postural drainage; IPPB
VASCULAR			
Congestive heart failure (Chapter 16)	Tachypnea, tachycardia, murmur, rales, wheezing, cyanosis, cardiomegaly, productive cough	Chest x-ray study; ABG; ECG	Diuretics, digitalis; evaluate underlying cause
Mitral stenosis	Dyspnea, cyanosis, pulmonary edema, CHF, hemoptysis	Chest x-ray study; ABG; ECG	Congenital or rheumatic; cardiology consultation
INTOXICATION			
Hydrocarbon ingestion (p. 379)	Initially asymptomatic, then in 12-24 hr tachypnea, fever; prolonged productive cough	Baseline and follow-up chest x-ray studies	Postural drainage; treat complications of secondary infection, central nervous system toxicity
CONGENITAL (Chapter 11)			
Cystic fibrosis	Chronic productive cough, recurrent pulmonary infection; frequent illness, poor weight gain; abnormal stools	Chest x-ray study; ABG, pulmonary functions; positive sweat test	Postural drainage; antibiotics for acute exacerbations; dietary supplement
Tracheoesophageal fistula	Variable cough with feedings; poor weight gain, vomiting	Barium swallow	Surgery
Diaphragmatic hernia	As newborn, acute-onset cyanosis, poor feeding, vomiting, nonproductive cough, respiratory distress	Chest x-ray study, barium swallow	Surgery
NEOPLASM			
Pulmonary or mediastinal	Insidious onset, variable cough, hemoptysis, weight loss, chronically ill	Chest x-ray study; nuclear scan, biopsy	Refer to oncologist

rhinorrhea, or rash. Allergic disease usually has accompanying eczema, boggy nasal mucosa, clear rhinorrhea, hypertrophic lymphoid follicles, or allergic shiners.

Ancillary data must be individualized and may include a complete blood count (CBC), chest x-ray study (inspiratory and expiratory films if a foreign body is suspected), examination of sputum, pulmonary function tests, and specific studies such as a sweat chloride analysis, sinus or neck x-ray studies, or barium swallow to explore diagnostic considerations. ABGs or oximetry may be useful in selected conditions.

Hemoptysis, or coughing up blood often mixed with sputum (appearing red and frothy), is an unusual pediatric condition, which may occur with a number of clinical entities.

1. Infection/inflammation
   a. Pneumonia: group A streptococci, tuberculosis
   b. Pertussis
   c. Pulmonary abscess
   d. Bronchiectasis, especially cystic fibrosis
   e. Viral infections: most common
2. Trauma: foreign body
3. Vascular: pulmonary hypertension, mitral stenosis, pulmonary embolism
4. Neoplasm: mediastinal or pulmonary
5. Bleeding diathesis
6. Idiopathic pulmonary hemosiderosis
7. Following acute asthmatic attack
8. Cystic fibrosis
9. *Pseudohemoptysis:* Munchausen syndrome or upper airway lesion such as epistaxis, gingival bleeding, or gastrointestinal bleeding

Most patients with coughing have only minimal signs and symptoms and may be discharged with an appropriate therapeutic regimen. Those with respiratory distress or significant hemoptysis should be hospitalized to define the underlying disease and facilitate treatment.

MANAGEMENT

The focus of management must be on determining the cause of the cough and instituting specific therapy for that condition. Beyond these specific steps, cough suppression may be necessary in older children if the cough is interfering significantly with activities, sleep, or eating or causing significant vomiting.

Therapeutic options for cough suppression, if desired, include mixtures of honey (corn syrup in children under 1 year), lemon concentrate, and liquor (for older children), medicines with dextromethorphan (DM), or antitussives with 10 mg codeine/5 ml and given as 1 mg codeine/kg/24 hr q4-6hr PO (adult: 10-20 mg codeine/dose PO). However, antitussive medications have limited use in pediatrics because a specific therapy (i.e., bronchodilator for asthma, sputum production) may be more important to minimize lower airway disease; furthermore, narcotics are sedating and reduce mucokinesis.

Parental Education

The following instructions apply to the child discharged with a cough, commonly after an upper respiratory tract infection.

1. Sucking on cough drops or hard candy may be useful for the older child. A good cough medicine can be made at home by mixing equal amounts of honey (corn syrup for children under 1 year of age), lemon concentrate, and liquor such as Scotch or bourbon. You may omit the liquor for younger children.
2. Cough syrups are rarely useful. Stronger cough medicines containing DM or codeine must be prescribed by a physician, but they have the danger of reducing the cough reflex that protects the lungs.
3. Humidifiers and pushing warm fluids may be helpful.
4. Call your physician if the following occur:
   a. Difficulty in breathing or shortness of breath develops.

b. Cough lasts more than 2 weeks.

c. Cough changes to croup ("barking-seal cough") or wheezing develops.

d. Child develops fever that lasts more than 72 hours.

e. Cough spasms occur that cause choking, passing out, a bluish color of lips, or persistent vomiting.

f. There is blood in the mucus.

g. Chest pain develops.

REFERENCES

Braman SS, Corrao WM: Cough: differential diagnosis and treatment, *Clin Chest Med* 8:177, 1987.

Denny F: Acute respiratory infections in children: etiology and epidemiology, *Pediatr Rev* 9:135, 1987.

Hannaway PJ, Hopper DK: Cough variant asthma in children, *JAMA* 247:206, 1982.

Morgan WJ, Taussig LM: The child with persistent cough, *Pediatr Rev* 8:249, 1987.

Reisman J, Canny GJ, Levinson H: The approach to chronic cough in childhood, *Ann Allergic* 61:163, 1988.

32 ACUTE DIARRHEA

ETIOLOGY

Acute diarrheal disease in childhood is primarily infectious in origin, resulting from a host of viral and bacterial agents delineated in Chapter 76. Acute gastroenteritis commonly leads to postinfectious malabsorption, secondary to lactose intolerance. Rarely do patients with peritoneal irritation, pneumonia, otitis media, or urinary tract infections have associated diarrhea. Antibiotics (e.g., ampicillin) are commonly associated with diarrhea (Table 32-1). When other obvious causes are ruled out, a patient probably has infectious diarrhea if there are unformed bowel movements at twice the normal rate, which are associated with one or more of the following: fever, nausea, vomiting, abdominal pain, cramps, blood or mucoid stools, or tenesmus.

Evaluation of more chronic diarrhea should account for inflammatory bowel disease, irritable bowel syndrome, malabsorption, secretory disorders, anatomic abnormality (especially Hirschsprung disease), parasites, systemic disease, overfeeding, antibiotics, toxins, and secondary lactase deficiency (Box 32-1).

DIAGNOSTIC FINDINGS

The onset of symptoms and the characteristics of bowel movements (consistency, mucus, blood, frequency) are important, with particu-lar attention to factors that increase (e.g., time, diet) or decrease (e.g., dietary elimination, withdrawal of drugs) elimination. Related signs and symptoms including fever, rash, and arthralgia must be assessed. Recurrence and exposures may be important clues. Urine output should be evaluated.

Bacterial gastroenteritis is more likely in children with a history of blood in the stool in combination with a fever greater than 38° C or at least 10 stools in 14 hours.

The physical examination should focus on the state of hydration, hemodynamic stability, and associated findings. Abdominal and rectal examination may be useful. Serial monitoring is essential.

Ancillary Data

Hydration status may require evaluation, including electrolytes, blood urea nitrogen (BUN), and urine specific gravity. Complete blood count (CBC) is variably helpful. Methylene blue smears for stool polyps are particularly useful in excluding a number of bacterial causes; for example, bacterial gastroenteritis is commonly associated with the presence of polymorphonuclear cells in the smear. Rapid tests for rotavirus may be diagnostic. On rare occasions, stool cultures and ova and parasite examination are appropriate.

TABLE 32-1 Acute Diarrhea: Diagnostic Considerations

Condition	Character of stool	Associated symptoms	Evaluation	Comments
INFECTION				
Acute gastroenteritis (p. 631)				
Virus	Loose; rare blood; rare WBC	Respiratory symptoms, vomiting	ELISA for rotavirus; electron microscopy	Acute onset
Bacteria	Loose/watery; variable blood; PMNs common	Vomiting; fever; seizure (*Shigella*); crampy abdominal pain	Culture; methylene blue for PMN	Acute onset; toxic; may be related to food poisoning
Parasite	Variable	Multisystem involvement; weight loss	Ova and parasite	May be insidious
Postinfectious malabsorption	Watery	Recovering from acute gastroenteritis	Reducing substance in stool (≥0.5%); pH <5.0	Usually lactose intolerant; may be primary
Food poisoning	Profuse	Abdominal pain, cramping, vomiting	Epidemiologic	Usually temporally related to food ingestion
Acute appendicitis (p. 648) or peritonitis	Loose	Reflects associated problems	Abdominal x-ray study; CBC	Surgical exploration
Extraintestinal				
Respiratory infection (p. 794)	Variable	Fever, rhinorrhea	Chest x-ray study, if needed	Antibiotics
Urinary tract infection (p. 815)	Variable	Dysuria, frequency, burning	Urinalysis, urine culture	Antibiotics
INTOXICATION				
Antibiotics	Loose; fat (variable)	Vomiting, anorexia; adverse reactions of medication	Withdrawal of drug	Clindamycin causes pseudomembranous enterocolitis
Iron (p. 381)				
Antimetabolites				
AUTOIMMUNE/ALLERGIC				
Ulcerative colitis	Mucus; pus; blood; nocturnal	Urgency; tenesmus, abdominal pain, fever, weight loss; systemic signs (e.g., arthritis)	Sigmoidoscopy; barium enema	Insidious; age: 10-19 yr; treatment: sulfasalazine, steroids

Continued

TABLE 32-1   Acute Diarrhea: Diagnostic Considerations—cont'd

Condition	Character of stool	Associated symptoms	Evaluation	Comments
AUTOIMMUNE/ALLERGIC—cont'd				
Regional enteritis (Crohn's disease)	Loose; blood (variable); nocturnal	Abdominal pain; weight loss, fever; perianal disease	Sigmoidoscopy; barium enema	Insidious; teenagers; treatment: surgery, sulfasalazine, steroids
Milk allergy	Watery; blood (occult or gross)	Vomiting, anemia	Dietary elimination	May also be caused by soy formula
Gluten sensitivity (celiac disease)	Profuse; bulky; pale; frothy	Failure to thrive, anemia, vomiting, abdominal pain	Peroral intestinal biopsy, stool fat	Onset reflects age of introduction of gluten (wheat, rye, oats); eliminate gluten foods
IRRITABLE BOWEL SYNDROME	Watery; mucus	None; normal growth	Therapeutic response	Treatment: bland diet; reduce snacks; peak: 6-36 mo; multiple inciting causes
INTRAPSYCHIC				
Fear/anxiety	Loose	Anxiety	History helpful	Stress-reducing activities; needs long-term therapy
Fecal impaction (encopresis) (Chapter 30)	Watery	Variable abdominal pain	History; rectal examination; x-ray study	Chronic constipation
CONGENITAL				
Cystic fibrosis	Fatty; bulky; foul-smelling	Respiratory infections; poor growth	Sweat test	Needs enzyme replacement; long-term follow-up
Hirschsprung's disease (p. 652)	Green; watery; foul-smelling	Abdominal distension; vomiting; fever; lethargy; poor growth	Barium enema; rectal biopsy	Surgical intervention
ENDOCRINE				
Hyperthyroid (p. 623)	Watery	Systemic signs	Thyroid studies	
NEOPLASM				
Lymphoma Carcinoma Neuroblastoma Zollinger-Ellison syndrome	Watery, variably severe	Associated problems	Variable	Important cause to exclude

Box 32-1

PRESENTATION AS DIAGNOSTIC CONSIDERATION FOR DIARRHEA

ACUTE ONSET

Fever common, ± vomiting/dehydration

Acute infectious gastroenteritis
  Viral (rotavirus, calicivirus, enteric adenovirus)
  Bacteria or toxin (*Campylobacter, Shigella, Salmonella, Staphylococcus* toxin)
"Parenteral" diarrhea (secondary to otitis, UTI)
Medication related
  Antibiotic-associated diarrhea
  Pseudomembranous colitis

Usually afebrile, hydrated

Transient malabsorption
  High fat intake
  Food intolerance/adverse reaction to food
Protozoal gastroenteritis *(Giardia, Entamoeba, Cryptosporidium)*
Psychogenic—anxiety/stress

CHRONIC COURSE

Failing to thrive, ± dehydration

Postinfectious diarrhea
  Starvation stools (prolonged liquid diet)
  Lactose intolerance postenteritis
Inflammatory bowel disease
Hirschsprung's disease
Chronic malabsorption
  Protein (celiac disease)
  Fat (cystic fibrosis, pancreatic diseases)
  Carbohydrates (acquired lactase deficiency)
Protozoal diarrhea (also cause of acute process)

Thriving, afebrile, hydrated

Age-specific variant of normal
  Breast-feeding stools (0-2 mo old infant)
  Chronic nonspecific diarrhea of infancy/childhood (up to age 3)
Medication related
  Laxative abuse in adolescents
  Sorbitol content of cough syrups/bronchodilators
Encopresis—overflow incontinence

From Boenning DA: Diarrhea. In Barkin RM, editor: *Pediatric emergency medicine: concepts and clinical practice,* ed 2, St Louis, 1997, Mosby.

More exhaustive evaluations are rarely indicated unless the diarrhea has been prolonged. Sigmoidoscopy, barium enema, rectal biopsy, and other studies are performed for severe disease in the absence of an infectious cause.

MANAGEMENT

Management must focus on correcting any fluid deficits (see Chapter 7) and treating the specific condition. Hospitalization should be considered when there is dehydration, intractable vomiting, young age (especially under 2 to 3 months), underlying disease, systemic toxicity, and disrupted social or physical environment. Patients with severe abdominal pain associated with bloody stools require immediate evaluation and surgical consultation.

The patient whose clinical status is stable can usually be followed at home. Clear liquids should be given until there is some resolution of the diarrhea or specific therapy can be instituted.

Parental Education

1. Give only clear liquids; give as much as your child wants. The following may be used during the first 24 hours:
   a. Rehydralyte during initial rehydration

followed by Pedialyte or Lytren is ideal

   b. Defizzed, room-temperature soda for older children (>2 years) if diarrhea is only mild

2. If your child is vomiting, give clear liquids *slowly.* In younger children, start with 1 teaspoonful and slowly increase the amount. If vomiting occurs, let your child rest for a while and then try again. About 8 hours after vomiting has stopped, the child can gradually return to a normal diet.

3. After 24 hours your child's diet may be advanced if the diarrhea has improved. If your child is taking only formula, mix the formula with twice as much water to make up half-strength formula, which should be given over the next 24 hours. Applesauce, bananas, and strained carrots may be given if your child is eating solids. If this is tolerated, your child may be advanced to a regular diet over the next 2 to 3 days.

4. If your child has had a prolonged course of diarrhea, it may be helpful in the young child to advance from clear liquids to a soy formula (Isomil, ProSobee, or Soyalac) for 1 to 2 weeks.

5. Do not use boiled milk. Kool-Aid and soda are not ideal liquids, particularly in younger infants, because they contain few electrolytes.

6. Call your physician if the following occur:

   a. The diarrhea or vomiting is increasing in frequency or amount.

   b. The diarrhea does not improve after 24 hours of clear liquids or resolve entirely after 3 to 4 days.

   c. Vomiting continues for more than 24 hours.

   d. The stool has blood, or the vomited material contains blood or turns green.

   e. Signs of dehydration develop, including decreased urination, less moisture in diapers, dry mouth, no tears, weight loss, lethargy, or irritability.

33 DYSPHAGIA

ALERT: After correcting hydration, diagnostic considerations should be evaluated before initiating definitive therapy.

Patients with dysphagia have difficulty swallowing because of pharyngeal, laryngeal, or esophageal lesions. Clinically, patients experience associated choking, regurgitation, pain and discomfort, and a sense of food sticking. When such symptoms are caused by esophageal lesions, the patient commonly has a subjective sensation of a bolus of food failing to pass, with accompanying pain and discomfort.

Dysphagia results from either anatomic obstruction or compression or a physiologic dysfunction of the neuromuscular process of swallowing; that is, swallowing requires coordination with sucking and breathing (Table 33-1). *Obstructive* or compressive lesions usually can be evaluated by careful physical examination and radiologic studies, including lateral neck film, barium swallow, or fluoroscopy. Such

TABLE 33-1   Dysphagia: Diagnostic Considerations

| Condition | Primary mechanism | | Comments |
	Obstruction/ compression (mechanical)	Physiologic dysfunction (motor)	
INFECTION/INFLAMMATION			
Tonsillitis (p. 604)	Yes		Group A streptococci, diphtheria, mononucleosis, etc.
Stomatitis (p. 593)	Yes		Herpes, apthous
Peritonsillar abscess (p. 603)	Yes		Direct visualization to define
Retropharyngeal abscess (p. 608)	Yes		Lateral neck
Epiglottitis, croup (p. 784)	Yes	Yes	Direct visualization imperative
Botulism, rabies, polio (Chapter 80)		Yes	Cranial nerves affected; also post polio
Guillain-Barré syndrome (Chapter 41)		Yes	Ascending paralysis
Esophagitis		Yes	Retrosternal discomfort (e.g., hiatal hernia, reflux)
Chalasia/gastroesophageal reflux	Yes	Yes	May be physiologic in infants
Pericarditis	Yes		Associated symptoms present

Continued

TABLE 33-1   Dysphagia: Diagnostic Considerations—cont'd

Condition	Obstruction/ compression (mechanical)	Physiologic dysfunction (motor)	Comments
INTOXICATION			
Caustic ingestion (p. 366)	Yes	Yes	Requires immediate intervention to minimize injury
Phenothiazine overdose (p. 387)		Yes	Associated with dystonia
CONGENITAL (Chapter 11)			
Cleft palate	Yes	Yes	
Macroglossia	Yes		Consider hypothyroidism, Beckwith syndrome
Esophageal web, atresia, stenosis	Yes		May be associated with tracheal anomaly (tracheal-esophageal fistula)
Riley-Day syndrome		Yes	
DEGENERATIVE			
Central nervous system disease		Yes	
Hypotonia		Yes	
Myasthenia gravis		Yes	Tensilon trial
INTRAPSYCHIC			
Globus hystericus		Yes	Psychiatry consult
TRAUMA			
Foreign body (p. 637)	Yes		History crucial
ENDOCRINE (p. 622)			
Goiter	Yes		Thyroid studies required
Hashimoto's thyroiditis	Yes		Thyroid studies required
NEOPLASM			
Carcinoma, Hodgkin's disease	Yes		Usually associated nodes, weight loss
VASCULAR			
Vascular ring	Yes		Chest x-ray study, ECG, catheterization
Heart disease	Yes		Chest x-ray study, ECG, echocardiogram, catheterization
Aortic aneurysm	Yes		Chest x-ray study, ECG, ultrasound, catheterization
AUTOIMMUNE			
Various collagen-vascular diseases (dermatomyositis)	Yes	Yes	Evaluate in detail

The "Primary mechanism" header spans the "Obstruction/compression (mechanical)" and "Physiologic dysfunction (motor)" columns.

patients usually have difficulty only in swallowing solids. *Physiologic* dysfunction, often associated with systemic disease, is rarely isolated to the alimentary tract. Patients commonly have difficulty with both solids and liquids.

The assessment of these patients must delineate the mechanism and degree of dysfunction. The rapidity of onset and recurrence and the nature of any progression are important diagnostic clues. Accompanying pain, discomfort, vomiting, and a preceding history of trauma should be noted. Systemic findings should be evaluated.

Laboratory studies may include cultures and measurement of drug levels and electrolytes. Manometry to measure the upper and lower esophageal pressures and peristaltic wave may provide physiologic information. Radiologic studies, including a barium swallow to exclude narrowing, stricture, and presence of a foreign body are essential, as is examining the swallowing mechanism. A lateral neck radiograph to look for masses and a computed tomography (CT) scan of the neck or head may be diagnostic.

A therapeutic trial of edrophonium (Tensilon) may be warranted.

Management of the patient must focus on stabilization by ensuring adequate vital signs and hydration, followed by diagnostic testing.

REFERENCES

Castell DO, Donner MW: Evaluation of dysphagia: a careful history is crucial, *Dysphagia* 2:2, 1987.

Sonies BC, Dalakas MC: Dysphagia in patients with post-polio syndrome, *N Engl J Med* 324:1162, 1991.

Weiss MH: Dysphagia in infants and children, *Otolaryngol Clin North Am* 21:4, 1988.

34 Fever in Children

ALERT: The acutely ill, febrile child requires a systematic approach to exclude serious systemic disease. Evaluation and management must reflect the child's age, medical history, examination, toxicity, environment, and family compliance

Fever is an important symptom of illness and is a frequent complaint in children, accounting for up to 20% of emergency department (ED) visits. Most children seeking medical care for evaluation of a fever can be easily diagnosed and have minor illnesses. The clinical challenge is to differentiate those with significant underlying infections.

Physiologic mechanisms to control body temperature include sweating and hyperventilation to lower temperature and vasoconstriction and shivering to raise temperature. Circulating interleukins, prostaglandins, and prostacyclins mediate the febrile response.

MEASUREMENTS

A child is generally considered febrile when the rectal temperature is 38.0° C (100.4° F). The reliability of other methods of temperature measurement is variable. There is a normal diurnal variation in children of up to 1.1° C; this is less pronounced in younger children. Seriously ill infants may be euthermic or hypothermic. The absence of fever is not reliable in eliminating the consideration of serious disease.

The *site* for temperature measurement must reflect proximity to major arteries, absence of inflammation, degree of precision required, safety, and insulation from external factors (e.g.,

drinking). *Rectal* temperatures provide precision and should be the technique in infants, especially infants less than 90 days old. Care should be exercised to avoid rectal perforation or emotional trauma. *Axillary* temperatures are appropriate in thermostable environments or when absolute precision is not mandatory, neither of which is present in the ED setting. The *oral or sublingual* site is useful in a cooperative older child who does not have a rapid respiratory rate. The *tympanic membrane* has been used with great reproducibility but appears to be less accurate in infants less than 6 months of age, yielding falsely low values. It measures the infrared radiation emitted by the tympanic membrane. Speed of measurement must be balanced by the relative inaccuracy of the method. When using the tympanic membrane approach, pulling posteriorly and superiorly on the external ear at the midpoint between the apex of the helix and the inferior border of the lobule may improve accuracy. Children less than 90 days of age should have the temperature taken rectally. Bundling has little impact on rectal temperature.

Although most underlying illness is infectious, the obligation is to ensure that children with significant and potentially life-threatening conditions are distinguished from those with self-limited problems. The nonspecific presentation in neonates and infants and their impaired immunocompetency require aggressive evaluation and treatment in children less than 90 days of age, but recent patterns of management have introduced greater support for individualizing treatment beyond 30 days.

DIAGNOSTIC FINDINGS

1. History usually reflects nonspecific observations related to behavior and associated signs and symptoms rather than data that permit an early focus on the involved system. The history is important in defining the nature of the illness, the height and duration of fever, dosage, frequency, and response to antipyretics and past medical problems. A measured elevated temperature within the previous 6 hours is usually considered significant. Associated symptoms and behavioral patterns should be reviewed, particularly looking for irritability, response to the environment, respiratory or gastrointestinal abnormalities, limpness, and other localizing findings. Exposures to other ill children or adults, immunizations, travel, and source of water may be useful. Preexisting medical conditions (e.g., sickle cell disease, immunodeficiency, respiratory, cardiac, renal disease) should be delineated. Prematurity and associated problems may affect the assessment and blur specific age parameters, especially during the first 6 months of life.

2. Physical examination should be systematic and thorough. While the child is distracted with play objects, obvious physical abnormalities such as limitations of limb movement, rashes, and points of tenderness should be defined. The chest, heart, and abdomen require a gentle hand and patience. Tachypnea disproportionate to fever (>59 breaths/min in a child <6 months, >52/min in those 6 to 11 months, and >42/min in children 1 to 2 years of age) may suggest underlying pneumonia. Once these areas have been assessed, a full examination of the eyes, ears, throat, neck, extremities, and skin is required to look for specific findings.

3. Behavioral observation of the child at play while encouraging the youngster to follow lights, bring objects to parents, and so forth:
   - Child looks and focuses on the clinician and spontaneously explores the room.
   - Child spontaneously makes sounds or talks in a playful manner.
   - Child plays and reaches for objects.
   - Child smiles and interacts with parent or practitioner.
   - Child quiets easily when held by parents.

4. Antipyretic therapy is imperative in facilitating observation. Many children who are irritable and uninterested in their environment improve markedly with antipyretic management. Acetaminophen (15 mg/kg/dose q4-6hr PO or PR) should be administered to children with temperatures greater than 38.5° to 39° C on arrival in the ED to ensure optimal observation by reducing temperature and permitting a more accurate assessment of the child. Ibuprofen (5-10 mg/kg/dose q6-8hr PO) may be useful as an ancillary agent. Children who are particularly uncomfortable may also benefit from a lukewarm water sponge bath. Studies have documented that the clinical response to antipyretics is not predictive of the nature of the illness; the response may facilitate evaluation.

5. In the first few months of life, studies have suggested that febrile children are far more likely to have serious illness. Fever may be the only early symptom; few signs and symptoms may exist. Children with serious disease, as mentioned, may be normothermic. The absence of specific

findings mandates complete laboratory evaluation, admission, and antibiotics in this age group.

The older the patient, the more reliable are the findings. Meningitis in youngsters may merely present with irritability or lethargy, whereas in the teenager, meningismus, pain on extension of the knee with the leg positioned in flexion at the hip (Kernig's sign), and reflex flexion at the knee and hip when the neck is flexed (Brudzunksi's sign) are noted.

Ancillary Data

1. No laboratory or historical factors definitively exclude serious underlying bacterial disease. The peripheral white blood cell count above 15,000 cells/mm^3 or below 5000 cells/mm^3 may indicate a serious infection. Meningococcemia, disseminated intravascular coagulation (DIC), or septic shock classically have low white blood cell counts. Studies have suggested that a ratio of bands to neutrophil of 0.2 is associated with bacterial infections.

2. Blood cultures for aerobic and anaerobic organisms should be obtained in patients suspected of having bacteremia.

3. Examination of urine for urinalysis in children with fever and no source. In the neonate, the urinalysis may be unremarkable in up to 80% of children with a documented positive culture. Of older children with urinary tract infections, 20% have a normal urinalysis with negative leukocyte esterase or nitrite. A Gram stain of the spun urine sediment is the most sensitive screening test. The only reliable methods to obtain a urine sample are straight catheterization or suprapubic bladder aspiration. Table 85-2 provides an interpretation of culture results. Bagged urine is useful to screen for dehydration, hematuria, proteinuria, or glucosuria. Urine cultures should be processed promptly.

4. Lumbar punctures (LPs) are appropriate to exclude meningitis when this diagnosis is considered. Febrile children with seizures deserve special consideration, especially those 12 months or younger in whom a spinal tap is generally done. The fluid should be cultured and studies should include cell count, Gram stain, protein, and glucose (with concurrent blood glucose) (see Table 81-3). Performing an LP on a bacteremic child does not significantly increase the risk of meningitis developing.

5. Erythrocyte sedimentation rate (ESR) is a nonspecific test for infection, inflammatory bowel disease, and collagen vascular disease. Its usefulness is limited by the length of time required for the study.

6. Stool smear examination for polymorphonuclear leukocyte cells is useful in children with diarrhea because 90% of infections with salmonella or shigella have accompanying cells; *Campylobacter,* toxigenic *Escherichia coli,* and *Yersinia* species may also have polymorphonuclear leukocytes.

7. Chest x-ray studies are recommended in young febrile children with evidence of lower respiratory tract disease such as coughing, wheezing, tachypnea, dyspnea, retractions, grunting, nasal flaring, or focally decreased breath sounds. Tachypnea disproportionate to the child's age as noted above may be an additional risk factor. An abnormal radiograph result in the absence of respiratory findings of cough, rales, or wheezing is unusual in children less than 8 weeks of age.

8. Coagulation studies, cultures, and radiographs as indicated.

SPECIFIC ENTITIES
Occult Bacteremia

Although bacteremia occurs in association with a host of clinical entities, including meningitis, septic arthritis, epiglottitis, cellulitis, pneumonia, and kidney infection, about 6% of febrile patients without a defined focus have positive blood culture results. The most common pathogen is *Streptococcus pneumoniae,* accounting for 85% of positive cultures. Most of the remaining cultures are *Haemophilus influenzae* type B infections, although this is decreasing with widespread immunization. *Neisseria meningitidis, Salmonella* species, and other pathogens may also be found.

The highest risk group are those 24 months of age or younger with a fever 39.4° C or greater and a white blood cell count of 15,000/mm^3 or greater. The differential does not increase predictive value. An ESR greater than 30 mm/hr may also be suggestive.

Each degree elevation above 39° C increases the risk; children with a temperature of 39.5° to 39.9° C have about a 3% incidence of bacteremia, those with a temperature of 40° to 40.9° C have a 4% risk, and those with a temperature greater than 41° C have a 10% risk.

It is essential to evaluate such children carefully to be certain no underlying disease exists. If pneumococcal bacteremia is suspected, consideration should be given to initiating prophylactic antibiotics, but the benefit is controversial. Retrospective review of *Haemophilus influenzae* and *Neisseria meningitidis* bacteremia suggested that children sent home taking oral antibiotics do better compared with those sent home without therapy; parenteral administration of antibiotics may have further benefit. Another study demonstrated enhanced defervescence when oral amoxicillin was started but questionably prevented major morbid events. A meta-analysis of studies involving *S. pneumoniae* bacteremia demonstrated similar findings; oral antibiotics decrease the incidence of serious bacterial infections but did not decrease the risk of meningitis. In general, children less than 60-90 days old with suspected occult bacteremia in whom empiric antibiotics are initiated should have a full sepsis evaluation including an LP.

Hyperpyrexia

True hyperpyrexia, defined as a temperature greater than 41° C (105.8° F), is rare but is more commonly associated with serious infections. About 20% of children with temperatures greater than 41° C will have convulsions. Ten percent of children less than 2 years old with temperatures greater than 41.1° C have bacterial meningitis, whereas an additional 7% have bacteremia without meningitis. Press noted that 8 of 15 (53%) children with temperatures over 41.1° C had serious disease (2 bacterial meningitis, 2 with bacteremia, 2 pneumonia, 1 pericarditis, and 1 Kawasaki syndrome).

Temperatures greater than 42° C often have noninfectious causes, such as hyperthermia, head injury, ingestion of psychotropic drugs, and malignant hyperthermia during anesthesia.

Antipyretic management is appropriate, and patients should receive a minimum of a complete blood count (CBC), urinalysis, and blood culture. LP should be considered and a chest x-ray obtained if there is any suggestion of respiratory findings.

Immunocompromise

Children with a history of recurrent serious bacterial infection should be evaluated for immunodeficiency. Children undergoing cancer chemotherapy or having a history of asplenia (e.g., congenital, trauma) are obviously at risk. Those with sickle cell disease have a 400-fold increased risk of pneumococcal septicemia if less than 5 years old and a fourfold risk of *H. influenzae* septicemia if less than 9 years of age.

Fever and Petechiae

Children with fever and petechiae may have a viral illness, Rocky Mountain spotted fever, or invasive bacterial disease. Rapid intervention is required. In one study of 190 patients with fever and petechiae, 15 had bacterial disease, half of which was meningitis. The most common pathogen was *Neisseria meningitidis,* accounting for 13 of the 15 patients with invasive disease; group A streptococcus and respiratory syncytial virus were the most common causes of noninvasive bacterial disease. Most well-appearing children do not have serious bacterial invasive infections.

Children with fever and petechiae who have a normal LP, a white blood cell count that is neither elevated nor decreased, a normal absolute neutrophil and band count, and a temperature less than 40° C are less likely to have a bacterial infection.

Fever of Unknown Origin

A fever of unknown origin (FUO) is commonly used to refer to a febrile illness of unknown cause lasting 14 days or more. Most children have actually had two or more febrile illnesses within a short period. When the prolonged fever is continuous, numerous causes need to be considered (Box 34-1). In a study of 100 children, 52 had an infectious origin, 20 had collagen inflammatory disease, 6 had a malignancy, and 12 were undiagnosed. A systematic approach to evaluation and referral for ongoing management is appropriate.

MANAGEMENT

A conservative yet responsible approach appears mandatory, recognizing the need to individualize assessment and care. Antibiotic sensitivity patterns constantly evolve with resistance to *H. influenzae* and *S. pneumoniae* being increasingly prevalent.

Box 34-1

ETIOLOGY OF PEDIATRIC PROLONGED FEVER OF UNKNOWN ORIGIN

INFECTION

Bacterial
  Sinusitis
  Pyelonephritis
  Mastoiditis
  Endocarditis
  Adenitis
Viral
  Infectious mononucleosis
  Hepatitis A, B, or C
  Cytomegalovirus
Chlamydial
Mycoplasma
Fungal
  Cysticercosis, blastomycosis, histoplasmosis
Rickettsial
  Q fever
  Rocky Mountain spotted fever
Parasitic
  Malaria
  Toxoplasmosis

COLLAGEN VASCULAR

Juvenile rheumatoid arthritis
Lupus erythematosus
Vasculitis, postinfectious
Acute rheumatic fever
Ulcerative colitis/regional enteritis

MALIGNANCY

Leukemia, lymphoma, neuroblastoma, Wilms' tumor

DRUG-INDUCED

Antineoplastic, anticonvulsants, antituberculosis agents
Quinidine, procainamide
Serum sickness

OTHER

Kawasaki syndrome
AIDS
Hypothalamic dysfunction
Factitious

From Fetter RA, Bower JR: Infectious diseases. In Barkin RM, editor: *Pediatric emergency medicine: concepts and clinical practice*, ed 2, St Louis , 1997, Mosby.

Infants Less Than 90 Days of Age

A rational and conservative approach is essential in infants. This history is rarely more specific than the triad of fever, irritability, and poor feeding. The physical examination may fail to reveal specific focal findings, despite the presence of systemic infections, which may be enteric, as well as the more common organisms infecting older children. Children less than 3 months of age with a temperature above 38.5° C have more than a 20-fold greater risk of having a serious infection than do older children with similar temperatures. High fever has some correlation with serious illness, but the absence of this finding does not exclude bacterial infections. Prematurity makes age cutoffs less distinct.

Prospective studies have demonstrated that clinical judgment alone is not adequate in the assessment of febrile infants. No clear factors are sensitive or specific enough to be relied on in decision making. However, factors that have been most consistently associated with bacterial disease include age below 1 month, breast feeding, history of lethargy, no contact with an ill person, polymorphonuclear neutrophil count above 10,000 cells/mm^3, and band count greater than 500 cells/mm^3. *No laboratory or historical factors should be used to exclude underlying bacterial infection.*

1. During the first 30 days of life, infants undergo tremendous developmental and immunologic change and are difficult to assess. In one study, one in nine neonates with serious bacterial infection appeared clinically well. Furthermore, the etiologic agents evolve from vaginal flora (*E. coli,* group B streptococcus, *Listeria monocytogenes,* herpes, and chlamydia) to more traditional community-acquired disease. Children in this age group require admission after a full sepsis work-up for administration of parenteral antibiotics and monitoring until culture results are negative at 48 to 72 hours. These children should have blood, urine, and cerebrospinal fluid (CSF) cultures, as well as consideration for other studies as indicated. Antibiotics should be initiated, including ampicillin, 100-200 mg/kg/24 hr q4-6hr IV, and cefotaxime, 50-100 mg/kg/24 hr q8hr IV. Gentamicin, 5-7.5 mg/kg/24 hr q8hr IV, or ceftriaxone, 50-100 mg/kg/24 hr q12hr IV, may substitute for cefotaxime, the latter in children older than 30 days of age.

2. From 30 to 60 days of age, the assessment has greater validity because of the enhanced developmental skills of the child and maturing of the immune system. Blood and urine cultures, CBC, and LP should be done in febrile children in this age group. An LP is indicated in children who have an abnormal examination or evaluation or in whom antibiotics are prescribed. Admission is indicated in children with systemic findings, toxic appearance, or any abnormal laboratory findings and those who do not meet the low-risk Rochester criteria delineated in Box 34-2. Children requiring treatment should be treated with antibiotics identical to those for children less than 30 days of age.

3. Children 60 to 90 days of age should have a CBC, urinalysis, and urine culture done. If any of these are abnormal, a blood culture should be done. An LP is appropriate if indicated by the examination of the child or if antibiotics are to be started. Admission is appropriate if the child is not low risk, appears toxic, or the physical or laboratory evaluation is abnormal in any aspect. Additional studies should be considered.

Children 90 Days to 36 Months

From 90 days to 36 months, the evaluation is more specific, and the examination may provide information about a specific diagnostic direction. Studies have shown that most children with serious infections can be identified by the

Box 34-2
LOW-RISK ROCHESTER CRITERIA

Well-appearing infant; normal vital signs; good hydration and perfusion
Healthy infant
    Term (≥37 weeks' gestation)
    No antibiotic therapy—antenatal or postnatal
    No unexplained hyperbilirubinemia
    No underlying illness
    No previous hospitalizations; discharged with mother as newborn
No focal infection (skin, soft tissue, bone/joint)
Good social situation
Laboratory criteria
    WBC count 5000 to 15,000/mm^3
    Band form count ≤1500/mm^3
    Normal urinalysis (<5 WBC/HPF)
    Normal stool (<5 WBC/HPF, if done)

WBC, White blood cell; *HPF,* high-power field.

initial evaluation. Furthermore, beyond the greater reliability of the examination, the mature immune status provides reassurance regarding the nature of infection, Clearly, toxic-appearing children need extensive evaluations, whereas children without specific findings who appear nontoxic can generally be managed by ambulatory observation. When the temperature is greater than 39.4° C or 103° F, a CBC is indicated; when the CBC is greater than 15,000/mm^3, a blood culture to exclude occult bacteremia is appropriate. For those who are to receive antibiotics, males less than 6 months of age, and girls, a urinalysis and culture should be obtained.

If blood cultures are obtained, empiric treatment with antibiotics may be considered; controversy exists about whether the incidence of significant complications is reduced. *Follow-up observation is essential,* usually in 12 to 24 hours, depending on clinical and logistical constraints. This is particularly important in children at high risk for bacteremia.

If the elevated temperature has been present for less than 24 hours and the child looks well without any high-risk factors, follow-up observation for 4 to 12 hours may substitute for laboratory evaluation at the time of the first encounter. Close follow-up is essential.

Children Older Than 3 Years of Age

Children older than 3 years of age require careful evaluation focused on specific findings. Although viral illness predominates, such organisms as group A streptococcus, mycoplasma, and Epstein-Barr virus become more common etiologic agents.

DISPOSITION

Obviously, close follow-up is essential in all discharged children with a febrile illness, usually within 24 hours either by phone or return visit to the ED or primary care physician. Children less than 30 days of age are routinely admitted, whereas those 30 to 60 days of age are often hospitalized. Changing clinical status, evolving foci, or other parameters should be evaluated as well as the cultures obtained initially checked for results.

If the blood culture remains negative, follow-up on an outpatient basis is appropriate if the patient remains well without any focal findings. Antibiotics, if started, should be stopped after 48 hours and the patient followed up until the illness resolves.

If the blood culture is positive, thereby documenting bacteremia, reexamination of the patient is essential. If the patient is totally normal and the culture is positive for a gram-positive organism, close follow-up and continuing antibiotics may be continued for a total 10-day course. If the child is febrile or toxic, has an evolving focus, or the organism is gram negative, admission and intravenous antibiotics are indicated.

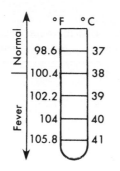

Fig. 34-1   Conversion scale.

Parental Education

Parental education is important in the management of the febrile infant. Obviously, instructions are indicated in the management of the specific diagnostic entity, but additional information about fever control must be provided. This is of utmost importance in the initial assessment of the child and may additionally make the child more comfortable throughout the duration of the illness. Fever is a means of fighting infection, and the degree of fever does not always reflect the severity of the illness.

1. Fever is a temperature over 99.7° F (37.6° C) orally or 100.4° F (38.0° C) rectally (Fig. 34-1). If the fever is between 100° F and 101° F orally or rectally, the temperature should be taken again in 1 hour. Temperatures may be temporarily elevated from too much clothing or exercise. Oral temperatures can be raised by recently eaten warm food. Teething does not cause marked elevations of temperature. Bundling has little impact on rectal temperature.

2. Take the rectal temperature:
   a. Shake the thermometer down to below 97° F (36° C).
   b. Lubricate the thermometer with petroleum jelly (Vaseline), cold cream, or cold water.
   c. Gently insert the thermometer ½ inch into the rectum. Often, holding the child stomach down on the parent's lap is helpful.
   d. Leave the thermometer in 3 minutes or until the silver line stops rising.
   e. Do not leave the child unattended. Hold the child still.
   f. Read by turning the sharp edge of the triangle toward you. Turn it slightly in each direction until you can see the end of the silver column.
   g. On the centigrade (Celsius) thermometer, each line is 0.1° C; on the Fahrenheit thermometer, each line is 0.2° F.
      NOTE: In unusual circumstances, axillary temperatures may be taken as a screen, holding the tip of the thermometer under the dry armpit for 4 minutes. The elbow should be held against the chest. If the temperature is above 99° F (37.2° C), recheck by taking a rectal temperature.

3. *Fever medicines* (see the table) should be used if the temperature is above 101.5° F (38.6° C) and your child is very uncomfortable, or if any fever is present at bedtime. If your child is acting normally, fever medicines may be delayed until the temperature is 102.2° F (39.0° C).
   a. If your child is older than 3 months of age, give fever medicine if the temperature is above 101.5° F (38.6° C). Acetaminophen (Tylenol or equivalent) is recommended every 4 to 6 hours in the dosage indicated on the table. Many use 10-15 mg/kg/dose. Younger febrile children should be evaluated immediately.
   b. Ibuprofen is a useful addition or single-agent antipyretic, usually given at a dosage of 10 mg/kg/dose PO QID. It is available over-the-counter in tablets of 200 mg or as a prescription suspension with 100 mg/5 ml.
   c. Do not use aspirin if your child has chickenpox or an influenza-like illness

Brand	Dose of fever medicine							
	0-3 mo	4-11 mo	12-23 mo	2-3 yr	4-5 yr	6-8 yr	9-10 yr	11-12 yr
Acetaminophen drops (80 mg/0.8 ml)	0.4 ml	0.8 ml	1.2 ml	1.6 ml	2.4 ml			
Acetaminophen elixir (160 mg/tsp)		½ tsp	¾ tsp	1 tsp	1½ tsp	2 tsp	2½ tsp	
Chewable tablet acetaminophen or aspirin (80 mg)			1½	2	3	4	5	6
Junior swallowable tablet (160 mg)				1	1½	2	2½	3
Adult tablet acetaminophen or aspirin (325 mg)						1	1	1½
Ibuprofen suspension (100 mg/5ml)	½ tsp	¾ tsp	1 tsp	1¼ tsp	1¾ tsp	2 tsp		
Ibuprofen capsule (200 mg)						1	1½	2

because of the association of Reye syndrome and aspirin.

4. *Sponging* is rarely needed but may be useful if the temperature remains over 104° F (40° C) after medicines and your child remains uncomfortable or irritable. Sponge or partially submerge your undressed child in *lukewarm* water (96° to 100° F). This can be done for 15 to 30 minutes as often as necessary. Some parents prefer laying the undressed child on a towel. Another towel or washcloth soaked in lukewarm water is placed over the child, changing the towel periodically every 1 to 2 minutes for 15 to 30 minutes.

5. Dress your child lightly. Push fluids.

6. Call your physician if the following occur:
   a. The fever goes above 105° F (40.5° C).
   b. The fever lasts beyond 48 to 72 hours.
   c. Your child is less than 3 months old and has a rectal temperature over 100.4° F (38° C).
   d. Your child has a seizure (convulsion) or abnormal movements of face, arms, or legs, stiff neck, purple spots, or fullness of the soft spot; looks sicker than expected; or has difficulty breathing, burning on urination, decreased urination, abdominal pain, marked change in behavior, or level of consciousness or activity.

REFERENCES

Baker RC, Tiller T, Bausher JC, et al: Severity of disease correlated with fever reduction in febrile infants, *Pediatrics* 83:1016-1019, 1989.

Baker RC, Sequin JH, Leslie N, et al: Fever and petechiae in children, *Pediatrics* 84:1051, 1989.

Baker MD, Bell LM, Avner JR: Outpatient management without antibiotics of fever in selected infants, *N Engl J Med* 329:1437-1441, 1993.

Baker D, Avner J, Bell J: Failure of infant observation scales in detecting serious illness in febrile four to eight-week-old infants, *Pediatrics* 85:1040-1043, 1990.

Baraff U, Bass JW, Fleisher GR, et al: Practice guidelines for the management of infants and children 0 to 36 months of age with fever without source, *Ann Emerg Med* 22:1198-1210, 1993.

Baraff U, Oslund SA, Schriger DL, et al: Probability of bacterial infections in febrile infants less than three months of age: a meta analysis, *Pediatr Infect Dis J* 11:257, 1992

Baskin MN, O'Rourke EJ, Fleisher GR: Outpatient treatment of febrile infants 28 to 89 days of age with intramuscular administration of ceftriaxone, *J Pediatr* 120:22, 1992.

Bonadio WA, Webster H, Wolfe A, et al: Correlating infectious outcome with clinical parameters of 1130 consecutive febrile infants aged zero to eight weeks, *Pediatr Emerg Care* 9:84, 1993.

Brannan DF, Falk JL, Rothrock SG, et al: Reliability of infra red tympanum thermometry in the determination of rectal temperature in children, *Ann Emerg Med* 25:21, 1995.

Cram E, Gershel J: Urinary tract infections in febrile infants younger than 8 weeks of age, *Pediatrics* 86:363, 1990.

Crain EF, Bulas D, Bijur PE, et al: Is a chest radiograph necessary in the evaluation of every febrile infant less than 8 weeks of age? *Pediatrics* 8:821, 1991.

Goldsmith B, Campo J: Comparison of urine dipstick, microscopy and culture for the detection of bacteriuria in children, *Clin Pediatr* 29:214, 1990.

Graneto JW, Soglin DF: Maternal screening of childhood fever by palpation, *Pediatric Emerg Care* 12:183, 1996.

Grover G: The effects of bundling on infant temperatures, *Pediatrics* 94:669, 1994.

Jaskiewicz JA, McCarthy CA, Richardson AC, et al: Febrile infants at low risk for serious bacterial infection: an appraisal of the Rochester criteria and implications for management, *Pediatrics* 94:390, 1994.

Klassen TP, Rowe PC: Selecting diagnostic tests to identify febrile infants less than 3 months of age as being at low risk for serious bacterial infection: a scientific overview, *J Pediatr* 121:671-176, 1992.

Kramer M, Lane D, Mills E: Should blood cultures be obtained in he evaluation of young febrile children without evident focus of bacterial infections? A decision analysis of diagnostic management strategies, *Pediatrics* 84:18, 1989.

Kramer MS, Shapiro ED: Management of the young febrile children: a commentary on recent practice guidelines, *Pediatrics* 100:128, 1997.

McCarthy P, Sharpe M, Spisel S, et al: Observation scales to identify serious illness in febrile children, *Pediatrics* 70:802, 1982.

Muma BK, Treloar DJ, Wurmlinger K, et al: Comparison of rectal, axillary and tympanic membrane temperatures in infants and young children, *Ann Emerg Med* 20:41, 1991.

Mandl KD, Stack AM, Fleisher GR: Incidence of bacteremia in infants and children with fever and petechiae, *J Pediatr* 131:398, 1997.

Nguyen QV, Nguyen EA, Weiner LB: Incidence of invasive bacterial disease in children with fever and petechiae, *Pediatrics* 74:77, 1984.

Pikis A, Akram S, Donkerscoot JA, et al: Penicillin resistant pneumococci from pediatric patients in the Washington DC area, *Ann Pediatr Adolesc Med* 149:30, 1995.

Pizzo PA, Rubin M, Freifeld A, et al: The child with cancer and infection. I. Empiric therapy for fever and neutropenia and preventive strategies, *J Pediatr* 119:679, 1991.

Pizzo PA, Lovejoy FH, Smith DH: Prolonged fever in children: review of 100 cases, *Pediatrics* 55:468, 1975.

Pollack CV, Pollack ES, Andrew ME: Suprapubic bladder aspiration versus urethral catheterization in ill infants: success, efficiency, and complication rates, *Ann Emerg Med* 23:225, 1994.

Rothrock SG, Harpee MB, Green SM, et al: Do oral antibiotics prevent meningitis and serious bacterial infections in children with *Streptococcus pneumoniae* occult bacteremia? A meta-analysis, *Pediatrics* 99:438, 1997.

Smart D, Baggoley C, Head J, et al: Effect of needle changing and intravenous cannula collection on blood culture contamination rates, *Ann Emerg Med* 22:1164, 1994.

Stewart JV, Webster D: Reevaluation of tympanic thermometer in the emergency department, *Ann Emerg Med* 21:158, 1992.

Walson PD, Galletta G, Chomilo F, et al: Comparison of multidose ibuprofen and acetaminophen therapy in febrile children, *Am J Dis Child* 146:626, 1992.

Williams JA, Flynn PM, Harris S, et al: A randomized study of outpatient treatment with ceftriaxone for selected febrile children with sickle cell disease, *N Engl J Med* 329:472-476, 1993.

35 Gastrointestinal Hemorrhage: Hematemesis and Rectal Bleeding

ALERT: The initial focus must be on assessing the severity of bleeding, initiating necessary stabilization measures, and determining diagnostic considerations.

Gastrointestinal (GI) hemorrhage, whether it be manifested by vomiting (hematemesis) or rectal bleeding (melena), reflects infectious, inflammatory, or anatomic abnormality (Tables 35-1 and 35-2). It must be differentiated from hemoptysis (p. 230), which is indicated by red, frothy material mixed with sputum.

ETIOLOGY

In the newborn, swallowed blood,* bleeding diathesis, and stress ulcers are the most common causes. Necrotizing enterocolitis (NEC) is occasionally noted in the nursery. During the first year of life, anal fissures and intussusception account for 70% of noninfectious gastrointestinal hemorrhage, with gangrenous bowel, peptic ulcers, and Meckel's diverticulum less common. Lesions in older children include colonic polyps (50%), anal fissures (13%), peptic ulcers (13%), intussusception (9%), and esophageal varices (9%). Infectious diarrhea is a frequent cause.

---

*Apt test for maternal blood: Mix 1 part bright red stool or vomitus with 5 to 10 parts water and centrifuge. Add 1 ml 0.2N NaOH to supernatant fluid. Pink color that develops in 2 to 5 minutes indicates fetal hemoglobin; brown color indicates adult hemoglobin.

DIAGNOSTIC FINDINGS

Initially, the urgency of intervention must reflect hemodynamic instability assessed by history and physical examination. The history should determine the onset, progression, character, frequency, and quality of bleeding. Associated vomiting, diarrhea, and abdominal pain should be noted. A history of drug ingestion, especially of aspirin, alcohol, caustic agents, and gastric irritants, should be delineated, as well as previous episodes of bleeding or family history of problems.

The physical should determine vital signs and abdominal tenderness, sounds, rebound, guarding, and rectal disease.

The diagnostic evaluation focuses on defining the site of hemorrhage with particular reference to whether it is proximal or distal to the ligament of Treitz after baseline laboratory data, including complete blood count (CBC), platelets, type and cross-match, and coagulation studies (platelets, prothrombin time [PT], partial thromboplastin time [PTT]), have been obtained (Fig. 35-1). The approach must be individualized.

1. Lesions proximal to the ligament of Treitz usually result in nasogastric (NG) aspirates positive for blood (see Fig. 56-1).

TABLE 35-1 Gastrointestinal Hemorrhage: Diagnostic Considerations by Age

Infant (<3 mo)	Toddler (<2 yr)	Preschooler (<5 yr)	School-age child (>5 yr)
UPPER GASTROINTESTINAL BLEEDING			
Swallowed maternal blood	Esophagitis	Esophagitis	Esophagitis
Gastritis	Gastritis	Gastritis	Gastritis
Ulcer, stress	Ulcer	Ulcer	Ulcer
Bleeding diathesis	Pyloric stenosis	Esophageal varices	Esophageal varices
Foreign body (NG tube)	Mallory-Weiss syndrome	Foreign body	Mallory-Weiss syndrome
Vascular malformation	Vascular malformation	Mallory-Weiss syndrome	Inflammatory bowel disease*
Duplication	Duplication	Hemophilia	Hemophilia
		Vascular malformation	Vascular malformation
LOWER GASTROINTESTINAL BLEEDING			
Swallowed maternal blood	Anal fissure	Infectious colitis*	Infectious colitis*
Infectious colitis*	Infectious colitis*	Anal fissure	Inflammatory bowel disease*
Milk allergy	Milk allergy	Polyp	Pseudomembranous enterocolitis*
Bleeding diathesis*	Colitis	Intussusception*	Polyp
Intussusception*	Intussusception*	Meckel's diverticulum	Hemolytic-uremic syndrome*
Midgut volvulus*	Meckel's diverticulum	Henoch-Schönlein purpura	Hemorrhoid
Meckel's diverticulum	Polyp	Hemolytic-uremic syndrome*	
Necrotizing enterocolitis (NEC)*	Duplication	Inflammatory bowel disease*	
	Hemolytic-uremic syndrome*	Pseudomembranous enterocolitis*	
	Inflammatory bowel disease*		
	Pseudomembranous enterocolitis*		

*Commonly associated with systemic illness involving multiple organ systems either primarily or secondarily.

a. Bright red hematemesis indicates that there is little or no contact with gastric juices; it results from an active bleeding site at or above the cardia. In children it is usually caused by varices or esophagitis and, rarely, Mallory-Weiss syndrome. Occasionally, duodenal or gastric bleeding may be so brisk that it is bright red.

b. Coffee-ground aspirate indicates that it has been altered by the gastric juices.

c. Melena may be present, indicating a blood loss in excess of 50-100 ml/24 hr.

d. Evaluation should involve endoscopy and an upper GI series, depending on the stability of the patient and the likely cause.

2. If rectal bleeding is the primary presentation, the stool should be examined for stool leukocytes and a culture obtained. The color of the blood in the stool reflects the amount and site of bleeding.

a. Hemorrhage proximal to the ileocecal valve produces tarry stools, but lower GI bleeding is red.

b. Streaks of blood on the outside of the stool indicate a lesion in the rectal

Text continued on p. 256

TABLE 35-2   Hematemesis and Rectal Bleeding: Diagnostic Considerations

Condition	Age	Character of bleeding	
		Gastric aspirate	Stool
INFECTION/INFLAMMATION			
Acute diarrhea (p. 631) Bacteria, virus, parasites	Any	—	Small (variable)
Gastritis (Chapter 44)	Any	Mild-moderate, coffee ground	Tarry
Ulcer			
Peptic	>6 yr	Small/large; red/coffee ground	Small/large; tarry
Duodenal	>6 yr	Small/large; red/coffee ground	Small/large; tarry
Stress	Any	Small/large; red/coffee ground	Small/large; tarry
Esophagitis	Any	Small	
Ulcerative colitis	Any	—	Small/large
Crohn's disease (regional enteritis)	10-19 yr	—	Variable, red
ANATOMIC			
Intussusception (p. 654)	<2 yr (5-12 mo)	—	"Currant jelly"
Volvulus (p. 659)	Neonate	—	Red/tarry
Rectal fissure (Chapter 30)	Infant	—	Blood-streaked stool
Polyps	2-10 yr	—	Small/moderate; red, intermittent
Meckel's diverticulum (p. 656)	4 mo-4 yr	—	Large; red and tarry
VASCULAR			
Esophageal varices	>2 yr (3-5 yr)	Large; red	Large, tarry
Hemangioma/hematoma/ telangiectasia	Any	—	Occult/large

Signs and symptoms	Evaluation	Comments
Fever, diarrhea, polymorpho-nuclear cells (bacterial)	Stool leukocytes, culture, CBC, ova and parasites	Dietary manipulation useful
Vomiting		Acute gastroenteritis, ASA, alcohol, *Helicobacter pylori*
Vomiting, pain, anemia	Endoscopy with biopsy/culture; upper GI series; exclude Zollinger-Ellison syndrome; determine diet, family history	May be life threatening; peptic ulcer often associated with *H. pylori* and treated with bismuth, amoxicillin, metroni-dazole, cimetidine/ranitidine for 14-28 days; cimetidine, ranitidine, or antacids (30 ml 1 and 3 hr after meals and before bed)
Vomiting, retrosternal pain	Upper GI, esophagoscopy	May be caused by hiatal hernia, chalasia; cimetidine
Insidious weight loss and pain	Proctoscopy, barium enema	Multiple complications
Insidious weight loss and pain	Proctoscopy, barium enema	
Acute onset, crampy, abdominal pain	Hydrostatic barium enema	Life threatening, requires immedi-ate surgery
Bile-stained vomit, shock, abdomi-nal distension	Barium enema	
Well child	Inspection of anus	Stool softener
Well, variable anemia	Proctoscopy, barium enema	Severe if Peutz-Jeghers syndrome; may be inflammatory, adenoma or hematoma
Well with acute, massive bleeding	Pertechnetate scan	
Painless, cirrhosis, portal vein thrombosis	Esophagoscopy, barium swallow	
Painless, mucocutaneous lesions	Angiography, laparotomy	Familial (Peutz-Jeghers syndrome)

Continued

TABLE 35-2   Hematemesis and Rectal Bleeding: Diagnostic Considerations—cont'd

Condition	Age	Character of bleeding	
		Gastric aspirate	Stool
TRAUMA			
Foreign body (p. 637)	2-6 hr	—	Variable, red
Mallory-Weiss syndrome		Large; red	
AUTOIMMUNE/ALLERGY			
Henoch-Schönlein purpura (p. 805)	3-10 yr		Small/large; red/tarry
Idiopathic thrombocytopenia purpura (p. 694)	Any		
Milk allergy (cow or soy)	<12 mo	—	Occult/small; red
CONGENITAL			
Hemophilia (p. 685)	Any (male)	Occult/large; red/coffee ground	Occult/large; red/tarry
DEGENERATIVE			
Vitamin K deficiency	1-2 days	Mild/large; red	Mild/large; red/tarry
ENDOCRINE			
Zollinger-Ellison syndrome	>7 yr	Small/large coffee ground	Tarry
NEOPLASM			
Esophageal/gastric carcinoma		Occult/large	Tarry; occult/large
MISCELLANEOUS			
Iron deficiency anemia (Chapter 26)	<18 mo	—	Occult/small
Swallowed blood	Any	Small/large; coffee ground	Occult/small

Signs and symptoms	Evaluation	Comments
History, rectal pain	Digital examination, proctoscopy	
History, vomiting	Esophagoscopy	
Abdominal pain, arthritis, hematuria, purpura	Physical examination, CBC, platelet count	Risk of intussusception
Recurrent vomiting, diarrhea, colic, failure to thrive; rarely, fulminant enterocolitis	Dietary change	
History of bleeding diasthesis	Coagulation screening	Factor replacement
Well or bleeding	PT	Vitamin K, 1-2 mg (infant), 5-10 mg (child, adult)
Vomiting, pain, anemia	Endoscopy, upper GI series, gastric acid	Recurrent ulcers
Variable with location and histology	Endoscopy, barium contrast study	Rare in infants
Well, pale	CBC	Iron supplementation
Usually obvious source	CBC, Apt (newborn)	Newborn—maternal blood, epistaxis, etc.

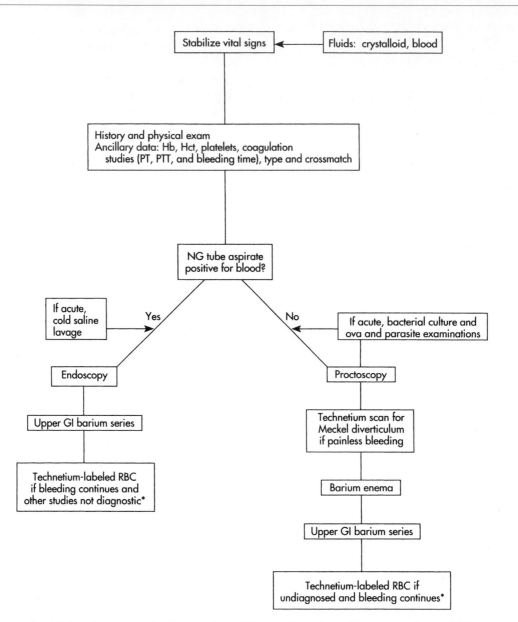

Fig. 35-1 Gastrointestinal hemorrhage. Diagnostic options. *Study may be useful in detecting and localizing sites of active bleeding. Assumes history, physical examination, and ancillary data do not indicate a cause. Consultation is generally indicated. If nondiagnostic and bleeding continues, arteriogram may be indicated.

ampulla or anal canal, most commonly fissures.

c. Depending on the suspected cause and clinical status, other evaluation can include anal inspection, sigmoidos-copy, colonoscopy, technetium scan, and double-contrast barium enema.

Occult blood may be identified by guaiac test (most conveniently supplied as Hemoccult packets), which produces a blue discoloration when positive. Stools may appear black from ingestion of iron, large numbers of chocolate sandwich cookies, bismuth, Pepto-Bismol, lead, licorice, charcoal, or coal, or they may be red from gelatin. False-positive findings may result from ingestion of iron, red fruit, and meats; false-negative findings occur when the fecal specimen is stored and dried or there has been recent ingestion of ascorbic acid. Hemoccult testing is not useful for detecting gastric bleeding. Gastroccult testing should be used for detecting occult blood in gastric juice.

MANAGEMENT

Management of significant GI bleeding involves stabilization of the patient, using crystalloid initially, followed by whole blood or packed red blood cells. Coagulopathies must be treated. Patients should be given oxygen, have an intravenous line or lines started, and be monitored closely from the time they enter the emergency department (ED). A hematocrit should be done immediately and blood sent for type and cross-matching. If upper GI bleeding is present, a large-caliber NG tube should be passed and the stomach lavaged with cooled saline solution to decrease mucosal blood flow while monitoring blood in the returned aspirate. Lavage is continued until the aspirate is clear. Consultation should usually be obtained, and if bleeding stops within 30 to 45 minutes, gastroduodenoscopy is often done to provide direct visualization. If the bleeding is massive or ongoing, endoscopy may not be useful, and scanning or arteriography may be required.

Vasopressin (Pitressin) may rarely be required with intractable variceal bleeding. After consultation, an initial bolus of 20 units/1.73 m^2 IV diluted in 2 ml/kg of D5W is given over 20 minutes followed by a continuous infusion of 0.2-0.4 units/1.73 m^2/min. If bleeding ceases,

infusion is maintained at the initial dosage for 12 hours and then is tapered over 24 to 36 hours. If it fails, sclerosing agents or a Sengstaken-Blakemore tube may be needed.

Surgical intervention is required if there is life-threatening hemorrhage, intussusception (if not reducible), volvulus, Meckel's diverticulum, ulcer (if perforated), or a neoplasm.

All patients require hospitalization for evaluation, monitoring, and intervention. After stabilization and diagnostic evaluation, a long-term management plan must be developed. Mucosal lesions may be treated with antacids containing magnesium hydroxide and aluminum hydroxide (e.g., Maalox, Mylanta). During an acute episode, patients are given 0.5 ml/kg (maximum: 30 ml/dose) q1-2hr PO to maintain gastric pH 5 or above. On a maintenance basis, the same dose is given at 1 and 3 hours after meals and before bedtime. Pharmacologic agents (histamine [H_2] receptor antagonist) that are equally effective include cimetidine (Tagamet), 20-30 mg/kg/24 hr q6hr PO (adult 600-1800 mg/24 hr PO) or 20-30 mg/kg/24 hr q4hr IV slowly as 15-minute infusion; ranitidine (Zantac) (adult: 150 mg q12hr PO or 50 mg q6-8hr IV); or Pepcid (adult: 40 mg q24hr PO or 20 mg q12hr IV). A pediatric dosage for ranitidine has not been established but is expected to range from 1-2 mg/kg/24 hr q12hr PO or IV.

REFERENCES

Hyams JS, Leichtner AM, Schwartz AN: Recent advances in diagnosis and treatment of gastrointestinal hemorrhage in infants and children, *J Pediatr* 106:1, 1985.

Jenkins HR, Pincott JR, Soothill JF, et al: Food allergy: the major cause of infantile colitis, *Arch Dis Child* 59:326, 1984.

Oldham KT, Lobe TE: Gastrointestinal hemorrhage in children: a pragmatic update, *Pediatr Clin North Am* 32:1247, 1985.

Steer ML, Silen W: Diagnostic procedures in gastrointestinal hemorrhage, *N Engl J Med* 309:646, 1983.

36 HEADACHE

Because the brain has no pain-sensitive structures, headaches secondary to intracranial disease arise from irritating pain fibers that innervate the dura or vessels of the pia-arachnoid. Headaches may also be extracranial, involving muscles, blood vessels, epithelial tissue of the sinuses, orbit, and eye. Nearly two thirds of headaches in children are associated with extracranial infections (viral syndrome, sinusitis, pharyngitis). The pain associated with headaches has several mechanisms:

1. Muscle contraction—tension
2. Vascular—migraine, cluster, hypertension
3. Traction—subarachnoid hemorrhage, mass lesion, postconcussive
4. Inflammatory—meningitis, sinusitis, arteritis
5. Secondary to extracranial structures—refractive error, sinusitis
6. Psychogenic—depression, conversion

DIAGNOSTIC FINDINGS

The initial evaluation of the patient with a headache who is otherwise stable must determine the characteristics with regard to location, nature of pain, age of onset, frequency, duration and progression, precipitating and ameliorating factors, pica, ingestions, exposures, associated signs and symptoms, medications, medical history (especially hypertension, sinusitis, heart disease, ear infections, and seizures), and family history. The temporal pattern is particularly important to determine whether the headache is acute (single event with no previous episodes), acute and recurrent, chronic and progressive (suggesting potential increased intracranial pressure with increasing severity and frequency), or chronic and nonprogressive (several times per day/week, with no change in severity or signs and symptoms). Recent stresses and emotional stability should be delineated. A careful physical examination must be performed with a complete neurologic evaluation, including visual acuity and fields, cerebellar signs, and auscultation for bruits.

Because children less than the age of 5 years rarely have headaches, an organic cause is highly likely. Increased intracranial pressure is suggested by a headache that awakens the patient from sleep, occurs in the morning, is associated with vomiting without nausea, or is related to a change in position from prone to supine or erect. Occipital pain is often associated with an anatomic abnormality. Presenting signs and symptoms are helpful in differentiating cause of the headache (Tables 36-1 and 36-2).

Ancillary Data

Ancillary data should reflect positive findings. Studies that may be useful under specific circumstances include skull x-ray studies,

TABLE 36-1   Differentiation of Headache Type By Signs and Symptoms

Clues	Type of headache
ASSOCIATED EVENTS	
Abrupt onset	Convulsive, subarachnoid hemorrhage
Afternoon	Muscle contraction
Present on arising	Convulsive (following nocturnal seizure), emotional depression, traction (tumor), vascular
Preceded by aura	Convulsive, vascular (migraine)
Exacerbated by coughing	Paranasal sinus, traction (tumor, increased intracranial pressure), vascular
Followed by lethargy	Convulsive, vascular
Followed by focal central nervous system deficit	Convulsive (Todd paresis), traction (tumor), vascular (hemiplegic migraine)
Fever, neck stiffness	Meningitis
Related to posture	Posttraumatic, traction (tumor and after lumbar puncture)
Related to stress	Muscle contraction, vascular (migraine)
Nausea and vomiting	Migraine, convulsive, traction (tumor)
Elevated diastolic pressure	Hypertensive encephalopathy
CHARACTER OF PAIN	
Steady	Emotional depression, muscle contraction, sinus, traction (tumor, increased intracranial pressure)
Throbbing	Convulsive, posttraumatic, traction (tumor, increased intracranial pressure), vascular (migraine, vasculitis, inflammatory)
LOCATION	
Frontal	Traction (supratentorial tumor), vascular
Occipital and neck	Muscle, contraction, sinus (ethmoid), traction (posterior fossa tumor)
Unilateral	Traction (lateralized supratentorial tumor), vascular (migraine), intracranial hemorrhage

Modified from Kriel RL: Headache. In Swaiman KF, Wright FS, editors: *The practice of pediatric neurology,* ed 2, vol 1, St Louis, 1982, Mosby.

TABLE 36-2   Headache: Diagnostic Considerations

Condition	Diagnostic findings	Comments
INTRAPSYCHIC		
Tension	Common; anxiety, stress, recurrent headache; pain—occipital, neck, or generalized, although it can be bifrontal or frontotemporal; sense of pressure or constriction; no prodrome, aura; spasm of muscles of neck and shoulder	Attempt to reduce anxiety; analgesia, stress control
Conversion reaction (p. 758)	Inconsistent findings	
Depression	Inciting event	
INFECTION		
Meningitis/encephalitis (p. 725)	Acute onset, infectious prodrome and associated findings; pain on movement; diffuse headache; lumbar puncture diagnostic	Hospitalize; antibiotics; support
Abscess, cerebral	Low grade fever; focal neurologic findings; localized headache; meningism; lumbar puncture: variable WBC, negative culture; CT scan	Neurosurgical referral
Sinusitis (p. 610)	Unilateral or bilateral frontal headache; pain on percussion of sinus; if sphenoid, may be occipital; purulent rhinorrhea; sinus x-ray studies	Antibiotics; rare drainage and referral; other ear, nose, and throat infections can cause headache including otitis media, mastoiditis, and retropharyngeal abscess
Dental abscess (p. 590)	Insidious onset; local pain; dental x-ray studies	Dental referral
VASCULAR		
Migraine (p. 734)	Unilateral recurrent headache (young children—generalized); throbbing; associated visual, sensory, motor deficit; abdominal pain, nausea, vomiting, positive family history; 25%-50% of chronic headaches	Supportive; analgesia, steroids, ergotamine (Cafergot); prophylaxis if frequent; sumatriptan useful in older children
Cluster	Paroxysmal, unilateral, explosive retroorbital, periorbital, or frontal headache; unilateral autonomic symptoms—nasal stuffiness, lacrimation, Horner syndrome; cluster in short period separated by long pain-free interval; rare in children; lasts 30-120 min but extremely severe; may occur several times in 24-hr period	Propranolol, steroids, indomethacin, lithium

TABLE 36-2   Headache: Diagnostic Considerations—cont'd

Condition	Diagnostic findings	Comments
VASCULAR—cont'd		
Subarachnoid or cerebral bleeding; AV malformation (Chapter 18)	Acute onset; intense headache; focal neurologic examination; obtundation; meningism; CT scan; lumbar puncture bloody	Predisposing factors: trauma, bleeding problem
Hypertensive encephalopathy	Diffuse headache, nausea, vomiting, confusion, seizure, focal neurologic finding; high blood pressure	Associated illness: acute glomerulonephritis, etc.
TRAUMA (Chapter 57)		
Postconcussive	Diffuse headache, often occiptal, neck, or generalized bifrontal; vertigo, dizziness, confusion, sensitivity to noise, movement, heat, light; emotional instability; normal neurologic finding	Observation; frequent examinations; analgesia, muscle relaxants
Subdural	Acute or insidious onset headache; CT scan	Neurosurgical intervention, observation; frequent examination
Fracture	Local tenderness and swelling; skull x-ray study	Neurosurgical consultation
INTOXICATION		
Carbon monoxide (p. 371)	Headache, weakness; dizziness; respiratory arrest, coma; carboxyhemoglobin level	Oxygen; hyperbaric chamber
Lead	Diffuse headache; weakness; irritability, personality change; ataxia; seizures, coma; pica; red cell δ-aminolevulinic acid dehydratase	Dimercaprol and EDTA; penicillamine
NEOPLASM		
Cerebral	Frontal unrelenting headache, unilateral or bilateral; usually worse on rising; papilledema; increased intracranial pressure	Neurosurgical consultation
Cerebellar	Occipital unrelenting headache; vomiting; ataxia	Neurosurgical consultation
Pseudotumor cerebri (p. 737)	Nausea, vomiting, diplopia, acute or insidious generalized headache; full fontanelle, variable papilledema, ↑ CSF pressure	Predisposing factors: viral illness, intoxication, head trauma, steroids, etc.

Continued

TABLE 36-2   Headache: Diagnostic Considerations—cont'd

Condition	Diagnostic findings	Comments
AUTOIMMUNE		
Temporal arteritis	Local headache with tenderness and pain over temporal artery	Steroids; rare; increased ESR
Trigeminal neuralgia	Unilateral, recurrent headache and pain over distribution of second branch, trigeminal nerve	Carbamazepine, phenytoin
MISCELLANEOUS		
Eye		
Glaucoma	Generalized headache; blurred vision, dilated pupil; tonometry	Miotic, osmotic, diuretic
Refractive error	Generalized headache	Glasses
Epilepsy (p. 738)	Paroxysmal onset of headache and abrupt termination; brief duration; loss of contact with environment; variable abdominal pain	Rare cause of headaches
High altitude (Chapter 49)	Diffuse headache; weakness	
Temporomandibular joint (TMJ) disease	Frontotemporal or temporal pain; bilateral or unilateral severe, steady ache; limited mandibular movement, tenderness in muscles of jaw and neck	Refer to dentist
S/P lumbar puncture	Diffuse headache following procedure; unusual in young children	Bed rest, supine

sinus series, computed tomography (CT) scan (elevated intracranial pressure, progressive or new neurologic signs, behavioral change, growth drop-off, reduced visual acuity, increasing frequency or severity of headaches, or increasing pain on awakening, coughing, straining, or changing position, focal electroencephalogram [EEG], meningismus, focal headache, seizures), electroencephalography, and lumbar puncture.

MANAGEMENT

Management should focus on suitable analgesia and treatment of the underlying condition. An empiric trial is sometimes indicated. Hospitalization is indicated if there is any evidence of increased intracranial pressure, progressive or new neurologic signs, or intractable pain.

REFERENCES

Burton LJ, Quinn B, Pratt-Cheney JL, et al: Headache etiology in a pediatric emergency department, *Pediatr Emerg Care* 13:1, 1997.

Cooper PJ, Bawden HN, Camfield PR, et al: Anxiety and life events in childhood migraine, *Pediatrics* 79:999, 1987.

Olness KN, MacDonald JT: Recurrent headaches in children: diagnosis and treatment, *Pediatr Rev* 8:307, 1987.

Shinnar S, D'Souza BJ: Diagnosis and management of headache in children, *Pediatr Clin North Am* 29:79, 1981.

Singer HS, Rowe S: Chronic recurrent headache in children, *Pediatr Ann* 21:369, 1992.

Stratton SJ: Sumatriptan: a clinical standard, *Ann Emerg Med* 25:538, 1995.

Svenson J, Cowen D, Rogers A: Headache in the emergency department: importance of history in identifying secondary etiologies, *J Emerg Med* 15:617, 1997.

37 HEMATURIA AND PROTEINURIA

ALERT: Hematuria and proteinuria require a systematic evaluation to exclude glomerular or extraglomerular disease.

Hematuria is present when there are 5 or more red blood cells/high-power field (RBCs/HPF) in a sediment of 10 ml of centrifuged urine.* It can result from nonrenal as well as glomerular and extraglomerular abnormality, which can often be clinically distinguished by urinalysis:

	Glomerular	Extra glomerular or nonrenal
Urine color	Brown, smoky "cola color"	Red, pink, or bright red blood
RBC casts	May be present	Absent
Blood clots	Absent	May be present

Hematuria in newborns results primarily from vascular disorders such as hypoxia, thrombosis, or circulatory compromise; in older children, urinary tract infections account for most cases, followed by glomerulonephritis and trauma. Hypercalciuria and nephrolithiasis also can cause hematuria.

Hemoglobinuria or myoglobinuria can cause false-positive test results, as can iodine. Obviously, a microscopic examination for RBC should be done. With myoglobinuria, the hematocrit is normal and the serum is clear (not pink). Common causes of hemoglobinuria include hemolytic anemia, incompatible blood transfusions, disseminated intravascular coagulation (DIC), hemolytic-uremic syndrome, infec-tion (sepsis, malaria), burns, exertion, cold, nocturnal and exertional hemoglobinuria, and drugs (carbon monoxide, sulfonamides, snake venom). Myoglobinuria may be caused by muscle injury (crush, burn), myositis, or rhab-domyolysis.

Drugs and other agents that cause a red or dark urine include aniline dyes, blackberries, phenolphthalein, phenazopyridine (Pyridium), rifampin, and urates (p. 359).

Proteinuria is clearly present when more than 200 mg/m^2/24 hr of protein is excreted in the urine. It is usually transient, occurring with fever, exercise, seizures, pneumonia, congestive heart failure (CHF), or environmental stress. Orthostatic proteinuria occurs when an individual is in an upright position; resolution occurs in 50% of patients by early adulthood. Evaluation of orthostatic proteinuria requires careful collection and comparison of standing and recumbent urinalyses. During a 24-hour collection, separate voids during the night and on awakening (recumbent position) from the remainder of the urine collected during the day.

Ideally this is done by fasting (NPO) after 9 PM and voiding before bed. Urine specimens are then collected at midnight and 5 AM without getting up, at 7 AM, and while active from then until bedtime.

Urine dipstick tests for hematuria change color with the oxidation of orthotolidine to

---

*See also Chapter 85.

263

TABLE 37-1 Hematuria and Proteinuria: Diagnostic Considerations*

Condition	Site of involvement	Diagnostic findings	Urinalysis Hematuria	Proteinuria	Comments
INFECTION					
Urinary tract infection (p. 815)	Nonrenal/extraglomerular	Acute onset fever, dysuria, frequency, burning; if pyelonephritis, may appear toxic, with CVA tenderness, WBC casts	Gross/microscopic	Positive	Cystitis or pyelonephritis; bacterial, viral, tuberculosis, other; culture
AUTOIMMUNE					
Glomerulonephritis, acute (p. 800)	Glomerular	Malaise, headache, vomiting, fever, abdominal pain; oliguria, edema, high BP	Gross/microscopic	Positive	Poststreptococci; high ASO titer; low complement
Membranoproliferative glomerulonephritis (p. 809)	Glomerular	Often insidious; malaise, headache, vomiting, edema, high BP	Gross/microscopic	Positive	Low complement; biopsy
Henoch-Schönlein purpura (p. 805)	Glomerular	Purpuric rash, arthritis, GI involvement	Microscopic	Variable	Variable involvement; may have elevated IgA level
Lupus nephritis	Glomerular	Associated signs and symptoms	Microscopic	Positive	Variable involvement; positive ANA result, low complement; biopsy
Nephritis Bacterial endocarditis (p. 559) Shunt	Glomerular	Acute illness, fever, toxicity, signs and symptoms of related disease	Microscopic	Positive	Low complement
Nephrotic syndrome (p. 806)	Glomerular	Periorbital swelling and oliguria followed by edema, malaise, abdominal pain	Rare (25%)	Positive	Low albumin, high lipid levels; cause unknown
TRAUMA (Chapter 64)					
Renal calculi	Nonrenal	Asymptomatic to severe back and abdominal pain, nausea, vomiting	Gross/microscopic	Negative	Idiopathic, UTI, ↑ Ca^{++}, cystinosis, hyperuricemia; IVP indicated
Foreign body	Nonrenal	Frequency, urgency, pain	Microscopic	Negative	Usually experimenting or masturbating

CHAPTER 37 • HEMATURIA AND PROTEINURIA

Condition		Clinical Features		Proteinuria	Comments
Direct trauma (Chapter 64)	Variable	History of trauma with variable complaints	Gross/microscopic	Negative	Usually renal contusion; if gross, laceration or rupture; IVP
Exercise	Nonrenal	Follows heavy exercise	Microscopic	Variable	
Meatal excoriation (p. 495)	Nonrenal	Local lesion	Gross/microscopic	Negative	Local treatment
CONGENITAL					
Hydronephrosis	Extraglomerular	Abdominal mass	Microscopic	Positive	Most common uretero-pelvic junction
Polycystic kidney	Extraglomerular	Large kidney, other cystic anomalies	Microscopic	Positive	Infant, adult types
Hemangioma/telangiectasis	Extraglomerular	Hemangioma, telangiectasia	Microscopic	Negative	Rendu-Osler-Weber disease
Hemoglobinopathy/ hemophilia Sickle cell trait, SC (p. 698)	Extraglomerular	Associated signs and symptoms	Microscopic	Negative	Difficulty concentrating urine; factor levels
Coagulopathy thrombocytopenia (p. 694)	Extraglomerular	Bleeding problems elsewhere	Gross/microscopic	Negative	Bleeding screen, platelets
Hereditary nephritis	Glomerular	Hearing deficit	Microscopic	Negative	Alport syndrome
Benign familial hematuria	Glomerular	Intermittent or persistent	Microscopic	Negative	Benign
INTOXICATION					
Anticoagulants Aspirin Methicillin Sulfonamides	Extraglomerular	Nephritis or crystalluria	Gross/microscopic	Variable	Temporally related to drug use
NEOPLASM					
Wilms' tumor	Extraglomerular	Abdominal mass	Gross/microscopic	Negative	Surgical consultation
Leukemia	Extraglomerular	Systemic disease	Microscopic	Variable	Oncology consultation
OTHER					
Renal vein thrombosis	Extraglomerular		Gross/microscopic	Variable	Occurs in acutely ill children
Congestive heart failure (Chapter 16)	Extraglomerular	Dyspnea, tachycardia, tachypnea	Microscopic	Negative	Accompanies cardiac disease

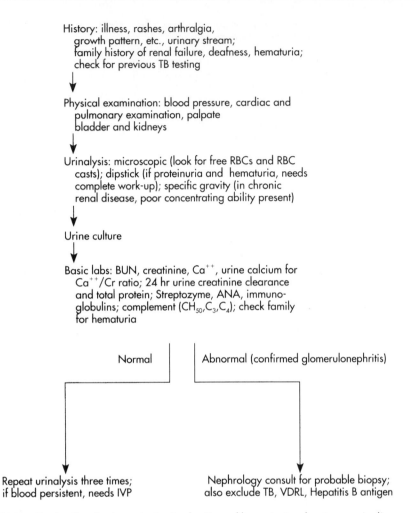

History: illness, rashes, arthralgia,
growth pattern, etc., urinary stream;
family history of renal failure, deafness, hematuria;
check for previous TB testing

Physical examination: blood pressure, cardiac and
pulmonary examination, palpate
bladder and kidneys

Urinalysis: microscopic (look for free RBCs and RBC
casts); dipstick (if proteinuria and hematuria, needs
complete work-up); specific gravity (in chronic
renal disease, poor concentrating ability present)

Urine culture

Basic labs: BUN, creatinine, Ca^{++}, urine calcium for
Ca^{++}/Cr ratio; 24 hr urine creatinine clearance
and total protein; Streptozyme, ANA, immunoglobulins; complement (CH_{50}, C_3, C_4); check family
for hematuria

Normal | Abnormal (confirmed glomerulonephritis)

Repeat urinalysis three times; | Nephrology consult for probable biopsy;
if blood persistent, needs IVP | also exclude TB, VDRL, Hepatitis B antigen

Fig. 37-1 Evaluation for hematuria. Evaluation of hematuria after trauma is discussed in Chapter 64.

cumene hyproperoxide with the catalysis of hemoglobin or myoglobin. Oxidizing agents such as povidine-iodine, hexachlorophene, or hypochlorite may cause false-positive results, as can markedly alkaline urine. False-negative findings can result from ascorbic acid.

Proteinuria may be read as 0 to 4+ (0 to >2000 mg/dl). Fifty percent of "trace" proteinurias have normal quantitation results. False-positive results occur with highly alkaline urine

(pH results >6.5) or contamination with benzalkonium.

A ratio may allow use of a single specimen. Quantitative protein excretion can be established by the following formula: total protein (gm/m²/24 hr) = 0.63 (urine protein/urine creatinine). The normal ratio is less than 0.5 in children less than 2 years old. A ratio greater than 1.5 indicates severe proteinuria, and 3.0 is seen in the nephrotic range.

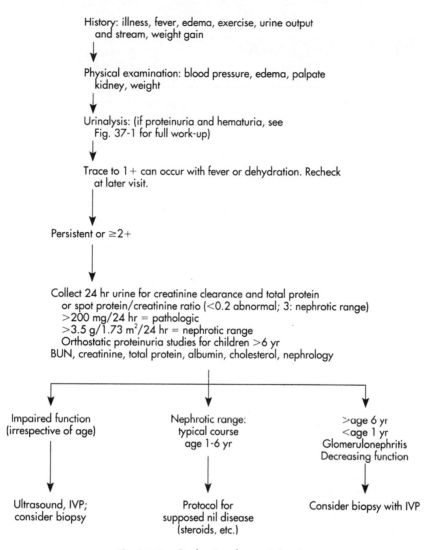

Fig. 37-2 Evaluation for proteinuria.

The evaluation is outlined in Figs. 37-1 and 37-2 and Table 37-1.

REFERENCES

Abitol C, Zilleruelo G, et al: Quantitation of proteinuria with urinary protein/creatinine ratios and random testing with dipstick in nephrotic children, *J Pediatr* 116:243, 1990.

Fitzwater DS, Wyatt RJ: Hematuria, *Pediatr Rev* 15:102, 1994.

Elises JS: Simplified quantification of urinary protein excretion in children, *Clin Nephrol* 30:225, 1988.

Feld LG: Evaluation of the child with asymptomatic proteinuria, *Pediatr Rev* 5:248, 1984.

White RHR: The investigation of hematuria, *Arch Dis Child* 64:259, 1989.

Yaden O: Hematuria in children, *Pediatr Ann* 23:474, 1994.

38 HYPOGLYCEMIA

ALERT: If signs and symptoms are consistent, an emergent therapeutic trial of glucose administration should be attempted after obtaining specimens for glucose determination.

Hypoglycemia is a blood sugar level of less than 40 mg/dl in the child, less than 30 mg/dl in the newborn, and less than 20 mg/dl in the preterm infant in the first 24 hours of life. These criteria are based on whole-blood determinations; the serum or plasma level is 15% to 20% higher. Initial use of Dextrostix or Chemstrips is helpful for emergency approximations before confirmation by clinical analysis in the laboratory.

Fasting hypoglycemia, which is related to an imbalance between glucose production and use, is most common in thin male children between 18 months and 5 years. Reactive hypoglycemia produces a low glucose level within 5 hours after eating; it accompanies increased insulin and is usually severe. Drugs also can cause hypoglycemia.

ETIOLOGY (Table 38-1)

Newborns experience transient hypoglycemia, often associated with perinatal complications caused by excessive insulin secretion, including maternal diabetes or erythroblastosis. After the first day of life, and often in association with hypoxia and intrauterine growth retardation, a more prolonged hypoglycemia produced by inadequate glycogen stores may develop. Congenital abnormalities of the central nervous system (CNS) or heart may cause hypoglycemia; sepsis and hypocalcemia may develop.

Inborn errors of carbohydrate and glycogen storage, amino acid and organic acid metabolism, and endocrine abnormalities may cause hypoglycemia during *infancy.* Hypoglycemia occurs shortly after the ingestion of protein in patients with idiopathic leucine sensitivity and defects in amino acid and organic acid metabolism. Ingestion of lactose may stimulate hypoglycemia associated with galactosemia; sucrose ingestion may produce hypoglycemia in the presence of hereditary fructose intolerance. Patients with medium-chain acyl-CoA dehydrogenase deficiency (MCADD) typically are seen between 3 months and 2 years of age with minor illnesses or when a baby first sleeps through the night. This disorder of fatty acid oxidation impairs ketogenesis.

In *childhood,* fasting hypoglycemia may result from ketotic hypoglycemia, as well as hormonal deficiencies, hyperinsulinism, glycogen storage disease, or fructose 1,6-diphosphatase deficiency. *Preschool* children may be symptomatic after prolonged fasting, exacerbating the physiologic response to starvation. Poisons and toxins may be contributory in other patients.

DIAGNOSTIC FINDINGS

The patient's history may be helpful in focusing on the appropriate cause. Onset; frequency; relationship to food (fruits and fructose

TABLE 38-1   Hypoglycemia: Diagnostic Considerations

Condition	Type	Hepatomegaly (variably abnormal liver function test)	Ketonuria/ketonemia
NEONATAL (TRANSIENT) (Chapter 11)			
Small-for-gestational age infant	Fasting	No	No
Hyperinsulinism	Fasting	No	No
Infant of diabetic mother			
Erythroblastosis			
Perinatal insult	Fasting	No	No
Asphyxia, infection			
HEPATIC ENZYME DEFICIENCY			
Glycogen storage disease (I, III, VI)	Fasting	Yes	Variable
Disorder of gluconeogenesis	Fasting	Yes	No
LIMITED SUBSTRATE			
Ketotic hypoglycemia (onset 1½-5 yr; resolves by 9-10 yr)	Fasting	No	Yes
Endocrine (Chapter 74)			
Panhypopituitarism	Fasting	No	Yes
Growth hormone deficiency			
ACTH deficiency			
Addison disease			
Hypothyroidism			
HYPERINSULINEMIA			
Beta-cell tumor, adenoma, hyperplasia	Fasting	No	No
Leucine sensitivity	Reactive	No	No
Extrapancreatic tumor	Fasting	No	No
Prediabetes	Fasting	No	No
INTOXICATION (Chapter 54)			
Salicylates		No	Yes
Ethanol		No	Variable
Propranolol		No	No
Insulin		No	No
MISCELLANEOUS			
Malnutrition	Fasting	Yes	Yes
Hepatic damage	Fasting	Variable	Variable
Reye syndrome (p. 646)			
Hepatitis (p. 639)			
Fructose intolerance, galactosemia	Reactive	Yes	No
Amino acid abnormalities	Fasting	No	No
Gastroenteritis	Fasting	No	No

intolerance, high-protein diet intolerance or leucine sensitive), drugs, or fasting; family history; and concurrent medical problems must be explored. Evidence of abnormalities in growth and development must be sought (Table 38-2).

The systemic response primarily reflects excessive catecholamine release. Clinically, patients have sweating, weakness, tachycardia, tachypnea, variable elevations of blood pressure and temperature, anxiety, tremulousness, and hunger. Neonates may be asymptomatic.

If the hypoglycemia is not treated, cerebral dysfunction may progress, the presentation and complications paralleling those of hypoxia. Patients may have headaches; disturbed mental status with confusion, irritability, and psychotic behavior; ataxia; seizures; and coma. The signs and symptoms of the underlying cause may also be present.

1. **Complications:** permanent brain damage from frequent or prolonged hypoglycemia

2. **Ancillary data**
   a. Serum insulin, serum, and urine glucose and ketone, lactate, and phosphate levels and liver function test results.
   b. Specific tolerance tests, response to ketogenic diet, enzymes in urine, liver biopsy, and so on, may all need to be considered, depending on the differential.

DIFFERENTIAL DIAGNOSIS

See Chapters 15 and 54.

MANAGEMENT

Concurrently with stabilization, the hypoglycemia must be treated. Patients with clinical

TABLE 38-2 Hypoglycemia: Etiologic Differentiation

	Inborn error of metabolism (carbohydrate/amino acid)	Hormonal deficiency	Hyperinsulinism
HISTORY			
Hypoglycemia			
Fasting (time after fasting)	Common* (many hours)	Common (few hours)	Common (few hours)
After lactose	Galactosemia	No	No
After sucrose	Hereditary fructose intolerance	No	No
After protein	Amino acid, organic acid	No	No
Family history	Common	Variable	Variable
PHYSICAL			
Hepatomegaly	Common	No	No
Failure to thrive	Common	Variable	Variable
LABORATORY			
Ketosis	Common†	Variable	No
Acidosis	Common	No	No
Nonglucose urine reducing substance	Galactosemia, hereditary fructose intolerance		
Hyperammonemia	Amino acid, organic acid		
Liver function abnormality	Common	No	No

*Glycogen storage disease. Fructose 16-diphosphatase deficiency.
†If no ketosis, consider 3-hydroxy-3-methylglutaric aciduria, glutaric aciduria type II, systemic carnitine deficiency, and carnitine palmitoyl transferase deficiency.

components of hypoglycemia require emergency intervention.

1. In the newborn, early, frequent feedings are often adequate.
2. In the older child, if there are no vital sign or central nervous system findings, oral sources of glucose may be attempted, with frequent feedings.
3. If the patient is unstable with altered mental status, glucose should be administered parenterally:
   a. Give 0.5-1.0 gm/kg/dose IV, usually administered as D25W (2-4 ml/kg/dose) slowly; a rapid response is to be expected if hypoglycemia is the prominent cause. D50W (1-2 ml/kg/dose) may be used for children older than 3 years of age; D10W for preterm infants. D10W has 10 gm of glucose/dl.
   b. Thereafter, maintain through adequate glucose homeostasis and fluid balance: 10% glucose in 0.2% normal saline (NS) solution at a rate of about 7 mg of dextrose/kg/min.
4. If glucose is unavailable, glucagon. 0.03-0.1 mg/kg/dose IM, IV (1 mg may be given at any age), will provide transient elevation of glucose level if liver stores are adequate. Dose may be repeated in 20 minutes.
5. Sources of 20 gm of glucose commonly available include Kool-Aid with sugar (13.4 oz), Coca Cola (13.3 oz), orange soda (10 oz), ginger ale (15.5 oz), Hershey's milk chocolate bar (2.5 oz bar), orange juice (12 oz), and apple juice (12 oz). Obviously, these may vary with variations in products or mixing technique.
6. In severe hyperinsulinemia, diazoxide, 6-12 mg/kg/24 hr q12hr PO, is usually required on an ongoing basis. Frequent feedings alone are often successful in preventing fasting types of hypoglycemia. Underlying diseases must receive prompt treatment.

DISPOSITION

Most patients with suspected hyperinsulinemia or any vital-sign abnormalities or cerebral dysfunction should be admitted to the hospital until the cause is clear and future episodes can be prevented. Patients with only minimal symptoms and a known cause can, with adequate follow-up observation, often be monitored as outpatients. The ultimate disposition and management must reflect the cause.

REFERENCES

Bonham JR: Investigation of hypoglycaemia during childhood, *Ann Clin Biochem* 30:238, 1993.
Bradows RG, Williams C, Amatruda JM: Treatment of insulin reactions in diabetes, *JAMA* 252:3378, 1984.
Haymond M: Hypoglycemia in infants and children, *Endocrinol Metab Clin North Am* 18:211, 1989.
LaFranchi S: Hypoglycemia of infancy and childhood, *Pediatr Clin North Am* 34:961, 1987.
Phillip M, Bashari N, Smith CPH, et al: An algorithm approach to diagnosis of hypoglycemia, *J Pediatr* 110:387, 1987.

39 IRRITABILITY

ALERT: Irritability may be the presenting complaint for a potentially life-threatening systemic disease. It is essential to consider such conditions in determining management.

Children tend to be irritable with acute infections, particularly those associated with fever. The febrile child needs careful evaluation to ensure that no underlying significant disorder is associated with the behavioral change. Chronic illnesses, such as juvenile rheumatoid arthritis, may cause a child to be irritable.

Most children tend to have some period of the day when they are most irritable, usually toward the evening. When this becomes marked, it is known as colic and occurs in as many as 10% of children. Irritability from teething usually begins at 6 months of age with the appearance of the first teeth. Because medications commonly cause irritability, this factor should be considered in prescribing drugs. Unrecognized trauma must also be excluded (Table 39-1).

The history and physical examination should focus on the pattern of irritability and contributing findings. Time and duration, frequency, and factors that reduce or exacerbate

TABLE 39-1   Irritability: Diagnostic Considerations

Condition	Diagnostic findings	Comments
INFECTIONS		
Minor acute infections		
Upper respiratory infections (p. 609)	Rhinorrhea, cough, variable fever, decreased activity, nontoxic	Irritability decreases with antipyretic therapy; must rule out other abnormality
Otitis media (p. 596)	Rhinorrhea, fever, ear pain	Irritability usually decreases with antipyretic therapy and local therapy (eardrops) if needed
Urinary tract infection (p. 815)	Fever, dysuria, frequency, burning	Irritability decreases in 24 hr with appropriate antibiotics
Other	Associated signs and symptoms	
Meningitis (p. 725)/encephalitis	Fever, anorexia, changed mental status, lethargy, variable stiff neck, headache	Important infection to consider in irritable child; may exist even in presence of other infection such as otitis media
Osteomyelitis (p. 753)	Bone pain, redness	Orthopedic consultation

TABLE 39-1   Irritability: Diagnostic Considerations—cont'd

Condition	Diagnostic findings	Comments
COLIC	Episodic, intense, persistent crying in an otherwise healthy child; usually occurs in late afternoon or evening	Usually begins at 2-3 wk and continues until 10-12 wk; must be certain no abnormality exists; advise soothing rhythmic activities (rocking, wind-up swing), avoiding stimulants coffee, tea, cola) if breast feeding, and minimizing daytime sleeping; soy or hydrolyzed casein formula may be transiently beneficial; make sure that mother gets adequate sleep and is handling stress; colic may have long-term impact on family; diagnosis of exclusion
TEETHING	Irritated, swollen gum; does *not* cause high fevers, significant diarrhea, or diaper rash	Advise teething ring, wet washcloth to chew on; rubbing gums with small amount of Scotch (or other liquor) or proprietary products; avoiding salty foods
INTRAPSYCHIC		
Parental anxiety	Insecure, anxious parents; overly responsive, irritable well child	Unstable or changing home environment, inconsistent parenting; attempt to support parents
INTOXICATION (Chapter 54)		
Phenobarbital Aminophylline Amphetamines Ephedrine	In therapeutic or high dosage may cause irritability as either a primary or paradoxical effect	May try different form of drug or substitute
Lead	Weakness, weight loss, vomiting, headache, abdominal pain, seizures, increased intracranial pressure	Dimercaprol, EDTA
Narcotics withdrawal in newborn (Chapter 11)	Yawning, sneezing, jitteriness, tremor, constant movement, seizures, vomiting, dehydration, collapse	Symptoms begin in first 48 hr but may be delayed; support child: phenobarbital 5 mg/kg/24 hr q8hr IM or PO with slow tapering over 1-3 wk
TRAUMA		
Foreign body, fracture, tourniquet (hair around digit) (Chapter 66)	Local tenderness, swelling, often following injury; thread or cloth around digit or penis	Splinter or other foreign body, hairline fracture; contusion; tourniquet around digit or penis

Continued

TABLE 39-1   Irritability: Diagnostic Considerations—cont'd

Conditions	Diagnostic findings	Comments
TRAUMA—cont'd		
Subdural hematoma (Chapter 57)	History of head trauma; progressively impaired mental status; vomiting, headache, seizures	May be acute or chronic; requires recognition, computed tomography scan; neurosurgical consultation
Epidural hematoma		
Corneal abrasion (p. 436)	May not have history; patch; fluorescein positive	
DEFICIENCY		
Iron deficiency anemia (Chapter 26)	Pallor, learning deficit, anorexic, poor diet, microcytic, hypochromic anemia	Peaks at 9 and 18 mo of age; diet insufficient; elemental iron 5 mg/kg/24 hr q8hr PO
Malnutrition	Wasted, distended abdomen	May be caused by neglect or poverty
ENDOCRINE/METABOLIC		
Hyponatremia/hypernatremia (Chapter 8)	Dehydration, edema, seizures, intracranial bleeding	Multiple causes
Hypocalcemia	Tetany, seizure, diarrhea	Multiple causes
Hypercalcemia	Abdominal pain, polyuria, nephrocalcinosis, constipation, pancreatitis	Multiple causes
Hypoglycemia (Chapter 38)	Sweating, tachycardia, weakness, tachypnea, anxiety, tremor; cerebral dysfunction	Multiple causes; dextrose 0.5-1.0 gm/kg/dose IV
Diabetes insipidus	Polydipsia, thirst, constipation, dehydration, collapse	May be hyponatremic; urine specific gravity <1.006; inability to concentrate urine on fluid restriction
VASCULAR		
Congenital heart disease	Cyanosis, other cardiac findings	Usually cyanotic
Congestive heart failure (Chapter 16)	Tachypnea, tachycardia, rales, pulmonary edema	Cardiac and noncardiogenic
Paroxysmal atrial tachycardia (Chapter 6)	Heart rate >180, restless, variably cyanotic, variable congestive heart failure	Irritability if prolonged
MISCELLANEOUS		
Incarcerated hernia	Specific abdominal findings	Surgical consultation; may be more common cause than expected
Intussusception		
Diphtheria-pertussis-tetanus reaction	Immunization within 48 hr	Analgesia

the behavior should be defined. The response to being consoled, fed, and rocked should be noted. Factors such as loud noises, hunger, wet diapers, or search for attention may impact behavior. Potential contributing conditions, including trauma, medication, infection, congenital anomalies, and metabolic abnormalities, should be excluded. The parent-child interaction should be evaluated. Tooth eruption should be noted.

Attempts must be made to ensure the child's comfort while ensuring that there is no significant disorder and that the parents are dealing with the child's irritability with appropriate perspective. In addition to specific therapeutic interventions, support, empathy, and frequent follow-up observation are essential.

REFERENCES

Forsythe BWC: Colic and the effect of changing formula: a double-blind multiple crossover study, *J Pediatr* 115: 521, 1989.

Harkness MJ: Corneal abrasion in infancy as a cause of inconsolable crying, *Pediatr Emerg Care* 5:242, 1989.

Harley LM: Fussing and crying in young infants, *Clin Pediatr* 8:138, 1969.

Honig PJ: Teething: are today's pediatricians using yesterday's notions? *J Pediatr* 87:415, 1975.

Rautava P, Lehtonen L, Helenius H, et al: Infantile colic: child and family three years later, *Pediatrics* 96:43, 1995.

Zuckerman B, Stevenson J, Bailey V: Sleep problems in early childhood: continuities, predictive factors, and behavior correlates, *Pediatrics* 80:664, 1987.

40 LIMP

The child with a limp requires a systematic assessment of gait to determine the functional problem and cause. In children, it is often difficult to isolate the abnormality on clinical grounds alone because of the difficulty in eliciting specific signs and symptoms.*

ETIOLOGY

By age group, the following conditions are most commonly associated with limping (Table 40-1):

1-5 year	5-10 years
Toxic synovitis	Toxic synovitis
Occult fracture	Legg-Calvé-Perthes disease
Osteomyelitis	
Septic arthritis	**10-15 years**
Juvenile rheumatoid arthritis	Slipped capital femoral epiphysis
	Osgood-Schlatter disease
	Osteochondroses

Limping may be associated with *back pain* and the differential considerations should consider additional conditions, including trauma resulting in musculoskeletal soft tissue injury (most common), fractures, and osteomyelitis. The diagnosis of low back pain in the adolescent should also consider the following:

1. Lumbar strain
2. Spondylolysis
3. Spondylolisthesis
4. Disc syndrome

5. Spinal cord tumor
6. Discitis
7. Scheuermann disease
8. Ankylosing spondylitis

DIAGNOSTIC FINDINGS

The history is particularly important in helping localize the exact site of abnormality. The progression of signs and symptoms, precipitating factors, relationship to trauma, and infection and systemic disease are crucial in the initial evaluation. Previous medical problems, exposures, family history, and patient's age are helpful in considering diagnostic entities.

In physically evaluating the child, it is important to watch the child walk, focusing on the components of gait. First, the hips, knees, and ankles should be examined for pain, warmth, effusion, asymmetry, and limitation of motion and then the femur, tibia, fibula, and foot and ankle bones. Length of legs from the anterior iliac crest to the medial malleolus should be compared. Circumference should also be measured. A complete neurologic examination of the lower extremities (motor strength, sensory, reflexes) and examination of the abdomen, rectum, and genitalia are required. Hip pain is often referred to the knee.

If the results of the physical examination and history are inconclusive, complete blood count (CBC), erythrocyte sedimentation rate (ESR),

---

*See also Chapters 27, 66-70, and 82.

TABLE 40-1   Limp: Diagnostic Considerations

Condition	Diagnostic findings	Ancillary data	Comments/management
TRAUMA (Chapters 66-70)			
Sprain/contusion	History of trauma; local pain, tenderness, swelling, ecchymosis; variably unstable	X-ray study result negative	Support, restrict weight bearing
Fracture	Variable history of trauma: local pain, tenderness, swelling; may be occult	X-ray study result may be positive; if negative, do serial studies, looking for buckle fracture in the cortex of tibia, fibula, or femur; be certain x-ray study includes all potentially involved areas; technetium bone scan rarely needed	Orthopedic consultation; stress fracture may occur after repeated indirect trivial injuries; consider child abuse
Periostitis	Minor trauma to tibia, femur; local tenderness, fullness	X-ray study for subperiosteal hemorrhage (may be delayed)	Periosteum is loosely attached, with minor trauma; may have periosteal hemorrhage
Foreign body/splinter in foot	Acute onset pain, local tenderness, variable erythema	X-ray study rarely needed, but foreign body may localize if radiopaque	Remove; location will dictate need for consult
Poorly fitting shoe	Limp disappears when shoe is removed		
Vertebral disk injury	Motor defect—weakness, asymmetric reflexes; sensory defect	X-ray study may show injury	Orthopedic and neurosurgical consultation
INFECTION/INFLAMMATION			
Toxic synovitis of hip (Chapter 69)	Preceding viral illness, nontoxic; hip rarely warm, tender, or limited range of motion	CBC, ESR: WNL; x-ray study: variable effusion; aspirate if question of septic arthritis	Self-limited; common in 1½- to 7-yr-old children
Osteomyelitis (p. 753)	Fever, variable systemic toxicity; local swelling, tenderness, warmth; monoarticular, long bones (femur, tibia)	↑ CBC, ↑ ESR; x-ray study; technetium bone scan; joint and bone aspirate	May have arthritis and osteomyelitis concurrently; antibiotics
Arthritis, septic (p. 751)	Febrile, monoarticular, large weight-bearing (knee, hip) joints; local swelling, warmth, tenderness	↑ WBC, ↑ ESR; x-ray study; bone scan; joint aspirate	Requires urgent drainage and antibiotics

Continued

TABLE 40-1 Limp: Diagnostic Considerations—cont'd

Condition	Diagnostic findings	Ancillary data	Comments/management
INFECTION/INFLAMMATION—cont'd			
Arthritis, viral Rubella Rubella vaccine Hepatitis Chickenpox	Local swelling, warmth, tenderness; polyarticular, particularly large joints (knee); associated symptoms	CBC, viral titers, liver functions; x-ray study: effusion; joint aspirate	Usually self-limited
Arthritis, uncommon Mycobacterium Fungal	Insidious, commonly hip with progression; leg is flexed, well abducted	Joint aspirate; CBC; variable syphilis serologic findings; tuberculin skin test	
Appendicitis (p. 648)	RLQ pain, psoas/obturator sign, limited hip movement	↑ WBC, variable pyuria	Important to consider in differential as well as other abdominal problems
Polio (Chapter 41)	Systemic disease with asymmetric flaccid paralysis, bulbar involvement	CSF pleocytosis; ↑ WBC; positive viral culture finding	Decreased incidence
Guillain-Barré syndrome (Chapter 41)	Ascending symmetric paralysis with pain, paresthesias and paralysis; may involve cranial nerves; preceding viral illness	CSF: high protein	Danger of respiratory insufficiency; associated with viral infection; supportive care with IV gamma globulin (? plasma exchange)
VASCULAR			
Legg-Calvé-Perthes disease (Chapter 69)	Insidious onset pain of hip with limp or limitation of motion	X-ray study: bulging capsule with widened joint space; technetium scan: ↓ uptake	Peak: 4:1 males, 4-10 yr; orthopedic consultation—treat hip in abduction and internal rotation
Discitis	Gait problem (<3 yr); local back, abdominal pain with limp (>3 yr); irritable, no systemic illness	X-ray study result normal for 4-8 wk; disc space may narrow by 3-4 wk; result of technetium scan abnormal after 7 days	Vascular disruption of epiphyseal end-plate of vertebrae; prognosis good; treatment: support, antibiotics controversial
DEGENERATIVE			
Slipped capital femoral epiphysis (Chapter 69)	Unilateral or bilateral pain in knee (referred) or in medial aspect of thigh; hip or knee made worse by activity; limitation of abduction and internal rotation	X-ray study: widening epiphyseal growth plate	Peak: 12-15 yr; orthopedic consultation; surgical immobilization; child obese or tall and thin, with rapid growth spurt
Osgood-Schlatter disease (Chapter 69)	Pain in knee caused by patellar tendonitis at insertion into tibial tubercle	X-ray study result: fragmentation of tibial tuberosity	Peak: 11-15 yr; symptomatic treatment, rest, avoid activities that cause pain

Osteochondroses

	Associated signs and symptoms	Laboratory/X-ray	Comments/treatment
Chondomalacia patellae	Irregularity of patella, pain on compression of patellar at inter-condylar notch with contraction of quadriceps	X-ray study result: WNL	Teenagers, female > males; symptomatic; treatment: quadriceps strengthening
Osteochondritis dissecans	Pain, stiffness, swelling, clicking of knee	X-ray study result: tunnel view shows demineralization of medial femoral condyle	Teenagers; decreased activity, muscle strengthening
Neuromuscular disease	Associated motor and sensory findings		Often progressive
CONGENITAL			
Hemophilia (p. 685)	Variable history of trauma; muscle bleeding; monoarticular joint swollen, tender with hemarthrosis	X-ray study result: variable bleeding screen	Factor replacement
Sickle cell disease (p. 698)	Systemic disease; bone pain; polyarticular joint involvement	X-ray study result; Hct; positive sickle preparation; variable technetium bone scan	May have concurrent infection; may be crisis or infarct
Dislocated hip	Normal newborn except for instability and range of motion of joint; positive hip click (abduction)	X-ray study	Orthopedic consult, splint hip in flexion and abduction
Unequal leg length	Unequal length from anterior iliac crest to medial malleolus		Orthopedic consultation
Testicular torsion (p. 663) Incarcerated hernia (p. 652)	Acute onset of scrotal or groin pain; mass, tender swollen		Surgical emergency
AUTOIMMUNE (Table 27-1)			
NEOPLASM			
Osteochondroma Leukemia Neuroblastoma Ewing Spinal cord tumor	Local pain with exostosis Systemic disease with associated symptoms		
INTRAPSYCHIC			
Attention getting	Inconsistent signs and symptoms		May be functional habit after resolution of physical problem, particularly in children under 5 yr

RLQ, Right lower quadrant.

and blood cultures may be useful in evaluating a potential infectious cause. X-ray studies for infection, trauma, neoplasm, congenital abnormalities, and degenerative problems are often diagnostic. A technetium bone scan may be obtained for further clarification. When infectious arthritis or osteomyelitis is suspected, an aspirate may be useful, with appropriate stains and cultures (pp. 751 and 753). If the initial evaluation is unrevealing, serial examinations with close follow-up may be required because an occult or stress fracture, osteomyelitis, infectious arthritis, or other condition may be delayed in developing objective signs and symptoms.

REFERENCES

Blatt SD, Rosenthal BM, Barnhart DC: Diagnostic utility of lower extremity radiographs of young children with gait disturbances, *Pediatrics* 87:138, 1991.

Hensinger RN: Limp, *Pediatr Clin North Am* 33:1355, 1986.

Illingworth CM: 128 limping children with no fracture, sprain or obvious cause, *Clin Pediatr* 17:139, 1978.

McCarthy PL, Wasserman D, Spiesel SZ, et al: Evaluation of arthritis and arthralgia in the pediatric patient, *Clin Pediatr* 19:183, 1980.

Olson TL, et al: The epidemiology of low back pain in an adolescent population, *Am J Public Health* 82:606, 1992.

Sills EM: What's causing the back pain? *Contemp Pediatr* 5:85, 1988.

41 PARALYSIS AND HEMIPLEGIA

ALERT: After assessment of respiratory and circulatory status, the diagnostic evaluation must quickly establish the underlying process to provide guidelines for support and therapy.

The acute onset of paralysis in children may be indicated by a youngster not wanting to walk. Infectious and inflammatory causes are most common (Table 41-1). In addition, spinal cord or central nervous system (CNS) injury resulting from trauma can cause transient or permanent deficits. Heavy metal intoxications can induce paralysis. Hysterical conversion reactions may mimic paralysis, but usually the examination is inconsistent.

CNS lesions generally are accompanied by a flaccid paralysis and loss of tone and deep tendon reflexes (DTRs). After about a week, the patient may become spastic with hyperactive reflexes. The evaluation should include a careful neurologic examination, as well as a check for associated symptoms. Spinal fluid should normally be examined.

The major complications encountered by these patients is respiratory failure (rarely requiring ventilatory support) and secondary bacterial infections. Treatment is generally supportive.

Rarely, patients have *acute hemiplegia,* secondary to emboli, thromboses, or intracerebral hemorrhage. Emboli produce a rapidly evolving clinical picture, but thromboses often evolve over hours to days. Predisposing factors include the following:

1. Infection
   a. Viral: herpes or coxsackievirus encephalitis
   b. Bacterial meningitis
2. Vascular—embolic
   a. Congenital heart disease
   b. Endocarditis
   c. Dysrhythmias: atrial fibrillation
   d. Arteriovenous malformations
   e. Acute infantile hemiplegia: seizure followed by coma, hemiplegia, and fever caused by occlusion of the middle cerebral artery
3. Vascular
   a. Hemiplegic migraine
   b. Vasculitis
4. Trauma
   a. Blunt trauma to the neck (or intraoral trauma): may produce delayed onset of symptoms in 24 to 48 hours
   b. Penetrating trauma: may produce immediate loss or vascular foreign body emboli
5. Congenital
   a. Sickle cell disease (thrombosis, spasm)
   b. Hemophilia (hemorrhage)
6. Todd paralysis: transient paralysis after seizures that resolve without therapy

Fig. 41-1 on p. 283 provides a summary of the anatomic and functional correlations in upper and lower motor neuron disease; Table 41-2 helps differentiate the site of injury. Treatment must focus on the underlying disorder as well as complicating conditions.

Bell's palsy is a seventh cranial nerve

TABLE 41-1   Paralysis: Diagnostic Considerations

	Guillain-Barré syndrome	Secondary polyneuropathy	Poliomyelitis	Tick-bite paralysis	Transverse myelitis/ neuromyelitis optica
Etiology	Unknown; role of viral, mycoplasm infections unknown	Infectious or inflammatory: viral, bacterial (diphtheria, botulism), immunizations; autoimmune; intoxication	Poliovirus	Toxin release by tick	Unknown but may be inflammatory and related to multiple sclerosis
Prodrome	Nonspecific respiratory or gastrointestinal symptoms 5-14 days before onset	Low-grade fever and other signs and symptoms reflecting the underlying disease	Fever, respiratory or gastrointestinal symptoms; may have meningism	1 wk after tick bites and remains attached; fatigue, irritability	
Neurologic findings	Symmetric flaccid ascending paralysis; greater involvement of lower extremities, greater proximally; facial diplegia, cranial nerve, bulbar involved; muscle tenderness; sensory-distal hyperesthesia with impaired position, vibration	Variable involvement; flaccid paralysis with loss of DTR and position and vibration senses; ataxia; cranial nerve involvement with dysphagia; generalized weakness	Flaccid, asymmetric paralysis with maximum deficit 3-5 days after onset; lower extremities more involved than upper; bulbar involvement may occur very early; sensory examination normal; marked muscle tenderness, pain, fasciculations, and twitching	Rapid progression of muscle pain with ascending flaccid symmetric paralysis; pain and paresthesias	Rapid progression; may have ataxia, weakness, multiple neurologic deficits; optic neuritis; paralysis develops with sensory loss below lesion and hyperesthesia above; bowel and bladder problems
Ancillary data	CSF: few WBC, high protein after 10 days	CSF: few monocytes with high protein; tests to determine underlying disease; nerve conduction velocity	CSF: pleocytosis (initially PMN, then monocytes), elevated protein level	CSF: normal	CSF: (not done routinely) pleocytosis, increased protein level; myelogram if indicated
Comments	Peaks in 5- to 9-yr-old children; usual recovery in 1-3 wk; supportive care and IV gamma globulin*	Major systemic illness reflects nature of underlying disease	May be asymptomatic or nonparalytic; summer epidemic; unimmunized individuals	Tick usually attached to head or neck; rapid improvement with removal of tick (Table 45-1)	Steroids (ACTH) may be useful in treatment

*Gamma globulin, 400 mg/kg/24 hr q24hr IV.

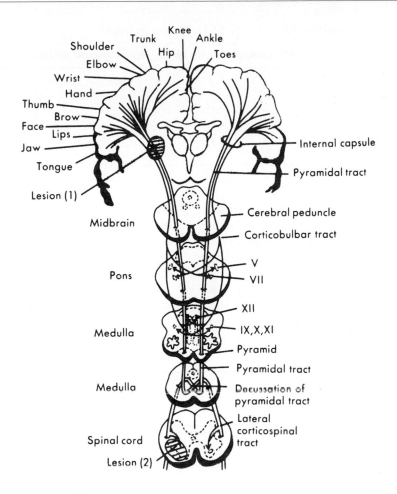

Lesion (1)

**Upper motor neuron
lesion**

Contralateral hemiparesis
Postural flexion of arm,
 extension of leg
Muscles hypertonic
Tendon reflexes hyperactive
Atrophy not prominent
No muscle fasciculations
Pathologic reflexes present

Lesion (2)

**Lower motor neuron
lesion**

Paresis limited to specific muscle groups
Gait depends on muscles
 affected; flail-like
 movements common
Muscles flaccid
Tendon reflexes absent
 or hypoactive
Atrophy prominent
Muscle fasciculations present
Contractures and skeletal
 deformities may develop

Fig. 41-1   The pyramidal system.

(From Gilman S, Newman SW, editors: *Essentials of clinical neuroanatomy and neurophysiology,* Philadelphia, 1987, FA Davis.)

TABLE 41-2   Differentiating Findings Noted by Level of Injury

	Motor neuron	Muscle	Neuromuscular junction	Nerve
Reflexes	−	−	−	−
Muscle bulk	↓	↓	↓	↓
Fasciculations	+	+	−	−
Tone	↓	↓	↓	↓
Strength	↓	↓	↓	↓
Sensation	WNL	↓	Variable	↓

−, Absent; +, present; ↓, decreased.

paralysis of sudden onset and unknown cause. The patient has a flattened nasolabial fold on the affected side and is unable to close the eyelids, pucker the lips, or wrinkle the brow. Recovery usually occurs over 3 to 6 weeks. Therapy should include protection of the cornea with artificial tears. Steroids may be useful if initiated within 2 days of onset of symptoms. Prednisone, 1 mg/kg/24 hr PO, can be initiated and tapered over 7 to 10 days.

REFERENCES

Birse GS, Strauss RW: Acute childhood hemiplegia, *Ann Emerg Med* 14:74, 1985.

Freeman JM: Diagnosis and evaluation of acute paraplegia, *Pediatr Rev* 4:327, 1983.

Gold AP, Carter S: Acute hemiplegia of infancy and childhood, *Pediatr Clin North Am* 23:413, 1976.

Van der Meché FGA, Schmitz PIM, Dutch Guillain-Barré Study Group: A randomized trial comparing intravenous immune globulin and plasma exchange in Guillain-Barré syndrome, *N Engl J Med* 326:1123, 1992.

42 RASH

Although rash is a common presenting complaint, the term requires careful definition.* The identification of a rash disease requires examination of the lesions, focusing on whether there are blisters, or if solid, whether the lesions are red or scaling (Table 42-1). It is important to define the configuration and distribution of findings and relate the chronology of the evolution with the development of systemic signs and symptoms.

Most urgent encounters related to rashes have an infectious origin. Tables 42-2, 42-3, and 42-4 divide the common exanthems into categories based on structure: maculopapular, vesicular, and petechial or purpuric.

The condition must be treated as an emergency if the lesions are purple or look like blood (purpura); do not blanch (petechiae); are

*See also Chapter 72.

TABLE 42-1   Rash: Evaluation

Appearance	Diagnostic considerations
BLISTER (FLUID-FILLED)	
Clear	*Vesicular* (Tables 42-2 and 42-4): herpes simplex, varicella-zoster, scabies
	Bullous: bullous impetigo, erythema multiforme, burn, contact dermatitis, friction blister
Pustular	Acne, folliculitis (bacterial, fungal), candidiasis, bacteremia (gonococcemia, meningococcemia)
SOLID (NONRED)	
Skin-colored	*Keratotic* (rough-surfaced lesion): wart, corn, callus
	Nonkeratotic (smooth lesion): wart, molluscum contagiosum, epidermoid (sebaceous) cyst, basal and squamous cell carcinoma, nevi
White	Pityriasis alba, vitiligo, pityriasis versicolor, postinflammatory hypopigmentation, milia, molluscum contagiosum
Brown	Café-au-lait patch, nevi, freckle, melanoma, hypopigmentation secondary to systemic disease, medication, or postinflammatory condition
Yellow	Jaundice, nevi sebaceous

Modified from Lynch PJ, Edminister SC: *Ann Emerg Med* 13:603, 1984; and Weston WL: *Primary Care* 11:469, 1984.

Continued

TABLE 42-1　Rash: Evaluation—cont'd

Appearance	Diagnostic considerations
SOLID (RED, NONSCALING)	
Inflammatory papule/nodule	*Papule (maculopapular):* (Tables 42-2 and 42-3): viral exanthem, erythema multiforme, insect bite, scarlet fever, angioma *Nodule:* furuncle, erythema nodosum
Vascular (flat-topped)	*Nonpurpuric:* toxic erythema (viral exanthem, medication, photosensitivity), urticaria (infection, medication), erythema multiforme, cellulitis (erysipelas) *Purpuric* (Table 42-2): vasculitis, petechiae, ecchymosis
SOLID (RED, SCALING)	
Papulosquamous disease	No epithelial disruption: pityrisis rosea, tinea corporis, capitus, pedis or cruris, lupus erythematosus, syphilis
Eczematous disease	Epithelial disruption: atopic (eczema); seborrheic, diaper, contact, or stasis dermatitis, tinea cruris, capitus or pedis, nummular eczema, impetigo, candidiasis

burnlike (scalded skin); are red, blue, or tender to the touch (cellulitis); have red streaking; or are pustular. Lesions that are pruritic, have associated fever more than 24 hours, may be related to a medication, or are pustular with a red or cola-colored urine should also be seen.

Chapter 72 provides a more detailed summary of the common dermatologic problems that require evaluation and treatment.

REFERENCES

American Academy of Pediatrics Committee on Infectious Diseases: Use of oral acyclovir in otherwise healthy children with varicella, *Pediatrics* 91:674, 1993.

American Academy of Pediatrics: *Report of the committee on infectious diseases*, Elk Grove Village, Ill, 1997, American Academy of Pediatrics.

Balfour HF, Rotbart HA, Feldman S, et al: Acyclovir treatment of varicella in otherwise healthy adolescents, *J Pediatr* 120:627, 1992.

Doctor A, Harper MB, Fleischer AR: Group A beta-hemolytic streptococcal bacteremia. historical overview, changing incidence, and recent association with varicella, *Pediatrics* 96:428, 1995.

Kraemer MJ, Smith AC: Rashes with ampicillin, *Pediatr Rev* 1:97, 1980.

Tyring S, Barbarash RA, Nahlik JE: Famciclovir for the treatment of acute herpes zoster: effects on acute disease and post herpetic neuroglia, *Ann Intern Med* 123:89, 1995.

Ware R: Human parvovirus infection, *J Pediatr* 114:343, 1989.

Weston WL: *Practical pediatric dermatology,* ed 2, Boston, 1985, Little, Brown.

Yoshiyama H, Suzuki E, Yoshida T, et al: Role of human herpesvirus 6 infection in infants with exanthema subitum, *Pediatr Infect Dis* 9:71, 1990.

TABLE 42-2   Acute Exanthems

	Maculopapular	Vesicular	Petechial or purpuric
Infection	Viral	Viral	Viral
	Measles ⎤	Chickenpox (Table 42-4)	Enterovirus
	Rubella ⎬ Table 42-3	Herpes zoster (Table 42-4)	Hemorrhagic measles
	Roseola ⎦	Herpes simplex	Rubeola (atypical)
	Enterovirus	Enterovirus (Table 42-2)	Chickenpox
	Infectious mononucleosis	Hand, foot, and mouth	
	(p. 714)	Herpangina	
	Pityriasis rosea (p. 584)	Molluscum contagiosum	
		(p. 589)	
		Historical: smallpox	
	Other	Other	Other
	Scarlet fever (Table 42-3)	Impetigo (p. 581)	Meningococcemia (p. 713)
	Staphylococcal scalded	Rickettsialpox	*Haemophilus influenzae*
	skin (p. 586)	Candidiasis	Pneumococcemia
	Toxic shock syndrome	Staphylcoccal scalded skin	Rocky Mountain spotted
	(p. 721)	syndrome (p. 586)	fever
	Kawasaki syndrome	Erythema multiforme	Sepsis (with thrombocyto-
	(p. 710)	(p. 580)	penia or DIC)
	Meningococcemia (p. 713)		Gonococcemia (p. 673)
	Mycoplasma pneumoniae		Endocarditis (p. 559)
	Tick diseases (Table 45-1)		Plague
	Rocky Mountain spotted		
	fever		
	Typhus		
Intoxication	Ampicillin		
	Penicillin		
	Barbiturates		
	Anticonvulsants		
	Sulfonamides		
Other	Sunburn (p. 587)	Insect bites (p. 306)	Henoch-Schönlein purpura
	Juvenile rheumatoid arthritis		(p. 805)
	Serum sickness		Idiopathic thrombocytopenic
			purpura (p. 694)
			Coagulation disorder
			Trauma
			Tourniquet (distal)
			Coughing (head and neck)
			Leukemia
			Aplastic anemia

TABLE 42-3   Common Maculopapular Exanthems

	Measles (rubeola)	Rubella (German, 3-day measles)	Roseola (exanthema subitum)
Incubation	10-14 days	14-21 days	10-14 days
Prodrome	3 days high fever, cough, conjunctivitis, and coryza; child appears toxic, lethargic	May be none; lymphadenopathy (especially postauricular, suboccipital), malaise, variable low-grade fever	3-4 days high fever in otherwise well child, preceding rash
Exanthem	Reddish-brown; begins on face and progresses downward; generalized by third day; confluent on face, neck, upper trunk; lasts 7-10 days; desquamates; atypical measles: maculopapular, purpuric, petechial, or vesicular rash	Pink; begins on face and progresses rapidly downward; generalized by second day; discrete; lasts 2-3 days; fades in order of appearance	Appears after defervescence; rose, discrete; initially on chest, spreads to involve face and extremities; fades quickly
Enanthem	Koplik spots (2 days before rash, on buccal mucosa opposite molars)	None	None
Complications	Pneumonia Encephalitis Otitis media Thrombocytopenia Hemorrhagic measles Pneumothorax Hepatitis Exacerbation of TB	Arthritis (common in women) beginning after 2-3 days illness; knee, wrist, finger Congenital rubella syndrome Encephalitis Thrombocytopenia	Febrile seizures Meningoencephalitis Pseudotumor cerebri
Management	Supportive; may require hospitalization; active immunization of contacts within 72 hr of exposure; immune serum globulin (0.25 ml/kg) for children <1 yr and pregnant women within 6 hr of exposure; reportable	Supportive; isolate from pregnant women; active immunization of contacts; reportable	Supportive; good fever control
Comments	Rare with immunization	Rare with immunization; serologic diagnosis	Usually 1- to 4-yr-old children Probably caused by human herpesvirus-6 (HHV-6)

Fifth disease (erythema infectiosum)	Enterovirus	Scarlet fever
7-14 days None	Variable (short) Variable; fever, malaise, vomiting, sore throat, rhinorrhea	2-4 days 1-2 days fever, vomiting, sore throat; often toxic
Erupts in 3 stages: (1) red-flushed cheeks with circumoral pallor (slapped cheek), (2) maculopapular eruption on extremities (lacelike), (3) may recur secondary to heat, sunlight, trauma	Maculopapular, discrete, nonpruritic, generalized; rubella like; hand, foot, and mouth distribution	Erythematous, punctate, sandpaper texture; appears first in flexion areas, then generalized; most intense on neck, axilla, inguinal, popliteal skin fold; circumoral pallor; lasts 7 days, then desquamates
Variable	Variable	Red pharynx, tonsils; palatal petechiae; strawberry tongue
Transient arthritis	Aseptic meningitis Myocarditis Hepatitis	Rheumatic fever Acute glomerulonephritis
Rarely needs care	Supportive	Penicillin
Caused by human parvovirus B19 associated with hypoplastic anemia, arthropathy, myocarditis, vasculitis, multiple organ failure; may be role for IVIG	Concurrent family illness, gastroenteritis, herpangina	Group A streptococci (p. 604)

TABLE 42-4   Vesicular Exanthems

	Varicella (chickenpox)	Herpes zoster (shingles)	Herpes simplex
Diagnostic findings	Rapid progression of erythematous macules, developing into papules and vesicles; vesicles are thin-walled and superficial, surrounded by an erythematous area; pruritic; distribution is central with relative sparing distally; marked variability in severity of exanthem—may only have a few lesions; usually febrile; enanthem—shallow mucosal ulcers; different ages of lesions; may initially resemble insect bites	Erythema followed by red papules that become vesicular in 12-24 hr, pustular in 72 hr, and crusts in 10-12 days; distribution is unilateral after peripheral dermatome or cranial nerve; preeruptive pain with hyperesthesia over involved skin	Multiple presentations **Gingivostomatitis:** fever, irritability, pain in mouth, throat, and with swallowing; shallow ulcers on mucosa (buccal, tonsillar, and pharyngeal); crusts on lips; cervical lymphoadenopathy; lasts 1-14 days **Vulvovaginitis:** similar shallow ulcers on vagina and vulva; pain on urination **Keratoconjunctivitis:** corneal ulceration
Complications	Pneumonia Secondary bacterial infections: cellulitis, bacterial pneumonia, especially group A streptococcus Encephalitis, myelitis Hepatitis Reye syndrome	Ophthalmic: neuralgia, corneal dendrites, iritis Postherpetic neuralgia and death	Ophthalmic: corneal ulceration Encephalitis Neonatal viremia with encephalitis
Management	Antipruritic agents Topical: calamine lotion; cold baths with small amount of baking soda (⅓ tsp) in water Systemic: diphenhydramine Antipyretics—*Do not use aspirin* Treatment of complications Acyclovir, 80 mg/kg/24 hr (maximum: 3200 mg/24 hr) PO QID for 5 days; begin within 24 hr of rash in high-risk patients* Zoster-immune globulin (VZIG) for exposure in high-risk patient; 125 units/10 kg (maximum: 625 units)	Support, analgesia Eye involvement needs ophthalmology consultation Famciclovir, 500-750 mg/dose TID for 7 days; decreases duration, accelerates lesion healing, and decreases duration of viral shedding Acyclovir may have a role in specific circumstances Steroids or amitriptyline may reduce postherpetic neuralgia	General support Gingival: topical analgesia—antacid or mixture of viscous lidocaine (Xylocaine), diphenhydramine, Kaopectate; acyclovir (Zovirax): topical IV, PO for initial and recurrent lesions
Comment	Incubation: 14-21 days Vaccine Particularly dangerous in newborns, pregnant females, immunosuppressed or immunodeficient individuals	Common history of chickenpox	Sexual spread of vulvovaginitis Potentially life threatening to newborn, immunodeficient, or immunosuppressed; consider systemic acyclovir IV probably indicated. (p. 675)

*Nonpregnant patients ≥13 yr, children >12 mo with chronic cutaneous or pulmonary disorder, and children receiving long-term salicylate therapy. Children receiving short, intermittent, or aerosoled corticosteroids are probably not immunocompromised, and the risk is unknown. If taking high-dose corticosteroids, acyclovir IV probably indicated.

43 VAGINAL BLEEDING

ALERT: Third-trimester bleeding requires immediate obstetric consultation. Dysfunctional uterine bleeding is most common in pubescent females, but ectopic pregnancy should be excluded; in younger girls the cause is commonly trauma or foreign bodies. Hypotension may develop.

Vaginal bleeding is most commonly related to menstruation in the pubescent female. The most common problem associated with vaginal bleeding is dysfunctional uterine bleeding because of anovulatory cycles in which the bleeding is scanty, watery, and irregular. Most young girls begin their cycles with anovulatory ones, and it may be several years before ovulation

TABLE 43-1   Vaginal Bleeding: Diagnostic Considerations*

Condition	Signs and symptoms	Evaluation/comments
ENDOCRINE		
Uterine dysfunction (p. 667)	Irregular menses, flow too frequent, heavy, or prolonged	Diagnosis of exclusion; anovulatory cycle
Pregnancy complications (p. 676)		
Abortion	First trimester; cervix variably dilated; various products of conception	Treatment depends on type of abortion
Placenta previa	Third trimester; painless; may have profuse bleeding	Ultrasound; avoid pelvic examination in ED; double setup; fetal monitor
Abruptio placentae	Third trimester; abdominal pain; tender uterus; bleeding may be concealed	Ultrasound; avoid pelvic examination in ED; double setup; fetal monitor; common in blunt trauma
Ectopic pregnancy	Missed menses, pelvic pain, rebound, adnexal mass; low Hct, hypotension	Culdocentesis or ultrasound; rapid pregnancy test; potentially life threatening
Following delivery	Bleeding without pain	Pharmacologic curettage (rarely mechanical); consider endometriosis
Thyroid disease (p. 622)	Associated signs and symptoms	Thyroid functions
Physiologic	Newborn may have bleeding at 5-10 days	Caused by withdrawal from maternal estrogens

*See also Chapter 78.

Continued

291

TABLE 43-1   Vaginal Bleeding: Diagnostic Considerations—cont'd

Condition	Signs and symptoms	Evaluation/comments
TRAUMA		
Foreign body	Foul-smelling discharge	Peak is 5-9 yr (may occur at any age); forgotten tampon common in adolescent; also IUD
Laceration	Signs of trauma	Secondary trauma, intercourse, heavy exercise, molestation
INFLAMMATION		
Vulvovaginitis (p. 671)	Characteristic discharge and inflamed introitus	Culture, wet and KOH preparation of discharge
Pelvic inflammatory disease (p. 669)	Abdominal, pelvic tenderness, fever, chills, nausea, vomiting	Elevated CBC and ESR, culture and Gram stain
INTOXICATION		
Birth control pills	Irregular intake or acute overdose	Adjust or control dosage
Anticoagulants	Bleeding sites elsewhere	Coagulation studies
DEFICIENCY		
Bleeding diathesis	Bleeding sites elsewhere	Coagulation studies
Idiopathic thrombocytopenic purpura (p. 694)	Bleeding elsewhere	Platelet count and coagulation studies
NEOPLASM		
Tumors, polyps, fibroid tumors	Physical examination reveals mass, spotty bleeding	Unusual; may occur in children with DES exposure; Pap smear

occurs. Other etiologies, including complications of pregnancy, trauma, vulvovaginitis, and pelvic inflammatory disease, must be considered (Table 43-1).

After assuring that there is no vascular instability, a thorough pelvic examination must be performed, including an evaluation of both the internal and external genitalia (p. 666). Appropriate cultures (*Neisseria gonorrhoeae* and *Chlamydia trachomatis*) and microscopic examination (potassium hydroxide and saline solution) are usually indicated if the bleeding is not caused by obvious trauma. If there is any question of potential pregnancy (and often even if there is no question), a serum pregnancy test should be performed. Ultrasound examination

may confirm an intrauterine pregnancy and identify pelvic abnormality. A hematocrit is usually indicated in the assessment if bleeding is significant. A bleeding screen may be helpful.

Pregnant women with third-trimester bleeding should be examined in the operating room, with preparations for a double setup whereby the baby can be delivered vaginally or by cesarean section. As appropriate, cultures of the cervical os and rectum (and pharynx), analysis of discharges, and a Papanicolaou smear should be done.

The prepubescent girl commonly has bleeding caused by foreign bodies or hymenal trauma. Vulvovaginitis may produce a bloody discharge. Tumors are uncommon unless the patient had an intrauterine exposure to diethylstilbestrol (DES). Vaginal bleeding may accompany endocrine and hematologic disorders.

REFERENCES

American College of Emergency Physicians, Clinical Policy Committee: Clinical policy in the initial approach to patients presenting with a chief complaint of vaginal bleeding, *Ann Emerg Med* 29:435, 1997.

Anderson M, Lewin CE, Sayder DL: Abnormal vaginal bleeding in adolescents, *Pediatr Ann* 15:696, 1986.

Baldwin DD, Landa HM: Common problems in pediatrics and gynecology, *Urol Clin North Am* 22:161, 1995.

Emans SJH, Goldstein DP: *Pediatric and adolescent gynecology,* ed 3, Boston, 1990, Little, Brown.

Litt I: Menstrual problems during adolescence, *Pediatr Rev* 7:203, 1983.

44 VOMITING

ALERT: Assessment initially must determine the child's hydration status and initiate stabilization. Cause must be determined.

Vomiting is the forceful ejection of the stomach contents into the esophagus and through the mouth. It may be caused by irritation of the peritoneum or mesentery, obstruction of the intestine, action of a toxin on the medulla, or primary central nervous system (CNS) disorder.*

ETIOLOGY

In children the most common cause of vomiting is acute gastroenteritis, as well as other infections, including otitis media, urinary tract infections, and meningitis. Infants often vomit as a result of faulty feeding techniques or chalasia. Other conditions that must be considered include congenital obstructions of the gastrointestinal tract, particularly pyloric stenosis; CNS lesions producing increased intracranial pressure; and a variety of endocrine, metabolic, and toxic problems. Newborns often have congenital obstructions.

Intestinal obstruction in the neonate should be suspected if there is more than 20 ml of fluid in the gastric aspirate (especially bile stained), he or she vomits and has abdominal distension in the first 24 to 36 hours of life, or meconium is not passed in the first 48 hours of life (Tables 44-1 and 44-2).

---

*See also Acute gastroenteritis, p. 631, and Chapter 32.

DIAGNOSTIC FINDINGS

The history must determine precipitating factors, including trauma, recent illness, medications, poor feeding techniques, and instability in the environment leading to emotional upheaval. Associated symptoms and family history are important. The nature of the vomiting must be determined: its color, composition, relationship to eating and position, onset, progression, and whether it was projectile. The expelled material should be examined.

1. Undigested food suggests an esophageal lesion at or above the cardia.
2. Nonbilious vomitus may result from lesions proximal to the pylorus.
3. Bile-containing material involves obstruction beyond the ampulla of Vater, or it may result from an adynamic ileus found in sepsis, significant other infections, or serious underlying disease. Bile turns green on exposure to air.
4. A fecal odor is consistent with peritonitis or a lower obstruction.
5. A bloody vomitus usually involves a lesion proximal to the ligament of Treitz. If it is bright red, there has been little contact with gastric juices and the site is at or above the cardia. Coffee-ground vomitus results from alteration by gastric juices.

The physical examination should include inspection of the abdomen for trauma, distension,

TABLE 44-1 Vomiting: Diagnostic Considerations

Condition	Diagnostic findings	Evaluation	Comments/management
INFECTION/INFLAMMATION			
Acute gastroenteritis (p. 631)	Acute onset with nausea, fever, diarrhea, and evidence of systemic illness	Fluid status, stool culture if needed	NPO, if indicated; clear liquids, advance slowly
Posttussive/posterior nasal drip	Follows vigorous coughing; may be greatest at night when recumbent; associated cough, rhinorrhea	Chest x-ray study if needed	Therapeutic trial: cough suppressant or decongestant
Otitis media (p. 596)	Fever, irritability, painful ear		Antibiotics; topical therapy for extreme pain
Esophagitis/gastritis (Chapter 35)	Variably coffee ground, bloody; epigastric or substernal pain, discomfort; reflux	Endoscopy; upper GI series	Associated reflux, hiatal hernia; drugs; trial of antacids
Ulcer, peptic/duodenal (Chapter 35)	Usually coffee ground; epigastric, abdominal pain; may be chronic or acute; possible anemia	Endoscopy; upper GI series	
Hepatitis (p. 639)	Associated liver tenderness; icterus	Liver function tests	May be life threatening
Peritonitis	Generalized or localized tenderness, guarding, rebound	WBC, x-ray studies UA	Usually infectious; viral, EB virus
Appendicitis (p. 648)			Surgical exploration usually needed
Cholecystitis			
Pancreatitis			
Cystitis	Associated fever, dysuria, frequency, burning, variable CVA tenderness	UA, urine culture	Initiate antibiotics pending culture results
Pyelonephritis (p. 815)			
Meningitis (p. 725)	Fever, systemic toxicity; changed mental status; local neurologic signs, variable signs of increased intracerebral pressure	Lumbar puncture; CT scan if needed	Antibiotics; neurosurgical consultation if indicated
CNS abscess			
Subdural effusion/empyema			
CONGENITAL			
Pyloric stenosis (p. 658)	Regurgitation progressing to projectile vomiting; palpable olive-sized tumor in RUQ; vigorous gastric peristalsis present; variable dehydration, poor weight gain	Upper GI series—delayed gastric emptying, narrow pyloric channel ("string sign"), ultrasound may substitute; electrolytes to assess hydration	Usually male, 4-6 wk of age; treat fluid deficits, then surgery (pyloromyotomy)

L/RUQ, Left/right upper quadrant; *UA,* urinalysis.

Continued

TABLE 44-1 Vomiting: Diagnostic Considerations—cont'd

Condition	Diagnostic findings	Evaluation	Comments/management
GI obstruction (Chapter 11) Intestinal obstruction/stenosis/bands Imperforate anus Malrotation Meconium ileus/plug Volvulus, sigmoid/midgut (p. 659) Intussusception	Obstructive pattern beginning in newborn period, >20 ml in gastric aspirate; if proximal to ampulla of Vater; distension epigastrium or LUQ and gastric peristaltic wave; if distal to ampulla of Vater, vomitus contains bile, generalized distension	Abdominal x-ray study with contrast studies if needed; electrolytes to assess fluid status	Immediate decompression; correction of fluid deficits; surgical consultation Associated with cystic fibrosis Life threatening
Hydrocephalus	Excessive growth of head circumference; irritability, lethargy, headache, budging of fontanelle	CT scan	Life threatening May involve blockage of ventricular shunt; neurosurgical consultation; urgent care
TRAUMA			
Concussion (Chapter 57)	Trauma; headache, minimally changed mental status; often projectile vomiting	Skull x-ray study, CT scan	Support; monitoring
Subdural hematoma (Chapter 57)	Marked change in mental status, signs of increased intracranial pressure: headache, ataxia, sixth-nerve palsy, seizures; focal neurologic signs	CT scan	Immediate neurosurgical consultation; support: intubate, hyperventilate, diuretics, etc.
Foreign body (p. 637)	History: may have dysphagia or total obstruction; may have respiratory distress	X-ray study; esophagoscopy	If esophagus, attempt to remove by use of Foley catheter under fluoroscopy; if elsewhere, endoscopy or surgery, depending on foreign body
Intramural duodenal hematoma (Chapter 63)	Following even minimal blunt trauma: nausea, bilious vomiting, pain, tenderness, ileus; may have abdominal mass	Upper GI series	May be delay in symptom presentation
Ruptured viscus (Chapter 63)	Trauma followed by abdominal tenderness, rebound, guarding	Peritoneal lavage; x-ray study for free air	Immediate surgical intervention; fluids, antibiotics
Subarachnoid hemorrhage (Chapter 18)	Headache, stiff neck, progressive loss of consciousness; focal neurologic signs	CT scan; bloody spinal fluid	Neurosurgical consultation; supportive care
Cerebral edema	Signs of increased intracranial pressure: headache, ataxia, sixth-nerve palsy; altered mental status	CT scan	Diuretics, steroids, hyperventilation, elevation

INTOXICATION (Chapter 54)

Cause	Clinical features	Evaluation	Treatment/Comments
Alkali burns	Associated mouth burns, difficulty swallowing	Endoscopy	Lye, bleaches most common; surgery consultation
Salicylates	Nausea, vomiting, tinnitus	Salicylate level	Stop medication; antacids, fluids
Iron	Hematemesis, shock, acidosis	Iron level, ABG, CBC	Urgent treatment with deferoxamine
Lead	Usually chronic exposure; signs of increased intracranial pressure	Lead level	Dimercaprol, EDTA
Digitalis	Underlying heart disease; nausea, dysrhythmias	Digitalis level; ECG	Stop digitalis; institute active treatment of dysrhythmia, etc.

VASCULAR

Cause	Clinical features	Evaluation	Treatment/Comments
Migraine (p. 734)	Unilateral, throbbing headache, aura; family history	Evaulation to exclude other etiology	Consider therapeutic trial of ergotamine; analgesia, steroids
Hypertensive encephalopathy (Chapter 18)	Rapid increase in BP; changed mental status; headache, nausea, anorexia	Evaluation of underlying disease	Rapid response when diastolic BP brought below 100 mm Hg

ENDOCRINE/METABOLIC

Acidosis (Chapter 8)

Cause	Clinical features	Evaluation	Treatment/Comments
Acidosis	Underlying cause; rapid, deep breathing	ABG	Correction
Diabetic ketoacidosis (p. 615)	Kussmaul breathing; history of diabetes; nausea, abdominal pain; ketones on breath	Electrolytes; ABG; glucose; ketone levels	Hydration, insulin, K^+
Uremia (p. 809)	Oliguria, often predisposing cause	BUN, creatinine levels; tests for underlying conditions	Evaluate and treat underlying cause
Inborn errors of metabolism Amino/organic acids	Associated acute-onset vomiting and acidosis, progressive deterioration or poor growth and development	Urine and blood for amino and organic acids; electrolytes, ABG: acidosis	Exacerbation precipitated by acute illness
Fructose intolerance	Associated with ingestion of sugar or fruits	Challenge test under controlled conditions	
Addison disease (p. 614)	Dehydration, circulatory collapse; if chronic: weakness, fatigue, pallor, diarrhea, increased pigmentation	Serum Na^+, K^+; urine adrenocorticoids low	Adrenal genital syndrome in newborns

Continued

TABLE 44-1   Vomiting: Diagnostic Considerations—cont'd

Condition	Diagnostic findings	Evaluation	Comments/management
Reye syndrome (p. 646)	Associated liver failure, with marked change in mental status (often combative)	Liver function test results and ammonia level elevated	
INTRAPSYCHIC			
Attention getting	Inconsistent history; times usually related to getting attention	Psychiatric evaluation	Organic causes must be ruled out
Hysteria/hyperventilation	Anxiety, nausea, and other psychosomatic symptoms; may hyperventilate	Psychiatric evaluation	Exclude organic causes
NEOPLASM			
GI	Related to location, type, and extent of neoplasm; insidious onset of symptoms	Specific for tissue considerations	Rare in children
Intracerebral			
MISCELLANEOUS			
Improper feeding techniques	Often regurgitation; bad nipple on bottle; improper position; usually occurs shortly after feeding; usually vomited material is undigested	Rarely need upper GI series to rule out abnormality	Implement support system; make sure child not overfed
Chalasia	May be small amounts; associated with feeding, usually within 30-45 min of feeding; child well, good growth	Upper GI series if needed	Trial of slow, careful, prone, upright feedings; child usually under 6 mo; avoid overfeeding
Pregnancy	Increased intraabdominal pressure; usually first trimester		
Epilepsy (p. 738)	Aura or seizure may involve vomiting	EEG	Requires good neurologic follow-up evaluation
Ascites	Increased intraabdominal pressure	As related to cause; total serum protein, albumin levels	
Environmental heat illness (hyperthermia) (Chapter 50)	Abnormal mental status; variably febrile, leg cramps, dehydrated	Electrolytes	Fluids, cooling
Superior mesenteric artery syndrome	Compression of duodenum in child (adolescent female) leading to obstruction; usually recent marked weight loss	Upper GI series	Usually requires psychiatric therapy for underlying problems; support

TABLE 44-2   Vomiting: Gastrointestinal Caused By Age

Newborn (0-28 days)	Infant	Child (>2 yr)
GASTROINTESTINAL—OBSTRUCTIVE		
Intestinal atresia/stenosis	Pyloric stenosis	Foreign body
Malrotation of bowel	Foreign body	Duodenal hematoma
Volvulus	Malrotation/volvulus	Intussusception
Meconium ileus/plug	Intussusception	Meckel's diverticulum
Hirschsprung's disease	Meckel's diverticulum	Hirschsprung's disease
Imperforate anus	Hirschsprung's disease	Incarcerated hernia
Incarcerated hernia	Incarcerated hernia	Adhesions
GASTROINTESTINAL—INFECTIOUS/INFLAMMATORY		
Necrotizing enterocolitis	Gastroenteritis	Gastroenteritis
Gastroesophageal reflux	Gastroesophageal reflux	Peptic ulcer disease
	Peritonitis	Appendicitis
	Milk allergy	Pancreatitis
		Paralytic ileus
		Peritonitis

Adapted from Fuchs S, Jaffe D: Vomiting, *Pediatr Emerg Care* 6:664, 1990.

hyperactivity of the bowel, and congenital abnormalities as well as systemic illness.

MANAGEMENT

Management should focus on correction of fluid deficits (see Chapter 7), as well as definitive treatment of underlying abnormality. The well-hydrated patient with a self-limited problem can usually be discharged and sent home to follow a clear-liquid regimen. Antiemetics are usually unnecessary for children. A good balance of efficacy and sedation is achieved by promethazine (Phenergan), 0.25-0.5 mg/kg/dose q4-6hr PO, PR, IM prn (adult: 12.5-25 mg/dose). An effective parenteral antiemetic is droperidol (Inapsine), 0.05-0.1 mg/kg/dose IV in children more than 2 years of age (adult: 1.25 mg or 0.5 ml/dose IV). Otherwise, hospitalization is indicated.

Parental Education

1. Give only clear liquids *slowly:* Pedialyte, Lytren, Gatorade, defizzed soda pop (cola, ginger ale), and so on. With younger children, start with a teaspoon and slowly advance the amount. If vomiting occurs, let your child rest for a while and then try again.

2. About 8 hours after vomiting has stopped, your child can gradually return to a normal diet. With older infants and children, give bland items (toast, crackers, clear soup) slowly.

3. Call your physician if the following occur:
   a. Vomiting continues for more than 24 hours or increases in frequency or amount.
   b. Signs of dehydration develop, including decreased urine level, less moisture in diapers, dry mouth, no tears, or weight loss.
   c. Child becomes sleepy, difficult to awaken, or irritable.
   d. Vomited material contains blood or turns green.

Many children will spit up *(regurgitate)* food, particularly during the first few months of life. This is normal in most children but may be exaggerated by faulty feeding techniques or gastroesophageal reflux **(chalasia).** If the child is well and growing normally, the problem may be reduced by careful attention to feeding techniques. Suggestions that may be useful include the following:

1. Keep your child in an upright position during feeding and prone for 30 to 45 minutes after feeding.
2. Feed your baby smaller amounts more often.
3. Burp your baby frequently.
4. Thickened liquids may be helpful.

REFERENCES

Fomon SJ, Filer LJ, Anderson TA, et al: Recommendation for feeding normal infants, *Pediatrics* 63:52, 1979.

Hargrove CB, Ulshen MH, Shub MD: Upper gastrointestinal endoscopy in infants: diagnostic usefulness and safety, *Pediatrics* 74:828, 1984.

Orenstein SR, Whittington PF, Orenstein DM: The infant seat as treatment for gastroesophageal reflux, *N Engl J Med* 309:760, 1983.

Osundwa VM, Dawod ST: Vomiting as the main presenting symptom of acute asthma, *Acta Pediatr* 78:968, 1989.

Swishuk LE: Acute vomiting and abdominal pain in an infant, *Pediatr Emerg Care* 2:201, 1986.

VII
ENVIRONMENTAL EMERGENCIES

45 BITES

JEFFREY RICHKER

ALERT: Bites must be evaluated to determine the extent of local tissue injury
and potential immediate and long-term systemic or local infectious
reactions.

ANIMAL AND HUMAN BITES

Children commonly experience animal bites, as many as 20% of which are dog bites. The peak age is 5 to 14 years of age, with the highest incidence among males during the spring and summer. Management involves minimizing skin and soft tissue injury to achieve a good cosmetic and functional result, while providing prophylaxis against infection in the initial encounter and adequate follow-up observation to ensure prompt treatment of delayed infection.

DOG AND CAT BITES

Large dogs are responsible for most animal bites, although smaller dogs and cats may bite and scratch. It is estimated that 0.5 to 2 million dog bites occur each year, representing about 1% of emergency department visits. Up to 5% of dog bites and 20% to 50% of cat bites become infected. In most cases, the dog belongs to the family or a neighbor.

Etiology

1. *Pasteurella multocida* is often involved in children with evolving cellulitis early;

Staphylococcus aureus, usually a common secondary infection beginning at 2 to 4 days, is cultured in as many as 50% of infected wounds. Mixed infections are common. Anaerobic bacteria are present in approximately one third of infected wounds.
2. Rabies virus is an unusual pathogen but must be considered. Rodents (e.g., rats, mice, gerbils, hamsters, squirrels) do not carry rabies virus (p. 717).

Diagnostic Findings

Patients commonly have soft tissue injuries, which are usually a combination of crush injury with lacerations. Injuries to the face, head, and neck are most common.

Complications

Cellulitis may develop with the onset of erythema, swelling, or tenderness. Lymphadenitis also may develop. If no signs of infection are present within 3 days of trauma, infection is unlikely to occur. Puncture wounds have a higher rate of infection than do lacerations because the bacterial inoculum is deeper and the wound more difficult to cleanse.

Cat-scratch disease may occur after a cat bite, producing regional lymphadenitis of an extremity 14 days (range: 3 to 50 days) after the scratch. Cats less than 1 year of age are more likely to be involved; 80% of cases occur in individuals younger than 21 years of age. *Bartonella henselae* (formerly *Rochalimaea henselae*) most commonly causes the disease.

All patients will have adenopathy, whereas half will have this as the only clinical feature. The most common site is the axilla. Perinaud oculoglandular syndrome (POGS), associated with cat scratches in 97% of cases, may include neuroretinitis, encephalopathy (headache, lethargy, transient hemiplegia, aphasia, hearing loss), thrombocytopenic purpura, angiomatous papules, hepatomegaly, and splenomegaly. Atypical cases in about 5% of patients may have prolonged fever, malaise, fatigue, myalgia, arthralgia, or POGS.

The immunofluorescent antibody (IFA) is 98% to 100% sensitive; the antibody titer peak occurs at 6 to 8 weeks after the onset of illness. The skin test is not generally recommended. Biopsy of the lymph notes may be useful in atypical disease.

Other complications include the following:
1. Crush injuries
2. Osteomyelitis (p. 753)
3. Septic arthritis (p. 751)
4. Tenosynovitis

Ancillary Data

Cultures and Gram stain are unnecessary with routine animal bites. However, if a wound becomes infected, cultures should be obtained, particularly if the infection has been unresponsive to previous therapy or if the patient either is taking prophylactic antibiotics or is immunosuppressed. IFA for cat scratch disease.

Management (see Chapter 65)

1. Mechanical irrigation and debridement are crucial to the treatment of animal bites.
   a. Adequate cleansing may require local or regional anesthesia.
   b. Irrigation should be done extensively with 1% povidone-iodine solution (Betadine), not scrub. Some prefer to use sterile saline solution, but the iodine solution is preferable. Peroxide and isopropyl alcohol may cause tissue damage. Using pressure is ideal. A 19-gauge needle attached to a 35-ml syringe can generate 7 pounds per square inch (PSI), whereas a standard bulb syringe creates only 0.05 PSI. Irrigation is best done at 7 PSI or greater using a 19-gauge or larger needle syringe system. The fluid is directed at various angles so that all surfaces are cleansed.
   c. Debridement of wound edges and devitalized tissues is essential to reduce nonvital tissue and facilitate a good plastic closure.
   d. Scrubbing (except for wounds with rabies potential) is usually harmful to tissues.
   e. Wounds with extensive damage require particular attention to irrigation and debridement.
2. Suturing is indicated for cosmetic and functional reasons.
   a. It should be done only after thorough irrigation and debridement.
   b. Hand injuries, those involving extensive soft tissue injury or damage to deep tissues, puncture wounds, and those older than 24 hours should not be sutured if any question exists regarding the extent of the wound, the adequacy of irrigation and debridement, and the completeness of follow-up. Steri-strips may be useful.

      A study of dog bites to the hand revealed a small difference in the infection rate between sutured and unsutured wounds (5.5% versus 4.5%). Human bites of the hand are not usually sutured.

3. Wounds that have a high risk of becoming infected include the following:
   a. Bites of the hand, wrist, or foot. On infants, the scalp and face are problematic.
   b. Extensive wounds, where devitalized tissue cannot be entirely debrided.
   c. Wounds older than 12 hours.
   d. Wounds involving tendons, joints, or bone.
   e. Sutured wounds.
   f. Puncture wounds.
   g. Crush injuries that cannot be debrided.
   h. Wounds in patients with peripheral vascular insufficiency (e.g., diabetes). Also asplenic, or immunocompromiscd patients and those older than 50 years of age. Cat bites are generally considered to be high risk.
4. Antibiotics may be considered prophylactically with high-risk injuries (as defined previously). About 14 patients are treated for every patient who has an infection prevented. The estimated relative risk of antibiotic-treated patients is 0.56% to develop an infection, whereas the risk is 16% if untreated.
   a. Penicillin VK, 25-50 mg/kg/24 hr q6hr PO, and cephalexin (Keflex) or cephradine (Velosef), 25-50 mg/kg/24 hr q6hr PO; or amoxicillin-clavulanic acid (Augmentin), 30-50 mg AMX/kg/24 hr q8hr PO.
   b. Wounds that become infected, particularly those in high-risk locations, generally require parenteral therapy:
      • Penicillin G, 100,000 U/kg/24 hr q4hr IV, and nafcillin (or equivalent), 100 mg/kg/24 hr q4hr IV; or less ideally a cephalosporin such as cefazolin (Ancef), 50-100 mg/kg/24 hr q6-8hr IV.
      • Infections in low-risk areas may be initially treated orally if the child is nontoxic and follow-up observation is good.

5. Although antibiotics are generally not recommended for cat scratch disease, they may be indicated if systemic disease is present. Oral rifampin, ciprofloxacin, or trimethoprim-sulfamethoxazole are effective in decreasing order; or parenteral gentamicin may be used.
6. Other considerations include the following:
   a. Tetanus toxoid should be administered as indicated (p. 718).
   b. Wounds with great soft tissue injury should be immobilized and, if on an extremity, elevated.
   c. If an abscess forms, surgical drainage is required.
   d. Sutured wounds that become infected should have the suture material removed.
   e. Rabies should be considered in some geographic areas, depending on the animal inflicting the scratch or bite, the location of the injury, and other factors outlined on p. 717.

Disposition

Patients with uncomplicated animal bites may be discharged, with careful instructions to monitor for infection. Those with high-risk bites should take antibiotics. Careful follow-up observation is essential. If a bite is sutured, it should be reexamined within 24 hours. Patients with high-risk category bites that become infected may require hospitalization for parenteral therapy.

Parental Education

1. Instruct children about playing with unfamiliar animals. Do not allow children to place face near dog; do not leave children unattended with dogs. Dogs may misinterpret human gestures that may be considered threatening. Obey leash laws and be particularly careful with large dogs. Dogs must be treated with respect, which

includes never hurting, teasing, or taking things from them.

2. Call your physician if the following occur:
   a. The wound gets red, tender, or swollen or develops a discharge.
   b. Child develops a fever.

REFERENCES

Bass JW, Vincent JM, Person DA: The expanding spectrum of *Bartonella* infections: II. Cat-scratch disease, *Pediatr Infect Dis* 16:163, 1997.

Brogan TV, Bratton SL, Dowd MD, et al: Severe dog bites in children, *Pediatrics* 96:5, 1995.

Cummings P: Antibiotics to prevent infections in patients with dog bite wounds: a meta-analysis of randomized trials, *Ann Emerg Med* 23:535, 1994.

Dire DJ, Hogan DE, Walker JS: Prophylactic oral antibiotics for low risk dog bite wounds, *Pediatr Emerg Care* 8:194, 1992.

Goldstein EJ: Bite wounds and infection, *Clin Infect Dis* 14:633, 1992.

Margileth AM: Antibiotic therapy for cat-scratch disease: clinical study of therapeutic outcome in 268 patients and a review of the literature, *Pediatr Infect Dis J* 11:474, 1992.

Midani S, Ayoub EM, Anderson B: Cat-scratch disease, *Adv Pediatr* 43:397, 1996.

Rosenkrans JA: Animal and human bites. In Barkin RM, editor: *Pediatric emergency medicine: concepts and clinical practice*, ed 2, St Louis, 1997, Mosby.

HUMAN BITES

Human bites have a greater risk of tissue damage and infection than do those inflicted by dogs and cats.

Etiology

More than 40 organisms have been identified as mouth flora and may be potential pathogens.

Diagnostic Findings

The most common injury involves a clenched fist striking an opponent's mouth, with potentially great tissue damage. Examination of damage to soft tissues and tendons must include repositioning of the hand in the clenched and neutral positions. Other tissues may be involved.

Infection produces cellulitis with potential closed-space infections and abscess formation, as well as osteomyelitis and septic arthritis.

Management

Irrigation and debridement are similar to treatment given animal bites (p. 304) and must be done with meticulous care. These wounds should never be sutured because of the high rate of infection.

1. Antibiotics should be administered as noted for animal bites (p. 305). Tetanus should be administered toxoid as indicated (p. 718).
2. Patients who have infections associated with human bites should usually be admitted to the hospital for parenteral therapy:
   Ampicillin, 100 mg/kg/24 hr q4hr IV, and nafcillin (or equivalent), 100 mg/kg/24 hr q4hr IV; or a cephalosporin such as cefazolin (Ancef), 50-100 mg/kg/24 hr q6-8hr IV

Disposition

Patients with uncomplicated human bites may be discharged with antibiotics and good follow-up monitoring. Patients with bites that are infected should be admitted to the hospital.

REFERENCE

Leung AKC, Robson WLM: Human bites in children, *Pediatr Emerg Care* 8:225, 1992.

ARTHROPOD (INSECT) BITES

BROWN RECLUSE SPIDER

The brown recluse spider *(Loxosceles reclusa)* is 1 inch long and is distinguished by violin-like markings on the dorsum of the thorax. The spider introduces a venom containing necrotizing, hemolytic, and spreading factors in the skin. It seeks out dry, warm habitats, spinning the webs in protected places, such as under stones and cliffs; in rarely disturbed areas such as attics, closets, and garages; and in corners and crevices of houses. It is not aggressive toward man and generally attacks only when trapped or crushed against the skin.

Diagnostic Findings

Local pain and erythema at the site develop 2 to 8 hours after the bite, followed by bleb or blister formation, with a surrounding area of pallor. The pain is out of proportion to the size of the lesion. Over the ensuing 48 to 72 hours, central induration occurs, and a dark violet color develops, surrounded by a larger area of reactive erythema. This "red, white, and blue" sign is typical of severe bites. The area then ulcerates, and a black eschar forms within a week, which heals over 6 to 8 weeks. If these changes have not occurred by 58 to 96 hours, patients will usually not have any significant necrosis. Bites in the fatty areas such as the abdomen, buttocks, and thighs develop necrosis with greater frequency than bites elsewhere.

Systemic signs develop in the initial 24 to 48 hours, including headache, fever, nausea, vomiting, joint pains, and very rarely, cyanosis, hypotension, and seizures. The variability of the response reflects the immune status of the patient, the amount of venom injected, and the location of the bite.

Complications

1. Hemolysis with hemoglobinemia, hemoglobinuria, and renal failure. Bites less than 1 cm in diameter rarely cause hemolysis. If the bite enlarges on serial examinations, continue to monitor urine. Bites larger than 1 cm require close monitoring of urine. If hemolysis occurs, hydrate and consider steroids.
2. Disseminated intravascular coagulation (DIC) (p. 683).
3. Seizures (see Chapter 21).
4. Rarely, death.

Ancillary Data

A complete blood count (CBC), prothrombin time (PT), partial thromboplastin time (PTT), platelet count, and urinalysis should be obtained.

Management

1. Assess airway and ventilation. Manage anaphylaxis (see Chapter 12).
2. Local care of the site of bite. Rest the bitten site, place ice compresses to the area, and elevate.
3. Give parenteral steroids. Hydrocortisone (Solu-Cortef), 5mg/kg/dose q6hr IV, administered for a minimum of 24 hours if any systemic signs develop.
4. Give analgesia for pain.
5. Excise, if the ulceration and necrotic area develop into an area greater than 1 cm (rarely needed).
6. Provide specific treatment for complications.
7. Studies suggest the efficacy of dapsone, 1-4 mg/kg/24 hr q12hr PO (adult: 50-100 mg/24 hr PO), for 3 days in reducing ulceration because of its leukocyte-inhibiting properties, but no randomized data are available. Potential adverse effects include hemolysis, agranulocytosis, aplastic anemia, methemoglobinemia, rashes, and toxic epidermal necrolysis.
8. Hyperbaric oxygen has been studied without clear benefit.

Disposition

Patients with evidence of systemic signs and symptoms should be admitted to the hospital; others may be followed closely as outpatients.

REFERENCES

Eitzen EM, Seward PN: Arthropod envenomations in children, *Pediatr Emerg Care* 4:266, 1988.

Phillips S, Kohn M, Baker D, et al: Therapy of brown spider envenomation: a controlled trial of hyperbaric oxygen, dapsone, and cyproheptadine, *Ann Emerg Med* 25:363, 1995.

Wright SW, Wrenn KD, Murray L, et al: Clinical presentation and outcome of brown recluse spider bite, *Ann Emerg Med* 30:28, 1997.

Wilson DC, King LE Jr: Spider and spider bites, *Dermatol Clin* 8:2, 1990.

BLACK WIDOW SPIDER

The black widow spider *(Latrodectus mactans)* is identified by a shiny, black button-shaped body with a red hourglass marking on the underside. The venom is a neurotoxin.

Diagnostic Findings

At the site of the bite, there is immediate pain with burning, swelling, and erythema. Double fang markings are located at the site. Other local features may include piloerection, mild edema, perspiration, and lymphangitis.

The degree of systemic signs and symptoms will reflect the number of bites, the amount of venom injected, and the toxicity of the spider's venom. Within 30 minutes of the bite, crampy abdominal pain, accompanied by dizziness, nausea, vomiting, headache, and sweating occur. The abdomen is characteristically board-like, mimicking an acute abdomen. Other findings may include salivation, lacrimation, tremors, tachycardia or bradycardia, and anxiety. The patient's condition usually resolves in 24 hours, but the bite is associated with hypertension rather than hypotension.

In one study, 79% of patients had pain at the bite site, 71% had abdominal pain, and 57% had lower extremity weakness.

Complications

1. Ascending motor paralysis (see Chapter 41)
2. Seizures (see Chapter 21)
3. Shock (see Chapter 5)
4. Coma, respiratory arrest, death

Management

Supportive therapy should be instituted at the first sign of systemic symptoms. Options include the following:

1. Muscle relaxant: diazepam (Valium), 0.1-0.3 mg/kg/dose IV; and
2. Analgesics: meperidine (Demerol), 1-2 mg/kg/dose q4-6hr IM, IV. Morphine, 0.1-0.2 mg/kg/dose q2hr IV, may be an alternative.
3. Calcium gluconate (10%), 50-100 mg (0.5-1.0 ml)/kg/dose IV (up to a maximum dose of 10 ml) slowly, has been reported to have a variable and transient efficacy. May need to be repeated. Controversial.

An equine antivenin, ethacrynate (Lyovac)—in a vial containing 2.5 ml—is administered, according to package directions, after negative skin test results for horse serum sensitivity have been obtained. It has a limited role, given efficacy of the preceding therapy but may be important for young children and individuals with hypertension and cardiac disease. Some have suggested that it is indicated if all of the following are present or three have been present for more than 12 hours: abdominal pain, hypertension, muscular pain, and agitation or irritability.

Disposition

All patients with known black widow spider bites require admission for observation and potential treatment.

REFERENCES

Clark RF, Wethern-Kestner S, Vance NV, et al: Clinical presentation and treatment of black widow spider envenomation: a review of 163 cases, *Ann Emerg Med* 21:782, 1992.

Moss HS, Binder LS: A retrospective review of black widow spider envenomation, *Ann Emerg Med* 16:188, 1987.

HYMENOPTERA

Hymenoptera (honey bees, wasps, yellow jackets, and hornets) produce a variety of systemic effects, reflecting individual sensitivity and the number of bites or stings inflicted by the offending insect.

Diagnostic Findings

1. Local reactions commonly produce edema and pain.
2. Toxic reactions occur with multiple stings (10 or more): vomiting, diarrhea, dizziness, muscle spasms, and rarely, convulsions.
3. Anaphylactic reactions, such as wheezing and urticaria (see Chapter 12), occur in sensitive individuals.
4. Delayed serum-sickness reaction occurs 10 to 14 days after the sting, with morbilliform rash, urticaria, myalgia, arthralgia, and fever.

Management

1. Local attention to the point of sting—cleansing, removing the stinger with a scraping motion, and cold compresses—may provide symptomatic relief. Local application of papain, found in meat tenderizer, is believed by some to relieve pain.
2. Diphenhydramine (Benadryl), 5 mg/kg/24 hr q6-8hr PO, IM, or IV, may reduce local, as well as systemic, signs and symptoms.
3. Systemic signs of anaphylaxis are treated with epinephrine, nebulized β-agonist agents, and steroids (see Chapter 12).

Disposition

1. Patients with only local reactions can usually be discharged with symptomatic treatment.
2. Those with severe reactions should be admitted for continuation of emergent care.
3. After resolution of severe systemic and anaphylactic reactions, the patient should be referred to an allergist for hyposensitization.
4. A bee sting kit containing epinephrine and syringes should be carried by those who have experienced severe local or systemic reactions (see Chapter 12). Children should be warned to avoid clothing with bright colors and flowery patterns, as well as perfumes, hairsprays, and colognes that attract insects.

TICKS

Most tick bites are benign and simply require removal of the tick. However, a number of diseases may be transmitted by ticks, with specific types serving as the vector (Table 45-1).

As indicated in the table, Lyme disease has three clinical phases. The first stage occurs within a few days up to weeks after the tick inoculation. Erythema chronicum migrans begins as a red papule/macule at the site and expands to an annular lesion with central clearing. Viral-like syndromes may be present. Stage 2, associated with spirochete dissemination, has neurologic, cardiac (AV nodal block), and ophthalmologic findings. Stage 3 may occur with ongoing neurologic findings and synovitis. Long-term sequelae may include neuropathy, encephalopathy, fibromyalgia, chronic fatigue syndrome, or recurrent arthralgia. An antibody response does not protect against subsequent infection. A vaccine is being developed.

Tick-bite paralysis presenting with an ascending paralysis is discussed on page 282. Embedded ticks usually can be withdrawn by covering the tick with alcohol, mineral oil, nail polish, or an ointment. Another suggested protocol for tick removal is the following:

1. Using a blunt, curved forceps or tweezer, grasp the tick close to the surface and pull upward in a steady motion.
2. If steady traction is unsuccessful, the tick

TABLE 45-1 Tick-Transmitted Diseases

	Tularemia	Relapsing fever	Rocky Mountain spotted fever (RMSF)	Colorado tick fever	Ehrlichiosis	Lyme disease
ETIOLOGY	*Francisella tularemia*	*Borrelia recurrentis*	*Rickettsia rickettsii*	Colorado tick fever virus	*Ehrlichia chaffeenis*	*Borrelia burgdorferi*
TICK VECTOR	*Dermacentor*	*Orinthodoros*	*Dermacentor*	*Dermacentor*	*Amblyomma americanum*	*Ixodes scapularis/pacificus*
INCUBATION	1-14 days	5-9 days	2-14 days	3-6 days	7-20 days	3-32 days
DIAGNOSTIC FINDINGS	Headache, persistent fever, malaise, anorexia, lymphadenopathy, conjunctivitis	Relapsing fever, occipital headache, malaise, myalgia, cough, meningismus, lymphadenopathy, leukocytosis	Resistant fever, headache, malaise, arthralgia, periorbital edema, conjunctivitis, meningismus, coma, centrifugal hemorrhagic rash, petechiae	Sudden onset of fever, retroorbital headache, myalgia, anorexia, meningismus, rash, conjunctivitis, leukopenia	Fever, headache, malaise, arthralgia, myalgia, nausea, rash (30% of cases); low platelet count and WBC	Erythema chronicum migrans (ECM) (macular/papular becoming annular), flulike symptoms (headache, anorexia, chills) during first stage; 15% progress to stage two with neurologic complications (encephalopathy, cranial neuropathy, peripheral radiculoneuropathy), joint complications, 50%-60% have pericarditis; stage three may occur with persistent central nervous system (CNS) findings, and arthritis (arthralgia); pericarditis; remissions; enzyme-linked immunosorbent assay (ELISA)
ANTIBIOTICS	Streptomycin, tetracycline,* chloramphenicol	Tetracycline*, penicillin, chloramphenicol	Tetracycline,* doxycycline,* chloramphenicol	None (support)	Tetracycline,* doxycycline,* chloramphenicol (less effective)	Tetracycline*, doxycycline,* cefuroxime, or amoxicillin for 10-30 days; late-stage or toxic child needs additional therapy (ceftriaxone)

*Do not use in children <9 yr.

and superficial attached skin can easily be cut away. Brief pressure will stop the bleeding.

3. Do not squeeze, squash, or puncture the body of the tick because fluids (saliva, hemolymph) may contain infective agents.

4. Do not handle the tick with bare hands.

Protective clothing should reduce potential exposure.

REFERENCES

Committee on Infectious Diseases, AAP: Treatment of Lyme borreliosis, *Pediatrics* 88:176, 1991.

Feder HM, Hunt MS: Pitfalls in the diagnosis and treatment of Lyme disease in children, *JAMA* 274:66, 1995.

Gerber MA, Shapiro ED: Prognosis of Lyme disease in children, *J Pediatr* 121:157, 1992.

Gerber MA, Shapiro ED, Burke GS, et al: Lyme disease in children in southeastern Connecticut, *N Engl J Med* 335:1270, 1996.

Jacobs RF, Schutze GE: Ehrlichiosis in children, *J Pediatr* 131:184, 1997.

Shadick NA, Phillips CB, Logigian EL, et al: The long-term clinical outcome of Lyme disease: a population based retrospective cohort study, *Ann Intern Med* 121:560, 1994.

Williams CL, Strabino B, Lee A, et al: Lyme disease in childhood: clinical and epidemiologic features of ninety cases, *Pediatr Infect Dis* 9:10, 1990.

SNAKE BITES

ALERT: It is crucial to determine rapidly whether a snake is potentially poisonous. If it is, urgent local treatment, support, and administration of antivenin are required.

Of the known species of snakes, only 5% are venomous. In the United States, the most commonly encountered venomous snakes are Crotalidae (pit vipers, water moccasins, and copperheads) and Elapidae (coral snakes). Their venom consists of multiple poisonous proteins and enzymes that are absorbed through the lymphatic system after envenomation. Most snake bites occur in the summer during the afternoon and evening hours.

The severity of injury from a poisonous snake bite reflects, among other factors, the amount of venom released and the size of the victim. The following factors should be considered:

1. Age, size, and health of the patient.

2. The size of the snake; larger snakes produce more venom. Juvenile snakes may produce a more lethal venom to compensate for their diminished venom volume. Not all strikes result in envenomation; thus the biting and envenomation can be distinct processes.

3. The location of the injury. Peripheral injuries account for more than 90% of bites and are usually less severe. Bites to the distal aspect of the digit may be associated with less severe clinical manifestations.

Distinguishing venomous from nonvenomous snakes is sometimes difficult. Venomous snakes usually have vertically elliptic pupils, a facial pit between eye and nostril, a rattle, fangs, and subcaudal plates behind oval plates—in pit vipers arranged in a single row. Nonvenomous snakes have round pupils; no pit, rattle, or fangs; and a double row of subcaudal plates.

DIAGNOSTIC FINDINGS

1. The site of the poisonous snake bite may display fang marks, with subsequent burning, pain or numbness, swelling, and erythema. This may progress rapidly to hemorrhage and necrosis. A compartment syndrome may develop, which is difficult to distinguish from the local effects of the venom.

2. Regional effects of extremity bites include edema of the arm or leg, ecchymoses, and lymphadenopathy.

3. Systemic signs and symptoms may develop within 15 minutes, depending on the severity of the injury.

   a. Nausea, vomiting, sweating, chills, numbness, and paresthesias of the tongue and perioral region may occur.

  b. Fasciculations, dysphagia, bleeding, and hypotension are common.

4. Nonpoisonous snake bites often leave the patient with major psychologic trauma, which may result in mild nonspecific symptoms similar to those of actual envenomation.

Complications

1. DIC and hemolysis (p. 683)
2. Respiratory failure caused by noncardiogenic pulmonary edema
3. Renal failure (p. 809)
4. Seizures (see Chapter 21)
5. Shock and death

Ancillary Data

1. CBC, platelets, coagulation studies (PT, PTT, fibrinogen, fibrin split products [FSPs]).
2. Urinalysis, blood urea nitrogen (BUN), serial electrolyte, creatinine levels.
3. Type and cross-match, which may be difficult once hemolysis occurs; should be done initially.
4. In moderate to severe cases, consider a chest radiograph, electrocardiogram (ECG), and arterial blood gas.

MANAGEMENT

1. If possible, the snake should be killed and identified, with careful handling of the head because it can still deliver venom for as long as 1 hour after death.
2. Initially, a broad, firm, constrictive bandage should be applied proximal to the bitten area and around the limb. It should be tight enough to reduce superficial lymphatic drainage.
3. The extremity should be splinted to reduce motion.
4. Activity of the patient should be mini-

mized and cooling, which can cause further tissue damage, avoided.

5. Surgical excision of the wound site or fasciotomy is probably unnecessary because the muscle necrosis is probably due to proteolytic enzymes rather than increased compartmental pressure. Incision and drainage are effective only if performed within 45 to 60 minutes of the bite.

6. Hyperbaric oxygen may be an adjunctive treatment if severe envenomation occurs with a large open wound and a significant volume of necrotic muscle.

Transport to the hospital should be expedited for support and administration of antivenin. First, skin tests for hypersensitivity to horse serum must be done. However, patients with serious bites must be given antivenin regardless of the sensitivity. Reactions can be managed by slowing down or temporarily stopping infusions and pretreatment with diphenhydramine (Benadryl) and histamine (H_2) blocker (cimetidine). The antivenin infusion should begin slowly at a dilution of 1:10 and be increased slowly if no reaction is noted. If anaphylactic reactions are noted despite pretreatment, it is possible to titrate with an epinephrine infusion after consultation (see Chapter 12). Monitoring is mandatory.

Antivenin should be administered intravenously. A history should be taken for allergy to horse serum. Smaller patients may get larger initial doses. The amount of antivenin administered relates to the category of the patient as determined by symptomatology. No therapy is required if no findings beyond fang marks are present. *Minimal* findings include local swelling with no systemic symptoms. *Moderate* or progressive symptoms are marked swelling and systemic signs, including metallic taste, paresthesias, or laboratory abnormalities. The moderate category also includes those patients who have had multiple or provoked bites of a large venomous snake or highly toxic species (Mojave, diamond back). *Severe* symptoms are marked, with rapid swelling, severe systemic symptoms (muscle fasciculations, hypotension, oliguria), and abnormal laboratory findings. These patients with severe symptoms may also have a history of a highly toxic snake, prolonged embedding of the fangs, and multiple bites. A snakebite severity scoring system has been proposed.

Severity	Antivenin administered (adult)
None	None required
Minimal	5 vials
Moderate	5-10 vials
Severe	10-20 vials

1. For rattlesnake, water moccasin, and copperhead bites: antivenin (Crotalidae) Polyvalent.*
2. For coral snake bites: antivenin (Micrurus fulvius). Usually give 3 to 5 vials.

Repeat infusion of 4 to 5 vials may be given every 1 to 2 hours if symptoms are progressing. Antivenin for rare species may be obtained from Oklahoma Poison Control Center: 405-271-5454.

Complications include anaphylactic shock, DIC, and serum sickness. Serum sickness (p. 216) may develop 7 to 14 days after antivenin administration. Treatment of complications is essential to the ultimate outcome. Tetanus toxoids should also be given, if indicated. A new antivenom has been developed consisting of an affinity purified, mixed, monospecific crotalid antivenom ovine Fab. Trials of progressive, serious envenomations were conducted in a small number of patients (mild to moderate copperhead bites were excluded) and showed beneficial response without any acute or delayed allergic reactions. Further studies are under way.

DISPOSITION

All patients with poisonous snake bites should be admitted to the hospital for supportive care. Patients with unidentified snake bites may be discharged if no signs and symptoms develop in 4 hours of observation. Reassurance may be necessary.

REFERENCES

Burgess JL, Dart RC, Egan NB, et al: Effects of constriction bands on rattlesnake venom absorption: a pharmacokinetic study, *Ann Emerg Med* 21:1086, 1992.

Dart RC, Seifert SA, Carroll L, et al: Affinity-purified mixed monospecific crotalid antivenom ovine Fab for the treatment of crotalid venom poisoning, *Ann Emerg Med* 30:33, 1997.

Dart RC, Hurlbut KM, Garcia R, et al: Validation of a severity score for the assessment of crotalid snakebites, *Ann Emerg Med* 27:321, 1996.

Moss ST, Bogen G, Dart RC: Association of rattlesnakes bite location with severity of clinical manifestations, *Ann Emerg Med* 30:58, 1997.

Seiler JG III, Sagerman SD, Geller RJ, et al: Venomous snake bite: current concepts of treatment, *Orthopedics* 17:8, 1994.

Tully SA, Wingert WA: Venomous animal bites and stings. In Barkin RM, editor: *Pediatric emergency medicine: concepts and clinical practice,* ed 2, St Louis, 1997, Mosby.

*Wyeth Laboratories: telephone 215-688-4400.

46 Burns, Thermal

ALERT: Rapid assessment of the depth, location, and extent of a burn should
          determine the severity of the injury. Airway and pulmonary status
          and associated trauma must be treated and volume deficits corrected.
          Specific burn therapy should be initiated immediately after stabilization.

ETIOLOGY

The mechanism of heat transfer and injury influences the type of burn.

1. Scald burns result from contact with a hot object or hot liquid. They are most commonly seen in children less than 3 years of age and may be sharply demarcated and of partial thickness, except in young infants, where full-thickness injury may be noted.
2. Flame burns occur with direct-flame exposure resulting from ignition of clothing. They are commonly seen in children older than 2 years of age who play with matches, fire, and flammable materials. The borders are irregular and may be of full thickness.
3. Flashburns are caused by exposure to an explosion, resulting in a uniform, partial-thickness burn.
4. Electrical burns are discussed in Chapter 48.

DIAGNOSTIC FINDINGS

Initial evaluation must include information about the mechanism of injury, duration since the burn, patient's age and weight, underlying disease, past medical problems, and associated injuries.

Body surface area (BSA) in children may be estimated to determine the extent of burns (Fig. 46-1). In adults, the rule of 9's is easily used for estimating involved body surface: head and neck (9%), anterior trunk (18%), posterior trunk (18%), each leg (18%), each arm (9%), and anorectal area (1%).

The patient should be thoroughly examined to ascertain other associated traumatic injuries, as well as signs of smoke inhalation, including hoarseness, cough, singed nasal hairs, oral burns, carbonaceous sputum, wheezing, rhonchi, and cyanosis (see Chapter 53).

Depth of burn is an important determinant of severity and potential complications.

1. Superficial partial-thickness (first-degree) burns involve only the epidermis and are characterized by erythema and local pain.
2. Partial-thickness (second-degree) burns involve the epidermis and corium.
   a. Partial-thickness burns produce erythema and blisters.
   b. Deep partial-thickness burns are white and dry and have reduced sensitivity to touch and pain. They blanch with pressure.
3. Full-thickness (third-degree) burns are numb, with a tough, brownish surface

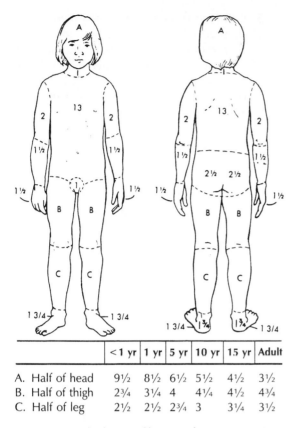

	<1 yr	1 yr	5 yr	10 yr	15 yr	Adult
A. Half of head	9½	8½	6½	5½	4½	3½
B. Half of thigh	2¾	3¼	4	4¼	4½	4¾
C. Half of leg	2½	2½	2¾	3	3¼	3½

Fig. 46-1   Calculation of burn surface area.

(After Lund and Browder.)

and a hard eschar. Spontaneous healing will not occur.

Severity of burns is determined by the depth of the burn, BSA involved, location of the injury, age and health of the patient, and associated injuries.

1. *Major* burn:
   a. Partial thickness: more than 25% BSA (adults); more than 15% to 20% BSA (children); or full thickness: more than 10% BSA
   b. Burns of the hands, face, eyes, ears, feet, or perineum
   c. Patients with inhalation injury, electrical burns, burns complicated by fractures or other major trauma
   d. Poor-risk patients, including those with underlying disease, associated major injuries, or suspicion of child abuse
2. *Moderate* uncomplicated burn: partial thickness: 15% to 25% BSA (adults); 10% to 15% BSA (children); or full thickness: 2% to 10% BSA
3. *Minor* burn: partial thickness: less than 15% BSA (adults); less than 10% BSA (children); or full thickness less than 2% BSA

Complications

1. Smoke inhalation. Direct inhalation of toxic particles or exposure to hot smoke and air may produce respiratory distress on the basis of upper or lower respiratory abnormality (see Chapter 53).
2. Carbon monoxide poisoning (p. 371).
3. Dehydration and shock from fluid losses and inadequate fluid therapy.
4. Renal failure secondary to myoglobinuria or dehydration.
5. Sepsis and death. Very young children (0 to 4 years) dying in house fires account for 47% of deaths.

Ancillary Data

1. Blood tests for moderate or major burns should include, when appropriate, complete blood count (CBC), electrolytes, blood urea nitrogen (BUN), and creatinine levels; arterial blood gas; type and cross-match; and carboxyhemoglobin level.
2. A chest x-ray film is useful for all patients with major burns and for those with any question of smoke inhalation. The initial film will be useful for comparison with later x-ray studies. Abnormal findings are often delayed up to 24 hours.
3. Urinalysis should be performed for specific gravity, sugar, protein, myoglobin, and hemoglobin. Urine output is useful in assessing fluid status.

MANAGEMENT OF MINOR AND SOME MODERATE BURNS

1. Burn wounds should initially be covered by a cloth cooled with saline solution. Minimize contact with nonsterile objects.
2. Intact blisters should be left unbroken unless they are at flexion creases. Ruptured vesicles should be debrided and the area cleansed gently.
3. Superficial partial-thickness burns require no topical therapy except for symptomatic relief.
4. Partial-thickness injuries may be treated with 1% silver sulfadiazine or by applying a fine-mesh gauze impregnated with a petroleum jelly (Xeroform, Adaptic, Vaseline). Very small burns, particularly those in difficult areas, may be left exposed.
5. The dressing should be changed in 24 hours and then every 2 to 3 days or sooner if an odor develops or if the area becomes painful.
6. Tetanus immunization should be given, if necessary.
7. Pain medication is rarely needed.
8. If the patient has evidence of group A streptococcal disease, penicillin (50,000 U/kg/24 hr q6hr PO or IV) should be given to prevent colonization of the burn.
9. Exclude child abuse in cases of inconsistent or suspicious injury.

Disposition

Patients with minor burns can routinely be sent home unless other medical problems, associated injuries, or suspicion of child abuse or lack of compliance preclude such management. Infants with more than 10% to 15% BSA involvement and adults with 25% BSA burns or burns qualifying as major burns should be admitted.

Parental Education

1. Keep the wound clean and dry.
2. Change the dressing in 24 hours and then every 2 to 3 days. Wash burn gently, apply cream, and dress as directed.

3. Call your physician if the following occur:
   a. Increasing redness or discolorations of the normal tissue around the burn site develop or the area becomes odorous or painful.
   b. Red streaks develop around the area.
   c. Fever and chills are present.
   d. Swelling or progressive inability to use fingers or toes (if extremities are involved) is noted.
   e. Shortness of breath, increased cough, or difficulty in swallowing is present.
   f. Blurred vision develops if face is involved.
4. Sunblock should be used for up to 6 months.

MANAGEMENT OF MAJOR AND MOST MODERATE BURNS

Assessment of airway and ventilation is crucial to seek evidence of respiratory distress or smoke-inhalation injury. Oxygen should be administered to all patients, and if respiratory distress or abnormal arterial blood gases are present, the patient should be intubated. Pulmonary disease may have a delayed onset of up to 24 hours, secondary to smoke inhalation or CO intoxication (see Chapter 53 and p. 371).

Intravenous fluid resuscitation must be initiated immediately with one to two large-bore catheters. Initial stabilization should include infusion of 20 ml/kg 0.9% normal saline (NS) or lactated Ringer's (LR) solution over 20 to 30 minutes. Although controversial, the following is then suggested as an initial guideline for fluid therapy:

1. *Day 1:* 4 ml lactated Ringer's solution with 5% dextrose × kg × (percentage of burn as number, e.g., 70% = 70) given over the first 24 hours, in addition to normal maintenance fluids (see Chapter 8). Half of the total volume of fluids should be given during the first 8 hours after the burn and the remainder over 16 hours.

   For instance, a 10-kg child with 20% BSA burn would require the following fluid management, with adjustments as necessitated by urine output:

a. Maintenance: 1000 ml H_2O with 30 mEq NaCl and 20 mEq KCl—approximately D5W 0.2% NS with 20 mEq KCl/L.

b. Replacement: 800 ml of D5WLR = 4 ml D5WLR × 10 (kg) × 20 (% BSA)

   • One half of replacement and one third of maintenance dose to be given during first 8 hours

2. *Day 2:* Crystalloid solution infused at about one half to three fourths of the previous day's needs. In addition, colloid is useful at this time when administered as a 5% albumin solution at 0.5 gm/kg/% BSA.

The following considerations should be kept in mind:

1. Potassium should generally not be added to the fluid.
2. If fluid management is difficult, a central venous pressure line should be inserted.
3. Urine output and vital signs are the most sensitive indicators of the adequacy of therapy. A Foley catheter should be inserted to monitor urine flow. Optimal flow output should be 2-3 ml/kg/hr, but a minimal level of 1 ml/kg/hr is acceptable.
4. A nasogastric tube should be inserted.

Wound Management

1. Initially, cover the wound with a cloth cooled in saline. Place the patient on a sterile sheet, and make sure those touching the patient wear sterile gloves, gowns, and a cap.
2. Gently scrub the wound, using povidone-iodine soap (Betadine) diluted in saline followed by irrigation. Cool saline or water may reduce pain.
3. Obtain surgical consultation.
4. Debride all dead material. Intact blisters should be left unbroken unless they are at flexion creases. Ruptured vesicles should be debrided.
5. Dress wounds with a liberal application of a 1% silver sulfadiazine cream. Apply an absorbent dressing of fine (36 × 44) mesh gauze or 4 × 4 fluffs, using several layers and a role of gauze to hold the dressing. Biobrane, a bilayer semisynthetic dressing, may decrease pain and total healing time in thermal partial-thickness fresh burns without contamination.

6. Leave the face and perineum open after applying antibiotic cream.
7. Escharotomy is indicated with full-thickness, circumferential burns of the extremities accompanied by impaired neurovascular function. Eschars of the chest may impair ventilation and thus require surgical intervention.
8. Depending on the depth and severity of the wounds, dressings may be left on for 24 hours. At each change, the wound can be cleansed with warm water and debrided, often facilitated by a whirlpool. The burns may then be redressed after application of silver sulfadiazine and fine mesh gauze.
9. Skin grafting after early (3 to 5 days) burn excision is useful in some injuries with large deep burns. Early excision may reduce mortality risk and hospital stay. Biologic and synthetic dressings have an increasing role in treatment.
10. A burn should be epithelialized in 2 to 3 weeks. If healing is not occurring by 14 days, consider excision and grafting. Superficial partial-thickness injuries should be examined for up to 6 weeks for hypertrophic scarring.

Other Considerations

1. Pain medication may be used once vital signs have normalized. Optimally, drugs such as morphine or meperidine should be given intravenously.
2. Update tetanus immunization if appropriate.
3. Initiate peptic ulcer (Curlings ulcer)

prophylaxis—antacid therapy, using antacids, cimetidine (20-30 mg/kg/24 hr q6hr IV or PO), or famotidine (Pepcid) (adult: 20 to 40 mg q24hr PO or 20 mg q12hr IV)—in the first 6 hours after burn.

4. Antibiotics should not be administered prophylactically but for specific signs and symptoms of infection after appropriate cultures. Give penicillin if there is evidence of a group A streptococcal infection.
5. Begin intravenous, tube, and oral nutrition after the stabilization period. An increased metabolic response is noted after a thermal injury.
6. Keep body temperature normal. Do not apply cold or ice dressings.
7. Provide psychologic support of the family when dealing with a major burn; this is imperative from the first encounter through the entire hospitalization. This is often complicated by concerns about potential child abuse.
8. Initiate rehabilitation after stabilization.
9. Exclude child abuse if the cause of injury is suspicious.

DISPOSITION

All patients with moderate or major burns should be admitted to the surgical service with appropriate consultation as necessary.

Major burns can often best be cared for in burn centers, where the burn team can deal with the patient's total needs on a more routine basis.

If transport is necessary, the initial stabilization should be achieved at the primary receiving hospital, often involving a surgical consultant at that time. The same level of care must be maintained throughout the transport process.

REFERENCES

Baxler CR, Waeckerle JF Jr: Emergency treatment of burn injury, *Ann Emerg Med* 17:1305, 1988.

Blinn DL, et al: Inhalation injury with burns: a lethal combination, *J Emerg Med* 6:471, 1988.

Carvasal HF: Fluid resuscitation of pediatric burn victims: a critical approach, *Pediatr Nephrol* 8:357, 1994.

Deitch EA: The management of burns, *N Engl J Med* 323:1249, 1990.

Gerding RL, Emerman CL, Effron D, et al: Outpatient management of partial thickness burns: Biobrane versus silver sulfadiazine, *Ann Emerg Med* 19:121, 1990.

Goldstein AM, Weber JM, Sheridan RL: Femoral venous access is safe in burned children: an analysis of 224 catheters, *J Pediatr* 130:442, 1997.

McLoughlin E, McGuire A: The causes, cost and prevention of childhood burn injuries, *Am J Dis Child* 144:677, 1990.

Parish RA: Thermal burns. In Barkin RM, editor: *Pediatric emergency medicine: concepts and clinical practice,* ed 2, St Louis, 1997, Mosby.

47 DROWNING AND NEAR-DROWNING

ALERT: After initial resuscitation, evaluate for associated injuries. Monitor patient for evolving pulmonary or cerebral edema.

The victim of a submersion episode may die immediately or within 24 hours of the hypoxic insult of complications (drowning) or may survive the incident but require intensive support (near-drowning). Most accidents occur in swimming pools, ponds, lakes, and bathtubs, with a peak incidence in children less than 4 years and 15 to 24 years old. Among boys 15 to 19 years old, 38% of drownings were alcohol related. Nearly two thirds of bathtub near-drownings have evidence of abuse or neglect.

Freshwater and saltwater drowning have distinct pathophysiologies leading to hypoxemia and similar clinical presentations. Freshwater drowning disrupts surfactant, causing atelectasis and ultimately pulmonary edema; saltwater drowning causes fluid movement along an osmotic gradient, producing flooding of alveoli with protein-rich plasma and pulmonary edema. Electrolyte and erythrocyte abnormalities may also develop in both cases; however, this rarely occurs because large amounts of water usually are not aspirated.

Prolonged immersion in cold water is associated with a better prognosis than prolonged immersion in warm water.

ETIOLOGY: PRECIPITATING FACTORS

1. Trauma
   a. Head or neck (see Chapters 57 and 61)
   b. Barotrauma: scuba diving
   c. Hypothermia (see Chapter 51)
   d. Child abuse (see Chapter 25)
2. Seizures (see Chapter 21)
3. Intoxication: alcohol, sedatives, phencyclidine (PCP), lysergic acid diethylamide (LSD) (see Chapter 54)
4. Exhaustion, boating accident, poor swimmer

DIAGNOSTIC FINDINGS

The signs and symptoms reflect pulmonary and cerebral hypoxic injury. The spectrum of illness may range from minimal or negative findings initially, with a delayed onset in 2 to 6 hours, to complete cardiac respiratory arrest. Vital signs and temperature must be determined. Hypothermia may be protective.

Pulmonary findings may include cyanosis, pallor with pulmonary edema, or aspiration pneumonitis often associated with intrapulmonary shunting. Patients may develop rales, frothy sputum, and rhonchi or wheezing and progress to respiratory failure or arrest. Seizures, changed mental status, and stupor or coma may be present with or without focal findings, reflecting hypoxia and cerebral edema. The patient may be postictal if a seizure precipitated the episode. Cardiac dysrhythmias and asystole are possible.

Evidence of trauma must be evaluated as possible precipitating factors, particularly head and neck injuries. Other unexplained signs may indicate child abuse.

Several researchers have defined factors that are *unfavorable* prognosticators in cases of pediatric near-drowning. Outcome is usually a reflection of hypoxia, not the toxicity of the water. Patients who are conscious or have only blunted levels of consciousness on arrival in the emergency department (ED) usually do well. Such patients usually have pupillary light responses, even if the reaction is slightly blunted.

Clinical indicators suggestive of a poor outcome include the following:

1. Patient is less than 3 years of age.
2. Maximum submersion time is more than 5 minutes.
3. Resuscitation efforts are not attempted for at least 10 minutes after rescue.
4. Seizures, fixed and dilated pupils, decerebrate posture, flaccid extremities, and coma are present.
5. Cardiopulmonary resuscitation required on admission in patients who are not hypothermic. Of those arriving at the ED with asystole, 76% died and the remainder remained vegetative.
6. Glasgow Coma Scale (see Table 57-1) score less than 5 is associated with an 80% mortality rate; scores of 6 or greater had no sequelae.
7. Arterial pH is 7.10 or less.
8. Initial blood glucose increased more than 200 mg/dl.

Children with an intracranial pressure (ICP) of 20 mm Hg or less and a cerebral perfusion pressure (CPP) (difference between systemic arterial and intracranial pressure) of 50 mm Hg or more had the best prognosis, with only an 8% mortality rate. Sustained late intracranial hypertension is more likely a sign of profound neurologic insult than its cause.

Complications

1. Pulmonary edema, respiratory failure, adult respiratory distress syndrome (ARDS), and cardiorespiratory arrest (see Chapters 4 and 19)
2. Aspiration pneumonia
3. Hypoxic encephalopathy and seizures
4. Acute tubular necrosis and renal failure (p. 809)
5. Spinal cord injury
6. Disseminated intravascular coagulation (DIC) (see Chapter 79)
7. On-site resuscitation complications: pneumothorax, abdominal visceral tears, etc.

Ancillary Data

1. Electrolytes: usually normal but when drowning occurs in water with high concentrations of electrolytes (i.e., Dead Sea), marked elevations of calcium and magnesium levels, as well as the more common electrolytes, may be noted
2. Complete blood count (CBC) and coagulation screen: usually normal
3. Arterial blood gas (ABG)
4. Chest x-ray film: result may be normal initially and have delayed onset of evidence of aspiration or pulmonary edema
5. Head, neck, and other x-ray studies as indicated by condition
6. Other studies, as indicated by possible precipitating factors

MANAGEMENT

In cases of significant near-drowning, initial management must focus on stabilization of the airway, removal of foreign material, maintenance of ventilation, and administration of oxygen and fluids. Vital signs must be meticulously monitored. A nasogastric (NG) tube and urinary catheter should be inserted. If the patient is febrile, antipyretics and a cooling mattress should be used. If the patient is hypothermic, normalize aggressively. Rapid prehospital intervention can improve outcome (p. 335). Furthermore, immediate resuscitation before arrival of prehospital personnel is associated with a better neurologic outcome.

Consideration must be directed toward precipitating conditions, with particular attention to head trauma, neck injury, hypothermia, and barotrauma. Trauma requires neck immobilization until the lateral neck x-ray film, and ultimately, the full cervical spine series is cleared. Patients should be rewarmed in accordance with the clinical protocol outlined in Chapter 51. Slow decompression* is required if the injury was secondary to barotrauma.

1. Pulmonary management.
   a. Oxygenation is essential. Humidified oxygen at 3-6 L/min is given by mask or nasal cannula until stabilization and evaluation are completed. Continuous positive airway pressure (CPAP) should be considered if an FiO_2 greater than 40% is needed. In the awake, cooperative patient, a CPAP of 10-12 cm H_2O can be administered by a tightly fitting face mask or other device. Otherwise, intubation may be required.
   b. Intubation and initiation of positive end-expiratory pressure (PEEP) or CPAP are indicated if there is clear evidence of progressive pulmonary edema with an FiO_2 greater than 40% required, particularly if CPAP delivered by mask has been unsuccessful. PEEP should be initiated at 5 cm H_2O and increased slowly, monitoring oxygenation and cardiac output. If the cardiac output decreases, increasing the intravascular volume may be useful.
   c. Intubation and mechanical ventilation are indicated if the patient is unable to handle secretions, if respiratory failure (PaO_2 less than 50 mm Hg and $PaCO_2$ greater than 50 mm Hg at room air at sea level) is present, if there is a severe metabolic acidosis, or if the patient has developed evidence of cerebral edema.

*Information about decompression chambers can be obtained from the Diver's Alert Network: telephone 919-684-8111.

d. Monitor ABGs and oximetry.
   e. Bronchospasm may require specific β-adrenergic (albuterol) therapy (p. 769).
2. Cerebral edema secondary to hypoxic injury (or head trauma): ICP monitor may be useful in measuring the therapeutic effect (p. 419). Optimally maintain ICP less than or equal to 20 mm Hg and CPP greater than or equal to 50 mm Hg. Measures to reduce ICP may include one or more of the following:
   a. Hyperventilate the patient to maintain a $PaCO_2$ of 22 to 27 mm Hg.
   b. Elevate the head of bed 30 degrees if vital signs, cervical spine, and head injuries from trauma are stable.
   c. Give furosemide (Lasix), 1 mg/kg/dose up to 3 mg/kg/dose q6hr, which may be repeated q2hr if indicated.
   d. Give mannitol, 0.5 gm/kg/dose over 30 minutes q3-4hr prn IV. Effect lasts 2 to 3 hours and there may be rebound. Use only when patient is symptomatic.
   e. Restrict fluids to 50% to 60% of maintenance rate while keeping CVP in the low to normal range (8 to 10 mm Hg) and urine output between 0.5 and 1.0 ml/kg/hr. Initial resuscitation may require a fluid bolus.
   f. Barbiturates are controversial. No evidence that they affect outcome independently of associated hyperthermia. Intracranial monitor necessary.
      • Pentobarbital (Nembutal): initial dose of 3-20 mg/kg IV slowly push while monitoring BP. Maintain infusion of 1-2 mg/kg/hr. Level should be maintained between 25 and 40 μg/ml. Levels above 30 μg/ml are associated with hypotension in as many as 60% of patients.
   g. Muscle relaxants may be required if the patient is symptomatic and requires ventilation. Intubate. Pancuronium (Pavulon), 0.1 mg/kg/dose q1hr or prn IV.
3. Other considerations.

a. Acidosis, if present, requires treatment. Sodium bicarbonate, 1 mEq/kg/dose IV, may be given. Subsequent doses may be required in response to changes in ABG.

b. Hypoxic seizures may be controlled by oxygen, ventilation, and diazepam (Valium), 0.2-0.3 mg/kg/dose IV, or lorazepam (Ativan), 0.05-0.15 mg/kg/dose IV over 1 to 3 minutes, until seizures cease. Control airway. Begin phenobarbital or phenytoin (Dilantin) (see Chapter 21).

c. Antibiotics are administered only with specific indications.

d. Steroids have no proven value beyond their controversial role in the treatment of cerebral edema or aspiration pneumonia after near-drowning.

e. Fevers may indicate that a secondary infection exists such as pneumonitis. It should be treated aggressively with appropriate antibiotics and antipyretics.

f. Maintain normal electrolyte, glucose, etc., levels.

g. Avoid procedures that may be poorly tolerated.

h. Emotional support for the family and friends is imperative.

DISPOSITION

All patients with significant episodes of near-drowning require admission to the hospital, particularly in view of the delayed onset of symptoms. Most require the monitoring available in an intensive care unit. Cessation of treatment may be guided by the prognostic factors that have been defined and clinical response to support.

Parental Education

1. Teach swimming and water safety techniques at an early age but probably not less than 3 years.

2. Define water areas the children cannot use. Fence them off.

3. Children require supervision near water and boats. Always have appropriate supervision. Keep rescue devices and first aid equipment near pools.

4. Children with seizure disorders may swim if they have been seizure free for 1 to 2 years but then only with supervision.

REFERENCES

American Academy of Pediatrics Council on Injury and Poison Prevention: Drowning in infants, children, and adolescents, *Pediatrics* 92:292, 1993.

Biggart MJ, Bohn D: Effect of hypothermia and cardiac arrest on outcome of near drowning accidents in children, *J Pediatr* 117:179, 1990.

Graf WD, Cummings P, Quan L, et al: Predicting outcome in pediatric submersion victims, *Ann Emerg Med* 26:312, 1995.

Griest KJ, Zumwalt RE: Child abuse by drowning, *Pediatrics* 83:41, 1989.

Habib DM, Tecklenburg FW, Webb SA, et al: Prediction of childhood drowning and near drowning morbidity and mortality, *Pediatr Emerg Care* 12:255, 1996.

Harley JR, Ochsenschlager DW: Near drowning. In Barkin RM, editor: *Pediatric emergency medicine: concepts and clinical practice*, ed 2, St Louis, 1997, Mosby.

Kyriacou DN, Arcinue EL, Peek C, et al: Effect of immediate resuscitation of children with submersion injury, *Pediatrics* 94:133, 1994.

LaVelle JM, Shaw KN, Seidl T, et al: Ten-year review of pediatric bathtub near-drownings: evaluation for child abuse and neglect, *Ann Emerg Med* 25:344, 1995.

Nichter MA, Everett PH: Childhood near-drowning: is cardiopulmonary resuscitation always indicated? *Crit Care Med* 17:993, 1989.

Orlowski JP, Abulleck MM, Phillips JM: The hemodynamic and cardiovascular effects of near drowning in hypotonic, isotonic or hypertonic solutions, *Ann Emerg Med* 18:1044, 1989.

Quan L, Wentz ICR, Gore EJ: Outcome and predictors of outcome in pediatric submersion receiving prehospital care in Kings County, Washington, *Pediatrics* 86:586, 1991.

Spack L, Gebeit R, Splaingard M, et al: Failure of aggressive therapy to alter outcome in pediatric near drowning, *Pediatr Emerg Care* 13:98, 1997.

Weinstein MD, Krieger BF: Near drowning: epidemiology, pathophysiology, and initial treatment, *J Emerg Med* 14:461, 1996.

Wintemute GJ: Childhood drowning and near-drowning in the United States, *Am J Dis Child* 144:663, 1990.

48 ELECTRICAL AND LIGHTNING INJURIES

ALERT: Extent of burns does not reflect severity of injury.

Electrical and lightning injuries have similar clinical presentations, both affecting the electrical charge of functional cells, particularly conductive tissue of the nervous system and heart, and causing cell death by intense heat. Individuals may have direct contact with electrical sources, such as high-tension wires or faulty wiring in a home, or they may be struck by lightning. The injury will reflect the resistance of the tissue, the path and type of current (alternating is three times more dangerous than direct current), the voltage, and the duration of contact.

Lightning acts as a massive DC countershock, instantly depolarizing the myocardium and causing asystole, whereas ventricular fibrillation occurs with a high-voltage electrical current. Injury may be caused by a direct hit, by a charge jumping from object to object, or by ground current.

DIAGNOSTIC FINDINGS

The patient may have only minor burns or may undergo full cardiac respiratory arrest. Most patients have some evidence of burns.

1. Entry-exit burns. The entry wound is ischemic, with a well-circumscribed area of whitish-yellow material and charred center. The exit wound is extensive, often with indistinct margins.
2. Arc burns, usually across joints.
3. Flame burn, resulting in direct thermal injury.
4. Mouth burns. In children they may look innocuous initially but often involve the labial artery, which, after some delay, may result in significant hemorrhage. This injury commonly results from a child biting on an electrical cord.

The extent of the burns rarely reflects the potential severity of the injury.

Cardiac dysrhythmias and even infarction may occur. Lower voltages produce ventricular fibrillation; higher voltage may produce asystole.

Neurologically, most patients have impaired mental status, with associated paresthesias, headache, aphasia, and paralysis. Abnormalities of memory, mood, and affect may persist for months. There may be permanent damage.

Additional findings include the following:
1. Pulmonary contusion and chest pain
2. Retinal detachment and burns; cataracts (a delayed sequela)
3. Tinnitus, hearing loss, and perforated tympanic membranes
4. Nonspecific abdominal pain, with nausea, vomiting, splenic rupture, intestinal perforation, stress ulcers, and pancreatitis (rarely noted)

Complications

Complications include the following:
1. Cardiac respiratory arrest caused by central respiratory apnea, dysrhythmias, or cardiac ischemia leading to death

323

2. Neurologic complications such as amnesia, headache, sensorineural deafness, visual blurring, sensory complaints, and cerebral edema and intracranial hemorrhages with seizures
3. Fractures, dislocations, cervical spine injury, and amputations secondary to falls, sustained muscle contraction, or direct cell death and neurovascular compromise
4. Acute tubular necrosis resulting from crush injury and myoglobinuria
5. Complications related to extensive burns
6. Vascular injury with thrombosis

Ancillary Data

1. Complete blood count (CBC) with elevated white blood cells (WBC), platelet level.
2. Electrolytes to check on potassium level, which may be elevated.
3. Blood urea nitrogen (BUN) and creatinine levels.
4. Urinalysis (myoglobinuria or hemoglobinuria).
5. Cardiac enzymes. Peak creatine kinase (CK) reduces the amount of muscle injury and the extent of injury.
6. Arterial blood gas (ABG).
7. Electrocardiogram (ECG).
8. X-ray films.
   a. Chest—to check for pulmonary contusion, cardiac decompensation
   b. Bones, cervical spine, and others as indicated

MANAGEMENT

The key to outcome is the adequacy of prehospital care, which must involve the rapid removal of the individual from the source, the institution of appropriate resuscitation, and immobilization of the cervical spine.

Stabilization in the emergency department (ED) should focus on airway and cardiac status and ensure that the cervical spine is stable:

1. Oxygen, IV fluids, nasogastric (NG) tube, and urinary catheter as indicated.
2. ECG and cardiac monitoring. This should be on a prolonged basis if the patient has a dysrhythmia, loss of consciousness, significant injury, chest pain, or hypoxia. Cardiac monitoring is also indicated if the skin was wet at the time of injury or the current flowed across the heart region.
3. Fluid resuscitation must be done empirically on the basis of vital signs and urinary output. Patients with significant myoglobinuria require diuresis. Alkalinization (urine pH ≥ 7.45) achieved by using fluids with one ampule of $NaHCO_3$/L of infusate increases the solubility of myoglobin in the urine.
4. Burn care should be initiated (see Chapter 46).

Lip burns should not be debrided. These patients should be observed for hemorrhage in the hospital for 3 to 4 days. Bleeding is controlled by pressure, with the area kept clean. Special feeding devices and splints may be needed to prevent microstomia. The patient is at risk for bleeding for 5 to 10 days after injury.

In cases of cerebral edema and seizures (p. 419), the following measures should be considered:

1. Hyperventilate to maintain $Paco_2$ at 25 mm Hg.
2. Elevate head of bed 30 degrees if possible.
3. Give furosemide (Lasix), 1 mg/kg/dose q4-6hr IV.
4. Give mannitol, 0.5 gm/kg/dose q3-4hr prn IV, if patient has neurologic symptoms or seizures.
5. Control seizure initially with diazepam (Valium), 0.2-0.3 mg/kg/dose q2-5min prn IV. Initiate other anticonvulsants (see Chapter 21).

Other management techniques include the following:

1. Insertion of NG tube
2. Treatment of associated complications
3. Tetanus immunization, if indicated

DISPOSITION

All patients with a high-voltage injury (>1000 volts) or with any evidence of cardiac, pulmonary, gastrointestinal, or neurologic abnormalities should be hospitalized. Patients with lip burns or those with potential neurovascular compromise require observation. Neurologic, ophthalmologic, otolaryngologic, and plastic surgery consultations may be useful in the management of the patient.

Asymptomatic patients may be discharged after a minimum of 4 hours of observation and after arranging for follow-up.

Parental Education

1. Instruct your child about the dangers of electrical injury.
2. Eliminate access to electrical plugs and wires.
3. In case of lightning, have your child stay indoors or seek shelter in a building away from windows and telephones. If there is no shelter, instruct your child to avoid the highest object in the area, hilltops, open spaces, metal clotheslines, and wire fences. Avoid contact with metal objects such as golf clubs. Remaining in a closed automobile may be protective. Lightning rods and streamer retardants may be useful.
4. If lightning does strike, initiate cardiopulmonary resuscitation (CPR) immediately, if necessary. If contact with an electrical source occurs, withdraw the patient from it without exposing the rescuer to potential injury.

REFERENCES

Bailey B, Guadreault P, Thirierge RL, et al: Cardiac monitoring of children with household electrical injuries, *Ann Emerg Med* 25:612, 1995.

Baker MD, Chiaviello C: Household electrical injuries in children, *Am J Dis Child* 143:59, 1989.

Cherington M: Lightning injuries, *Ann Emerg Med* 25:516, 1995.

Dado DV, Polley W, Kernahan DA: Splinting of oral commissure electrical burns in children, *J Pediatr* 107:92, 1985.

Epperly TD, Stewart JR: The physical effects of lightning injury, *J Fam Pract* 29:267, 1989.

Fish R: Electrical shock, *J Emerg Med* 11:457, 599, 1993.

Hall ML, Sills RM: Electrical and lightning injuries. In Barkin RM, editor: *Pediatric emergency medicine: concepts and clinical practice,* ed 2, St Louis, 1997, Mosby.

Kotagal S, Rawlings CA, Chen S: Neurologic, psychiatric, and cardiovascular complications in children struck by lightning, *Pediatrics* 70:190, 1982.

Thompson JC, Ashwai S: Electrical injuries in children, *Am J Dis Child* 137:231, 1983.

49 HIGH-ALTITUDE SICKNESS AND DYSBARISM

ADAM Z. BARKIN

ALERT: Acute onset of fatigue, respiratory distress, headache, or confusion when adapting to a high altitude requires interventions. Diving injuries require carefully controlled recompression with significant clinical findings.

People often have difficulty making the physiologic adaptation to altitudes above 7500 ft (2500 m), particularly on the initial exposure to the low oxygen content of the air at that height. In up to 25%, evidence of acute mountain sickness develops at 2000 m, whereas 50% of non-acclimated people who ascend rapidly to 10,000 ft develop acute mountain sickness within 6 to 8 hours and respond well to conservative therapy. Most symptoms of hypoxia occur within 48 to 96 hours of arrival at high altitudes and are characterized by one of three clinical presentations (Table 49-1).

The adaptation to increasing altitude is inadequate when symptoms occur. People may have only self-limited fatigue and mild headaches. High-altitude illnesses are characterized by one of three typical clinical presentations (see Table 49-1). It may be rapid in onset, affect the young and healthy, and be life threatening if not promptly recognized and treated.

Factors predisposing individuals to high-altitude sickness include the following:

1. Rapid ascent (airplane versus car versus walking)
2. Return of a high-altitude resident after a period of being at a lower altitude
3. Exercise
4. Preexisting infection
5. Preexisting pulmonary disease
6. Previous episodes

The underlying pathogenesis is a response to relative or absolute hypoxia.

High-altitude retinal hemorrhage (HARH) is rare, occurring in 50% of climbers who ascend to 16,500 ft and 100% of those who ascend to 21,000 ft, usually within 2 to 3 days of arrival at these altitudes. HARH findings include increased dilation of the retinal veins and arteries, retinal hemorrhages, and papilledema without pain. It may be a warning sign of impending high-altitude pulmonary edema (HAPE). If visual changes occur, descent is recommended. Prevention is key, achieved by acclimatization.

Patients with sickle cell (SC) disease may be affected by the hypoxemia of altitudes above 5000 ft. Oxygen is recommended, even for air travelers who have SC disease.

Caution is usually advised for women from low altitudes who wish to travel above 13,000 ft and for women who reside at high altitudes for prolonged periods because of concerns of potential fetal growth retardation and hypoxemia.

Treatment for HAPE is descent to a lower altitude. Nifedipine may be useful, particularly when descent is not readily possible. The adult protocol that has been shown to be efficacious is 10 mg of nifedipine sublingually and 20 mg of

TABLE 49-1   High-Altitude Sickness

	Acute mountain sickness (AMS)	High-altitude pulmonary edema (HAPE)	High-altitude cerebral edema (HACE)
Diagnostic findings	Nausea, vomiting, headache, lethargy, sleep disturbance, tinnitus, vertigo	Shortness of breath, tachypnea, tachycardia, cough, variable cyanosis	Headache, mental confusion, delirium, ataxia, hallucination, seizure, focal neurologic signs, coma
Onset	4-6 hr after reaching high altitude	24-96 hr	48-72 hr
Altitude	>8000 ft	8000-14,000 ft	Usually >12,000 ft
Ancillary data (in addition to those indicated for diagnostic evaluation)	ABG, Chest x-ray study, Electrolytes	ABG, Chest x-ray study, ECG, Bleeding screen	ABG, Electrolytes, CT head
Differential considerations			
Trauma	Concussion, Gastroenteritis	Pulmonary contusion	Head, Meningitis
Infection	Respiratory or CNS infection	Pneumonia	Encephalitis
Metabolic		Uremia	Diabetic ketoacidosis, Uremia, Encephalopathy, $\downarrow\uparrow Na^+$, $\uparrow Ca^{++}$
Intoxication	Salicylates	Multiple	Narcotics
Vascular		CHF	Subarachnoid hemorrhage
Management (all respond to descent)			
Admit	Variable	Yes	Yes
Oxygen	Yes	Yes	Yes
Acetazolamide	Prophylactic	Prophylactic	Prophylactic
Bronchodilator	No	Yes	No
Steroids	Controversial	Yes	Yes
Ventilation with PEEP	No	Yes, if severe	Hyperventilation

slow-release nifedipine. If the systolic blood pressure does not drop more than 10 mm Hg within 10 minutes, the sublingual dose is repeated after 15 minutes. Subsequently, 20 mg of slow-release nifedipine is administered every 6 hours for the period at high altitude.

Dexamethasone has been demonstrated to decrease the symptoms of acute mountain sickness and is specifically recommended when descent is impossible or when it is necessary to facilitate cooperation in the evacuation process.

Prevention must be emphasized. Acclimatization is essential, with attention to the rate of ascent and initiation of a graded exercise program. Acetazolamide (Diamox) is useful in preventing high-altitude sickness (5-10 mg/

TABLE 49-2   Dysbarism Syndrome: Diagnostic Findings

	Barotrauma			Nitrogen necrosis	Decompression sickness
	Otolaryngolic, dental, gastrointestinal	Pulmonary overpressurization syndrome (POPS)	Dysbaric air embolism (DAE)		
Ascent or descent	Both	Ascent	Ascent	Descent	Ascent
Onset	Variable	Before surfacing or at the surface	Within 10 min of surfacing	Variable depths	>10 min after surfacing
Diagnostic findings	Pain in the sinuses, ears, teeth, and abdomen; vertigo; flatulence; hearing impairment	Hoarseness, subcutaneous emphysema, dyspnea, cyanosis, neurologic deterioration, hemoptysis	Seizures, visual impairment, aphasia, altered mental status, multiplegia, hemoptysis, chest pain, cardiac arrest	Incoordination, altered mental status, obtundation	Pruritus, lymph node pain, joint pain, vertigo, deafness, paralysis, seizures, headache, respiratory failure, shock
Ancillary data	Electronystagmogram, audiogram	ABG, chest x-ray film	ABG, electrolytes, coagulation profile, chest x-ray film	None	ABG, electrolytes, coagulation profile, urinalysis, ECG, chest x-ray film
Differential considerations	Otitis media, labyrinthitis, sinusitis, head trauma, gastroenteritis	Pulmonary contusion, head trauma, coagulopathy, pneumonitis, spontaneous pneumothorax	Cerebrovascular disease, coronary vascular disease, cerebral AVM or aneurysm, stroke due to cyanotic heart disease	Metabolic derangement drugs or ethanol intoxication, CNS hemorrhage or infection	Barotrauma, POPS, DAE, exhaustion, dermatitis, muscle strain
Management:					
Admit	Variable	Yes	Yes	Immediate ascent	Yes
Oxygen	No	Yes	Yes	No	Yes
IV hydration	No		Yes	No	Yes
Recompression	No	Yes	Yes	No	Yes

From Smith KM: High altitude illness and dysbarism. In Barkin RM, editor: *Pediatric emergency medicine: concepts and clinical practice*, ed 2, St Louis, 1997, Mosby.

kg/24 hr PO q12hr or in an adult either 250 mg q12hr PO or 500 mg in sustained-release form/24 hr). It should be taken 1 to 2 days before ascent (it is not useful once illness has commenced) and should be continued during ascent. Dexamethasone (initially 8 mg PO followed by 4 mg q6hr PO for at least six doses) may reduce the incidence of acute mountain sickness by 50% in those ascending to 2700 m or above.

DYSBARIC DIVING INJURIES

Divers are subject to barotrauma resulting from barometric pressure changes within body structures. Inadequate pressure adaptation between air-containing cavities and ambient atmosphere causes tissue damage, most commonly in the ear, paranasal sinuses, gastrointestinal (GI) tract, and chest. Problems may also be caused by breathing gases of elevated partial pressure (i.e., nitrogen narcosis and decompression sickness).

The diagnostic findings are presented in Table 49-2. Help with the treatment of diving-related incidents may be obtained from the U.S. Diving Accident Network (919-684-8111).

REFERENCES

Arthur DC, Margulies RA: A short course in diving medicine, *Ann Emerg Med* 16:689, 1987.

Dembert ML, Keith JF: Evaluating the potential pediatric scuba diver, *Am J Dis Child* 140:1135, 1986.

Foulke GE: Altitude-related illness, *Am J Emerg Med* 3:217, 1985.

Hackett PH, Roach RC: Medical therapy of altitude illness, *Ann Emerg Med* 16:980, 1987.

Larson EB, Roach RC, Schoene RB, et al: Acute mountain sickness and acetazolamide: clinical efficacy and effects on ventilation, *JAMA* 248:328, 1982.

Levine BD, Yoshimura K, Kobayasizi J, et al: Dexamethasone in the treatment of acute mountain sickness, *N Engl J Med* 321: 1907, 1989.

Montgomery AB, Luce JM, Michael P, et al: Effects of dexamethasone on the incidence of acute mountain sickness at two intermediate altitudes, *JAMA* 261:734, 1989.

Oelz O, Ritter M, Jenni R, et al: Nifedipine for high altitude pulmonary edema, *Lancet* 867(2):1241, 1989.

Shupak A, Doweck I, Greenberg E, et al: Diving-related inner ear injuries, Laryngoscope 101:173, 1991.

Theis MK, Honigman B, Yip R, et al: Acute mountain sickness in children at 2835 meters. Am J Dis Child 147:143, 1993.

Tso E: High-altitude illness. Emerg Med Clin North Am 10:231, 1992.

50 HYPERTHERMIA

ALERT: Prompt attention must be given to fluid management and cooling.

Exposure to environmental heat without appropriate acclimatization, equipment, or fluid replacement may lead to a variety of clinical presentations that are usually preventable. Particularly at risk are athletes, laborers, soldiers, the chronically ill, and the very young or old when the air temperature exceeds the skin temperature (Table 50-1).

Children acclimatize more slowly than adults to exercise in the heat. Youngsters have a greater surface area/mass ratio than adults and produce more metabolic heat per mass unit when walking or running. Sweating capacity is not as great in children as adults, nor is the ability to convey heat by blood from the body core to the periphery.

HEAT CRAMPS
Etiology

Heat cramps are caused by sodium depletion from prolonged or excessive exercise, accompanied by profuse sweating, in an environment with high temperature and low humidity. Thirst is relieved by fluids that do not contain salt.

Diagnostic Findings

Patients are alert and oriented, with normal or slightly elevated temperatures. They experience severe cramps in those skeletal muscles subjected to intense exercise, most commonly the legs.

Ancillary Data

Low serum sodium level indicates heat cramps.

Differential Diagnosis

1. Intrapsychic: hyperventilation
2. Metabolic: hypokalemia
3. Trauma: black widow spider bite

Management

1. Hydration
   a. If severe, 0.9% normal saline (NS) solution at 20 ml/kg/hr over 1 to 2 hours
   b. If mild, oral salt solution: 1 tsp NaCl (4 gm) in 500 ml of water administered at same rate as in *(a)*
2. Rest

HEAT EXHAUSTION
Etiology

Heat exhaustion is caused by exposure to a high-temperature environment, with continuous sweating and lack of appropriate replenishment of water or salt.

Diagnostic Findings

Many individuals have a combination of the following:

1. *Water depletion:* inadequate water replacement (see Chapter 7 for hyperna-

TABLE 50-1 Environmental Heat Illnesses: Clinical Presentation

Condition	Predisposing cause	Central nervous system	Skin	Muscle cramps	Thirst	Rectal temperature	Blood pressure	Pulse	Management
Heat cramps	Muscle work, sodium depletion, drinking large quantities of water	WNL	Sweating	Severe	WNL	<40° C	WNL	WNL	Replace salt
Heat exhaustion	Heat exposure: (1) without access to water, (2) with replacement of sweat loss with water only	Fatigue, weakness, headache, anxiety	Sweating	Variable	Variable	<40° C	Tends to be low	Tends to be low	Replace salt or water
Heat stroke	Heat exposure, K^-–Na^+ depletion, impaired sweating, increased heat production	Headache, listlessness, confusion, seizure, psychosis, coma	Hot, dry	Variable	Abnormal	>40° C	Abnormal (high or low)	Elevated	Cooling and support

tremic dehydration). Signs and symptoms of dehydration are thirst, irritability, fatigue, anxiety, and disorientation. Temperature is usually normal.

2. *Salt depletion:* inadequate salt replacement—the more common type of heat exhaustion. Signs and symptoms of salt depletion are fatigue, headache, nausea, vomiting, diarrhea, and muscle cramps. Temperature is normal or slightly increased. An acclimatized individual has a lower salt content of sweat.

Complications
1. Shock
2. Seizures and coma

Ancillary Data
Serum sodium level may be high (water depletion) or low (salt depletion).

Management

Necessary stabilization must be provided. Management must reflect the underlying cause. In patients with only modest elevations in body temperature, oral fluids and sprinkling water over the body to increase evaporative losses may be adequate. In severe disease with obtundation, intravenous fluid should be initiated. If water depletion is accompanied by hypernatremic dehydration, fluid should be instituted slowly in accordance with the protocol in Chapter 7. With salt depletion and isotonic or hypotonic dehydration:

• Initiate 20 ml/kg of 0.9% NS over 30 minutes; then follow protocol for dehydration (see Chapter 7).

Disposition

Patients with significant dehydration should be admitted for fluid management and monitoring. Those with no metabolic abnormalities and only mild symptoms may be discharged after initial fluid push.

Prevention requires the availability and intake of appropriate fluids.

HEAT STROKE
Etiology

The body's heat dissipation system (sweating, radiation, and convection) is overwhelmed by production and absorption of heat. Underlying conditions may contribute to this imbalance.

1. Trauma/physical
   a. Environment: particularly in the newborn, who has immature thermoregulation and is more dependent on the environment
   b. Burns (see Chapter 46)
2. Congenital
   a. Cystic fibrosis—excessive sweating and salt loss
   b. Dermatologic: anhidrotic ectodermal dysplasia, ichthyosis
3. Intoxication (see Table 54-1)
   a. Decreased sweating—antihistamines, phenothiazines, anticholinergics, and cardiac β blockers
   b. Increased heat production and impaired sweating—amphetamines, lysergic acid diethylamide (LSD), phencyclidine (PCP), and thyroid replacements
   c. Increased heat absorption—ethanol

Diagnostic Findings

Heat stroke may be caused by the following:
1. Exertion, which has a rapid course
2. A preexisting condition that has a slow onset (nonexertional)
3. Intoxication

Symptoms include the following:
1. Anorexia, nausea, vomiting, headache, fatigue, and confusion or disorientation, possibly progressing to coma and posturing
2. Skin that is red, hot, and dry
3. High temperatures (>40° C), accompanied by tachycardia and hypotension

Complications
1. Coma with permanent neurologic sequelae
2. Acute tubular necrosis (p. 809)
3. Acidosis
4. Dysrhythmias (see Chapter 6)

5. Rhabdomyolysis and myoglobinuria
6. Hepatic damage
7. Coagulopathy with disseminated intravascular coagulation (DIC) and thrombocytopenia (see Chapter 79)
8. Death

Ancillary Data
1. Arterial blood gas. Changes in body temperature alter true values. For each degree greater than 37° C, the following adjustments to the measured value should be made:

pH	↓ 0.015
Pa_{CO_2}	↑ 4.4%
Pa_{O_2}	↑ 7.2%

NOTE: The opposite adjustment should be made for each less than 37° C.

2. Electrolytes (hyperkalemia, hypokalemia, hyponatremia, hypernatremia), blood urea nitrogen (BUN) (increased), and glucose (hyperglycemia)
3. Complete blood count and platelets
4. Electrocardiogram: ST depression, nonspecific T-wave changes, premature ventricular complex (PVC), supraventricular tachycardia
5. Bleeding and disseminated intravascular coagulation screen, if appropriate
6. Other studies to evaluate nature of underlying condition

Differential Diagnosis

1. Infection: meningitis or encephalitis; rickettsial disease: typhus, Rocky Mountain spotted fever; malaria
2. Endocrine: hypothalamic disorder

Management

Heat stroke is life threatening and requires rapid intervention. Initial stabilization in the field should include removing the patient from the heat and drenching or immersing the individual in cool water. The airway should be stabilized and oxygen administered. Circulatory status should be assessed and intravenous fluids initiated. Patients require ongoing cardiac and rectal temperature probe monitoring.

Other management techniques include the following:

1. Ice bath (if unavailable, fan patient while sprinkling water or use ice packs) until patient reaches 38.5° C. Simultaneously massage extremities.
2. Intravenous fluids appropriate to the patient's electrolyte levels and fluid balance. Initially, give 0.9% NS at 20 ml/kg over 45 to 60 minutes. If cardiac status is unstable, insert a central venous line.
3. Foley catheter, with nasogastric tube to minimize aspiration.
4. Diazepam, 0.2-0.3 mg/kg/dose IV for treatment of shivering.

Disposition

All patients should be admitted to an intensive care unit (ICU).

Prevention includes ensurance of adequate water and salt intake during heat exposure. The intensity of activities that last more than 30 minutes should be reduced when there is relatively high humidity and air temperature. A warm-up period may be useful. Children should not be left unattended in automobiles.

Individuals with cystic fibrosis or a dermatologic problem should avoid prolonged exposure. Response to predisposing drugs should be monitored.

Runners in hot weather should drink 100 to 300 ml of water 10 to 15 minutes before a race and drink about 250 ml of water every 3 to 4 km. Fluid losses may exceed electrolyte abnormalities. Clothing should be lightweight.

REFERENCES

Gentile DA, Kennedy BC: Wilderness medicine in children, *Pediatrics* 88:967, 1991.

Mellor MFA: Heat-induced illnesses. In Barkin RM, editor: *Pediatric emergency medicine: concepts and clinical practice,* ed 2, St Louis, 1997, Mosby.

Robinson MD, Seward PN: Heat injury in children, *Pediatr Emerg Care* 3:114, 1987.

Sessler DI: Malignant hyperthermia, *J Pediatr* 109:9, 1986.

Rek D, Olshaker JS: Heat illness, *Emerg Med Clin North Am* 10:299, 1992.

Tomarken JL, Britt BA: Malignant hyperthermia, *Ann Emerg Med* 16:1253, 1987.

51 HYPOTHERMIA AND FROSTBITE

ADAM Z. BARKIN

ALERT: Resuscitation must continue in the pulseless, apneic patient until the core temperature is at least 30° C.

Hypothermia exists when a patient's core temperature is 35° C or less. It results from prolonged exposure, conditions that secondarily contribute to hypothermia, or systemic diseases that interfere with thermoregulation.

Temperature control is a balance of heat loss and heat production. Loss is associated with heat flow from hot to cold by radiation or conduction, the latter including convection and evaporation. Heat dissipation results from blood flow, sweating, excretion of warm urine and feces, and exhalation of air. Voluntary muscle exercise, eating, and shivering produce heat.

Neonates are particularly at risk because of their relatively large surface area and small percentage of subcutaneous fat.

Progressive decrease in core temperature initially produces changes in basal metabolic rate, vasoconstriction, increased antidiuretic hormone (ADH), and impaired cerebral blood flow. Below 29° C, thermoregulation is lost; this is accompanied by vasodilation, impaired cardiac and central nervous system (CNS) function, slowed nerve conduction, and cardiac irritability. Eventually apnea and asystole become prominent.

ETIOLOGY (AND ASSOCIATED CONDITIONS)

1. Trauma/physical
   a. Exposure
   b. Near-drowning (see Chapter 47)
   c. Head or spinal cord injury (see Chapter 57)
   d. Subdural hematoma (see Chapter 57)
2. Infection
   a. Bacterial meningitis (p. 725)
   b. Encephalitis
   c. Respiratory infection (p. 794)
   d. Gram-negative septicemia
3. Endocrine/metabolic factors
   a. Hypoglycemia (see Chapter 38)
   b. Diabetic ketoacidosis (p. 615)
   c. Hypopituitarism
   d. Myxedema (p. 624)
   e. Addison's disease (see Chapter 74)
   f. Uremia (p. 809)
4. Intoxication (see Table 54-1)
   a. Alcohol
   b. Barbiturates
   c. Carbon monoxide
   d. Narcotics
   e. Phenothiazines
   f. Anesthetics, general
   g. Cyclic antidepressants
5. Degenerative/deficiencies
   a. CNS disease
   b. Malnutrition and kwashiorkor
6. Vascular factors
   a. Shock (see Chapter 5)
   b. Subarachnoid hemorrhage (see Chapter 18)
   c. Pulmonary embolism (p. 568)
   d. Cerebrovascular accident

335

7. Intrapsychic: anorexia nervosa
8. Neoplasm, intracranial

DIAGNOSTIC FINDINGS

The severity of the findings reflect the degree and duration of hypothermia and the nature of any underlying or predisposing condition. Special low-reading thermometers are required.

In general, the progression of signs and symptoms reflect the degree of hypothermia:

Core temperature	Common signs and symptoms
35° C (95° F)	Slurred speech, lapse of memory, shivering maximum.
32° C (89° F)	Diminished mental status: drowsy, amnesic, confused, disoriented. Muscle rigidity, poor muscle coordination.
30° C (86° F)	Skin cyanotic, edematous. Stuporous, irritable. Progressive decline in basal metabolic state. Shivering stops. Myocardial irritability, bradycardia. J (or Osborne) waves on electrocardiogram (ECG), decreased cardiac output, and hypotension. Decreased minute ventilation.
28° C (82° F)	Dysrhythmias common. Bradycardia in up to 50%, refractory to atropine with progression to ventricular fibrillation and asystole. This is the cardiac fibrillatory threshold at which ventricular fibrillation can be induced by cardiac stimulation.
26° C (79° F)	Loss of consciousness, areflexive.
25° C (77° F)	Respirations cease, dead appearance.

General Findings

1. Patients will initially have tachycardia, progressing to bradycardia associated with a decreased respiratory rate, tidal volume, and hypoxia at 30° C. Blood pressure declines with decreased cardiac output. On rewarming, patients may exhibit shock secondary to the initial vasodilation.
2. Myocardial irritability and impaired pacemaker function lead to atrial and ventricular dysrhythmias and bradycardia. Asystole and electromechanical dissociation (or pulseless electrical activity [PEA]) develop at 20° C.
3. Neurologic status progresses from slight ataxia, slurred speech, and hyperesthesias to frank coma. Recovery on warming may be slow.
4. Body heat is partially maintained by shivering, which ceases somewhere between 30° and 33° C. Pallor and cyanosis are noted. Muscular rigidity develops.
5. Renal function is diminished with poor renal perfusion. Oliguria may be noted.
6. With profound hypothermia (often <25° C), the patient will appear apneic, rigid, pulseless, areflexive, and unresponsive, with fixed, dilated pupils.
7. Infants with hypothermia have decreased feeding, lethargy, edema of the limbs, and cold, erythematous, and scleremic (hardened) skin. Bradycardia and abdominal distension may be observed. Metabolic acidosis, hypoglycemia, and hyperkalemia are usually present.

Complications

Frostbite

1. Ice crystallization in the cells associated with vasoconstriction
2. Fingers, hands, feet, toes, ears, and nose most common sites
3. Severity of injury depends on temperature, duration of exposure, wind-chill factor, immobility, tightness of clothing, and dampness of environment
4. Classification

Degree	Clinical presentation
First	Skin is mottled, edematous, hyperemic, with burning and tingling. Peaks in 24 to 48 hours and may persist for 1 to 2 weeks.
Second	Blister formation with paresthesia and anesthesia.

Degree	Clinical presentation
Third (deep)	Necrosis of skin with ulceration and edema. Involves subcutaneous tissue.
Fourth (deep)	Necrosis with gangrene. Vesicle followed by eschar and ulceration. Progression over 24 to 36 hours. Demarcation may take several weeks.

5. The initial evaluation may be faulty because involvement is dynamic.

Other Complications

1. Metabolic abnormalities: metabolic acidosis, hypoglycemia, hyperkalemia
2. Gastrointestinal bleeding (see Chapter 35)
3. Acute renal failure (p. 809)
4. Pancreatitis (p. 644)
5. Hypovolemia secondary to shift of fluids into extracellular spaces
6. Sepsis
7. Dysrhythmias
8. Deep vein thrombosis (p. 568)
9. Coagulopathy, disseminated intravascular coagulation (DIC), thrombocytopenia, leukopenia (see Chapter 79)
10. Pulmonary edema (see Chapter 19)

Ancillary Data

1. Arterial blood gas. Changes in body temperature alter true values. For each degree below 37° C, the following adjustment to the measured value should be made.

pH	↑ 0.015
P_{CO_2}(mm Hg)	↓ 4.4%
P_{O_2} (mm Hg)	↓ 7.2%

Recent studies suggest that measurements should be reported uncorrected after the blood sample is warmed to 37.1° C (98.6° F) for analysis.

NOTE: The opposite adjustment should be made for each degree greater than 37° C.

2. ECG: Dysrhythmias are noted with progression—for example, J (or Osborne) wave at about 30° C. It appears as a "camel-humped" deflection of the QRS-ST junction.

3. Chemical evaluation.
   a. Hyperkalemia secondary to metabolic acidosis, renal failure, or rhabdomyolysis.
   b. Blood urea nitrogen (BUN) and creatinine levels increased.
   c. Increased amylase level.
   d. Glucose level increased when patient is cold and decreased during rewarming. Liver function test results elevated with hepatitis.
4. Hematologic evaluation.
   a. Possible coagulopathy with DIC
   b. Thrombocytopenia and leukopenia secondary to sequestration; possible hemoconcentration
5. Studies to assess status of underlying conditions.

MANAGEMENT

Initial management must stabilize the patient's condition and treat underlying conditions. In addition to standard resuscitation regimens, the patient should be moved to a warm environment and clothing should be removed. Handling of the patient should be minimized to avoid precipitating a dysrhythmia. Cardiac and rectal probe monitors are necessary. Hypoglycemia and hypoxia should be corrected with administration of oxygen, glucose, and warmed IV solutions. Underlying conditions need prompt attention. A low-reading thermometer is needed. Closed-chest compressions maintain neurologic viability in hypothermic patients hours longer than in normothermic patients. Prehospital misdiagnosis of cardiac arrest is a hazard.

Temperatures >32° C (Mild/Moderate)

1. Initiate passive external rewarming by warming the patient in blankets, optimally in a warm room to maintain peripheral vasoconstrictors.
2. Attempt to raise the temperature 0.5° to 2.0° C/hr.

3. If no increase in temperature is seen in 2 hours, evaluate for underlying disease and initiate active rewarming.

Temperature <32° C (Moderate/Severe)

1. Begin active rewarming at 0.5° C/hr. Patient may experience rewarming shock during treatment (vasodilation may cause transient fall in blood pressure).
2. Monitor at all times. Handle patient carefully.
3. Avoid inserting intracardiac monitors and administering adrenergic drugs until the temperature is greater than 28° C, if possible. If necessary, preoxygenate patient before performing invasive procedures.
4. Administer oxygen, humidified and heated if possible. If intubation is required, preoxygenate well.

If the cardiovascular system is *stable,* active external rewarming is appropriate, using a radiant heater, warmed blankets, chemical hot packs, and heated objects (e.g., water bottle) applied primarily to the trunk. With temperature below 28° C, emergency intervention is needed.

If the cardiovascular system is *unstable,* the patient experiences diabetic ketoacidosis (insulin inactive at <30° C), endocrinologic insufficiency, peripheral vasodilation due to trauma or ingestion, or spinal cord injury or external rewarming is ineffective, initiate active core rewarming, which may be used in conjunction with active external rewarming procedures. Techniques that may be used individually or in combination include the following:

1. Humidified oxygen delivered at about 40.5° C (105° F) to 42° C (107.6° F) by either mask or endotracheal tube.
2. Warmed (36° to 40° C) intravenous fluids: D5W 0.9% NS without potassium is preferred.
3. Peritoneal dialysis using K^+-free dialysate heated to 40.5° to 42.5° C. Warmed lavage (gastric enema, bladder, pleural) fluid may be useful.
4. Hemodialysis and extracorporeal blood rewarming. These are controversial but may be attempted if other approaches are unsuccessful. It is clearly indicated in the arrested, unresponsive patient or the non-arrested, stable patient with concomitant significant drug overdose, infection, or trauma. It should be continued until a core temperature of 30° to 32° C is achieved. It is logistically difficult and may produce complications, including bleeding.
5. Active rewarming should generally be discontinued when the core temperature reaches 32° to 34° C to prevent overheating.

Dysrhythmias

Lidocaine and bretylium are effective in treatment of hypothermic ventricular dysrhythmias. Defibrillation is usually not effective at less than 29.4° C (85° F). If ventricular fibrillation occurs at greater than 29.4° C, one attempt at defibrillation is warranted. If this fails, a single intravenous bolus of lidocaine or bretylium may be useful. Bradycardia and atrial fibrillation usually revert with warming.

Frostbite

1. Initial treatment in the field must include careful handling with rewarming only if there is no chance of a second freezing during transport. Superficial first- and second-degree injuries of the hand may be treated in the field by holding the fingers in the armpits or blowing on them with hot air. Once warmed they should be covered with a dry, clean cloth.
2. Deep frostbite should be treated definitively by immersion of the extremity or part in tepid water (40.5° to 43.3° C) for 20 minutes after core rewarming is well under way. Protect the involved tissue from

further damage. After warming, apply sterile gauze and elevate for 40 minutes.

3. Amputation of fourth-degree injuries must be delayed until there is good demarcation of necrotic tissue. Gentle debridement may be done.
4. Hyperbaric oxygen (HBO) therapy may be useful.
5. Analgesics may be required. Handle involved area gently.
6. Tetanus prophylaxis may be appropriate.

DISPOSITION

Patients with hypothermia require hospitalization, and those with core temperatures less than 32° C should be admitted to an intensive care unit (ICU). The best predictors of outcome are the underlying disease and response to therapy. Patients with only superficial frostbite may be sent home.

Patients should be informed about the importance of appropriate clothing. Layering allows air trapping (air is an effective insulator), which reduces heat loss by conduction and convection. Wicking facilitates movement of sweat from the surface of the skin to outer layers of clothing. Garments should be nonconstricting and provide special protection of hands, face, and feet.

REFERENCES

Cornelli HM: Accidental hypothermia, *J Pediatr* 120:671, 1992.

Danzl DF, Pozos RS: Accidental hypothermia, *N Engl J Med* 331:1756, 1994.

Delaney KA, Howland MA, Vassallo S, et al: Assessment of acid base disturbances in hypothermia and their physiologic consequences, *Ann Emerg Med* 18:72, 1989.

Heggers JP, Phillips LG, McCauley RL, et al: Frostbite: experimental and clinical evolutions of treatment, *J Wilderness Med* 1:27, 1990.

Hofstrand HT: Accidental hypothermia and frostbite. In Barkin RM, editor: *Pediatric emergency medicine: concepts and clinical practice,* ed 2, St Louis, 1997, Mosby.

Jolly BT, Ghezzi KT: Accidental hypothermia, *Emerg Med Clin North Am* 10:311, 1992.

Otto RJ, Metzler MH: Rewarming from experimental hypothermia: comparison of heated aerosol inhalation, peritoneal lavage, and pleural lavage, *Crit Care Med* 16:869, 1988.

Weinberg AD: Hypothermia, *Ann Emerg Med* 22:374, 1993.

Zell SC, Kurtz KJ: Severe exposure hypothermia: a resuscitation protocol, *Ann Emerg Med* 14:339, 1985.

52 RADIATION INJURIES

Radiation injuries most commonly result from transportation, nuclear facility, or industrial accidents. Ionizing radiation may consist of alpha (noninjurious), beta (minimal surface injury), or gamma (penetrates deeply, causing acute radiation injury) exposure. Injury depends on the amount of body surface exposed, the length of exposure, the distance from the source, the type of radiation, and shielding techniques.

The normal background annual radiation exposure is 110 mrem/year. A chest radiogram has about 10 mrem/study.

The clinical presentation is delineated in relation to dose in Table 52-1. It reflects the type and amount of radiation, length of exposure, distance of source to victim, amount and type of shields, and continuous nature of exposure.

From the perspective of the receiving hospital, the following steps should be taken:

1. Advance notification of arrival should be received.
2. Treatment areas, with specific entrance, should be designated.
3. Personnel should wear operating room attire with gloves.
4. Life-saving measures should be performed first.
5. Contamination should be defined with radiation detectors.
6. Patient should be washed with washcloths, soap, and water.
7. After the patient's condition is medically stable, exposure should be evaluated.
   a. External contamination: Clothing should be removed with proper disposal. Swabs of orifices should be obtained for sampling and the patient washed with warm water and soap. Eyes are irrigated and open wounds

TABLE 52-1   Radiation Dose-Effect Relationship

Whole body radiation dose (RAD)	Clinical manifestations
<150	Asymptomatic or mild symptoms (anorexia, nausea, vomiting) Mild depression of white cells and platelets
400	Mild nausea and vomiting Hematologic change with lymphocyte depression within 48 hr
400-600	Serious symptoms; nausea, vomiting, diarrhea, bleeding, infection Hematologic depression of about 75% within 48 hr Mortality >50%
600-1500	Severe nausea, vomiting, diarrhea, progressing to coma Severe hematologic changes Mortality up to 100%
>5000	Fulminant course with GI, cardiovascular, and CNS complications Death within 48 hr

are irrigated. All waste water must be collected and placed in appropriate containers.

b. Internal contamination: Prevent absorption and increase elimination. Gastric lavage is followed by administration of antacids to precipitate heavy metals. Chelation may be useful.

c. Partial body exposure whereby part of body receives large dose of radiation.

d. Acute radiation syndrome (ARS).

8. Expert medical consultation is usually necessary to assist in management. Routine steps for symptomatic patients with significant exposure include isolation; fluids; bowel sterilization with antibiotics; red blood cell (RBC), platelet, and granulocyte infusions; and infection control and monitoring.

REFERENCES

Asch SM, Cosimi L: Radiation exposures. In Barkin RM, editor: *Pediatric emergency medicine: concepts and clinical practice,* ed 2, St Louis, 1997, Mosby.

Mettler FD: Emergency management of radiation accidents, *J Am Coll Emerg Phys* 7:302, 1978.

Vyas DR, Dick RM, Crawford J: Management of radiation accident and exposure, *Pediatr Emerg Care* 10:232, 1994.

53 SMOKE INHALATION

ALERT: Airway stabilization is imperative.

Smoke inhalation most commonly accompanies major burns and is considered to be the major respiratory complication of thermal burns (see Chapter 46). Several factors affect toxicity:

1. Heat of gases. Inhalation of heated gas at 150° C may result in injuries to the face, nasal mucosa, oropharynx, and upper airway. Adding moisture to the air increases injury to the upper airway. Air is rapidly cooled after reaching the vocal cords.
2. Particulate matter. Particulate matter deposition with adsorbed toxins may lead to chemical injury, tracheobronchitis, and pulmonary edema.
3. Toxic gases. Most common is carbon monoxide (CO). Others include hydrogen cyanide, aldehydes, ammonia, chlorine, and hydrochloric acid.

ETIOLOGY

1. Direct thermal injury to respiratory tract, often associated with flame burns in a closed room
   a. Major burns
   b. Nasopharyngeal—circumoral burns
      (1) Singed nasal hairs
      (2) Singed eyelids and eyebrows
2. Inhalation of toxins, often secondary to noxious fumes that may be the products of combustion

   a. Acetic acid (petroleum products)
   b. Formic acid or aldehydes (wood, cotton, paper, petroleum products)
   c. Chlorine (polyvinylchloride)
   d. Hydrochloric acid or HCN (hydrocyanic acid) (plastics)
3. CO poisoning
4. Hypoxia, usually secondary to closed-space fire

DIAGNOSTIC FINDINGS

1. Patients usually demonstrate thermal burns (see Chapter 46) and may have evidence of CO poisoning (p. 371).
2. Patients demonstrate evidence of direct thermal damage to the upper respiratory tract (which may be delayed up to 24 hours), for example, stridor, hoarseness, and black or brown carbonaceous sputum.
3. Lower airway findings reflect the irritant effects of noxious gases and particulate matter, alveolar-capillary membrane damage, and ultimately pulmonary edema/infiltrates from impaired mucociliary transport, diminished surfactant production, and macrophage dysfunction.
4. Concurrently patients may have CO poisoning, hypoxia, and upper airway obstruction. The relative hypoxia may cause confusion and agitation; rare cases progress to coma.

Complications

1. Upper airway obstruction, secondary to mucosal injury, similar to croup
2. Pulmonary edema (see Chapter 19), usually developing 1 to 4 days after injury: dyspnea, cough, wheezing, rales, and respiratory distress may be noted
3. Bacterial pneumonia about 1 week after injury

Ancillary Data

All patients require arterial blood gas (ABG), carboxyhemoglobin level, and chest x-ray film.

DIFFERENTIAL DIAGNOSIS

See Chapters 19 and 20.

MANAGEMENT

Humidified oxygen should be administered to all patients. This is appropriate treatment for CO poisoning (p. 371) and direct respiratory tract injury.

1. Manage airway.
   a. If the patient's airway is compromised, intubate and initiate active control. Positive end-expiratory pressure (PEEP) and constant positive airway pressure (CPAP) improve oxygen exchange in the lungs. Indications include the following:
      (1) Respiratory failure (Pao_2 <50 mm Hg and $Paco_2$ >50 mm Hg)
      (2) Severe acidosis
      (3) Laryngeal obstruction
      (4) Difficulty with secretions
   b. If bronchospasm is present, useful bronchodilators include inhaled β agonists (see Chapter 84).
   c. Early bronchoscopy is indicated for significant secretions or direct evaluation of injury when pulmonary lesion is suspected.

2. Manage associated burn, if present (see Chapter 46).
3. Corticosteroids, which increase the mortality rate, are not indicated.

DISPOSITION

All patients with the following findings should be hospitalized:

1. Respiratory failure
2. Carboxyhemoglobin level elevation requiring admission (p. 371)
3. High-risk category: major and most moderate burns, as well as facial or nasal burn
4. Upper airway signs of involvement (hoarseness, stridor)
5. Lower airway involvement (bronchospasm, dyspnea)

Patients with none of these factors may be discharged if follow-up care and observation can be ensured and there is no question of child abuse. Parents must watch for any changes in respiratory status.

Parental Education

1. Call your physician immediately if your child develops any of the following:
   a. Increasing difficulty in breathing
   b. Hoarseness, stridor, cough, or wheezing
   c. Lethargy, agitation, or other behavioral changes
   d. Fever
2. Read information about fire prevention.

REFERENCES

Beeley MJ, et al: Mortality and lung histopathology after inhalation lung injury—the effect of corticosteroids, *Am Rev Respir Dis* 133:191, 1986.

Blinn DL, Slater H, Goldfarb IW: Inhalation injury with burns: a lethal combination, *J Emerg Med* 6:471, 1988.

Lee MJ, O'Connell DJ: The plain chest radiograph after acute smoke inhalation, *Clin Radiol* 39:33, 1988.

Parish RA: Smoke inhalation and carbon monoxide poisoning in children, *Pediatr Emerg Care* 2:36, 1986.

VIII

POISONING AND OVERDOSE

KENNETH W. KULIG and ROGER M. BARKIN

54 MANAGEMENT PRINCIPLES

Poisoning is a significant cause of morbidity and mortality in the United States; it is the fourth most common cause of death in children. Approximately 80% of accidental ingestions occur in children less than 5 years of age, the peak incidence being between 1 and 3 years. In children less than 1 year old, poisoning usually results from therapeutic misuse of drugs. The preschooler is adventuresome and curious and will ingest any accessible household product or medication. The adolescent may experiment with mind-altering drugs, often with peers; manipulative behavior and suicide become important motivators. Family turmoil is commonly present, and the poisoning tends to be recurrent.

Children less than 6 years old ingest a wide variety of substances, most commonly involving cosmetics, cleaning substances, analgesics, plants, cough and cold preparations, foreign bodies, topicals, pesticides, antimicrobials, vitamins, gastrointestinal preparations, arts/crafts/office supplies, hydrocarbons, hormones, and food products. The most significant exposures commonly involve salicylates, alkaline corrosives, acetaminophen, iron, petroleum products, antihistamines, cardiac medications, street drugs, alcohols, cyclic antidepressants, benzodiazepines, barbiturates, pesticides, carbon monoxide, and opiates. Of childhood poisonings, 87% occur in the home. The volume of a normal swallow in an infant is about 0.21 ml/kg, 1 teaspoon (4.5 to 5 ml) in a child 18 to 36 months old, and 15 ml in an adult.

INITIAL CONTACT WITH THE POISONED PATIENT

1. Determine that the ABCs (airway, breathing, and circulation) are being maintained.
2. *Basic information* is essential. Obtain name, weight, and age. Address and telephone number provide a means for later contact.
3. Determine the *type of ingestion*. Define the product name, exact ingredients, amount consumed, and any current symptoms. Always relate the amount taken to the patient's weight. If any question exists about the medication, ask for a prescription number, the dispensing pharmacy, or prescribing physician. Always request that the product be taken to the emergency department (ED) if the patient gets there. The history is often inaccurate.
4. Determine *when ingestion occurred.*
5. Are there any other possible poisoning victims in the home?

INITIATION OF THERAPY AT HOME

Many accidental ingestions may be treated at home without an ED visit if the substance or the amount ingested is nontoxic (Box 54-1).

1. Be certain to cover the areas of poison prevention. Dangerous substances that are often found in the household include medications, dishwasher soap and cleaning supplies, drain-cleaning crystals or liquids, paints and thinners, automobile products, and garden sprays.
2. Regional poison control centers provide

347

Box 54-1
LOW-TOXICITY INGESTIONS*

Abrasives
Adhesives
Antacids
Antibiotics
Baby product cosmetics
Ballpoint pen inks
Bathtub floating toys
Birth control pills
Calamine lotion
Candles (beeswax or paraffin)
Chalk (calcium carbonate)
Clay (modeling or Play Doh)
Corticosteroids
Cosmetics (most, except perfumes)
Crayons marked AP or CP
Dehumidifying packets (silica)
Deodorants and deodorizers
Etch-A-Sketch
Fabric softener
Fish bowl additives
Glues and pastes
Greases
Gums
Hair products (dyes, sprays, tonics)
Hand lotions and creams

Ink (black, blue, indelible, felt-tip markers)
Kaolin
Lanolin
Linoleic acid
Linseed oil
Lipstick
Lubricants and lubricating oils
Newspapers
Paint (indoor and latex)
Pencil (graphite)
Petroleum jelly (Vaseline)
Polaroid picture coating fluid
Putty (<2 oz)
Sachets (essential oils, powder)
Shampoos and soap (bubble baths, soap bar)
Shoe polish (not containing aniline dyes)
Spackle
Suntan preparations
Sweetening agents (saccharin, cyclamate)
Teething rings
Thermometers (mercury)
Tooth paste (without fluoride)
Vitamins without iron
Zinc oxide

*These materials generally do not produce significant toxicity except in large doses. Substances such as cologne, after-shave lotion, deodorant, fabric softeners, and oral contraceptives may be toxic in large amounts. Toxicity is altered if the patient is pregnant or has an underlying disease.

an effective means of disseminating information, providing medical consultation, and arranging for follow-up. Unnecessary hospital visits may therefore be decreased.

3. If specific social problems are noted, initiate referral to a public health nurse. Any nonaccidental ingestions or potential child abuse must be seen in a health care facility despite the seemingly benign nature of the exposure.

Prevention of Absorption

Techniques to prevent further absorption can and should be initiated before the patient arrives at the ED.

1. External
   a. Skin exposed to insecticides (organophosphates or carbamates), hydrocarbons, or acid or alkali agents should be flooded with water and washed well with soap and a soft washcloth or sponge. Remove clothing.

b. Eyes must be irrigated immediately, before any transport or other therapy is discussed. Have the patient hold head under the sink or shower, or pour water into the eye from a pitcher or glass. Irrigation should be continued for a steady 15 to 20 minutes.

2. Internal

a. Dilute any acid or alkali ingestions with milk or water; do *not* induce emesis.

b. For other agents, and if so advised by the regional poison control center, emesis with *syrup of ipecac* may be induced in children older than 6 months, if indicated. Do not use for children less than 6 months of age. Give 10 ml (child less than 1 year); 15 ml (child 1 to 12 years); or 30 ml (child older than 12 years), followed by 15 ml/kg of fluid (up to 250 ml or 8 oz of water). Do not use milk or heavily sugared liquids. Ambulate the patient and wait for vomiting, which usually occurs in the next 20 minutes. Pharyngeal stimulation may be useful. If the patient does not vomit, repeat dose in 20 minutes if child is older than 12 months.

The shelf-life of syrup of ipecac is probably longer than indicated by the expiration date.

NOTE: Contraindicated in the home setting if the following are true:

(1) Patient is comatose, stuporous, seizing, has no gag reflex, is less than 6 months of age, or has a bleeding diathesis.

(2) Ingestion involves acid or alkali substances (p. 366).

(3) Ingestion involves hydrocarbons that do not contain camphor, halogenated or aromatic products, heavy metals, or pesticides ("CHAMP") (p. 379).

(4) Ingestion involves rapid-acting central nervous system (CNS) depressant or convulsant.

c. The value of home administration of activated charcoal has been explored. Sixty percent of children between the ages of 8 months and 5 years in one study drank the entire recommended dose. This may ultimately replace the home use of syrup of ipecac.

Transport to Hospital

All patients who require evaluation or treatment should be transported. The ED to receive the patient should be notified and given information about the treatment plan initiated and the means of transport. The parent or patient should be reminded to bring the ingested material for identification.

Other Considerations

If a potentially toxic ingestion is treated at home, arrangements should be made for the patient to be called back. Asking the older patient to call back is risky because of the possibility of the patient becoming obtunded or confused. Poison control centers can often facilitate this follow-up. All suicidal patients must be sent to a health care facility.

Records of all poison calls should be kept, including basic information, the type of ingestion, and therapy initiated.

Treatment information is available from multiple sources. *Poisindex* is a comprehensive information system available on microfiche or computer in many EDs. Poison control centers are a further source of data and management advice.

MANAGEMENT IN THE EMERGENCY DEPARTMENT

Stabilization and assessment are required of these potentially critically ill patients. Often an associated ingestion may change the clinical presentation and treatment plan. Dilution of acid and alkali ingestions with milk or water is of immediate priority, even before patient arrival in the ED. Patients usually fast (NPO) after initial evaluation.

Cardiopulmonary Status

1. Ensure that airway, ventilation, and circulation are adequate.
2. Establish intravenous lines in potentially serious ingestions.
3. In any patient with altered mental status, seizures, or coma, simultaneously administer the following:
   a. Oxygen at 4-6 L/min
   b. Dextrose, 0.5-1.0 gm (1-2 ml D50W)/kg/dose IV (or STAT documentation of a normal blood sugar)
   c. Naloxone (Narcan), 0.1 mg/kg/dose up to 2 mg IV

Other Considerations

1. Focus the physical examination on the cardiopulmonary and neurologic status. A specific toxic syndrome may be identified.
2. Place patients on a cardiac monitor and perform an electrocardiogram (ECG) if the ingested drug or chemical might precipitate dysrhythmias.
3. Evaluate electrolytes and acid-base status.

Toxicologic Screen

Blood analysis provides quantitative levels of specific drugs. Urine toxicology screening can provide rapid qualitative information about the presence of certain drug classes but does not provide quantitation.

Agents requiring emergency quantitative laboratory analysis include acetaminophen, salicylates, alcohols (methanol, ethylene glycol), iron, theophylline, lithium, and carbon monoxide.

The timing of drug concentration determinations may be complicated by the ingestion of large amounts; absorption may be prolonged. Modified-release agents may also delay and prolong toxicity.

The toxicology laboratory alone should not be relied on to make the diagnosis. Patient history and physical examination are far more important and timely (Tables 54-1 and 54-2).

1. Always let the laboratory personnel know what drugs are suspected.
2. Because a negative toxicologic screen result does not exclude a drug overdose, knowing which drugs the laboratory has screened for in its analysis is a must.

Prevention of Absorption

1. External.
   a. Skin—as described on p. 348.
   b. Ocular exposures, particularly to caustic agents, require immediate irrigation before examination. Each eye should be washed with a minimum of 1 L of saline solution; eversion of eyelids and cleaning of the fornices increases effectiveness.
2. Internal. Emesis or lavage is unlikely to be of benefit unless it is performed very quickly (<1 hour) after ingestion or the ingested drug delays gastric emptying. Beyond this period, administration of charcoal is probably the most beneficial approach.
   a. *Emesis* with syrup of ipecac, if indicated. Do *not* give if patient is comatose, stuporous, seizing, has no gag reflex, is less than 6 months old, has a bleeding diathesis, or has ingested an acid, alkali, or a hydrocarbon that does not contain camphor, halogenated or aromatic products, heavy metal, or pesticides. Ipecac also should not be given if the ingested substance can rapidly cause seizures or coma (i.e., cyclic antidepressants) (p. 352).

Age	Amount of ipecac administered
6-12 mo	10 ml (do not repeat)
1-12 yr	15 ml
>12 yr	30 ml

If emesis does not occur in 20 minutes, repeat the dose if the child is older than 12 months.

TABLE 54-1 Clues to Diagnosis of Unknown Poison: Vital-Sign Changes

DYSRHYTHMIAS	CYANOSIS (secondary to methemoglobinemia; does not respond to oxygen)
Anticholinergics	Anesthetics, local
β Blockers (e.g., propranolol)	Aniline dyes
Carbon monoxide	Nitrates
Cardiovascular drugs	Nitrites
Chloral hydrate	Phenacetin
Cyclic antidepressants (CADs)	Pyridium
Digitalis	Sulfonamides
Phenothiazines	
Quinidine	
Sympathomimetics (e.g., cocaine)	
Theophylline	

Increased	Decreased
BLOOD PRESSURE	
Amphetamines	Antihypertensives
Anticholinergics (antihistamines, CAD)	Cyanide
Sympathomimetics (phencyclidine, lysergic acid diethylamide, caffeine, cocaine, theophylline)	Narcotics
	Sedatives/hypnotics (see Table 54-2, Coma)
HEART RATE	
Alcohol	Barbiturates
Anticholinergics	β Blockers
Sympathomimetics (e.g., caffeine, amphetamines, cocaine)	Calcium channel blockers
Theophylline	Cholinergics
Hallucinogens	Digitalis
	Narcotics
	Sedatives/hypnotics
RESPIRATORY RATE	
Amphetamines	Alcohols (ethanol, isopropyl, methanol)
Anticholinergics	Barbiturates
Hydrocarbons	Central nervous system depressants
Nicotine	Narcotics
Secondary to metabolic acidosis ("MUDPILES") (p. 359)	Sedatives/hypnotics
Secondary to noncardiogenic pulmonary edema	
Carbon monoxide	
Hydrocarbons	
Narcotics	
Organophosphates	
Salicylates	
Sedatives/hypnotics	
TEMPERATURE	
Anticholinergics	Alcohol (ethanol)
Atropine	Anesthetic, general
β Blockers	Barbiturates
Cyclic antidepressants	Carbon monoxide
Phenothiazines	Narcotics
Salicylates	Phenothiazines
Selective serotonin reuptake inhibitors	Sedatives/hypnotics
Sympathomimetics (e.g., cocaine, amphetamines)	Cyclic antidepressants

TABLE 54-2   Clues to Diagnosis of Unknown Poison: Neurologic Alterations

	Findings associated with coma		
	Seizures, myoclonus, hyperreflexia	Hyporeflexia, hypotension	Pulmonary edema, hypotension
COMA			
Amphetamines	+		
Anticholinergics	+		
Barbiturates		+	+
Benzodiazepines		+	
Carbamazepine	+		
Carbon monoxide	+		
Chloral hydrate		+	
Cocaine	+		
Cyclic antidepressants (CAD)	+		
Ethanol, isopropyl		+	+
Haloperidol	+		
Narcotics		+	+
Phencyclidine (PCP)	+		
Phenothiazines	+		
Phenytoin	+		
Salicylates			+
Sedatives/hypnotics			+

SEIZURES ("CAP")

Camphor	Aminophylline	Pesticides (organophosphates)
Carbon monoxide	Amphetamines and sympathomimetics	Phencyclidine (PCP)
Cocaine	Anticholinergics	Phenol
Cyanide	Aspirin	Propoxyphene

Also lead, isoniazid, drug withdrawal, carbamazepine (Tegretol), lithium, strychnine, cyclic antidepressants, sympathomimetics, and organophosphates

BEHAVIOR DISORDERS

Toxic psychosis: hallucinogens (lysergic acid diethylamide [LSD], phencyclidine [PCP]), sympathomimetics (cocaine, amphetamines), anticholinergics, heavy metals
Paranoid, violent reactions: phencyclidine
Depression, paranoid hallucinations, emotional lability: sympathomimetics (cocaine, amphetamines)
Hallucinations, delirium, anxiety: anticholinergics, hallucinogens

MOVEMENT DISORDERS

Choreoathetosis, orofacial dyskinesis, nystagmus, ataxia: phenytoin
Extrapyramidal: anticholinergics, phenothiazines, haloperidol
Choreoathetoid movements: cyclic antidepressants, carbamazepine
Ataxia, choreiform movements: heavy metals
Ataxia, tremors: lithium
Nystagmus: SALEMTIP (sedative, alcohol, lithium, ethanol/ethylene glycol, methanol, thiamine depletion/Tegretol, isopropanol, phencyclidine/phenytoin/primidone)

PUPILS

Pinpoint (miosis)	**Dilated** (mydriasis)	Meperidine
Barbiturates (late)	Alcohol	Phenytoin
Cholinergics	Anticholinergics	Sympathomimetics (e.g., amphetamines,
Narcotics (except meperidine)	Antihistamines	cocaine, ephedrine, LSD, PCP)
Organophosphates	Barbiturates	

b. *Lavage.*

    (1) Indicated for patients who have ingested a potentially toxic substance and are seen within 1 to 2 hours of ingestion and are seizing, comatose, uncooperative, or have lost their gag reflex. The procedure also facilitates later administration of activated charcoal and cathartics.

    (2) Contraindicated for caustic or acid ingestions.

    (3) A 24- to 36-Fr tube (36 to 40 Fr in adults) inserted orally with the patient tilted slightly to the left side in Trendelenburg position. Saline or half-normal saline solution at 200 to 300 ml per pass in adult (proportionatcly smaller in child) is administered and repeated until the return is clear. Often a funnel or other device attached to the tube facilitates the procedure.

    If the patient is seen more than 1 to 2 hours after ingestion, administration of a single dose of activated charcoal may be the preferred approach to preventing absorption rather than lavage or emesis being performed first.

    (4) In comatose patients or those who lack protective reflexes (gag, cough, swallow), intubation is usually indicated before insertion of the lavage tube.

    (5) The procedure is performed with the patient on the left side in the Trendelenburg (head down) position.

c. *Activated charcoal* can be given without a prior gastric emptying procedure (syrup of ipecac or lavage). If emesis has been induced, wait 30 to 60 minutes after vomiting; in patients who have had lavage, charcoal can be administered through the tube. Often a 12- to 16-Fr nasogastric tube may be inserted to facilitate administration if a patient is unable to take the charcoal orally and lavage is not indicated. Verification of tube placement in the stomach clinically or radiographically is mandatory to prevent charcoal administration in the lungs.

Commonly 1 gm/kg body weight is the dose. Adults usually receive 50 to 100 gm and children 15 to 50 gm orally. It can be mixed in 35% to 70% sorbitol in children older than 1 year of age to allow simultaneous administration of a cathartic.

The efficacy is greatest when given early. Ingestions that reduce gastric motility (i.e., anticholinergics) may continue to be absorbed up to 12 to 24 hours after ingestion and are usually treated with activated charcoal as well as more specific measures.

Almost all drugs are absorbed by activated charcoal and include the following:

    (1) Analgesic/antiinflammatory agents: acetaminophen, salicylates, nonsteroidals, morphine, propoxyphene

    (2) Anticonvulsants/sedatives: barbiturates, carbamazepine, chlordiazepoxide, diazepam, phenytoin, sodium valproate

    (3) Other: amphetamines, atropine, chlorpheniramine, cocaine, digitalis, quinine, theophylline, cyclic antidepressants

Drugs that are not absorbed by activated charcoal include simple ions (iron, lithium, cyanide), strong acids or bases (hydrochloric acid and sodium hydroxide), and simple alcohols (ethanol and methanol).

Multiple-dose activated charcoal (adult: 20 to 50 gm q2-4hr PO; child: 1 gm/kg/dose q2-4hr PO) increases the clearance of carbamazepine, meprobamate, phenobarbital, phenytoin, salicylates, theophylline, and others. Do not mix charcoal with cathartic (including sorbitol) after the first dose in multiple-dose charcoal regimen.

d. *Catharsis,* with magnesium sulfate, 250 mg/kg/dose PO (adults 20 gm PO), should be given to increase transit time. It is contraindicated in patients with renal failure, severe diarrhea, adynamic ileus, or abdominal trauma. Do not use multiple doses. Sodium sulfate, sorbitol (2 ml/kg of 70% sorbitol [1-2 gm/kg]; do not give repeated doses), or magnesium citrate (4-8 ml/kg [maximum: 300 ml]) also may serve as a cathartic. Use one dose only.

e. *Whole-bowel irrigation.* Rapid administration of a specialized fluid solution (polyethylene glycol electrolyte or GoLYTELY) can be useful in cases when iron, packets of street drugs, or large amounts of sustained-release drugs have been ingested. Patients must be alert and be able to protect the airway. Adults and adolescents receive 1.5-2.0 L/hr; toddlers and preschoolers may receive 500 ml/hr until the rectal effluent is similar in appearance to the infusate.

Enhancement of Excretion (Table 54-3)

1. *Diuresis* can hasten the excretion of a few substances—namely, those with small volumes of distribution that are excreted by the kidneys. When a drug is ionizable, intracellular and CNS drug levels may be reduced and renal excretion increased by ion-trapping. Ionizable drugs cross lipid membranes (cell wall or blood barrier) only in a nonionized state. Alkaline pH favors dissociation (ion-trapping) of weakly acidic drugs (phenobarbital, salicylates). Potassium depletion may prevent excretion of salicylates. Substances whose excretion may be definitely enhanced by diuresis include phenobarbital (alkaline) and salicylates (alkaline) (see Table 54-3).

TABLE 54-3   Volume of Distribution and Efficacy of Diuresis and Dialysis

Drug	Volume of distribution (L/kg)*	Diuresis	Dialysis
Acetaminophen	1.0	No	No
Amphetamine	0.6	No	No
Benzodiazepines	>10	No	No
Caffeine	0.9	No	No
Cyclic antidepressants	>8	No	No
Digoxin	7.5-15	No	No
Ethanol	0.6	No	No
Ethylene glycol	0.6	No	Yes
Lithium	0.7	Yes	Yes
Methanol	0.6	No	Yes
Narcotics	>5	No	No
Phencyclidine	8.5	No	No
Phenobarbital	0.75	Alkaline	Yes
Phenothiazines	>30	No	No
Phenytoin	0.75	No	No
Salicylates	0.3-0.6	Alkaline	Yes
Theophylline	0.46	No	Yes†

*Dose (mg/kg)/plasma concentration (mg/L).

†Theophylline overdoses of significance may be treated with hemoperfusion. Dialysis may be useful if hemoperfusion is unavailable or patient is small child.

The goal of alkaline diuresis is to increase urinary pH to 7.5 or higher and to maintain brisk urine flow (2-5 ml/kg/hr). It is imperative to prevent fluid overload; hourly assessment of volume status is mandatory.

  a. Alkaline diuresis is achieved by giving NaHCO$_3$, 1-2 mEq/kg/dose IV over 1 hour, with K$^+$ supplement as necessary. Adding two to three adult ampules (44.5 mEq NaHCO$_3$ per ampule) to 1 L of D5W will result in a solution that is not hypertonic and that facilitates alkalinization. Urine pH should be equal to or greater than 7.5. Monitor electrolytes. Potassium usually must be given in concentrations of 30-50 mEq/L. It is contraindicated if pulmonary or cerebral edema or renal failure is present.

  b. Acid diuresis is no longer recommended.

2. *Dialysis*, usually considered after failure of conservative medical treatment, may be useful in only a few circumstances. It is indicated if life-threatening symptoms are present with markedly elevated serum levels of phenobarbital, salicylates, theophylline, methanol, ethylene glycol, or lithium. Immediate dialysis should be performed for unresponsive patients, significant acidosis, renal failure, visual symptoms, or peak levels (measured or extrapolated) greater than 50 mg/dl after methanol ingestion.

3. *Hemoperfusion* with charcoal or resin-filled devices has been helpful but is still controversial. Hemoperfusion appears particularly useful for significant theophylline overdoses, but because of the greater availability of hemodialysis, the latter is usually preferred.

Antidotes (Table 54-4)

Specific antidotes are useful when used appropriately. The antiquated "universal antidote" (burned toast, magnesium oxide, and tannic acid) has no place in modern therapy.

Disposition

1. Discharge from the ED must reflect the severity of the ingestion and potential life-threatening medical and psychiatric considerations.
2. Before discharging the patient, specific attention must be focused on poison prevention, with emphasis on discarding old medications and placing needed drugs and toxic household substances in locked cabinets.
3. Children and their families should be cautioned about accident prevention. Families with 2- to 6-year-old children who have a possible poison exposure are at an increased risk of subsequent injury. Injury prevention education is essential.
4. Patients overdosing as suicide gestures or environmental manipulation should receive *psychiatric evaluation* before discharge (p. 757).
5. Incidents of child abuse must be referred to the appropriate child welfare authorities (see Chapter 25).

TOXIC SYNDROMES

While a patient's history is being obtained and the physical examination performed, certain toxic syndromes may become evident. This can assist the physician by focusing on a class of toxins to which the patient may have been exposed.

Narcotics and Sedative-Hypnotics (p. 383)

These drugs, which cause associated cardiorespiratory depression, can result in coma.

Diagnostic Findings

1. Narcotics (except meperidine) may produce miosis, noncardiogenic pulmonary edema, and seizures, especially with propoxyphene or meperidine.
  a. Anticholinergic findings—diphenoxylate (Lomotil) and atropine.
  b. Treatment: naloxone (Narcan), 0.4 to 2 mg IV. Propoxyphene (Darvon) and

TABLE 54-4   Common Antidotes (See Chapter 55)

Drug	Diagnostic findings requiring treatment	Antidote	Dosage
Acetaminophen	History of ingestion and toxic serum level	N-acetylcysteine	140 mg/kg/dose PO, then 70 mg/kg/dose q4hr PO × 17
Anticholinergics Antihistamines Atropine Phenothiazines Cyclic antidepressants	Supraventricular tachycardia (hemodynamic compromise) Unresponsive ventricular dysrhythmia, seizures, pronounced hallucinations or agitation	Physostigmine	Child: 0.02 mg/kg/dose up to 0.5 mg/dose IV slowly (over 3 min) q10min prn (maximum total dose: 2 mg) Adult: 1-2 mg IV slowly q10min prn (maximum: 4 mg in 30 min)
Benzodiazepines	Respiratory depression, coma	Flumazenil	10 µg/kg IV for 2 doses; adult: 0.2, 0.3, then 0.5 mg separated by 30 seconds, up to total of 3 mg
Cholinergics Physostigmine Insecticides	Cholinergic crisis: salivation, lacrimation, urination, defecation, convulsions, fasciculations	Atropine sulfate	0.05 mg/kg/dose (usual dose 1-5 mg; test dose for child 0.01 mg/kg) q4-6hr IV or more frequently prn Also pralidoxime (see below)
Carbon monoxide	Headache, seizure, coma, dysrhythmias	Oxygen, hyperbaric oxygen	100% oxygen (half-life 40 min); consider hyperbaric chamber
Cyanide	Cyanosis, seizures, cardiopulmonary arrest, coma	Amyl nitrite Sodium nitrite (3%) Sodium thiosulfate (25%) Also consider hyperbaric oxygen	Inhale perle q60-120sec 0.27 ml (8.7 mg)/kg (adult: 10 ml [300 ml]) IV slowly (Hb 10 g) 1.35 ml (325 mg)/kg (adult: 12.5 gm) IV slowly (Hb 10 gm)

Poison	Signs/Symptoms	Antidote	Dosage
Ethylene glycol	Metabolic acidosis, urine Ca^{++} oxalate crystals	Ethanol (100% absolute, 1 ml-790 mg)	1 ml/kg in D5W IV over 15 min, then 0.15 ml (125 mg)/kg/hr IV; maintain ethanol level of 100 mg/dl
Iron	Hypotension, shock, coma, serum iron level toxic	Deferoxamine	Shock or coma: 15 mg/kg/hr IV for 8 hr; if no shock or coma 90 mg/kg/dose IM q8hr
Phenothiazines Chlorpromazine Thioridazine	Extrapyramidal dyskinesis, oculogyric crisis	Diphenhydramine (Benadryl)	1-2 mg/kg/dose (maximum: 50 mg/dose) q6hr IV, PO
Methanol	Metabolic acidosis, blurred vision; level >20 mg/dl	Ethanol (100% absolute)	1 ml/kg in D5W over 15 min, then 0.15 ml (125 mg)/kg/hr IV
Methemoglobin Nitrate Nitrite Sulfonamide	Cyanosis, methemoglobin level >30%, dyspnea	Methylene blue (1% solution)	1-2 mg (0.1-0.2 ml)/kg/dose IV: repeat in 4 hr if necessary
Narcotics Heroin Codeine Propoxyphene	Respiratory depression, hypotension, coma	Naloxone (Narcan)	0.4-2 mg/dose IV; repeat as necessary
Organophosphates Malathion Parathion	Cholinergic crisis: salivation, lacrimation, urination, defecation, convulsions, fasciculations	Atropine sulfate	0.05 mg/kg/dose (usual dose 1-5 mg) IV prn or q4-6hr
		Pralidoxime	After atropine, 20-50 mg/kg/dose (maximum: 2000 mg) IV slowly or 500 mg/hr IV infusion

pentazocine (Talwin) ingestion may require larger doses for reversal. The use of naloxone is both therapeutic and diagnostic. Occasionally, a continuous infusion may be required.

2. Sedative-hypnotics: benzodiazepines (e.g., diazepam), barbiturates, methaqualone (Quāālude), meprobamate (Miltown), glutethimide (Doriden), ethchlorvynol (Placidyl), and methyprylon (Noludar).

   a. Management: prevention of absorption and supportive care (alkaline diuresis for phenobarbital)

   b. Benzodiazepine respiratory depression or coma reversed by flumazenil (Mazicon) in a dose of 10 μg/kg × 2 IV. Adult: 0.2 mg/dose, 0.3 mg/dose, and then 0.5 mg/dose IV separated by 30 seconds between doses, up to a cumulative dose of 3.0 mg.

Anticholinergics (p. 369)

Classes of drugs include the following:

1. Antihistamines
2. Antiparkinsonian—benztropine (Cogentin)
3. Belladonna alkaloids (atropine)
4. Butyrophenones (haloperidol)
5. Gastrointestinal (GI) and genitourinary (GU) antispasmodics
6. Over-the-counter (OTC) analgesics (Midol, Excedrin)
7. OTC cold remedies
8. OTC sleeping preparations
9. Phenothiazines
10. Cyclic antidepressants

Plants may also be sources, such as *Amanita muscaria.*

Diagnostic Findings

Peripheral signs include the following:

1. Tachycardia
2. Dry, flushed skin
3. Dry mucous membranes
4. Dilated pupils
5. Hyperpyrexia
6. Urinary retention
7. Decreased bowel sounds
8. Dysrhythmias
9. Hypertension
10. Hypotension (late)

Central anticholinergic syndrome causes:

1. Delirium—organic brain syndrome
   a. Disorientation
   b. Agitation
   c. Hallucinations
   d. Psychosis
   e. Loss of memory
2. Extrapyramidal movements
3. Ataxia
4. Picking or grasping movements
5. Seizures
6. Coma
7. Respiratory failure
8. Cardiovascular collapse

Phenothiazines may result in pronounced hypotension resulting from α-blocking action (p. 387).

Treatment

1. Seizures: diazepam (Valium) or phenobarbital; for the unresponsive or psychotic patient, physostigmine
2. Dysrhythmias (cyclic antidepressants): alkalinization, phenytoin, lidocaine; for the psychotic patient, physostigmine (p. 371)
3. Pronounced hallucinations and agitation (in which patient may be in danger of harming self or others) may require physostigmine
   • Physostigmine, 0.02 mg/kg/dose up to 0.5 mg/dose IV (children) or 1 to 2 mg IV (adults) slowly

Cholinergics

Cholinergics include organophosphates and carbamate pesticides (p. 385), physostigmine, neostigmine, pyridostigmine, and edrophonium (Tensilon).

Diagnostic Findings

1. "SLUDGE": *s*alivation, *l*acrimation, *u*rination, *d*efecation (diarrhea), *G*I cramping, and *e*mesis. Patients appear "wet."
2. CNS effects: headache, restlessness, and

Box 54-2

CLUES TO DIAGNOSIS OF UNKNOWN POISONS AND CONDITIONS: LABORATORY AND OTHER ALTERATIONS

TOXIC METABOLIC ACIDOSIS ("MUDPILES")

Methanol

Uremia

Diabetes ketocidosis

Paraldehyde

Isoniazid, iron, ibuprofen,
   inhalant (CO, cyanide)

Lactic acidosis

Ethanol, ethylene glycol

Salicylates, starvation, strychnine,
   solvent (benzene, toluene)

NOTE: Metabolic acidosis may be caused by any drug, chemical, or condition that causes hypotension, seizures, or cellular metabolism dysfunction.

GLUCOSE

Increased

Salicylates

Isoniazid

Iron

Isopropyl alcohol

Decreased

Acetaminophen (if hepatic failure)

Isoniazid

Salicylates

Methanol

Insulin

Ethanol

URINE COLOR

Red: hematuria, hemoglobinuria, myoglobinuria, pyrvinium (Povan), phenytoin (Dilantin), phenothiazines, mercury, lead, iron, anthrocycan (food pigment in beets and blackberries)

Brown-black: hemoglobin pigments, melanin, methyldopa (Aldomet), cascara, rhubarb, methocarbamol (Robaxin)

Blue, blue-green, green: amitryptyline, methylene blue, indigo blue, triamterene (Dyazide), Clorets, *Pseudomonas*

Brown, red-brown: porphyria, urobilinogen, nitrofurantoin, furazolidone, metronidazole, aloe (seaweed)

Orange: dehydration, rifampin, phenazopyridine (Pyridium), sulfasalazine (Azulfidine)

X-RAY STUDY (radiopaque medications and chemicals: "CHIPE," i.e., heavy metals and enteric-coated tablets)

Chloral hydrate, cocaine, "condos," calcium

Heavy metals (arsenic, lead)

Iron, iodides

Phenothiazines, psychotropics (CAD)

Enteric coated tablets, slow-release capsules

NOTE: Factors affecting radiopacity include the size of patient, the arrangement of the pills in the stomach, air-contrasting pills, and the composition of the enteric coating or pill matrix.

BREATH ODOR

Alcohol: ethanol, chloral hydrate, phenols

Acetone: acetone, salicylates, isopropyl alcohol, paraldehyde

Bitter almond: cyanide

Burned rope: marijuana

Garlic: arsenic, phosphorus, organophosphates

Oil of wintergreen: methylsalicylates

Rotten eggs: disulfiram, *N*-acetylcystine

anxiety progressing to confusion, coma, and seizures.
3. Sweating, miosis, muscle fasciculations and weakness, bradycardia, bronchorrhea, and bronchospasm. Tachycardia is also common.

Treatment
1. Decontamination and support.
2. Atropine (blocks acetylcholine), 0.05 mg/kg/dose (usual dose 1 to 5 mg) q10min prn or q4-6hr IV. The end-point of atropinization should be drying of pulmonary secretions. Pupil size is unsatisfactory because the pupils may initially be dilated.
3. Pralidoxime 2-PAM (cholinesterase reactivator), 20-50 mg/kg/dose IV slowly q8hr IV prn (three times), after atropine.

Sympathomimetics (p. 391)

Sympathomimetics include amphetamines, phenylpropanolamine, ephedrine, and cocaine.

Diagnostic Findings
Findings are similar to those of anticholinergic syndrome:
1. Psychoses, hallucinations, delirium
2. Nausea, vomiting, and abdominal pain
3. Possibly prominent piloerection
4. Tachycardia and cardiac dysrhythmias
5. Severe hypertension

Treatment
1. Supportive care after gastric emptying.
2. Diazepam (Valium), 0.1-0.2 mg/kg/dose q4-6hr IV or PO for sedation.
3. Haloperidol (Haldol), 0.05-0.15 mg/kg/24 hr q8-12hr PO; begin 0.5 mg/24 hr; dose not well established in children; adult: 0.05 to 2.0 mg (maximum: 5 mg) q8-12hr PO; may also be given parenterally if patient is extremity agitated. Adult emergent dose is 5 to 20 mg IV prn.

Drug-induced psychosis requires a reassuring attitude and maintaining verbal contact with the patient. Physical restraints should be avoided.

Classic Manifestations of Toxicity

See Tables 54-1 and 54-2 and Box 54-2.

Although tremendous variability exists in clinical presentations, certain manifestations of toxicity are commonly recognized and are particularly helpful in identifying unknown poisons.

REFERENCES

Albertson TE, Derlet RW, Foulke GE, et al: Superiority of activated charcoal alone compared with ipecac and activated charcoal in the treatment of acute toxic ingestions, *Ann Emerg Med* 18:56, 1989.

Baraff LF, Guterman JJ, Bayer MJ: The relationship of poison center contact and injury in children 2 to 6 years old, *Ann Emerg Med* 21:153, 1992.

Clark RF, Sage TA, Tunget C, et al: Delayed onset lorazepam poisoning successfully reversed by flumazenil in a child, *Pediatr Emerg Care* 11:32, 1995.

Fazen LE, Lovejoy FH, Crone RK: Acute poisoning in a children's hospital: a 2-year experience, *Pediatrics* 77:144, 1986.

Grbcich PA, Lacouture PG, Lovejoy FH: Effect of fluid volume on ipecac-induced emesis, *J Pediatr* 110:970, 1987.

Hoffman JR, Schriger DL, Luo JS: The empiric use of naloxone in patients with altered mental status, *Ann Emerg Med* 20:246, 1991.

James LP, Nichols MH, King WD: A comparison of cathartics in pediatric ingestion, *Pediatrics* 96:235, 1995.

Kaczorowski JM, Wax PM: Five days of whole-bowel irrigation in a case of pediatric iron ingestion, *Ann Emerg Med* 27:258, 1996.

Keller RE, Schwab RS, Krenzelok EP: Contribution of sorbitol combined with activated charcoal in prevention of salicylate absorption, *Ann Emerg Med* 19:654, 1990.

Kelley MT, Werman HA, Rund DA: Use of activated charcoal in the treatment of drug overdoses, *Am J Emerg Med* 3:280, 1985.

Kornberg AE, Dolgin J: Pediatric ingestions: charcoal alone versus ipecac and charcoal, *Ann Emerg Med* 20:648, 1991.

Kulig K: Initial management of ingestions of toxic substances, *N Engl J Med* 326:1677, 1992.

Kulig K, Bar-Or D, Cantrill SV, et al: Management of acutely poisoned patients without gastric-emptying, *Ann Emerg Med* 14:562, 1985.

Lewander WJ, Lacouture PG: Office management of acute pediatric poisoning, *Pediatr Emerg Care* 5:262, 1989.

Litovitz T, Manoquerra A: Comparison of pediatric poisoning hazards: an analysis of 3.8 million exposure incidents, *Pediatrics* 89:999, 1992.

Litovitz TL, Smilkstein M, Felberg L, et al: 1996 Annual Report of the American Association of Poison Control Centers Toxic Exposure Surveillance System, *Am J Emerg Med* 15:447, 1997.

Lovejoy FH, Robertson WO, Woolf AD: Poison centers, poison prevention, and the pediatrician, *Pediatrics* 94:220, 1994.

Mauro LS, Mauro VF, Brown DL, et al: Enhancement of phenytoin elimination by multiple-dose activated charcoal, *Ann Emerg Med* 16:1132, 1987.

McDuffee AT, Tobias JD: Seizure after flumazenil administration in a pediatric patient, *Pediatr Emerg Care* 11:186, 1995.

McNamara RM, Aaron CK, Gemborys M, et al: Efficacy of charcoal and cathartic versus ipecac in reducing serum acetaminophen in a stimulated overdose, *Ann Emerg Med* 18:934, 1989.

Merigian KS, Woodard M, Hedges JR, et al: Prospective evaluation of gastric emptying in the self-poisoned patient, *Am J Emerg Med* 9:479, 1990.

Olson KR, Pentel PR, Kelley MT: Physical assessment and differential diagnosis of the poisoned patient, *Med Toxicol* 2:52, 1987.

Osterloh JD: Utility and reliability of emergency toxicologic testing, *Emerg Med Clin North Am* 8:693, 1990.

Pond SM, Lewis-Driver DJ, Williams GM, et al: Gastric emptying in acute overdose: a prospective randomised controlled trial, *Med J Aust* 163:345, 1995.

Rosenberg PJ, Livingston DJ, McLellan BA: Effect of whole bowel irrigation on the efficacy of oral activated charcoal, *Ann Emerg Med* 17:681, 1988.

Savitt DL, Hawkins HH, Roberts JR: The radiopacity of ingested medications, *Ann Emerg Med* 16:331, 1987.

Shannon M, Amitai Y, Lovejoy FH: Multiple dose activated charcoal for theophylline poisoning in young infants, *Pediatrics* 80:368, 1987.

Sugarman JM, Paul RI: Flumazenil: a review, *Pediatr Emerg Care* 10:37, 1994.

Sugarman JM, Rodgers GC, Paul RI: Utility of toxicity screening in a pediatric emergency department, *Pediatr Emerg Care* 13:194, 1997.

Tenenbein M: General management principles in poisoning. In Barkin RM, editor: *Pediatric emergency medicine: concepts and clinical practice*, ed 2, St Louis, 1997, Mosby.

Tenenbein M: Multiple doses of charcoal: time for reappraisal? *Ann Emerg Med* 20:529, 1991.

Tenenbein M, Cohen S, Sitar DS: Efficacy of ipecac induced emesis, orogastric lavage, and activated charcoal for acute drug overdose, *Ann Emerg Med* 16:838, 1987.

55 SPECIFIC INGESTIONS

ACETAMINOPHEN

ALERT: History and plasma level determine the need for therapy.

Acetaminophen is a widely used antipyretic and analgesic that is metabolized in the liver in part by conjugation with glutathione. After an acetaminophen overdose, the glutathione substrate can be overwhelmed, and a toxic metabolite is formed via an alternate pathway. The toxic metabolite may bind covalently to hepatic macromolecules, producing cellular necrosis.

In adults, 150 mg/kg is considered a toxic overdose, but the same dose may produce only minor changes in children less than 10 years of age; children appear less susceptible to injury. Both children and adults, however, are susceptible to chronic overdose of acetaminophen causing hepatic damage. Chronic ingestion of alcohol, as well as malnutrition, appears to be a risk factor. Therapeutic levels are 10-20 µg/ml, whereas toxic levels are 150 µg/ml at 4 hours and 37.5 µg/ml at 12 hours.

DIAGNOSTIC FINDINGS

The history of ingestion is usually inadequate and often bears little correlation to the blood levels. Patients may develop hepatic failure secondary to necrosis of the centrilobular type. Encephalopathy, coma, and death may follow. Children are unlikely to have toxic levels if they experienced early, spontaneous emesis.

1. Initially, gastrointestinal (GI) symptoms and diaphoresis may develop 6 to 12 hours after ingestion. Many remain asymptomatic.

2. An asymptomatic period follows for 12 to 48 hours after ingestion, although hepatic enzyme levels begin to rise.
3. After about 48 hours, evidence of liver injury becomes apparent, with markedly elevated levels of hepatic enzymes, which usually then normalize over the ensuing 4 to 7 days.

Ancillary Data

1. Acetaminophen level obtained 4 hours after ingestion and plotted on nomogram (Fig. 55-1)
2. Liver function tests, including serum glutamic oxaloacetic transaminase (SGOT), serum glutamic pyruvic transaminase (SGPT), bilirubin, and prothrombin time (PT)
3. Arterial blood gas (ABG) and other evaluations as indicated by central nervous system (CNS) findings
4. Blood glucose if hepatic damage occurs

DIFFERENTIAL DIAGNOSIS

1. Infection: acute gastroenteritis (see Chapter 76) and hepatitis (p. 639)
2. Encephalopathy (p. 136)
3. Chemical hepatitis from other drugs or chemicals (e.g., solvents, mushrooms)

MANAGEMENT

The decision regarding intervention is made on the basis of the presumed history of ingestion and, ideally, an acetaminophen level. Information regarding the treatment protocol can be

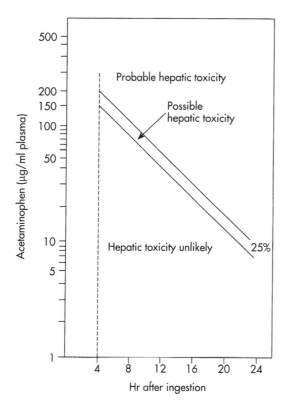

Fig. 55-1 Rumack-Matthew nomogram for acetaminophen poisoning.

(From Rumack BH, Matthew H: *Pediatrics* 55:871, 1975. Copyright American Academy of Pediatrics, 1975.)

obtained from your local poison center or the Rocky Mountain Poison Control Center at 303-629-1123.

1. Initial stabilization of the patient. Emesis or lavage may be indicated if these can be performed very soon after ingestion. Do not give syrup of ipecac to a patient who is already vomiting. Give charcoal as soon as possible, preferably without prior syrup of ipecac or lavage. If given less than 4 hours after ingestion, charcoal may prevent a toxic acetaminophen level from developing. Charcoal will not interfere with the absorption or efficacy of Mucomyst, although some clinicians suggest increasing the initial dose to 235 mg/kg orally.

2. *N*-acetylcysteine 20% (Mucomyst) (NAC): diluted fourfold to a 5% solution in grapefruit juice, water, or cola. An IV preparation also is available. It is ideally indicated within 8 hours of ingestion but is still somewhat effective up to 24 hours after the ingestion.

   a. Indicated if the serum acetaminophen level is in the toxic range and less than 24 hours has elapsed since ingestion. Toxic levels are considered to be those levels above the possible toxicity line on the nomogram. Levels obtained less than 4 hours after ingestion may not be interpretable because acetaminophen has a two-compartment kinetic pattern. Children appear to have more resistance to toxicity.

   b. If no levels are immediately available and the ingestion is considered to be toxic (>150 mg/kg), therapy should be initiated and may be stopped later if the level is determined to be in the nontoxic range. It is unclear whether ingestion of the new sustained-relief form of acetaminophen should be managed differently than the regular form regarding use of the nomogram. A certified regional poison center should be contacted for the most current information.

   c. Dosage. Load with 140 mg/kg/dose PO followed by 70 mg/kg/dose q4hr PO for 17 doses. An IV preparation also is available on an experimental basis and currently is given as an initial load of 140 mg/kg followed by 12 doses of 10 mg/kg/dose q4hr IV for 24 hours.

      Some toxicologists are now recommending a shorter course of oral Mucomyst, stopping treatment at 24 hours if the acetaminophen level is nondetectable and hepatic transaminases are normal. The safety of this protocol is uncertain. If the patient vomits within 1 hour of administration of the dose, repeat the dose. If vomiting persists, give by nasogastric (NG) or duodenal tube as slow drip or consider IV preparation. Metoclopramide (Reglan), 1 mg/kg IV up to 10 mg, 30 minutes before NAC may be useful. Inapsine (Droperidol) may also be useful.

DISPOSITION

All patients requiring treatment with NAC should be admitted for treatment and monitoring. Long-term follow-up observation will be required.

REFERENCES

Chamberlain JM, Gorman RL, Oderda GM, et al: Use of activated charcoal in a simulated poisoning with acetaminophen: a new loading dose for *N*-acetylcysteine, *Ann Emerg Med* 22:1398, 1993.

Smilkstein MJ, Bronstein AC, Linden C, et al: Acetaminophen overdose: a 48-hour intravenous n-acetyl cysteine treatment protocol, *Ann Emerg Med* 20:1058, 1991.

Smilkstein MJ, Knapp GI, Kulig KW, et al: Efficacy of *N*-acetylcysteine in the treatment of acetaminophen overdose, *N Engl J Med* 319:1557, 1988.

ALCOHOLS: ETHANOL, ISOPROPYL, METHANOL, ETHYLENE GLYCOL

Ethanol is becoming an increasingly popular drug among adolescents. The immediate medical problems, as well as the long-term psychiatric ones, must be treated.

DIAGNOSTIC FINDINGS (Table 55-1)

Classically, the progression of findings in nontolerant intoxicated individuals is related to the blood alcohol level (Table 55-2). A progressive change is seen in mental status and sensory impairment, ultimately leading to respiratory failure and death.

1. *Ethanol* equivalents: Approximately four

TABLE 55-1   Alcohol Ingestion and Overdose

Alcohol (uses)	"Toxic dose" (toxic level)	Central nervous system depression	Acidosis	Ketonemia	Increased osmolality at level of 50 mg/dl
Ethanol (beverages, mouthwash, perfumes)	3-5 gm/kg (>100 mg/dl)	+	±	±	11 mOsm/kg H_2O
Isopropyl (rubbing alcohol, solvent)	2-3 gm/kg (>50 mg/dl)	+	+	++	8.5 mOsm/kg H_2O
Methanol (canned heat, antifreeze, solvent, denaturant)	1-2 ml/kg (>20 mg/dl)		+++	±	15.5 mOsm/kg H_2O
Ethylene glycol (antifreeze, deicer)	1-2 ml/kg (>20 mg/dl)	+	+++	−	8 mOsm/kg H_2O

Modified from Goldfrank LR, Starke CL: Metabolic acidosis in the alcoholic. In Goldfrank LR: *Toxicologic emergencies*, ed 6, New York, 1998, Appleton-Century-Crofts.

drinks ingested quickly on an empty stomach will result in a peak blood level of about 100 mg/dl.

2. *Isopropyl* alcohol is considered to be more of a CNS depressant and GI irritant than ethanol. There may be a smell of acetone on the breath after ingestion.

3. *Methanol* ingestion results in a nonintoxicated, acidotic patient with visual symptoms 3 to 24 hours after ingestion.

4. *Ethylene glycol* produces an intoxicated patient with severe acidosis, rapid progression of CNS signs, renal dysfunction commonly associated with calcium oxalate crystalluria, pulmonary edema, and shock.

Often, an associated ingestion of a drug or another alcohol is present and there are many alcohol drug interactions.

Ancillary Data

1. Ethanol, methanol, ethylene glycol, and isopropanol levels.

2. Blood glucose, electrolytes, osmolality (by freezing point depression), and ABG. Osmolal gap may not be a reliable screen for methanol or ethyl glycol ingestion.

DIFFERENTIAL DIAGNOSIS

Differentiation of the alcohols may be made on the basis of blood levels, acid-base status, breath odor, and diagnostic findings.

• Metabolic acidosis: "MUDPILES" (*m*ethanol, *u*remia, *d*iabetes mellitus, *p*araldehyde, *i*ron, *i*soniazide, *l*actic acidosis, *e*thanol, *e*thylene glycol, *s*alicylates, and *s*tarvation). Acidosis is caused by these agents, as well as those that cause seizures, hypotension, and all cellular poisons (e.g., iron, cyanide, carbon monoxide).

MANAGEMENT

1. *Supportive care* with particular attention to the airway and fluids. Treatment of acidosis, hypoglycemia, hypocalcemia, res-

Diagnostic findings	Odor on breath	Treatment
Intoxication with nausea, vomiting, ataxia, uncoordination, slurred speech progressing to seizures, coma, hypothermia, respiratory failure, death	Ethanol	Gastric emptying, fluids, glucose support; blood level declines at 10-50 mg/dl/hr; consider dialysis if life threatening
Intoxication with significant CNS depression, hemorrhagic tracheobronchitis, gastritis; twice toxicity of ethanol	Acetone	Gastric emptying, fluid support; dialysis if life threatening
Not intoxicated; delayed onset; slight CNS depression initially may become severe; intractable acidosis; blurred vision with pink edema of optic disc in 12-24 hr; abdominal pain (pancreatitis)	None	Gastric emptying, fluid support; ethanol (100%) 1 ml/kg over 15 min, then 0.15 ml (125 mg)/kg/hr IV; dialysis if peak level >50 mg/dl, visual symptoms, or severe acidosis
Intoxicated; stupor, ataxia progressing to seizures, coma; severe acidosis; ocular nystagmus; CHF and pulmonary edema; shock; renal failure, calcium oxalate crystalluria, oliguria, hypocalcemia	None	Gastric emptying, fluid support; calcium prn; ethanol (100%) 1 ml/kg over 15 min, then 0.15 ml (125 mg)/kg/hr IV; dialysis if renal failure, severe acidosis or peak level >50 mg/dl

TABLE 55-2 Blood Ethanol Levels and Clinical Findings in the Nontolerant Adult

Blood ethanol level (mg/dl)	Clinical findings
≤99	Changes in mood, personality, behavior
	Progressive muscular incoordination
	Impaired sensory function
100-199	Marked mental and sensory impairment
	Incoordination, ataxia
	Prolonged reaction time
	Grossly intoxicated
200-299	Nausea, vomiting, diplopia, marked ataxia
300-399	Amnesia, dysarthria, hypothermia
400-700	Coma, respiratory failure, death

piratory and renal failure, or pulmonary edema.

2. *Gastric emptying* if soon after ingestion or if any question of associated ingestion exists.

3. *Ethanol,* as outlined in Table 55-1, for methanol or ethylene glycol ingestions. Maintain ethanol level at 100 mg/dl or greater.

   a. Fomepizole, a competitive inhibitor of alcohol dehydrogenase, may be useful to treat ethylene glycol ingestions. A loading dose of 15 mg/kg/dose IV (over 30 minutes) is followed by 10 mg/kg/dose q12hr IV for four doses and then increased to 15 mg/kg/dose q12hr until the ethylene glycol concentration is below 20 mg/dl. Forced diuresis is recommended. This may also be of value in patients after methanol poisoning as well.

4. Dialysis is indicated early in the treatment of methanol and ethylene glycol ingestions with peak levels that are or could have been above 50 mg/dl or accompanying severe acidosis, but only in life-threatening intoxication of ethanol and isopropyl alcohol.

5. Adolescents and adults undergoing alcohol withdrawal and the hyperkinetic state associated with chronic use of ethanol may be partially controlled with clorazepate (Tranxene), 15 mg q6hr PO, lorazepam (Ativan), 0.5 to 1.0 mg q6hr PO, or chlordiazepoxide (Librium), 50 to 100 mg IM or IV in adult. Diazepam (Valium) also may be useful.

DISPOSITION

All pediatric patients with significant methanol or ethylene glycol ingestions should be admitted, as well as those with toxic levels of ethanol and isopropyl alcohol.

Long-term psychiatric follow-up care usually is indicated.

REFERENCES

Burns MJ, Graudins A, Aaron CK, et al: Treatment of methanol poisoning with intravenous 4-methylpyrazole, *Ann Emerg Med* 30:829, 1997.

Chabali R: Diagnostic use of anion and osmolal gaps in pediatric emergency medicine, *Pediatr Emerg Care* 13:204, 1997.

Glaser DS: Utility of the serum osmol gap in the diagnosis of methanol or ethylene glycol ingestion, *Ann Emerg Med* 25:343, 1996.

Roth A, Norman SA, Manoguerra AS, et al: Short-term hemodialysis in childhood ethylene glycol poisoning, *J Pediatr* 18:153, 1986.

Shannon M: Fomepizole—a new antidote, *Pediatr Emerg Care* 14:170, 1998.

ALKALIS AND ACIDS

ALERT: Immediate dilution with milk or water should be initiated.

A large number of household products contain alkali or acid and may be ingested by the curious child. Accidental ingestions usually occur in children less than 4 years of age, whereas older individuals may be attempting suicide or self-mutilation.

ETIOLOGY

1. Common alkalis
   a. Sodium or potassium hydroxide (lye), washing powders, paint removers, drain pipe and toilet bowl cleaners, Clinitest tablets
   b. Liquids: drain (Liquid Plumber, Drāno) and oven cleaners
   c. Solid: Drāno (granular), Clinitest (tablets)
   d. Other: sodium hypochlorite bleach (if >5%), some detergents, electric dishwashing agents
   e. Button (disk) batteries
2. Common acids
   a. Hydrochloric acid: metal, swimming pool, and toilet bowl cleaners
   b. Sulfuric acid: battery acid, toilet bowl cleaners, industrial drain cleaners
   c. Other: slate cleaners, soldering flux

DIAGNOSTIC FINDINGS

The nature of the ingestion must be defined. Specific attention should be directed to the material ingested (solid or liquid, acid or alkali), to its volume, to the length of contact (when? was there emesis? was diluent used?), to the volume of liquids or solids in the stomach at the time of ingestion, and to the presence of pain, dysphagia, drooling, or other symptoms.

Physical examination should include a check for drooling, respiratory distress, oral or pharyngeal burns, evidence of chest abnormality or mediastinitis, and abdominal pain, guarding, or tenderness.

1. *Alkalis* primarily produce liquefaction necrosis and thermal injury, with deep tissue penetration and a high risk of perforation. Skin burns and major ocular injury may occur (see Chapters 46 and 59). Initially, esophageal burn is characterized by erythema followed by shallow ulceration within 24 hours. Edema may lead to narrowing in 48 to 72 hours and eventually scar tissue and strictures 4 to 6 weeks after the initial injury.
   a. Oropharyngeal burns with associated drooling, dysphagia, vomiting, and chest pain are common. Crystalline caustics tend to attach to the oral mucosa and produce severe burns of the mouth rather than the esophagus. Gulping caustic liquids may spare the oral and pharyngeal mucosa and cause severe burns of the esophagus. Solid alkali, particularly lye, may lodge in the oropharynx or esophagus. Clinitest tablets cause a high incidence of esophageal burns with stricture, intestinal perforation, and laryngeal edema.
   b. The absence of oropharyngeal burns does not exclude esophageal injury. Esophageal injury is most commonly present if two or more of the following are present: vomiting, drooling, or stridor. Esophageal perforation may result in mediastinitis and shock. Stricture may develop as a delayed complication.
   c. Soft tissue swelling of the upper airway caused by involvement of the larynx, epiglottis, or vocal cords or by tracheal aspiration may produce respiratory distress.
2. *Acid* substances cause coagulation necrosis and thermal injury. The skin may be burned by exposure, and a major ocular emergency may result from acid exposure (see Chapters 46 and 59). There may be associated soft tissue swelling, with potential respiratory obstruction. Specific effects may include the following:
   a. Oropharyngeal burns with significant ingestions; rare esophageal perforation
   b. Perforation of the stomach or small intestine, acute peritonitis, and shock
3. Bleach in combination with acids (HCl) may produce chlorine gas, resulting in pulmonary damage if inhaled. Household

bleach ingestion (about 3% concentration), rarely causes esophageal burns.

Ancillary Data

1. Complete blood count (CBC), type and cross-match, and oximetry or ABGs with significant exposure.
2. X-ray films. Lateral neck may be useful in evaluating upper respiratory edema; chest and abdominal films are needed if there are extensive complications.

MANAGEMENT

The first priority must be to assess the airway and ensure that any obstruction, if present, is relieved. If extensive burns of the oropharynx are present, a cricothyrotomy may be indicated. Ventilation and circulatory insufficiency must be treated.

1. Administer oxygen, particularly if the exposure has been to chlorine gas.
2. Dilute ingested material with milk or water as soon as possible. This should optimally be initiated at home before leaving for the emergency department (ED). Do not use weak acids or alkalis for neutralization because a tremendous amount of heat can be produced. If involved, the skin should be washed well; each eye is irrigated with 1 to 2 L saline solution for at least 20 minutes when exposed (see Chapter 59).

   NOTE: Dilution of ingested material is contraindicated if perforation, shock, or upper airway compromise is present.
3. Do not initiate emesis, lavage, or catharsis or give charcoal.

Other Considerations

1. Steroids may have a role in deep or circumferential esophageal burns, but their role is controversial. If used, they should be initiated as soon after injury as possible

and continued for at least 3 weeks, usually in consultation with a surgeon.
   • Hydrocortisone (Solu-Cortef), 4-5 mg/kg/dose q6hr IV, or methylprednisolone (Solu-Medrol), 2 mg/kg/dose q6hr IV
2. Antibiotics are not indicated prophylactically but may be required if mediastinitis or perforation develops.
3. A surgeon should be involved early in the evaluation. Surgery is immediately required if perforation or mediastinitis develops.
4. Esophagoscopy should be performed in the first 24 to 48 hours after ingestion in all patients with any oropharyngeal burns, symptoms, or history of significant ingestion.
   a. Should be performed only to the point of major burn and not beyond
   b. Contraindicated with respiratory obstruction, perforation, shock, or third-degree burns of the oropharynx
5. Button (disk) batteries require special considerations. For children with a history of ingestion, perform radiographs to localize the battery. If it is lodged in the *esophagus,* removal should be considered an emergency. Batteries less than 18 mm (penny size) are rarely stopped in the esophagus. When beyond the esophagus, it needs to be retrieved if there are any signs or symptoms of GI injury. Batteries larger than 15 mm, although rare, when ingested by children less than 6 years old may have a delayed transit time and are unlikely to pass if they have not passed within 48 hours of ingestion; camera batteries larger than 23 mm ingested by any age group need similar management. Follow-up in 4 to 7 days for all batteries if the object has not been found in the stool. The National Button Battery Ingestion Hotline (202-625-3333) can provide chemical content of batteries with the imprint code and update clinical management approaches.

6. The timing of esophageal dilation and bougienage is controversial; most prefer to wait until several weeks after injury. Serial barium swallows may provide evidence of developing esophageal stricture; if present, discontinue steroids and begin dilation.

7. Intraluminal shunt may be indicated for patients with documented second- and third-degree esophageal burns.

DISPOSITION

All patients with oropharyngeal burns should be admitted for fluid management and observation of respiratory and GI complications, as well as for esophagoscopy. Nutrition must be maintained.

Long-term follow-up observation is essential to monitor the development of esophageal or gastric stenosis, with esophagoscopy or barium studies. Dilation and bougienage may be necessary. In patients in whom complete obliteration of the esophagus develops from stricture or who have not responded to dilation, colon interposition may be considered.

Psychiatric involvement is required in self-inflicted injuries, and poison-prevention counseling is essential in all families.

REFERENCES

Anderson KD, Rouse TM, Randolph JG: A controlled trial of corticosteroids in children with corrosive injury of the esophagus, *N Engl J Med* 323:637, 1990.

Brent J, Lucas M, Kulig K, et al: Methanol poisoning in a 6-week old infant, *J Pediatr* 118:644, 1991.

Burkhart K, Kulig K: The other alcohols: methanol, ethylene glycol, and isopropanol. In Harwood-Nuss A, editor: *Emergency medicine clinics of North America,* Philadelphia, 1990, WB Saunders.

Crain EF, Gershel JC, Mezey AP: Caustic ingestion: symptoms as predictors of esophageal injury, *Am J Dis Child* 138:863, 1984.

Estrera A, Taylor W, Mills LJ, et al: Corrosive burns of the esophagus and stomach: a recommendation for an aggressive surgical approach, *Ann Thorac Surg* 41:276, 1986.

Howell JM, Dalsey WC, Hartsell FW, et al: Steroid for the treatment of corrosive esophageal injury: a statistical analysis of past studies, *Am J Emerg Med* 10:421, 1992.

Krenzelok EP: Caustic esophageal and gastric erosion without evidence of oral burns following detergent ingestion, *JACEP* 8:194, 1979.

Kulig K, Rumack CM, Rumack BH, et al: Disk battery ingestion: elevated urine mercury levels and enema removal of battery fragments, *JAMA* 249:2502, 1983.

Litovitz TL, Butterfield AB, Holloway RR, et al: Button battery ingestion: assessment of therapeutic modalities and battery discharge state, *J Pediatr* 105:868, 1984.

Litovitz T, Schmitz BF: Ingestion of cylindrical and button batteries: an analysis of 2382 cases, *Pediatrics* 89:747, 1992.

ANTICHOLINERGICS

ALERT: Peripheral and central effects are prominent. Physostigmine is indicated for unresponsive seizures and dangerous psychoses.

A wide spectrum of drugs possess anticholinergic properties. For most of these agents, there is good GI absorption with a peak effect at 1 to 2 hours.

PHARMACEUTICS WITH ANTICHOLINERGIC PROPERTIES

1. Antihistamines: diphenhydramine (Benadryl), tripelennamine (Pyribenzamine)

2. Belladonna alkaloids and related synthetic compounds: atropine, scopolamine, glycopyrrolate

3. Phenothiazines: chlorpromazine (Thorazine), thioridazine (Mellaril), prochlorperazine (Compazine), trifluoperazine (Stelazine)

4. Butyrophenones: haloperidol (Haldol)

5. Thioxanthenes: chlorprothixene (Taractan), thiothixene (Navane)

6. Cyclic antidepressants: amitriptyline (Elavil), nortriptyline (Pamelor), imipramine (Tofranil), desipramine (Norpramin), doxepin (Sinequan)

7. GI and genitourinary (GU) antispasmodics: dicyclomine (Bentyl), propantheline bromide (Pro-Banthine)
8. Local mydriatics: tropicamide (Mydriacyl), cyclopentolate (Cyclogyl)
9. Over-the-counter (OTC) analgesics: pyrilamine (Excedrin P.M.), cinnamedrine (Midol)
10. OTC cold remedies
11. OTC sleep aids: pyrilamine (Sominex, Sleep-Eze), doxylamine (Unisom)
12. Antiparkinsonian medications: benztropine (Cogentin), trihexyphenidyl (Artane)

PLANTS CONTAINING ANTICHOLINERGIC ALKALOIDS

1. *Amanita muscaria* (fly agaric)
2. *Amanita pantherina* (panther mushroom)
3. *Datura stramonium* (jimsonweed)
4. *Myristica fragrans* (nutmeg)
5. *Solanum carolinense* (wild tomato)
6. *Solanum dulcamara* (bittersweet)
7. *Solan tuberosum* (potato)
8. *Lantana camara* (wild sage)

DIAGNOSTIC FINDINGS

Anticholinergics present a consistent clinical picture, although some variability exists in findings with specific drugs. Patients with diphenoxylate and atropine (Lomotil) overdoses primarily have anticholinergic (atropine) findings initially, but many hours after ingestion they may have cardiopulmonary depression, miosis, hypotension, and coma consistent with a narcotic overdose.

1. *Peripheral* signs and symptoms of anticholinergic overdose result primarily from muscarinic blockage:
   a. Vital sign alterations: tachycardia, hyperpyrexia, hypertension. Hypotension may be a late finding (phenothiazines may cause hypotension because of their α-blocking action)
   b. Dry flushed skin and dry mucous membranes.
   c. Dilated pupils (mydriasis).
   d. Urinary retention and decreased bowel sounds.
   e. Dysrhythmias, primarily as a result of direct myocardial depressant effect. Only cyclic antidepressants predictably cause ventricular dysrhythmias. Cyclic antidepressants also prolong atrioventricular (AV) conduction and prevent reuptake of norepinephrine, leading to ventricular dysrhythmias and heart block. Thioridazine (Mellaril) may have a similar effect.
2. *Central* anticholinergic syndrome: a delirium characteristic of an evolving organic brain syndrome. Signs are as follows:
   a. Disorientation, uncontrolled agitation, impaired long-term memory, and hallucinations. The patient is rarely violent or self-mutilating.
   b. Movement disorders.
      (1) Phenothiazines and cyclic antidepressants often cause extrapyramidal reactions, including myoclonus and choreoathetosis.
      (2) Picking and grasping movements are common with overdoses of most of the anticholinergics.
   c. Seizures, coma, respiratory failure, and cardiovascular collapse.

Ancillary Data

1. Urine toxicology screen may be useful, but the laboratory should be notified of which agents are suspected.
2. Glucose, electrocardiogram (ECG), and ABG as indicated.
3. X-ray films. Abdominal film taken before tablets dissolve may show phenothiazines.

MANAGEMENT

Supportive care (airway management and maintaining vital signs) is of highest priority. All comatose patients should receive 0.5-1.0 gm/kg IV dextrose and 0.1 mg/kg up to 2 mg IV of naloxone.

Physostigmine is a naturally occurring alkaloid that is a reversible cholinesterase inhibitor.

Centrally, it crosses the blood-brain barrier and is capable of reversing coma, delirium, seizures, and extrapyramidal signs. Peripherally, it is effective in reversing the muscarinic blockage.

1. Indications for physostigmine.
   a. Supraventricular dysrhythmias resulting in hemodynamic instability.
   b. Pronounced hallucinations and agitation in which the patient may be a danger to self or others.
   c. Coma caused by anticholinergic overdose. Physostigmine should be used as a diagnostic test and not given just "to wake the patient up."
      NOTE: It is best to reserve physostigmine for life-threatening situations because safer agents are available for treatment of seizures (phenytoin, phenobarbital, and diazepam) and dysrhythmias (alkalinization, phenytoin, lidocaine).
2. Dosage (administer slowly).
   a. Children: 0.02 mg/kg/dose up to 0.5 mg/dose IV slowly over 3 minutes q10min up to a total dose of 2 mg.
   b. Adults: 1 to 2 mg IV slowly over 3 minutes q10min until cessation of life-threatening condition or until it appears ineffective. Maximum dose: 4 mg in 30 minutes.
3. Side effects include seizures, brady-dysrhythmia, asystole, and cholinergic crisis (hypersalivation, bradycardia, and hypotension).
4. Contraindications. Patients with asthma, gangrene, cardiovascular disease, or obstruction of the GI or GU tracts.

Other management techniques include the following:

1. Initial treatment of seizures with diazepam (Valium), 0.2-0.3 mg/kg/dose IV, followed by phenobarbital (see Chapter 21)
2. Treatment of cyclic antidepressant overdoses. If the QRS is prolonged or ventricular dysrhythmias are present, treat with sodium bicarbonate, 1-2 mEq/kg/dose q10-20min IV, to achieve alkalinization (plasma pH >7.5), as well as phenytoin or lidocaine (p. 61)
3. Sedation. May usually be achieved by treatment with diazepam (Valium)
4. Large amounts of naloxone (Narcan), 0.8 to 2.0 mg prn IV, with some cases of diphenoxylate (Lomotil) overdoses

DISPOSITION

All symptomatic patients require inpatient treatment and observation, usually in an intensive care unit (ICU) capable of cardiac and neurologic monitoring.

REFERENCES

Amitai Y, Singer R, Almog S, et al: Atropine poisoning in children from automatic injectors during the Gulf Crisis, *Vet Hum Toxicol* 33:360, 1991.
Sennhauser FGH, Schwarz HP: Toxic psychosis from transdermal scopolamine in a child, *Lancet* 2.1033, 1986.

CARBON MONOXIDE

ALERT: Several members of the same household with headache, nausea, or shortness of breath should be evaluated for exposure.

Carbon monoxide is an odorless, colorless gas produced by internal combustion engines and by combustion of natural gas, charcoal, and coal gas. Fire victims often have high levels after exposure. Methylene chloride (a solvent used in paint strippers) is metabolized to carbon monoxide. Carbon monoxide binds to hemoglobin 210 times more avidly than does oxygen.

DIAGNOSTIC FINDINGS

All potential cases should be evaluated, especially if several members of the same household are experiencing similar symptoms.

Signs and symptoms progress with increased exposure, reflecting the levels of carboxyhemoglobin in the blood. The levels listed below are from data about adults. Children may have an increased susceptibility to CO toxicity. Children with levels greater than 25% carboxyhemoglobin (HgCO) consistently showed syncope and lethargy in a recent study. Symptoms in all patients may correlate more closely with the length of exposure than with the actual, measured carboxyhemoglobin levels. Furthermore, levels may be influenced by significant delays between exposure and presentation, particularly if oxygen therapy has been administered en route.

Complications

1. Cardiac
   a. Dysrhythmias (see Chapter 6)
   b. Myocardial ischemia with ST-T wave changes (usually only in adults)
2. Pulmonary edema and hemorrhage either immediately or as delayed finding (see Chapter 19)
3. Renal failure secondary to myoglobinuria
4. CNS
   a. Encephalopathy with associated agitation, seizures, and coma (see Chapters 15 and 21)
   b. Cerebral edema
   c. Long-term neuropsychiatric changes and memory defects

Ancillary Data

1. HgCO level. Normally this is less than 1%, although it has been reported to be as high as 5% after driving on busy freeways. Heavy smokers may have levels up to 15%. Fetal hemoglobin can contribute to a falsely elevated level of HgCO in infants less than 30 months of age.

2. ABG with a measured, not calculated, oxygen saturation. Oximetry is not a reliable indicator of CO poisoning or lack thereof.
3. ECG with any evidence of myocardial ischemia, chest pain, or shortness of breath.
4. Chest x-ray film, with smoke inhalation. Often normal in first 24 hours (see Chapter 53).

MANAGEMENT

Although it is clear that hyperbaric oxygen is the treatment of choice for patients in coma from CO poisoning, it is controversial what levels of HgCO require such treatment if the patient has minimal symptoms and should not be the only criteria unless greater than 25%. Some factors that may be considered include transient loss of consciousness, ischemic changes on ECG, focal neurologic defects, or abnormal psychometric testing. Hyperbaric oxygen may decrease the long-term neurologic sequelae in these patients. Some experts have suggested that patients with HgCO levels greater than 20% to 25% at the point of exposure, a history of altered level of consciousness or persistent neurologic defect, cardiac abnormality, acidosis, or syncope should be treated in the hyperbaric chamber. The data regarding an absolute level are not available; symptoms may be more important than a specific level.

Carboxyhemoglobin level in the blood (%)	Common clinical findings
10-20	No apparent findings
20-30	Dyspnea (vigorous exertion)
30-40	Dyspnea (moderate exertion)
40-50	Intermittent throbbing headache
50-60	Throbbing headache, dyspnea, irritability, fatigue, dizziness, blurred vision
>60	Headache, confusion, syncope, tachycardia, tachypnea Stupor, seizures, coma Unconsciousness, fibrillation, tachycardia, death

1. Remove the patient from the source of combustion and immediately administer high-flow oxygen while continuing resuscitation. 100% oxygen can be delivered through a mask or an endotracheal tube.

   NOTE: The half-life of HgCO at room air is approximately 4 hours, and with 100% oxygen it is approximately 40 minutes. With hyperbaric oxygen (2 atm), this is reduced to less than 20 minutes.

2. Monitor for evolving complications and treat aggressively.

Patients who are pregnant at the time of exposure place the fetus at great risk. Fetus is at relatively increased risk from elevated carbon monoxide levels. Treatment should be continued for at least three times as long as the time recommended for the mother alone. Consultation should be obtained.

DISPOSITION

Patients who require admission for prolonged observation and treatment include the following:

1. Those with HgCO greater than 20% to 25%. This decision must be individualized.
2. Those with abnormal neurologic examination, ECG findings, or acidosis.
3. Pregnant women with HgCO greater than 15%. They require more prolonged oxygen therapy (approximately three times the amount calculated).

Before the patient is discharged, the source of CO must be eliminated in the household or car. The clinician who suspects CO poisoning should evaluate all household residents.

REFERENCES

Buckley RG, Aks SE, Eshom Jl, et al: The pulse oximetry gap in carbon monoxide intoxication, *Ann Emerg Med* 24:252, 1994.

Bozeman WP, Myers RA, Barish RA: Confirmation of the pulse oximetry gap in carbon monoxide poisoning, *Ann Emerg Med* 30:608, 1997.

Hampson NB, Norkool DM: Carbon monoxide poisoning in children riding in the back of pickup trucks, *JAMA* 267:538, 1992.

Olson KR, Seger D: Hyperbaric oxygen from carbon monoxide poisoning: does it really work? *Ann Emerg Med* 25:535, 1995.

Parish RA: Smoke inhalation and carbon monoxide poisoning in children, *Pediatr Emerg Care* 2:36, 1986.

Seger D, Welch L: Carbon monoxide controversies: neuropsychologic testing, mechanisms and toxicity and hyperbaric oxygen, *Ann Emerg Med* 24:242, 1994.

Sloan EP, Murphy DG, Hart R, et al: Complications and protocol considerations in carbon monoxide: poisoned patients require hyperbaric oxygen therapy: report from a 10-year experience, *Ann Emerg Med* 18:629, 1989.

Tibbles PM, Perrotta PL: Treatment of carbon monoxide poisoning: a critical review of human outcome studies comparing normobaric oxygen with hyperbaric oxygen, *Ann Emerg Med* 24:269, 1994.

Thom SR, Taver RL, Mendiguren IL, et al: Delayed neuropsychologic sequelae after carbon monoxide poisoning prevention by treatment with hyperbaric oxygen, *Ann Emerg Med* 25:474, 1995.

Weaver LK, Hopkins RO, Larson-Lohr V: Neuropsychologic and functional recovery from severe carbon monoxide poisoning without hyperbaric oxygen therapy, *Ann Emerg Med* 27:736, 1996.

CARDIOVASCULAR DRUGS

β-ADRENERGIC BLOCKING AGENTS

The primary indications for β-adrenergic blocking agents include angina, dysrhythmias, hypertension, migraines, glaucoma, and thyrotoxicosis. β-Adrenergic stimulation increases heart rate and cardiac inotropy (β_1) and relaxes bronchial and vascular smooth muscle (β_2). Blockade inhibits these effects and may have a direct myocardial depressant effect as well. Therapeutic doses vary with the individual drug but may include bradycardia, AV conduction defects, hypotension, congestive heart failure, bronchospasm, hypoglycemia, as well as fatigue, depression, and sexual dysfunction. Cardioselective agents (acebutolol, atenolol, metoprolol) cause little bronchospasm; pindolol is rarely associated with bradycardia and hypotension. However, after significant overdose, selectivity is lost and the toxicities of nonselective and selective agents are similar.

Diagnostic Findings

Signs and symptoms occur with impaired cardiovascular function. Dizziness, syncope, and collapse may occur along with impaired mental status, lethargy, coma, and seizures. Bradycardia and hypotension may be present. Pulmonary edema may be noted.

The ECG may reveal sinus bradycardia and AV conduction defects. Asystole, disappearance of P waves, and QRS widening may be associated with massive overdose. Serum drug levels do not correlate with the severity of intoxication.

Management

1. Supportive care and monitoring are essential. Evaluate airway and breathing and manage as appropriate. Gastric lavage may be performed initially in the patient. Administer charcoal as early as possible.
2. Treat symptomatic bradycardia initially with atropine, 0.02 mg/kg/dose IV.
3. Hypotension responds to fluids and dopamine, the latter often at very high dosages.
4. Seizures are best managed by diazepam, 0.2-0.3 mg/kg/dose IV, followed by standard management (p. 183).
5. Glucagon at high dosages and diluted is effective in a dose of 0.05-0.1 mg/kg IV (adult 3-5 mg/dose IV q5min up to a total dose of 10 to 15 mg). Response is rapid but lasts only 10 to 20 minutes and may require a continuous infusion, using the initial successful dose as the determinant of the rate of infusion, usually in the range of 0.05-0.1 mg/kg/hr.

Disposition

Patients who are asymptomatic 6 hours after a trivial ingestion may be discharged. Those with any evidence of cardiovascular or CNS findings and those who have ingested a time-release formulation should usually be admitted.

CALCIUM CHANNEL BLOCKERS

Becoming increasingly used in the management of angina, hypertension, and tachydysrhythmias, calcium channel blocking agents are available for ingestion. These calcium antagonists interfere with the entry of calcium into cells through the slow-calcium voltage-dependent channels. Toxicity is due to hypoperfusion associated with vasodilation, negative inotropism, and cardiac dysrhythmia.

Diagnostic Findings

Myocardial hypoperfusion may cause angina and evidence of ischemia. Mental status may be altered; focal neurologic findings (including hemiparesis) have been noted. Coma and seizures may occur.

ECG may demonstrate bradycardia, asystole, inverted P waves, tachycardia, conduction abnormalities, QRS prolongation, and nonspecific ST and T changes.

Management

1. Stabilize patient and begin lavage if ingestion was very recent. Charcoal should be given as quickly as possible. Patients require constant monitoring.
2. Intravenous calcium chloride (10% solution), 25 mg/kg (maximum: 1 gm) over 3 to 5 minutes, may be used in unstable patients.
3. Vasodilation may respond to fluids and dopamine.

Disposition

Patients who are asymptomatic 8 hours after a trivial ingestion of a nonmodified-release agent may be discharged. All others require ongoing monitoring.

CLONIDINE

Clonidine (Catapres) is the most common cardiovascular drug associated with pediatric ingestions. It is a central and peripheral α_2-adrenergic agonist used in the management of hypertension. The half-life is 9 hours.

Diagnostic Findings

Signs and symptoms that usually develop within 1 hour of ingestion include impaired level of consciousness, bradycardia, respiratory depression, miosis, hypotension, hypertension, and hypothermia. Hypotension may develop as a delayed finding. Symptoms and signs may mimic a narcotic overdose.

Laboratory studies are not useful except those obtained to maximize supportive care.

Management

Supportive care, gastric lavage (if done very early), and charcoal should be initiated. Hypotension may respond to fluids and dopamine; hypertension is transient and usually does not require therapy. In severe cases, it may be treated with a short-acting vasodilator such as nitroprusside, 0.5-10 µg/kg/min IV. Naloxone, 2 mg IV, supplemented by an IV infusion may have a beneficial role.

All children require monitoring for at least 4 hours. Symptomatic patients should be admitted.

DIGITALIS

Digoxin is widely used in the effort to improve cardiac inotropy, concurrently affecting electrical activity. Digitalis increases the level of intracellular calcium, promoting the initiation of muscle contraction. Excessive levels may result from dosing problems, decreased digoxin elimination (renal failure or drug interaction with quinidine, calcium channel blockers, or spironolactone), or decreased volume of distribution (starvation, muscle wasting). Toxicity can occur at therapeutic levels associated with hypokalemia, hypercalcemia, hypernatremia, alkalosis, hypoxia, hypomagnesemia, nodal disease, and primary cardiac disease such as ischemia, cor pulmonale, and cardiac trauma/surgery.

Clinical presentation and management are discussed on p. 150.

REFERENCES

Heidemann SM, Sarnaik AP: Clonidine poisoning in children, *Crit Care Med* 18:618, 1990.

Love JN: Beta blocker toxicity: a clinical diagnosis, *Am J Emerg Med* 12:356, 1994.

Weiner DA: Calcium channel blockers, *Med Clin North Am* 72:83, 1988.

Wiley JF, Wiley CC, Torrey SB, et al: Clonidine poisoning in young children, *J Pediatr* 116:654, 1990.

Woolf AD, Wendger T, Smith TW, et al: The use of digoxin-specific Fab fragments for severe digitalis intoxication in children, *N Engl J Med* 326:1734, 1992.

Zaritsky AL, Horowitz M, Chernow B: Glucagon antagonism of calcium channel blocker-induced myocardial dysfunction, *Crit Care Med* 16:246, 1988.

COCAINE (P. 391)

ALERT: Cardiovascular dysrhythmias and CNS stimulation must be monitored.

Cocaine may be used as an anesthetic, but it is often abused, causing sympathomimetic effects, CNS stimulation, and euphoria. Administration may occur through insufflation (30% to 60% absorption), intravenously, smoking free base (onset of symptoms is in seconds), or orally. Cocaine may be teratogenic.

DIAGNOSTIC FINDINGS (Table 55-3)

The major findings reflect sympathomimetic stimulation producing dilated pupils, tachycardia, dysphoric agitation, and respiratory stimulation.

TABLE 55-3 Sympathomimetic Syndrome: Common Clinical Findings

Clinical findings	Amphetamines	Cocaine (p. 391)	β-Adrenergic agents
Central nervous system			
Stimulation	Yes	Yes	Yes
Hallucination	Yes	Yes	Yes
Seizures	Yes	Yes	
Coma	Yes	Yes	
Cardiovascular			
Tachycardia	Yes	Yes	
Dysrhythmias	Yes	Yes	Yes
Hypertension	Yes	Yes	Yes
Nausea, vomiting, abdominal pain	Yes		Yes
Mydriasis	Yes	Yes	Yes
Hyperthermia	Yes	Yes	
Other	Intracranial hemorrhage, self-destructive behavior		

Complications

1. Cardiovascular dysrhythmias, myocardial ischemia
2. Intestinal ischemia
3. Pneumomediastinum
4. Intracranial hemorrhage
5. Rhabdomyolysis
6. Seizures
7. Cardiovascular collapse

MANAGEMENT

After stabilization and initiation of monitoring, specific problems may also need to be treated:

1. Seizures (see Chapter 21): Use diazepam (Valium), lorazepam (Ativan), or phenytoin.
2. Dysrhythmias (see Chapter 6): Use phenytoin initially. Consider cardioversion. Tachydysrhythmic patients with hypertension may be treated with labetalol (0.25 mg/kg IV over 2 minutes and titrated). Esmolol may also be helpful.
3. Decontamination.
   a. Nasal: Clean nasal passage with cotton applicator dipped in a non–water-soluble product such as petrolatum.
   b. GI: Give activated charcoal.

REFERENCES

Cravey RH: Cocaine deaths in infants, *J Anal Toxicol* 12:354, 1988.

Derlet RW, Albertson TE: Emergency department presentation of cocaine intoxication, *Ann Emerg Med* 18:182, 1989.

Garland JS, Smith DS, Rice TB, et al: Accidental cocaine intoxication in a nine-month old infant: Presentation and treatment, *Pediatr Emerg Care* 5:245, 1989.

Lyons Jones K: Developmental pathogenesis of defects associated with prenatal cocaine exposure: fetal vascular disruption, *Clin Perinatol* 18:139, 1991.

Mathias DW: Cocaine-associated myocardial ischemia: review of clinical and angiographic findings, *Am J Med* 81:675, 1986.

CYCLIC ANTIDEPRESSANTS

ALERT: Anticholinergic effects and cardiotoxicity are prominent. Immediate intervention is necessary.

Cyclic antidepressants (CADs) are a widely used class of medications. Beyond their use as antidepressants they are popular in the treatment of enuresis (e.g., imipramine). Their major toxicity is from their anticholinergic and quinidine-like effects. Plasma CAD levels do not correlate with toxicity. Tricyclic antidepressants (TCAs), one type of this class of drugs, are lipophilic. TCAs may cross the placental barrier, although teratogenicity is not documented.

ETIOLOGY

Imipramine (Tofranil), amitriptyline (Elavil), desipramine (Norpramine), doxepin (Sinequan), and nortriptyline (Pamelor) are commonly used.

DIAGNOSTIC FINDINGS

Anticholinergic, both peripheral and central, effects may be prominent and usually develop within 6 hours (p. 369).

1. Peripheral findings include dry, flushed skin and dry mucous membranes, dilated pupils, and urinary retention, with decreased bowel sounds. Tachycardia, dysrhythmias, hyperpyrexia, and hypertension may be present.
2. Centrally, patients have delirium with disorientation, agitation, hallucinations, and movement disorders. Seizures and coma are common.

Dysrhythmias result from the anticholinergic effects of tricyclics and from direct cardiotoxicity, blockage of norepinephrine uptake, and a quinidine-like action (myocardial depression and AV conduction delay). Supraventricular tachydysrhythmias, conduction blocks, and ventricular dysrhythmias are common, although their onset may be delayed. The best correlate with risk of seizures is a QRS equal to or greater than 0.10 second, whereas ventricular dysrhythmias occur when the QRS is 0.16 second or more.

Hypotension is common, secondary to myocardial depression and alpha blockade. Patients with fatal ingestion may exhibit trivial signs and symptoms that may have rapidly progressed to coma, conduction defects, dysrhythmias, hypotension, and seizures.

Ancillary Data

1. Cyclic antidepressant level. Although unreliable as an indicator of potential toxicity, documentation of the drug's presence by toxicology screens may be important. Toxicology screens are not of predictive value regarding complications.
2. ECG on all patients; oximetry, ABG, and glucose as indicated.

DIFFERENTIAL DIAGNOSIS

Intoxications must be differentiated from anticholinergic and quinidine reactions.

MANAGEMENT

1. Life support is crucial because of the potential findings of respiratory depression and hemodynamic compromise. Patients should receive oxygen, IVs, and cardiac monitoring on arrival. Administer dextrose and naloxone as indicated by mental status.
2. Perform gastric emptying (only by lavage, and only if done very early); give charcoal as soon as possible.
3. Physostigmine is effective as a treatment for the anticholinergic effects; its use should be reserved for situations where other modalities have failed (p. 371).
   a. Dosage—children: 0.02 mg/kg/dose up to 0.5 mg/dose IV slowly over 3 minutes q10min up to a total dose of 2 mg; adult: 1 to 2 mg IV slowly over 3 minutes q10min until cessation of life-threatening condition or ineffective. Maximum dose: 4 mg in 30 minutes.
   b. Indicated with hemodynamically unstable supraventricular dysrhythmias and also behavior that is potentially harmful. It is best to reserve physostigmine for life-threatening situations because there are safer agents for treatment of seizures (phenytoin, phenobarbital, diazepam) and dysrhythmias (phenytoin, alkalinization, lidocaine).
4. Seizures should initially be treated with diazepam (Valium), 0.25 mg/kg/dose IV q10min prn (see Chapter 21).

5. Patients with prolongation of the QRS or ventricular dysrhythmias should be alkalinized with $NaHCO_3$ 1-2 mEq/kg/dose IV q10-20min prn to maintain plasma pH of 7.5 or greater. This appears to be prophylactic in preventing progression of dysrhythmias.

- Ventricular dysrhythmias or conduction delays (QRS >0.16 second) should be treated with phenytoin (Dilantin), 5 mg/kg loading dose IV and then with maintenance dose. It also has the advantage of being an anticonvulsant. Lidocaine also may be used (see Chapter 6).

6. Coma usually requires supportive care but is self-limited and not an indication for physostigmine.

7. Hypotension may respond to fluid challenge. If unsuccessful, use norepinephrine as the pressor agent (see Chapter 5).

DISPOSITION

All patients require monitoring for at least 6 hours after ingestion. Significant ingestions or symptomatic patients with CAD overdose require admission to an ICU for treatment and cardiac monitoring. Those with minimal ingestions who after 6 hours are asymptomatic may be discharged if there are bowel sounds and cathartics and charcoal have been administered. Appropriate psychiatric evaluation should also be completed if ingestion was deliberate. Follow-up observation is necessary.

REFERENCES

Boehnert MT, Lovejoy RH: Value of QRS duration versus serum drug level in predicting seizures and ventricular arrhythmia after an acute overdose of tricyclic antidepressants, *N Engl J Med* 313:474, 1985.

Callaham M, Kassel D: Epidemiology of fatal tricyclic antidepressant ingestion: implications for management, *Ann Emerg Med* 14:1, 1985.

Ellison DR, Pentel PR: Clinical features and consequences of seizures due to cyclic antidepressant overdose, *Am J Emerg Med* 7:5, 1989.

Pellinen TJ et al: Electrocardiographic and clinical features of tricyclic antidepressant intoxication, *Ann Clin Res* 19: 12, 1987.

Sasyniuk BI, Jhamandas V, Valois M: Experimental amitriptyline intoxication: treatment of cardiac toxicity with sodium bicarbonate, *Ann Emerg Med* 15:1052, 1986.

Stremski ES, Brady WB, Prasad K, et al: Pediatric carbamazepine, *Ann Emerg Med* 25:624, 1995.

Tokarski GF, Young MJ: Criteria for admitting patients with tricyclic antidepressant overdose, *J Emerg Med* 6:121, 1988.

HALLUCINOGENS: PHENCYCLIDINE, LSD, MESCALINE

ALERT: Differentiate from other entities causing hallucinations

A wide variety of agents produce hallucinogenic states. Phencyclidine (PCP, angel dust), lysergic acid diethylamine (LSD, acid), and mescaline (buttons, peyote, cactus) produce similar behavioral changes, although the systemic effects are markedly different. Of the three, PCP is most widely used at present, although there is significant geographic variability to this pattern. Hallucinogens may be ingested along with other drugs, altering the presentation markedly.

DIAGNOSTIC FINDINGS
Phencyclidine (PCP)

Children less than 5 years old have symptoms different from those of older patients:

1. Bizarre behavior, including lethargy, staring spells, intermittent unresponsiveness, irritability, and poor feeding
2. CNS findings that may progress to coma—commonly ataxia, nystagmus, opisthotonos, and hyperreflexia
3. Tachypnea, tachycardia, and hypertension

Older patients have a progression of symptoms with increasing dosage.

1. Low doses (<5 mg): induce associated agitation, excitement, disorganized thought process, incoordination, nystagmus, blank-

stare appearance, and intoxication with drowsiness and apathy

2. Moderate doses (5-10 mg or 0.1-0.2 mg/kg): often induce stupor or coma, decreased peripheral sensation, muscular rigidity, myoclonus, nystagmus, flushing, hypersalivation, and vomiting

3. Large doses (>10 mg): cause coma with scizures, decerebrate posturing, hypertension, nystagmus, opisthotonos, hypersalivation, and diaphoresis

Lysergic Acid (LSD)

Effect lasts for 4 to 12 hours with an accompanying hallucinogenic state. The pupils are usually massively dilated. LSD may produce permanent psychosis in susceptible individuals and flashbacks months after the initial ingestion.

Ancillary Data

1. Do urine toxicology, analysis for PCP, and other studies indicated for support.
2. Let the laboratory know if phencyclidine is suspected because many urine screens do not specifically examine for it.

DIFFERENTIAL DIAGNOSIS

1. Intoxication
   a. Sedative: Hypnotics do not generally cause hypertension or hyperreflexia. Respirations are usually decreased.
   b. Anticholinergics: There are prominent peripheral and central findings. May cause hallucinations.
   c. Stimulants: Tachycardia, hypertension, and piloerection are more prominent.
2. Encephalitis, meningitis, Reye syndrome, or high fever
3. Acute psychosis

MANAGEMENT

Supportive care is essential, and associated drug ingestion should be considered.

1. Administration of dextrose and naloxone as indicated.
2. Activated charcoal.
3. Diuresis: Acidifying the urine is not recommended because it may increase the risk of precipitating myoglobin crystals in the urine if rhabdomyolysis has occurred.

With agitated and hallucinating patients:

1. Avoid physical restraints if possible.
2. With PCP, reduce stimuli.
3. Try to maintain verbal contact and reassure the patient.
4. Consult a psychiatrist for acute and long-term care.

If sedation is necessary, use diazepam (Valium) or midazolam (Versed). Hypertensive crisis may require treatment (see Chapter 18).

DISPOSITION

Most patients with significant findings require hospitalization for medical or psychiatric management.

REFERENCES

Farrar HC, Kearns GL: Cocaine: clinical pharmacology and toxicology, *J Pediatr* 115:665, 1989.

Kulig K: LSD. In Augenstein WL, editor: *Emergency medicine clinics of North America,* Philadelphia, 1990, WB Saunders.

Lange RA: Cocaine-induced coronary artery vasoconstriction, *N Engl J Med* 321:1553, 1989.

Tokarsk GF, Paganussi P, Urbanski R, et al: An evaluation of cocaine-induced chest pain, *Ann Emerg Med* 19:1088, 1990.

Woodward GA: Chest pain secondary to cocaine use, *Pediatr Emerg Care* 3:153, 1987.

HYDROCARBONS

ALERT: Pulmonary and CNS findings predominate, and specific guidelines for emesis or lavage should be followed.

The ingestion of hydrocarbons is a common occurrence in children, but management remains controversial. The toxicity of hydrocarbons varies with the relative viscosity (SSU: seconds for a quantity of liquid to pass through a standard aperture) and additives. The lower the viscosity, the higher the risk of pulmonary aspiration; certain additives have significant toxicity of their own.

ETIOLOGY

1. Viscosity (SSU)
   a. Less than 60 SSU: gasoline, turpentine, benzene, kerosene, mineral seal oil (furniture polish)
   b. Less than 100 SSU: lubricating grease, diesel oil, mothballs, paraffin
2. Toxic additives: "CHAMP"
   a. *C*amphor causes CNS excitement or depression.
   b. *H*alogenated hydrocarbons (i.e., carbon tetrachloride) produce hepatitis, nephritis, diarrhea, and CNS excitement or depression.
   c. *A*romatic (benzene) results in aplastic anemia, dysrhythmias, and CNS and respiratory depression.
   d. *M*etals (heavy metals such as mercury) result in GI bleeding, renal failure, and neurologic sequelae.
   e. *P*esticides, primarily organophosphates, also cause cholinergic signs and symptoms (p. 358).

DIAGNOSTIC FINDINGS

These depend on the history of the amount ingested (one swallow in a child is about 4 ml), the material (container should be examined), and the time elapsed. Findings include the following:

1. Coughing, dyspnea, and choking accompanying the initial ingestion.
2. Pulmonary symptoms. May be delayed up to 6 hours and include tachypnea, wheezing, and respiratory distress. The pneumonitis produces a fever that does not necessarily reflect a bacterial infection.
3. CNS depression or excitement.

4. Nausea, vomiting, and abdominal pain.
5. Pulmonary edema and dysrhythmias (see Chapter 6 and 19).
6. Cyanosis developing shortly after ingestion. May be associated with a toxin that causes methemoglobinemia.
7. Toluene (glue or paint sniffing). Produces psychiatric disturbances, CNS depression, abdominal pain, dysrhythmias, or renal tubular acidosis with associated hypokalemia and acidosis.

Ancillary Data

1. CBC. May demonstrate leukocytosis. Electrolytes are indicated if toluene inhalation is suspected.
2. ABG or pulse oximetry.
3. X-ray studies. Chest film results are usually abnormal in 90% of symptomatic patients, usually with a multilobar fluffy infiltrate. These findings may be delayed. Pulmonary edema may be present.
4. Other studies as indicated, including red cell cholinesterase and ECG.

MANAGEMENT

Initial management should include stabilization, with administration of oxygen, and decontamination of the patient by removal of clothing and washing the skin. Associated findings require treatment.

Indications for gastric emptying are controversial. At present they include the following: severe gastrointestinal or CNS symptoms, or hydrocarbon that contains one of the "CHAMP" additives (Fig. 55-2). Intubation and protection of the airway should be considered before lavage.

Steroids and antibiotics are not indicated prophylactically.

DISPOSITION

Patients require admission in accordance with the protocol outlined in Fig. 55-2. Before the

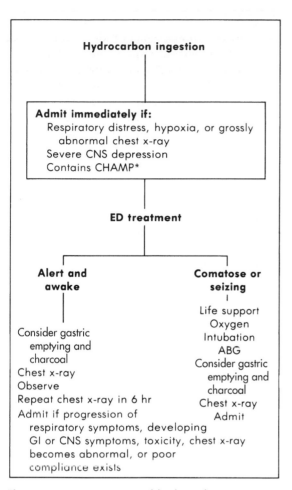

Fig. 55-2 Management of hydrocarbon ingestion. *Camphor, halogenated, aromatic (Benzene), metals (heavy), pesticides (organophosphates). Most of the common hydrocarbons ingested (e.g., gasoline, kerosene, oil) need not be removed regardless of the volume swallowed.

patient is discharged, poison-prevention counseling is required, and long-term follow-up observation of pulmonary status should be arranged.

REFERENCE

Zucker AR, Berger S, Wood LD: Management of kerosene induced pulmonary injury, *Crit Care Med* 14:303, 1986.

IRON

ALERT: GI symptoms are followed by shock, acidosis, and liver failure. Rapid treatment is required.

Normal daily dietary iron intake is about 15 mg, of which 10% is absorbed. It is then transported in the plasma bound to ferritin. The elemental iron content of the ingested substance is a good measure of potential toxicity. Ferrous sulfate contains 20% elemental iron; ferrous gluconate, 12%; and ferrous fumarate, 33%. Normally the serum iron (SI) is 50-100 µg/dl, and the total iron-binding capacity (TIBC) of ferritin is 300-400 µg/dl. An ingestion of 60 mg/kg of elemental iron is considered dangerous. Ingestions less than 20 mg/kg of elementary iron rarely are symptomatic.

DIAGNOSTIC FINDINGS

Toxicity from an iron ingestion has a fairly classic pattern of progression unless intervention is timely.

1. Stage 1: initial period (to 6 hours after ingestion). Vomiting, hematemesis, diarrhea, hematochezia, and abdominal pain occur.
2. Stage 2: latent period (2 to 12 hours). The patient improves.
3. Stage 3: systemic toxicity 4 to 24 hours after ingestion. Shock, metabolic acidosis, fever, hyperglycemia, bleeding, and death may occur.
4. Stage 4: hepatic failure beginning at 48 to 96 hours. This is associated with seizures and coma, and the patient has a poor prognosis.
5. Stage 5: late sequelae of pyloric stenosis may develop at 2 to 5 weeks.

Ancillary Data

Levels of SI and TIBC should be ascertained.

1. Peak SI less than 350 µg/dl is rarely symptomatic.

2. Peak levels greater than 500 µg/dl are considered toxic; patient should be chelated.

The presence of diarrhea, vomiting, leukocytosis, hyperglycemia, or a positive abdominal radiograph result is predictive of an SI level greater than 300 µg/dl.

Recent evidence suggests that the relative relationship between the SI and the TIBC should not be solely used as a basis for deciding to use deferoxamine because the TIBC is artificially increased in the presence of iron poisoning, although patients with a serum iron level greater than the TIBC require careful evaluation for chelation.

Immediate release products peak at 2 to 4 hours; modified-release preparations may have a later peak.

If an SI level is not readily obtainable, the deferoxamine provocation test may be useful for asymptomatic patients. A dose of 90 mg/kg given IM, or 1 hour of IV infusion at 15 mg/kg/hr IV, is given. The urine turning rose colored within 1 to 3 hours indicates the presence of free iron and feroxamine complex and is an indication for further treatment with deferoxamine.

Critically ill patients may be given higher doses of IV deferoxamine.

Other data include the following:

1. CBC, electrolyte and glucose levels, liver function tests, and ABG with significant ingestion.
2. Abdominal flat plate. Should be obtained as soon as possible. The presence of intact tablets in the stomach mandates aggressive therapy for removal.

DIFFERENTIAL DIAGNOSIS

1. Infection
   a. Acute gastroenteritis (see Chapter 76)
   b. Hepatitis (p. 639)
2. Gastrointestinal bleeding (see Chapter 35)
3. Shock (see Chapter 5)

MANAGEMENT

Management should reflect the amount of iron ingested; the clinical status of the child in terms of GI, CNS, and vital signs problems; and laboratory data.

Initial fluid and acid-base resuscitation is imperative when it is indicated. Shock, GI hemorrhage, and significant metabolic acidosis may be present. After initial measures are taken, the patient should be lavaged. Emesis or lavage to reduce or eliminate absorption is important. Some recommend adding some bicarbonate or deferoxamine to the lavage solution, although the efficacy is controversial. Radiographs should be taken as soon as possible to detect undissolved tablets (repeat radiograph after lavage if tablets are present initially).

1. Patients with peak levels less than 350 µg/dl require no further treatment if TIBC is greater than 350 µg/dl.
2. Patients with SI greater than TIBC (see above note) or SI greater than 350 µg/dl and TIBC unavailable should be treated with IV or IM deferoxamine if symptomatic.

Patients with levels of greater than or equal to 500 µg/dl must be treated immediately, with monitoring of electrolytes, hematocrit, and ABG.

1. For patients in shock or coma, give deferoxamine at 15 mg/kg/hr for 8 hours IV or as long as the urine remains colored. Start slowly and work up to this infusion rate over the first 15 to 30 minutes. In some cases, a higher dosage of IV deferoxamine may be used.
2. If patient is less seriously ill, give 90 mg/kg/dose IM q8hr.

Deferoxamine, 100 mg, can chelate 8.5 mg of elemental iron. It is contraindicated in renal failure and in patients shown to be sensitive to it.

1. Rapid IV administration of deferoxamine may cause hypotension, facial flushing, rash, urticaria, tachycardia, and shock.

2. If an SI level is unavailable or delayed and the patient is symptomatic, give deferoxamine, 90 mg/kg/dose IM and repeat q8hr.
3. An exchange transfusion may be indicated in cases of life-threatening iron toxicity.

If the x-ray study result is positive for iron past the pylorus, whole bowel irrigation can be useful with such solutions as polyethylene glycol electrolyte lavage solution. Surgical removal is rarely needed.

DISPOSITION

Asymptomatic patients with peak levels less than 350 µg/dl may be discharged after poison-prevention counseling.

All patients treated with deferoxamine should be admitted for observation and treatment. Such patients require follow-up observation after discharge to monitor long-term sequelae.

REFERENCES

Burkhart KK, Kulig KW, Hammond KB, et al: The rise in the total iron binding capacity after iron overdose, *Ann Emerg Med* 20:532, 1991.

Gomez III, McClafferty HH, Flory D, et al: Prevention of gastrointestinal iron absorption by chelation from an orally administered premixed deferoxamine/charcoal slurry, *Ann Emerg Med* 30:587, 1997.

Schaubein JL, Augestein L, Cox J, et al: Iron poisoning: report of three cases and a review of therapeutic intervention, *J Emerg Med* 8:309, 1990.

Tenenbein M: Whole bowel irrigation in iron poisoning, *J Pediatr* 111:142, 1987.

Tenenbein M, Yatschoff RW: The total iron binding capacity in iron poisoning, *Am J Dis Child* 145:437, 1991.

NARCOTICS AND SEDATIVE-HYPNOTICS

ALERT: CNS and respiratory depression and hypotension are prominent.

Narcotics and sedative-hypnotics in overdoses consistently produce CNS and respiratory depression, along with hypotension. Aggressive supportive care is the key to treatment.

ETIOLOGY

1. Narcotics
   a. Heroin (skag, dope, horse)
   b. Morphine
   c. Codeine
   d. Meperidine (Demerol)
   e. Methadone
   f. Propoxyphene (Darvon)
   g. Diphenoxylate (Lomotil)
2. Barbiturates
   a. Long acting (onset: 1 hour; peak: 6 hours; duration: days)—phenobarbital
   b. Intermediate acting (onset: 1 hour; peak: 3 to 6 hours; duration: 6 to 8 hours)—amobarbital, butabarbital
   c. Short acting (onset: minutes; peak: 3 hours; duration: 4 to 8 hours)—pentobarbital, secobarbital
   d. Ultra-short acting (onset: seconds; peak: seconds; duration: minutes)—thiopental
3. Sedative-hypnotics
   a. Benzodiazepines: chlordiazepoxide (Librium), diazepam (Valium)
   b. Cyclic ether: paraldehyde (Paral)
   c. Alcohols: chloral hydrate, ethchlorvynol (Placidyl)
   d. Propanediol carbamates: meprobamate (Miltown, Equanil)
   e. Piperidinediones: glutethimide (Doriden), methyprylon (Noludar)
   f. Quinazolines: methaqualone (Quäälude)

DIAGNOSTIC FINDINGS (Table 55-4)

Patients with overdoses of these drugs demonstrate variable levels of CNS depression with associated respiratory impairment. Other findings are outlined in Table 55-3. Associated ingestions may change the presentation.

TABLE 55-4   Narcotics and Sedative-Hypnotic Overdose: Clinical Findings and Treatment*

	Narcotics	Sedative-hypnotics	Barbiturates
FINDINGS			
CNS			
Depressed/coma	Yes	Yes	Yes
Seizures (associated drugs)	Meperidine, propoxyphene	Methaqualone, meprobamate	Butabarbital, pentobarbital, secobarbital
Cardiovascular			
Hypotension/shock	Yes	Yes	Yes
Dysrhythmias	No	Chloral hydrate, haloperidol, meprobamate	No
Miosis	Yes (not meperidine)	Variable	Variable
Respiratory			
Depression	Yes	Yes	Yes
Pulmonary edema	Yes	Meprobamate, ethchlorvynol, paraldehyde	Yes
Anticholinergic	Lomotil (early)	Glutethimide, OTC sleep medications	No
Other	Analgesia (GI, GU motility; bronchoconstriction)	Paraldehyde—acute renal failure	Cutaneous bullae
MANAGEMENT			
Support	Yes	Yes	Yes
Charcoal	Yes	Yes	Yes
Antidote	Naloxone	No*	No
Diuresis	No	No	Phenobarbital (alkaline)
Dialysis	No	No	Phenobarbital

*Flumazenil for benzodiazepines.

Ancillary Data

1. Toxicologic levels. Send urine and blood to analysis for all patients whose diagnosis is uncertain. Notify the laboratory which drugs are suspected.
2. Electrolytes, glucose, CBC, and ABG as indicated.
3. X-ray film: abdominal flat plate if chloral hydrate is suspected (radiopaque).
4. Other studies to exclude differential diagnostic considerations.

DIFFERENTIAL DIAGNOSIS

See Chapter 15.

MANAGEMENT

1. Good supportive care is of primary importance, with particular attention to the airway, ventilation, and circulation.
   a. All patients with impaired mental status or respiratory function should have oxygen, cardiac monitor, and IV in place.
   b. D50W, 0.5-1.0 gm dextrose (1-2 ml)/kg/dose IV; and naloxone, 0.1 mg/kg/dose up to 2 mg/dose. If no response, 2 mg (5 adult vials) IV should be given to all patients with altered mental status.
2. Gastric emptying, usually by lavage, may

be indicated with impaired mental status after oral overdose. Give activated charcoal as early as possible.

3. For narcotic overdoses, administer naloxone (Narcan 0.1 mg/kg/dose up to 2 mg) IV. Propoxyphene (Darvon) and pentazocine (Talwin) overdoses may require larger than usual amounts of naloxone for adequate reversal. If a response to naloxone occurs, a continuous infusion may be indicated. After the initial bolus, begin an infusion (2 ml in 500 ml D5W or 0.9% NS equaling 4 μg/ml). Start at 1-4 μg/kg/min (adult: 0.4 mg/hr) IV and titrate. Naloxone infusion should never replace careful observation and support. Use with caution after oral overdose; the effective half-life of naloxone is 30 to 60 minutes.

4. Benzodiazepine-induced respiratory depression and coma may be reversed by the antidote flumazenil (Mazicon) with an onset of effect of 1 to 2 minutes and an effective duration of 1 to 4 hours. The adult dose is 0.2 mg; repeating dose up to a total cumulative dose of 3 mg. May increase the total dose to 5 mg if only partial response. The dose in children has not been established but doses of 10 μg/kg for two doses have been suggested.

5. Alkaline diuresis may enhance excretion of phenobarbital. Urine flow should be established at 3 to 6 ml/kg/hr by giving an initial flush of 0.9% NS or LR at 20 ml/kg and then NaHCO$_3$ 1-2 mEq/kg/dose over 60 minutes with K$^+$ supplements as necessary. Fluids should be infused at twice the maintenance level. Urine pH should be 7.5 or greater. Dialysis or hemoperfusion is rarely required. Hourly intake and output should be measured.

6. Serial doses of activated charcoal (adults: 20 to 50 gm q2-4hr PO) in 70% sorbitol increase the elimination of oral or intravenous phenobarbital, but the effect on clinical course is unclear. Mixing every other dose with a cathartic may be beneficial.

7. Dialysis may be useful in severe phenobarbital ingestions.

8. Associated ingestions should be treated as necessary.

DISPOSITION

All patients with significant overdoses should be hospitalized, and after medical clearance, psychiatric consultation should be sought.

REFERENCES

Lewis JM, Klein-Schwartz W, Benson BE, et al: Continuous naloxone infusion in pediatric narcotic overdose, *Am J Dis Child* 138:944, 1984.

Pond SM, Olson ICR, Osterloah JD, et al: Randomized study of the treatment of phenobarbital overdose with repeated doses of activated charcoal, *JAMA* 251:3104, 1984.

ORGANOPHOSPHATES AND CARBAMATES

ALERT: The classic cholinergic syndrome is recognized by the mnemonic SLUDGE (salivation, lacrimation, urination, defecation, GI cramping, and emesis).

Organophosphate pesticides are widely used and produce the classic cholinergic syndrome by the inhibition of acetylcholinesterase. There are many different organophosphates with widely varying toxicities, including chlorthion, parathion, diazinon, malathion, TEPP, OMPA, and systox. Parathion is 600 times more toxic than malathion, the latter being used for household purposes. Carbamates have similar uses as insecticides but are less toxic partially because the carbamate-cholinesterase bond is reversible; symptoms are of shorter duration (about 24 hours). Absorption is primarily through the skin and gastrointestinal tract.

DIAGNOSTIC FINDINGS

The symptoms of cholinergic syndrome are usually evident within hours of exposure (Table 55-5).

Specific findings reflect excessive acetylcholine.

1. *Muscarinic* (parasympathomimetic) findings
   a. Sweat glands: increased sweating
   b. Lacrimal glands: increased lacrimation
   c. GU: urinary incontinence
   d. GI: anorexia, nausea, emesis, diarrhea, fecal incontinence
   e. Eye: miosis, blurred vision
   f. Bronchial: bronchoconstriction, pulmonary edema
   g. Cardiovascular: bradycardia, hypotension
2. *Nicotinic* (motor) findings
   a. Striated muscle: fasciculations, cramping, weakness, hyperreflexia
   b. Long-term peripheral neuropathy may be seen after serious exposure.
3. CNS: restlessness, ataxia, seizures, depression of respiratory and cardiovascular centers, emotional lability, impaired memory, confusion, coma

Ancillary Data

1. Blood CBC, electrolytes, blood urea nitrogen (BUN), glucose, liver function tests, PT, and ABG.
2. Chest x-ray film with evidence of pulmonary edema and ECG for dysrhythmias.
3. Serum cholinesterase is a more sensitive but a less specific indicator of organophosphate poisoning than is red blood cell (RBC) cholinesterase and will return to normal without treatment weeks after exposure. RBC cholinesterase regenerates at 1% or less per day and can require 3 to 4 months to regenerate.

   However, the levels are only rarely available to the physician soon enough to make a difference in treatment and may not correlate directly with the clinical status of the patient. Such determinations are particularly useful in cases of chronic exposure, when it is desirable to know whether further protection from the organophosphate is needed.

DIFFERENTIAL DIAGNOSIS

1. Intoxication: physostigmine, neostigmine, pyridostigmine, edrophonium (Tensilon)
2. Noncardiogenic pulmonary edema

TABLE 55-5   Organophosphate Exposure: Clinical Manifestations and Management

Serum cholinesterase level*	Clinical manifestations	Management
>50%	Usually none	Observe 6 hr
20%-50%	Fatigue, headache, numbness, salivation, wheezing, abdominal pain	Atropine Pralidoxime (2-PAM)
10%-20%	Weakness, dysarthria, muscle fasciculations, plus above	Atropinization Pralidoxime (2-PAM)
<10%	Miosis, loss of pupillary reflex, flaccid paralysis, pulmonary edema, plus above	Atropinization Pralidoxime (2-PAM) (multiple doses)

*Clinical manifestations rather than the serum cholinesterase level should be used in determining management in acute situations. Percentages best compared to baseline.

MANAGEMENT

Stabilization of the airway and resuscitation are imperative. Additional measures include decontamination by removal of clothing and washing of skin for contact exposure and emesis or lavage and administration of charcoal and cathartic for ingestion. Health care workers must be protected.

Organophosphate and carbamate insecticides are rapidly absorbed through the clothes and skin. Contaminated clothes must be removed, and skin must be decontaminated. This is optimally done outside a medical facility by personnel wearing gloves, rubber apron, and so on. Two separate water/detergent washes remove a total of 91% to 94% of organophosphates, even when performed up to 6 hours after exposure. Hospital personnel must be protected during and after decontamination.

Specific treatment involves administration of anticholinergic medications to the symptomatic patient.

1. Atropine binds at muscarinic receptors and is given first: 0.05 mg/kg/dose (maximum: 2-5 mg/dose) IV. Test dose (child: 0.01 mg/kg IV; adult: 2 mg IV) is usually given. This may be repeated every 5 minutes until atropinization is achieved, with drying of pulmonary secretions. Mydriasis is not an adequate endpoint. Some advocate a continuous infusion of atropine of 0.02-0.05 mg/kg/hr IV.
   • Should be given for the first 24 hours as needed to maintain atropinization. Average adult dose is 40 mg/day. Adults may need 100 mg in the first 24 hours of therapy.
2. Pralidoxime (2-PAM) reactivates acetylcholinesterase and reverses cholinergic nicotinic stimulation. It is useful if given within 36 hours of exposure. It should be administered after adequate atropinization.
   a. Dosage: pralidoxime, 20-50 mg/kg/dose (maximum: 2 gm/dose) IV slowly. In the adult, 1 gm is mixed with 250 ml 0.9% NS and given over 30 to 60 minutes. If symptoms of weakness and fasciculations persist, it may be repeated in 1 hour and then every 8 hours for additional doses.
   b. No serious side effects noted from pralidoxime.

Carbamates have lower toxicity of shorter duration.

DISPOSITION

All symptomatic patients with exposure or ingestion require admission and usually consultation with a poison control center for guidance in drug therapy.

REFERENCES

Tafuri J, Roberts J: Organophosphate poisoning, *Ann Emerg Med* 16:193, 1987.

Zwiener RJ, Ginsburg CM: Organophosphate and carbamate poisoning in infants and children, *Pediatrics* 81:121, 1988.

PHENOTHIAZINES

ALERT: Symptoms include sedation and anticholinergic findings; occasionally there may be prominent dystonic reactions.

Phenothiazines are widely used antipsychotics as well as antinauseants. They have anticholinergic, antidopaminergic, and α-blocking actions.

ETIOLOGY

See Table 55-6.

DIAGNOSTIC FINDINGS

The major finding in overdoses reflects anticholinergic and antidopaminergic effects. An inverse relationship exists between the anticholinergic potency and extrapyramidal side effects (p. 369).

TABLE 55-6 Phenothiazines: Related Side Effects*

	Sedation	Extrapyramidal	Hypotension
PHENOTHIAZINES			
Chlorpromazine (Thorazine)	+++	++	IM +++ PO ++
Triflupromazine (Vesprin)	++	+++	++
Thioridazine (Mellaril)	+++	+	++
Trifluoperazine (Stelazine)	+	+++	+
Prochlorperazine (Compazine)	++	+++	
THIOXANTHENE			
Thiothixene (Navane)	+ or ++	++	++
BUTYROPHENONES			
Haloperidol (Haldol)	+	+++	+

Modified from Gilman AG, Goodman LS, Gilman A: *The pharmacological basis of therapeutics,* ed 8, New York, 1989, Macmillan, Inc. Copyright © 1989, Macmillan, Inc.
*+, ++, +++, Relative prominence.

Extrapyramidal dystonic reactions may be divided into several categories, although clinically different patterns may appear simultaneously. Dystonia is not necessarily dose related.

1. Oculogyric: upward-gaze paralysis, bizarre tics
2. Torticollis: may involve one side, often with arm involvement
3. Buccolingual: facial grimacing with dysphagia, mutism, trismus
4. Opisthotonic
5. Tortipelvic: abdominal wall spasms, bizarre gait, lordosis, kyphosis

Other side effects include the following.

1. Seizure threshold is reduced.
2. Anticholinergic findings.
3. Hypothermia may occur early, but the patient with sufficient thermal exposure may have hyperthermia.
4. Tachycardia and orthostatic hypotension are common.
5. Non–life-threatening side effects include hepatitis, photosensitivity, visual blurring, hirsutism, and gynecomastia. Thioridazine has been associated with retinal pigment degeneration.

Ancillary Data

1. Granulocytopenia, hyperglycemia, and acetonemia are reported.
2. Other studies should include toxicology screen (in seriously ill patients), ECG, and x-ray film.
3. A few drops of 10% ferric chloride added to 5 ml of urine will turn urine purple-brown. Urine turns purple in presence of salicylates.

MANAGEMENT

Initial attention must be given to stabilization, with particular attention to airway, ventilation, and circulation. Obtunded patients should receive oxygen, dextrose, and naloxone. Hypotension should be treated initially with IV fluids. Rhythm should be monitored and dysrhythmias treated as appropriate.

Emesis in a child may remove some small amount of drug if done within 30 minutes of ingestion. Lavage may be necessary, followed by charcoal and catharsis.

Extrapyramidal dystonic reactions should be treated with diphenhydramine (Benadryl), 1-2

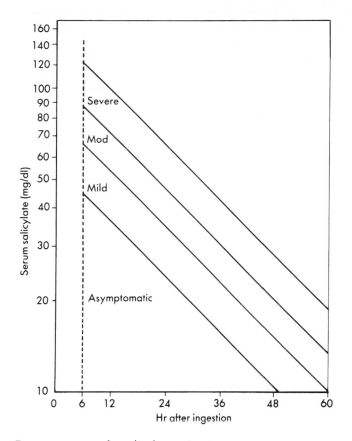

Fig. 55-3   Done nomogram for salicylate poisoning.

(From Done AK: *Pediatrics* 26:805, 1960. Copyright American Academy of Pediatrcis, 1960.)

mg/kg/dose IV. Benztropine (Cogentin), 1-4 mg/dose (adult) IV, may cause anticholinergic effects because of atropine component. Patients are maintained with one of these drugs for 1 to 2 days.

DISPOSITION

Disposition must reflect the severity of symptoms. Those with adequately treated extrapyramidal findings can usually be discharged with follow-up observation. Others often require hospitalization. Depending on the nature of the ingestion, psychiatric counseling or poison prevention should be stressed.

SALICYLATES (ASPIRIN)

ALERT: Consider if patient has tachypnea, hyperthermia, or metabolic acidosis.

Ingestion of salicylates is common but has decreased with the widespread use of safety lids on medication bottles and the popularity of acetaminophen-containing products. A wide variety of products contain salicylates, and an acute, single ingestion of 250 mg/kg may produce toxicity. Signs and symptoms are related to the salicylate levels diagrammed in the Done nomogram (Fig. 55-3). Therapeutic levels are 15 to 30 mg/dl in arthritic conditions. The

Done nomogram cannot be used in cases in which chronic ingestion produces symptoms at levels less than those normally considered to be toxic or for overdose of sustained-release aspirin products. Methyl salicylate (oil of wintergreen) is particularly toxic, having 1365 mg salicylate/ml.

DIAGNOSTIC FINDINGS

Patients with significant ingestions initially may have tachypnea and deep, labored respirations, hyperthermia, tinnitus, and vomiting. Mental status changes may develop with moderate ingestions, ranging from lethargy or excitability and progressing to seizures and coma. Slurred speech, hallucinations, vertigo, pulmonary edema, and cardiovascular collapse may develop.

Chronic salicylism is associated with accentuated CNS findings and less prominent acid-base abnormalities. Thus levels do not indicate the seriousness of ingestion.

Complications

1. Metabolic
   a. Hypoglycemia, sometimes preceded by an initial hyperglycemia.
   b. Metabolic acidosis and respiratory alkalosis. In children less than 4 years of age metabolic acidosis develops more rapidly, without the concurrent respiratory alkalosis. This is often the predominant presentation.
   c. Electrolyte abnormalities.
      (1) Potassium deficit secondary to acidosis with urinary losses
      (2) Hyponatremia because of inappropriate antidiuretic hormone (ADH)
2. Noncardiogenic pulmonary edema (see Chapter 19)
3. CNS findings in moderate to severe ingestions
   a. Seizures from hypoglycemia, hyponatremia, cerebral edema, or decreased

ionized calcium caused by alkali therapy.
   b. Coma. May occur in acute ingestions when the level is very high or the patient has ingested more than one agent. Coma is more common with chronic salicylism (see Chapter 15).
4. Bleeding from hypothrombinemia and platelet dysfunction
5. Chemical hepatitis
6. Allergic manifestations, particularly wheezing

Ancillary Data

A qualitative test for the presence of aspirin in urine may be performed by adding 5 ml of urine to a few drops of 10% ferric chloride. The urine will turn purple and remain stable if salicylates are present, purple-brown with phenothiazines, purple-red (fades in minutes) with ketosis, and yellowish green with isoniazid. Normal urine turns brownish, whitish, or yellowish.

To provide a semiquantitative measure of salicylate level, one drop of serum may be applied to a Phenistix. A tan color is consistent with a level of less than 40 mg/dl, brown with a level of 40-90 mg/dl, and purple with a level greater than 90 mg/dl.

1. A quantitative salicylate level may be done and interpreted by the Done nomogram (see Fig. 55-3). It is not useful in chronic ingestions. Therapeutic: 15-30 mg/dl. The value of the Done nomogram is only as a general reference. The clinical condition of the patient is far more important than where the salicylate level falls on the nomogram. It is unnecessary to wait until 6 hours after ingestion to get a salicylate level in a symptomatic patient.
2. Electrolytes, glucose, and ABG as indicated.
3. Coagulation studies if indicated. Prolonged PT and bleeding time.
4. ECG, if severe electrolyte problems are suspected.

DIFFERENTIAL DIAGNOSIS

1. Metabolic acidosis ("MUDPILES")
   a. Ingestions: methanol, paraldehyde, iron, isoniazid, lactic acid, ethanol, ethylene glycol, salicylates, strychnine.
   b. Metabolic: uremia, diabetes mellitus, starvation.

      NOTE: In general, metabolic acidosis results from ingestions of the specific drugs listed above, as well as cellular poisons (e.g., iron, cyanide) and drugs that cause seizures. In addition, poor perfusion, ischemia or cellular death produces metabolic acidosis.

2. Infection: meningitis, encephalitis, pneumonia, Reye syndrome

MANAGEMENT

After stabilization, oral absorption should be reduced by emesis (syrup of ipecac) if within 30 minutes of ingestion or gastric lavage, activated charcoal, and catharsis. Mild ingestions require no additional therapy.

Moderate or severe ingestions require parenteral therapy with forced alkaline diuresis. Salicylates are weak acids (pKa = 3), and elimination may be facilitated by alkalinization of the urine to pH of 7 to 8 and correction of potassium and acid-base abnormalities. Ancillary data should be monitored.

1. If the patient is initially dehydrated, expand the vascular volume by D5W 0.45% NS, adding 60 mEq/L $NaHCO_3$. Infuse at 10-20 ml/kg over 1 hour.
2. After the resuscitation and establishment of good urine flow (>2 ml/kg/hr), infuse D5W with 88-132 mEq (2-3 ampules)/L $NaHCO_3$, and 30-40 mEq/L KCl at a rate of 4-8 ml/kg/hr. May also use D5W 0.45% NS with 40-60 mEq/L $NaHCO_3$, and 30 mEq/L KCl. Hypokalemia is very common.
   • If a severe metabolic acidosis is present, give an additional 1-2 mEq/kg $NaHCO_3$ IV slowly.
3. Multiple-dose activated charcoal may enhance elimination. Give 1-2 gm/kg/dose (adult: 30-100 gm/dose) q4hr PO.
4. Treat hyperpyrexia with cooling blanket.
5. For seizures give diazepam (Valium), 0.2-0.3 mg/kg/dose IV q10min prn. Treat metabolic problems, if any.
6. For bleeding diathesis: vitamin K (infants—1-2 mg/dose IV; children and adults—5-10 mg/dose IV).

Dialysis is indicated for the following conditions:

1. Renal failure
2. CNS deterioration or poor response, particularly with chronic salicylism
3. Unchanging high salicylate level or level greater than 130 mg/dl at 6 hours
4. Severe, unresolving metabolic acidosis
5. Pulmonary edema

Hemodialysis is more effective than peritoneal dialysis.

DISPOSITION

Patients with mild ingestions may be discharged with appropriate poison-prevention counseling. Patients who are significantly symptomatic, have serum levels equal to or greater than 60 mg/dl at 6 hours, have ingested methyl salicylates, or have chronic or sustained-release ingestions that are potentially toxic should be hospitalized.

REFERENCE

Burton RT, Bayer MJ, Barron L, et al: Comparison of activated charcoal and gastric lavage in the prevention of aspirin absorption, *J Emerg Med* 1:411, 1984.

SYMPATHOMIMETICS

ALERT: CNS and cardiovascular stimulants may produce ventricular dysrhythmias or sudden death.

The sympathomimetics are a diverse group of stimulant drugs with primarily CNS and cardiovascular toxicity.

TYPES

1. Amphetamines: methamphetamine, phenmetrazine (Preludin) (much greater toxicity intravenously than orally).
2. Cocaine (street names: snow, gold dust, coke, speed ball—when combined with heroin) (p. 375).
3. β-Adrenergic agents. Ephedrine (available alone or in combination with theophylline), pseudoephedrine, phenylpropanolamine, terbutaline, albuterol.

DIAGNOSTIC FINDINGS (see Table 55-3)

Ancillary data should include CBC, electrolytes, glucose, BUN, oximetry or ABG, ECG, and toxicology screens as indicated.

DIFFERENTIAL DIAGNOSIS

The diagnosis must be differentiated from intoxication caused by phencyclidine, hallucinogens, anticholinergics, sedative-hypnotics, alcohol, theophylline, caffeine, and camphor.

MANAGEMENT

1. Supportive care is important, focusing particularly on potential cardiovascular instability and altered mental status.
   a. Patients should receive oxygen, dextrose, and naloxone if mental status is altered.
   b. Hyperthermia must be aggressively treated with cooling blankets.
   c. Hypoglycemia should be suspected and treated.
   d. Hypokalemia may be seen with β agonists.
2. Gastric emptying should be achieved either by emesis or lavage (if done very soon after ingestion), as well as by charcoal and catharsis as outlined earlier.
3. A calming, reassuring approach to the patient with an acute psychosis or hallucinations is important, as is an attempt to reduce stimuli.
4. Sedation, if necessary, may be achieved with diazepam (Valium), 0.2-0.8 mg/kg/24 hr q6-8hr PO (adult: 5-10 mg/dose). Titrate response.
5. For behavioral changes caused by amphetamines not responsive to benzodiazepine haloperidol (Haldol), 2 to 10 mg IV may be used.

REFERENCES

Pentel P: Toxicity of over-the-counter stimulants, *JAMA* 252:1898, 1984.

Spiler HA, Ramoska EA, Henretig FM, et al: A two year retrospective study of accidental pediatric albuterol ingestions, *Pediatr Emerg Care* 9:338, 1993.

Wasserman D, Amitai Y: Hypoglycemia following albuterol overdose in a child, *Am J Emerg Med* 10:556, 1992.

THEOPHYLLINE (P. 776)

ALERT: Seizures and cardiac dysrhythmias may occur with toxicity.

Theophylline overdoses are less common in children with decreased uses.

DIAGNOSTIC FINDINGS

Effects are primarily sympathomimetic in action, resulting in irritability and seizures as well as tachycardia, dysrhythmias (atrial fibrillation and ventricular tachycardia), and hypertension. Patients may be restless and agitated. Nausea, vomiting, diarrhea, and abdominal pain are seen frequently, even at nontoxic levels (p. 778).

Overdoses with sustained release preparations can produce severe and prolonged CNS and cardiovascular toxicity.

In one study, the mean theophylline level of patients who had seizures was 45 µg/dl.

Ancillary Data

Theophylline levels are commonly available and should be obtained for all patients who are considered to have potentially toxic levels. Rapid office assays may also be used for measuring levels. An ECG should usually be obtained.

MANAGEMENT

1. Supportive care is essential with ongoing cardiac monitoring. Gastric emptying either by emesis or lavage (reflecting level of consciousness, seizures, or absence of gag reflex) if done very soon after ingestion followed by charcoal and catharsis as outlined earlier.
2. In the asymptomatic patient with minimal overdoses, withholding drug and monitoring are usually adequate.
3. Significant theophylline overdoses may initially be treated with serial doses of activated charcoal (adult: 10 gm q1hr or 20 gm q2hr to total dose of 120 gm; children: proportionately less). This approach markedly decreases the half-life of elimination. If the level is greater than 50 μg/dl, dialysis (and rarely, hemoperfusion) should be considered.

4. Whole-bowel irrigation may be useful, especially if long-acting medication is involved.
5. Seizures are treated initially with diazepam (Valium), 0.2-0.3 mg/kg/dose IV q2-5min prn (see Chapter 21), and dysrhythmias treated with specific drugs (see Chapter 6).

DISPOSITION

Patients who are symptomatic or have levels greater than 30 mg/dl should generally be admitted for observation and treatment.

REFERENCES

Gal P, Miller A, McCue JD: Oral-activated charcoal to enhance theophylline elimination in an acute overdose, *JAMA* 251:3130, 1984.

Jain R, Tholl DA: Activated charcoal for theophylline toxicity in a premature infant on the second day of life, *Dev Pharmacol Ther* 19:106, 1992.

Paloucek FP, Rodvoid KA: Evaluation of theophylline overdoses and toxicities, *Ann Emerg Med* 17:135, 1988.

Park GD, Spector F, Roberts RJ, et al: Use of hemoperfusion for treatment of theophylline intoxication, *Am J Med* 74:961, 1983.

IX

TRAUMA

56 Evaluation and Stabilization of the Multiply Traumatized Patient

PAUL A. KOZAK, ROBERT C. JORDEN, and ROGER M. BARKIN

ALERT: An aggressive, highly prioritized approach must be immediately implemented, using a team approach to the stabilization of airway, ventilation, the spine, shock, and external hemorrhage. A multiply injured patient may be able to respond only to one major painful stimulus at a time. Thus a careful identification of all sites of injury is important.

The traumatized pediatric patient presents unique challenges to the physician, but the principles of establishing treatment priorities are identical to those for older patients. However, beyond the principles of immediate stabilization, the psychologic impact on a child and family are immense and must be addressed with appropriate urgency through communication, support, and understanding. Furthermore, the pediatric patient presents logistic problems with respect to ensuring intravenous access, adjusting to limitations of equipment, monitoring and determining vital signs, and assessing fluid requirements.

Fatal childhood injury patterns suggest that one third of deaths are due to homicides in an urban setting. House fires (34%), firearms (19%), drowning (11%), and motor vehicle accidents (7%) account for most fatal injuries.

In caring for the infant, it is important to recognize that they depend on others for care, placing them in a uniquely vulnerable position. Of trauma victims less than 3 months of age, 28% were injured under neglectful or abusive conditions. Peak incidence occurs from June to September. Many injuries are sustained in falls.

These infants are unable to roll; falls from a height less than 90 cm rarely result in fractures or serious injury. A fracture explained by a fall from a low height is suspicious for abuse as are injuries with multiple or stellate skull fractures and spiral long bone extremity fractures.

PRINCIPLES OF MANAGEMENT
Organization

For optimal treatment, trauma care requires organizational structure and coordination at several levels: the region and prehospital system, the hospital, and crucial health care professionals. Although this text focuses on the hospital-based physician-centered organization, to be effective the physician must understand the other components of the emergency medical services (EMS) system and be able to communicate effectively with the prehospital system.

Triage

Trauma patients are often triaged to a trauma center, reflecting the specific local guidelines and protocols. The familiarity with trauma and a multidisciplinary approach to managing traumatized patients is generally present in such settings. The triage criteria used by the American College of Surgeons Committee on Trauma purposely overtriages patients by 30%. The Florida Triage Study suggests that undertriage in the pediatric population occurs approximately 33% of the time, and triage criteria specific to the pediatric population need to be developed. At present, a debate about the benefits of destination policies including pediatric and general trauma centers is ongoing, reflecting the substantive data that support the importance of personnel, resources, responsiveness, and system commitment.

Team Approach

Effective trauma resuscitation requires a trauma team led by a senior member designated as the trauma captain. Although the exact composition of the team varies with the institution and availability of personnel, the need for some type of organized team approach is essential. Trauma injuries are complex, requiring multiple procedures and frequent reassessment in a timely fashion. Only through a team effort, orchestrated by a team captain, can optimal care be provided.

The team organization must reflect the resources and expertise of a specific institution, the clinical needs of the specific patient, and other resource demands at a specific moment. Prioritization of specific resources and manpower is always essential. The structure must be predetermined to enhance efficiency, define responsibilities, and assure completeness of assessment and treatment. A suggested structure might include the following:

Trauma captain
Overall direction and assessment
Coordination of resuscitation
First assistant (clavicles and up)
Airway stabilization
C-spine immobilization
Breathing and oxygen
Examination of scalp and cranial nerves
Hemorrhage control

2nd and 3rd assistants (each arm)
Vascular access
Laboratory tests, type and cross-match
Monitor vital signs
4th assistant (pelvic and below)
Vascular access
Splint
Foley catheter
Rectal

Aggressive Management

Because the multiply injured child has a high potential for rapid deterioration, an aggressive approach must be the foundation for determining treatment priorities.

Treatment Based on Clinical Findings

Diagnosis need not always be confirmed by x-ray study or laboratory work before treatment is initiated. Such delays in treatment may prove detrimental to patient survival. For example, the treatment urgency of a tension pneumothorax, diagnosed by clinical findings of diminished breath sounds, subcutaneous emphysema, or hemodynamic compromise, necessitates immediate placement of a chest tube without x-ray study confirmation of the diagnosis.

Assuming the Most Serious Diagnosis

When a number of diagnostic possibilities explain a physical finding, the most serious of these possibilities should be assumed and appropriate treatment instituted until that diagnosis can be excluded.

Consideration of the Nature of the Accident (i.e., the mechanism)

Victims of potentially serious accidents should be considered seriously injured until proved stable. For example, the victim of a fall or auto-pedestrian accident should have IV lines started and be carefully monitored despite an initial stable appearance and absence of complaints.

Assessment of Priorities

Evaluation of the trauma victim must be conducted in a prioritized and systematic fashion to guarantee that life-sustaining functions are addressed and maintained first.

Thorough Examination

The trauma team rapidly ensures that the airway, ventilation, and circulation are adequate; obtains a history; and then does a more complete examination.

1. Remove all clothing to prevent overlooking an injury.
2. Perform a concise and systematic, yet thorough, examination to ensure detection of all injuries.
3. Do not stop looking for injuries after one serious injury has been detected.
4. Examine the patient's back. If there is potential cervical spine injury, obtain an x-ray film before examining the back if the patient's condition permits. Otherwise, the patient may be logrolled.

Frequent Reassessments

Trauma victims are dynamic in their clinical presentation and thus subject to sudden deterioration. Frequent assessment of vital signs and indicators of vital function (e.g., level of consciousness, pupils, ventilation) is essential. Vigilance in monitoring intake and output and correlation with vital signs is impera-tive in determining additional fluid or blood requirements.

Technical Steps

Technical procedures should be accomplished early to facilitate monitoring and intervention in seriously ill patients. *Intravenous (IV) lines* should be placed, oxygen administered, *urinary catheter* (6 months: 8 Fr; 2 to 3 years: 10 Fr; 6 to 8 years: 10 to 12 Fr; 8 to 10 years: 12 Fr) inserted, and urine examined for blood and monitored for volume of output. *Nasogastric (NG) tube* (6 months: 8 Fr; 2 to 3 years: 10 Fr; 6 to 8 years: 10 to 12 Fr; 8 to 10 years: 14 to 18 Fr) should be inserted (after cervical spine is cleared), and *cardiac monitor* applied. Fig. 56-1 provides guidelines for length of insertion of gastric tubes. *Laboratory and x-ray studies* are ordered as discussed later. Five tubes are virtually always required in situations where major trauma is suspected: two IV tubes, an NG tube, a bladder tube, and tubes of blood for hematocrit (Hct) and type and cross-match determinations.

NOTE: Insertion of the NG tube is usually delayed in patients with significant facial fractures.

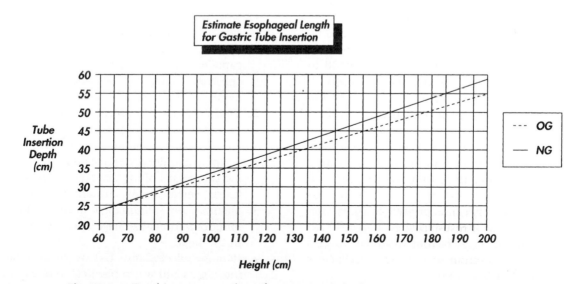

Estimate Esophageal Length for Gastric Tube Insertion

Fig. 56-1 Graphic representation of recommended tube insertion depths based on patient length. OG, orogastric tube; NG, nasogastric tube.

(From Scalzo AJ, Tominack RL, Thompson MN: *J Emerg Med* 10:581, 1992).

If prehospital IV cannulation is achieved, it is essential to ensure that it is clinically useful in the field by initiating adequate fluid resuscitation. On arrival in the emergency department (ED), the cannula should be reassessed and fluids continued with adequate monitoring of the rates and response.

The practice of type and cross-matching every trauma patient has come under close scrutiny. Obtaining a type and screen is a cost-effective alternative that will not put blood out of circulation in the blood bank and save resources. Cross-matching should take only an additional 5 minutes after the type and screen has been completed. Studies suggest that type and cross-match should be done initially in cases of hypotension or obviously severely injured children with a Pediatric Trauma Score of less than 7.

AGE AND SIZE CONSIDERATIONS

Age and size-specific issues must be considered in management. The child's relatively large surface area increases the risk of heat loss, whereas abdominal distension may impede diaphragmatic breathing.

1. Vital signs, including respiratory rates, vary by age (see Appendix B-2). Systolic blood pressure (BP) may be estimated by adding twice the patient's age to 80. The heart rate varies with age (infant: 100 to 160, child: 60 to 150, adult: 59 to 90).
2. Fluid replacement should be done on the basis of the patient's blood volume (70-80 ml/kg), the vital signs, the nature of the injury, and the presence of ongoing hemorrhage. Unless the patient is in profound shock, the initial approach is to give a fourth of the patient's blood volume (20 ml/kg) as crystalloid (0.9% normal saline [NS] or lactated Ringer's [LR] solution). Gear further treatment toward the initial response and the other factors mentioned.
3. Venous access is somewhat more difficult in children, particularly if the youngsters are hypovolemic. If establishing a percutaneous line is impossible, establish a venous cutdown in the distal saphenous or external jugular vein. Intraosseous infusion during the initial fluid resuscitation may be particularly useful for transient venous access if access is difficult through traditional routes (see Appendix A-3). Central venous lines are rarely used in children because of the increased risk of pneumothorax and vascular injury, but they may be used, ideally with a Seldinger wire approach. If a central line is desired, the internal jugular or femoral veins may be cannulated by the customary approaches.
4. Tube placement, including thoracostomy and endotracheal (ET), NG, and urinary catheters, should be accomplished with the largest tube that the child can accommodate.
5. Administer medications on an age-specific basis. The Broselow tape may be useful in relating height to dose.

ASSESSMENT BY PRIORITIES
Preliminaries

1. Assemble the trauma team, which will vary, depending on the number and type of people available in the ED. A team captain must be identified who can orchestrate the resuscitation and task assignments on the basis of ambulance reports.
2. Take an updated report from ambulance personnel while the patient is being transferred from the ambulance stretcher. Attempt to acquire additional history, including the details of the accident, significant history, medications, and allergies.
3. Maintain any splinting and head and neck immobilization that have been instituted in the field.
4. Remove all clothing. Use overhead heating, lights and warm blankets to maintain body temperature, especially in smaller children. Hypothermia may occur be-

cause of the relatively large body surface area of children.

5. Attach the patient to a cardiac monitor and oximeter and administer oxygen. Initiate IV lines.

6. *AMPLE* history is essential: *a*llergy, *m*edications, *p*ast medical history, time of *l*ast meal, and *e*vents leading to injury.

Approach

Initial management can be divided into stabilization of immediate life-threatening conditions and a subsequent brief but systematic head-to-toe evaluation. Life-threatening conditions include five high-priority factors: airway, ventilation, the spine, shock, and level of consciousness. These five factors require rapid assessment and intervention to permit survival (see Chapter 4).

The second phase of management is a complete evaluation of other potentially injured systems. A reassessment of the high-priority factors and evaluation of neurologic status, abdomen, heart, musculoskeletal system, and soft tissue injuries is essential. Although of lower priority, these elements do have the potential for causing serious morbidity and mortality and must be addressed expeditiously.

PRIMARY SURVEY AND RESUSCITATION
Airway

1. Check for patency. If there is any question, open the airway, suction secretions, remove foreign debris, and insert an oral or nasal airway. High-flow oxygen should be applied, often using a mask while monitoring with an oximeter.

2. Check for adequacy of air exchange; if insufficient, active intervention is necessary.

   a. If urgent airway management is needed before the cervical spine can be cleared, the decision to orally or nasally intubate must be made. The comfort level and experience of the physician will dictate the choice; both methods are safe and effective.

   (1) Nasotracheal intubation in a spontaneously breathing patient may be attempted unless there is a severe facial injury (which may allow the tube to pass into the cranium). Apnea is a contraindication because the breath sounds are used to guide tube placement.

   (2) In patients at risk for cervical spine injury in whom nasal intubation is contraindicated or unsuccessful, the preferred technique is oral intubation while maintaining in-line stabilization of the head and neck. Please note that in-line stabilization is not in-line traction. Most authorities prefer the in-line stabilization approach to a surgical airway, which is difficult in young children. In cases of significant head trauma, rapid sequence induction with oral intubation is the preferred technique. Blind nasotracheal intubation is discouraged in these cases because it can increase intracranial pressure. The lower incidence of unstable neck fractures in children further supports this recommendation. If a surgical airway is performed, cricothyroidotomy because of simpler anatomy is preferred over tracheostomy. However, size limitation precludes cricothyroidotomy in small children. Although recommendations vary, most suggest that children less than 12 years of age undergo tracheostomy. Other options to consider include digital intubation, intubation guided by fiberoptic laryngoscopy, or transtracheal needle jet insufflation.

b. If no evidence of cervical spine injury is present (conscious patient with no nerve deficit or neck pain and normal cervical spine x-ray studies), standard oral intubation may be performed with caution while minimizing motion. Remember that normal C-spine films do not rule out an unstable ligamentous injury.

Ventilation

1. Inspection. Look for signs of respiratory distress, including dyspnea, tachycardia, tachypnea, cyanosis, diaphoresis, retractions, flail segments, external evidence of trauma and tracheal deviation.
2. Palpation. Feel for bony crepitus, subcutaneous emphysema, chest wall tenderness, and tracheal deviation.
3. Auscultation. Determine presence, character, and symmetry of breath sounds.
4. Management.
    a. Evidence of inadequate ventilation indicates the need for active airway management or tube thoracostomy.
    b. Airway management may be achieved as outlined previously. If necessary, *rapid sequence induction* (RSI) may be used for specific patients to maintain adequate oxygenation, protect the airway, and reduce adverse cardiovascular or intracranial pressure responses to intubation (see Chapter 4).
    The patient's anatomy is initially evaluated, looking for oral or dental abnormalities, trauma to the neck or face, and systemic abnormalities. Equipment is checked.
    (1) The patient is preoxygenated. If the patient is hypoventilating, hyperventilate while the Sellick maneuver is performed.
    (2) Administer a nonparalyzing dose of nondepolarizing agent (i.e., vecuronium [Norcuron], 0.01 mg/kg IV [adult: 1 mg IV]), to reduce

fasciculations. Allow 3 to 5 minutes before proceeding with succinylcholine. This step is unnecessary in children less than 5 years old, and many believe it can be left out entirely unless fasciculations may cause injury. With extensive burns or crush injury more than 72 hours old, fasciculations may release potassium from damaged cells and cause a dangerous hyperkalemia. In those cases, a nondepolarizing agent should be used.
    (3) Atropine, 0.01-0.02 mg/kg IV (minimum: 0.10 mg/dose), may be given to prevent bradycardia caused by vagal stimulation and to reduce secretions. This was previously given to all children less than 7 years of age but may also be beneficial into the preteen years. A minimum dose will prevent a paradoxical bradycardia. In the presence of significant head injury, administer lidocaine, 1.5 mg/kg IV, to blunt the rise in intracranial pressure caused by the stimulation of intubation and allow 2 minutes before giving succinylcholine.
    (4) Sedate patient with thiopental, 3-5 mg/kg IV, if the patient is not hypotensive or in status asthmaticus. Alternatives include midazolam, 0.1-0.3 mg/kg IV (maximum: 4 mg), or ketamine, 1-2 mg/kg IV, if there is no head injury.
    (5) Give succinylcholine, 1.0-1.5 mg/kg IV to adults and 2 mg/kg IV to children less than 10 kg. Allow 45 to 60 seconds for muscle relaxation. Cricoid pressure should be maintained.
    (6) Orally intubate the patient, verify position, and release cricoid pressure. When paralysis wears off, may use vecuronium, 0.1 mg/kg IV, if needed.

(7) The use of RSI before intubation has been shown to reduce the complication rate of intubation. All facilities dealing with pediatric trauma should have protocols for its use in place, and the physicians should be comfortable with the use of these medications. Remember to continue to keep the patient sedated and comfortable after the initial medicines are given. Children are often undertreated with sedative and analgesic agents.

c. Perform chest tube insertion if there are any signs of pneumothorax or hemothorax (see Chapter 62). If the patient is relatively stable, tube thoracostomy may obviate the need for active airway management.

Cervical Spine (see Chapter 61)

1. The cervical spine of every multiply traumatized patient should be considered fractured beyond infancy until proved otherwise. This has direct bearing on airway management. Fracture or dislocation is unusual in the patient less than 3 years old without neurologic defect.

2. In the awake, alert, and cooperative older child, palpation to detect misalignment or tenderness may be all that is needed to rule out injury. If any doubt exists, particularly in the younger, uncooperative child or in those with an impaired sensorium, a portable cross-table lateral view of the neck should be taken. This study, to be adequate, must include all seven cervical vertebrae and the top of the first thoracic vertebral body. One person should maintain axial traction while a second pulls the patient's arms caudad from the foot of the bed, thus lowering the shoulders enough to expose the lower cervical vertebrae (p. 454).

   The criteria for obtaining a cervical spine series in the traumatized child are undefined. Factors that may be useful in defining high-risk patients include those with neck pain, tenderness, or limited mobility; involvement in a vehicular accident with head trauma; a history of trauma to the neck; or abnormalities of reflexes, strength, sensation, or mental status.

3. Management.
   a. Immobilize the head and neck with sandbags and tape and a semirigid collar, if possible, until the entire cervical spine series is completed. Agitated or combative patients may also require manual immobilization by one of the trauma team members.
   b. If dislocation or fractures are detected or suspected, immobilize with a Philadelphia or 4-poster collar with tape and sandbags. Products such as the Stif Neck and Baby No-Neck (California Medical Products) are available. Request immediate neurosurgical consultation.

Thoracic and Lumbar Spine (see Chapter 61)

1. Thoracic or lumbar fractures are easily overlooked in the confused or obtunded child or in one with other painful injuries.

2. Palpation of the spinal column often localizes tenderness and step offs or, on logrolling, one may see ecchymoses.

3. Cross-table lateral views may not be easily obtainable anywhere but in the x-ray suite, but anteroposterior views often show thoracic or lumbar fractures. Moreover, it is the view from which to assess stability if there is a fracture and also to obtain important information about other structures in the chest, abdomen, and pelvis.

4. Management.
   a. Maintain the patient in a supine position on a hard stretcher. If it is necessary to move the patient, use a backboard or scoop stretcher rather than the logroll maneuver.

b. Insert an NG tube and urinary catheter if the cervical spine is clear and no major facial trauma or meatal bleeding is present.

Shock (see Chapter 5)

1. Up to 25% to 30% of blood volume can be lost before a child exhibits hypotension in the supine position. More subtle findings of tachycardia, a narrowed pulse pressure, or poor perfusion should be sought and treated aggressively.

2. Normal age-specific values of pulse and blood pressure must be considered in the evaluation of the patient. Normal systolic blood pressure in individuals 1 to 18 years of age can be estimated by adding twice the age in years (yr) plus 80. Diastolic blood pressure is usually two thirds of the systolic blood pressure (see Appendix B-2).

3. The initial hematocrit done in the ED usually produces a normal result in acute hemorrhages and is therefore a poor indicator of volume status. If it is low, it may indicate preexisting anemia, chronic hemorrhage, or a massive acute hemorrhage.

4. The presence of shock demands a thorough, rapid evaluation to determine the source of bleeding. In the absence of external musculoskeletal hemorrhage, three cavity spaces must be evaluated: chest, abdomen, and retroperitoneum. Except in the small infant, isolated head trauma does not cause shock. Therefore another concurrent source of shock must be aggressively investigated in the presence of head trauma.

5. Management.
    a. Significant external hemorrhage should be controlled by direct pressure. If an isolated bleeding vessel can be identified, it may be clamped, but blind clamping in the depths of a wound is never indicated.
    b. Establish IV lines. Large-bore, peripherally placed, over-the-needle catheters are optimal for rapid fluid infusion. Larger catheters permit greater flow rates. Resistance is increased by longer catheters. The flow of whole blood (at 300 mm Hg pressure) through a 16-gauge subclavian line is 60 ml/min; this increases to 149 ml/min when using a 16-gauge short catheter. In the case of shock, if intravenous access cannot be obtained within the first 5 minutes, the intraosseous route should be considered.

    On occasion, central venous pressure (CVP) lines may be helpful, particularly if pericardial tamponade is suspected or if there is poor response to fluid administration.

    c. Initially, administer a bolus of LR solution or 0.9% NS solution, 20 ml/kg IV, as rapidly as possible. Subsequent crystalloid solution and blood administration should reflect the response to the initial infusion and ongoing hemorrhage. Once 40-50 ml/kg of crystalloid has been infused during the initial resuscitation, blood should be considered if evidence of hypovolemia persists.

    d. Monitor urine output and titrate crystalloid solution infusion to maintain output at 1-2 ml/kg/hr.

    e. If completely cross-matched blood is not available, administer type-specific blood. It is usually available 10 to 15 minutes after delivery of a clot to the blood bank. O negative blood should be reserved for those patients who are in profound shock or cardiac arrest. Warm, fresh blood is optimal when available.

    f. If massive transfusions are necessary (equivalent to one total blood volume), use blood warmers and micropore filters and also consider administration of fresh-frozen plasma and platelets.

g. *MAST suits* are available for pediatric patients, but their effectiveness is controversial, particularly for the major trauma patient. It may also be useful in stabilizing large-bone fractures and in controlling hemorrhage caused by intraabdominal injury or pelvic fractures. Efficacy is controversial and controlled data are not available to demonstrate an improved outcome.

The MAST suit is contraindicated in patients with pulmonary edema and cardiogenic shock. The abdominal compartment should not be inflated in pregnant patients or in patients with evisceration or abdominal impalements. Complications include compartment syndromes and metabolic acidosis.

h. Thoracotomy permits cross clamping of the aorta and shunting of available blood to the cerebral and coronary circulations. It also permits immediate relief of pericardial tamponade and temporary control of certain cardiothoracic injuries.

ED thoracotomy should be selectively applied to trauma arrest patients. The prognosis for survival is best among victims of penetrating trauma with signs of life (palpable pulse, spontaneous respirations, reactive pupils) at the scene who subsequently arrest and undergo thoracotomy within 10 minutes of initiation of cardiopulmonary resuscitation (CPR). Conversely, blunt trauma victims who present to the ED in pulseless cardiac arrest or with severe hypotension (systolic BP <50 mm Hg) have virtually a 100% mortality and should generally not undergo resuscitative thoracotomy. A 7-year study of pediatric blunt trauma arrest patients yielded no functional survivors. The only survivor was neurologically devastated. Blunt trauma patients who lose their vital signs and penetrating trauma victims with no signs of life at the scene have a dismal prognosis.

Fortunately, the incidence of pediatric trauma arrest is low, and any extrapolation of pediatric trauma arrest data from the general population should be made with caution. Furthermore, an initial full resuscitation may stabilize the patient enough to make it to the intensive care unit (ICU) for consideration as an organ transplant donor. It is doubtful that thoracotomy will improve outcome and the risk to the physician performing the procedure, in the form of blood exposure, must be considered.

Loss of Consciousness and Pupillary Response

A detailed neurologic examination is not conducted at this point, but findings requiring immediate intervention are investigated. Specifically, the level of consciousness, as indicated by response to verbal and painful stimuli, is determined. Likewise, pupillary symmetry and reactivity to light are noted in an effort to identify an impending herniation. Patients with persisting coma and certainly those with evidence of herniation should be promptly intubated and hyperventilated and should undergo neurologic evaluation. The use of furosemide (Lasix), 1 mg/kg/dose IV, and mannitol, 0.25-1.0 gm/kg/dose IV, should be individualized and if possible given in conjunction with neurosurgical consultation. Generally, these agents are reserved for patients who show signs of developing herniation while under evaluation.

REASSESSMENT AND SECONDARY SURVEY

Once the high-priority factors listed on pp. 400-405 have been evaluated and appropriate treatment administered, reassessment of vital signs, urine output, perfusion, saturation, and overall status should be done. If no further actions are necessary beyond those already initiated, a complete secondary survey, including a thorough examination and a more detailed history, should be initiated.

Neurologic Considerations (see Chapter 57)

Level of consciousness is the most important indicator of prognosis. The Glasgow Coma Scale (GCS) (see Table 57-1; p. 414) provides an objective, reproducible means of assessing level of consciousness. A numerical score is given on the basis of motor and verbal responses and eye movement. Because the head is relatively large in children in relation to the trunk, it is often the primary point of contact.

1. **Head.** Inspect and palpate the head for any hematomas, ecchymoses, lacerations, or bony instability. When possible, examine deep lacerations digitally, using sterile gloves.
2. **Eyes.** Evaluation includes the size, shape, symmetry, and reactivity of pupils; the fundus; the fullness of extraocular movements; and any evidence of obvious trauma.
3. **Nose and ears.** Hemotympanum, otorrhea, and rhinorrhea indicate a basilar skull fracture and often represent the only means of making that diagnosis.
4. **Movement of extremities.** Note spontaneous movement or movement of all extremities in response to pain. Is movement symmetric? Any evidence of posturing?
5. **Rectal tone.** The presence of rectal tone in a patient paralyzed from spinal cord injury may indicate a central cord syndrome, which has a good prognosis. Absence of rectal tone in a comatose patient may be the only discernible clue to spinal cord injury.
6. **Reflexes.** Absent deep tendon reflexes are consistent with a cord injury; upward flexion of the toes (positive Babinski

reflex) is consistent with upper motor neuron damage.

Management

Any alteration of consciousness or abnormal neurologic findings warrant close and repeated observation, neurosurgical consultation, and consideration of a computed tomography (CT) scan. Intubation is usually indicated for a GCS score of 8 or less.

Persistent loss of consciousness requires intubation and hyperventilation if there is evidence of cerebral herniation; also use furosemide (Lasix), 1 mg/kg/dose IV, or mannitol, 0.25-1.0 gm/kg/dose IV, if the patient is hemodynamically stable. A neurosurgeon should be consulted.

Cardiac Considerations (see Chapter 62)

Although usually not very enlightening in trauma cases, a cardiac examination should be performed, and cardiac monitoring is imperative. A full 12-lead electrocardiogram (ECG) should be obtained on all patients with chest wall trauma and dysrhythmias, hypotension, or other signs of cardiac dysfunction.

1. Inspect for signs of anterior chest wall trauma that suggest the possibility of cardiac contusion. Persistent tachycardia may be the only sign of myocardial contusion.
2. Auscultate to determine the character of the heart sounds and the presence of rubs or murmurs.
3. In penetrating chest trauma, exclude cardiac tamponade. Inspect for evidence of hypotension, tachycardia, dilated (full) jugular veins (elevated CVP), and muffled heart sounds. A pericardiocentesis may be indicated.

Management

1. Cardiac tamponade requires immediate pericardiocentesis or thoracotomy, depending on the status of the vital signs.
2. Myocardial contusion requires ICU monitoring because of the potential for dys-

rhythmias and even hemodynamic compromise in cases of severe contusion. Serial cardiac isoenzymes should also be determined.

The Abdomen (see Chapter 63)

The abdomen is difficult to examine. Older, cooperative children without evidence of injury or unexplained hemodynamic instability may require no further evaluation. Younger children and those with any alteration in mental status should undergo a diagnostic evaluation by CT scan if there is any indication of abdominal injury or unexplained vital sign abnormalities. The patient's stability is an important factor in deciding the diagnostic approach, with unstable patients more likely to undergo laparotomy or lavage. Ultrasound may become an increasingly important modality for evaluation and treatment, with laparoscopy as another option.

Examination of the Abdomen

1. Inspect for signs of trauma, distension, or surgical scars.
2. Auscultate to determine the presence or absence of bowel sounds.
3. Palpate to elicit tenderness and rebound and to define any masses.
4. Do a rectal examination to evaluate tone, the prostate, and the presence of blood in stool.
5. Palpate, compress, and rock the pelvis over the iliac crest and pubis to detect movement, tenderness, or crepitus suggestive of pelvic fracture.
6. Examine the genitalia for obvious trauma. Blood at the urethral meatus precludes the insertion of a urinary catheter and requires investigation.
7. Do a dipstick examination of urine for blood; if present, do a microscopic analysis. If more than 20 red blood cells/high-powered field (RBC/HPF), further investigation should be considered, including an intravenous pyelogram (IVP),

although the indications are somewhat controversial and are evolving (p. 488). A CT scan with contrast may substitute. With a pelvic fracture, a cystogram should be done. In males, blood at the urethra indicates the need to do a retrograde urethrogram after urologic consultation.

Management

Management of blunt abdominal trauma in children is controversial. Although persistent unexplained shock requires a laparotomy, the presence of hemoperitoneum is not uniformly managed. Some centers recommend laparotomy, whereas others favor a conservative, nonoperative approach in the hemodynamically stable child employing ICU observation and hemodynamic support, including limited blood transfusion. A CT scan is usually indicated in this later group to define the nature of the injury. Both approaches have merit; the point to stress is consistency and careful adherence to the protocol followed in a given institution. Laparoscopy may also have a role. Early surgical consultation is imperative to oversee and guide diagnostic and therapeutic interventions.

Musculoskeletal Injuries (see Chapters 66-70)

These are relatively low-priority injuries. Obvious extremity injuries require splinting and referral for a more detailed examination. Nevertheless, major bone fractures can contribute significantly to hypovolemic shock.

Examinations

1. Inspect and palpate all extremities for deformity, tenderness, bony crepitus, and joint laxity.
2. Assess distal pulses and neurovascular integrity distal to the injury.
3. Inspect and palpate the spine for deformity and tenderness.

Management

This involves appropriate x-ray studies, temporary splinting, and orthopedic consultation.

Facial and Soft Tissue Injuries
(see Chapters 58, 60, and 65)

Facial injuries, unless massive, are not life threatening and require little initial treatment, although they do affect airway management. Severe hemorrhage and distortion are indications for active intervention.

1. Define contusions and lacerations of the soft tissues and apply pressure to control hemorrhage. Assess neurovascular function, and when time permits, place sutures as needed.
2. Carefully explore the depth and severity of penetrating or significant soft tissue injuries to the neck. A surgeon should be involved in evaluation and management if there is penetration of the platysma or extensive blunt soft tissue involvement.

X-RAY AND LABORATORY EVALUATION
X-Ray Studies

1. Essential roentgenograms during the initial evaluation of any victim of multiple trauma include a chest, pelvis, and cross-table, lateral view of the cervical spine. The spine film is essential in diagnosing fractures and dislocations, and the chest and pelvic films may identify serious abnormality requiring further assessment and treatment, as well as defining a source of blood loss.
2. Obtain portable films. Do not transport unstable patients to the radiology department. After stabilization, additional films can be obtained while the patient is being appropriately monitored.
3. CT scans and angiography may be necessary. Exercise great care and judgment in obtaining these studies in the unstable patient. Other priorities of care such as a laparotomy must be carefully weighed before obtaining diagnostic x-ray studies. Careful monitoring must be maintained throughout the examination.

Laboratory

1. Studies that should be done in the ED include a spun hematocrit, urinalysis, and perhaps an oximetry or arterial blood gas (ABG) determination.
2. Type and cross-match are essential in all significant trauma cases.
3. Routine studies include a complete blood count (CBC), platelet count, electrolytes, blood urea nitrogen (BUN), glucose, amylase (with abdominal abnormality), and coagulation studies (prothrombin time [PT] and partial thromboplastin time [PTT]).

   Coagulation disorders are most common in patients with severe head trauma and less common in cases of gunshot wounds, blunt trauma, and stab wounds. A rapid bedside screen may be done by observing for clot formation in blood drawn into a clean tube. Normally, the blood will clot and then retract within 10 minutes. The absence of clotting indicates a major coagulopathy, whereas abnormal clot retraction suggests thrombocytopenia. If the blood clots and subsequently lyses, fibrinolysis is occurring.
4. Consider a urine drug screen (unfortunately drug use is increasing in every young population).
5. Perform an ECG if indicated by the nature of the injury.
6. Test for pregnancy in menstruating females.

SCORING PEDIATRIC TRAUMA

A number of scoring systems have been developed to facilitate consistency of evaluation. Using the pediatric trauma score (Table 56-1), 28% of patients with a score of 6 or less died, whereas only 1% of those with a score of 7 or more died. All children with a score less than 2 died.

The revised trauma score (Table 56-2), which can be used in both adults and children, has

TABLE 56-1   Pediatric Trauma Score*

| Component | Score for each variable* | | |
	+2	+1	−1
Weight	≥20 kg	10-20 kg	<10 kg
Airway patency	Normal	Maintainable	Unmaintainable
Systolic blood pressure	≥90 mm Hg	90-50 mm Hg	<50 mm Hg
CNS status	Awake	Obtunded/loss of consciousness	Coma/decerebrate
Open wound	None	Minor	Major/penetrating
Skeletal injury	None	Closed fracture	Open/multiple fractures

From Tepas JJ, Mollitt DL, Talbert JL, et al: *J Pediatr Surg* 22:14, 1987.
*A score of +2, +1, or −1 is given to each variable and then added (range, −6 to 12). A score ≤8 indicates potentially important trauma.

TABLE 56-2   Revised Trauma Score*

Revised trauma score	Glasgow Coma Scale score (Table 57-1)	Systolic blood pressure (mm Hg)	Respiratory rate (breaths/min)
4	13-15	>89	10-29
3	9-12	76-89	>29
2	6-8	50-75	6-9
1	4-5	1-49	1-5
0	3	0	0

From Wesson DE, Spence LJ, Williams JI, et al: *Can J Surg* 30:398, 1987.
*A score of 0-4 is given for each variable, then added (range, 1-12). A score ≤11 indicates potentially important trauma.

been shown to be a valid predictor of severity. It may define severity of injury from the prehospital environment through the hospital stay.

After blunt trauma, patients who present to an ED with pulseless cardiac arrest have little chance of functional survival.

CONSULTATION

1. Notify a trauma surgeon as soon as the facility is alerted that a patient with serious trauma is en route to the hospital. Depending on the reliability of the prehospital care assessment, this initial surgical contact may await arrival and primary assessment if the surgeon is not in the hospital.
2. Notify a neurosurgeon if significant head injury is present.
3. Orthopedic, plastic surgery, and urology personnel may be notified after sta-

bilization. Premature consultation may add chaos and confusion to the initial resuscitation.

PSYCHOLOGIC CONCERNS

For many reasons, the child who is the victim of trauma may be terrified and crying hysterically on arrival in the ED. Pain is present from either the injuries or their treatment. The child is separated from parents and is in a strange environment and surrounded by unfamiliar doctors and nurses.

Support is essential for the conscious child. Time must be taken to explain in a reassuring way that the youngster has been injured, is in the hospital, and is going to be all right. Touching the child in a soothing manner as well as speaking in a calm, controlled tone may be helpful in winning confidence and establishing rapport. Procedures should be explained if possible and the child warned that there may be accompanying pain. The patient should not be surprised.

Parents should be allowed to stay with the child whenever possible. This may not be feasible when the youngster is critically ill, requiring major resuscitative efforts, or when the parents are so upset that they are actually contributing to the patient's hysteria. If parents are unavailable, a member of the resuscitation team should be designated to support the child as a surrogate parent in these circumstances; make sure that there is adequate communication and support for the family when contact is made.

Long-term follow-up is probably indicated to monitor for the evolution of poststress anxiety reactions. These may develop in children who have experienced a life-threatening event or witnessed such an episode in a family member or friend.

DISPOSITION

Patients with multiple serious injuries should be admitted to the trauma service, with coordination of the appropriate consulting services.

Transfer to another institution is indicated only if definitive care cannot be provided at the initial facility. Lines of referral for specific types of injury (i.e., burns, amputation) should be established in advance to facilitate communication and transfer.

Before transfer, the patient's condition must be stabilized. During transfer, the same levels of monitoring and treatment established in the ED should be maintained. All records, x-ray films, and laboratory data should accompany the patient (see Chapter 3).

COST OF TRAUMA

In 1985 alone, among children age 0 to 14 years the estimated direct and indirect costs of traumatic injury approached $14 billion. Trauma results in costs not just in terms of recovery after the initial injury but also in loss of future productivity of the child throughout his or her life, damage to parental marital relationships, and the financial impact on the family.

Jacobs' study of adults and children with severe head injuries found 28% of families reporting use of all or most of their fiscal resources to recover after an injury. Harris also studied severely injured children and estimated 32% of families experienced marital difficulties and 60% had new social and financial problems. Osberg found that even among children who are only mildly injured, 60% of the families reported at least one financial or work-related problem at 1 month after discharge and 40% still reported at least one problem 6 months after discharge.

Families need to be counseled about the impending stresses that they can expect in the recovery phase and they need to be aware of any resources that they may have at their disposal.

REFERENCES

American College of Emergency Physicians: Clinical policy for the initial approach to patients presenting with acute blunt trauma, *Ann Emerg Med* 31:422, 1998.

Agran PF, Dunkle DE, Winn DG: Motor vehicle childhood injuries caused by non-crash falls and ejections, *JAMA* 253:2530, 1985.

Agran PF, Dunkle DE, Winn DG: Injuries in a sample of seat-belted children evaluated and treated in a hospital emergency room, *J Trauma* 27:58, 1987.

American College of Emergency Physicians: Guidelines for trauma care systems, *Ann Emerg Med* 22:1079, 1993.

American College of Surgeons Committee on Trauma: *Advanced trauma life support program for physicians*, Chicago, 1993, American College of Surgeons.

Boulanger BR, McLellan BA, Brenneman FD, et al: Emergent abdominal sonography as a screening test in a new diagnostic algorithm for blunt trauma, *J Trauma* 40:867, 1996

Civil ID, Ross GE, Botehlo G: Routine pelvic radiography in severe blunt trauma: is it necessary? *Ann Emerg Med* 17:488, 1988.

Durham LA, Richardson RJ, Wall JM, et al: Emergency center thoracotomy: impact of prehospital resuscitation, *Trauma* 32:775, 1992

Esposito TJ, Jurkovich GJ, Rice CL, et al: Reappraisal of emergency room thoracotomy in a changing environment, *J Trauma* 31:881, 1991

Fitzmaurice LS: Approach to multiple trauma. In Barkin RM, editor: *Pediatric emergency medicine: concepts and clinical practice,* ed 2, St Louis, 1997, Mosby.

Gerardi MI, Sacchetti AD, Kantor RM, et al: Rapid sequence intubation of the pediatric patient, *Ann Emerg Med* 28:55, 1996.

Gin-Shaw SL, Jorden RC: Multiple trauma. In Rosen P, editor: *Emergency medicine, concepts and clinical practice,* ed 4, St Louis, 1998, Mosby.

Gnauck K, Lungo JB, Scalzo A, et al: Emergency intubation of the pediatric medical patient: use of anesthetic agents in the emergency department, *Ann Emerg Med* 23: 1242, 1994.

Grupp-Phelan J, Tanz RR: How rational is the crossmatching of blood in a pediatric emergency department? *Arch Pediatr Adolesc Med* 150:1140, 1996.

Guyer B, Lescohier I, Gallagher SS, et al: Intentional injuries among children and adolescents in Massachusetts, *N Engl J Med* 321:1584, 1989.

Harris BH, Schwaitzberg SD, Seman TM, et al: Hidden morbidity of pediatric trauma, *J Pediatr Surg* 24:103, 1989.

Hazinski MF, Chahine AA, Holcomb GW, et al: Outcome of cardiovascular collapse in pediatric blunt trauma, *Ann Emerg Med* 23:1229, 1994.

Honigman B, Lowenstein SR, Moore EE, et al: The role of the pneumatic antishock garment in penetrating cardiac wounds, *JAMA* 266:2398, 1991.

Hooker EA, Miller FB, Holanderi R, et al: Do all trauma patients need early crossmatching for blood? *J Emerg Med* 12:447, 1994.

Ivatury RR, Kazigo J, Rohman M, et al: Directed emergency room thoracotomy: a prognostic prerequisite for survival, *J Trauma* 31:1076, 1991.

Jacobs HE: The Los Angeles head injury survey: procedures and initial findings, *Arch Phys Med Rehabil* 69:425, 1988.

Jaffe D, Wesson D: Emergency management of blunt trauma in children, *N Engl J Med* 324:1477, 1991.

King BR, Baker MD, Braitman LE, et al: Endotracheal tube selection in children: a comparison of four methods, *Ann Emerg Med* 22:530, 1993.

Lowenstein SR, Yaron M, Carrero R: Vertical trauma: injuries to patients who fall and land on their feet, *Ann Emerg Med* 18:161, 1989.

Mattox KL, Moore EE, Feliciano DV: *Trauma,* Norwalk, Conn, 1987, Appleton & Lange.

Nakayama DK, Waggoner T, Venkataraman ST, et al: The use of drugs in emergency airway management in pediatric trauma, *Ann Surg* 216:205, 1992.

Ordog GJ, Wasserberger J, Balasubramanium M: Coagulation abnormalities in traumatic shock, *Ann Emerg Med* 14:650, 1985.

Ordog GI, Wasserberger J, Schwartz I, et al: Gunshot wounds in children under 10 years of age, *Am J Dis Child* 142:618, 1988.

Osberg JS, Kahn P, Rowe K, et al: Pediatric trauma: impact on work and family finances, *Pediatrics* 98:890, 1996.

Pearlman MD, Tintinalli JE, Lorenz RP: Blunt trauma during pregnancy, *N Engl J Med* 323:1609, 1990.

Phillips S, Rond PC, Kelly SM, et al: The need for pediatric-specific triage criteria: results from the Florida Trauma Triage Study, *Pediatr Emerg Care* 12:394, 1996.

Rice DP, MacKenzie EJ, et al: *Cost of injury in the United States: a report to Congress,* San Francisco, CA, Institute for Health and Aging, University of California and Injury Prevention Center, Baltimore: Johns Hopkins University, 1989:68.

Rothenberg SS, Moore EE, Moore FA, et al: Emergency department thoracotomy in children: a critical analysis, *J Trauma* 29:1322, 1989.

Selbst SM, Alexander D, Ruddy R: Bicycle-related injuries, *Am J Dis Child* 141:140, 1987.

Stewart G, Meert K, Rosenberg N: Trauma in infants less than three months of age, *Pediatr Emerg Care* 9:199, 1993.

Teech SJ, Antosia RE, Luno DF, et al: Prehospital fluid therapy in pediatric trauma patients. *Pediatr Emerg Care* 17:5, 1995.

Thomas B, Falcone RE, Vasquez D, et al: Ultrasound evaluation of blunt abdominal trauma: program implementation, initial experience, and learning curve, *J Trauma* 42:384, 1997.

Trunkey D: Initial treatment of patients with extensive trauma, *N Engl J Med* 324:1259, 1991.

Trunkey D, Federle MP: Computed tomography in perspective, *J Trauma* 26(7):660, 1986 (editorial).

Walls RM: Rapid-sequence intubation in head trauma, *Ann Emerg Med* 22:1008, 1993.

Weesner CL, Hargarfen SW, Aprakamian C, et al: Fatal childhood injury patterns in an urban setting, *Ann Emerg Med* 23:231, 1994.

Woolard DJ, Terndrup TE: Sedative-analgesic agent administration in children: analysis of use and complications in the emergency department, *J Emerg Med* 12:453, 1994.

Yamamoto LG, Yim GK, Britten AG: Rapid sequence anesthesia induction for emergency intubation, *Pediatr Emerg Care* 6:200, 1990.

Yurt RW: Triage, initial assessment and early treatment of the pediatric trauma patient, *Pediatr Clin North Am* 39: 1083, 1992.

57 HEAD TRAUMA

PETER T. PONS

ALERT: Any patient with head trauma must be considered to have spinal trauma and other associated injuries. Initial evaluation must focus on airway, ventilation, circulation, and immobilization of the cervical spine. Head injury as an isolated finding very rarely causes shock.

Auto accidents account for most head trauma. The primary insult is the injury to the brain that occurs at the time of impact. This results from translational or rotational forces. Translational forces produce compressive and tensile strains on the skull and brain, leading to focal brain injuries such as linear skull fractures, cerebral contusions, epidural hematomas, acute subdural hematomas, or contrecoup cerebral contusions. Rotational forces can be more devastating, resulting in a shearing stress that causes diffuse brain injuries, including mild contusion, cerebral concussion, or diffuse cerebral injury. Significant distortion of the skull can occur in infants less than 2 years of age because of the open sutures and relative elasticity of the skull. This distortion can be transmitted to the underlying meninges, cortical vessels, and brain, leading to a high incidence of hematomas, tentorial and dural lesions, and shearing.

The secondary insult is the progressive deficit caused by cerebral ischemia, hypoxia, hypercapnia, hypotension, and increased intracranial pressure. Brain swelling is the most common cause of death in patients with severe head injuries. Brain swelling compromises oxygen and glucose delivery to neurons.

Child abuse should be considered in cases of intracranial injuries or skull fractures in children less than 1 year if there is no history of significant accidental trauma, such as a motor vehicle accident.

Aggressive early resuscitation, encompassing the establishment of the integrity of the airway, ventilation, and circulation and the immobilization of the spine, largely determines the outcome. Careful examination, evaluation, and treatment of associated injuries is crucial. This is followed by systematic, definitive care of neurologic and other injuries.

DIAGNOSTIC FINDINGS
History

The mechanism of trauma and associated signs and symptoms must be determined following initial resuscitation:

1. Mechanism of injury: direct blow (define implement) or acceleration/deceleration
2. Circumstances of accident: motor vehicle accident, diving accident, fall, or blow (any inconsistencies that might suggest abuse)
3. Chronology
   a. Loss of consciousness immediately or shortly after accident

b. Period of lucidity
c. Progression of deficits
4. Associated findings
  a. Amnesia
  b. Disorientation
  c. Sensorimotor abnormalities
  d. Visual disturbances
  e. Dizziness
  f. Vomiting or nausea
  g. Seizures
5. Medications at the time of the incident including alcohol, drugs, and prescribed treatments
6. Medical history and allergies
Associated injuries, especially facial and neck, are often present.

GENERAL PHYSICAL EXAMINATION

In addition to specific evaluation of the head and back, examination of the cervical spine and other areas of trauma should be defined.

Frequent repetition of the examination is essential to detect any signs of deterioration, as well as to monitor improvement. Specific consideration must be given to determining the extent of neurologic injury, the presence of a mass lesion effect, and the course of the injury.

Vital Signs

1. Airway. Often occluded by blood, mucus, fractures, or foreign bodies, leading to respiratory distress.
2. Hypotension. Acute head trauma does not produce hypotension except in infants with open sutures and massive intracranial bleeding or in individuals with large scalp lacerations. If shock is present, look for other associated injuries.
3. Dysrhythmias: ventricular and atrial. Prolonged QT interval and large T and prominent U waves have been noted without cardiac abnormality.
4. Cushing's reflex. Produces elevated blood pressure, slowed pulse, and irregular res-

pirations. Usually a late finding of increased intracranial pressure.
5. Cheyne-Stokes respiration. Characterized by crescendo-decrescendo patterns of hyperventilation, followed by periods of apnea. Often accompanies decorticate posturing caused by cerebral hemispheric lesions and incipient temporal lobe herniation. May be seen during normal infant sleep.
6. Central neurogenic hyperventilation with deep, rapid ventilation. May accompany decerebrate posturing and is indicative of brainstem dysfunction, either as a primary injury or secondary to supratentorial herniation.

Neurologic Examination (see Table 15-3)

Level of Consciousness
1. Maximal depression in the level of consciousness usually occurs at the time of impact and should subsequently improve. Failure to improve indicates that additional or massive injury has occurred.
2. The level of consciousness may be recorded in a descriptive (mnemonic: AVPU) narrative indicating the patient's response to stimuli:
  • A: awake verbal child
  • V: in a nonverbal child, denotes a child who is responsive to verbal stimuli; clues include behavioral signs such as eye opening, quieting, or calming
  • P: response to painful stimuli such as moaning or crying
  • U: unresponsive to any stimuli
  Another descriptive approach includes *alert* (awake and responds verbally to questions), *lethargic* (sleeps when undisturbed but is incoherent when awakened), *semicomatose* (responds to painful stimuli in a purposeful, decorticate, or decerebrate posture), and *comatose* (no response to stimuli).
3. The Glasgow Coma Scale (GCS) for

responsiveness (Table 57-1) standardizes assessment, predicts outcome, and is useful in monitoring patient. A pediatric modification has been developed.

A GCS score of 3 to 8 on presentation to the emergency department (ED) indicates severe head trauma and is predictive of past traumatic seizures. Children with a GCS score of 15 and a normal neurologic examination are generally not reported to have intracranial hemorrhage.

Posturing
Decerebrate posturing and flaccidity are associated with the worst prognosis.

Pupils: Size, Equality, and Reactivity
1. Unilateral pupillary dilation strongly suggests a mass lesion with actual or incipient herniation requiring immediate intervention. A dilated and fixed pupil is the most reliable sign of the side of the lesion. It results from pressure on the third cranial nerve (oculomotor).
2. Examination must exclude previous eye trauma, topical medications, or congenital anisocoria.

NOTE: Retinal hemorrhage in children less than 1 year is usually associated with shaking injuries.

TABLE 57-1   Pediatric Modification of Glasgow Coma Scale (GCS) by Age of Patient*

Glasgow Coma Scale score	Pediatric modification	
EYE OPENING		
≥1 year	**0-1 year**	
4 Spontaneously	4 Spontaneously	
3 To verbal command	3 To shout	
2 To pain	2 To pain	
1 No response	1 No response	
BEST MOTOR RESPONSE		
≥1 year	**0-1 year**	
6 Obeys		
5 Localizes pain	5 Localizes pain	
4 Flexion withdrawal	4 Flexion withdrawal	
3 Flexion abnormal (decorticate)	3 Flexion abnormal (decorticate)	
2 Extension (decerebrate)	2 Extension (decerebrate)	
1 No response	1 No response	
BEST VERBAL RESPONSE		
>5 years	**0-2 years**	**2-5 years**
5 Oriented and converses	5 Cries appropriately, smiles, coos	5 Appropriate words and phrases
4 Disoriented and converses	4 Cries	4 Inappropriate words
3 Inappropriate words	3 Inappropriate crying/screaming	3 Cries/screams
2 Incomprehensible sounds	2 Grunts	2 Grunts
1 No response	1 No response	1 No response

*Score is the sum of the individual scores from eye opening, best verbal response, and best motor response, using age-specific criteria. GCS score of 13-15 indicates mild head injury, GCS score of 9-12 indicates moderate head injury, and GCS score of ≤8 indicates severe head injury.

3. Hemorrhaging into the retina with a decrease in visual acuity may be noted after trauma.

Eye Movements

1. Destructive lesions in the occipital or frontal lobes cause deviation of the eyes toward the lesion. Injury to the brainstem causes deviation away from the lesion.
2. Oculocephalic reflex (doll's eye) demonstrates intactness of the brainstem, as does the oculovestibular reflex. These should be tested only after the cervical spine has been cleared.
   a. *Oculocephalic reflex* (doll's eyes) is performed with the eyes held open and the head turned quickly from side to side. A comatose patient with an intact brainstem will respond by the eyes moving in the direction opposite to that which the head is turned as if still gazing ahead in the initial position. Comatose patients with midbrain or pons lesions have random eye movements.
   b. *Oculovestibular reflex* with caloric stimulation is done with the head elevated 30 degrees in the patient with an intact eardrum. Ice water is then injected through a small catheter lying in the ear canal (up to 200 ml is used in an adult). Comatose patients with an intact brainstem respond by conjugate deviation of the eyes toward the irrigated ear, whereas those with a brainstem lesion demonstrate no response.
   c. *Corneal reflex* is elicited by gently stroking the cornea with sterile cotton. A blink response demonstrates an intact brainstem and nucleus of cranial nerves V, VI, and VII.

Sensory and Motor Response

1. Motor responses may be determined by response to verbal commands, painful stimuli, and spontaneous movements. Tone and symmetry should be evaluated.
2. Sensory examination should include light touch and pain.

Reflexes

1. Presence, absence, and equality of reflexes should be ascertained.
2. The presence of Babinski reflex (dorsiflexive plantar response) is indicative of an upper motor neuron lesion.

Rectal Examination

This must be performed to check for spinal cord integrity, indicated by the presence of sphincter tone.

Other Findings

For a careful assessment the following signs are important:
1. Bulging fontanelle.
2. Palpable depression or crepitus of skull; unusual hematoma, particularly longitudinal ones.
3. Evidence of basilar skull fracture:
   a. Battle signs (ecchymosis posterior to ear) or raccoon (bilateral black eyes) eye sign
   b. Cerebrospinal fluid (CSF) rhinorrhea or otorrhea
   c. Hemotympanum or bleeding from middle ear
4. Diabetes insipidus; polyuria, nocturia, and polydipsia.
5. *Cortical* blindness may occur after minor head injury from vascular hyperactivity (similar to migraine equivalent). Typically, children sustain trauma without loss of consciousness. Blindness develops after a latent period of 15 to 45 minutes and may last a few hours up to 10 days, usually with total recovery. Pupillary light reflexes are normal.

Increased Intracranial Pressure

Increased intracranial pressure should be suspected in patients with trauma who have a GCS score of less than 8, difficult to control seizures, abnormal vital signs (hypertension, bradycardia, abnormal respirations), dilated and unreactive pupils, and decerebrate/decorticate posturing.

As the intracranial pressure rises, a relatively

well-defined series of events will occur, ultimately leading to the patient's death unless
appropriate actions are performed to slow or
reverse the process. As the pressure rises in the
supratentorial compartment, the brain (usually
the uncus or medial temporal lobe) is pushed
against and through the opening of the tento-
rium. This produces compression of the ipsilateral third cranial nerve, leading to a fixed,
dilated pupil. Occasionally, the contralateral
third nerve will be compromised.

Progression of the herniation leads to compression of the pyramidal tract, usually resulting
in contralateral weakness or paralysis. Simultaneously, pressure on the reticular activating
system results in impaired consciousness,
which may be the first sign of deterioration.

In the infant with an open fontanelle, initial
findings may include a bulging fontanelle, irritability, and listlessness, eventually progressing to
focal findings. Those with closed fontanelles
present a more classic picture.

In patients with cerebellar tonsillar herniation, the midline force causes the low brainstem
and cerebellar tonsils to herniate through the
foramen magnum, leading to Cushing's reflex
(bradycardia, hypertension, and apnea).

Prognostic Factors

Prognostic factors in severe head trauma may be
useful in the management of children's injuries.
Severe head trauma is defined as unconsciousness more than 6 hours and inability to obey
commands, utter recognizable words, or open
the eyes.

Children less than 10 years of age generally
have the best prognosis. Those with a GCS
score of 5 to 8 usually do not die, and only 20%
have permanent focal deficits. Those with
scores of 3 to 5 can achieve independent
function. Higher scores are associated with
even fewer sequelae. The recovery to consciousness and function is usually complete
within 3 weeks, and 77% of the children in one
study returned to a regular school setting.

The worst prognosis is for those children
with flaccidity or decerebrate posturing. Although children with prolonged coma tend to
have a poor outcome, in one study 9 of 14
children in coma for more than 2 weeks had
little or no handicapping neurologic sequelae.

Complications

Several other findings secondary to complications of the initial mechanical injury, as well as
hypoxia, increased intracranial pressure, hypotension, and hypercapnia, may be noted.

1. Altered neurologic examination result as
   noted.
2. Seizures within 1 week of injury occur in
   approximately 5% of children hospitalized
   after head trauma. Another 5% of these
   hospitalized children have a seizure after
   the first week. Half of these children
   eventually stop having seizures; 25% have
   occasional seizures, and the remainder
   have more than 10 per year. Patients in
   coma longer than 6 hours have almost a
   50% incidence of seizures. Other findings
   associated with seizures include a GCS
   score of 3 to 8 and an abnormal computed
   tomography (CT) scan. Children with
   these findings have a 35% to 40% incidence of seizure, whereas without these
   abnormalities the overall incidence is approximately 5%.
3. Psychosocial and behavioral findings after
   mild head trauma may include disinhibi-
   tion, depression, emotional lability, and
   irritability.
4. Noncardiogenic pulmonary edema.
5. Apnea. Posttraumatic apnea is due to
   transient impairment of the reticular activating system along the brainstem. It
   usually is self-limited or requires limited
   stimulation. Prolonged apnea implies a
   more serious injury.
6. Shock is generally not associated with
   isolated head trauma. However, in children less than 1 year of age, an expanding

epidural hematoma may lead to significant blood loss. A subgaleal hematoma or scalp avulsion may also cause major blood loss.

7. Death resulting from the primary process or secondary complications.

Ancillary Data

X-Ray Film of the Cervical Spine
(see Chapter 61)

This should be obtained routinely on all patients older than 3 years of age with a posttraumatic altered mental status, neurologic deficit, neck or back pain, and mechanism of injury consistent with causing a spine injury or for those who give incomplete histories, such as younger children and drug abusers. Younger infants should be studied selectively.

A cross-table lateral cervical spine view should be the first radiograph obtained.

Skull X-Ray Film

This is usually not needed in the initial management because a bone fracture is not the critical injury; intracranial injury must be defined. Thus CT scan is the preferred diagnostic study.

Patients for whom there is a high risk of fracture include those with the following:

1. Documented loss of consciousness longer than 5 minutes or lack of consciousness at the time of the evaluation.
2. The possibility of a depressed skull fracture (palpable defect, crepitus) or a suggestive history (blunt injury with head of hammer or heel of high-heeled shoe). Tangential views may be required.
3. Focal neurologic signs.
4. Penetrating trauma.
5. Evidence of basilar skull fracture (Battle or raccoon-eye sign, CSF from nose or ear, hemotympanum).
6. Head trauma where child abuse is suspected, particularly in children less than 1 year.

Important findings are as follows:

1. Fracture that crosses the middle meningeal artery groove associated with increased incidence of epidural hematoma
2. Depressed skull fracture
3. Open fracture

The absence of a fracture does not exclude significant intracranial pathologic conditions. The presence of a skull fracture may be a valuable marker in the early identification of pediatric patients with moderate head injury who are at greatly increased risk of an intracranial injury.

Computed Tomography (CT) Scan

CT scan is the definitive diagnostic procedure of choice. A noncontrast study of the *acutely* traumatized patient, including bone and subdural windows, is usually sufficient, but a contrast study (3 ml/kg) may be useful for chronic subdural hematoma 7 days of age or older. Generalized cerebral swelling is common. If a CT scan is immediately available, a skull roentgenogram may be selectively omitted.

Indications for obtaining a CT scan include but are not limited to the following:

1. Unconsciousness at the time of evaluation
2. Focal neurologic deficits
3. Depressed skull fracture or fracture crossing middle meningeal artery groove; suspected depressed skull fracture
4. Deterioration of mental status or neurologic function
5. Delayed posttraumatic seizure
6. Children less than 1 year with bradycardia, diastasis of sutures on skull x-ray study, or full fontanelle
7. Progressive or ongoing symptoms such as headache or vomiting

However, no clinical findings accurately identify all patients with abnormal CT scan findings. Clinical findings that have been associated with abnormal CT scan results include a GCS score of 12 or less, altered mental status on admission, and focal abnormalities indicated on neurologic examination.

Another study indicated that four variables (nausea, vomiting, severe headache, skull depression) identified patients with minor head trauma and a GCS score of 15 who ultimately required neurosurgical intervention. These clinical parameters may be useful in screening patients who require CT scans. Prospective studies are still required.

Assessing the patient with head trauma requires a systematic approach to radiologic evaluation (Table 57-2). Magnetic resonance imaging (MRI) may offer detection of more subtle changes indicating subtle contusions and non-hemorrhagic injuries. More planes of visualization are available without patient manipulation, and evaluation of extracerebral fluid collections is improved. Time availability, and patient instability usually preclude use of this technology in the emergency setting.

Other Data

1. Arterial blood gas (ABG) and oximetry are important to ensure that the patient is being adequately ventilated and oxygenated and that hyperventilation is maintaining $Paco_2$ at about 28 mm Hg. Exclude pulmonary edema.
2. Lumbar puncture (LP) is not indicated. If infection is considered, LP should be done only after a negative CT scan finding when there is preceding trauma. Empiric administration of antibiotics after appropriate cultures should be considered.
3. Electroencephalogram (EEG) rarely provides any information that is useful either therapeutically or prognostically.

TABLE 57-2 Radiographic Imaging Strategy in Patients with Head Trauma*

Low-risk group	Moderate-risk group	High-risk group
FINDINGS		
Asymptomatic	History of change of consciousness at the time of injury or subsequently	Deteriorating or depressed level of consciousness not caused by alcohol, drugs, or other cause (e.g., metabolic and seizure disorders)
Headache	History of progressive headache	Focal neurologic signs
Dizziness	Alcohol or drug intoxication	Penetrating skull injury or palpable depressed fracture‡
Scalp hematoma	Posttraumatic seizure or amnesia	
Scalp contusion, abrasion, or laceration	Persistent vomiting	
Absence of moderate-risk or high-risk criteria	Serious facial injury	
	Signs of basilar fracture†	
	Possible skull penetration or depressed fracture‡	
	Suspected child abuse	
MANAGEMENT		
Observation alone: discharge patients with head-injury information sheet (listing subdural precautions) and a second person to observe them	Extended close observation (watch for signs of high-risk group) Consider CT examination and neurosurgical consultation	Neurosurgical consultation and emergency CT examination

Modified from Masters SJ, McClean PM, Acarese JS, et al: *N Engl J Med* 315:84, 1987.
*Physician assessment of the severity of injury may warrant reassignment to a higher risk group. Any single criterion from a higher-risk group warrants assignment of the patient to the highest risk group applicable.
†Signs of basilar fracture include drainage from ear, drainage of cerebrospinal fluid from nose, hemotympanum, Battle sign, and "raccoon eyes."
‡Factors associated with open and depressed fracture include gunshot, missile, or shrapnel wounds; scalp injury from firm, pointed object (including animal teeth); penetrating injury of eyelid or globe; object stuck in the head; assault (definite or suspected) with any object; leakage of cerebrospinal fluid; and sign of basilar fracture.

4. Check electrolytes if evidence of diabetes insipidus is present.
5. Perform a chest x-ray study to exclude pulmonary edema.

MANAGEMENT
Initial Management

The initial management of severe head trauma is directed not at therapy of the head trauma but rather at immediate or potential life threats. Minimal head trauma requires a careful examination, appropriate laboratory studies, a short period of observation, and good follow-up observation and instructions.

Airway
1. Oxygenate.
2. Suction blood and secretions, and remove foreign material from airway.
3. If the patient is unable to maintain a patent airway, active management is essential while attempting to maintain cervical spine precautions, if necessary. Orotracheal intubation while maintaining in-line cervical spine immobilization may be attempted.
4. Acutely unconscious patients secondary to trauma, particularly those requiring prolonged diagnostic evaluation or transport, should generally be considered for intubation on a prophylactic basis, as well as to initiate hyperventilation.
5. If time permits, administer lidocaine (1.5 mg/kg IV) 1 minute before intubation to prevent an acute rise in intracranial pressure. Administration of atropine (0.01 mg/kg/dose; minimum: 0.1 mg; maximum: 1 mg) may reduce potential bradycardia. Rapid sequence induction is outlined in Chapter 56.

Respirations
Supplemental oxygen and assisted ventilation should be administered as necessary.

Circulatory Status (see Chapter 5)
Fluids are generally administered at a rate of two thirds of maintenance. Intake and output must be closely monitored. Cerebral perfusion pressure depends on an adequate blood pressure.

Shock must be managed aggressively with crystalloid infused into large-bore IV lines. If shock is present, associated injuries should be delineated while hemodynamic stability is being achieved.

Immobilization of Cervical Spine
See Chapter 61.

Reduction of Intracranial Pressure (ICP)
1. Hyperventilation is the most rapid method of decreasing ICP and is usually indicated if the GCS score is less than or equal to 8 (see Table 57-1, p. 414).
   a. Hyperventilate the patient to maintain a $Paco_2$ (ABG) of about 25 to 28 mm Hg. Decreasing the $Paco_2$ from 40 to 20 mm Hg reduces cerebral blood flow by nearly 60% of normal.
   b. Maintain Pao_2 of at least 90 mm Hg. Supplemental oxygen and PEEP may be required.
2. Elevate head to approximately 30 degrees if patient is not in shock.
3. Administer one or more of the following:
   a. Furosemide (Lasix), 1 mg/kg/dose q4-6hr IV. Adult: 20-40 mg/dose q4-6hr IV.
   b. Mannitol:
      (1) Dosage: 0.25 gm/kg/dose over 10 to 15 minutes q3-4hr IV prn.
      (2) Not used in routine management but useful if there are signs of increased ICP.
      (3) Risks: fluid and electrolyte imbalance, hyperosmolality, volume overload, and rebound cerebral edema. Not to be used for patients with renal failure. Role in patients with evidence of shock is controversial.
4. Monitor ICP in consultation with a neurosurgeon in cases of severe head trauma. Optimally, maintain ICP at 20 mm Hg or less and cerebral perfusion pressure (CPP) at 50 mm Hg or more. An ICP above 40 mm Hg is associated with a poor outcome.

5. Barbiturates are useful for significant cerebral edema associated with elevated and poorly responsive intracranial pressure. They decrease ICP and cerebral metabolism and stabilize cell membranes. Because the ability to evaluate neurologic status is lost, barbiturates should be given only in consultation with a neurosurgeon.
   • Pentobarbital (Nembutal) dosage is 3-20 mg/kg IV slow push while monitoring blood pressure. Infusion is maintained at 1-2 mg/kg/hr to maintain level of 25-40 μg/ml. Levels above 30 μg/ml may be associated with hypotension in as many as 60% of patients.
6. The use of anticonvulsants prophylactically such as phenytoin or phenobarbital is controversial and should be discussed with the consultant neurosurgeon. Anticonvulsants should be initiated if there is seizure activity and should be considered in patients with significant neurologic deficit, penetrating brain injuries, and depressed fractures with true penetration.
7. Maintain hypothermia if already present. Induce hypothermia (see Chapter 51) only as a last resort in patients whose ICP remains elevated despite other measures and after consultation.
   a. It reduces cerebral metabolism and vulnerability to hypoxemia.
   b. In consultation with a neurosurgeon, temperature may be gradually reduced to 32° to 33° C.
8. The potential role of calcium channel blockers is under investigation; they may help reduce cerebral damage after head trauma. Studies are also exploring the effects of a vasoactive analog of adrenocorticotropic hormone (GMM$_2$).

SPECIFIC CLINICAL ENTITIES (Fig. 57-1)
Contusion of Scalp, Forehead, or Face

Diagnostic Findings
1. Localized swelling and tenderness; variable hematoma or ecchymosis

2. No neurologic deficit

Management
1. Discharge patient.
2. Prescribe ice packs for swelling and analgesia (aspirin or acetaminophen) for pain.
3. Discuss head injury precautions.
4. Do not aspirate (commonly liquefies in children).

Concussion

Diagnostic Findings
1. Transient neurologic dysfunction, which disappears within minutes to days, leaving a neurologically normal patient
2. May include transient loss of consciousness, as well as isolated findings of dizziness, nausea, vomiting, amnesia, or confusion
3. CT scan indicated with dysfunction more than 5 minutes

Management
1. Observation. When there has been persistent symptoms or inadequate home environment, hospitalization is recommended.
2. Aspirin or acetaminophen analgesia. Narcotics should be avoided.

Skull Fracture

Diagnostic Findings
1. Pain, tenderness, and swelling over fracture site. Isolated skull fractures rarely present without local signs such as palpable fracture, soft tissue swelling, or signs of basilar skull fracture. May be associated with other severe injuries.
2. Significance related not to bony defect but to intensity of injury and possible damage to underlying structures.
3. Basilar skull fracture is suggested by findings of hemotympanum, Battle sign (bilateral postauricular ecchymoses), raccoon-eye sign (bilateral periorbital ecchymoses), or CSF rhinorrhea or otorrhea. Anosmia may indicate involvement

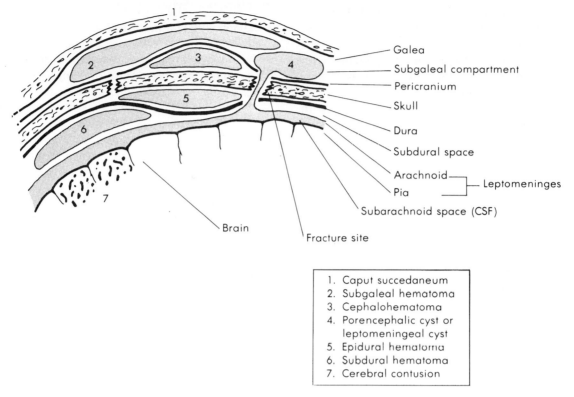

Galea
Subgaleal compartment
Pericranium
Skull
Dura
Subdural space
Arachnoid — ⎤
                ⎬ Leptomeninges
Pia — ⎦
Subarachnoid space (CSF)
Brain
Fracture site

| 1. Caput succedaneum |
| 2. Subgaleal hematoma |
| 3. Cephalohematoma |
| 4. Porencephalic cyst or leptomeningeal cyst |
| 5. Epidural hematoma |
| 6. Subdural hematoma |
| 7. Cerebral contusion |

Fig. 57-1   Traumatic head injuries.

of cranial nerve I via damage to the cribriform plate.

4. Clinical characteristics suggesting an intracranial injury associated with a parietal skull fracture include neurologic dysfunction or a bilateral, depressed, or diastatic skull fracture.

5. X-ray study (p. 417). The CT scan is preferred because intracranial injury, as well as the skull fracture, will be demonstrated.

   a. Linear fractures may be noted involving the flat bones of the skull (frontal, temporal, parietal, or occipital).

      (1) Fractures crossing the middle meningeal artery have the potential of causing epidural hematoma.

      (2) Fractures of the occiput, particularly if stellate or comminuted, are associated with child's being re-

peatedly struck against object (child abuse).

   b. Depressed fractures are recognized on skull x-rays by areas of lucency adjacent to an area of increased density. This represents a double density of bone caused by depressed segment overlapping a nondepressed segment. Tangential views or CT scan may be helpful.

   c. Basilar skull fracture is commonly not detectable by plain roentgenogram. Rarely, a blood-air level may be noted on sphenoid sinus (with patient supine as film is taken), often visualized on a cross-table lateral corneal spine x-ray. CT scan is the most sensitive diagnostic tool.

6. A local swelling with increased transillumination overlying a fracture suggests a

porencephalic or leptomeningeal cyst associated with a "growing" fracture.

Management

1. Generally, hospitalize all patients with skull fractures for observation, with neurosurgical consultation.
2. Perform early CT scan in patients with fractures detected on plain films or if there is any degree of neurologic dysfunction, especially if progressive.
3. Prescribe aspirin or acetaminophen analgesia (no narcotics).
4. Use of antibiotics for patients with basilar skull fractures is controversial, and the ultimate decision should rest with the neurosurgeon. Intracranial contamination by foreign bodies is often treated with ampicillin and chloramphenicol or other agents providing gram-positive and anaerobic coverage.
5. Depressed fractures often require elevation of a fragment surgically.

Cerebral Contusion

Diagnostic Findings

1. Decreased level of consciousness is usually present.
2. Associated neurologic deficits, if any, reflect the contused area of brain. Pathologically, this represents an injury to the brain and is marked by hemorrhage and swelling.
3. CT scan demonstrates an area of cortex with both increased and decreased density.

Management

1. Hospitalization and close observation are required.
2. Principles of head trauma management, including stabilization of airway, ventilation, circulation, and cervical spine, should be used, depending on the degree of injury and neurologic impairment. Other measures outlined previously should be implemented when appropriate.

Intracranial Hemorrhage

Diagnostic Findings (see Fig. 57-1)

1. *Subdural hematomas* are more common than epidural hematomas and usually result from laceration of bridging veins.
2. *Epidural hematoma* is usually associated with a skull fracture and associated meningeal artery bleeding. The classic history of loss of consciousness followed by a lucid period and then deepening coma is rare (10%). In children less than 5 years old, it usually follows a fall.
3. *Intracerebral hemorrhage* is usually associated with a brain laceration. The anterior frontotemporal region is most common. Progression of findings may be gradual.

Because the clinical presentation of these entities is similar, it is impossible to differentiate them clinically without radiologic confirmation. They show signs of a space-occupying lesion, with progressive increase in ICP. Hemiparesis, unequal pupils, hyperactive deep tendon reflexes, and positive Babinski sign may be noted. Drowsiness may progress to stupor, coma, and convulsions. In rare cases, the signs and symptoms may progress insidiously, with irritability, anorexia, and failure to thrive seen.

Ancillary Data

An x-ray film may demonstrate a fracture, particularly with epidural hematomas, whereas a CT scan differentiates the location of hemorrhage.

1. Subdural hematomas appear as an increased density spread over the entire cerebral cortex. There is often cerebral edema on the side of the injury, with a midline shift.
2. Epidural hematoma appears as a lens-shaped (biconvex) area of increased density. The size of the hematoma is limited by the dural attachments at the sutures.
3. Intracerebral hemorrhage has increased density within the cortex and is surrounded by small areas of decreased density, representing edema.

An individual with a history of head trauma and coma or an abnormal neurologic examination result should be presumed to have an intracranial injury even if the initial CT scan does not confirm its presence. Follow-up scan may be required.

Management

1. Resuscitation and head trauma management are urgently required. Emergency intervention is mandatory. Suspicion and recognition determine the ultimate outcome.
2. Neurosurgical consultation is required with an immediate CT scan to define the lesion and then to evacuate the hematoma.
3. On occasion, emergency trephination without CT scan is required. This may be performed by trained physicians for patients with a coning syndrome and a dilated pupil who do not respond to intubation and hyperventilation or who have other injuries that need operative intervention.

DISPOSITION

Obviously, the decision regarding discharge or admission must be individualized, reflecting the mechanism of injury, clinical condition, progression of findings, and follow-up observation. Children with a GCS score of 14 or 15, minor head trauma, and a normal CT scan result can usually be observed at home. Those with a lower GCS score are usually observed in the hospital.

The criteria for hospitalization must be individualized, but indications may include the following:

1. Documented, prolonged loss of consciousness
2. Coma, altered mental status, or seizure
3. Focal neurologic deficit
4. Persistent vomiting or severe and persistent headache
5. Abnormal CT scan
6. Presence of recent linear skull fracture

7. Alcohol or drug intoxication interfering with a reliable examination
8. Suspicion of child abuse or unreliable caregiver
9. High-risk individuals, including children less than 2 years of age and patients with underlying hydrocephalus or coagulopathy

Studies of children with less significant head trauma indicate that some may be observed at home by a responsible adult after a period of monitoring. Criteria may include the following:

1. Loss of consciousness less than 5 minutes
2. Normal examination
3. Absence of severe or progressive symptoms of headaches or vomiting
4. Absence of clinical evidence of basilar skull fracture

Follow-up observation should be arranged because even a minor head trauma may cause mild, long-term problems, such as inability to learn new material or behavioral problems (increased irritability and wide emotional swings).

Parental Education

All children who are discharged from the hospital after head trauma must be released to the care of a responsible adult who has been carefully and explicitly instructed in head precautions.

1. Limit activities and restrict the patient to a light diet. If trauma is recent, apply an ice pack to reduce swelling.
2. Waken child every 2 hours and observe.
3. Call your physician immediately with any of the following:
   a. Increasing sleepiness, drowsiness, or inability to awaken patient from sleep
   b. Change in equality of pupils (black center of eye) or if blurred vision, peculiar movements of the eyes, or difficulty focusing develops
   c. Stumbling, unusual weakness, or difficulty using arms or legs or change in normal gait or crawl

    d. Seizures

    e. Change in personality or behavior, such as increasing irritability, confusion, unusual restlessness, or inability to concentrate

    f. Persistent vomiting (more than three times)

    g. Drainage of blood or fluid from nose or ears

    h. Severe headache

  4. Aspirin or acetaminophen may be given for pain. Do not use narcotics.

REFERENCES

Ampel L, Hott KA, Sielaff GW, et al: An approach to airway management in the acutely head-injured patient, *J Emerg Med* 6:1, 1988.

Bernard B, Zimmerman RA, Bilaniuk LT: Neuroradiologic evaluation of pediatric craniocerebral trauma, *Top Magn Reson Imaging* 5:161, 1993.

Billmire ME, Myers PA: Serious head injury in infants: accident or abuse, *Pediatrics* 75:340, 1985.

Bonadio WA, Smith DS, Hillman S: Clinical indicators of intracranial lesion on computed tomographic scan in children with parietal skull fracture, *Am J Dis Child* 143:194, 1989.

Brock BF, Krause GS, White BC, et al: Neurotrauma: concepts, current practice, and emergency therapies, *Ann Emerg Med* 22:957, 1993.

Davis RL, Mullen N, Makela M, et al: Cranial computed tomography scans in children after minimal head injury with loss of consciousness, *Ann Emerg Med* 24:640, 1994.

Davis RL, Hughes M, Gubler D, et al: The use of cranial CT scans in the triage of pediatric patients with mild head injury, *Pediatrics* 95:345, 1995.

Dietrich AM, Bowman MJ, Ginn-Pease ME, et al: Pediatric head injures: can clinical factors reliably predict an abnormality on computed tomography? *Ann Emerg Med* 22:1535, 1993.

Dolan M: Head trauma. In Barkin RM, editor: *Pediatric emergency medicine: concepts and clinical practice,* ed 2, St Louis, 1997, Mosby.

Duhaime AC, Alario AJ, Lewander WJ, et al: Head injury in very young children: mechanisms, injury types and ophthalmologic findings in 100 hospitalized patients younger than 2 years of age, *Pediatrics* 90:179, 1992.

Feldman JA, Fish S: Resuscitation fluid for a patient with head injury and hypovolemic shock, *J Emerg Med* 9:465, 1991.

Goldman H, Morehead M, Murphy S: Use of adrenocorticotrophic hormone analog to minimize brain injury, *Ann Emerg Med* 22:1035, 1993.

Greenes DS, Schutzman SA: Infants with isolated skull fracture: what are their clinical characteristics and do they require hospitalization? *Ann Emerg Med* 30:253, 1997.

Hamill JF, Bedford RF, Weaver DC, et al: Lidocaine before endotracheal intubation: intravenous or laryngotracheal? *Anesthesiology* 55:578, 1981.

Harrison DW, Walls RM: Blindness following minor head trauma in children: a report of two cases with a review of the literature, *J Emerg Med* 8:21, 1990.

Hennes H, Lee M, Smith D, et al: Clinical predictors of severe head trauma in children, *Am J Dis Child* 142:1045, 1988.

Jacobson MS, Rubenstein EM, Bohannon WE, et al: Follow-up of adolescent trauma victims: a new model of care, *Pediatrics* 77:236, 1986.

Kadish HA, Schunk JE: Pediatric basilar skull fracture: do children with normal neurologic findings and no intracranial injury require hospitalization? *Ann Emerg Med* 26:37, 1995.

Kraus JF, Fife D, Conroy C: Pediatric brain injuries: the nature, clinical course, and early outcomes in a defined U.S. population, *Pediatrics* 79:501, 1987.

Kraus JF, Rock A, Hemyari P: Brain injuries among infants, children, adolescents, and young adults, *Am J Dis Child* 144:684, 1990.

Lewis RJ, Yee L, Inkelis SH, et al: Clinical predictors of post-traumatic seizures in children with head trauma, *Ann Emerg Med* 22:1114, 1993.

Lieh-Lai MW, Theodorou AA, Sarnaik AP, et al: Limitations of the Glasgow Coma Scale in predicting outcome in children with traumatic brain injury, *J Pediatr* 120:195, 1992.

Mahoney WJ, D'Souza BJ, Haller JA, et al: Long-term outcome of children with severe head trauma and prolonged coma, *Pediatrics* 71:756, 1983.

Miller EC, Holmes JF, Derlet RN: Utilizing clinical factors to reduce head CT ordering for minor head trauma patients, *J Emerg Med* 15:453, 1997.

Ramvndo ML, McKnight T, Kempf J, et al: Clinical predictors of computed tomographic abnormalities following pediatric traumatic brain injury, *Pediatr Emerg Care* 11:1, 1995.

Rhee KJ, Muntz CB, Donald PJ, et al: Does nasotracheal intubation increase complication in patients with skull bone fracture? *Ann Emerg Med* 22:1145, 1993.

Rivara F, Tanaquichi D, Parish RA, et al: Poor prediction of positive computed tomographic scans by clinical content in symptomatic pediatric head trauma, *Pediatrics* 80:579, 1987.

Roddy SP, Cohn SM, Moller BA, et al: Minimal head trauma in children revisited: is routine hospitalization required? *Pediatrics* 101:575, 1998.

Ros SP, Ros MA: Should patients with normal cranial CT scans following minor head injury be hospitalized for observation? *Pediatr Emerg Care* 5:216, 1989.

Rosenthal BW, Bergman I: Intracranial injury after moderate head trauma in children, *J Pediatr* 115:346, 1989.

Schunk JE, Rodgerson JD, Woodward GA: The utility of head computed tomographic scanning in pediatric patients with normal neurologic examination in the emergency department, *Pediatr Emerg Care* 12:160, 1996.

Schutzman SA, Barnes PD, Mantello M, et al: Epidural hematomas in children, *Ann Emerg Med* 22:535, 1993.

Shahar E, Sagy M, Koren G, et al: Calcium block agents in pediatric emergency care, *Pediatr Emerg Care* 6:52, 1990.

Shane SA, Fuchs SM: Skull fracture in infants and predictors of associated intracranial injury, *Pediatr Emerg Care* 13:198, 1997.

Stein SC, Ross SE: The value of computer tomography scans in patients with low-risk head injuries, *Neurosurgery* 26:638, 1990.

Stein SC, O'Malley KF, Ross SE: Is routine computed tomography scanning too expensive for mild head injury, *Ann Emerg Med* 20:1286, 1991.

Stein SC, Ross SE: Mild head injury: a plea for routine early CT scanning, *J Trauma* 33:11, 1992.

Tannebaum RD, Sloan EP: Non-hemorrhagic pontine infarct in a child following mild head trauma, *Acad Emerg Med* 2:523, 1995.

Tecklenburg FW, Wright MS: Minor head trauma in the pediatric patient, *Pediatr Emerg Care* 7:40, 1991.

Tempkin NR, Dikmen SS, Wilensky AJ, et al: A randomized, double-blind study of phenytoin for the prevention of posttraumatic seizures, *N Engl J Med* 323:497, 1990.

Woodward GA: Posttraumatic cortical blindness: are we missing the diagnosis in children? *Pediatr Emerg Care* 6:289, 1990.

58 FACIAL TRAUMA

ALERT: Protection of the airway is essential after facial trauma and often requires active intervention. Cervical spine and other associated injuries must be excluded.

Facial trauma in children is most commonly associated with vehicular accidents, usually because of failure to use restraints, as well as falls and child abuse. Home accidents, athletic injuries, bites (animal and human), child abuse, playground accidents, and altercations are also sources of facial trauma.

As a result of the disproportionate size of the cranium with respect to the face, skull fractures are more common than facial fractures in children less than 12 years. The period of maximal enlargement of the face occurs during the sixth and seventh years. Facial proportions at that time are primarily influenced by the development of the midface and eruption of teeth. Therefore the development and treatment of the preadolescent must reflect the stage of facial development.

DIAGNOSTIC FINDINGS

Patients with facial trauma often have involvement of other organ systems, especially the head, chest, and abdomen. Facial trauma rarely represents a life threat, and therefore its evaluation and treatment should be deferred until the other, more serious injuries are evaluated and treated.

1. A complete appraisal of facial trauma includes careful evaluation of soft tissue,
bony structures, innervation, eyes, ears, and mouth. Specific attention to the eye is required as outlined in Chapter 59.
2. Inspection of the face must include assessment for deformity, asymmetry, dental malocclusion or displacement, cerebrospinal fluid (CSF) rhinorrhea, nasal septal hematoma, and examination of any obvious wounds.
3. Palpation of the face should include the infraorbital and supraorbital ridges, zygomas and zygomatic arches, nasal bones, maxilla (grasp the upper central incisors and attempt to move), and mandible. Examine for tenderness, bony defects, crepitus, and false motion.
4. Neuromuscular evaluation consists of evaluation of the facial nerves, trigeminal nerves, extraocular movements, visual acuity, and hearing. The facial nerves may be tested by having the patient wrinkle the forehead, smile, bare the teeth, and tightly close the eyes. All three branches of the trigeminal nerve (sensory) should be tested on each side of the face. Anesthesia in any area implies a disruption of that branch until proved otherwise. Extraocular movements are tested to uncover diplopia or entrapment, both signs of a blow-out fracture.

Complications

1. Disfigurement.
2. Loss of function.
3. Infection.
4. Airway obstruction.
5. Hemorrhage.
6. Ocular injuries occur in as many as 67% of facial fractures, especially those that are midfacial.

Ancillary Data

X-Ray Study

The selection of radiographic studies should be based on physical findings, the clinician's suspicions, and the patient's overall status. If there is any possibility of cervical spine trauma, cervical spine x-ray films must be ordered and evaluated to exclude abnormalities before any other radiographic investigations.

A Water's view is the single most helpful x-ray film for the evaluation of facial fractures. Specific views are outlined in Table 58-1 for common injuries. Findings may include fractures, air-fluid levels in the sphenoid sinus (implies basilar skull fracture), opacification or air-fluid levels in the maxillary sinus (implies blow-out fracture), and subcutaneous air (implies occult fracture until proved otherwise).

Computed axial tomography (CT scan) is useful in defining fractures in selected patients after stabilization. It is usually more sensitive than routine tomography.

MANAGEMENT

Management procedures for specific soft tissue and bony injuries follow. However, several general principles must be carefully considered, as partially outlined in Chapter 65.

1. Provide adequate airway and ventilation. Administer oxygen at 3-6 L/min while determining the necessity to intervene actively. Intubation may be required on either an emergency or a prophylactic basis. Cricothyrotomy is necessary with massive facial injury and airway obstruction.
2. Evaluate cervical spine (see Chapter 61).
3. Begin stabilization of the cardiovascular system. Control hemorrhage.
4. Administer tetanus prophylaxis as indicated.
5. Arrange for specific management of the fracture in consultation with otolaryngologists, oral surgeons, or plastic surgeons.
6. Initiate antibiotics in patients with open facial fractures. Penicillin and cephalosporins are often used unless there is central nervous system (CNS) involvement (orbital floor or maxillary or frontal sinuses), in which case nafcillin (or equivalent) and chloramphenicol or other alternative agents are used.
7. Stimulate prevention programs that encourage use of seat belts and motorcycle full-face helmets.

TABLE 58-1 Optimal Views for Specific Facial Injuries

Injury	Radiologic view
Nasal	Water's, lateral nose
Orbital	Caldwell, Water's, lateral and oblique facial CT scan
Zygomatic/maxillary	
Tripod	Water's, CT scan
Zygomatic arch	Towne, Water's, PA facial, CT scan
LeFort	CT scan
Mandible	Towne, Caldwell, panoramic, CT scan
Alveolar arch	Panoramic
Temporomandibular joint	Oblique and lateral (open and closed mouth), Towne
Teeth	Panoramic, bite wings

From Rahman WM, O'Connor TJ: Facial trauma. In Barkin RM, editor: *Pediatric emergency medicine: concepts and clinical practice,* ed 2, St Louis, 1997, Mosby.
CT, Computed tomography.

SPECIAL CONCERNS IN THE MANAGEMENT OF FACIAL SOFT TISSUE INJURIES

The general principles of management of soft tissue injuries are summarized in Chapter 65. Bony injuries usually require attention first, followed by management of soft tissue damage. All involved structures must be identified and bleeding controlled. The injury should be repaired within 24 hours. Anesthesia (local or regional), cleansing with copious irrigation, debridement, and removal of all imbedded particles are imperative.

Lip Lacerations

Lacerations of the lips require extra attention because a displacement of 1 to 2 mm in the vermilion border (the mucocutaneous junction) is quite noticeable. Little, if any, wound revision should be done in this area. If there is significant loss of tissue, the patient should be referred.

1. The vermilion border, if violated, should be marked on both sides of the laceration before injection of anesthetic because injection causes distortion of landmarks. This may be done with a needle scratch or a needle dipped in methylene blue. Unless the laceration is very superficial, a layered closure should be done to prevent tissue defects.

2. The first skin stitch placed to repair a facial laceration extending beyond the vermilion border should be at the vermilion border. The cutaneous component is then closed with nonabsorbable synthetic suture. The vermilion section is closed with 5-0 or 6-0 silk for patient comfort.

3. Lower lip anesthesia may be achieved by injecting 1 to 2 ml of 2% lidocaine with epinephrine in close proximity to the neurovascular bundle of the mental nerve intraorally at the point just posterior to the first premolar.

Lip Burn, Electrical

Burns to the lips from biting power cords deserve special consideration. They may initially appear localized but may become more extensive over the subsequent 3 to 5 days.

Lip burns should not be debrided. Hemorrhage may occur in the subsequent 5 to 10 days, and close observation is essential, often in the hospital. Bleeding is controlled by pressure, with the area kept clean. Special feeding devices and arm splints may be necessary. Delayed revision may be required after 6 to 12 months.

Mouth and Tongue

1. Through-and-through lacerations of the mouth require a careful, layered closure. The inner mucosa should first be closed with 4-0 or 5-0 absorbable suture to give a watertight seal. The wound is then irrigated from the exterior and closed in layers. Some recommend that these lacerations be covered with antibiotics because of the degree of contamination. Penicillin VK, 40,000 units (25 mg)/kg/24 hr q6hr PO for 10 days, is adequate for these wounds.

2. Lacerations in the area of the submandibular or parotid salivary ducts require the physician to demonstrate patency of these structures before closure. If there is any doubt, a consultant should be used.

3. Superficial lacerations of the tongue need not be closed. However, larger lacerations should be repaired in a layered fashion with the mucosal layer closed with a synthetic absorbable suture so it need not be removed later. Exposure of a tongue laceration may be improved by having an assistant grasp the tongue with a piece of gauze and apply gentle traction. Anesthesia is difficult for these lacerations, and sedation may be required (p. 507).

4. Local care for mouth wounds should

include rinsing the mouth three to four times a day with a mild antiseptic such as half-strength hydrogen peroxide.

Nose

Any nasal injury requires an examination for a septal hematoma, a large, purple, grapelike swelling over the septum, which should be drained through a vertical incision to avoid eventual septal necrosis. An anterior nasal pack should then be placed to prevent reaccumulation of blood. The patient should be treated with penicillin and referred to a consultant for follow-up observation.

Through-and-through lacerations of the nose require a careful layered closure and antibiotic treatment.

Ear

1. Adequate anesthesia of the ear may be achieved by raising a wheal with lidocaine (Xylocaine) 1% without epinephrine about the entire base of the ear. Injuries to the ear require approximation of the cartilaginous structures with fine absorbable suture. The lateral skin should be closed with fine nonabsorbable suture; the medial skin may be closed with absorbable suture to prevent bending the ear back for suture removal. Ear canal injuries require alternative anesthesia.
2. All significant injuries to the cartilage of the ear should be splinted with moist cotton balls medially and laterally and then dressed with a circumferential bandage about the head. These injuries, if at all contaminated, should be treated with antibiotics to prevent the complication of a smoldering chondritis.
3. Subperichondrial hematomas of the ear, usually caused by direct blunt trauma, often require aspiration and a compression dressing applied to avoid the development of a "cauliflower" ear. Careful

follow-up and possible reaspiration are indicated.

Eyelid (see Chapter 59)

1. Lacerations involving the lid margin should be referred to an ophthalmologist. If the injury prevents the cornea from being bathed by tears, artificial tears should be instilled on a regular basis until repair is achieved.
2. Lacerations not involving the lid margin should be carefully closed in layers, with the skin sutured with fine silk for comfort.
3. Wounds near the medial canthus may violate the lacrimal apparatus and require probing of the tear duct by an ophthalmologist to demonstrate its integrity.

Eyebrow

1. Debridement of lacerations to the eyebrow should be kept to an absolute minimum and should be done parallel to the hair follicles, not perpendicular to the skin, to minimize the scar.
2. The eyebrow should not be shaved, because the margins are important landmarks to observe in the closure.

Scalp

It is imperative to explore all scalp lacerations with the finger to exclude fractures and debris. There may be a great deal of blood loss. Lacerations may involve the skin, subcutaneous tissue, galea, subgalea, and periosteum or pericranium. Anesthetic agents should be administered above the galea where most of the nerves and vessels rest. When involved, the galea is closed separately.

Neck

Penetrating injuries of the neck involving the platysma or deeper structures or extensive blunt soft tissue damage require surgical consultation and in-hospital observation for a minimum of 24 to 48 hours.

Missile injuries to the neck produce major injury. High-velocity bullets cause significant pathology in 90% of victims, whereas buckshots or birdshots inflicted at a distance less than 5 meters, as well as high-velocity shrapnel, routinely cause major damage.

Three zones of the anterior neck are commonly identified:

I. Below the level of the top of the sternal notch
II. Between the angle of the mandible and the sternal notch
III. The region cephalad to the angle of the mandible

Airway stabilization and ventilation must be considered along with fluid resuscitation and direct pressure (not clamping) for control of hemorrhage. Anterior neck injuries from striking the steering wheel or a wire or board cause laryngotracheal damage making airway management difficult. Chest x-ray films, arteriography, endoscopy, and water-soluble contrast studies may assist in defining the extent of the injury. In the stable patient, cervical spine films and soft tissue films of the neck may be useful. Angiography often is indicated in asymptomatic level I injuries to identify damage to thoracic outlet vessels, whereas it may be done in level III wounds to exclude a high internal carotid injury at the base of the skull.

The necessity for mandatory versus selective surgical exploration is controversial. Findings requiring surgery include shock; active bleeding; moderate, large, or expanding hematomas; pulse deficits; bruits; neurologic deficits; dyspnea; hoarseness; stridor; dysphonia; hemoptysis; difficulty or pain on swallowing; subcutaneous crepitations or air; or hematemesis. If these do not exist, the edges of the wound can be spread apart gently to prevent dislodging a clot. If the platysma has been penetrated, the patient should be admitted for observation. The need for surgical exploration and repair must reflect individual experience and preference and the

ability of the facility to provide close monitoring for the patient.

FACIAL FRACTURES AND DISLOCATIONS

Facial fractures are rare in the pediatric age group because of the elasticity of the child's facial bones and the protection offered by the relatively large skull in children. Any facial fractures in children should increase the physician's suspicion of child abuse (see Chapter 25).

Facial fractures are often associated with other, more severe injuries that require emergent attention of a higher priority (e.g., closed head and cervical spine injuries) (see Chapter 56). As many as 55% of facial fractures have associated closed head injuries.

The emphasis here is on diagnosis. Manual palpation of the facial skeleton is particularly helpful, especially of the orbital rim, zygomatic arch, nasal bridge, and inferior border of the mandible. Ocular injuries are often associated with facial fractures, and it is imperative to exclude injuries to the eye, as well as associated injuries to the head, cervical spine, and so on.

Facial fractures cannot be definitively treated in the emergency department (ED) but require referral to a consultant. However, if the fracture is not initially diagnosed, the child may suffer permanent impaired function, disability, and disfigurement. Delay in treatment may be required because of the patient's general condition and associated injuries. The outcome still can be excellent without extensive complications. Appropriate antibiotic therapy should be considered. Uncomplicated mandibular and maxillary fractures can be managed by routine methods with good outcome even after a delay of weeks. Cosmetic complications, however, are more likely to occur with prolonged delay in treatment of zygoma fractures.

Nasal Fractures

Nasal fractures may be difficult to diagnose in children because of the relative immaturity of the nasal pyramid, which makes an adequate physical examination difficult. X-ray films may be of help in making the diagnosis, especially if there is a displaced fracture. Intranasal inspection should be done, searching for a septal hematoma or a fracture dislocation of the septal cartilage. A septal hematoma should be treated as outlined on p. 429 to avoid a "saddle nose" deformity.

1. Any continuing epistaxis should be controlled by an anterior nasal pack.
2. Because of the growth potential of a child's nose, any fracture should be reduced accurately to avoid future disfigurement. Therefore any child with significant posttraumatic epistaxis, tenderness, and swelling is assumed to have a nasal fracture until proved otherwise.
3. Any child with a documented or suspected nasal fracture should be referred to a consultant for reevaluation in 4 to 6 days (after the swelling has subsided).
4. Trauma to the bridge of the nose may result in an ethmoidal fracture with possible violation of the cribriform plate followed by CSF rhinorrhea. This may be disguised by epistaxis. Patients with ethmoidal fractures with suspected CSF rhinorrhea should be admitted for observation and placed in a head-up position. If a CSF leak is proved, prophylactic antibiotics may be used according to the recommendation of the neurosurgical consultant.

Mandibular Fractures

The pediatric mandible is more susceptible to fracture than the adult mandible because of its inherent weakness from multiple tooth buds. The subcondylar area is the most common site of fracture, especially in children less than 10 years old.

1. Patients with mandibular fractures have mandibular pain and tenderness, often exacerbated by movement of the mandible. Malocclusion, a step-off in dentition, or a sublingual hematoma may be present and is highly suggestive of a mandibular fracture. Ecchymosis on the floor of the mouth is pathognomonic. Laceration of the chin associated with hyperextension also may be noted. Crepitus felt by the fingers placed in the auditory meatus during mandibular movement may indicate a condylar fracture.
2. Because the mandible is a ring structure, multiple fractures are very common, with the fracture sites possibly distant from the point of trauma. Mandibular fractures involving the teeth are considered open fractures.
3. Mandibular x-ray films, especially a panoramic view, will assist in the diagnosis.
4. Almost all of these patients require admission for fixation by a consultant. Usually, closed immobilization for 3 to 4 weeks is adequate.

Zygomatic Fractures

In children the frontozygomatic suture is weak and may be a common site of fracture. Severe trauma may result in a tripod or trimalar fracture with fracture lines at the frontozygomatic suture and the temporozygomatic suture and through the infraorbital foramen. Patients with this complex fracture often have flatness of the cheek, anesthesia over the infraorbital nerve (cheek and ala of nose and upper lip), a palpable step defect, or change in consensual gaze.

A zygomatic arch fracture may be sustained by lateral force over the area of the arch. These patients may have a palpable defect over the arch or difficulty with mandibular movement caused by impingement of the defect on movement of the coronoid process of the mandible. X-ray studies, specifically the Water's (occipitomental) and the submental-vertex views, are helpful in diagnosing these fractures.

These patients usually do not require immediate hospitalization, but the case should be discussed with a consultant because open reduction and fixation are frequently required.

Orbital Floor Fractures (Blow-Out Fractures) (see Chapter 59)

Isolated fractures of the orbital floor are most often caused by the direct application of pressure to the globe of the eye with subsequent fracture at the weakest area of the orbit, the floor. This often results in herniation of orbital contents and flow of blood into the maxillary sinus.

These patients have impaired ocular motility with diplopia, secondary to entrapment of the inferior rectus muscle, infraorbital hypesthesia, and enophthalmos. The impaired motility may be difficult to see in a child and may require a forced-traction examination under anesthesia by a consultant. Periorbital crepitus is highly suggestive of a fracture.

- The Water's view and tomograms are most helpful in radiographically diagnosing this injury. Presence of orbital contents or opacification of the maxillary sinus is presumptive evidence of an orbital-floor fracture until proved otherwise. An exaggerated Water's view may be helpful. The patient's head is angled so that the orbitomeatal line forms a 37-degree angle with the plane of the cassette. The beam is angled at 10 degrees, 20 degrees, and 30 degrees caudad.

These patients do not usually require admission but should be referred to a consultant for follow-up observation in 3 to 5 days. Definitive therapy remains controversial. Many delay the decision on selective repair for 10 to 14 days.

Maxillary Fractures

Maxillary fractures are most often the result of massive facial trauma, such as that caused by a deceleration injury. These patients have midface mobility, as demonstrated by movement of the hard palate and upper incisors during examination. They also have massive facial soft tissue injury and malocclusion. In addition, CSF rhinorrhea may be present.

An idealized classification scheme of maxillary fractures follows (however, fractures rarely appear in pure form).

LeFort I: fracture at the level of the nasal fossa

LeFort II: pyramidal disjunction involving fractures of the maxilla, nasal bones, and medial aspects of the orbits

LeFort III: craniofacial disjunction involving fractures to the maxilla, zygomas, nasal bones, ethmoids, and vomer

Because of the configuration of the child's head, LeFort II and III fractures are rare in children, and when present, they are usually accompanied by other head trauma inconsistent with survival. LeFort I fractures may often be seen in conjunction with dentoalveolar injuries. Radiographically, these fractures are diagnosed by the lateral facial bones and Water's views.

Immediate care of these injuries requires aggressive airway maintenance and intensive care monitoring. Patients with these injuries must also be suspected of having cervical spine injuries, especially those with an altered sensorium. In these cases, a CT scan is indicated, and a consultant should be immediately used (e.g., a neurosurgeon if the patient is comatose).

Temporomandibular Joint Dislocations

Dislocation of the temporomandibular joint may be the result of trauma or be caused merely by the patient opening his or her mouth widely. In these cases, the mandible dislocates forward and superiorly. The dislocation may be unilateral or bilateral.

These patients have moderate discomfort and inability to close the mouth. X-ray films are indicated before reduction to rule out fracture if the dislocation is posttraumatic.

1. Reduction is performed by placing the thumbs (wrapped in gauze for protection) on the third molars of the mandible with the fingers curled under the mandibular symphysis. The condyles are levered downward and posteriorly by applying downward pressure on the molars and slight upward pressure on the symphysis.

In cases of severe spasm, IV diazepam may facilitate reduction.

2. Postreduction x-ray studies are indicated for the first occurrence of this dislocation if it is not trauma related.

Admission for occlusal fixation is indicated if severe pain, tenderness, or spasm is present after reduction. Otherwise the patient may be discharged and placed on a soft diet with instructions to avoid yawning or otherwise stressing the temporomandibular joints for several days.

REFERENCES

Rahman WH, O'Connor TJ: Facial trauma. In Barkin RM, editor: *Pediatric emergency medicine: concepts and clinical practice,* ed 2, St Louis, 1997, Mosby.

Carducci B, Springs C, Lower RA, et al: Penetrating neck trauma: consensus and controversies, *Ann Emerg Med* 15:208, 1986.

Cooper A, Barton B, Nienirska M, et al: Fifteen year's experience with penetrating trauma to the head and neck in children, *J Pediatr Surg* 22:24, 1987.

Crockett DM, Mungo RP, Thompson RE: Maxillofacial trauma, *Pediatr Clin North Am* 20:1471, 1989.

East CA, O'Donaghue GO: Acute nasal trauma in children, *J Pediatr Surg* 22:308, 1987.

Holt GR, Holt JE: Incidence of eye injuries in facial fractures: an analysis of 727 cases, *Otolaryngol Head Neck Surg* 91:276, 1983.

Keene J, Doris PE: A simple radiographic diagnosis of occult blow-out fracture, *Ann Emerg Med* 14:335, 1985.

Maniglia AJ, Kline SN: Maxillofacial trauma in the pediatric age group, *Otolaryngol Clin North Am* 16:717, 1983.

Narrod JA, Moore EE: Initial management of penetrating neck wounds: a selective approach, *J Emerg Med* 2:17, 1984.

Ordog GJ: Penetrating neck trauma, *J Trauma* 27:543, 1987.

Press BHJ, Boies LR, Shons AR: Facial fractures in trauma victims: the influence of treatment delay on ultimate outcome, *Ann Plast Surg* 11:121, 1983.

Ramba J: Fractures of the facial bones in children, *Int J Oral Surg* 14:472, 1985.

Rao PM, Bhatti FK, Gaudino J: Penetrating injuries of the neck: criteria for exploration, *J Trauma* 23:47, 1983.

Sinclair D, Schwartz M, Gruss J, et al: A retrospective review of the relationship between facial fractures, head injuries and cervical spine injuries, *J Emerg Med* 6:109, 1988.

Walton RL, Hagan KF, Parry SH, et al. Maxillofacial trauma, *Surg Clin North Am* 62:73, 1982.

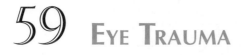

59 EYE TRAUMA

JAMES B. SPRAGUE

ALERT: Visual acuity must be screened. If it is found to be abnormal, referral to
          an ophthalmologist is essential. Associated injuries, especially facial
          fractures, must be excluded.

Eye injuries in children commonly result from sports injuries or projectiles. Baseball is the leading cause of sports-related injuries, followed by basketball. There are often associated facial fractures. Injuries to the eye may be divided as follows:

- Intraocular (82%)
    Perforating: cornea, sclera, lens, retina, intraocular foreign body
    Nonperforating: hyphema, traumatic cataract, vitreous hemorrhage, retinal detachment
- Extraocular (15%): lid laceration, canalicular laceration, foreign body of the lid
- Intraorbital (2%): hemorrhage, foreign body
- Orbital wall fracture (1%)

The traumatized eye requires prompt attention because of potential damage and the high level of anxiety for the patient. Both can be reduced by a systematic approach emphasizing visual acuity and external examination. Visual acuity determination is often neglected or is done in a cursory fashion. It is helpful to remember that an injured eye with good acuity, regardless of its appearance, is unlikely to have sustained an injury requiring immediate referral or surgery.

The following equipment facilitates examination and treatment of the eye:

1. Visual acuity chart
2. Bright pen light
3. Ophthalmoscope
4. Irrigation setup, including irrigating ocular lens, saline solution, and intravenous (IV) tubing
5. Fluorescein strips (and Wood or cobalt blue light)
6. Topical anesthetics
7. Topical antibiotics
8. Lid retractor
9. Foreign body spud
10. Patch (gauze and fox metal)
11. Paper/plastic tape
12. Contact lens removal suction cup
13. Slit lamp

GENERAL EXAMINATION
Visual Acuity

Visual acuity should be assessed first. The only exception is an acute chemical injury to the eye, which requires immediate irrigation.

1. For children less than 3 years of age, use HOTV letter charts, a picture-card test

that is easy to administer. Older preschool children can usually do the "E" test. By 7 years, most children can use the Snellen chart.

2. Each eye should be checked individually, with the patient wearing eyeglasses, if previously prescribed.

3. Many preschool children do not have $20/20$ acuity, despite normal examination findings. Some may have delayed myelination of the optic nerve. Useful age-specific acuity levels for screening are as follows:

3 yr	20/50
4 yr	20/40
5 yr	20/30

The numerator is the distance in feet at which the patient reads the chart, and the denominator is the distance at which a normal adult reads the same line.

A difference of more than two lines between the eyes is probably more significant than the absolute acuity and suggests unequal refractive error, amblyopia, or trauma. A pinhole testing device may compensate for visual acuity impairment caused by a refractive error.

In patients who are unable to cooperate in reading the eye chart, the following assessments may be helpful: light perception by watching response to light source (blinking, aversion, discomfort, identifying of two lights) or ability to recognize movement of an object, count fingers, distinguish faces, or recognize objects or pictures. These subjective responses should be recorded.

External Examination

1. Orbital bones. Palpate the orbital rim for a step-off or marked local tenderness. Press on the zygomatic arch; if it is not tender, it is usually intact.

2. Infraorbital nerve. Compare sensation on both cheeks. Hypesthesia points to a fracture of the orbital floor, which the nerve traverses.

3. Lids. Retract lids with a lid retractor. If

unavailable, use two paper clips shaped like a U. Instill topical anesthetic drops to anesthetize the cornea.

4. Position of the globe: exophthalmos or enophthalmos.

5. Cornea: clarity and absence of fluorescein staining.

6. Anterior chamber: clarity and depth.

7. Pupil: size, reactivity, symmetry, regularity.

8. Ocular motility. Test in all nine positions (primary, up, down, down to both sides, and up to both sides) for limitation or diplopia.

Funduscopic Examination

This examination is performed to evaluate for optic nerve pallor, papilledema, retinal or vitreous hemorrhage, and macular abnormalities.

Fluorescein Stains

Fluorescein stain shows corneal epithelial defects and should be used if there is a question of abrasion. A fluorescein strip is moistened (sterile saline or water) and applied to the conjunctiva. A staining area appears green with white light. A cobalt blue flashlight or Wood light will cause the dye to fluoresce, which facilitates the examination.

X-Ray Studies

1. Water's view to evaluate the orbital rim and maxillary sinus

2. CT scan for localization of a foreign body and for facial fractures

3. Tomography of the orbital floor to define an orbital floor blow-out fracture, if surgery is contemplated

TOPICAL MEDICATIONS

1. Mydriatics/cycloplegics.
   a. Tropicamide (Mydriacyl): onset, 15 to

20 minutes; duration, 2 to 6 hours (useful for ocular examination)

  b. Homatropine 2% to 5%: onset, 30 minutes; duration, 24 to 48 hours (useful for more prolonged action, as with corneal abrasion)

2. Anesthetic: proparacaine 0.5% (Alcaine, Ophthaine, Ophthetic); 1 to 2 drops provides immediate corneal anesthesia. Not for home use.

3. Topical steroids: indicated for some allergic conditions, iritis, and phlyctenular disease. Should be prescribed in consultation with an ophthalmologist if available. Complications include exacerbation of herpes, glaucoma, and impaired healing.

4. Topical antibiotics for bacterial conjunctivitis are normally given four times per day for 3 days (a patient who does not respond should be seen again):

  a. Sulfa (sulfisoxazole 4% [Gantrisin], sulfacetamide 10% [Sulamyd]): may cause burning

  b. Polymyxin B-bacitracin (Polysporin): if patient is allergic to sulfa

  c. Polymyxin B-bacitracin-neomycin (Neosporin): may cause local sensitization with prolonged use

  d. Erythromycin: minimal corneal activity

EYE PATCHES

Eye patches keep the lid closed over a corneal surface defect and promote healing. Use two patches/pads to fill the depth of the orbital recess. Secure with a single piece of paper tape. Place strips of tape from the hairline to the angle of the jaw. Patching is indicated in treatment of corneal epithelial defects of any cause. Do not patch eye infections.

Although the pressure eye patch has traditionally been used in management of traumatic corneal defects, a number of studies have not substantiated a difference between a patched and nonpatched group.

Because corneal abrasions can become infected, a patched eye should be examined every 24 hours; patching should be continued until fluorescein staining is gone. Usually the patch should be left in place for that time without supplemental medication; removing the patch to instill topical medication usually results in inadequate patching. In addition, children can lose central nervous system (CNS) fusional mechanisms rapidly. After only 1 to 2 days, esotropia may develop. Therefore long-term, unsupervised patching of children is ill advised.

Cycloplegics may be useful in reducing photophobia and surface pain caused by secondary iritis and ciliary spasm. Medium-acting cycloplegics prevent pupillary movement and put the ciliary body to rest. Cyclogen, 2%, homatropine, 2% to 5%, and scopolamine, 0.25%, usually last 24 hours or longer. Atropine, 1%, lasts 7 to 10 days and should be avoided.

Antibiotic ointment such as erythromycin is usually recommended.

TYPES OF INJURIES
Corneal Abrasion, Foreign Body, Radiation/Solar Keratitis, Chemical Burn (Table 59-1)

Most ocular injuries damage the corneal epithelium with resulting pain and photophobia. Frequently, the pain is so intense that examination is difficult or impossible without topical anesthetics.

Chemical Injuries

Chemical injuries are a true ophthalmologic emergency and must be triaged for immediate care. Alkali burns are usually much worse than acid injuries; it is important to find out the pH of the chemical agent. The eye should be lavaged as soon as possible, preferably at the site of injury. If the pH of the tears is abnormal, lavage should be continued in the emergency department (ED) with normal saline solution. Extensive lavage is easier with an irrigating contact lens (Mediflow lens). Lavage should be continued until tear pH is normal. The cul-de-sacs must be swept to ensure that foreign material is not left in contact with the globe. Referral is

TABLE 59-1   Corneal Abrasion, Burn, and Foreign Body

	Corneal abrasion	Foreign body	Radiation burn	Chemical burn
Cause	Direct trauma, contact lens, foreign body		Sun lamp, snow reflection	Alkali much worse than acid
Diagnostic findings	Pain, photophobia, lacrimation, fluorescein positive; small, vertical linear abrasion suggests foreign body beneath upper lid	Pain, photophobia, lacrimation, fluorescein finding positive; may see foreign body*	Pain, photophobia, lacrimation, fluorescein positive Punctate keratitis or diffuse abrasion; stain may be difficult to see without magnification	Pain, photophobia, lacrimation Cornea: hazy to opacified Conjunctiva/sclera: no ischemic change to blanched
Visual acuity	WNL	Usually WNL	Decreased	Markedly decreased
Complications	Infection	Penetration, infection	Infection	Corneal opacification, necrosis
Treatment	Remove contact lens, if present Visual acuity check Topical anesthetic† Topical antibiotic Cycloplegic (homatropine 5%) if >40% involved Eye patch‡ Systemic analgesia Recheck in 24 hrs§ Avoid contact lens for 4-5 days	Visual acuity check Topical anesthetic† Remove with spud or 25-gauge needle if superficial; otherwise refer Topical art biotics Topical cycloplegic Eye patch Recheck in 24 hr	Visual acuity check Topical anesthetic,† eye patch, analgesia Recheck in 24-48 hr	Irrigate with 1-2 L saline solution per eye *immediately* Evert eyelids Clear fornices Refer to ophthalmologist

WNL, Within normal limits.

*If there is any question of intraocular foreign body, particularly after hammering metal on metal, orbital x-ray studies and direct ophthalmoscopy should be performed. Penetrating injuries require immediate repair by an ophthalmologist.

†Topical anesthetics facilitate examination. They should not be dispensed for prn use.

‡Although traditionally recommended, efficacy may be controversial.

§On reevaluation in 24 hr, check to make certain that staining and edema have decreased. If not, refer.

usually indicated unless the history suggests only minimal exposure, the vision is completely normal, and there is no corneal staining or corneal clouding.

Foreign Bodies

Corneal foreign bodies typically are painful but may be asymptomatic for a prolonged time. Long-standing ferrous foreign bodies usually rust, leaving a "rust ring" when removed. The rust is usually easier to remove in 24 to 48 hours. Many children are difficult enough to examine at the slit lamp, let alone to approach with a needle or foreign body spud. These children are best managed with immobilization (often with a papoose board), topical anesthetic, and lid speculum. When restrained, many children watch the physician and the foreign body can be quickly removed. While the child is still restrained, topical antibiotic can be instilled and the eye patched. It is important to remember that the topical anesthetic will wear off in 15 to 30 minutes and that systemic analgesics and ice packs will help.

Perforation/Rupture

Ocular perforation usually causes decreased vision and intraocular hemorrhage. If the anterior chamber has been entered, it is often flat or shallow compared with the normal side. The pupil is often irregular. To minimize further injury, the patient should be moved with the eye shielded to prevent pressure on the globe and with instructions to avoid any Valsalva maneuvers, which increase intraocular pressure. If x-ray films are obtained to look for a retained foreign body, the patient should be assisted in sitting up on the stretcher or on the x-ray study table.

Rupture must be recognized because pressure on the eyeball can cause extrusion of intraocular contents. Such injuries have intraocular blood that appears as a brown/blue spot or line on the white of the eye, which may plug the wound and preserve the appearance of the eye. A teardrop pupil may be noted. Such patients require immediate ophthalmologic evaluation but should be shielded and kept in bed with the head elevated 40 degrees until treatment is initiated.

Hyphema

Hyphema is blood in the anterior chamber compared with the subconjunctival space and represents a severe ocular injury. Although it may complicate a penetrating injury, it usually follows blunt trauma with an object small enough to fit within the ocular rim such as a knuckle, bottle, small ball, or pool cue.

Diagnostic Findings

Vision is immediately impaired but may have returned to normal by the time the patient enters the ED. After recording the visual acuity, the examiner should look at the iris for blood or a meniscus. Unclotted blood in suspension in the aqueous humor may be suspected if the iris color or the detail of the iris stroma is not the same as that of the uninjured eye. If a patient has been supine, the blood may not layer out until x-ray studies in the seated position are made, leading to a distinct meniscus. However, the most common cause of overlooking the diagnosis is failure to look carefully, particularly in patients with a brown iris.

Complications

Complications include the following:

1. Associated injuries, such as corneal abrasion, orbital rim or floor fracture, vitreous hemorrhage, or retinal edema, may be present.
2. Increased intraocular pressure may be present initially and requires careful monitoring. This examination should not be done with the Schiotz tonometer; the applanation unit should be used. Patients with sickle cell disease may have dramatic glaucomatous changes with a mild pressure increase.
3. Secondary hemorrhage occurs in as many

as 30% of patients with a hyphema and is associated with glaucoma, corneal blood staining, and optic atrophy. It typically occurs 3 to 5 days after injury.

Management

Care of the patient with hyphema is directed to reducing the incidence of secondary hemorrhage. There are many treatment regimens, depending on the patient's general health, age, family availability, and physician preference.

1. Bed rest with no Valsalva maneuver. This can be done at home if social circumstances allow it. No reading is allowed, although television is permitted. The head of the bed is elevated. Sedation is given as needed.
2. Metal shield for involved eye. Patch under the shield for comfort or treatment of an associated corneal abrasion. Bilateral patching is not required.
3. Pupillary dilation may be necessary to see the fundus. If so, the pupil can be kept dilated with 0.25% scopolamine, 5% homatropine, or 1% atropine. Allowing the pupil to constrict and then dilating it may cause secondary hemorrhage.
4. Oral prednisone, 1 mg/kg/24 hr, may decrease the incidence of secondary hemorrhage.
5. Aminocaproic acid used prophylactically may reduce secondary hemorrhage. The initial dosage of 200 mg/kg/dose (maximum: 6 gm) PO is followed by 50-100 mg/kg/dose q6hr PO for 3 to 7 days.
6. Intraocular pressure must be carefully monitored in sickle cell disease.
7. The anterior chamber angle should be examined by gonioscopy 4 to 6 weeks after injury. If there is an angle recession, annual examinations for late-onset glaucoma are indicated. Dilated fundal examination with scleral depression ideally should be done when possible to rule out traumatic retinal tear or detachment; these conditions are rare in children.

Blow-Out Fracture

Blunt trauma may fracture the orbital floor as a result of being hit with something small enough to enter between the orbital rims. The eyeball absorbs the force of the blow and is compressed backward into the orbit. The marked increase in intraorbital pressure results in a blow-out fracture of the orbital floor, which is thin.

Diagnostic Findings

1. Pain is related to the injury, periorbital swelling and ecchymosis, subcutaneous emphysema, and ipsilateral epistaxis.
2. Associated injuries include corneal abrasions, traumatic cataracts, hyphema, vitreous hemorrhage, and retinal damage in 15% to 40% of patients.

Complications

Several problems may be noted:

1. Hypesthesia in the distribution of the intraorbital nerve, which is best tested by evaluating sensation of the upper lip and cheek. Regeneration usually occurs.
2. Limitation of upward gaze with vertical diplopia, caused by entrapment of the inferior rectus muscle and orbital fat in the orbital floor break.
3. Enophthalmos of the injured eye, which becomes obvious as the swelling resolves.

Ancillary Data

Helpful imaging studies include the following:

1. X-ray film: Water's view shows antral clouding.
2. Tomograms may be needed.

Differential Diagnosis

1. Restriction of vertical motion may result from mechanical entrapment of the inferior rectus muscle or damage to the nerve of that muscle. This distinction can be made by a forced traction test.
2. Posttraumatic diplopia occurring with entrapment must be considered in the differential of a number of entities:
   a. Orbital fracture
   b. Extraocular muscle avulsion, contusion, transection, or hematoma

c. Palsy of the third, fourth, or sixth cranial nerves

Management

1. A careful examination to exclude intraocular damage and other entities in the differential diagnosis must be conducted.
2. An ophthalmologist should be involved in the acute and long-term care of the patient.
3. If the vision is normal and there are no associated facial or other major injuries, the patient can usually be followed as an outpatient. Analgesics, ice packs, elevation, and bed rest are indicated.
4. If the motility defect persists or there is frank enophthalmos initially, surgical exploration is usually necessary. The timing of surgery is controversial. Some of the restrictions in eye movement may result from hemorrhage and edema in the orbital fat, which typically resolve and may not require surgery. However, some consider it important to explore the orbital floor early and remove any orbital material in the defect.

Subconjunctival Hemorrhage

The subconjunctival space is defined by the conjunctiva anteriorly, the sclera posteriorly, the cul-de-sac above and below, and the limbus centrally. The conjunctiva lines the inside of the eyelid and then is reflected in the cul-de-sac before it spreads over the globe and inserts at the corneal-scleral limbus. This space is therefore extraocular. Subconjunctival hemorrhage is associated with trauma, coughing, Valsalva maneuver, or a coagulation disorder.

Diagnostic Findings

1. The symptoms are usually those associated with the initial trauma.
2. Vision is normal if there is no damage to the intraocular contents. The hemorrhage spreads out as a thin sheet and appears bright red and homogeneous. It comes up to the limbus. Usually conjunctival vessels are not involved in areas where hemorrhage is not present.
3. The condition resolves in 1 to 2 weeks without sequelae.
4. Cases of trauma to the eye followed by a 360-degree subconjunctival hemorrhage should be referred, especially if associated with anterior chamber or vitreous hemorrhage because of the potential of posterior rupture of the globe.

Management

If there is conjunctival prolapse, sterile ointment prevents keratinization.

Lid and Lacrimal Laceration

Lid lacerations may be associated with ocular injuries and lead to other complications if improperly treated. The eyelids provide protection and lubrication of the eye.

1. Full-thickness lacerations of the lid may be associated with perforating injuries of the globe.
2. Improper repair of the eyelid may result in poor lacrimal function, with secondary irritation and lacrimation.
3. Laceration of the medial aspect of the lid may involve the lacrimal system, which, if not treated, may lead to poor lacrimal drainage and epiphora.

Management

1. Examine the eye. Be certain there is no penetration of the globe. If there is any suspicion, avoid direct pressure or excessive manipulation. Immediate ophthalmologic consultation is indicated. If there is any doubt, treat as a penetration. In general, start systemic antibiotics, keep the patient in a fasting state (NPO), and apply a loose patch and metal shield until the patient can be seen. With question of a foreign body penetration, obtain a computed tomography (CT) scan or soft tissue globe film.

2. Irrigate all wounds carefully. Minimize debridement.

3. Careful apposition of the lid margins is essential in vertical lacerations, usually requiring general anesthesia in children and involvement of an ophthalmologist.

   a. Lid avulsion requires reattachment of the eyelid to the canthal tendons.

   b. Interruption of the lacrimal system necessitates intubation of the lacrimal system and suturing of the canaliculus. The medial portion of the lid includes the lacrimal drainage canaliculi, whereas the lacrimal duct runs along the outer third of the upper lid.

4. Horizontal lacerations may disrupt the levator palpebra, causing ptosis. Careful apposition is essential. A through-and-through laceration requires a three-layered closure (conjunctiva, levator aponeurosis, and skin). Consult an ophthalmologist.

Ecchymosis of the Eyelid ("Black Eye")

Ecchymosis requires examination to exclude more significant abnormalities such as an orbital fracture or hyphema. It is treated with cold compresses, analgesics, and head elevation.

Other Blunt Ocular Injuries

Several other findings may be noted. Traumatic iritis may present with photophobia, blurred vision, or headache. Traumatic cataracts, subluxation and dislocation of the lens, and retinal tears/detachment/hemorrhage are reported after trauma and require referral.

REFERENCES

Agapitos PJ, Noel LP, Clarke WN: Traumatic hyphema in children, *Ophthalmology* 94:1238, 1987.

Brinkley JR: Emergency management of ocular trauma, *Top Emerg Med* 6:35, 1984.

Campanile TM, St. Clair DA, Benaim M: The evaluation of eye patching in the treatment of traumatic corneal epithelial defects, *J Emerg Med* 15:769, 1997.

Dejaun E, Sternberg P, Michels RG: Penetrating ocular injuries: types of injuries and visual results, *Ophthalmology* 90:1318, 1983.

DeRespinis PA, Caputo AR, Fiore PM, et al: A survey of severe eye injuries in children, *Am J Dis Child* 143:711, 1989.

Farber MD, Fiscella R, Goldberg MF: Aminocaproic acid versus prednisone for the treatment of traumatic hyphema, *Ophthalmology* 98:279, 1991.

Grin TR, Nelson LB, Jeffers JB: Eye injuries in childhood, *Pediatrics* 80:13, 1987.

Juang PSC, Rosen P: Ocular examination techniques for the emergency department, *J Emerg Med* 15:793, 1997.

Klein BR, Sears MZ: Pediatric ocular injuries, *Pediatr Rev* 13:422, 1992.

Kraft SP, Christianson MD, Crawford JS, et al: Traumatic hyphema in children, *Ophthalmology* 94:1233, 1987.

Nelson LB, Wilson TW, Jeffers JB: Eye injuries in childhood: demography, etiology and prevention, *Pediatrics* 84: 438, 1989.

Shingleton BJ: Eye injuries, *N Engl J Med* 325:408, 1991.

Sternberg PJ, Dejaun E, Michels RG: Penetrating ocular injuries in young patients: initial injuries and visual results, *Retina* 4:5, 1984.

Turturro MA, Paris PA, Arffa R, et al: Contact lens complications, *Am J Emerg Med* 8:228, 1990.

60 DENTAL INJURIES

GARY K. BELANGER

ALERT: After management of associated injuries, traumatic dental problems usually require referral.

The examination of the oral cavity requires a systematic approach to the soft tissues and teeth. The mechanism and time of traumatic injuries must be determined, as well as the onset and nature of other complaints and complicating medical problems (e.g., cardiac disease, which may require antibiotic prophylaxis, or bleeding diatheses). The status of tetanus immunizations should be assessed.

BASIC CONSIDERATIONS

Soft Tissues

1. Lips: pink, moist, continuous vermilion border, possible glandular inclusions (Fordyce granules)
   - Abnormal: tenderness, ulcers, swelling, lacerations, hemorrhage, hematoma, burn
2. Mucosa: pink, moist, possible glandular inclusions, major salivary duct openings, possible areas of hyperkeratosis associated with chewing
   - Abnormal: same as for lips; possible torn frenulum
3. Tongue: pink, papillated dorsum (possibly coated), smooth ventral surface, normal range of motion and strength
   - Abnormal: same as for lips; weakness, loss of function
4. Palate: *hard palate*—pink, firm, rugae normal in anterior half; *soft palate*—pink, mobile, functional
   - Abnormal: same as for lips; for soft palate, abnormal function or loss of function
5. Floor of the mouth: pink with areas of high vascularization (varices) appearing blue-gray; moist, major salivary duct openings, tissue tags
   - Abnormal: same as for lips; excessive firmness or elevation may indicate cellulitis or mucus-retention phenomenon

Teeth

See Fig. 60-1.
1. Color: white (permanent can appear slightly more yellow than primary)
   - Abnormal: caries, pulp degeneration; environmental and genetic defects can cause range-of-color changes
2. Integrity: complete crown without interruptions of surface structure
   - Abnormal: caries, fractures, hypoplasias, anomalous crown forms
3. Mobility: lateral and anteroposterior (AP) movement slight to imperceptible; vertical movement nonexistent; exfoliating primary teeth may normally be very mobile
   - Abnormal: displacement by light finger pressure
4. Position: upper teeth overlap lower teeth;

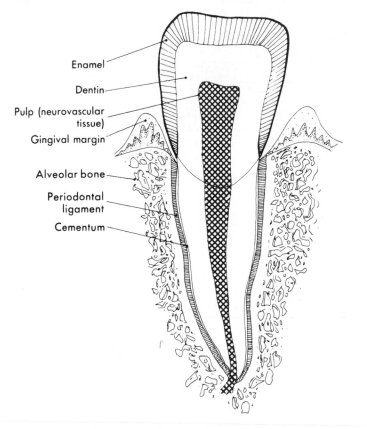

Enamel

Dentin

Pulp (neurovascular tissue)

Gingival margin

Alveolar bone

Periodontal ligament

Cementum

Fig. 60-1   Basic dental anatomy.

mirror imaging of teeth left to right; teeth in each arch arranged in arch form
- Abnormal: asymmetry and obvious displacements

5. Pain and sensitivity: ascertained by questioning patients about abnormal pain on percussion or sensitivity to air, cold, heat, or chewing in both involved and uninvolved areas
6. Development status (Fig. 60-2)
- Abnormal: more than 1 year deviation from chart

Mandible

See Chapter 58.

1. Observe opening and closing of mouth.
2. Check bite for malocclusion.

3. Palpate for tenderness, crepitus, deformity, asymmetry, and mental nerve anesthesia.

TRAUMATIC INJURIES TO THE TEETH

Tooth fractures are usually caused by a blow to the tooth from a fall, sports, fight, or abuse. It is important to define whether the injury is to a primary or permanent tooth.

Diagnostic Findings

The signs and symptoms vary with the site of fracture. Cracks, loss of tooth structures, hemorrhage at the gingival margin or from an exposed pulp, pain, and sensitivity to stimuli can all result.

Dental age   Erupting   Exfoliating

0-1

1-2

2-3

3-4

4-5

5-6

6-7

7-8

8-9

9-10

10-11

11-12

12-13

16-24

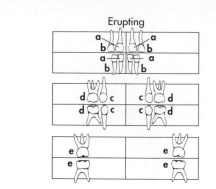
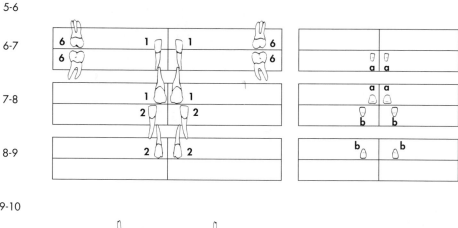
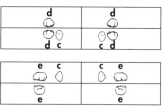
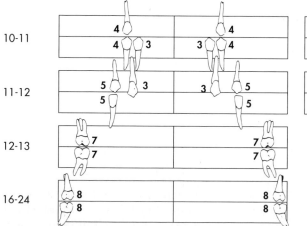

Fig. 60-2   Most common pattern of dental development. **a** to **e,** A quadrant's primary teeth. **1-8,** A quadrant's' secondary (permanent) teeth. Within each age box, the vertical line represents the dental midline, and the horizontal line represents upper/lower dentitions.

1. Crown cracks (crazing), which are incomplete fractures of the enamel without loss of tooth structure, may be associated with other injuries to the tooth.
2. Uncomplicated crown fractures involve the enamel or dentin. If the dentin is involved, a yellow area appears at the center of the fracture site and may demonstrate sensitivity to thermal or direct stimuli (air, heat, cold) because of proximity of the pulp.
3. Complicated crown fractures extending through the pulp almost uniformly produce sensitivity to thermal or direct stimuli (e.g., touch, air, ice). There is usually hemorrhage from the exposed dental pulp. Pulp injuries may lead to subsequent inflammation, necrosis, and abscess formation.
4. Crown-root fractures appear as a "split tooth" and involve the enamel, dentin, cementum, and almost always the pulp. There is usually hemorrhage at the gingival margin, and if the fracture extends through the pulp, there is bleeding along the fracture line as well.
5. Root fractures are rare in the anterior primary teeth before 18 months of age. They involve the cementum, dentin, and pulp and, on physical examination, may be associated with movement of the tooth.
6. Periodontal injuries are often found with dental fractures.

Complications
1. Imbedding of tooth fragments into the soft tissue (tongue, lips)
2. Aspiration of tooth fragment
3. Damage to the pulp, resulting in subsequent inflammation, necrosis, or abscess formation; may be secondary to initial injury to the neurovascular bundle at time of trauma or to secondary bacterial contamination and inflammatory response
4. Dentoalveolar abscess

5. Damage to underlying permanent tooth bud
6. Death of tooth nerve or eventual loss

Ancillary Data

Dental x-ray films, if available, are particularly important in evaluating all injuries involving fractures of the dentin, pulp, or roots. X-ray evaluation is a required diagnostic modality for root fractures.

Differential Diagnosis

1. Dental attrition (normal wear)
2. Loss or fracture of a previously placed restoration

Management

Life-threatening conditions must be stabilized and take precedence over dental injuries. Management of specific injuries reflects the nature of the findings and whether a primary or secondary tooth is involved.

1. Uncomplicated crown fractures or cracks not involving the pulp
   a. Primary tooth: nonurgent referral to a dentist for follow-up for definitive treatment
   b. Secondary tooth: dental referral within 24 hours for the following:
      (1) Smoothing of sharp, jagged edges of the remaining surface to prevent damage to soft tissues
      (2) Restoring tooth appearance, using composite resin material
      (3) Initial data gathering for long-term follow-up to monitor for pulp death
2. Complicated crown fracture involving the pulp
   a. Primary tooth: urgent dental referral within 24 hours
   b. Secondary tooth: immediate referral to minimize bacterial contamination of the pulp, minimize pain, and provide

subsequent endodontic therapy and crown

3. Crown-root fracture
   a. Primary tooth: urgent referral within 24 hours, usually for extraction
   b. Secondary tooth; immediate referral
4. Root fractures
   • Immediate referral to a dentist for stabilization or extraction of the fracture segment. Primary teeth may be removed.
5. Long-term goals of the dentist include the following:
   a. Maintenance of vitality of the tooth, if possible
   b. Treatment of the pulp and its complications, often requiring root canal therapy and a crown
   c. Restoration of a clinical crown
   d. Extraction and prosthesis if other goals are not achieved

Disposition

Close dental follow-up is essential for all patients with dental trauma and for any findings on physical examination—for both acute management and long-term monitoring of dental health. Some dental injuries develop signs or symptoms years after the original trauma.

TRAUMATIC PERIODONTAL INJURIES

Periodontal injuries involving the alveolar bone or socket and the periodontal ligament are almost always caused by a blow. Teeth are abnormally mobile or displaced.

Diagnostic Findings

The extent of mobility or displacement reflects the severity of the injury. Pain and increased sensitivity are commonly present.

1. Concussion results in minimal damage to the periodontal ligament. The tooth is sensitive to percussion or pressure such as chewing, biting, or mobility testing but is not displaced or excessively mobile.
2. Subluxation produces abnormal looseness and mobility (<2 mm of displacement) of the tooth from moderate damage to the periodontal ligament with slight displacement. The tooth is displaced out of the socket. Hemorrhage at the gingival margin may be noted.
3. Intrusive or traumatic impaction displacement is common in primary teeth and involves the tooth being driven into the socket. The tooth may appear avulsed. Compression fractures of the alveolar socket are common.
4. Extrusive displacement occurs with relocation of the tooth outside of the alveolar socket into an abnormal position and is often associated with a fracture of the alveolar socket and tear of the periodontal ligament.
5. Avulsion of a tooth is common, particularly in 7- to 10-year-old children. The tooth is completely detached from the alveolar socket and the periodontal ligament is severed.
6. Periodontal injuries may be associated with dental fractures.

Complications
1. Those involving traumatic injuries to the teeth
2. Root resorption
3. Ankylosis (fusion of tooth to bone)
4. Eruption problem for a permanent successor tooth (i.e., delays, displacement, space loss)

Ancillary Data
Dental x-ray films, if available, are particularly important to identify associated root fractures.

Differential Diagnosis

1. Root fracture
2. Normally exfoliating primary tooth (variably mobile, possibility of slight bleeding)

3. Newly erupting primary and secondary teeth (slightly mobile, possibility of being malpositioned)
4. Dentoalveolar infection
5. Systemic disease with bone loss (e.g., hypothyroidism, diabetes, leukemia)

Management

First priority must be given to stabilization of life-threatening conditions.

1. Concussion. No immediate therapy indicated but requires long-term follow-up observation to ensure that complications of root resorption, pulp injury, and ankylosis do not occur.
2. Subluxation. Usually requires immobilization with an acrylic splint and long-term follow-up observation.
3. Intrusive displacement.
   a. Primary tooth: urgent referral to dentist within 24 hours. Unaffected permanent tooth will be allowed to erupt with careful observation and close follow-up observation.
   b. Secondary tooth: initial care giver should attempt to reposition, particularly in adolescents. Younger patients' secondary teeth may be allowed to erupt. Immediate dental referral for stabilization.
4. Extrusive displacement.
   a. Primary tooth: urgent referral to dentist within 24 hours (usually extracted).
   b. Secondary tooth: immediate dental referral for stabilization and positioning.
      (1) Initial caregiver should attempt to reposition, using gentle pressure.
      (2) Delays in repositioning the tooth increase the chance that the tooth will stabilize in an ectopic position.
5. Avulsion.
   a. Primary tooth: nonurgent dental referral (usually omitted).
   b. Secondary tooth: immediate dental referral and careful handling of the tooth and rapid reimplantation to maximize the success of replacement. Periodontal ligament fibers are best preserved if reimplanted within 30 minutes. Dentists immobilize the tooth with nonrigid acrylic splint and arrange close follow-up observation.
      (1) Hold the tooth carefully by the crown. Do not touch the roots!
      (2) Wash the tooth with saline solution or milk. Plug the drain to prevent loss of the tooth. Rinse off foreign material.
      (3) Irrigate the socket and suction lightly to remove clots. Insert the tooth slowly but firmly into the socket as soon as possible (lacerations should be cared for after reimplantation if bleeding is controlled). Maintain compression for several minutes.
      (4) See a dentist immediately. In the interim, have the child hold the tooth in place with a finger or bite on a gauze to stabilize the tooth.
      (5) If immediate reimplantation is impossible, place the tooth under the child's or parent's tongue to bathe in saliva until seen by a dentist. Other options include soaking in milk or normal saline solution.
6. Long-term goals of dentist include the following:
   a. Maintaining the tooth in the dentition; stabilizing the tooth via interdental acrylic splinting immediately after the injury
   b. Monitoring and treating later pulp and root resorption problems
   c. Considering possible later orthodontic repositioning
   d. Extracting tooth and inserting prosthesis if other goals are not achieved

Disposition

Dental follow-up observation is essential.

REFERENCES

Andreasen JO, Andreasen FM, editors: *Textbook and color atlas of traumatic injuries to the teeth,* ed 3, St Louis, 1994, Mosby.

Crona-Larsson G, Noren JG: Luxation injuries to permanent teeth: a retrospective study of etiological factors, *Endodont Dent Traumatol* 5:176, 1989.

Harding AM, Camp JH: Traumatic injuries in the preschool child, *Dental Clin North Am* 39:817, 1995.

Harrington MS, Eberhart AF, Knapp JF: Dentofacial trauma in children, *J Dent Child* 55:334, 1988.

Josell SD, Abrams RG: Managing common dental problems and emergencies, *Pediatr Clin North Am* 38:1325, 1991.

Josell SD, Abrams RG: Traumatic injuries to the dentition and its supporting structures, *Pediatr Clin North Am* 29: 717, 1982.

Wilson CFG: Management of trauma to primary and developing teeth, *Dent Clin North Am* 39:133, 1995.

61 SPINE AND SPINAL CORD TRAUMA

RONALD D. LINDZON

ALERT: Exercise extreme caution when the type and mechanism of injury are sufficient to cause spinal or spinal cord trauma.

Most trauma spinal cord injuries are partial or incomplete. With care from the onset of trauma, substantial recovery may ensue, thereby preventing the catastrophic physical and psychologic disorders associated with major neurologic involvement. Motor vehicle accidents remain the single most common cause of spinal and spinal cord trauma, followed by falls, diving accidents, electrical injuries, and in newborns, birth trauma.

Initial stabilization of the spine in all major trauma, particularly of the head and face, with collar, sandbags, and tape is imperative in the interval before the cervical spine can be evaluated. This stabilization is maintained until x-ray studies have excluded injury or appropriate intervention has been initiated if abnormality is present.

The case fatality rate of cervical spine injuries is 59%, in contrast to a 6% fatality rate associated with head injuries. Children less than 8 years old tend to sustain injury to the upper (C1-C3) cervical spine.

ETIOLOGY
Mechanisms of Injury

1. Flexion
   a. Stretching of the posterior ligamentous complex produces tears or spinous process avulsions.
   b. Wedge fractures of vertebral bodies result from mechanical pressure of one vertebral body on the next.
   c. Ligamentous disruptions result in variable degree of subluxation and dislocation of bony spinal elements.
2. Rotation
   a. Simultaneous flexion and rotation about one of the facet joints may cause unilateral facet-joint dislocation.
   b. Rotational forces produce unstable articular process fractures in the lumbar region.
3. Extension
   a. With extension, compression of the posterior neural arch of C1 or the pedicles of C2 secondary to the heavy occiput above can result in fractures of these elements. The latter is known as a hangman fracture.
   b. Stretching of the anterior longitudinal ligament can produce ligamentous tears or avulsion (tear-drop) fractures of the vertebral body.
   c. Buckling of the ligamentum flavum into the posterior spinal canal can produce central or posterior cord syndromes.
4. Vertical compression/axial loading
   • The cervical and lumbar spines straighten at the time of impact from above or below, potentially compress-

ing the nucleus pulposus (disc matter) into the vertebral body, with compromise of the anterior spinal canal, causing the anterior cord syndrome.

Generally, children less than 6 years of age who fall less than 5 feet have clinical evidence of injury on history or physical examination.

DIAGNOSTIC FINDINGS

At high risk for spinal injuries are those patients with the following:

1. Injury compatible with causing spinal injury as outlined above
2. Posttraumatic neck or back pain
3. Posttraumatic neurologic complaints or deficits, whether stable or progressive
4. Posttraumatic impaired level of consciousness or an inability to give an accurate history (e.g., infants, alcohol or drug abusers, and those who have had a concussion or are postictal)
5. Breathing difficulty
6. Presence of severe associated injuries or shock

The ability to ambulate after an accident does not exclude spine or spinal cord trauma because 15% to 20% of patients may be able to walk initially. Severe head and facial injuries carry a 15% to 20% risk of concomitant spine or spinal cord trauma. Other associated injuries must be defined. The neck and back should be palpated for tenderness, step deformity, crepitus, and paraspinous spasm.

Vital Signs

1. Breathing pattern may indicate loss of diaphragmatic breathing and hypoventilation or apnea with injuries to C3, C4, and C5, which supply the phrenic nerve. Although lower cervical lesions preserve diaphragmatic function, there may be a loss of abdominal and intercostal breathing.
2. Hypotension may exist with spinal shock. Hypovolemic shock must be excluded.
3. Temperature regulation is impaired with associated hypothermia or hyperthermia.

Neurologic Findings (see Chapters 15 and 57)

1. Determine mental status and level of consciousness.
2. Cranial nerves. Assess for associated intracranial injury.
3. Motor:
   a. Tone
      (1) Flaccid: lower motor neuron (LMN) lesion or spinal shock (with areflexia)
      (2) Spastic: upper motor neuron (UMN) lesion (with hyperreflexia)
   b. Power (Table 61-1)
      (1) Comparison of strength of upper to lower extremities and right to left. Muscles that are essential for maintaining normal posture usually have bilateral innervation and are not useful in lateralizing weakness. The best muscle groups to use for rapid examination are the following:
         (a) Upper extremity: dorsiflexion of wrist and extension of forearm
         (b) Lower extremity: dorsiflexion of great toe and flexion of lower leg at knee
      (2) Mass flexion withdrawal movements in response to stimulation may occur in infants with paralyzed limbs and may be indistinguishable from normal movements.
4. Sensation. Upper level of sensory impairment is best guide to accurate localization (Table 61-1 and Fig. 61-1).
   a. Light-touch sense tests ipsilateral posterior spinal column and contralateral anterior column.

TABLE 61-1   Spinal Cord Injuries: Motor, Sensory, and Reflex Deficits

Level of lesion	Motor function lost	Sensation lost at and below	Reflex
C2	Breathing	Occiput	
C3	Spontaneous breathing and trapezius function	Thyroid cartilage	
C4		Suprasternal notch	
C5	Shoulder flexion and abduction	Infraclavicular +/– lateral arm sparing	Biceps brachialis*
C6		Infraclavicular +/– lateral arm, forearm sparing	Brachioradialis*
C7	Elbow and wrist extension	Infraclavicular with sparing as above to middle finger	Triceps*
C8	Small muscles of hand (lumbricales and interossei)	Infraclavicular with sparing as above to little finger	
T1		Infraclavicular with upper extremity sparing to axilla	
T4		Nipple line	
T7	Intercostal and abdominal musculature	Inferior costal margin	Upper abdominal†
T10		Umbilicus	Lower abdominal†
T12			
L1	Hip flexion	Groin	
L2		Anteromedial thigh	
L3	Hip adduction and knee extension	Medial knee	Knee/patellar*
L4	Hip abduction and knee extension	Anterior knee and medial calf	
L5	Foot and great toe dorsiflexion	Lateral dorsum foot and lateral sole foot	
S1	Foot and great toe plantar flexion	Lateral dorsum foot and lateral sole foot	Ankle/Achilles*
S2	Perianal and rectal sphincter tone	Perianal and rectal sensation	
S3			
S4			

*Deep tendon.
†Superficial.

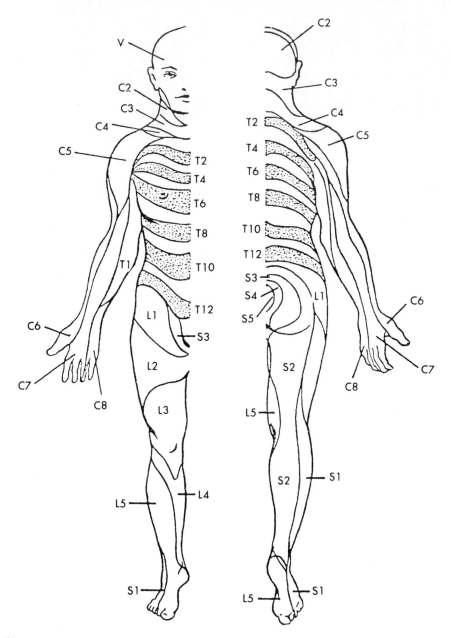

Fig. 61-1   Segmental area of innervation of the skin. Overlapping of one segment occurs between adjacent dermatomes.

(From Gilman S, Newman SW, editors: *Essentials of clinical neuroanatomy and neurophysiology,* Philadelphia, 1987, FA Davis.)

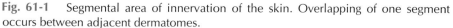

b. Pain sense (pinprick) tests contralateral anterolateral spinal column.

c. Position sense tests ipsilateral posterior spinal column.

5. Reflexes.

  a. Deep tendon, superficial (see Table 61-1)

  b. Primitive: Babinski reflex, Hoffmann reflex, and others, if present beyond 4 weeks of life, may indicate a UMN lesion.

  c. Rectal. Very important prognostically to assess rectal tone in children with quadriplegia or paraplegia. If rectal tone is present, sacral sparing is implied, with subsequent partial or complete neurologic recovery in up to 30% to 50%. Absence of rectal tone implies only a 2% to 3% chance of partial or complete recovery.

  d. Bulbocavernous reflex is performed by pressing the glans penis or pulling on urinary catheter. An intact reflex results in distinct rectal sphincter contraction. The absence of an intact reflex indicates the presence of spinal shock. No accurate estimate of prognosis can be made until this reflex has returned.

  e. Autonomic reflex paralysis produces vasomotor paralysis with flushed, warm, dry skin, loss of temperature regulation (if lesion above T8), hypotension, and bradycardia.

6. Mental status changes, craniofacial injuries, range of motion abnormalities, and focal neurologic findings are not always present in acute cervical spine injuries.

Cervical Spine Injury Stability

1. Intact anterior structures with disrupted posterior elements often are unstable.

2. Intact posterior elements with disrupted anterior elements are occasionally unstable.

3. Disruption of both anterior and posterior structures usually causes instability.

4. Mechanically stable fractures may still coexist with neurologic defects.

Spinal stability can be assessed by using a three-column technique. The *anterior* column includes the anterior longitudinal ligament, the anterior two thirds of the vertebral body, the anulus fibrosus, and the disc. The *middle* column includes the posterior one third of the vertebral body, the anulus fibrosus, the disc, and the posterior longitudinal ligament. The posterior column includes the remaining posterior components: the pedicles, lateral masses, intertransverse ligaments, facet capsular ligaments, lamina, ligamentum flavum, spinous processes, interspinous and supraspinous ligaments, and ligamentum nuchae. To be unstable, the injury generally involves two of these columns.

Spinal Cord Injury without Radiographic Abnormality

Spinal cord injury without radiographic abnormality (SCIWORA) may occur in as many as 50% to 60% of children with traumatic spinal cord injuries, not commonly in children less than 8 years of age. This results from a nondisruptive and self-reducing intersegmental deformation. Hyperextension with inward bulging of interlaminal ligaments, reversible disc prolapse, flexion compression of the cord, longitudinal distraction of the cord, and vertebral artery spasm or thrombosis may all contribute.

Paresthesia may be the only clinical finding and it is essential to address the presence of transient paresthesias at the time of the accident. The diagnosis can then only be made after occult fractures and ligament/disc damage have been excluded by computed tomographic (CT) scanning, flexion-extension views, and myelography.

The cord injuries may have a delayed onset of deficit, presenting with central cord, partial cord, and complete cord syndromes days after the event. The prognosis reflects the abnormality.

Complications

1. Quadriplegia or paraplegia; paralysis.
2. Spinal shock. Flaccid paralysis, areflexia, and sensory loss distal to lesion. Impaired temperature control. Hypotension with bradycardia. Skin is warm, flushed, and dry as a result of loss of sympathetic tone and decreased peripheral vascular resistance. Priapism.
3. Acute urinary retention or incontinence.
4. Paralytic ileus with potential for aspiration.
5. Gastric stress ulcer.
6. Incomplete spinal cord syndromes.
   a. Anterior cord (contusion of the anterior cord or laceration/thrombosis of the anterior spinal artery). Complete paralysis and hypalgesia with preservation of touch and proprioception. Flexion or vertical compression injury with anterior spinal cord compressed by bony fragments, disc material, or hematoma.
   b. Central cord (damage to central gray matter and most central regions of the pyramidal and spinothalamic tracts). Motor weakness in arms greater than in legs, with variable bladder and sensory involvement. Extension injury, with buckling of the ligamentum flavum into posterior spinal canal.
   c. Posterior cord. Loss of proprioception with variable paresis. Extension injury as in (b). Rare.
   d. Brown-Séquard syndrome. Cord hemisection with ipsilateral motor, proprioception, and light-touch deficit, with contralateral pain and temperature impairment. Usually penetrating injury.
   e. Horner's syndrome. Unilateral ptosis, miosis, anhidrosis, facial flushing with apparent enophthalmos. Disruption of the cervical sympathetic chain arising at C7-T2.
7. Vertical trauma in addition to spinal injury may have associated pelvic fractures, as well as urinary and thoracic injuries.
8. Death secondary to respiratory failure, cardiovascular collapse, hypothermia or hyperthermia, or associated injuries.
9. Long-term sequelae, including psychologic trauma, repeated pulmonary and genitourinary infections, muscle contractures, progressive spinal deformity, and decubitus ulcers.

Ancillary Data

Cervical X-Ray Studies (Fig. 61-2)

The criteria for obtaining a cervical spine series in the traumatized child are undefined. Indications for radiography after spinal trauma generally include the following:

1. Acute neurologic deficit or altered mental status
2. Intoxication from alcohol or drugs
3. Head or back/neck pain or tenderness
4. High-risk mechanism of injury: high-speed motor vehicle accident, fall of more than 10 feet, or injury associated with near-drowning
5. Severe associated injuries of head, face, or musculoskeletal system
6. Competitive pain from a nonspinal injury

All cervical vertebrae except C1 have a body. C1 moves in union with the occiput. C1 (axis) has the odontoid process (dens) protruding from its body to rest posterior to the anterior arch of C1 and anterior to the transverse atlantal ligament, allowing for rotation of the neck. The atlas is formed from three ossification centers (body and two neural arches), whereas the axis forms from four centers (odontoid, body, and two neural arches).

The most important initial x-ray film is the *cross-table lateral cervical spine.* This film identifies more than 75% to 95% of cervical spine fractures, dislocations, and subluxations.

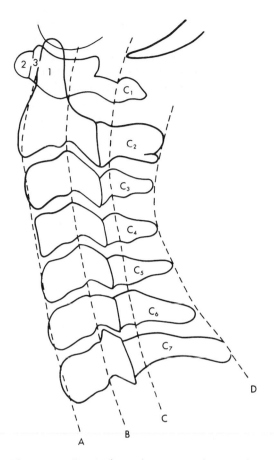

Fig. 61-2 Cervical vertebrae. Lateral cervical spine: **A,** anterior vertebral bodies; **B,** posterior vertebral bodies and anterior spinal canal; **C,** spinolaminal line and posterior spinal canal; **D,** spinous process tips C2-C7. *1,* Odontoid process of dens of C2; *2,* anterior arch of C1; *3,* predental space between posterior surface of anterior arch of C1 and anterior surface of odontoid process.

It should be obtained early in the resuscitation, and the cervical spine should be immobilized during this phase.

All seven cervical vertebrae must be included. To visualize C7-T1, it may be necessary to have one person hold the patient's head, applying in-line traction, while another pulls gently down on the arms from the foot of the bed. This is particularly useful in heavy patients. Lead aprons should be worn by care providers.

Swimmer's (transaxillary) view should be obtained if C7-T1 is not visualized by the preceding technique.

Complete cervical spine trauma series must include, as a minimum, the cross-table lateral view, anteroposterior view, and open-mouth odontoid study. Some recommend oblique views as well.

- Assessment of the lateral cervical spine (ABC)
 1. Alignment: four continuous curvilinear lines without step-offs. Loss of the normal lordotic curve is seen in 20% of normal patients with spasm, or it may be the only evidence of severe spinal injury (see Fig. 61-2).
 2. Bony integrity. Compare uniformity, shape, mineralization, density. Look for fracture lines, displacements, subluxations, or dislocations in systematic manner by first assessing each vertebral body and then each pedicle, facet joint, lamina, and spinous process.
 3. Cartilaginous spaces.
   a. Assessment of disc-space uniformity. Isolated disc-space narrowing in a child with the appropriate type and mechanism of injury is suggestive of acute disc herniation. Lengthening of the disc space implies disruption of the anulus fibrosus and possibly the longitudinal ligaments.
   b. The inferior articular facets above and the superior facet below articulate and must line up in parallel. Widening, facet overriding, or vertebral body rotation more than 11 degrees above the facet joint is pathologic.
   c. Interspinous widening is suggestive of ligamentous disruption of the interspinous and supraspinous ligaments.
 4. Soft tissue spaces.
   a. Predental space (space between the posterior aspect of the anterior arch of C1 and the anterior aspect of the odontoid process of C2 on lateral

view) should be 5 mm or less in children less than 8 years of age and 3 mm or less in adults. Greater distance may represent odontoid fractures with posterior displacement or transverse atlantal ligament tear.

b. Normal prevertebral spaces:

(1) Anterior to C2: 7 mm or less in children and adults

(2) Anterior to C3, C4: 5 mm or less in children and adults or less than 40% of the AP diameter of the C3 and C4 vertebral bodies

(3) Between C6 and trachea: 14 mm or less in children (under 15 years) and 22 mm or less in adults

NOTE: Nasogastric (NG) or endotracheal (ET) tubes may invalidate these measurements. Soft tissue swelling may be secondary to hemorrhage, abscess, infection, foreign body, tumor, air, or bony injury. Using these measurements as sole criteria for injury is not reliable as the only basis for determination of an injury.

c. Because the retropharyngeal space may be widened during expiration, inspiratory film should be attempted.

d. The body of the hyoid bone should normally lie entirely below a line that is parallel to the top of C3. The hyoid bone crosses the epiglottis and is helpful in identifying an inflamed epiglottis.

• Other considerations

1. The odontoid film (open-mouth view preferable) ensures that the dens is centered between the lateral masses of the atlas, and the anteroposterior (AP) view is useful in assessing C3-C7. Both should be obtained after initial stabilization of the patient and after confirmation that the lateral view is normal.

2. Oblique, flexion, and extension views and tomograms are occasionally required although practice varies. They should be done with supervision.

3. Epiphyseal growth plates may resemble fractures. Other developmental changes must be considered in interpreting films.

a. Pseudosubluxation of C2 occurs anterior to C3, particularly in children less than 8 years old and, in rare cases, at C3-C4. Maximum normal: 2.7 mm although it is more than 3 mm and up to 5 mm in 20% in children less than 8 years of age. If the posterior cervical line (the line drawn from the anterior aspect of the spinous process of C1 to the anterior aspect of the spinous process of C3) misses the anterior aspect of the C2 spinous process by 2 mm or more, a hangman fracture with subluxation may be present. This finding is useful only if C2 is displaced anterior to C3. Normally, the posterior cervical line misses the anterior aspect of the C2 spinal process by 2 mm or more.

b. The posterior arch of C1 (three ossification centers) fuses around 3 years and the anterior arch at 7 to 10 years.

c. The epiphyseal plate at the base of the odontoid fuses with the body of C2 at 3 to 6 years.

4. A widened anteroposterior dimension of C2 in relation to C3 may indicate a fracture.

5. The minimal wedge shape of the body of C3 may be normal. The anterior wedging of immature vertebral bodies may appear as compression fractures. Similar-appearing adjacent vertebral bodies suggest a normal variant.

6. A CT scan often is preferred in selected circumstances when routine film findings are negative and a fracture is still suspected. The anatomy can be well documented without unnecessary movement of the patient, and it is particularly important in patients with abnormal neurologic findings who have normal cervical x-ray studies.

7. Magnetic resonance imaging (MRI) is superior to CT in demonstrating spinal cord

injury (edema, hemorrhage, compression, and transection) and intervertebral disc herniation. CT is better in defining bony injury. Limitations of availability and image degradation caused by resuscitation and monitoring equipment restrict MRI's usefulness in evaluating acutely injured patients. Experience in pediatric trauma is limited.

Thoracic and Lumbar Spine X-Ray Studies

1. A cross-table lateral view of the thoracic or lumbar spine should be obtained first, with the patient immobilized on a firm backboard.
2. An AP view is taken next (obliques periodically needed).
3. Interpedicular space must be assessed, as well as the *ABCs* delineated on p. 455.
4. The distance between the medial aspects of the two pedicles overlying each vertebral body (on the AP view) gradually increases in a caudal (cervical-to-lumbar) direction. A marked increase in this distance is indicative of posterior disruption and probable instability.
5. Most fractures of the lower spine occur in the region of T10-L4 although in the multiply injured patient, injuries are common at T2-T7. In multiple level, noncontiguous fractures, the secondary lesions commonly occur at L4-L5 and C1-C2.
6. Fractures of T1-T5 may produce mediastinal hematomas with widening of the mediastinum.
7. Thoracolumbar compression fractures in children may appear as beaklike projections on the anterior margin of the vertebral body, usually superior.

DIFFERENTIAL DIAGNOSIS

1. Hysterical paralysis
2. Trauma
   a. Bilateral brachial plexus injury
   b. Nerve root injury
   c. Cauda equina syndrome
3. Vascular: ischemia resulting from atherosclerosis, thromboembolic disease, thoracic aorta dissection, or epidural hematoma
4. Spinal tumor

MANAGEMENT

Initial attention must be paid to resuscitation and support while immobilizing the spine at the levels of suspected injury. Immediate consultation with a neurosurgeon is necessary.

1. Airway stabilization, with ventilatory support as necessary and administration of oxygen.
   a. Bag-valve-mask ventilation, nasotracheal intubation, or cricothyroidotomy in patients with severe respiratory compromise.
   b. Oral ET intubation may be contraindicated because excessive C-spine motion may occur.
   c. Forced vital capacity determination may be useful in the evaluation.
2. Circulation (see Chapter 5).
   a. If shock is present, treat initially as hypovolemic. Look for source of internal hemorrhage. Excessive transfusion of crystalloid in the presence of spinal shock may precipitate pulmonary edema. Urinary output rather than blood pressure is the best monitor.
   b. Once hypovolemic shock has been excluded, neurogenic shock should be considered. Patients are hypotensive with bradycardia and have warm, flushed, dry skin—in contrast to hypovolemic shock.
      (1) May use pneumatic antishock trousers, military antishock trousers (MAST) to potentially increase peripheral vascular resistance, although there is no clear evidence related to efficacy. Trendelenburg position. Ensure adequate ventilation and oxygenation.
      (2) To treat decreased sympathetic tone: low-dose norepinephrine

(Levophed) drip infusion at 0.1-1.0 µg/kg/min IV, with close attention to vital signs.

(3) To treat increased parasympathetic tone: atropine, 0.01-0.02 mg/kg/dose IV repeated q5-10min as necessary, used alternatively or concurrently with norepinephrine

(4) Insert NG tube once neck stabilized and Foley catheter in place. Consider cimetidine, 20-40 mg/kg/24 hr (maximum: 300 mg) q6hr IV.

3. Immobilization and stabilization of neck from the outset.

   a. Place in neutral position with sandbags and 1- to 2-inch tape across the forehead and chin with the patient on a rigid backboard or scoop.

   b. Apply gentle in-line traction with neurologic abnormalities. Cervical spine stabilization can be achieved with a semi-hard Stif Neck, Philadelphia collar, or four-poster collar. Tape and sandbags or supplemental device in combination with an immobilizer is most effective. Soft collars offer no demonstrable stability.

   c. Much attention is given to the cervical spine; thoracic and lumbar fractures are equally possible, even in the young child. These must be diligently sought.

4. When there is cervical neurologic impairment, *skeletal traction* is indicated on an emergent basis. Traction can be applied by using halo, Gardner-Wells, Crutchfield, or Vinke tongs. A neurosurgeon is best involved in these procedures.

   a. The patient is then transferred to a suitable frame and 1 to 5 lb of weight/interspace (adult) is applied. Lateral spine roentgenograms are repeated to assess alignment. If alignment is not achieved, muscle relaxants are often required.

   b. Thoracic and lumbar injuries are treated by immobilizing the patient to allow for postural reduction. Concurrent stabilization of other life-threatening injuries with appropriate consultations is essential.

5. *Steroids* have generally been demonstrated to reduce neurologic function at all levels of injury when begun within 8 hours. Very-high-dose methylprednisolone, 30 mg/kg IV, followed by an infusion of 5.4 mg/kg/hr for the subsequent 23 hours is beneficial. However, children less than 13 years of age were excluded from the initial studies, as were patients with gunshot wounds, nerve root impairment, or cauda equina syndrome. Significant improvement in motor function and pin and touch sensation were seen in treated patients at 6 weeks and 6 months after injury.

6. Gangliosides are a complex acidic glycolipid present in the central nervous system (CNS) as a component of the cell membrane. Administration of GM_1 ganglioside may enhance recovery after injury.

7. *Surgical decompression,* when required, should be done in a timely fashion. When performed more than 8 hours after injury, it is significantly less successful. The indications include progressive neurologic deterioration, penetrating injuries of the spinal cord, and a foreign body within the spinal canal. Surgical stabilization and realignment may be necessary for potentially unstable injuries or for relief of pain.

DISPOSITION

All patients with spine or spinal cord injury require hospitalization and immediate neurosurgical consultation. A team approach to the management of such patients is mandatory. After they are stabilized, patients often require transfer to neurosurgical spinal trauma centers.

Parental Education

Prevention

1. Automobile restraints should always be used.
2. Swimming and diving in uncontrolled areas should be avoided.
3. Trampolines should be forbidden.

REFERENCES

Anderson DK, Hall ED: Pathophysiology of spinal cord trauma, *Ann Emerg Med* 22:987, 1993.

Blahd WH, Iserson KV, Bjelland JC: Efficacy of the post-traumatic cross-table lateral view of the cervical spine, *Ann Emerg Med* 2:243, 1983.

Bohn D, Armstrong D, Becker L, et al: Cervical spine injuries in children, *J Trauma* 30:463, 1990.

Bracken MB, Shepard MJ, Collins WF, et al: A randomized controlled trial of methylprednisolone or naloxone in the treatment of acute spinal cord injury: results of the Second National Acute Spinal Cord Injury Study, *N Engl J Med* 322:1405, 1990.

Cadoux CG, White JD, Hedberg MC: High-yield roentgenographic criteria for cervical spine injuries, *Ann Emerg Med* 16:738, 1987.

Dachling P, Pollack IF: Spinal cord injury without radiographic abnormality in children: the seaworld syndrome, *J Trauma* 29:654, 1989.

DeBehn DJ, Havel CG: Utility of pre-cervical soft tissue measurements in identifying patients with cervical spine fracture, *Ann Emerg Med* 24:1119, 1994.

Fesmire FM, Luten RC: The pediatric cervical spine: developmental anatomy and clinical aspects, *J Emerg Med* 7:133, 1989.

Felsberg GJ, et al: Utility of MR imaging in pediatric spinal cord injury, *Pediatr Radiol* 25:131, 1995.

Geisler FH, Dorsey FC, Coleman WP: Recovery of motor function after spinal cord injury: a randomized placebo controlled trial with GN-1 ganglioside, *N Engl J Med* 324:1829, 1991.

Geisler FH, Dorsey FC, Coleman WP: Past and current clinical studies with GM-1 ganglioside in acute spinal cord injury, *Ann Emerg Med* 22:1041, 1993.

Hockberger RS, Kirshenbaum K, Doris PE: Spinal injury. In Rosen P, editor: *Emergency medicine: concepts and clinical practice*, ed 4, St Louis, 1998, Mosby.

Huerta C, Griffith R, Joyce SM: Cervical spine stabilization in pediatric patients: evaluation of current techniques, *Ann Emerg Med* 16:1121, 1987.

Jaffe DM, Binns H, Radkowski MA, et al: Developing a clinical algorithm for early management of cervical spine injury in child trauma victims, *Ann Emerg Med* 16:270, 1987.

Kelen GD, Noji EK, Doris PE: Guidelines for use of lumbar spine radiography, *Ann Emerg Med* 15:245, 1986.

Kriss VM, Kriss TC: Imaging of the cervical spine in infants, *Pediatr Emerg Care* 13:44, 1996.

Medina FA: Neck and spinal cord trauma. In Barkin RM, editor: *Pediatric emergency medicine: concepts and clinical practice,* ed 2, St Louis, 1997, Mosby.

Pang D, Pollock IF: Spinal cord injury without radiographic abnormality in children: the SCIWORA syndrome, *J Trauma* 29:654, 1989.

Podolsky S: Efficacy of cervical spine immobilization methods, *J Trauma* 23:461, 1983.

Prendergast MA, Saxe JM, Ledgerwood AM, et al: Massive steroids do not reduce the zone of injury after penetrating spinal cord injury, *J Trauma* 37:576, 1994.

Rachesky I, Boyce WT, Duncan B, et al: Clinical prediction of cervical spinal injuries in children, *Am J Dis Child* 141:199, 1987.

Schwartz GR, Wright SW, Fein JA, et al: Pediatric cervical spine injury sustained in falls from low heights, *Ann Emerg Care* 30:249, 1997.

Turetsky DB, Vines FS, Clayman DA, et al: Technique and use of supine oblique views in acute cervical spine trauma, *Ann Emerg Med* 22:685, 1993.

Walter J, Doris PE, Shaffer MA: Clinical presentation of patients with acute cervical spine injury, *Ann Emerg Med* 3:512, 1984.

62 THORACIC TRAUMA

VINCENT J. MARKOVCHICK and BENJAMIN HONIGMAN

ALERT: Blunt or penetrating thoracic trauma requires a rapid assessment of pulmonary, cardiac, and mediastinal injuries. These may necessitate lifesaving procedures without a complete database.

Traumatic injuries of the chest are common and require urgent attention to therapy and diagnosis. More than with any other anatomic area, the physician must rapidly assess the patients' status and may have to intervene without a full diagnosis. Delays in management are often life threatening, whereas lifesaving procedures such as pericardiocentesis and the insertion of a chest tube are associated with relatively minimal complications.

The initial evaluation of the patient must take into consideration all aspects of the injuries (see Chapter 56). The airway, ventilation, and circulation are of primary concern. Specific attention must be focused on the mechanism and severity of the injury and the progression of signs and symptoms since the trauma.

1. *Blunt trauma* is associated with chest-wall injuries (rib fractures or flail chest), hemothorax, pneumothorax, pulmonary contusion, myocardial contusion, aortic tears, diaphragmatic rupture, and esophageal rupture (Box 62-1).
2. *Penetrating injuries* cause hemothorax, pneumothorax, penetrating cardiac injuries and tamponade, direct vessel damage, esophageal, and diaphragmatic injuries. The amount of time elapsed since injury and the patients' current status provide some indication of the urgency of intervention.

Diagnostic findings by a quick physical examination must include blood pressure (including an evaluation for pulsus paradoxus), respiratory rate and pattern, and heart sounds. Evidence of upper airway obstruction must be sought, including stridor and facial and neck injuries, with active intervention initiated when indicated. If the upper airway appears intact, lower airway compromise must be excluded by evaluating chest wall stability, symmetry and adequacy of air movement, and presence of subcutaneous emphysema.

If the patient is in obvious respiratory distress, immediate therapy is required. Oxygen should be administered by a nonrebreathing bag reservoir mask, and simultaneously, an airway ensured. Unilateral or bilateral chest tubes may be required, often solely on the basis of the physical examination.

Shock must be treated. With isolated thoracic injuries, shock is most commonly caused by massive pulmonary hemorrhage, pericardial tamponade, or tension pneumothorax. With multiple trauma, other causes must be excluded.

Ancillary data that are mandatory in any thoracic injury include chest x-ray film (portable supine if the patient is unstable), electrocardiogram (ECG), arterial blood gas (ABG), oximetry, and complete blood count (CBC) (hematocrit [Hct] done in the emergency department [ED]). Patients with major injuries also should have a type and cross-match performed immediately. However, these studies should not delay intervention in the patient with respiratory distress after a traumatic injury.

RIB FRACTURE

ALERT: Rib fractures are rare in children because of the child's highly elastic chest wall; therefore, when a rib fracture is noted, significant underlying organ injury (e.g., liver, lung, spleen) must be suspected. Upper rib fractures are associated with pulmonary and major vessel injuries; lower rib injuries are associated with potential liver, spleen, lung, and kidney injury. Conversely, the absence of a rib fracture does not preclude serious injury to the underlying soft tissue structures. Child abuse may need to be considered.

Fractured ribs are caused by blunt trauma resulting from motor vehicle accidents, falls,

blows with blunt objects, child abuse, and athletic injuries and are the most common significant findings after blunt trauma. Rib fracture is unlikely in minor trauma; however, a rib fracture from major trauma may lacerate underlying structures. Child abuse may need to be considered.

Diagnostic Findings

The mechanism of injury and an estimate of the force of impact may predict the type of injury.

1. Dyspnea and chest pain are common symptoms with isolated rib fractures.
2. Point tenderness over the rib is uniformly present. Anterior-posterior and lateral-lateral compression is painful. Referred pain is present on proximal or distal compression of the fractured rib.
3. Tachypnea, tachycardia, and shock are associated with underlying organ damage and respiratory failure.

Complications

1. **Pneumothorax** occurs in more than one third of patients.
2. Hemothorax is noted in 13% of patients.
3. Pulmonary laceration or contusion.
4. Myocardial contusion.
5. Solid visceral damage (liver, spleen, kidney), particularly with fractures of ribs 9 to 12.
6. Neurovascular tears (e.g., subclavian, brachial plexus, aorta) with fractures of ribs 1 and 2.

Ancillary Data

1. Chest x-ray studies. Most useful in evaluating status of pulmonary parenchyma and mediastinum. More than 50% of single-rib fractures are overlooked on the initial chest x-ray film.
2. Hct (to be done in ED) and urinalysis.
3. ABG with any respiratory distress or complications. Oximetry.
4. ECG for major blunt chest injury.
5. Angiogram or dynamic computed tomography (CT) scan as an initial screen before

angiogram for widened mediastinum (aortic tear) or fractures of the first or second rib, particularly if displaced (vascular injury).

Differential Diagnosis

1. Infectious/inflammatory: pleurisy, pneumonia, perichondritis, pericarditis
2. Trauma: rib contusion, costochondral separation (snapping sound with breathing)

Management

1. Treatment of any complications
2. Simple rib fractures without complications
   a. Analgesia.
   b. Intercostal nerve block, using long-acting local anesthetic agent such as bupivacaine (Marcaine) with epinephrine. Inject 1 to 2 ml in the subcostal space at the posterior axillary line. The intercostal nerve above and below the fracture should be blocked.
3. Instructions to patients
   a. Patients should be taught deep-breathing exercises.
   b. Patients should not use binders or rib belts because they inhibit adequate ventilation.

Disposition

1. Hospitalization should be strongly considered for young children and infants with any rib fracture because of the extreme force necessary to break a rib in this age group and, therefore, the high probability of complications and the high possibility of child abuse.
2. Hospitalization for observation should be strongly considered for older children and adolescents who sustain multiple (more than two) fractures.
3. All children with any complications require admission.

Parental Education

1. Continue deep-breathing exercises.
2. Call your physician if cough, fever, dyspnea, or increased pain develop.

FLAIL CHEST

ALERT: Flail chest is invariably associated with pulmonary contusion and abnormal respiratory physiology.

Flail chest results from blunt trauma when three or more adjacent ribs are fractured at two points, resulting in a freely movable chest wall segment. This results in paradoxic movement on respiration (inward with inspiration and outward with expiration), which may compress lung tissue, decrease ventilation on the ipsilateral side, and cause mediastinal shift to the opposite side. Venous return is decreased secondary to lung compression. More important, the underlying pulmonary contusion contributes to hypoxia and increasing respiratory distress.

Diagnostic Findings

1. Usually associated with multiple trauma.
2. Tenderness over ribs with crepitus and ecchymoses.
3. Commonly associated with increased heart and respiratory rates. Shock may occur secondary to complications or related injuries.
4. Visible or palpable paradoxic movement, which may require a tangential light to see. Up to 30% of cases are missed on the initial examination in the first 6 hours.
5. Decreased oxygen saturation as increased by oximetry secondary to underlying pulmonary contusion.

Complications

Complications are commonly associated with flail chest. Respiratory insufficiency is caused by pulmonary contusion, atelectasis, and decreased tidal volume and vital capacity, with resultant hypoxia, atrioventricular (AV) shunting, and ultimately, shock. Mortality is increased when associated head injuries are present.

The respiratory embarrassment results primarily not from the paradoxic movement of the chest but from the underlying injury to lung parenchyma.

Ancillary Data

Chest x-ray studies, ABG, and oximetry are required.

Management

1. For multiple trauma management, treat and diagnose complications and associated life-threatening injuries: oxygen, IV, chest x-ray film, ABG, and Hct.
2. Place on bag reservoir mask, oxygen, and oxygen saturation monitor.
3. Stabilize flail chest with sandbags and pressure over the unstable segment, or position the patient on side of injury, if possible.
4. Correct associated respiratory complications (e.g., thoracostomy for pneumothorax or hemothorax). If respiratory distress continues, intubate and internally stabilize with positive-pressure ventilation.
5. Intubate if flail chest is associated with the following:
   a. Shock
   b. Three or more related injuries
   c. Five or more rib fractures
   d. Underlying pulmonary disease
   e. Respiratory failure, with Pao_2 less than 50 mm Hg and $Paco_2$ greater than 50 mm Hg
      (1) Relative indications include increasing respiratory rate, restlessness, anxiety, abnormal A-a oxygen gradient, or decreasing Pao_2 or oxygen saturation.
      (2) Some clinicians recommend intubation only when flail chest is associated with respiratory failure.

6. Strongly consider thoracostomy if the patient is to have general anesthesia or if the patient requires ventilator support (especially if positive end-expiratory pressure [PEEP] is to be used). In addition, thoracostomy is required for hemothorax or pneumothorax (see Appendix A-9).
7. Do not give antibiotics prophylactically. Steroids are not indicated.

Disposition

All patients require admission to an intensive care unit (ICU).

STERNAL FRACTURE

ALERT: Sternal fractures and dislocations in children are unusual but when present suggest underlying myocardial contusion, cardiac rupture, pericardial tamponade, pulmonary contusion, or aortic rupture. The mortality rate is 25% to 45%.

Diagnostic Findings

Simple sternal fractures, which are unusual, are accompanied by anterior chest pain with point tenderness and ecchymoses over the sternum. More commonly, there are associated problems.

Complications

1. Flail chest and other contiguous injuries
2. Myocardial contusion or rupture, pericardial tamponade, or vascular injury
3. Pulmonary contusion
4. Traumatic aortic dissection

Ancillary Data

1. Chest x-ray study. Reveals fractures on lateral view, although special sternal views may be necessary. Differentiate from non-ossified cartilage of sternum. Will not be seen on posteroanterior (PA) or rib films.
2. ECG reveals nonspecific ST-T wave changes and a persistent tachycardia. Dysrhythmias may be seen.

Management

1. Treat life-threatening injuries and complications with oxygen, IV, cardiac monitor, and specific intervention.
2. Give analgesia.
3. Surgery may be required if the fracture is displaced.

Disposition

All patients require admission to an ICU for continuous monitoring.

TRAUMATIC PNEUMOTHORAX

ALERT: A simple pneumothorax may cause respiratory distress. Bilateral or tension pneumothoraxes are life threatening and require immediate intervention.

A *simple* pneumothorax occurs when air accumulates in the pleural space without mediastinal shift. It is invariably present with penetrating chest injuries and in 15% to 50% of blunt trauma chest injuries. A *tension* pneumothorax is produced when there is progressive accumulation of air in the pleural space with shift of mediastinal structures to the opposite hemithorax and compression of the mediastinum and contralateral lung. Tension pneumothorax can progressively decrease cardiac output. Massive shunting of blood occurs from perfused but nonventilated areas, resulting from lung compression, atelectasis, and collapse.

Open pneumothorax accompanies sucking chest wounds when there is a free bidirectional flow of air between the atmosphere and pleural space. It requires a large enough penetrating wound to result in a loss of a portion of the chest wall that approaches the size of the bronchial lumen.

Etiology

1. Blunt trauma: complication of fractured ribs, cardiopulmonary resuscitation, violent chest impact with closed glottis, or bronchial disruption
2. Penetrating trauma: complication of stab, gunshot, or other penetrating wounds or complication of insertion of a central venous catheter

Diagnostic Findings

1. Patients have dyspnea, chest pain, and a history of trauma.
2. With a small, uncomplicated pneumothorax, patients have normal vital signs, although respiratory and heart rates may be increased. Large defects are associated with respiratory distress and sometimes cyanosis.
3. Tension pneumothorax is accompanied by respiratory distress, hypotension, tachycardia, and absent breath sounds. Other signs that may be present include pulsus paradoxus, increased jugular venous pressure (JVP), tracheal shift, altered mental status, and at times, cyanosis. Air hunger is usually marked.
   a. If the patient is being ventilated with bag-valve-mask, an early indication of tension pneumothorax is an increasing resistance to bag ventilation. If the patient is being mechanically ventilated, increasing airway pressure may be needed to deliver the same volume of air.
   b. Other clues are increased central venous pressure (CVP), decreased blood pressure (BP), electromechanical dissociation, and marked intercostal and supraclavicular retractions.
4. Absent or markedly decreased breath sounds and hyperresonance to percussion may be present. Subcutaneous emphysema with crepitus is common, increasing rapidly if positive-pressure ventilation is being used.
   NOTE: Soon after penetrating injuries, and in children with small chests, transmission

of breath sounds from the unaffected lung may simulate normal breath sounds, making clinical diagnosis more difficult.

5. Pneumomediastinum may accompany pneumothorax.

Complications

Complications include respiratory distress, hypotension, and cardiac arrest.

Ancillary Data

1. Chest x-ray film for simple pneumothorax
   a. Definitive diagnostic procedure
   b. On occasion, may only be found in an expiratory view, which increases intrapleural pressure, pushing the lung and visceral pleura away from the chest wall
   c. Classification: small (<10%), moderate (10% to 50%), large (>50%)
      NOTE: Tension pneumothorax should be a clinical diagnosis and not await x-ray confirmation. X-ray film shows marked lung compression with mediastinal shift away from the affected side.
2. Arterial blood gases (ABGs) and oximetry after patient is stabilized

Differential Diagnosis

Many other entities besides trauma cause pneumothorax:

1. Asthma and other reactive airway diseases with hyperexpansion
2. Spontaneous pneumothorax secondary to apical blebs in adolescents
3. Meconium aspiration and hyaline membrane disease in the newborn (see Chapter 11)

Management

Life-threatening injuries must be treated immediately.

1. Tube thoracostomy is the treatment of choice for pneumothorax, sometimes before making a definitive diagnosis (see Appendix A-9).
   a. Indications for insertion of a chest tube include the following:
      (1) Tension pneumothorax
      (2) Traumatic cause, especially penetrating injuries
      (3) Any pneumothorax with respiratory symptoms
      (4) Increasing pneumothorax after initial conservative therapy
      (5) Pneumothorax with need for mechanical ventilation or general anesthesia
      (6) Associated hemothorax
      (7) Bilateral pneumothorax
         NOTE: Small (<10%), simple pneumothorax—one that shows no increase on repeat x-ray study—in a symptom-free patient who does not require general anesthesia or mechanical ventilation may be observed in the hospital without a chest tube.
   b. Position for chest tube.
      (1) Insert in fourth or fifth intercostal space in midaxillary line directed posteriorly and apically.
      (2) Insert superior to rib because neurovascular bundle runs inferior to rib in the lateral interspaces.
   c. Size. As large a tube as possible should be inserted, particularly with a hemothorax.
      • Newborn (10 to 12 Fr), infants (14 to 20 Fr), children (20 to 28 Fr), adolescents (28 to 42 Fr)
   d. Use tube with radiopaque line (for placement verification by roentgenogram) and make certain that the last hole is within the pleural cavity.
   e. Drainage. All chest tubes should be connected to an underwater seal drainage. Patients with continuous air leaks or associated hemothorax may require suction (15 to 25 cm H_2O).
2. Chest venting may be required as an initial, transient therapeutic maneuver when tension pneumothorax is suspected

and there is some delay in placement of a chest tube.

   a. Venting can be done with a needle, angiocath, or one-way flutter valve.

   b. Venting necessitates the eventual use of a chest tube.

   c. Venting should be done in the second or third intercostal space at the midclavicular line of the anterior chest wall or in the fourth or fifth intercostal space midaxillary line. Care must be taken to prevent the vent from being dislodged before the chest tube is placed.

3. Emergency management focuses on conversion to a simple pneumothorax, followed by immediate evacuation of entrapped air and reexpansion of the lung by means of a tube thoracostomy. It is usually effective.

Disposition

All patients with traumatic pneumothorax require hospitalization. The level of monitoring depends on the degree of respiratory distress and associated injuries.

PULMONARY CONTUSION

ALERT: Pulmonary contusion is a significant cause of respiratory failure after major blunt trauma injury in children, particularly rapid deceleration injuries.

Pulmonary contusion occurs when there is lung parenchymal damage with intraalveolar hemorrhage and edema. This is secondary to increased capillary membrane permeability, which impairs gas exchange.

Pulmonary contusion is usually associated with high-impact trauma; most occur at age 5years or older. Most patients have multiple trauma and at least one other major organ system involved. There is often a relative absence of external chest wall injury.

Diagnostic Findings

Patients who have experienced a rapid-deceleration injury may arrive with dyspnea and cyanosis, particularly those older than 5 years of age. Hemoptysis is rare in children. Tachycardia, tachypnea, anxiety, restlessness, labored respiration, and hypotension may be present. Localized rales or wheezing, with decreased breath sounds, also may be present. Significant hypoxia may be delayed 4 to 6 hours from the time of injury.

Obvious evidence of external trauma may not be present. Approximately 80% to 90% of patients have associated injuries.

Complications

Pneumonia is a complication. Intrathoracic effusion and hemothorax may develop over 48 hours.

Ancillary Data

1. Chest x-ray film. For all patients with increased respiratory or heart rate after trauma even if there is no external evidence of injury. Serial x-ray studies may be required.

   a. Findings vary from patchy areas of alveolar infiltrates to frank consolidation. They may be delayed 4 to 6 hours or they may be rapid in onset.

   b. Usually clear in 48 to 60 hours.

2. ABG.

   a. Hypoxemia is invariable but may be delayed in onset for 4 to 6 hours (deteriorates over the ensuing 24 hours). Continuous oximetry is appropriate.

   b. The $A\text{-}ao_2$ difference (gradient) at room air ($A\text{-}ao_2 = 150 - Pao_2 - 1.2\ Paco_2$), which is normally 15 or less, is the first to increase.

   c. Respiratory rate will increase and is a noninvasive clue to onset of insufficiency when followed serially.

Differential Diagnosis

1. Trauma: multiple causes of acute respiratory distress syndrome (ARDS) in children include smoke inhalation and fat emboli (fracture, penetrating chest wound). ARDS is usually delayed in onset, beginning 24 to 48 hours after the injury, and it has diffuse involvement (p. 44).

2. Medical causes of infiltrates and hypoxia: congestive heart failure (CHF), embolism, pneumonia.

Management

1. Treat associated life-threatening injuries.
2. Maintain oxygenation and ventilation.
   a. Intubation and ventilation are indicated if PaO_2 is less than 50 mm Hg at 100% O_2 (sea level).
   b. PEEP or continuous positive airway pressure (CPAP) may shorten the length of ventilatory assistance. Begin at 5 cm H_2O and increase slowly, monitoring oxygenation and cardiac output.
3. Give intravenous fluids.
   a. Patients with pulmonary contusion benefit from low levels of fluid administration. However, associated injuries may require high volumes of crystalloid solution. This infusion may increase pulmonary interstitial fluid, worsening the respiratory status.
   b. Ideally, the goal is to combine blood products and crystalloid solution to maintain adequate perfusion, CVP, and urinary output.
4. Steroids should not be used.
5. Analgesics may be required but must be used sparingly in view of the potential respiratory compromise. Intercostal nerve blocks may produce comfort and allow easier respirations in patients with rib fractures.
6. Antibiotics are reserved for demonstrated infections.

Disposition

All patients require admission to an ICU.

HEMOTHORAX

ALERT: Hemothorax can cause hypovolemic shock and respiratory failure from compression of the lung.

As a result of blunt or penetrating trauma, large amounts of blood can accumulate in the pleural space, secondary to injury to intercostal and internal mammary arteries, the heart, great vessels, or the hilar vessels. Lung lacerations usually have self-limited bleeding. Hemostasis eventually occurs in hemothorax as a result of low pulmonary arterial pressures, large concentrations of thromboplastin in lung tissue, and the compressive effects of the pleural blood volume.

Diagnostic Findings

1. With small amounts of blood loss (<10% of blood volume), diagnosis may be difficult in an isolated injury; however, more than 75% are associated with extrathoracic injuries. The physical examination usually demonstrates evidence of trauma.
2. Larger accumulations of blood (>25% of blood volume) produce pallor, restlessness, anxiety, tachycardia, vasoconstriction, and eventually, orthostatic and resting hypotension.
3. Chest examination demonstrates evidence of external trauma and decreased breath sounds. Pneumothorax is often an associated finding.

Complications
1. Respiratory failure, hypotension, and shock
2. Infection with empyema

Ancillary Data
1. Chest x-ray study demonstrates blunting of the costophrenic angle on an upright film when more than 175 ml of blood accumulates in the adolescent.
   a. A supine chest film demonstrates haziness of the affected side.
   b. Pneumothorax may be present.
   c. A lateral decubitus film may be helpful

if an upright film cannot be obtained or interpreted.

2. ABG and oximetry reflect the degree of respiratory compromise.

3. Bedside ED ultrasound has been reported to be extremely sensitive and specific in detecting the presence of fluid in the pleural cavity.

Differential Diagnosis

1. Pleural effusion of any origin, for example, CHF, pneumonia, empyema, chylothorax, or hydrothorax (from improperly placed CVP catheter)

2. Trauma: pulmonary contusion (upright or decubitus chest x-ray film should differentiate)

Management

1. Priorities should be established with respect to concurrent life-threatening injuries; that is, maintenance of oxygenation and ventilation. Fluid resuscitation is commonly needed.

2. Tube thoracostomy is the treatment required immediately, sometimes solely on the basis of respiratory distress and physical examination (see Appendix A-9).
   a. Indications:
      (1) Penetrating injury with obvious or suspected hemothorax, respiratory distress, or shock. Treatment is required immediately, before chest x-ray film.
      (2) Blunt injuries with suspected hemothorax (e.g., decreased breath sounds, multiple rib fractures), respiratory failure, or shock. Treatment is required immediately.
      (3) Unsuspected thoracic injuries in a child with multiple trauma. A chest x-ray film is usually indicated before intervention but may not always be possible.
      (4) The child in hemorrhagic shock with no evidence of internal blood loss from the abdomen, retroperitoneal space, pelvis, or external blood loss. In these patients, bilateral chest tubes may be required as a diagnostic and therapeutic modality if hemothorax is present on the chest x-ray film or if instability prevents a chest x-ray film.
   b. Size. Large-bore Silastic tubes should be used for blood drainage: newborn (8 to 12 Fr), infants (16 to 20 Fr), children (20 to 28 Fr), adolescents (28 to 42 Fr).
   c. Position: fourth or fifth intercostal space in midaxillary line directed superiorly and posteriorly. If large amounts of blood return or if the tube becomes clotted, a second chest tube one or two interspaces below the first may be required.
      NOTE: The chest tube should be connected to an underwater seal drain and 15 to 25 cm H_2O suction.

3. Autotransfusions are useful if appropriate equipment is available.

4. Thoracotomy is only rarely needed but may be lifesaving in rare circumstances:
   a. When the blood drainage from the initial thoracostomy tube is more than one third of the patient's blood volume (blood volume in child: 80 ml/kg; in adult: 70 ml/kg)
   b. With persistent bleeding more than 10% blood volume/hr
   c. With increasing hemothorax on chest x-ray film, despite therapy
   d. With persistent hypotension despite adequate crystalloid solution and blood replacement and when other areas of blood loss have been excluded
   e. Vital signs deteriorate after initial successful resuscitation
   f. Salvage is greatest in patients with penetrating chest injuries whose con-

dition does not deteriorate until arrival in the ED or is stable throughout

Disposition

All patients require admission to an ICU.

SUBCUTANEOUS EMPHYSEMA AND PNEUMOMEDIASTINUM

ALERT: The presence of subcutaneous emphysema or pneumomediastinum in a trauma patient requires a careful search for laryngeal fracture, esophageal tear, or tracheobronchial injury, as well as pneumothorax.

Air in the subcutaneous tissue or mediastinum after trauma may be caused by an underlying intrapleural leak from a pneumothorax or bronchial tear or may be secondary to a penetrating injury with spread through the fascial planes.

Traumatic bronchial disruption is rare but may result from chest compression during expiration against a closed glottis or direct shearing associated with a crushing injury. Although rare, esophageal rupture can result from a blow to the upper abdomen forceful enough to eject gastric contents into the lower esophagus under high pressure.

Etiology

1. Trauma: blunt or penetrating (usually secondary to laryngeal tear). May involve pulmonary or mediastinal structures. May be secondary to foreign body.
2. Infection: respiratory.
3. Allergy: asthma.
4. Intoxication: marijuana inhalation, smoking or inhalation of cocaine, or heroin injection—may cause increased intrathoracic pressure from Valsalva maneuver and bronchial tear.
5. Valsalva maneuver from any mechanism, including yelling, coughing, emesis.
6. Iatrogenic: after intubation of trachea or esophagus.

Diagnostic Findings

1. History of trauma or excessive Valsalva maneuver
2. Pain and crepitus overlying the upper thorax and neck
3. "Hamman crunch" on auscultation in 50% to 80% of patients

Complications

Complications are directly related to the cause (e.g., mediastinitis from perforation of esophagus secondary to contamination with gastrointestinal contents)—in contrast to the benign course of only a pneumomediastinum caused by a simple Valsalva maneuver.

Ancillary Data

1. Chest x-ray film reveals air in the tissue planes of the thorax, neck, or mediastinum.
2. Laryngoscopy, bronchoscopy, or an esophagram may be indicated to determine the cause.

Differential Diagnosis

There may be infection by gas gangrene.

Management

1. Treat underlying cause. May need surgical intervention with certain entities. Bronchial disruption may require thoracostomy or intrathoracic control of the airway reflecting the stability of the patient. Esophageal rupture necessitates a transthoracic exposure and mediastinal drainage.
2. Administer 100% oxygen to facilitate resorption secondary to nitrogen washout.
3. Administer antibiotics (penicillin or cephalosporin) if an esophageal tear is present.

Disposition

1. Hospitalize the patient to evaluate causes and facilitate nitrogen washout.
2. Follow those with benign causes as outpatients (e.g., marijuana, simple Valsalva

maneuver) if there are no complications.

DIAPHRAGMATIC RUPTURE

ALERT: Often overlooked, diaphragmatic rupture may be an asymptomatic lesion or a large herniation accompanied by severe respiratory distress. Presentation may be acute or delayed in onset. The possibility of a diaphragmatic injury should be considered in any penetrating injury to the lower chest or upper abdomen.

Diaphragmatic tears may result from blunt or penetrating forces and most often (>90%) are on the left side. Blunt abdominal compression generates increased intraabdominal pressure, which can tear the diaphragm, with herniation of the stomach, colon, small bowel, spleen, or liver. The negative intrathoracic pressures create a gradient that keeps the diaphragmatic rupture open and facilitates herniation of abdominal contents into the thorax.

Diagnostic Findings

1. Presentation varies considerably, depending on whether the signs and symptoms are acute or delayed in onset, on the side of the defect, and on the degree of herniation of abdominal organs.
2. In acute cases, patients complain of abdominal and chest pain with dyspnea, nausea, and vomiting. Delayed presentation may be accompanied by nausea, vomiting, abdominal pain, and intermittent episodes of abdominal cramping and colic, with radiation to the associated shoulder.
3. Vital signs may be normal, or there may be tachycardia, hypotension, and tachypnea.
4. A large herniation produces cardiac dullness, with displacement of the point of maximal impulse (PMI) to the right, decreased breath sounds and tympany in the left chest, and bowel sounds or borborygmi in the chest. The abdomen may be distended with obstruction or scaphoid if large amounts of abdominal contents are in the thoracic cavity.

Complication

The complication is bowel obstruction with strangulation of herniated bowel. This may be delayed in those patients with a small diaphragmatic defect secondary to penetrating injury.

Ancillary Data

1. Chest x-ray film demonstrates an elevated diaphragm (usually on the left), pleural effusion, silhouetting of the diaphragm, and bowel or viscus in the chest. There may be a mediastinal shift to the right, atelectasis, and an air-fluid bubble, or the nasogastric (NG) tube may be above the diaphragm.

   NOTE: From 20% to 40% of films are read as normal because of misinterpretation of the findings. A common error is to misread the herniated bowel and other abdominal organs as a hemopneumothorax.

2. Laparotomy for associated injuries may reveal an unsuspected diaphragmatic tear.
3. Contrast studies (diluted upper gastrointestinal [GI] or barium enema) may reveal intrathoracic abdominal contents. Usually performed in stable cases with delayed presentation.
4. Peritoneal lavage. A low red blood cell (RBC) count (>5000 RBC/ml) in the peritoneal fluid is indicative of diaphragmatic injury associated with a penetrating wound of the lower thorax and is considered positive (see Chapter 63).

Differential Diagnosis

See Chapters 14, 20, and 63.

Management

1. Stabilize the patient, with particular attention to airway management, oxygen, IV lines, and cardiac monitor. Treat life-threatening conditions and hypovolemic shock.
2. Place an NG tube for decompression of

the stomach. An NG tube may be a useful aid in diagnosis if it is visualized within the chest on x-ray film.

3. Surgery is the definitive treatment. Acute herniated bowel must be reduced and vascular compromise prevented. With delayed presentation, resection for strangulated bowel is commonly needed. The diaphragmatic surface should be explored at surgery for blunt trauma to the chest.

Disposition

Patients must be hospitalized for fluid resuscitation and surgery.

MYOCARDIAL CONTUSION

ALERT: Children with major blunt trauma to the chest and persistent tachycardia or other ECG changes require monitoring and admission for cardiac evaluation.

Myocardial contusion results from blunt trauma to the anterior midchest from auto accidents, falls, or blunt objects. Most myocardial contusions involve the right ventricle. The injury may cause a cardiac concussion with sudden disruption of cardiac activity, ventricular fibrillation, or dysrhythmias and cellular injury from edema leading to necrosis, ischemia, valvular or ventricular rupture, or pericardial tamponade.

In the multiply traumatized patient, the diagnosis can be difficult or impossible because of the more obvious presentation of associated problems such as hypovolemic shock, pneumothorax, and head trauma. The condition must be suspected in any young patient without previous heart disease who has sustained chest trauma and has a persistent, unexplained tachycardia or dysrhythmia.

Diagnostic Findings

1. Chest pain is often present with associated chest-wall trauma. Unfortunately, the pain may be delayed until several days after the injury, when cellular swelling and ischemia ensue. Chest pain is unrelieved by nitrates.

2. Patients have a persistent tachycardia and may have tachypnea caused by associated pulmonary injuries or hypotension from ventricular dysfunction.

3. Contusions or tenderness over the precordium may be present, but associated rib and sternal fractures are unusual in children because of the compliance of a child's chest wall.

4. A new murmur may be present secondary to disruption of the septum, cardiac valve, or papillary muscle. Rales may be a later finding associated with left ventricular failure or pulmonary contusion.

Complications

1. Low cardiac output state secondary to ventricular dysfunction
2. Increased sensitivity to fluid overload
3. Cardiac tamponade (muffled sounds, hypotension, and pulsus paradoxus)
4. Dysrhythmias

Ancillary Data

1. ECG.
   a. Any new finding, including persistent, unexplained sinus tachycardia and nonspecific ST-T wave changes
   b. Acute ST segment elevation or T wave inversion
   c. Any dysrhythmia (e.g., premature atrial or ventricular contractions, atrial fibrillation, or atrial flutter)
   d. New bundle branch block
2. Chest x-ray studies. May demonstrate rib or sternal fracture and associated pulmonary injury. A lateral chest view must be obtained.
3. Isoenzymes. Creatine phosphokinase (CPK-MB) band peaks within 24 hours but may not rise until days after injury at the point at which edema and ischemia occur; therefore it is not very useful and not diagnostic.
4. Radionuclide studies (ventricular angiography) have been inconsistently demon-

strated to be useful in detecting myocardial dysfunction after blunt trauma to the
chest.

5. Echocardiography (two-dimensional) is
   useful to assess wall motion and exclude
   pericardial effusion.

Management

1. Stabilize life-threatening conditions. Administer oxygen and fluids and initiate
   cardiac monitoring. Prevent overzealous
   fluid administration, which may precipitate left ventricular failure.
2. Give analgesics as required.
3. Treat dysrhythmias (see Chapter 6).
4. Treat cardiogenic shock if present (see
   Chapter 5).

Disposition

1. Patients with myocardial contusion should
   be hospitalized for at least 24 to 72 hours
   for monitoring in the following situations:
   a. Anterior chest wall injury secondary to
      violent blunt trauma
   b. Persistent tachycardia when other
      causes have been ruled out
   c. Any changes on ECG or signs of dys-
      rhythmia
   d. As required by associated injuries
2. If tachycardia has subsided and if the
   home environment is adequate, the patient with no signs of cardiac dysfunction
   need not be hospitalized.
3. Long-term resolution usually occurs within a year of injury.

PERICARDIAL TAMPONADE

ALERT: With an overlying penetrating wound, hypotension, distended neck veins (increased CVP),
tachycardia, and muffled or faint heart sounds require
immediate pericardiocentesis after tension pneumothorax has been ruled out. If vital signs are unstable,
thoracotomy should be considered.

Penetrating wounds of the chest may injure the
pericardium or myocardium, resulting in pericardial pressure and volume with resultant
impaired diastolic filling, increased CVP, hypotension, and tachycardia.

Diagnostic Findings

Patients are agitated and hypoxic and have
poor peripheral circulation, elevated CVP,
tachycardia, and hypotension. A penetrating wound to any area of the thorax, epigas-
trium, or supraclavicular area may result in
tamponade.

1. A paradoxical pulse greater than 10 mm
   Hg is usually present.
2. If hypovolemic shock is present, the neck
   veins may not be distended until the
   patient is resuscitated with fluid.
3. Beck's triad (hypotension, increased venous pressure with distended neck veins,
   and muffled, distant heart sounds) is not
   usually present in the acutely traumatized
   patient.
4. If bradycardia occurs, the patient is about
   to arrest. Tamponade must be relieved
   immediately.

Complications are hypovolemic and cardiogenic shock and death.

Ancillary Data

1. Chest x-ray film is usually nondiagnostic.
2. ECG may have nonspecific ST-T wave
   changes and low voltage. ECG has no
   pathognomonic changes. In rare cases,
   pulsus alternans may be seen with chronic
   effusion.
3. Echocardiography demonstrates pericardial fluid. It is often useful on an emergency basis to diagnose the tamponade
   and provide bedside direction of the
   pericardiocentesis needle.

Differential Diagnosis

1. Constrictive pericarditis (p. 564)
2. Tension pneumothorax

Management

1. Initiate resuscitation, including oxygen, fluids, and cardiac monitoring. Consider active airway and ventilatory support.
2. Obtain immediate ED bedside cardiac ultrasound if available.
3. Insert CVP catheter.
4. An initial fluid push of 0.9% normal saline (NS) solution, 10-20 ml/kg over 20 minutes, may provide support of blood pressure while preparing for a pericardiocentesis.
5. Pericardiocentesis may be a lifesaving procedure that permits temporary improvement in cardiac output. Rarely is a patient stable enough to permit a diagnostic evaluation such as an echocardiogram before pericardiocentesis; this technology is becoming increasingly available on an emergency basis (see Appendix A-5).
   a. An 18-gauge metal spinal needle is attached to a syringe by a three-way stopcock. If a rhythm is present, one end of an alligator clip is fastened to the needle's base and the other end to chest lead V of the ECG with the limb leads attached normally.
   b. The needle is introduced into the left subxiphoid region and aimed cephalad and backward, toward the tip of the right scapula, exerting constant negative pressure on the attached syringe.
   c. On contact with the epicardium, the ECG will demonstrate an injury current, and the needle should be withdrawn slightly. This should be the pericardial space.
   d. Aspiration of even a few milliliters of blood may provide temporary decompression.
   e. A negative pericardiocentesis does not exclude the possibility of a pericardial tamponade.
6. Thoracotomy is indicated in the arrested patient, particularly in the presence of electromechanical dissociation, or if the patient has become bradycardic or has lost vital signs. The pericardial sac may be very tense if it is filled with blood and may require pericardiotomy with a scalpel rather than a scissors.

   NOTE: A tense tamponade should not be mistaken for adhesive pericarditis.
7. Definitive surgical care is the ultimate treatment. The patient should be moved expeditiously to the operating room once the diagnosis is made and the patient is temporarily stabilized.
8. If pericardiocentesis is positive, it may help to leave a catheter in the pericardial space. Even if the catheter does not drain, it may relieve the pressure in the pericardial space. If the patient's condition deteriorates again, the pericardiocentesis should be immediately repeated and subxiphoid pericardiotomy considered.

Disposition

1. Immediately transport the patient to the operating room.
2. If a thoracic surgeon or trauma surgeon is not available, repeated pericardiocentesis may be needed to allow transfer to an appropriate facility.

AORTIC INJURY

ALERT: Violent acceleration-deceleration injuries with associated chest trauma, upper rib fractures, or widened mediastinum require emergent evaluation.

Injury to the aorta may result from acceleration-deceleration injuries occurring in automobile accidents (usually front seat occupants), falls from heights, or from sudden massive compression injuries, resulting in a shearing force on the mobile aorta at points of fixation, most commonly at the isthmus distal to the left subclavian artery. Injury may also result from pressure waves generated in the aorta by the compression and decompression.

High-risk injuries include those at high speed (>45 mph accident), where there is chest trauma, fractured first or second ribs, or damage caused by the steering wheel.

Diagnostic Findings

1. Patients complain initially of retrosternal or interscapular pain, although the location may change with progression of the dissection. Dyspnea, stridor, and dysphagia occur secondary to pressure of a hematoma on the left recurrent laryngeal nerve, trachea, and esophagus. Ischemic extremity pain may be present.
2. A harsh systolic murmur of the precordium and interscapular area develops.
   a. A pseudocoarctation syndrome with upper extremity hypertension and decreased femoral pulses may be noted. Carotid bruits may be present with decreased carotid pulse and a pulsatile mass at the base of the neck.
   b. Generalized hypertension may occur.

Complications

Hypovolemic shock and death are common (80% to 90%) secondary to rupture.

Ancillary Data

1. Standard upright chest x-ray film if the patient is stable enough (supine chest film result may be falsely positive and normalize when repeated as an upright)
   a. Widened or indistinct mediastinum (in adult >8 cm at superior margin of anterior fourth rib and proportionately less in children) present in 50% to 85% of patients (exclude upper thoracic spinal fracture)
   b. Blurring of the aortic knob with loss of sharp aortic outline
   c. Depression of the left mainstem bronchus
   d. Left pleural effusion
   e. Deviation of an NG tube to the right at the T4 level
   f. A left apical pleural cap

2. Diagnostic studies
   a. Aortography is the definitive study in establishing the diagnosis. It is indicated if the patient is stable enough to tolerate it. If abdominal CT scan is positive for intraabdominal injury and the patient is hemodynamically unstable, an aortogram is usually done after laparotomy.
   b. A dynamic CT scan may be obtained to ascertain the presence of a periaortic hematoma.
   c. Transesophageal ultrasonography may be helpful in the diagnosis of aortic dissection.

Management

1. Supportive resuscitation measures, including oxygen, fluids, blood.
2. Immediate thoracic surgical consultation.
   a. Obtain thoracic aortogram or dynamic chest CT scan.
   b. If the patient is unstable, immediate surgery is indicated, sometimes without aortography.
3. Exclusion of concomitant intraabdominal injuries. If the result of peritoneal lavage or abdominal CT scan is positive, the abdomen should be explored before aortography.
4. Problem of concomitant head injury. Aortic evaluation needs to follow resuscitation of the abdomen and head.

REFERENCES

Bonodio WA, Hellmich T: Post-traumatic pulmonary contusion in children, *Ann Emerg Med* 18:1050, 1989.

Cooper A, Foltin GL: Thoracic trauma. In Barkin RM, editor: *Pediatric emergency medicine: concepts and clinical practice,* ed 2, St Louis, 1997, Mosby.

Eddy AC, Rusch VW, Fligner CL, et al: The epidemiology of traumatic rupture of the thoracic aorta in children: a 13-year review, *J Trauma* 30:989, 1990.

Garcia VF, Gotschall LS, Eichelberger MR, et al: Rib fractures in children: a marker of severe trauma, *J Trauma* 30:695, 1990.

Helling TS, Duke P, Beggs CW, et al: A prospective evaluation of 68 patients suffering blunt chest trauma for cardiac injury, *J Trauma* 29:961, 1989.

Kearney PA, Rouhana SW, Burney RE: Blunt rupture of the diaphragm: mechanism, diagnosis and treatment, *Ann Emerg Med* 18:1326, 1989.

Ma JO, Mateer JR: Trauma ultrasound examination versus chest radiography in the detection of hemothorax, *Ann Emerg Med* 29:312, 1997.

Marnocha KE, Maglinte DDT, Woods J, et al: Blunt chest trauma and suspected aortic rupture: reliability of chest radiograph findings, *Ann Emerg Med* 14:644, 1985.

Mattox KL, Bickell W, Pepe PE, et al: Prospective MAST study in 911 patients, *J Trauma* 29:1104, 1989.

Mellner JL, Little AG, Shermata DW: Thoracic trauma in children, *Pediatrics* 74:813, 1984.

Nakayama DK, Ramenofsky ML: Chest injuries in children, *Ann Surg* 210:770, 1989.

Rothenberg SS, Moore EE, Moore FA, et al: Emergency department thoracotomy in children: a critical analysis, *J Trauma* 29:1322, 1989.

Shapiro MJ, Yanofsky SD, Trupp J, et al: Cardiovascular evaluation in blunt thoracic trauma using transesophageal echocardiography (TEE), *J Trauma* 31:835, 1991.

Tenzer ML: The spectrum of myocardial contusion: a review, *J Trauma* 25:620, 1985.

Vukich DJ, Markovchick VJ: Thoracic trauma. In Rosen P, editor: *Emergency medicine: concepts and clinical practice,* ed 4, St Louis, 1998, Mosby.

63 ABDOMINAL TRAUMA

ROGER M. BARKIN and JOHN A. MARX

ALERT: Intraabdominal trauma poses an immediate threat to life. Aggressive volume resuscitation and timely peritoneal lavage, surgical consultation, and laparotomy are the foundations of therapy. Multisystem involvement is common.

In 80% to 90% of trauma cases, intraabdominal injuries are the result of blunt trauma. Hypovolemia in the presence of significant blunt trauma requires that intraperitoneal hemorrhage be excluded.

MECHANISM OF INJURY
Blunt Trauma

Blunt trauma injuries are caused primarily by motor vehicles, falls, contact sports, and child abuse. With infants and small children, pedestrian accidents predominate because of the child's limited ability to avoid or respond to potentially dangerous traffic situations. Passenger injuries are more common among adolescents. Auto accidents involving a shoulder-lap belt cause rib and lumbar spine fractures and duodenal and jejunal perforations; injuries involving a lap belt produce contusion or perforation of the intestine or mesentery. The use of motor bikes poses an increasing hazard. Inflicted injury may present a diagnostic dilemma.

The spleen and then the liver are the most likely organs to be injured, whereas small-bowel contusions and perforations are the most frequent type of damage to the hollow viscus. The rib cage in the child, although resilient and less prone to fracture, affords only partial protection for the liver and spleen. Intraabdominal injuries are often part of a multisystem disorder resulting from vehicular accidents. Injury to two or more intraabdominal organs occurs in up to 30% of blunt trauma victims.

Type of Injury
1. Crush injuries occur with compression of organs between external forces and the posterior thoracic cage or spine, resulting in contusions, lacerations, or disruption.
2. Shear injuries occur when acceleration and deceleration forces cause tearing of viscera and vascular pedicles, particularly at relatively fixed points of attachment.
3. Burst injury of hollow viscera follows the generation of sudden and pronounced increases in intraabdominal pressure (e.g., by seat belts).

Penetrating Injuries

In children less than 13 years old, penetrating injuries are likely to be caused by accidental impalement on objects such as scissors or picket fences or by accidental discharge of a weapon. In patients older than 13 years, 75% of penetrating trauma injuries are knife or handgun wounds inflicted by an assailant.

1. *Stab wounds* to the abdomen cause intraperitoneal organ damage in 30% of cases. Penetration of the peritoneum occurs 50% to 60% of the time.
2. *Gunshot wounds* enter the peritoneal cavity in 85% of cases, causing visceral injury in 95% to 99% of patients who have intraperitoneal penetration.
3. Penetrating trauma to the lower chest (below the fourth intercostal space anteriorly and the sixth to the seventh space laterally and posteriorly) places the abdomen and diaphragm at risk. In those with lower chest penetration, coincident injury to the diaphragm or peritoneal cavity occurs in 25% to 40% of cases. The peritoneal cavity may also be entered via back or flank wounds.

DIAGNOSTIC FINDINGS
History

The ability to obtain an accurate history may be compromised by the urgency of the situation, communication skills of the child, concomitant intracranial injuries, reluctance of parents, and interfering toxic agents (e.g., drugs or alcohol). Information about underlying cardiorespiratory disease, coagulopathies, and medication usage will help guide volume resuscitation.

With vehicular trauma it is helpful to know the amount of damage to the automobile and what, if any, restraint systems were used for the child. With penetrating injuries the type of weapon, number of shots or stabs inflicted, and blood loss at the scene should be ascertained.

Child abuse should be suspected when the child has difficulty or fear relating the circumstances of the injury or if the history is inconsistent with the injuries.

1. Volume loss secondary to acute hemorrhage (solid viscera or vascular) or later development of bacterial or chemical peritonitis (hollow viscus or pancreas) leads to inadequate perfusion, causing dizziness and confusion. With orthostatic hypotension, these may only be seen with the assumption of upright posture.
2. Pain is usually caused by hematic, infectious, or enzymatic irritation of the peritoneum. It may be localized or diffuse. Diminished ability to sense pain (e.g., because of alcohol, concussion, or spinal injury), ineffectual communication, or significant injury elsewhere may impair the recognition of abdominal pain.
   - Splenic and liver injury can cause diaphragmatic irritation and radiation of pain to the ipsilateral shoulder, especially when the patient is in the Trendelenburg position.
3. Nausea and vomiting are nonspecific (e.g., peritoneal irritation or obstruction caused by a duodenal hematoma).

Physical Findings

Physical findings are unreliable in 30% to 40% of cases, particularly in those in which central nervous system (CNS) trauma coexists. Serial examinations by a single observer are invaluable, especially with the patient whose sensorium is clearing.

1. All clothing must be removed to allow careful inspection of axilla, skin folds, and scalp for entrance and exit wounds.
2. Inspection may reveal superficial abrasions or contusions, which are often deceptively unremarkable in most cases of intraabdominal injury.
3. Acute hypotension is caused by hemorrhage from a solid organ or by major vessel injury. Hypotension may be delayed when there is third spacing or significant vomiting with pancreatitis or hollow-viscus damage. Delayed findings occur hours to days after trauma. Splenic injuries are usually obvious immediately but in rare cases may also have delayed presentations.
4. Tenderness is found in up to 90% of patients with intraabdominal abnormality and alert mental status. It may be localized

to the quadrant of injury (e.g., spleen, liver), or it may be diffuse. Abdominal rebound, tenderness, and rigidity are more specific but less common.

5. Bowel sounds may be decreased or absent and can be helpful in predicting intraperitoneal injury. However, they may be present with significant injury or absent as a result of vertebral fractures, electrolyte disturbances, or other pathologic conditions.

6. Gastrointestinal (GI) hemorrhage may follow blunt or penetrating trauma and is identified with nasogastric (NG) tube placement and rectal examination.

7. Acute distension secondary to hemorrhage requires extreme intravascular volume loss and is accompanied by profound shock. It may occur gradually secondary to third spacing from peritonitis.

8. Pregnant patients with major trauma or obstetric problems, such as vaginal bleeding, uterine tenderness, uterine contractions, or ruptured membrane, should be observed for at least 24 hours with cardiotocographic monitoring. Pregnant patients with a gestational age greater than 24 weeks experiencing deceleration injuries, falls, or abdominal trauma should undergo cardiotocographic monitoring for at least 4 hours.

Ancillary Data

Laboratory evaluation should reflect routine management of multisystem trauma as outlined in Chapter 56.

1. Hematocrit (Hct) must be obtained early and followed throughout the period of observation. If hemorrhage has been acute, a normal initial Hct finding may be misleading. Changes reflect the baseline Hct, volume, and rate of blood loss, endogenous plasma refill, and parenteral fluid administration.

2. White blood cell (WBC) elevation occurs within several hours and may last for several days; it is a nonspecific response to injury. A prolonged leukocytosis may be seen with visceral injury and bacterial or chemical peritonitis.

3. Elevated serum amylase level is an insensitive and nonspecific marker of pancreatic or proximal small bowel injury. Persistently high or increasing values may be suggestive.

4. Other routine laboratory studies should reflect clinical condition and mechanism of injury but may include type and cross-match, platelet count, electrolytes, blood urea nitrogen (BUN), liver enzymes, arterial blood gas (ABG), and toxicologic screen. Hematuria should be excluded (see Chapter 64).

Diagnostic Peritoneal Lavage

Diagnostic peritoneal lavage (DPL) is a safe and extremely sensitive (98%) method of detecting intraperitoneal hemorrhage. However, it is neither organ- or injury-specific and is not useful in assessing retroperitoneal injury. It is particularly valuable in triaging the blunt trauma patient with hemodynamic instability to urgent laparotomy. It is reliable in clinical settings with limited imaging or monitoring capacity or without experience in the nonoperative management of trauma. A positive DPL by red blood cell (RBC) criterion or gross aspirate should be supplemented by an abdominal computed tomography (CT) scan if the patient is stable and the institution is capable of expectant (i.e., nonoperative) management. DPL is also useful in patients who are unconscious, are intoxicated, or require immediate general anesthesia for repair of life-threatening intracranial or axial skeletal injury. Patients in whom the integrity of the bowel is at risk, usually as a result of a penetrating mechanism, may be more accurately and expeditiously evaluated by DPL. DPL is relatively insensitive for small bowel and pancreatic injuries. A positive DPL result is often supplemented by an abdominal CT scan in stable patients.

1. Blunt trauma
   a. Acutely injured and unstable patients

with multiple trauma who have sustained a major mechanism of injury.

(1) Unreliable examination because of CNS or spinal cord injury, alcohol or drug intoxication, or communication barriers.

(2) Unexplained hypotension in the field or emergency department (ED).

(3) General anesthesia is required for immediate repair of life-threatening intracranial or axial skeletal injury.

b. Penetrating injury.

(1) Local stab wound exploration that is:

(a) Positive or equivocal

(b) Contraindicated or technically difficult because of low chest penetration or multiple stab wounds

(2) Gunshot wound with questionable peritoneal cavity penetration.

2. Contraindications

a. Absolute: Indications for laparotomy already exist.

b. Relative: Technically difficult because of previous abdominal surgery or intraperitoneal infection and adhesions, pregnancy, or massive obesity.

3. Procedures

a. A decompressive NG tube and urinary catheter should be placed.

b. Percutaneous entry via the Seldinger (guide wire) technique is more rapidly performed, may have comparable accuracy and incidence of complications, and is becoming more popular in the evaluation of children.

The semiopen method involves establishing a sterile field and injecting local anesthesia. Entry is done infraumbilically through the anterior rectus sheath. The catheter tip is directed through the peritoneum toward the pelvis. The fully open technique requires direct visualization of the peritoneum and is used when technical obstacles are considerable to ensure safety and accuracy.

Aspiration of 10 ml or more of free blood in adults (lesser amounts may be positive in pediatric patients) is positive. If this does not occur, 15 ml/kg (adult: 1 L) of normal saline solution should be instilled and recovered by gravity drainage. This procedure is usually done after surgical consultation.

4. Results of studies on the recovered peritoneal fluid that are indicative of a positive tap and intraperitoneal hemorrhage in adults:

a. RBC criterion is the most accurate parameter of peritoneal lavage fluid.

Type of trauma	RBC (per mm³) in peritoneal fluid
Blunt	>100,000
Penetrating stab wound	(20,000-1,000,000: equivocal)
	>100,000
Anterior abdomen*	(20,000-100,000: equivocal)
Lower chest†	>5000
Flank/back	>100,000 (20,000-100,000: equivocal)
Penetrating gunshot wound	>5000

*Inferior to costal margin to groin creases between anterior axillary lines.
†Between the fourth intercostal space anteriorly; seventh intercostal space posteriorly; and the costal margins. This incorporates the area of possible diaphragmatic excursion. Lavage in patients with possible diaphragmatic injury is considered to yield a positive finding at more than 5000 RBC/mm³.

b. Elevated lavage amylase (>20 IU/L) and alkaline phosphatase (>3 IU/L) may occur immediately after injury of the small bowel. A positive lavage WBC count (>500/mm³) is insensitive for 4 to 6 hours after injury, nonspecific, and should not be a sole indicator for laparotomy. Bile and Gram stains are of relatively little use in acute trauma.

c. If the initial results are equivocal, a repeat lavage in 4 to 6 hours may be diagnostic.

NOTE: Few data exist for children. These guidelines attempt to minimize missed significant injury, accepting a low rate of negative laparotomy.

Radiologic Studies

X-ray studies should be performed only after initial stabilization and when additional diagnostic data are necessary for management. Patients suspected of having serious injuries must be monitored by experienced personnel in the radiology suite.

1. Plain films are useful to detect small quantities of free intraperitoneal air, but normal study findings do not exclude a perforation. Patients should be maintained in the upright or left-lateral decubitus position, if possible, for 10 to 15 minutes before the x-ray film is taken to mobilize air. Peritoneal lavage causes iatrogenic pneumoperitoneum. Retroperitoneal rupture of a hollow viscus reveals a stippling pattern, outlining the duodenum, kidney, or psoas margins. Foreign bodies and missiles, hemoperitoneum, and skeletal fractures may be visualized or localized.

    NOTE: The incidence of free air caused by acute injury is so rare that one need not delay peritoneal lavage to obtain a negative preliminary film finding.

2. Ultrasound is of value in quickly discerning free intraperitoneal hemorrhage. Lesions that are easily identified include pancreatic pseudocyst, viable fetus, and enlargement of the pancreas, liver, or spleen. It is more limited in defining solid visceral injury and retroperitoneal injury. It may be of value in evaluating cardiac function. It does not show anatomic detail.

3. CT scan offers simultaneous visualization of all organs in the peritoneal cavity and retroperitoneum. It defines intra-

abdominal hemorrhage and the extent of damage to solid viscera. It may also facilitate concurrent intracranial evaluation.

A double-contrast (intravenous [IV] and enteral) CT scan provides a valuable adjunct in determining the presence and extent of hepatosplenic and retroperitoneal compartment injury and is commonly done when this modality is selected. Oral contrast may improve sensitivity for pancreatic injury but does not help identify injuries requiring surgical treatment. However, it is insensitive for GI perforation and intraluminal lesions even with oral contrast. Diaphragmatic injury and significant pancreatic pathology can also be missed.

CT scan alone is probably sufficient in patients with hemodynamic stability and no alteration in responsiveness. It may also be useful in stable patients undergoing DPL who have a positive DPL red cell count finding and an associated pelvic fracture or suspected isolated solid visceral injury, equivocal DPL results, or technical difficulties in performing the DPL.

On CT scan, solid organ injuries appear as a loss of homogeneity or disruption of the cortex. Hematoma appears as a nonenhanced collection of fluids that displaces normal anatomic relationships. Hollow-organ perforation may be identified by intraabdominal free air or extravasated contrast. An organ's failure to be enhanced with IV contrast material may suggest that a vascular injury has occurred.

4. Contrast studies may be useful in stable patients without life-threatening conditions. Intramural duodenal hematomas are best diagnosed with barium. Water-soluble contrast (Gastrografin) medium should be used for suspected gastric,

duodenal, and rectal perforations. An intravenous pyelogram (IVP) is indicated in the blunt trauma patient with significant posttraumatic hematuria if CT has not been performed or is unavailable. With a penetrating mechanism an IVP is necessary for entry proximate to the genitourinary (GU) tract irrespective of the presence of hematuria (see Chapter 64). Only limited studies may be indicated before laparotomy in the compensated but unstable patient.

5. Radionuclide studies. Liver-spleen studies are accurate in detecting subcapsular hematomas, parenchymal damage, lacerations, and intraparenchymal hematomas and may be particularly useful in the stable patient with these suspected injuries. CT scans, because of the additional information provided, have largely supplanted this technique for acute evaluation. Ongoing management of conservatively managed splenic injuries may be monitored by this modality.

6. Angiography is the most accurate method for visualizing vascular injury and active bleeding but has limited application in acute trauma.

7. Laparoscopy is a promising tool in experienced hands for the investigation of penetrating trauma, particularly to the low chest, flank, and back.

MANAGEMENT
General Principles

Resuscitation of the injured child must be tailored to the specific requirements of the patient and the nature of the trauma. Aggressive and systematic treatment, as outlined in Chapter 56, becomes crucial in view of the frequency of associated injuries in abdominal trauma. Delivery of adequate replacement fluid is critical. In the stable patient, extensive evaluation and diagnostic studies may be appropriately performed to establish the nature of the injuries and the patient's status. Immediate thoracotomy or laparotomy may be indicated under the following circumstances:

1. Blunt trauma
   a. Hemodynamic instability despite adequate volume resuscitation with strongly suspected or documented intraperitoneal hemorrhage
   b. Transfusion requirement greater than 50% of estimated blood volume
   c. Physical signs of peritonitis
   d. Positive peritoneal lavage (see earlier discussion)
   e. Radiologic evidence of pneumoperitoneum, diaphragmatic injury, intraperitoneal bladder rupture, or renovascular pedicle injury

2. Penetrating trauma
   a. Gunshot wounds with hemodynamic instability or suspected intraperitoneal penetration.
   b. All stab wounds with hemodynamic instability; positive DPL; GI blood; radiologic evidence of retroperitoneal air; implement in-situ; positive laparoscopy. Evisceration is a relative indication for operation.

Certain general principles apply. The emergency physician must make the initial assessment and stabilization while organizing resources within the ED. Assignment of specific tasks to members of the team should be rapid, preferably before the patient's arrival. Surgical staff should be contacted as early as possible to assist in the management of the patient.

Primary Assessment

This must ensure an adequate airway and ventilation and treatment of shock, when appropriate. The spine requires immobilization in multiply traumatized patients with suspected spinal injury and in those with altered mental status from blunt trauma injuries (pending spine films) (see Chapter 61).

1. All patients require oxygen and cardiac monitoring on arrival. Initiate airway intervention, as appropriate.
2. Remove clothing while vital signs are being obtained.
3. Hemorrhage is the immediate threat to life. Place large-bore catheters as dictated by the clinical situation. A central line may be required for monitoring if there is intercurrent cardiothoracic pathology or if it is necessary to gain rapid venous access.

   Initially, give a rapid bolus of 0.9% NS or lactated Ringer's (LR) solution, 20 ml/kg IV. Additional administration of crystalloid solution must reflect the response to the initial infusion and the presence of ongoing hemorrhage. In general, once 40-50 ml/kg of crystalloid solution has been infused during the initial resuscitation, blood should be administered if evidence of hypovolemia persists.
4. Initial laboratory studies are required. Do a hematocrit in the ED, and send a clot of blood for type and cross-match. An ABG determination may be helpful.
5. Other considerations.
   a. An NG tube will decompress the stomach, permitting improved ventilation and a more reliable examination. It will assist in determining whether there is upper GI hemorrhage.
   b. A urinary catheter is required to monitor urinary output and to help monitor fluid management. The urethral meatus should be examined for blood. The presence of blood precludes insertion.
   c. Reassessment is constantly required, with ongoing measures of vital signs and serial examinations by the same examiner. Once the primary assessment has been completed, a more extensive physical examination should be done and history obtained.
6. Perform an early rectal examination to assess the integrity of spinal cord function, exclude GI bleeding, and evaluate the prostate.
7. It is easy to overlook trauma to the thoracic or lumbar spine and the bony pelvis. These should be cleared with chest, abdomen, and pelvic x-ray studies as required.

Blunt Trauma (Fig. 63-1)

Certain victims of blunt trauma are candidates for immediate laparotomy after the initial resuscitation. In hemodynamically stable patients, further diagnostic evaluations and expectant management may be suitable.

1. Perform urgent laparotomy (as above) after stabilizing measures.
2. Conservative management is appropriate when physicians experienced in pediatric abdominal trauma are present and the facilities and personnel necessary for intensive observation of the child are available. Onset of instability, progressive abdominal findings, or the need for extensive blood transfusions (>40 ml/kg) to supplement crystalloid solution mandate operative intervention. Criteria for observation in a nontrauma center should be more stringent, favoring earlier surgical intervention or transfer with trained personnel to a better-equipped facility.
3. Pregnancy presents unique problems. By 12 weeks of pregnancy, the uterus grows out of the protective pelvis. Unique complications may include uterine rupture and abruptio placentae. Management should include resuscitation and prolonged fetal monitoring usually in consultation with an obstetrician.

Splenic Injury

This is associated with variable intraabdominal bleeding. Some patients may have massive bleeding. Left upper quadrant pain, guarding, and rigidity, as well as left shoulder pain, may be present.

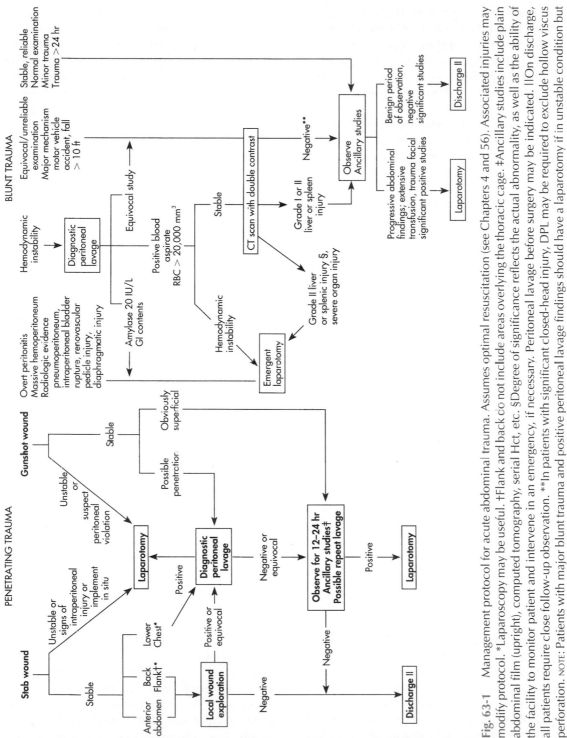

Fig. 63-1 Management protocol for acute abdominal trauma. Assumes optimal resuscitation (see Chapters 4 and 56). Associated injuries may modify protocol. *Laparoscopy may be useful. †Flank and back do not include areas overlying the thoracic cage. ‡Ancillary studies include plain abdominal film (upright), computed tomography; serial Hct, etc. §Degree of significance reflects the actual abnormality, as well as the ability of the facility to monitor patient and intervene in an emergency, if necessary. Peritoneal lavage before surgery may be indicated. ‖On discharge, all patients require close follow-up observation. **In patients with significant closed-head injury, DPL may be required to exclude hollow viscus perforation. NOTE: Patients with major blunt trauma and positive peritoneal lavage findings should have a laparotomy if in unstable condition but may be considered for observation and ancillary studies if in stable condition if adequate support services are available.

1. Splenectomy increases a patient's risk of overwhelming infection 65-fold. Therefore maximal splenic preservation is attempted whenever possible, using splenoplasty, partial splenectomy, hemostatic agents, and more recently, autotransplantation. Stable patients with defined injuries after blunt trauma may be managed in a nonoperative fashion with close monitoring. Patients with penetrating abdominal trauma are not candidates for nonoperative management because of the high incidence of associated injuries. Total splenectomy rarely is required and is reserved for the pulverized, nonsalvageable organ.

2. Laparotomy is indicated for the unstable patient with suspected splenic trauma.

3. A CT scan should be obtained in stable patients with suspected splenic trauma. The need for laparotomy (major laceration or hematoma), for close intensive observation with serial Hct (minor laceration), or for minimal observation (normal study) is dictated by the clinical status and results of the scan.

    NOTE: Children with positive scan findings who do not require surgery should be maintained at bed rest with daily Hct for 1 week. During this period, the rate of bleeding and the results of physical examination and monitoring parameters are the main determinants of the need for laparotomy.

    It is essential not to be lulled into a false sense of security; splenic lacerations that have ceased active bleeding and previously contained subcapsular hematomas may subsequently leak or rupture, classically on days 3 to 5 after injury.

    More than 4 units of blood in adults (or relative equivalent in children) over 48 hours or progressive peritoneal irritation necessitates laparotomy. Patients may return to full activity after 2 to 6 months of convalescence and a normal study finding on repeat CT or liver-spleen scan.

4. If splenectomy must be performed, it should optimally be accompanied by omental implantation of splenic remnants. Patients should receive vaccine to provide prophylaxis against *Streptococcus pneumoniae* and *Haemophilus influenzae* as soon as possible before (or after if necessary) operation.

Liver Injury

The liver is the second major source of hemorrhage from blunt trauma but tends to result in more massive hemorrhage; one third of patients die before transport. It is the major cause of immediate mortality related to abdominal trauma. With significant injury, patients may be in shock or have protuberant abdomens and right upper quadrant or diffuse abdominal pain.

The same basic principles of splenic management apply to injuries to the liver, although there is rarely time for diagnostic studies beyond peritoneal lavage.

Pancreatic and Duodenal Injuries

Because these structures have a retroperitoneal location, signs and symptoms may be obscure and delayed.

Pancreatic contusions, the most common type of injury to the pancreas, cause variable degrees of midepigastric, diffuse abdominal, or back pain. Lacerations cause focal hemorrhage and release of enzymatic contents toxic to the surrounding tissues. If this contamination is contained within the lesser sac, severe localized abdominal and back pain may be present. With leakage, there is diffuse chemical peritonitis. Elevated or rising serum or peritoneal lavage amylase levels may be seen. Conservative therapy with NG suction and parenteral nutrition is helpful. Worsening clinical signs may prompt surgical exploration.

Trauma is the leading cause of pancreatic pseudocysts in children and may occur days to months after injury. Capsulized collections of pancreatic secretions and debris form in the lesser sac, causing chronic, intermittent attacks of abdominal pain, nausea, vomiting, and weight loss. Ultrasound and CT scans are valuable in securing the diagnosis. Resolution may occur spontaneously. Otherwise, surgery is required.

Duodenal intramural hematoma causes signs and symptoms of proximal intestinal obstruction. The diagnosis is confirmed by barium contrast studies. Transection of the duodenum should be specifically considered if the barium does not at least partially pass, if extravasation has occurred, or if there is unexplained diffuse abdominal tenderness. The hematoma often resolves after 8 to 10 days of conservative management, including an NG tube and parenteral nutrition. Surgery is necessary if this approach fails. Duodenal perforations cause a range of abdominal pain and tenderness, often developing hours after injury. Intraabdominal or retroperitoneal free air may be demonstrated radiographically. Surgery is necessary.

Bowel Injuries

Injury to the remainder of the small bowel or colon may also lead to subtle or delayed findings. Perforation usually results in signs of peritonitis 4 to 12 hours after injury and radiologic evidence of free air. Elevations in peritoneal lavage enzymatic markers may be diagnostic immediately after injury.

Penetrating Wounds (see Fig. 63-1)

Stab Wounds

1. Immediate exploration is required for hemodynamically unstable patients or for those with clear physical or radiographic evidence of intraperitoneal injury (peritoneal irritation, significant GI bleeding, evisceration, evidence of diaphragmatic injury, or positive peritoneal lavage finding).

2. In the stable, cooperative child, local wound exploration with meticulous hemostasis and possible extension of the wound to facilitate inspection are used to assess the extent of the penetration. An equivocal examination result must be considered positive.

    a. If the end of the wound tract is clearly demonstrated superficial to the posterior rectus fascia, wound care is pro-

vided and the patient may be safely discharged if the stab wound was an isolated injury.

    b. If the end cannot be clearly seen or if the peritoneum is violated, peritoneal lavage or laparoscopy should be performed. If results are negative or equivocal, observation for 12 to 24 hours with additional studies and possible repeat lavage are indicated. Positive lavage results are an indication for laparotomy.

3. The care of flank and back wounds (excluding areas overlying the thoracic cage) should be individualized. Because retroperitoneal structures are at greater risk, peritoneal lavage may not be diagnostic, and other ancillary diagnostic techniques such as CT scan with contrast or laparoscopy may be helpful. Local wound exploration is useful for superficial entry.

4. Penetrating injury from lower chest (below the fourth intercostal space anteriorly or sixth to seventh posteriorly) wounds places the abdomen at risk. However, deep local wound exploration over the rib cage is hazardous and contraindicated because of the risk of causing a pneumothorax. Peritoneal lavage is the most accurate determinant of diaphragmatic injury and should be performed unless other clinical evidence dictates the need for laparotomy.

Gunshot Wounds

The incidence of intraabdominal injury exceeds 95% when the missile has entered the peritoneal cavity. Therefore the criteria for selective management are greatly restricted as compared with stab wounds.

1. Unstable patients are immediately explored. When peritoneal violation is suspected on the basis of entrance and exit wounds or radiographic findings or if other evidence of intraabdominal injury exists (peritoneal irritation, evisceration, evidence of diaphragmatic injury, free

intraperitoneal air, or positive peritoneal lavage finding), perform laparotomy.

2. Local wound exploration is technically more difficult and less reliable. It is not generally used. Observe patients with obviously superficial injuries. For those in whom an intraabdominal penetration is unclear, perform peritoneal lavage.

3. If the situation permits, perform peritoneal lavage in patients with lower chest gunshot wounds to ascertain existence of concomitant diaphragmatic or intraabdominal injury. Many times these patients require immediate thoracic surgery, which precludes the need for peritoneal lavage.

4. There is limited experience with laparoscopy in gunshot wounds. It may be useful in the determination of intraperitoneal penetration and injury as well as diaphragmatic entry.

REFERENCES

Bocka J, Courtney J, Pearlman M, et al: Trauma in pregnancy, *Ann Emerg Med* 17:829, 1988.

Bresler MJ: Computed tomography of the abdomen, *Ann Emerg Med* 15:280, 1986.

Foltin GL, Cooper AP: Abdominal trauma. In Barkin RM, editor: *Pediatric emergency medicine: concepts and clinical practice*, ed 2, St Louis, 1997, Mosby.

Giacomantonio M, Filler RM, Rich RH: Blunt hepatic trauma in children: experience with operative and nonoperative management, *J Pediatr Surg* 19:519, 1984.

Graham JS, Wong AT: A review of computed tomography in the diagnosis of intestinal and mesenteric injury in pediatric blunt abdominal trauma, *J Pediatr Surg* 31:754, 1996.

Harris BH, Barlow BA, Ballantine TV, et al: American Pediatric Surgical Association: principles of trauma care, *J Pediatr Surg* 27:423, 1992.

Healy M, Simon R, Winchell R, et al: A prospective evaluation of abdominal ultrasound in blunt trauma: is it useful? *J Trauma* 42:220, 1996.

Henneman P, Marx JA, Cantrill SC, et al: The use of an emergency department observation unit in the management of abdominal trauma, *Ann Emerg Med* 18:647, 1989.

Kane NM, Cronan JJ, Dorfman GS, et al: Pediatric abdominal trauma: evaluation by computed tomography, *Pediatrics* 82:11, 1988.

Karp MP, Cooney DR, Pros GA, et al: The non-operative management of pediatric hepatic trauma, *J Pediatr Surg* 18:512, 1983.

Katz S, Lazar L, Rathaus V, et al: Can ultrasonography replace computed tomography in the initial assessment of children with abdominal trauma? *Pediatr Surg* 31:649, 1996.

Kearney PA: Blunt trauma to the abdomen: CT imaging is unreliable for detection of bowel injury, *Ann Emerg Med* 18:1322, 1989.

Konradsen HB, Hemrichsen J: Pneumococcal infections in splenectomized children are preventable, *Acta Paediatr Scand* 80:423, 1991.

Kothenberg S, et al: Selective management of blunt abdominal trauma in children: the triage role of peritoneal lavage, *J Trauma* 27:1101, 1987.

Kuhn JP: Diagnostic imaging for the evaluation of abdominal trauma in children, *Pediatr Clin North Am* 32:1427, 1985.

Marx JA: Abdominal injuries. In Rosen P, editor: *Emergency medicine; concepts and clinical practice*, ed 3, St Louis, 1992, Mosby.

McAnena OJ, Marx JA, Moore EE: Contribution of peritoneal lavage enzyme determinations to the management of isolated hollow visceral abdominal injuries, *Ann Emerg Med* 20:834, 1991.

Moore EE, Marx JA: Penetrating abdominal wounds: rationale for exploratory laparotomy, *JAMA* 253:2705, 1985.

Moore EE, Mattox KL, Feliciano D: *Trauma*, Norwalk, Conn, 1991, Appleton & Lange.

Moore JB, Moore EE, Markovchick VJ, et al: Diagnostic peritoneal lavage for abdominal trauma: superiority of the open technique at the infraumbilical ring, *J Trauma* 21:570, 1981.

Neufeld JDG: Trauma in pregnancy, *Emerg Clin North Am* 11:207, 1993.

Nordenholz KE, Rubin MA, Gularte GG, et al: Ultrasound with evaluation and management of blunt abdominal trauma, *Ann Emerg Med* 29:357, 1997.

Pearl RH, Wesson DE, Spence LJ, et al: Splenic injury: a 5-year update with improved results and changing criteria for conservative management, *J Pediatr Surg* 24:121, 1989.

Pearl WS, Todd KH: Ultrasonography for the initial evaluation of blunt abdominal trauma: a review of prospective trials, *Ann Emerg Med* 27:353, 1996.

Porter RS, Nester BA, Dalsey WC, et al: Use of ultrasound to determine need for laparotomy in trauma patients, *Ann Emerg Med* 29:323, 1997.

Powell RW, Green JB, Ochsner MG, et al: Peritoneal lavage in pediatric patients sustaining blunt abdominal trauma: a reappraisal, *J Trauma* 27:6, 1987.

Reid MM: Splenectomy, sepsis, immunization, and guidelines, *Lancet* 344:970, 1992.

Saladino R, Lund D, Fleisher G: The spectrum of liver and spleen injuries in children: failure of the pediatric trauma score and clinical signs to predict isolated injuries, *Ann Emerg Med* 6:636, 1991.

Sivit CJ, Taylor GA, Newman KD: Safety belt injuries in children with lap-belt ecchymoses, *Am J Radiol* 157: 111, 1991.

Taylor GA, Eichelberger MR, O'Donnel R, et al: Indications for computed tomography in children with blunt abdominal trauma, *Ann Surg* 213:212, 1991.

Tsang BD, Panacek EA, Brant WE, et al: Effect of oral contrast administration for abdominal computed tomography in the evaluation of acute blunt trauma, *Ann Emerg Med* 30:7, 1997.

Turnock RR, Sprigg A, Lloyd DA: Computed tomography in the management of blunt abdominal trauma in children, *Br J Surg* 80:982, 1993.

Zucker R, Browns K, Rossman D, et al: Non-operative management of splenic trauma: conservative or radical treatment, *Arch Surg* 119:400, 1984.

64 GENITOURINARY TRAUMA

SUSAN B. KIRELIK

ALERT: Anyone with trauma to the perineum, back, abdomen, flank, or genitalia should be suspected of having genitourinary (GU) trauma. Hematuria, oliguria, tenderness, pain, masses, or lower rib fractures must be carefully evaluated for associated abnormality.

Auto accidents, sports injuries, or falls cause 75% of genitourinary (GU) trauma. After the brain, the kidney is the most commonly injured internal organ in children. The kidney, primarily an intraabdominal organ in younger children, is more mobile and not protected by perinephric fat. Although most urogenital injuries are caused by blunt trauma, the incidence of penetrating trauma in the pediatric population has increased dramatically in the past several years.

The diagnosis of GU trauma must be entertained anytime a patient has hematuria (more than 5 red blood cells/high-powered field [RBC/HPF]), decreased urinary output, an unexplained abdominal mass or pain and tenderness, penetrating trauma, a fractured pelvis, fractures of lower ribs, thoracic or lumbar vertebral fractures, blood at the urethral meatus, or scrotal swelling and hematoma.

Preexisting congenital anomalies such as hydronephrosis and polycystic disease make renal injury more likely and are present in 10% of children evaluated for renal trauma. Other causes of hematuria (see Chapter 37) and infection (p. 815) must also be considered in the initial evaluation. Epididymitis, testicular tor-

sion, and penile disorders are discussed in Chapter 77.

EVALUATION

Evaluation must include a careful urinalysis and radiographic studies when appropriate. Indications for imaging and choice of radiographic study are still somewhat controversial. The most commonly used modalities are computed tomography (CT) and intravenous pyelography (IVP).

1. Urinalysis.
   a. Dipstik shows positive value if hemoglobin or myoglobin is in the urine. False-positive values occur when urine is contaminated with povidone-iodine (Betadine) or hexachlorophene. Drugs and chemicals may turn the urine dark or red (p. 359).
   b. Microscopic examination for red cells is mandatory if the Dipstik result is positive.
   c. The absence of hematuria does not exclude significant renal injury. Renal vascular thrombosis, renal pedicle injury, and complete transection of the

ureter are common causes of false-negative values.

2. Abdominal flat plate and chest x-ray film. May have a variety of findings associated with GU injuries requiring further evaluation:
   a. Fracture of lower rib.
   b. Fractured vertebrae or transverse process in lower thoracic or lumbar vertebrae.
   c. Pelvic fracture.
   d. Other findings, including ileus, scoliosis of vertebral column toward injured side, unilateral enlarged kidney shadow, loss of psoas muscle margin, displaced bowel secondary to hemorrhage or urine extravasation, or an elevated ipsilateral hemidiaphragm.
3. CT scan enhanced by intravenous (IV) contrast medium can be useful in the identification of renal injuries. Some studies suggest that sensitivity may approach that of IVP. It clearly has the benefit of identifying associated ultraabdominal injuries in the multiply injured patient (see Chapter 63). It provides good anatomic detail and is not dependent on renal vasculature. It is useful for staging or renal injuries in blunt trauma. The role of CT in staging penetrating renal trauma is still undetermined. CT has limited sensitivity in identifying minor parenchymal fractures and minimal degrees of extravasation seldom critical to accurate therapeutic decisions.

   Indications for use of this modality include a stable patient with gross or microscopic hematuria (>20 RBC/HPF), who has had multiple trauma, a mechanism suggesting intraabdominal or renal injury, or an equivocal IVP result.
4. Excretory urography (IVP) is a common method for initial appraisal of suspected renal injury or traumatic hematuria. Its sensitivity has been reported to be as high as 90%. It can provide a determination of urologic function. The study cannot provide imaging of other intraabdominal organs, which may have associated injuries. Urologic function, regardless of delay or diminution, usually indicates that the injury is amenable to self-repair. Parenchymal laceration or urinary extravasation usually resolves in patients uncompromised by hemorrhagic complications, with the exception of apparent polar or hemirenal nonfunction; this suggests a parenchymal avulsion, which requires surgery or selective embolization.

   Persistent urographic nonfunction reflects either parenchymal shattering or pedicle interruption (avulsion, thrombosis).
   a. Indications after trauma:
      (1) GU injury alone suspected
      (2) Flank pain or fullness, hematoma, or ecchymosis
      (3) Suspected ureteral injury
      (4) Microscopic hematuria finding exceeding 20 RBC/HPF
      (5) Gross hematuria
   b. The indications for IVP are somewhat controversial at present. Patients with gross hematuria or microscopic hematuria and shock after blunt trauma require study, as do those with penetrating trauma when there is concern about renal involvement.

      Increasing data suggest that routine evaluation of children with microscopic hematuria less than 20 RBC/HPF and no other suggestive findings is probably not routinely justified solely to evaluate traumatic injuries because of the low incidence of such problems requiring surgical intervention (i.e., IVPs demonstrate either contusion or normal kidneys and rarely have more significant injuries). Although an IVP is usually suggested in adults with more than 50 RBC/HPF, the lower threshold in children is suggested to exclude congenital abnormalities that may result in hematuria without significant trauma.

Radiographic evaluation of the kidney should be undertaken as noted. A patient in whom hematuria develops after a minor mechanism should be considered for radiographic evaluation to exclude underlying congenital abnormality or tumor.

c. Procedure: sodium diatrizoate (Conray) 60% (or equivalent) IV at 2 ml/kg (<4.5 kg: 4 ml/kg) (adult: 50 to 100 ml). Films at 1, 5, 10, and 20 minutes if possible. A "single film IVP" with imaging 10 minutes after administration of contrast may help determine renal function in the unstable patient who is being taken to the operating room (OR) for laparotomy.

d. Reactions to IV contrast material may be reduced in patients with a questionable history by pretreatment with corticosteroids. Optimally, give methylprednisolone (Solu-Medrol), 0.5-1.0 mg/kg/dose (adult: 32 mg/dose), 12 and 2 hours before contrast material is injected or one dose 2 hours after challenge.

5. Retrograde urethrogram should be done before urethral instrumentation or catheterization, if indicated.

   a. Indications include the following:
      (1) Blood at meatus
      (2) Significant scrotal or perineal hematoma
      (3) Obvious urethral trauma (penetrating or foreign body)

   b. Procedure: 10 to 30 ml of standard water-soluble Renografin is drawn into a catheter-tipped syringe, the tip of which is inserted into the urethral meatus. Anterior, posterior, and oblique x-ray films are obtained as the dye is injected. Patient sedation may be required.

6. Cystogram. Indicated when the injury and findings are consistent with bladder injury, pelvic fracture, inadequate urine production, or gross hematuria.

   a. If indicated, performed after urethrogram.

   b. Procedures: 150 to 300 ml (depending on size of child) of 10% solution water-soluble Renografin is placed in bladder through urethral catheter by gravity. Smaller volumes may be required in infants to fill bladder. Anteroposterior (AP) and oblique views are required with filled and postevacuation films.

7. Isotopic renal scanning has limitations similar to those of CT. It may be used to monitor patients with known renal injury and to detect recovery or loss of function of renal parenchyma.

8. The renal arteriogram has been largely supplanted by CT. Indications for an arteriogram include assessment of the nature of persistent, fresh hemorrhage or of delayed or intermittent hematuria and evaluation of renal shattering. Digital subtraction angiography is preferable in evaluating renovascular injury.

9. Ultrasonography has been studied as a modality for evaluation of GU trauma and has been found to have sensitivity of only 40% to 70% when compared with CT. It may also fail to diagnose associated injuries and is therefore rarely used in the acute trauma setting.

10. Magnetic resonance imaging (MRI) has been shown to be very similar to CT in renal trauma. Because it is not readily available, its use in the acute trauma setting is limited. It may have a role in staging the renal injuries of the patient with iodine allergy who is unable to undergo a contrast-enhanced CT.

RENAL TRAUMA

More than 90% of direct renal trauma is caused by blunt injuries from auto accidents or significant falls. Males, particularly less than 30 years of age, are at greatest risk. The kidney can move on the pedicle and can therefore be contused or lacerated by ribs or spinal transverse process. Gerota's fascia surrounding the kidney may restrict bleeding.

Diagnostic Findings

Signs or symptoms, such as abrasion, ecchymosis, pain or tenderness to the chest, back, abdomen, or flank, should raise suspicion of renal injury.

Classification of Degree of Renal Trauma

Class I: renal contusions or hematomas that are small, subcapsular, and nonexpanding. Hematuria with no evidence of decreased renal function, extravasation, or pelvical-iceal injury on IVP.

Class II: contained renal cortical lacerations less than 1 cm in depth and hematomas confined to the retroperitoneum without urinary extravasation.

Class III: lacerations into the perirenal fat more than 1 cm in depth but not penetrating into the collecting system. No urinary extravasation.

Class IV: deep lacerations into the collecting system and renal vascular injury with contained hemorrhage.

Class V: shattered or fractured kidney and renal pedicle injuries that devascularize the kidney.

Complications

1. Extravasation of urine is variably associated with infection or obstruction.
2. Vascular compromise of the kidney.
3. Acute tubular necrosis (ATN) with renal failure.
4. Hemorrhage with hypovolemic shock.

5. Delayed complications, including hypertension, chronic infection, hydronephrosis, calculus formation, chronic renal failure, arteriovenous fistula, pseudocyst formation, and nonfunction.

Ancillary Data

Data include complete blood count (CBC), urinalysis, abdominal flat plate, and IVP or contrast CT scan. If the renal unit is not seen, selective arteriogram is performed and then, for follow-up evaluation, renal scan and sonography.

The urinalysis result may be normal, especially in pedicle injury or renal vascular thrombosis.

Management (Fig. 64-1)

1. Class I, II, and III injuries account for about 85% of renal injuries. Conservative treatment is appropriate, and these patients do well with good follow-up care. Patients are placed on bed rest with frequent monitoring of vital signs and urinalysis.
2. Moderate injuries noted in class IV injuries may require surgical intervention, depending on the degree of extravasation, stability of the patient, underlying renal anatomy, and degree of renal impairment. Many of these patients are managed nonsurgically with close monitoring of vital signs and serial hematocrits while the patient is treated with IV antibiotics. It is crucial that these patients are attended to by a surgeon who is capable of intervening surgically should the patient's condition deteriorate. These patients must be followed closely after discharge for the development of hypertension or the need for delayed nephrectomy.
3. Severe class V injuries are rare (3%). Exploration and either nephrectomy of the fractured kidney or repair of the renal pedicle injury are recommended. Results

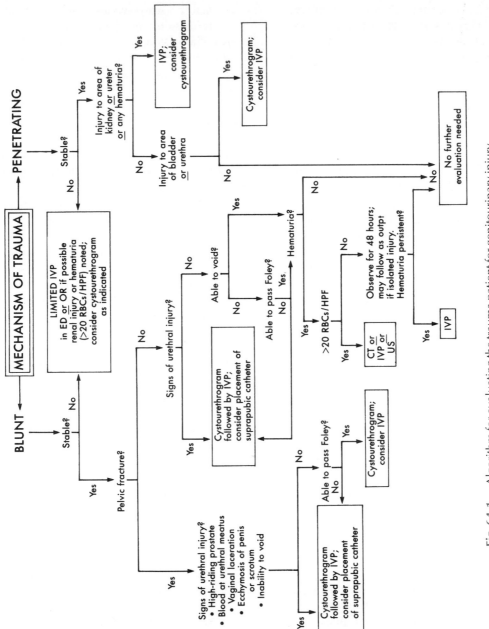

Fig. 64-1 Algorithm for evaluating the trauma patient for genitourinary injury.
(From Barkin RM: *Pediatric emergency medicine: concepts and clinical practice,* ed 2, St Louis, 1997, Mosby.)

of revascularization are usually poor. Penetrating renal trauma is generally treated surgically.

URETERAL TRAUMA

Blunt injuries result from a hyperextension, with bowstringing of the ureter, causing complete or partial laceration. Although rare, ureteral injury is more common in children than adults. Ureteral injuries are common in children after auto-pedestrian accidents because of the flexibility of the torso and limited retroperitoneal fat for protection. The tear almost always occurs at the ureteropelvic junction (UPJ). Penetrating ureteral injuries and surgical damage are more common in adults.

Diagnostic Findings

Patients may have lumboiliac pain from a blow, a flank mass from extravasated urine or blood, frequency of urination, hematuria, or pyuria. The diagnosis is often missed because of the severity of other associated multiple injuries and the subtlety of the findings. The prognosis is better with early repair.

Delayed retroperitoneal mass, back pain, unexplained fever, or urine drainage from a wound or operative incision site may be noted. More than 50% of patients with delayed repair lose ureter and kidney function.

Complications
1. Extravasated urine may cause peritonitis if the peritoneum is damaged or empyema if the diaphragm is involved.
2. Ureteral strictures secondary to obstruction or infection may occur.

Ancillary Data
1. Hematuria is present in 66% of cases but may not be noted with complete transection of the ureter.
2. IVP demonstrates extravasation of dye. If the injury is near the UPJ, the dye may travel up and around the kidney, simulating a lacerated renal cortex or pelvis. A retrograde pyelogram may later be used to more accurately diagnose the level of injury to the ureter.
3. A CT scan may be used in multiple trauma cases but is no better than IVP in demonstrating ureteral injuries.

Management

1. A urologist should be consulted for primary repair and cutaneous ureterostomy as indicated. A nephroureterectomy may be necessary if the diagnosis is delayed.
2. Long-term follow-up observation must include monitoring of blood pressure and ensuring that a ureteral stricture or obstruction does not develop.

BLADDER TRAUMA

Most bladder ruptures result from blunt trauma to patients with full bladders, often during automobile or auto-pedestrian accidents. Inappropriate use of lap belts may increase the risk of bladder injury. Penetrating injuries may be caused by guns, knives, or fractured pelvic bones.

Diagnostic Findings

1. Bladder contusion is a bruise to the bladder wall.
2. Intraperitoneal bladder rupture is more common in younger children than in adults because the pediatric bladder is an abdominal organ. The break is usually at the bladder dome.
   a. Suprapubic tenderness, abdominal pain, ileus, extreme desire but inability to void, hematuria, pallor, tachycardia, hypotension
   b. Delayed symptoms 24 to 72 hours after rupture, including fever, abdominal tenderness, vomiting
3. Extraperitoneal bladder rupture is less common, occurring more often in the

older child and adolescent with pelvic injury.

    a. Symptoms are similar to those associated with intraperitoneal injury except that the patient may pass a small amount of urine, and a hematoma may be palpated in the suprapubic region. Urine can dissect up to the kidney or down into the legs, scrotum, and buttock.

    b. A red, indurated suprapubic area may develop if diagnosis is delayed.

4. Intraperitoneal and extraperitoneal rupture may occur.

5. Urethral injuries and associated abdominal or pelvic abnormalities are common.

Complications

Complications include peritonitis, abscess, sepsis, ileus, osteomyelitis, bladder neck contractures, and poor bladder muscle function.

Ancillary Data

Hematuria is present in more than 95% of patients. The degree of hematuria does not correlate with the severity of injury.

1. Retrograde cystogram.

    a. A cystogram is indicated when penetrating trauma and suspected lower GU injury, pelvic fracture, lower abdominal or perineal trauma with hematuria, or inability to void is present. The upper urinary system must first be evaluated.

    b. Contused bladder will show normal vesicle outline and a teardrop shape if bilateral hematomas are present or a half-moon shape with unilateral hematoma.

    c. Intraperitoneal rupture may have intraperitoneal organs outlined by dye.

    d. Extraperitoneal rupture demonstrates dye in contact areas after dye is drained from bladder on postevacuation film.

2. A CT scan may be useful in multiple trauma but may not detect bladder injury.

Management

1. Bladder contusion is treated by hospitalizing patient and placing indwelling catheter for 7 to 10 days. Minor contusions can be observed at home without catheter placement. Close follow-up observation is essential. Contact sports should be avoided for 2 to 6 weeks. Prognosis is good.

2. Bladder ruptures may be evaluated by cystoscopy and, if small, treated with indwelling catheter for 7 to 14 days. Larger deficits require operative repair and suprapubic cystoscopy.

3. A urologist should be consulted when the diagnosis is first suspected.

URETHRAL INJURIES

Urethral injuries commonly follow blunt trauma and are associated with pelvic fractures. Pelvic fractures, however, are rare in children and generally not as severe as in adults. They may be a complication of urethral catheterization.

Diagnostic Findings

Injury to the urethra in children most commonly occurs at the bladder neck. Although injury at the prostate membranous location is common in adult males, in young boys there is laxity in this region, and injury to this site is much less common.

- Signs include blood at urethral meatus and inability to void. In patients close to adulthood, the prostate may be boggy and high riding.

Injury to the bulbous and pendulous or penile urethra may result from a straddle fall or from foreign bodies.

- Perineal pain is prominent. There is blood at the meatus, but a good urinary stream when voiding. If patient is seen late after injury, penile and perineal edema, necrosis, and ecchymosis may be present.

Complications

These include stricture, impotence, or urinary incontinence.

Ancillary Data

These include urinalysis and retrograde urethrogram before urinary catheter is placed.

Management

1. A urologist must be consulted immediately on identifying blood at the meatus or on defining the abnormality.
2. Anterior injuries, if small, may be treated with a urethral catheter; otherwise operative repair is needed.
3. Posterior injuries are controversial. There is question about whether immediate or delayed intervention provides the best repair.
4. Because urethral injuries may be iatrogenic, careful technique in catheterization is advisable. The catheter should never be forced.

EXTERNAL GENITALIA TRAUMA (p. 662)

Penile, scrotal, and testicular injuries may result from missiles (bullet or knife); from strangulation secondary to a condom, string, hair, or constricting metal band; from blunt injury to an erect penis during intercourse or fall; from being caught in a zipper; or from amputation. Vulvar lesions usually follow blunt trauma. Vaginal injuries must raise suspicion of child abuse.

Diagnostic Findings

Penile swelling, ecchymosis, and other direct injury can be present. With a constricting band, close inspection is necessary because edema can hide a small constricting band such as hair.

Ancillary Data

Data include urinalysis to evaluate for blood, which indicates urethral injury requiring a retrograde urethrogram. Ultrasonography may be useful in the assessment of significant blunt scrotal and testicular trauma.

Management

Urology consultation is necessary.

Lacerations of the Penile Skin

These can be sutured with absorbable suture.

1. If the wound is not deep beyond the Colles fascia, it can be closed in the emergency department (ED) with two layers of Vicryl or Dexon sutures. If deeper, it should be explored in the OR.
2. If the corpus cavernosum penis is violated, it should be explored in the operating room.
3. Constricting devices should be removed as soon as possible. The distal penis that appears necrotic should be treated conservatively. Often, an apparently nonviable penis will survive.

Zipper Injuries

These are best treated by breaking or cutting the small bridge (U-shaped bar) between the anterior and posterior faceplates of the zipper fastener with a bone cutter. Others recommend local anesthetic of the involved skin and then unzipping by moving one tooth at a time, alternating sides.

Amputation of the Penis

This requires immediate consultation.

Lacerations of the Scrotum

1. Laceration of scrotal skin alone: debridement and closure with absorbable suture.
2. Scrotal skin and dartos layer only: debridement and two-layered closure with absorbable suture to reduce the chance of hematoma formation.
3. Penetrating wound or major blunt trauma: exploration in the OR. Conservative treatment leads to a high incidence of atrophied testes and loss of viability.

Blunt Injuries to the Scrotum

1. Usually can be managed with ice, elevation, and analgesia.

2. Scrotal ultrasonography should be done if a testicular rupture is suspected. This test is highly accurate. It can differentiate testicular rupture, scrotal hematoma, extratesticular fluid collection, and epididymal hematomas. A ruptured testicle requires surgical repair. The other injuries are often treated conservatively.

3. If there is a large or expanding hematoma, it may need to be explored in the OR. A urology consultation must be obtained.

Injury to Vulva

Vulva injury requires examination (often under anesthesia) to exclude extension of injury to the vagina, rectum, bladder, and urethra. Lacerations in the perineal area in prepubertal girls are more likely to involve the vagina. Because the extent of the injury is easily underestimated, examination under anesthesia must be considered if there is any concern of vaginal trauma.

Vulvar hematomas are usually treated conservatively and commonly result from handlebar or crossbar injuries. Patients may be placed on strict bed rest, ice packs, analgesia, stool softener, and close monitoring of urinary output. Rarely is a urinary catheter needed. Abuse should be excluded.

REFERENCES

Abou-Jaoude WA, Sugarman JM, Fallat ME, et al: Indicators of genitourinary tract injury or anomaly in cases of pediatric blunt trauma, *J Pediatr Surg* 31:86, 1996.

Fleisher G: Prospective evaluation of selective criteria for imaging among children with suspected blunt renal trauma, *Pediatr Emerg Care* 5:8, 1989.

Gausche M: Genitourinary trauma. In Barkin RM, editor: *Pediatric emergency medicine: concepts and clinical practice*, ed 2, St Louis, 1997, Mosby.

Guerriero WG: Etiology, classification and management of renal trauma, *Surg Clin North Am* 68:1071, 1988.

Halsell RD, Vines FS, Shatney CH, et al: The reliability of excretory urography as a screening examination for blunt trauma, *Ann Emerg Med* 16:1236, 1987.

Kane NM, Cronan JJ, Dorfman GS, et al: Pediatric abdominal trauma: evaluation by computed tomography, *Pediatrics* 82:11, 1988.

Kurn JP, Berger PE: Computerized tomography in the evaluation of blunt abdominal trauma in children, *Radiol Clin North Am* 19:503, 1981.

Lappäniemi A, Lamminen A, Tervanartiala P, et al: Comparison of high field magnetic resonance imaging with computed tomography in the evaluation of blunt renal trauma, *J Trauma* 38:420, 1995.

Lasser EC, Berry CC, Talner LB, et al: Pretreatment with corticosteroids to alleviate reaction to intravenous contrast material, *N Engl J Med* 317:845, 1987.

Levitt MA, Criss E, Kobernick M: Should the emergency IVP be used more selectively in blunt trauma? *Ann Emerg Med* 14:959, 1985.

Lieu TA, Fleisher GR, Mahboubi S, et al: Hematuria and clinical findings as indications for intravenous pyelography in pediatric blunt renal trauma, *Pediatrics* 82:216, 1988.

Mayor B, Gudinchet F, Wicky S, et al: Imaging evaluation of blunt renal trauma in children: diagnostic accuracy of intravenous pyelography and ultrasonography, *Pediatr Radiol* 25:214, 1995.

McAleer IM, Kaplan GW: Pediatric genitourinary trauma, *Urol Clin North Am* 22:177, 1995.

McAleer IM, Kaplan GW, Scherz HC, et al: Genitourinary trauma in the pediatric patient, *Urology* 42:563, 1993.

Morey AF, Bruce JE, McAninch JW: Efficacy of radiographic imaging in pediatric blunt renal trauma, *J Urol* 156:2014, 1996.

Munter DW, Faleske EJ: Blunt scrotal trauma: emergency department evaluation and management, *Am J Emerg Med* 7:227, 1989.

Nicolaisein GS, McAninch JW, Marshall GA, et al: Renal trauma: reevaluation of the indication for radiographic assessment, *J Urol* 133:183, 1985.

Nolan JF, Stillwell TJ, Sands JP: Acute management of the zipper-trapped penis, *J Emerg Med* 8:305, 1990.

Palmer JK, Benson GS, Corriere JN: Diagnosis and initial management of urologic injuries associated with 200 consecutive pelvic fractures, *J Urol* 130:712, 1983.

Peterson NE, Pfister RR: Renal trauma. In Barkin RM, editor: *The emergently ill child*, Rockville, Md, 1987, Aspen Publishing.

Stein JP, Kaji DM, Eastham J, et al: Blunt renal trauma in the pediatric population: indications for radiographic evaluation, *Urology* 44:406, 1994.

Uehara DT, Eisner RF: Indications for intravenous pyelography in trauma, *Ann Emerg Med* 15:266, 1986.

65 SOFT TISSUE INJURIES

VINCENT J. MARKOVCHICK

$\mathcal{S}$oft tissue injuries are common in children. They often are caused by falls, contact with sharp objects, or motor vehicle accidents. Because many involved areas are visible, such as the face (see Chapter 58), it is imperative that the principles of meticulous wound care and repair be practiced to maximize cosmetic and functional results.

DIAGNOSTIC FINDINGS

The following should be ascertained: the mechanism (cut, fall, crush, bite, or electrical injury) and the time of injury, whether the wound was clean or dirty, the amount of blood loss, the history of foreign body sensation, and the degree of paresthesia or impaired motor function distal to the wound. Child abuse must be considered in cases where the history and injury are inconsistent.

The status of tetanus immunization, as well as allergies to antibiotics, local anesthetic agents, and other medications, in addition to underlying medical problems, should be noted. True allergies to local anesthetics are extremely rare.

Local pain and swelling are common with all soft tissue trauma. Furthermore, children tend to be fearful and anxious.

All wounds must be carefully inspected to determine the depth of injury and involvement of underlying tissues, including vessels, nerves, muscles, tendons, ligaments, bone, joints, and ducts.

1. Attention must be given to the physical examination and to documentation of an accurate description of the wound for the record. The wound may be described with respect to location, length, depth, nature of the edges, cleanliness, and involvement of any underlying structures.

2. The integrity of arterial circulation is determined by palpation of peripheral pulses, skin color, temperature, and capillary filling. Contusions over the forearm and leg may lead to delayed onset of compartment syndromes.

3. Sensory deficits are tested by determination of distal sensation, often requiring measurement of two-point discrimination distal to the lesion. This can easily be done by using a paper clip and separating the ends by 8 mm.

   • Nerve injuries are classified as neuropraxia (nerve continuity maintained and no axonal degeneration secondary to compression or contusion), axonotmesis (preservation of anatomic continuity of nerve with axonal degeneration), or neurotmesis (complete division of nerve).

4. After a careful sensory examination, infiltration of local anesthesia may be provided for a painless yet accurate examination, cleansing, debridement, and definitive treatment.

5. Tendons, ligaments, and muscles should be tested distal to the injury individually and by muscle group.

6. Foreign bodies should be identified and removed.
7. Injuries of the hand or foot require very careful assessment. The examination of the hand, which is commonly injured in children, is outlined in Chapter 68. Open wounds require direct visualization with hemostasis and the tendon must be visualized throughout full range of motion because motor function may remain normal with partial laceration of tendons or ligaments.

Complications

Infections can be minimized by meticulous wound preparation, irrigation and debridement, careful closure of the wound, and application of appropriate dressings and splints.

Other complications include the following:
1. Failure to recognize deep structure injury to nerve, tendon, bone, or joint capsule with sensory or motor deficits (fractures underlying lacerations must be considered open fractures)
2. Delayed recognition of a foreign body
3. Cosmetic deformity

Ancillary Data

X-ray studies should be obtained when appropriate before testing motor function or range of motion:
1. For injuries secondary to blunt trauma or crush injury.
2. To exclude a radiopaque foreign body. The relative qualities of wound contaminants are as follows:
   a. Highly radiopaque: bone, metal (lead, steel, copper), gravel, or stone chips
   b. Slightly radiopaque: bone (birds), metal (aluminum), glass, some plastics
   c. Water density: plants, wood in situ more than 24 hours, some plastics
   d. Radiolucent: air, gas, wood in situ less than 24 hours, some plastics
      NOTE: Glass fragments usually can be

seen on a standard x-ray film. Small (0.5 to 1.0 mm) or thin glass fragments are more difficult to see but can be detected if no underlying bone is present.

MANAGEMENT (See Appendix to Chapter 65 on Analgesia and Sedation and Chapter 58 on Facial Injuries)

Although unusual, massive hypovolemia from a vascular injury or extensive laceration of the scalp or face may cause hypotension, which is usually responsive to crystalloid solution administration (0.9% normal saline [NS] or lactated Ringer's [LR] solution at 20 ml/kg over 20 to 30 minutes). Stabilization of life-threatening conditions has the greatest priority.

1. If hypotension is present, other injuries, in addition to the soft tissue damage, should be considered.
2. Hemorrhage can usually be controlled by direct pressure or local injection of lidocaine with epinephrine. If placement of hemostats is required for control of hemorrhage, this must always be done under direct vision (never blindly) to prevent iatrogenic injury to nerves, vessels, or tendons. Uncontrolled outgoing hemorrhage from an extremity should be controlled by application of a tourniquet.
3. Tetanus immunizations must be updated (p. 718).

Immediate consultation should be requested if the injury is very complex or if extensive follow-up evaluation will be required.

Analgesia and Sedation

Appropriate attention must be directed to reducing discomfort and anxiety as discussed in the appendix at the end of this chapter.

Restraint, Position, and Draping

Wounds in small children are most easily repaired if the child is appropriately sedated (see

Appendix to Chapter 65) or restrained (e.g., on a papoose board*). This must be individualized and necessitates careful attention to the child's respiratory status and the potential for aspiration of vomitus. A sterile field should be created by the use of drapes. However, the face should not generally be totally draped.

If extensive bleeding is associated with a finger laceration, an excellent field and tourniquet can be achieved by cleansing the patient's finger and then slipping the hand into a sterile glove, snipping the end of the glove on the involved finger, and then rolling the finger of the glove back to provide exposure and tourniquet. Careful scrubbing is then done.

Wound Exploration

This should be performed on all injuries so that the extent of the damage may be fully appreciated, violation of underlying structures realized, undetected fractures and tendon lacerations discovered, and removal of all foreign bodies ensured. Optimally, the wound is explored after injection of local anesthesia, hemostasis is obtained, and sensory examination.

Embedded, inert foreign bodies such as glass or metal should be removed if possible. X-ray films are often helpful in localization. The precise location of an embedded object can be identified by taping paper clips or a flexible radiopaque marker such as wire to the skin overlying the suspected location and getting an anteroposterior (AP) and a lateral view at 90 degrees to each other. However, if foreign bodies are small and if they are embedded deeply into muscle and cannot be easily removed, they may be left in place. The patient should be informed of the presence of the foreign body and follow-up observation should be arranged.

NOTE: Organic foreign bodies such as wood should be removed whenever possible to prevent local inflammatory reactions. Xeroradiography may be necessary to localize some foreign

bodies not seen on standard soft tissue radiographs. Surgical consultation should usually be obtained unless the material is superficial; deeper objects may require controlled removal in the operating room.

Wound Cleansing and Irrigation

Cleansing and irrigation are best done after local anesthesia has been injected; 1% povidone-iodine solution (Betadine) is an excellent cleansing agent. The "scrub" should not be used because it causes extensive tissue necrosis. If hair must be removed, this is ideally done by clipping rather than shaving, the latter increasing the incidence of wound infections. Moistening the hair with lubricating jelly (KY or Surgilube) may keep it out of the way. Eyebrows should not be shaved or clipped; they are important landmarks in aligning the wound.

Irrigation assists in the removal of particulate material in a *contaminated* wound. The efficacy is related to the force of the irrigating stream: A higher pressure is more efficient. Larger particles are more easily removed than smaller ones. High-pressure irrigation is accomplished by attaching an 18-gauge angiocath or 18- or 19-gauge needle to a 35-ml syringe and pressing down firmly on the plunger while keeping the tip 3 to 4 mm above the wound while flushing. A 500 to 1000 ml bag of normal saline solution fitted with blood administering tubing in a pressure sleeve may facilitate this process. Saline solution in pressurized canisters delivering 8 to 10 pounds per square inch (psi) is also effective. Irrigation before primary closure of a *clean, noncontaminated* facial or scalp laceration is of less importance.

Foreign material in an abrasion must be removed within 24 hours to prevent the creation of a permanent traumatic tattoo, particularly in such cosmetically important areas as the face. Anesthesia of the abrasion may be achieved by direct application of a cotton ball/swab to the wound that has been saturated in 4% lidocaine or TAC. The abrasion should then be scrubbed with a scrub brush or toothbrush. An 11-blade

---

*Available from Olympic Surgical Co., Seattle, Wash.

or 18-gauge needle may be used for material not removed by the scrubbing process.

Hemostasis

Direct pressure and tourniquets occasionally are needed for hemostasis. Vessels should not be sutured or clamped blindly because of the risk of injury to other underlying tissues.

Wound Revision and Debridement

This may require very conservative debridement, after anesthesia, of devitalized or severely contaminated tissue. Ragged and uneven edges may need to be incised using a scalpel or iris scissors to improve the wound configuration. Most wounds do well with little or no revision. It should be explained to the parents that the wound may leave a noticeable scar, which may be further revised by a consultant after 12 to 18 months of healing.

Associated abrasions can lead to permanent tattooing if foreign particulate material is not removed. Scrubbing and selective debridement are important.

Wound Closure

Wounds should be closed as soon as possible. In general, wounds more than 8 to 12 hours old should not be closed. Clean wounds on the face and scalp may be closed, if necessary, up to 24 hours after the injury because of the excellent vasculature.

1. Contaminated or dirty wounds are optimally treated with vigorous cleansing, appropriate dressing, and a delayed primary closure at 72 to 96 hours.
2. Puncture wounds should not be closed. Debridement and irrigation with close follow-up evaluation are essential.
3. Most bites on the face should be closed primarily after careful cleansing, irrigation, and debridement. Serious consideration should be given to delayed primary closure for bites in other areas of the body. However, if in the judgment of the clinician this would result in a serious cosmetic or functional deficit, such wounds may be closed primarily (p. 303).

Wound-Closure Techniques (Table 65-1)

The location of the injury and the goal of closure influence closure techniques. If the primary goal is a good cosmetic closure, deep or large wounds often require multilayer closure. The top sutures should be removed within 5 days to minimize the possibility of suture marks being part of the scar.

If a good functional result is the primary goal as on the head, arm or leg, then a single layer closure is usually adequate.

A sterile scalpel blade or stitch cutter facilitates removal, which must be done at the appropriate time to reduce suture marks.

Specific suturing techniques are beyond the scope of this book but several principles are important to emphasize:

1. Subcutaneous sutures should be placed equal in depth and distance from the wound edges.
2. Extrinsic tension should be reduced by using buried sutures or undermining the subcutaneous layers. This is often required in cases of extensive loss of tissue because of trauma or revision.

    Undermine areas of loose tissue at the level of subcutaneous fat or fascia to a width equal to the gap of the wound at its widest point.
3. To aid edge eversion, the base of the suture loop should be as wide or wider than the top of the suture loop. Enter the skin perpendicular to the skin plane rather than tangentially (less important with shallow sutures).
4. The closer the suture is to the wound edge, the better the control of the edge. Space the sutures an equal distance apart at the same depth on both sides of the

TABLE 65-1   Suture Repair of Soft Tissue Injuries

Location	Anesthetic	Suture material*	Technique of closure and dressing	Suture removal	Pitfalls
Scalp	Lidocaine 1% with epinephrine	3-0 or 4-0 nonabsorbable monofilament	Interrupted in galea; single tight layer in scalp—horizontal mattress if bleeding not well controlled by simple sutures	7-12 days	Failure to explore wound for fracture; hematoma formation secondary to "loose" closure
Face	Lidocaine 1% with epinephrine or use field block	4-0 or 5-0 synthetic absorbable or 6-0 nonabsorbable monofilament	If full-thickness laceration, layered closure is desirable	3-5 days	Failure to recognize and examine for damage to underlying structures, i.e., facial nerve or parotid duct
Pinna (ear)	Lidocaine 1% (field block)	6-0 nonabsorbable monofilament or 5-0 synthetic absorbable	Close perichondrium with 5-0 synthetic absorbable; close skin with nonabsorbable interrupted sutures—stint dressing	4-6 days	Hematoma formation secondary to improper or no dressing
Eyebrow	Lidocaine 1% with epinephrine	4-0 or 5-0 synthetic absorbable and 6-0 nonabsorbable monofilament	Layered closure	4-5 days	Perpendicular excision rather than one parallel to direction of hair follicles; shaving of eyebrows not indicated
Eyelid	Lidocaine 1%	6-0 nonabsorbable monofilament	Single-layer horizontal mattress, interrupted or running	3-5 days	Failure to examine for globe injury or to appreciate injury to tarsal plate
Lip	Lidocaine 1% with epinephrine or use field block	4-0 or 5-0 synthetic absorbable in mucosa, muscle and intradermal layer; 6-0 nonabsorbable monofilament	Three layers (mucosa, muscle, and skin) if through and through, otherwise two layers	3-5 days	1 mm or greater malalignment of the vermilion border causing cosmetic deformity

Continued

TABLE 65-1   Suture Repair of Soft Tissue Injuries—cont'd

Location	Anesthetic	Suture material*	Technique of closure and dressing	Suture removal	Pitfalls
Oral cavity	Lidocaine 1% with epinephrine or IV sedation may be necessary in children	4-0 synthetic absorbable	Simple interrupted or horizontal mattress; layered closure if muscularis of tongue involved	7-8 days or allow to dissolve	Inadequate sedation and exposure (particularly in children) for necessary procedure
Neck	Lidocaine 1% with epinephrine	4-0 synthetic absorbable intradermal 5-0 nonabsorbable monofilament	Two-layered closure for best cosmetic results	4-6 days	Failure to appreciate implication of zone I or zone III injuries; delay in airway management
Abdomen	Lidocaine 1% with epinephrine	4-0 synthetic absorbable 4-0 or 5-0 nonabsorbable monofilament	Single or layered closure	6-12 days	Failure to use local wound exploration as an initial screen and aggressively follow-up with further diagnostic procedures
Back	Lidocaine 1% with epinephrine	4-0 synthetic absorbable 4-0 or 5-0 nonabsorbable monofilament	Single or layered closure	6-12 days	Failure to appreciate possibility of renal or diaphragmatic injury
Chest	Lidocaine 1% with epinephrine	4-0 synthetic absorbable 4-0 or 5-0 nonabsorbable monofilament	Single or layered closure	6-12 days	Exploration of wound may cause hemorrhage or pneumothorax, failure to consider possibility of diaphragmatic penetration in low chest wounds and pericardial tamponade in wounds near midline

Location	Anesthetic	Suture material	Closure technique	Suture removal	Pitfalls
Extremity	Lidocaine 1% with epinephrine	3-0 or 4-0 synthetic absorbable (muscle) 4-0 or 5-0 nonabsorbable monofilament	Single-layered closure is adequate although layered or running SC closure may give better cosmetic result; apply splint if wound over a joint	6-14 days	Failure to make sensory examination before anesthesia; failure to explore wound visually after hemostasis, unrecognized foreign body left in wound
Hands and feet	Lidocaine 1% (if field block use 2% lidocaine or 0.25% bipivacaine)	4-0 or 5-0 nonabsorbable monofilament	Single-layered closure only with simple or horizontal mattress interrupted suture, at least 5 mm from cut wound edges; horizontal mattress sutures should be used if tension on wound edges; apply splint if wound over a joint	7-12 days	Use of subcuticular sutures, failure to explore wound visually with digit in original position at time of injury
Nailbeds	Lidocaine 2% or bipivacaine 0.25% digital nerve block	5-0 synthetic absorbable	Gentle, meticulous placement to obtain even edges; stint dressing with original nail or aluminum foil between cuticle and nail matrix to prevent adhesions	Allow to absorb	Loss of suture by tying too tightly and having it cut through friable nailbed suture; adhesions caused by failure to place stint between cuticle and matrix

*Tape may be used for surface or epidermal closure if buried intradermal closure results in perfectly even wound edges and no propensity for differential swelling of wound edges exists. Tape may also be used for tiny laceration with minimal or no tension on wound edges.
Synthetic absorbable sutures: polyglycolic acid, polyglactin 910, polydiaxone, glycolide trimethylene carbonate.
Synthetic nonabsorbable monofilament: nylon, polypropylene, polybutester.

wound. Tighten sutures to bring edges of the skin together; do not strangulate.

5. Cutaneous tape closure may occasionally be used for superficial wounds in areas without motion where meticulous closure is not required. The area should be dried, tincture of benzoin applied, and the edges approximated without tension or underlying dead space.

6. Longitudinal alignment of relatively straight lacerations may be achieved by selecting the midpoint of the laceration for the first suture and continuing to bisect each section. Place the sutures at the same depth on both sides and close the wound with the least amount of tension.

7. In the management of a flap, if it is proximal to the blood supply, especially on an extremity, the tip usually survives unless the base is narrow. Proximal flaps usually survive if the base is three times as long as the height. Distally based flaps have an increased risk of necrosis.

8. Staples may be used for lacerations of the scalp, trunk, or extremity.

9. Considerations regarding lacerations of the lip, eyelid, eyebrow, nose, ear, scalp, and neck are discussed in Chapter 58.

10. Histoacryl blue, a tissue adhesive, is suitable for closure of small lacerations with minimal tension and may replace tape and sutures for closure of these small wounds when approved for use by the FDA. It has been found to be useful in facial lacerations less than 4 cm long and less than 0.5 cm wide. Wounds that should be avoided include those that are deep, require multiple closure layers, result from animal bites, or involve mucocutaneous or hair-containing surfaces.

    The adhesive is applied using a 27-gauge needle and edges held together for approximately 30 seconds. The wound must be kept dry.

11. Horizontal mattress sutures should be considered for all wounds with significant tension that are to be closed in a single layer (i.e., wounds overlying joints).

Primary Repair of Nerve Injuries

Repair is more effective in children than in adults. Neuropraxia or axonotmesis should be observed for 3 to 6 months along with electrodiagnostic studies before surgical repair is performed. Neurotmesis requires an early epineural repair by a surgeon.

Dressing and Splints of the Hands and Feet

1. A large bulky dressing of the hand or foot is optimal for most children, particularly when immobilization will only be necessary for several days.

2. Injuries of the hand requiring immobilization usually involve wounds over the joints and are best dressed in the "hooded cobra" position. The wrist is in neutral position, the metacarpophalangeal (MCP) joints are flexed at about 60 to 70 degrees, the interphalangeal (IP) joints are flexed at 10 to 20 degrees, and the thumb abducted. A volar plaster splint may be incorporated over the dressing for additional immobilization.

3. The foot may require temporary immobilization if extensive injuries are present, particularly those involving tendons. This may be achieved by maintaining the ankle at 90 degrees with a posterior plaster splint.

4. Strong consideration should be given to splinting all full-thickness lacerations over joints for 1 to 2 weeks.

Antibiotics

Antibiotics are not required for clean lacerations. Grossly contaminated wounds are best left open and treated with delayed closure after copious irrigation.

The use of prophylactic antibiotics in animal bites remains controversial. Their use should be left to the judgment and discretion of the treating physician (see Chapter 45).

Oral penicillin may reduce the incidence of infection of intraoral and through-and-through lip lacerations. Topical antibacterial ointment may be used.

Puncture Wounds

Puncture wounds, usually of the foot, are common in children. These injuries have a higher infection rate because foreign material is easily trapped and the small size of the wound impedes irrigation. Simple puncture wounds can usually be treated with simple local irrigation with normal saline solution and close observation.

Wounds that possibly have a retained foreign material, are grossly contaminated, or develop local tenderness 2 to 3 days after the injury often need more aggressive medical and surgical therapy. After local anesthesia (without epinephrine), enlargement of the wound up to 4 to 5 mm using a No. 11 scalpel blade may be helpful in removing foreign material and irrigating the wound.

Osteomyelitis after punctures of the foot (usually through a sneaker) is most commonly due to *Pseudomonas aeruginosa* (see p. 753).

Fishhooks

Fishhooks commonly become embedded in fingers and other areas. Techniques for removal after anesthesia is achieved include the following:

1. Advance the tip of the hook through the skin past the barb and cut the distal hook and barb off. The remaining hook can be removed along its track of entry.
2. An 18-gauge needle is introduced along the barbed side of the hook at the entrance side of the wound, with the bevel toward the inside of the hook curve. Apply slight pressure upward on the hook shank to disengage it from the soft tissues. Push the needle upward and rotate until the lumen locks firmly over the barb. Keep the needle locked on the barb with gentle pressure. Then, with a slight rotation of the hook shank upward, the hook and needle can be removed through the original wound with a slight downward movement.
3. Newer devices have been introduced to specifically remove fishhooks.

Splinters, Subungual/Hematomas, and Paronychia

See discussion on these problems in Chapter 68, p. 541.

PARENTAL EDUCATION

Parental education and follow-up should be specifically delineated on a printed instruction sheet.

1. Mild bleeding and some discomfort may occur after suturing as anesthesia wears off.
2. Keep the wound clean and dry for 2 days. Then begin gentle cleaning of the wound with soap and water. If scab formation is significant, peroxide may be useful to facilitate suture removal.
3. Call your physician if the wound becomes red, painful, swollen, drains pus, or if red streaks appear.
4. Change dressing as directed.
5. Return for suture removal as instructed.
6. Apply sunscreen (SPF 15 or greater) over scar for 6 months after injury.

REFERENCES

Applebaum JS, Zalut T, Applebaum D: The use of tissue adhesion for traumatic laceration repair in the emergency department, *Ann Emerg Med* 22:1190, 1993.

Berk WA, Welch RD, Bock BF: Controversial issues in clinical management of the simple wound, *Ann Emerg Med* 21:72, 1992.

Brinkman KR, Lambert RW: Evaluation of skin stapling for wound closure in the emergency department, *Ann Emerg Med* 18:1122, 1989.

Chisholm CD, Cordell WH, Rogers K, et al: Comparison of a new pressurized saline canister versus syringe irrigation for laceration cleansing in the emergency department, *Ann Emerg Med* 21:1364, 1992.

Doser C, Cooper WL, Ediger WM, et al: Fishhook injuries: a prospective evaluation, *Am J Emerg Med* 9:413, 1991.

Edlich RF, Rodeheaver GT, Morgan RF, et al: Principles of emergency wound management, *Ann Emerg Med* 17:1284, 1988.

Grisham JE, Zukin DD: Suture selection for the pediatrician, *Pediatr Emerg Care* 6:301, 1990.

Hollander JE, Richman PB, Werblud M, et al: Irrigation in facial and scalp lacerations: does it alter outcome? *Ann Emerg Med* 31:73, 1998.

Hunt TK: The physiology of wound healing, *Ann Emerg Med* 17:1265, 1988.

Inaba AS, Zukin DD, Perro M: An update on the evaluation and management of plantar puncture wounds and *Pseudomonas* osteomyelitis, *Pediatr Emerg Care* 8:38, 1992.

Jacobs RF, McCarthy RE, Elser JM: *Pseudomonas* osteochondritis complicating puncture wounds of the foot in children: a 10-year evaluation, *J Infect Dis* 160:657, 1989.

Langsam A: Solid foreign bodies in the soft tissues: diagnosis and management, *Del Med J* 57:693, 1985.

Quinn JV, Drzewieck A, Limm, et al: A randomized controlled trial comparing a tissue adhesive with suturing in the repair of pediatric facial lacerations, *Ann Emerg Med* 22:1130, 1993.

Simon B: Principles of wound management. In Rosen P, editor: *Emergency medicine: concepts and clinical practice*, ed 4, St Louis, 1998, Mosby.

Simon HK, McLaird DJ, Bruns TB, et al: Long-term appearance of lacerations repaired using tissue adhesive, *Pediatrics* 99:193, 1997.

Singer AJ, Hollanger JE, Quinn JV: Evaluation and management of traumatic lacerations, *N Engl J Med* 337:1142, 1997.

Steele MT, Sainsbury CR, Robinson WA, et al: Prophylactic penicillin for intraoral wounds, *Ann Emerg Med* 18:847, 1989.

Tandberg D: Glass in the hand and foot: will an x-ray film show it? *JAMA* 248:1872, 1982.

Zukin DD, Inaba AS, Wuerker C: Minor wounds. In Barkin RM, editor: *Pediatric emergency medicine: concepts and clinical practice*, ed 2, St Louis, 1997, Mosby.

65 Appendix to Chapter: Analgesia and Sedation

Approaching the child who requires analgesia or sedation for a procedure must be done systematically, considering a number of factors:

1. What response is required—analgesia, sedation, or both?
2. What level of titration of analgesia or sedation is required? IV administration provides the most rapid onset of activity and controlled titration of effect. Other routes reflective of mucosal absorption and gastrointestinal absorption, motility.
3. What route(s) are available or potentially available?
4. Is immediate reversal of potential side effects necessary? Agents are available for narcotics (naloxone) and benzodiazepines (flumazenil).
5. Is the child at particular risk for a specific side effect?

    Infants younger than 1 month are particularly sensitive to morphine-induced respiratory depression. Do underlying medical problems or medications enhance the risk?

6. What monitoring equipment, personnel, and capabilities are available? Many agents have a dose-dependent relationship to ventilation. The P_{CO_2} may rise before the P_{O_2} drops.
7. What level of resuscitation capabilities is available?
8. What is the clinician's personal experience with the agent?

The answers to these questions will largely determine the therapeutic alternatives that are outlined in this Appendix. It is essential to be sensitive to the needs of the child in providing optimal analgesia and sedation within the bounds of appropriately balancing the risks and benefits. Children receiving systemic agents require monitoring if any anticipated risk of impacting airway, breathing, or circulation exists.

In addition to pharmacologic approaches, psychologic measures such as hypnosis and distraction may be useful with appropriate preparation. Parental participation can be helpful in reducing anxiety, communicating truthfully with the patient, and supporting the child through the procedure. A positive attitude will reduce anxiety. Letting children make choices (e.g., site of IV access, selection of stickers) is important.

A number of measurement tools exist to assess pain in adults and children older than 7 years. These include the use of cognitive (i.e., self-reporting, faces) and behavioral scales (Children's Hospital of Eastern Ontario Pain Scale [CHEOPS]).

ANALGESIA (see Table 65-2)

Pain control may be approached with systemic narcotic and other agents for longer or more complicated procedures while monitoring the patient. Localized anesthesia may be useful

TABLE 65-2　Recommended Sedative and Analgesic Agents for Pediatric Emergency Department Patients

Indication	Agent	Route	Initial dosage (mg/kg)	Maximum initial dose*	Onset	Duration
ANALGESIA						
Mild-moderate	Acetaminophen	PO, PR	10-15	1000 mg		
Moderate	Ibuprofen	PO	10	800 mg		
Severe	Morphine sulfate	IV, SC	0.1	10 mg	5-6 min	3-4 hr
	Ketorolac	IM, IV	0.5-1.0	60 mg		
	Meperidine	IM	2	100 mg	30-60 min	2-3 hr
	plus promethazine	IM	1	50 mg		
SEDATION						
Moderate	Midazolam	PO, PR, IN	0.5	10 mg	10-20 min	1 hr
	Chloral hydrate	PR, PO	50-80	2000 mg	30-90 min	2-4 hr
Deep	Midazolam	IV	0.1	5 mg	2-5 min	30 min
	Diazepam	IV	0.2	10 mg	5-10 min	1-2 hr
	Lorazepam	IV	0.02-0.05	2 mg	5-6 min	2-3 hr
	Pentobarbital	IV	2-5	200 mg	1 min	15 min
ANALGESIA AND SEDATION						
No IV	Codeine	PO	1-2	60 mg	1 hr	3-4 hr
	Hydrocodone	PO	0.2	7.5 mg	1 hr	3-4 hr
	Morphine	IM	0.1	10 mg	5-10 min	4-5 hr
	plus midazolam	IM	0.1	5 mg		
	Ketamine†	IM	4	50 mg	2-10 min	1 hr
	Meperidine	IM	2	50 mg	30-60 min	1-3 hr
	plus promethazine	IM	1	25 mg		
	plus chlorpromazine (MPC/DPT)	IM	1	25 mg		
With IV	Morphine	IV	0.1	10 mg	5-6 min	3-4 hr
	Morphine	IV	0.1	10 mg		
	plus midazolam	IV	0.1	5 mg		
	Fentanyl‡	IV (slow)	0.001-0.002	0.005 mg/kg (0.05-0.1 mg)	2-3 min	1 hr
	Fentanyl‡	IV	0.001-0.002	0.005 mg/kg (0.05-0.1 mg)	2-3 min	1 hr
	plus midazolam	IV	0.1	5 mg	2-5 min	30 min
	Ketamine†	IV	1	100 mg	1 min	10 min

IN, Intranasal; *PO*, oral; *PR*, rectal.

*Therapeutic doses may vary with individual patients. If higher dosages are required, they should be titrated while monitoring patient.

†Atropine is often given in the same syringe to reduce excess secretions associated with ketamine.

‡One-third dose in children <6 mo.

for procedures involving only limited areas through various routes: topical (TAC, cryoanesthesia), local infiltration (subcutaneous [SC], intradermal, field), regional block, or nerve block.

Topical

Topical mixtures may be useful for superficial injuries, particularly in young children. Do not use on mucosal lesions or where epinephrine is contraindicated.

1. TAC: Topical tetracaine, 1%, topical adrenaline (epinephrine) (1:4000), cocaine HCl solution 4%. TAC should *never* be used on mucosal injuries because of the potential absorption of cocaine. Most effective on face; inconsistently useful on extremities. Cardiac arrest has been reported. Solutions with other concentrations, including one that has half of the above amount of cocaine, have proven to be equally effective. Tetracaine and adrenaline (TA) applied topically is also useful. Studies have demonstrated the relative efficacy of prilocaine (3.56%) with 0.99% phenylephrine, 1.0% tetracaine with 5.0% phenylephrine, and 1.0% tetracaine with 1.0% lidocaine and 2.5% phenylephrine.

   For anesthesia, 2 to 3 ml of TAC may be instilled within the inner margins of the laceration until the cavity is filled. An equal amount of TAC is applied by using a cotton ball or swab (not gauze) over the wound for 10 to 15 minutes. The individual holding the cotton ball/swab should wear gloves.

   One study has reported the safety of careful application of TAC to an oral laceration with a cotton-tipped applicator applied directly to the wound for 5 minutes.

2. LET/XAP: Viscous Xylocaine (Lidocaine), 2%. 15 ml, topical adrenaline (epinephrine) (1:1000), 7.5 ml, and topical tetracaine, 2%, 7.5 ml. Has been shown to be as effective as TAC on facial wounds without potential complications. Same application technique as TAC.

3. EMLA (eutectic mixture of local anesthetics) cream is a commercially available mixture of lidocaine, 2.5%, and prilocaine, 2.5%, suspended in oil-in-water emulsion that is effective on uncomplicated extremity wounds; 2.5 to 5.0 gm is applied on skin and sealed at least 1 hour before procedure. It is more effective than TAC on extremity wounds.

4. Transient anesthesia can also be obtained by topical application for 5 to 15 minutes of gauze saturated with 2% to 4% of lidocaine.

5. Other transdermal drug delivery systems are being developed.

Infiltrative

Lidocaine (Xylocaine), 1% or 2%, is adequate for most infiltrative and regional anesthetics. Infiltration is done with a small needle (25 or 27 gauge) directly through the wound margins. Onset of anesthesia is 5 to 15 minutes with a duration of 1 to 2 hours.

1. Discomfort may be reduced by *buffering* the lidocaine. Sodium bicarbonate is added to the lidocaine in a ratio by volume of 1:10 to neutralize the pH. The shelf-life of buffered lidocaine is 1 week. *Slow injection* (30 seconds) through a 27-gauge needle minimizes pain. *Warming* the lidocaine (storing in fluid warmer at 98.6° F) may also be helpful. A slow rate of administration probably has the greatest impact on reducing pain.

2. Before injection, a small amount of 4% lidocaine or other topical anesthetic may be applied to the wound to decrease the pain of injection.

3. Toxic levels may result from local administration of more than 4 mg/kg plain lidocaine or more than 7 mg/kg of lidocaine with epinephrine. Toxicity includes sinus

arrest, bradycardia, hypotension, atrioventricular (AV) block, irritability, respiratory depression, seizures, and coma.

4. Lidocaine containing epinephrine at a ratio of 1:100,000 may assist with hemostasis but should only be used in areas of good perfusion and *never* on the digits, hands, feet, ear, tarsal plate of the eye, bridge of the nose, nipple, or penis.

5. Regional anesthesia may be achieved by using proper anatomic landmarks but may require additional local infiltration as well. It minimizes distortion.

6. The ear may be adequately anesthetized by raising a wheal with lidocaine 1% without epinephrine about the entire base of the ear. This will anesthetize all but the external canal.

7. Bupivacaine (Marcaine) is an alternative agent with onset of 10 to 30 minutes and a duration of anesthesia of 4 to 6 hours. The maximum dose (without epinephrine) is 2-3 mg/kg/dose.

Systemic Nonnarcotic

1. Aspirin and acetaminophen.
2. Nonsteroidal antiinflammatory drugs (NSAIDs) are potent analgesic and antiinflammatory agents. Ibuprofen is widely used. It may be a more effective antipyretic than acetaminophen.
   a. Ketorolac is the only available parenteral NSAID available in the United States. Available PO, IM, and IV, 0.5 mg/kg q6hr IV for 48 to 72 hours (maximum: 30 mg q6hr IV).

Systemic narcotic agent selection should be made on the basis of the required duration of action, dose, route of administration, patient's weight and clinical stability, and use of narcotic potentiators.

1. Fentanyl (Sublimaze), 1-2 µg/kg up to a total dose of 5 µg/kg IV slowly over 3 to 5 minutes, has been used with great success. It has a half-life of 20 minutes and can be easily reversed using naloxone (Narcan). Older children often require less than the calculated dose. Oral transmucosal fentanyl incorporated into a candy matrix may be a useful premedication.

2. Meperidine (Demerol) is used in a number of mixtures.
   a. Meperidine, 1 mg/kg/dose (maximum: 50 mg/dose) IM; or
   b. Meperidine, 1 mg/kg/dose (maximum: 50 mg/dose), and hydroxyzine (Atarax, Vistaril), 0.5-1 mg/kg/dose IM; or
   c. Meperidine, 1-2 mg/kg/dose (maximum: 50 mg/dose), and promethazine (Phenergan), 0.25-0.5 mg/kg/dose (maximum: 12.5 mg/dose), and chlorpromazine (Thorazine), 0.25-0.5 mg/kg/dose (maximum: 12.5 mg/dose) IM. Usually mixed in ratio of 1:0.25:0.25 (DPT cocktail).

      Meperidine has an increased risk of seizures associated with repeated use.

3. Morphine, 1 mg/kg/dose IV, is a potent narcotic that should be titrated slowly. It should not be used in hemodynamically or neurologically unstable patients.

4. Codeine is an oral opioid with a potency of one-sixth that of parenteral morphine.

5. Patient-controlled analgesia (PCA), although not typically begun in the emergency department (ED) setting, may be considered on admission for children who will be in substantial ongoing pain.

SEDATION (see Table 65-2)

Sedation is not required for most injuries and procedures. There are, however, specific circumstances when it is appropriate and will expedite the procedure. If a child is sedated, the face and chest should be uncovered (if not directly involved in procedure) when possible during the procedure to permit monitoring of color and respiratory effort. Oximetry must be monitored concurrently.

1. Midazolam (Versed), 0.05-0.10 mg/kg/dose IV over 1 to 2 minutes up to a maximum dose of 4-5 mg, may be given to an end-point of a drowsy patient with slurred speech. Efficacy of more than 98% causing antegrade amnesia. Flumazenil is a specific antagonist of benzodiazepines.

   Intranasal (IN) administration of the parenteral solution in a dose of 0.3-0.5 mg/kg/dose IN is effective.

   Oral midazolam, 0.3-0.7 mg/kg/dose PO, may reduce anxiety when given 30 to 45 minutes before a procedure.

   Rectal midazolam, 0.45 mg/kg/dose PR, may be useful when given 15 minutes before a procedure.

2. Chloral hydrate is a useful oral agent, particularly for nonpainful procedures such as radiologic imaging. The duration is variable but is generally 2 to 3 hours when given in a dose of 50-80 mg/kg/dose (maximum: 2000 mg) PO. Lower dosages are usually inadequate; higher dosages are more than 90% successful in children less than 4 years and greater than 80% in older children.

3. Pentobarbital (Nembutal) has been particularly effective in imaging and other nonpainful procedures. The starting dose is generally 2.5 mg/kg IV with supplemental doses of 1.25 mg/kg IV as needed up to a total maximum dose of 10-12 mg/kg IV.

   Often sedation can be avoided by creating a positive environment for the child. Avoid verbal and nonverbal communication that adds to the child's anxiety. Also, distracting the child is often useful.

OTHER AGENTS

1. Ketamine sedation may be used for facial lacerations requiring cooperation when close monitoring and observation are possible. A dosage of 1-5 mg/kg/dose IM is given 10 minutes after atropine, 0.01 mg/kg, the latter to reduce secretions. The ketamine IV dose is 0.5-1 mg/kg/dose IV. The oral dose of 10 mg/kg/dose PO may reduce anxiety. Patients must be observed carefully until fully awake, with equipment to manage the airway and ventilation if necessary. Combined ketamine (1-2 mg/kg/dose IV) and midazolam (0.05-0.10 mg/kg/dose IV) have been effectively used in procedures such as lumbar punctures and imaging studies.

   Ketamine should not be used in those 3 months of age or less, children who are to have procedures requiring stimulation of posterior pharynx, and patients with acute pulmonary infections or disease, cardiovascular disease, head injury, glaucoma, or psychosis. Those older than 1 to 5 years are more likely to have psychosis; the ideal age for use of the drug is 3 months to 10 years.

2. Propofol is a parenteral anesthetic with antiemetic, antipruritic, anticonvulsant, anxiolytic, hypnotic, and analgesic properties. The dosage in children is 1-2 mg/kg/dose IV followed by an infusion of 0.025-0.130 mg/kg/min IV because of the rapid clearance. Hypotension is not uncommon.

3. Nitrous oxide (30% to 50% mixture) is a useful supplement to local anesthetics.

SEQUENTIAL COMBINATION THERAPY—MIDAZOLAM (1 MG/ML) AND FENTANYL (50 µG/ML)

This sequential approach systematically provides analgesia and sedation if the previous step was not effective and requires continuous monitoring of individual responses. Oxygen should generally be administered. Pharmacologic antagonists should be readily available.

Step 1: Give fentanyl, 1 µg/kg IV, over 60 to 90 seconds.

Step 2: Give midazolam, 0.035 mg/kg IV.

Step 3: Repeat fentanyl, 1 µg/kg IV over 2 minutes, if patient is not drowsy and tranquil.

Step 4: Repeat one half of the first dose of midazolam if adequate sedation not achieved.

Step 5: Consider additional slow bolus of midazolam, 0.017 mg/kg IV.

The maximum doses are fentanyl, 5 µg/kg/hr IV, and midazolam, 0.15 mg/kg given stepwise with careful monitoring.

REVERSAL AGENTS

Naloxone (Narcan) is an opioid antagonist. The dosage is 0.1 mg/kg/dose IV/IM up to 2 mg/dose. It may be repeated every 2 to 3 minutes to a maximum total dose of 10 mg. Onset IV is 1 to 2 minutes with a duration of 20 to 40 minutes.

Flumazenil (Romazicon) is a pure benzodiazepine antagonist. The dosage is 0.02 mg/kg/dose IV/IM up to 0.2 mg/dose over 15 seconds. May repeat dose at 60-second intervals to a maximum total dose of 1 mg. Onset IV is 1 to 2 minutes with a duration of 20 to 40 minutes.

DISCHARGE GUIDELINES

After sedation and completion of the procedure, the child should be monitored until all vital signs are normal, mental status and muscular control/function have returned to baseline, and no support is required.

Specific instructions are required to be followed by responsible person:

- Monitor change in mental status and motor function. Watch for any difficulty with breathing.
- Provide dietary instructions, if any. Limit for the first 1 to 2 hours after discharge.
- Contact person.
- Arrange for observation. Return if any concerns, including recurrent vomiting, change in behavior, or other new problems, arise.

- Set activity limitations. Generally, no playing that requires coordination (biking, skating, swimming) for next 24 hours.

REFERENCES

Algren JT, Algren CC: Sedation and analgesia for minor pediatric procedures, *Pediatr Emerg Care* 12:435, 1996.

American Academy of Pediatrics, Committee on Drugs: Guidelines for monitoring and management of pediatric patients during and after sedation for diagnostic and therapeutic procedures, *Pediatrics* 89:1110, 1992.

American Academy of Pediatrics, Committee on Drugs: Reappraisal of lytic cocktail (Demerol, Phenergan and Thorazine[DPT]) for sedation of children, *Pediatrics* 95:598, 1995.

American College of Emergency Physicians: Clinical policy for procedural sedation and analgesia in the emergency department, *Ann Emerg Med* 31:663, 1998.

Bonadio WA: Safe and effective method for application of tetracaine, adrenaline and cocaine to oral lacerations, *Ann Emerg Med* 28:396, 1996.

Brogan GX, Giarrusso E, Hollander JE, et al: Comparison of plain, warmed and buffered lidocaine for anesthesia of traumatic wounds, *Ann Emerg Med* 26:2, 1995.

Connors K, Terndrup T: Nasal versus oral midazolam for sedation of anxious children undergoing laceration repair, *Ann Emerg Med* 24:1074, 1994.

Emslander HC: Local and topical anesthesia for pediatric wound repair: a review of selected aspects, *Pediatr Emerg Care* 14:123, 1998.

Fatovich DM, Jacobs IG: A randomized controlled trial of oral midazolam and buffered lidocaine for suturing lacerations in children, *Ann Emerg Med* 215:209, 1995.

Gamis AS, Knapp IF, Glenski JA: Nitrous oxide analgesia in a pediatric emergency department, *Ann Emerg Med* 18:177, 1989.

Green SM, Johnson NE: Ketamine sedation for pediatric procedures. 2. Pediatric procedures, *Ann Emerg Med* 19:1033, 1990.

Houck CS, Wilder RT, McDermott IS, et al: Safety of intravenous ketorolac therapy in children and cost savings from a unit dosing system, *J Pediatr* 129:292, 1996.

Orlinsky M, Hudson C, Chan L, et al: Pain comparison of unbuffered versus buffered lidocaine in local wound infiltration, *J Emerg Med* 10:44, 1992.

Parker R, Mahan RA, Giugliano D, et al: Efficacy and safety of intravenous midazolam and ketamine for therapeutic and diagnostic procedures in children, *Pediatrics* 99:427, 1997.

Scarfone RJ, Jasani M, Gracely EJ: Pain of local anesthetics: rate of administration and buffering, *Ann Emerg Med* 31:36, 1998.

Schechter NL, Weisman SI, Rosenblum M, et al: The use of oral transmucosal fentanyl citrate in children, *Pediatrics* 95:335, 1995.

Schilling CG, Bank DE, Borchart BA, et al: Tetracaine, epinephrine (adrenaline) and cocaine (TAC) versus lidocaine, epinephrine and tetracaine (LET) for anesthesia of lacerations in children, *Ann Emerg Med* 25:203, 1995.

Shane JA, Fuchs SM, Khine H: Rectal midazolam for the sedation of preschool children undergoing laceration repair, *Ann Emerg Med* 24:1065, 1994.

Smith GA, Strausbaugh SD, Harbeck-Weber C, et al: New non-cocaine containing topical anesthetics compared with tetracaine-adrenaline-cocaine during repair of lacerations, *Pediatrics* 100:825, 1997.

Smith GA, Strausbaugh SD, Harbeck-Weber C: Comparison of topical anesthetics without cocaine to tetracaine-cocaine and lidocaine infiltration during repair of lacerations: bupivacaine-norepinephrine is an effective new topical anesthetic agent, *Pediatrics* 97:301, 1996.

Smith SM, Barry RC: A comparison of three formulations of TAC (tetracaine, adrenaline, cocaine) for anesthesia of minor lacerations in children, *Pediatr Emerg Care* 6:266, 1990.

Steinberg AD: Should chloral hydrate be banned? *Pediatrics* 92:442, 1993.

Steward DI: Management of childhood pain: new approaches to procedure related pain, *J Pediatr* 122:51, 1993.

Terndrup TE, D'Agostino I: Pain control, analgesia and sedation. In Barkin RM, editor: *Pediatric emergency medicine: concepts and clinical practice*, ed 2, St Louis, 1997, Mosby.

Terndrup TE, Dire DI, Madden CM, et al: Comparison of intramuscular meperidine and promethazine with and without chlorpromazine: a randomized, prospective double; blind trial, *Ann Emerg Med* 22:206, 1993.

Theroux MC, West DW, Corddry DH, et al: Efficacy of intranasal midazolam in facilitating suturing of lacerations in preschool children in the emergency department, *Pediatrics* 91:624, 1993.

Waldbilig DK, Quinn JV, Stiell IG, et al: Randomized double-blind controlled trail comparing room temperature and heated lidocaine for digital nerve block, *Ann Emerg Med* 26:677, 1995.

Wase RE, Cardwell P: XAP: an alternative to cocaine for topical anesthesia, *Ann Emerg Med* 22:1 59, 1993.

Yaster M, Tobin JR, Fisher QA, et al: Local anesthetics in the management of acute pain in children, *Pediatrics* 124: 165, 1994.

Zempsky WT, Karasic RB: EMLA versus TAC for topical anesthesia of extremity wounds in children, *Ann Emerg Med* 30:163, 1997.

X

ORTHOPEDIC INJURIES

66 MANAGEMENT PRINCIPLES

DOUGLAS V. MAYEDA

ALERT: Management of orthopedic injuries must follow stabilization of the patient. The unique growth characteristics of the child affect the nature of potential injuries.

Most orthopedic injuries seen in the emergency department (ED) are not life threatening. However, those involving multiple trauma must be appropriately prioritized, and when the pelvis or femur is broken, vascular support may be required (spinal injuries are discussed in Chapter 61). For all patients, the diagnosis and management must be precise to maximize permanent function.

Children's bones differ from those of adults. They bend, buckle, and sustain greenstick fractures; fractures heal rapidly, and nonunions are rare. A child's periosteum is thicker and more resistant to disruption, potentially serving as a hinge to assist in reduction. Ligaments are more resistant to injury than are growth plates. Injury of the growth plate and buckle fractures are by far more common than sprains, which are uncommon in children.

The elasticity of children's bones allows the bone to deform before breaking and may result in a greenstick or torus fracture. Children's bones are able to absorb more energy and force before breaking when compared with a mature adult skeleton. A *greenstick* fracture involves the diaphysis of one side of a long bone, thus resulting in a fracture of one side of the cortex with an intact opposite side. A *torus* fracture is a buckling of one side of the cortex without an actual fracture line. This is usually seen in the metaphysis. The cortex in the developing skeleton and the microstructure and macrostructure dictate that the pattern of failure will be a torus deformation rather than a complete transverse fracture. A torus fracture is one of the most common patterns affecting the developing skeleton.

DIAGNOSTIC FINDINGS

An accurate history of the time of the event, mechanism of injury, and direction of forces and any history of previous injury and aggravating disease processes or bleeding diatheses should be obtained. The mechanism of injury is particularly important in defining the potential and type of injury and may assist in developing treatment plans by reducing a fracture or dislocation using a force that is opposite to that which led to the injury. Often, the injury was not witnessed and the child may be either unable (because of age) or too frightened to give a reliable history. Pseudoparalysis secondary to pain is common in the younger child. Children rarely complain persistently unless there is an abnormality. It is particularly important to recognize that pain may be referred, the classic example being hip injuries presenting as

---

Box 66-1

DIAGNOSTIC FINDINGS SUGGESTIVE OF A PATIENT HAVING A POSITIVE EXTREMITY RADIOGRAPH

UPPER EXTREMITY

Gross deformity
Activity restricted
Bone point tenderness
Pain on motion
Swelling moderate
   or severe
Time since injury >6 hr

LOWER EXTREMITY

Gross deformity
Activity restricted
Bone point tenderness
Pain on motion
Knee injury
Foot injury

---

knee pain. Histories that are vague or inconsistent with injuries or delay in seeking medical care suggest child abuse. Approximately 15% to 25% of fractures in children less than 3 years of age are caused by nonaccidental trauma (NAT) (see Chapter 25).

Observation and examination for obvious deformities, swelling, ecchymoses, and point tenderness should be performed. In addition, evaluation of skin integrity, neurovascular status, muscle and tendon function, and pretreatment x-ray films are required.

Because of difficulty with physical evaluation and the lack of history in many cases, if any suspicion of an underlying fracture exists, x-ray studies should be obtained (see Box 66-1). Routine anteroposterior (AP) and lateral views, with inclusion of the joints above and below the suspected fracture site, help ensure that all potentially involved areas are studied. If any doubt exists because of the growth plates, *comparison views* may be obtained on a selective basis. Gonadal shields should be used. Those fractures missed most commonly by x-ray study include fractures of the ribs, elbow, and periarticular regions of the phalanges. Other problem areas include fractures of the navicular and calcaneous.

The age of fractures may be estimated by the following radiologic guidelines:

4-10 days	Resolution of soft tissues
10-14 days	Periosteal elevation
14-21 days	Soft callus
21-42 days	Hard callus
1 year	Remodeling

MANAGEMENT

Fracture remodeling and growth are rapid with particular stimulation of longitudinal growth and therefore may lead to overgrowth of an extremity when they occur between 2 and 10 years of age. Greater degrees of angulation are accepted in the pediatric population when it involves metaphyseal fractures. However, angulation should be reduced as much as possible. It is tolerated better in children less than 2 years with fractures near the ends of bones, where there is bayonet opposition, or if the deformity is in the plane of motion of the joint. Displaced intraarticular fractures; fractures that are grossly shortened, angulated, or rotated; fractures at marked angles to the plane of motion of a joint; or fractures that cross the growth plate need accurate reduction. It is unusual for children to need open reductions, but early orthopedic consultation is usually desirable.

Dislocations are rare, and when they do occur, they most commonly involve the radial head or patella. *Fractures often accompany dislocations because the ligamentous structures are more resistant to trauma than the epiphyseal plates.* In general, the dislocation should be reduced before treatment of the fracture. An orthopedist should be involved. Neurologic function should be evaluated and, in most instances, x-ray studies obtained before and after reduction. Open dislocations or those with neurovascular compromise are true emergencies. A deformity is best corrected by an orthopedic consultant with gentle, steady, inline traction, if such traction does not further impede circulation, increase pain significantly, or result in increased resistance with correction.

Patients with any fracture or dislocation involving a potential for vascular compromise (e.g., supracondylar, humerus, posterior knee dislocation) should be generally admitted to the hospital after immediate ED orthopedic consultation and management. Should there be any suggestion of vascular compromise, it is also wise to have an immediate vascular consultation to assist in making a decision about angiography or surgery. The absence of a pulse does not always indicate that the vascular status is compromised nor does the presence of a pulse ensure adequate circulation. Severe pain in the forearm or calf, pain with passive stretching of the fingers or toes, or a sensory deficit in the distal extremity are more sensitive indicators of ischemia, which may be caused by arterial injury or a compartment syndrome.

Analgesia is usually required before reduction in treating dislocations or poorly aligned fractures. As discussed in the Appendix to Chapter 65, there are many alternatives, partially reflecting the clinician's preference. Analgesia should be provided only after careful evaluation of the entire patient and the injured site. There is no reason to withhold analgesia after evaluation for isolated orthopedic injuries. Primary concern with good reduction of pain should be to immobilize and stabilize a fracture site. All require careful monitoring of the patient. Fentanyl (Sublimaze), 1-5 μg/kg over 1 to 2 minutes up to a total dose of about 100 μg, may be given with the upper limit requiring titration. Older children may require a smaller dose than calculated. The half-life is 20 minutes. Midazolam (Versed), 0.05-0.10 mg/kg/dose IV, may be used as the sole agent or as an adjunct to fentanyl because of its rapid onset of action and short half-life. Midazolam, 0.3-0.7 mg/kg, may also be used orally and 0.4 mg/kg intranasally. Meperidine (Demerol), 1 mg/kg/dose intramuscular (IM) or IV (maximum: 50 mg/dose), and muscle relaxation (diazepam [Valium], 0.1-0.2 mg/kg/

dose PO or IV) is another useful alternative. Flumazenil (Mazicon) should be available. Conscious sedation protocols and guidelines need to be followed judiciously. Ketamine and nitrous oxide are alternatives. Patient-controlled anesthesia (PCA) may be useful in the postoperative setting under institutional specific protocols. The Bier block has been used for upper extremity reductions, usually in conjunction with an orthopedist. A double-cuff pneumatic pressure cuff is placed above the elbow on the affected arm. The limb is exsanguinated by using a pneumatic splint or Esmarch bandage on the affected limb, and the upper cuff is inflated to 200 to 250 mm Hg. Administer 1.5-3.0 mg/kg of a 0.5% solution of lidocaine intravenously in the involved limb over 30 to 60 seconds. Inflate the lower cuff to 100 mm Hg above systolic pressure and deflate the upper cuff. Anesthesia is generally achieved in 5 minutes. The tourniquet may be left in place for 60 to 90 minutes or 15 minutes after infusion of lidocaine. The block may be terminated by deflating slowly. Patients should have a second line placed in the unaffected arm in case dysrhythmias are noted as a result of systemic absorption of lidocaine; monitoring is essential.

Local analgesia may be achieved for closed reduction by "hematoma" block with 1% to 2% lidocaine solution injected directly into the hematoma.

Although stiffness is unusual, long-term care is essential for children to monitor growth and development. Communication with parents regarding treatment, home care, and possible complications is essential in initiating the management plan. In general, sprains and strains should be elevated, with use of ice packs for 12 to 24 hours. Elevation can reduce swelling and pain. Ice packs are best prepared by crushing ice and placing it with some water in a plastic bag and applying for 15 to 20 minutes every 3 to 4 hours with continuing use of an elastic bandage in between. The elastic ACE bandage, if used, should be rewrapped as necessary if too loose or too tight. If a cast is applied, it should be kept dry. Parents should call immediately if there is severe pressure or pain within the cast, increasing blueness, coldness, tingling, swelling, or decreased motion of the toes or fingers. Oral analgesics and antiinflammatory agents may be useful for ongoing care.

Long-term sequelae of fractures that should be monitored include nonunion, avascular necrosis, angulation deformities, shortening, overgrowth, infection, joint stiffness, and posttraumatic arthritis.

SPLINTS

All suspected fractures should be splinted when the patient arrives at the ED. Splinting can be performed in the position of function with firm materials, slings, and tape and is used primarily as an initial treatment to rest an injured area. Casts are often not applied for at least 48 hours after acute injuries because of swelling. Acute injuries should be splinted over adequate padding (e.g., Webril, stockinette) with plaster or fiberglass (10 layers for upper extremities and 20 layers for lower extremities). The splint is affixed with cotton or elastic bandages. An alternative is to place a circular cast and immediately bivalve it. Commercial splints and fiberglass casting material are also available.

Swelling during this period can cause neurovascular compromise if confined to a compartment. One joint above and one below should be incorporated. Delayed casting is particularly important in children, who are often unable to follow after-care instructions of elevation, rest, and cool packs. They can then be immobilized and followed by an orthopedist.

Those with obvious deformities should be stabilized on arrival before complete evaluation unless there is compromised sensation or circulation distal to the injury, indicated by pain, pallor, pulselessness, paralysis, paresthesias, and pain with passive movement. If neurovascular deficits exist, gentle longitudinal traction in line with the extremity should be performed.

Fractures of the femur are usually immobilized using a Thomas splint or Hare or Buck traction.

Commonly used splints include the following:

Sling and Swathe

This is used for injuries between the sternoclavicular joint and elbow. It is made by placing the arm at 90 degrees of flexion with a sling and immobilizing it against the chest using a swathe wrapped around the body.

Long-Arm Splint

This is used for injuries between the elbow and wrist, most commonly involving fractures of the forearm and distal radius.

Posterior Long-Arm Splint

This splint is used for elbow and forearm injuries, as well as wrist injuries, in which forearm rotation and elbow flexion must be eliminated. The plaster is applied from the dorsal aspect of the mid-upper arm, across the olecranon, and down the ulnar aspect of the forearm to the distal palmar flexion crease. In addition, seven to eight layers of plaster are positioned from the upper part of the humerus across the radial side of the elbow as a cross support. The elbow should be at 90 degrees of flexion with the forearm in neutral position.

Sugar-Tong Splint

The *brachial humerus* splint is applied from above the acromioclavicular (AC) joint, over the humerus, around the elbow, and up to the axillary crease. A collar and cuff provide support. The *forearm* splint goes from the distal palmar flexion crease to the elbow. The plaster is brought around the elbow to the dorsum of the hand just proximal to the metacarpophalangeal (MCP) joint.

Hand and Wrist Splints

Hand and wrist splints are used for injuries between the wrist and the tips of the fingers. In general, the position of function is the "hooded cobra." The wrist is in neutral position (the long axis of the forearm roughly lines up with the long axis of the thumb), the MCP joints are flexed to about 60 to 70 degrees, the interphalangeal (IP) joints are flexed 10 to 20 degrees, and the thumb is widely abducted (p. 534). The tips of the fingers must be visible for neurovascular examination. Other types of hand-wrist splints include the following:

Ulnar gutter splints: useful for nondisplaced fractures of the fourth and fifth digits. The fourth and fifth fingers should be kept at about 35 to 40 degrees of flexion at the MCP joint and 20 to 30 degrees at the IP joints.

Dorsal extension splints: used for nonrotated finger injuries involving the phalanges, metacarpals, MCP, and proximal interphalangeal (PIP) joints. A foam-padded aluminum splint is taped to the dorsum of the hand and wrist and bent to keep the MCP joint at 90 degrees of flexion. Bend the PIP joint to 45 degrees.

Thumb spicas: used for scaphoid injuries to the wrist, for ligamentous damage, and for injuries to the thumb. Plaster is cut in half longitudinally into two tails. The splint is applied to the radial aspect of the forearm, and one tail is wrapped around the thenar eminence and onto the palm and hand across the distal palmar crease. The second flap is wrapped around the thumb and up to the base of the nail.

Long-Leg Posterior Splint

This is used for injuries between the knee and ankle and is applied from the groin to the toes, with the ankle in neutral position of function.

Short-Leg Posterior Splint

This is used for injuries between the ankle and tips of the toes and is applied from just below the knee over the back of the leg to the toes, with the ankle at a 90-degree angle. The toes must remain visible. A stirrup or air splint available commercially provides support along the lateral and medial aspects of the ankle and distal leg.

SPRAINS AND STRAINS

The diagnosis of sprain or ligamentous tears, as an isolated injury, is unusual in children. A *sprain* is a tear of a ligament joining bone to bone around the joint and is caused most commonly by outside forces, especially contact sports. *Strains* are tears of the muscle or of fascia joining muscle to bone (musculotendinous unit), often resulting from a dynamic injury and usually not a contact sport.

Buckle fractures or epiphyseal injuries, rather than sprains and ligamentous injuries, often occur in young children because of the ease of injury to the epiphysis. However, adolescents do suffer ligamentous injuries.

First-Degree Sprain

First-degree sprain consists of minimal tearing of a ligament. There is point tenderness with neither abnormal motion nor joint instability and little or no swelling. The patient can bear weight.

Second-Degree Sprain

Second-degree sprain consists of appreciable tearing of a ligament (5% to 99% of fibers disrupted). There is point tenderness with moderate loss of function and variable presence of abnormal motion and joint instability. Weight bearing is painful, there is localized soft tissue hemorrhage, and hemarthrosis is present. Pain is evoked by testing of joint stability, and instability may be persistent.

Third-Degree Sprain

Third-degree sprain consists of complete disruption of the ligament surrounding a joint. There is extreme pain, loss of function, abnormal motion with absolute joint instability, deformity with tenderness and swelling, and diffuse hemorrhage. The patient is unable to bear weight, and there is persistent instability without surgical repair.

The patient may complain of little discomfort after the initial insult, and testing of the stability of the joint may cause little pain. Dislocations may have reduced spontaneously (common in fracture dislocation of the knee). The only clue may be the patient's unwillingness or inability to bear weight across the joint.

Strains

Strains are classified as sprains are. First-degree strains involve minimal tearing of a musculotendinous unit, whereas second-degree strains involve more significant tears. Third-degree strains are marked by complete tears and may be painless initially. Injuries are marked by tenderness and pain, usually accompanied by no evidence of joint instability.

Management

Elevation, ice, and analgesia may reduce symptoms. Splint immobilization may be used after x-ray studies have excluded a fracture and before consultation for second- and third-degree injuries. Support and crutches may be helpful.

EPIPHYSEAL FRACTURES (Fig. 66-1)

A long bone can be divided into four parts. The first part is the shaft of the bone, known as the diaphysis. The second part, the metaphysis, is adjacent to the growth plate. The third part is the growth or epiphyseal plate, a radiolucent horizontal line near the end of the bone where longitudinal growth occurs. The fourth part, the epiphysis, is the end of the bone near a joint and is separated from the metaphysis by the epiphyseal plate.

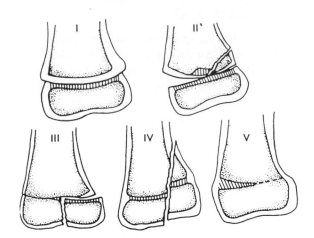

Fig. 66-1   Epiphyseal fractures: Salter classification.

Five types of epiphyseal fractures are identified by Salter and Harris, with the risk of growth disturbance increasing from a type I to a type V fracture.

Type I

Type I fracture consists of separation of the epiphysis from the metaphysis without displacement or injury to the growth plate. There is tenderness and pain at the point of the growth plate without other findings. The x-ray film result is initially normal but when repeated 7 to 10 days later may show calcification and new bone formation at the site of injury. The fracture should be immobilized for 3 weeks. Growth disturbance is rare.

Type II

Type II fracture consists of an epiphyseal plate slip with fracture through the metaphysis, producing a triangular metaphyseal fragment. It is the most common type of fracture. Treatment is achieved with a closed reduction and immobilization for 3 weeks (upper extremity) to 6 weeks (lower extremity). Growth disturbances are rare.

Type III

Type III fracture consists of an epiphyseal plate slip with an intraarticular fracture involving the epiphysis. The most common site is the distal tibial epiphysis. Accurate reduction (often surgical) with maintenance of blood supply is essential to reducing the risk of growth disturbance.

Type IV

Type IV fracture consists of an intraarticular fracture extending through the epiphysis, epiphyseal plate, and metaphysis. The lateral condyle of the humerus is the most common site. It requires surgical open reduction and internal fixation, and the prognosis regarding growth is guarded.

Type V

Type V fracture consists of a crush injury to the epiphyseal plate, producing growth arrest. This usually occurs in joints that move in one plane (flexion-extension), such as a knee, when a force in another plane is applied (abduction or adduction), such as smashing a dashboard or a direct-crush injury. The x-ray film may initially be normal. Despite treatment (no weight bearing for 3 weeks), the prognosis for normal growth is poor. Therefore this type of injury must be treated with immobilization and early follow-up. It is important to advise parents of growth problems. Early orthopedic consultation is vital.

OPEN FRACTURES

Open fractures require immediate treatment unless life-threatening injuries supersede. It is important to note how much bone is exposed and if it is comminuted, the degree of soft tissue damage, and the extent of contamination and bleeding. The only clue to an open fracture may be the collection of blood with fat globules from what is thought to be a small puncture wound. Regardless of the exposure of bone, the injury should be considered an open fracture and cleaned, debrided, cultured, covered, and immobilized. A sterile dressing soaked in antiseptic solution is applied to the wound. Tetanus toxoid or antitoxin should be given, when appropriate (p. 718). Cefazolin (Ancef), 75-125 mg/kg/24 hr q6-8hr IV, should be initiated, with an initial dose of 25-50 mg/kg IV. Anaerobic coverage may need to be considered.

The goal is to convert an open wound to a clean, closed wound as much as possible before definitive surgery.

REFERENCES

Berde CB, Lehn BM, Yee YD, et al: Patient controlled analgesia in children and adolescents: a randomized, prospective comparison with intramuscular administration of morphine for post-operative analgesia, *J Pediatr* 118:460, 1991.

Farrell RG: Safe and effective IV regional anesthesia for use in the emergency department, *Ann Emerg Med* 14:288, 1985.

Freed HA, Shields NN: Most frequently overlooked radiographically apparent fractures in a teaching hospital emergency department, *Ann Emerg Med* 13:900, 1984.

Hodge D III: Management principles: musculoskeletal and soft tissue injuries. In Barkin RM, editor: *Pediatric emergency medicine: concepts and clinical practice*, ed 2, St Louis, 1997, Mosby.

Jackimczyk KC, Goy W: Musculoskeletal trauma. In Rosen P, Doris PE, Barkin RM, et al, editors: *Diagnostic radiology in emergency medicine*, St. Louis, 1992, Mosby.

67 UPPER EXTREMITY INJURIES

MICHELE CHETHAM

CLAVICULAR FRACTURE

Clavicular fracture is the most common childhood fracture, including newborns. It may be associated with chest or shoulder trauma. In preschool children it is usually a greenstick fracture, with middle-third fracture most common.

Mechanism of Injury

A fall or blow to the shoulder or extended arm is the common cause.

Diagnostic Findings

1. Pain on movement of the affected arm or shoulder.
2. Tenderness and possibly deformity at the point of fracture. Comparison examination for the normal contralateral side may be useful.
3. Possible injury to the subclavian vessels. It is important to examine for this possibility. Clues include the presence of an unusual degree of swelling or ecchymosis, pulse changes, and occasionally a bruit over the involved vessel, which may radiate down the arm or to the heart.

X-Ray Film

A clavicular view is indicated.

Management

1. Fractures should generally be immobilized for 3 to 6 weeks in a figure-of-8 splint to maintain abduction of the shoulder. A commercial clavicular strap or one made of tubular stockinette filled with felt or cotton padding may be used. A sling may provide additional comfort. Some clinicians believe that little significant difference exists in the outcome in patients treated with a figure-of-8 splint and a simple sling. With this technique it is possible to do the following:
    a. Prevent skin maceration with a powdered pad in the axilla.
    b. Tighten to maintain abduction of the shoulder (may have to be adjusted occasionally).
    c. Observe frequently for axillary artery or brachial plexus compression.
    d. Caution parents that a residual bump will develop as the clavicle heals, which will subside in 6 to 12 months.
2. Fractures of the distal (outer) tip of the clavicle should be treated as acromioclavicular separations.
3. Fractures of the proximal (inner) third may be treated with a simple sling if the figure-of-8 splint distracts the pieces.
4. Follow-up visits every 2 to 3 weeks, with repeat radiograph when clinical healing achieved to assess callus formation.
5. Orthopedic referral if neurovascular or soft tissue compromise.

ACROMIOCLAVICULAR SEPARATION

Acromioclavicular separation is partial to complete disruption of the acromioclavicular (AC) ligaments.

Mechanism of Injury

Falling or a blow to the point of the acromion of the shoulder produces the injury.

Diagnostic Findings

1. Tenderness over the AC articulation
2. Limited abduction of the arm
3. If third-degree, step-off with upward displacement of the clavicle, representing complete rupture of the sternoclavicular and costoclavicular ligaments

X-Ray Film

An AC joint view is indicated. Traditionally, this is done initially without weights, but if normal, weight-bearing films are obtained by some. Comparison views of the opposite shoulder are necessary in all but third-degree separations.

1. First-degree: no evidence of displacement or joint subluxation
2. Second-degree: with weight bearing, less than 1 cm of upward displacement of the distal clavicle, indicating partial subluxation
3. Third-degree: with weight bearing, more than 1 cm of upward displacement

With the increasingly conservative approach to even the most significant AC injuries, some clinicians have suggested that weight-bearing films are no longer essential, preferring a new classification:

1. First-degree: less than 3 mm (or less than 50%) increase in AC joint width comparing the injured and uninjured sides with normal coracoclavicular (CC) distance (less than 5 mm or less than 50% difference between injured and uninjured sides)
2. Second-degree: 3 mm or greater (or greater than 50%) increase of injured versus uninjured AC joint width and normal CC distance
3. Third-degree: 5 mm or more (or 50% or more) increase of injured versus uninjured CC distance with or without AC widening and with or without clavicular elevation

Management

1. First- and second-degree separations require immobilization with sling and swathe or shoulder immobilizer and follow-up with an orthopedist.
2. Third-degree separation requires emergency department (ED) consultation.

SHOULDER DISLOCATION: ANTERIOR

Anterior dislocation accounts for 95% of cases of shoulder dislocations.

Mechanism of Injury

A blow to or fall on the arm while it is in external rotation, abduction, and extension produces this dislocation.

Diagnostic Findings

1. Prominent acromion process with flattening of the deltoid muscle
2. Head of the humerus palpable anterior, inferior, and medial to the glenoid fossa
3. Limitation of abduction and absence of external rotation

Complications

1. Greater tuberosity fractures or others secondary to manipulation
2. Associated abnormality of the glenoid (labrum detachment, tear of anterior capsule and subscapularis muscle, or Hill-Sachs lesion, the latter representing a compression fracture of the posterior humeral head)
3. Axillary nerve (lack of sensation over the lateral portion of the shoulder and upper arm with deltoid muscle palsy) and distal vascular compromise

X-Ray Films

Anteroposterior (AP) and axillary views are indicated. The humeral head lies inferior to the coracoid process. Fractures should be excluded. Postreduction x-ray films may reveal a fracture not seen initially or one that is secondary to reduction.

Management

1. Provide intravenous narcotic analgesia and muscle relaxation for patient comfort; also optimize the patient's condition for reduction. Morphine, 0.1 mg/kg/dose, or meperidine, 1.0 mg/kg/dose, may be used with diazepam (Valium), 0.1 mg/kg/dose, as discussed in the Appendix to Chapter 65.
2. Reduction of dislocation.
   a. With the patient prone and the involved arm and shoulder hanging in a dependent position over the table, have the patient hold a weight (about 1 lb weight/7 kg body weight). Reduction is usually achieved in 20 to 30 minutes. With younger children, the weight may have to be taped.
   b. In older children, especially when it is desirable to avoid large doses of opiates (e.g., long trip from point of injury to definitive medical care), or in recalcitrant dislocations, an alternative reduction technique is to help the child reach behind the head (as if to scratch the head). Then, with an assistant supporting the trunk, outward traction is applied in the line of the long axis of the humerus while the head of the humerus is pushed up into the fossa using pressure applied in the axilla.
   c. Another method is to have the child sit and have an assistant apply countertraction with a sheet by pulling with the sheet from the axilla toward the child's opposite shoulder. The shoulder is then reduced with a gentle, constant traction in a longitudinal manner with the shoulder abducted approximately 45 degrees. If this is unsuccessful, the abduction may be increased to 90 degrees while traction is maintained.
   d. Scapular manipulation has been used as well. With the patient prone and the arm hanging down, exert traction on the affected extremity scapula manipulated by pushing the inferior tip medially using thumb pressure while stabilizing or laterally rotating the superior aspect.

   A second approach with the patient seated involves placing the unaffected shoulder against an immobile support as a wall or the raised head of a stretcher. Facing the patient, a physician or assistant grasps the wrist of the patient's affected side and slowly raises this to the horizontal plane. Firm but gentle forward traction is applied with counterbalance provided by placing the palm of the extended free arm over the patient's midclavicular region. The force required in applying the traction is not great. Once traction is applied, a second physician manipulates the scapula as above.
3. Other considerations.
   a. The arm should be examined by physical assessment and an x-ray film should be taken before and after reduction.
   b. After reduction, treat any fractures. These often require surgery.
   c. Have patient use a sling and swathe or shoulder immobilizer (splinted in internal rotation) for 4 weeks to allow the capsule to heal.
   d. There is a 70% recurrence rate for those less than 20 years of age with this dislocation. Surgery may be required.

SHOULDER DISLOCATION: POSTERIOR

Posterior dislocations are uncommon.

Mechanism of Injury

Violent internal rotation motion of the shoulder, such as a seizure or electrical shock, or direct trauma to the shoulder joint when the arm is outstretched can produce a posterior dislocation.

Diagnostic Findings

1. There is an inability to abduct or externally rotate the arm.
2. The affected shoulder is flat anteriorly or full posteriorly. There is a defect in the position of the humeral head, which is felt as a vague prominence behind and below the acromion. The injury may be bilateral.
3. There may be associated fracture.

X-Ray Films

The AP view may be normal, but the dislocation will be apparent on an axillary or transthoracic view. The humeral head may overlie the glenoid rim. Prereduction and postreduction x-ray studies should be obtained.

Management

1. Muscle relaxation and analgesia usually are required, sometimes necessitating general anesthesia.
2. Reduction of dislocation.
   a. Orthopedic consultation is advisable.
   b. Exert pressure on the posterior aspect of the shoulder joint with the arm in external rotation.
   c. With a two-person approach, one person applies traction along the long axis of the humerus while it is in 45 degrees of abduction or backward extension with the elbow flexed to 90 degrees; the second person then pushes on the humeral head from behind.
   d. Anterior shoulder dislocation techniques also may be used.
3. Other considerations.
   a. Treat any associated fractures after reduction.
   b. Reexamine by physical assessment and x-ray film after reduction.

c. Immobilize with sling and swathe for 4 to 6 weeks.

ROTATOR CUFF INJURY
Mechanism of Injury

Strenuous shoulder motion, such as in throwing, heavy lifting, or falling on the shoulder, causes injury to the rotator cuff.

NOTE: The rotator cuff (*SIT:* *s*upraspinatus, *i*nfraspinatus, and *t*eres minor) stabilizes shoulder in the glenoid fossa in abduction and allows shoulder to abduct and externally rotate.

Diagnostic Findings

1. Severe pain worsening with attempts at abduction or external rotation. Abduction of the shoulder may not be possible. Passive range of motion of the shoulder joint may be normal.
2. Tenderness over the insertion of the rotator cuff into the tuberosities.
3. May be only a partial tear, with painful, weak abduction and a lack of endurance.

X-Ray Films

AP and lateral views of the shoulder may be normal or show a fracture of tuberosity. If significant with persistent weakness, magnetic resonance imaging (MRI) scan demonstrates soft tissue shoulder joint injury.

Management

1. Treat minimal tears with initial immobilization while maintaining good passive range of motion. Give analgesia.
2. Large tears require surgical intervention after confirmation. Early repair also is required in cases of an avulsion fracture of the tuberosity.

BRACHIAL PLEXUS
Mechanism of Injury

There is traction on the brachial plexus during delivery, particularly in nulliparous mothers with large babies. This injury may also result from major trauma such as a fall from a height or a motor vehicle accident, whereby traction forces the head and neck laterally and the shoulder is forced downward.

Diagnostic Findings

1. Arm held loosely at side of thorax in internal rotation with extension of the elbow, pronation of the forearm, and flexion at the wrist
2. Swelling in the region of the shoulder
X-Ray Films
Upper extremity and clavicle are indicated to exclude fractured clavicle, humerus, or dislocated shoulder. Cervical spine injury is also a consideration.

Management

1. Prescribe physical therapy to prevent contractures.
2. Consider neurosurgical consultation.

Most children have at least partial recovery by 18 months of age but may respond less fully if the injury occurs in older children.

SCAPULAR FRACTURE
Mechanism of Injury

Severe blunt trauma produces scapular injuries.

Diagnostic Findings

1. Swelling and localized tenderness are seen.
2. Severe associated injuries to the head, neck, and intrathoracic structures are possible because of the force required to produce this injury.
X-Ray Films
Scapular views are indicated. A chest x-ray film and other indicated studies are important in cases of severe trauma (see Chapter 56).

Management

A sling and swathe are indicated after caring for other injuries. Orthopedic follow-up is recommended.

PROXIMAL HUMERAL EPIPHYSEAL FRACTURE
Mechanism of Injury

Blunt trauma to the arm or shoulder may cause the fracture.

Diagnostic Findings

1. Shoulder deformed by pain and tenderness
2. Possible associated neurovascular injury
X-Ray Films
A Salter type II epiphyseal slip is most commonly seen. With infants, a Salter type I may be found. Such fractures may be classified by the amount of displacement.

Management

1. Treat separation (<1 cm) with angulation of less than 40 degrees and absence of malrotation with a shoulder immobilizer or sling and swathe. Greater angulation requires closed reduction.
2. Surgically correct fractures involving three pieces; four-piece fractures often involve replacement with a prosthesis.
3. Arrange orthopedic consultation.

HUMERAL SHAFT FRACTURE

A middle-third fracture is the most common.

Mechanism of Injury

1. Spiral fractures result from a twisting motion. Consider nonaccidental trauma when a young child presents with this injury.
2. Transverse fractures result from a direct blow.

Diagnostic Findings

Tenderness with or without deformity is noted.

Complications

Complications are associated with arterial and radial nerve injury, particularly mid- or distal humeral shaft injuries. Sensation (first dorsal web space) and motor function (extension of wrist and metacarpophalangeal [MCP] joint) should be assessed.

X-Ray Films

AP and lateral views of the humerus, including the shoulder and elbow, are indicated.

Management

1. In the younger child with minimal displacement and angulation, sling and swathe may be sufficient. In the older child, immobilization in a long-arm splint (sugar tong) from the axilla to the wrist with flexion of the elbow at 90 degrees may be required. Place in a sling and swathe.
2. Radial nerve involvement mandates early and frequent reassessment. Splint patients in position of function. May need traction or surgical repair to release entrapped radial nerve.

CONDYLAR AND SUPRACONDYLAR FRACTURES OF DISTAL HUMERUS

These are the most common fractures of the elbow.

Mechanism of Injury

1. A fall on the outstretched hand with the elbow extended or a fall on the flexed elbow
2. May also occur from snapping force, as in throwing a baseball too hard

Diagnostic Findings

1. Tenderness and deformity of the distal humerus. Distal fragment displaced upward, posterior, and medial.

2. Pain with flexion of the elbow.
3. May have associated dislocation of the elbow (see next topic).
4. Lateral condyle fracture is more common than medial type, which is commonly associated with ulnar nerve injury.

Complications

1. Nerve injury is associated with 20% of supracondylar fractures.
2. Pain with extension of fingers is an early sign of Volkmann's ischemia, which results from a volar-compartment syndrome of the forearm, leading to permanent hand disability.
3. In addition to neuromuscular complications, condylar fractures pose a risk for malunion and nonunion.

X-Ray Films

AP, lateral, and possibly oblique views are indicated. Posterior displacement is recognized by extending a line down the anterior of the cortex of the distal humerus on the lateral x-ray film. Normally, this line intersects the middle third of the capitellum. With posterior displacement accompanying a supracondylar fracture, the line intersects anterior to the capitellum or the anterior third.

A subtle sign of a nondisplaced fracture is the "fat-pad sign." The sign is nonspecific and reflects hemorrhage into the elbow joint. This may be related to injury of the radial head, capitellum, trochlear, olecranon, or coronoid process. The fat-pad sign is an area of radiolucency seen on the lateral x-ray view of the elbow just above the olecranon process posteriorly or above the radial head anteriorly. The posterior fat-pad sign is of greatest importance because the anterior sign may be seen normally (see discussion following on elbow dislocation: posterior).

Management

1. Orthopedic consultation in the ED.
   a. Early reduction if necessary, and immobilization with the elbow held at

90-degree flexion. Test radial pulse before and after flexion.

   b. If there is any question of neurovascular compromise, immediate reduction is mandatory (traction, supination of the forearm, and flexion with direct pressure to align the displaced segment).

   c. Open reduction may be required with condylar fracture.

2. Hospitalization. Neurovascular compromise must be closely monitored for at least 24 hours. Patients with undisplaced supracondylar fractures may be followed as outpatients if flexion is adequate and good follow-up and observation are feasible.

ELBOW DISLOCATION: POSTERIOR

This is the second most common dislocation in children.

Mechanism of Injury

A fall on a hyperextended arm causes the dislocation.

Diagnostic Findings

There is obvious deformity, swelling, and effusion. The two epicondyles and the tip of the olecranon normally form an isosceles triangle. In a dislocation, the sides of the triangle are unequal, whereas in a nondisplaced supracondylar fracture, they remain equal.

There may be associated fracture, often supracondylar (see preceding topic).

Complications

Neurovascular compromise is common. There is nerve injury (median) in as many as 5% to 10% of patients.

X-Ray Films

AP, lateral, and oblique views of the elbow are indicated. There may be associated fracture. A posterior fat-pad sign is pathognomonic for elbow injury (dislocation, fracture, or possibly a sign of spontaneous reduction of elbow). An anterior fat-pad sign may be normal or pathologic (see condylar and supracondylar fractures of distal humerus).

Management

1. Administer narcotic morphine or analgesia (meperidine [Demerol]) or muscle relaxation (diazepam [Valium]) (p. 507).

2. With the patient prone and the arm in a dependent position over the edge of the bed, apply gentle traction, with guidance of the olecranon process into normal position.

   NOTE: Ensure that there is no trapped medial epicondyle fracture, which requires open surgery.

3. Order postreduction x-ray films, and perform a physical examination to check neurovascular and motor function and to exclude fractures.

4. Immobilize in a splint with the elbow flexed 90 degrees for 14 to 16 days. Test radial pulse before and after flexion.

5. Arrange for close follow-up to monitor range of motion and to exclude compartment syndrome or myositis ossificans.

6. Arrange for ED orthopedic consultation.

RADIAL HEAD DISLOCATION OR SUBLUXATION (NURSEMAID ELBOW)

It occurs more often in younger children (<5 years) than in older ones. Recurrent radial head subluxation occurs frequently, with patients 24 months or younger at great risk.

Mechanism of Injury

1. Sudden longitudinal pull on the forearm while the arm is pronated

2. Reported in children less than 6 months after rolling over

Diagnostic Findings

1. The arm is in passive pronation. The child usually will not move the arm.
2. Resistance to the pain with full supination.
3. Pain over the head of the radius.
4. In rare cases, the anterior dislocation of the radial head is associated with a fracture of the proximal ulna *(Monteggia fracture)*.

X-Ray Films

Radiographs are usually normal. X-ray diagnosis is usually not required unless the mechanism of injury is unusual, the physical findings atypical, or the patient does not become rapidly asymptomatic after reduction. In fact, if pre-reduction films are obtained, reduction is usually achieved by the radiology technician in the process of supinating the forearm for x-ray films.

1. A line drawn along the proximal shaft of the radius should pass through the capitellum. If it does not, there is a dislocation.
2. If x-ray films are obtained, the forearm should be evaluated to rule out Monteggia fracture.

Management

Orthopedic consultation is usually unnecessary.

1. Reduction by supination of the forearm while feeling the head of the radius (anulus) and, in a continuous motion, flexing the elbow. There is usually a palpable click over the radial head.
   a. The patient should be asymptomatic after 5 to 10 minutes, although in patients who have been subluxed for several hours, return of function may take 6 to 12 hours.
   b. Patients not rapidly asymptomatic should have x-ray studies.
2. An alternate reduction technique is by pronation of the forearm, with flexion at the elbow.

3. Sling is usually not required except for comfort.
4. With Monteggia fracture, after reduction the forearm is casted in neutral position with flexion of more than 90 degrees at the elbow; cast remains for at least 6 weeks. Orthopedic consultation should be obtained for this fracture.

RADIAL HEAD FRACTURE

Mechanism of Injury

A fall on an outstretched hand produces a fracture of the radial head. This is relatively uncommon in children.

Diagnostic Findings

1. There may be tenderness over the radial head.
2. May be associated with supracondylar, olecranon, or epicondyle fracture.
3. Compartment syndrome of the forearm has been described with minimally displaced or angulated radial head fractures.

X-Ray Films

AP and lateral views are indicated.

Management

1. Nondisplaced fracture: long-arm splint, including immobilization of wrist, and a sling.
2. If more than one third of the articular surface is displaced, excision is required. Angulation does not require reduction with displacement less than 20 degrees. Greater angulation requires reduction to prevent limitation of movement.

DISTAL ONE THIRD RADIUS AND ULNAR FRACTURES

This is common in school-age children and adolescents.

Mechanism of Injury

A fall on the palm of the hand or a blow to forearm causes forearm fractures.

Diagnostic Findings

There is swelling and tenderness over the fracture site.

1. If a single bone is fractured and there is overriding, there must be a radial head dislocation *(Monteggia fracture)* or a distal radioulnar dislocation *(Galeazzi fracture).*

2. *Torus fracture:* common in children—a buckling or angulation of the cortex with no actual fracture line. A torus fracture usually is seen in the metaphyseal area.

3. *Greenstick fracture:* involves the diaphysis of a long bone—a fracture of one side of the cortex.

4. *Colles fracture:* transverse fracture of the distal radius with dorsal angulation and loss or reversal of volar tilt of distal radial articular surface; patient may have an accompanying fracture of the ulnar styloid. Usually Salter II epiphyseal injury.

5. *Smith fracture:* fracture of distal radius with increase in the volar tilt of the distal radial articular surface; reverse of Colles fracture. Caused by a blow on the dorsum of the wrist or distal radius with the forearm in pronation.

6. *Barton fracture:* marginal fracture of the dorsal or volar surface of the radius with dorsal or volar (corresponding to involved surface) dislocation of the carpal bones and hand.

7. *Hutchinson or chauffeur fracture:* fracture of the radial styloid process secondary to direct trauma or from impact of the styloid process against the navicular bone. Typically nondisplaced.

Occasionally, median or ulnar nerve injury occurs, with self-limited neuropraxia.

Management

Rotational deformities must be eliminated. Angulated fractures greater than 15 degrees (especially proximal) in children lead to decreased function. Potential for longitudinal bone growth depends on the distance from the growth plates, especially the distal one, where 80% of forearm growth occurs. Most pediatric distal forearm fractures can be treated nonoperatively. The fracture should be immobilized for 4 to 6 weeks. If both the radius and ulna are broken or dislocated, alignment is more difficult to attain and hold; therefore surgical stabilization may be necessary. Indirect or limited open reduction with fixation tools, such as Kirschner wires, is very successful, as is open reduction and internal fixation.

Torus Fracture

It is immobilized for 4 to 6 weeks in a long-arm splint.

Colles Fracture

1. Reduce by traction in the line of the deformity to disimpact the fragments; follow by pressure on the dorsal aspect of the distal fragment and volar aspect of the proximal fragment. Also apply pressure on the radial aspect of the distal fragment to correct radial deviation.

2. Test for reduction by palpation, lack of recurrence of deformity, and x-ray film.

3. Immobilize the hand in maximum ulnar deviation, the wrist neutral and the forearm in full pronation. (If markedly displaced, immobilization in supination may be helpful.) Use anterior and posterior splints wrapped in place or an immediately bivalved cast. The cast should extend from the knuckles to midhumerus. Some orthopedists prefer a short-arm cast. Once swelling resolves, a circular cast may be applied.

4. Ensure that there is no neurovascular compromise.

5. Consult with an orthopedist in the ED.

Smith Fracture

1. Reduce by longitudinal traction until the fragments are distracted. Supinate and apply dorsal pressure on the distal fragment.
2. Immobilize with an anterior and posterior splint (sugar tong), with the forearm in supination and the wrist in extension.
3. Consult with an orthopedist in the ED.

Barton Fracture

This usually requires open reduction.

REFERENCES

Anderson K, Jensen PO, Lauritzen J: Treatment of clavicular fractures: figure-of-eight bandage versus a simple sling, *Acta Orthop Scand* 57:71, 1987.

Chacon D, Kissoon N, Brown T, et al: Use of comparison radiographs in the diagnosis of traumatic injuries with the elbow, *Ann Emerg Med* 21:895, 1992.

Hendey GW, Kinlaw K: Clinically significant abnormalities in post reduction radiographs after anterior shoulder dislocation, *Ann Emerg Med* 28:399, 1996.

McNamara EM: Reduction of anterior shoulder dislocation by scapular manipulation, *Emerg Med* 21:1140, 1993.

Schunk JE: Radial head subluxation: epidemiology and treatment of 87 episodes, *Ann Emerg Med* 19:1029, 1990.

Skaggs D, Pershad J: Pediatric elbow trauma, *Pediatr Emerg Care* 13:425, 1997.

Snyder HS: Radiographic changes of radial head subluxation in children, *J Emerg Med* 8:265, 1990.

68 HAND AND WRIST INJURIES

DIANE M. BOURLIER

Hand and wrist injuries are common in children, and it is imperative to recognize their extent. A seemingly benign injury, if inappropriately managed, can lead to significant functional deficit. Historical data must include the time and mechanism of injury, defining whether it was a crush or puncture wound, whether it is dirty or clean, if there is tissue loss, the location of the injury, whether it is the patient's dominant hand, immunization status, allergies, history of previous hand injuries, and if possible, subjective motor and sensory deficits.

The physical examination is often more difficult because of decreased cooperation by the frightened child, as well as the size of the structures. Skin, nerves, vessels, tendons, bone, joints, and ligaments must be evaluated. The nomenclature of the fingers is thumb, index, long, ring, and little fingers. The bones of the hand are depicted in Fig. 68-1.

BASIC HAND EXAMINATION

This must be systematically and rapidly performed.

Observation

The hand should be observed at rest, looking for tendon injuries and obvious deformities. Fingers on flexion should normally point toward the scaphoid tubercle. If they deviate, there is a rotational injury. Digital cyanosis and capillary filling should be assessed.

Sensation

The hand should be observed for sweating, which should be present if the digital nerve (sympathetics) is intact. Finger skin should wrinkle in warm water. This does not require the active participation of the young or intoxicated patient. Systematically assess sensation:

1. Radial nerve: dorsal thumb—web space
2. Median nerve: tip of the index finger
3. Ulnar nerve: tip of the little finger

Sensation distal to the injury should be examined. Two-point discrimination is particularly useful. It can be performed by determining discrimination at 8-mm separation, using a paper clip.

Motor Function

Each individual tendon should be checked for function in the fingers and as part of the group in the hand and wrist:

1. Flexor digitorum profundus. Stabilize the proximal interphalangeal (PIP) and metacarpophalangeal (MCP) joints while asking the patient to flex the distal interphalangeal (DIP) joint.
2. Flexor digitorum sublimis. Hold the fingers extended and ask the patient to flex only the PIP joint. Some recommend that for testing of the small finger, the index and longer fingers can be held extended and the MCP joints of the ring and small finger be flexed at least 45 degrees. The PIP joints of the ring and

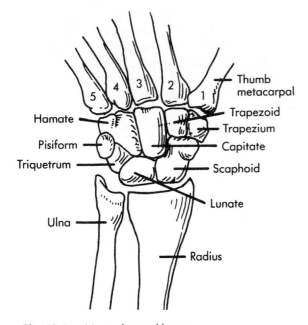

Fig. 68-1 Normal carpal bones.

(From Rosen P, et al: *Diagnostic radiology in emergency medicine,* St Louis, 1992, Mosby.)

small fingers are flexed to test the flexor function.

3. Extensor tendons. Extend each joint individually.
4. Flexor tendons. Flex each joint individually.

The following nerves should be checked:

1. Radial nerve: extension of the wrist and digits at the MCP joint
2. Median nerve: pointing the thumb upward or pinching the thumb and little finger tips together
3. Ulnar nerve: interossei muscles are tested by having patient abduct and adduct the long finger from midline

Other Considerations

1. If there is injury around a joint, check it for stability.
2. X-ray films are useful in showing fractures, foreign bodies, and air in the joint. A true

anteroposterior (AP) and lateral view of involved digits must be obtained, using the fingernail as a landmark.

3. Fractures are less common in children than in adults. In children, fractures usually heal rapidly because of the thick periosteum. Surgical repair is rarely needed, and early functional use is essential.

PERILUNATE DISLOCATION

Mechanism of Injury

A fall on an outstretched hand produces the dislocation.

Diagnostic Findings

There is pain and tenderness in the wrist, possibly accompanied by minimal swelling or deformity.

X-Ray Films

On a lateral roentgenogram, the long finger metacarpal, capitate, lunate, and radius normally line up in a straight line, and the lunate and navicular form an angle no greater than 50 degrees. This normal alignment is disrupted with a dislocation. A true lateral x-ray film is necessary because dislocation is easily missed on an AP view (Fig. 68-2).

If the dislocation is missed, the patient will have long-term disability. Thus the injury must not be passed off as a sprain.

Management

1. Immediate orthopedic consultation.
2. Open reduction is often required.

NAVICULAR (SCAPHOID) BONE FRACTURE

This is the most common carpal fracture and is the most commonly misdiagnosed orthopedic injury in the emergency department (ED). Other fractures of the carpal bones are rare in children.

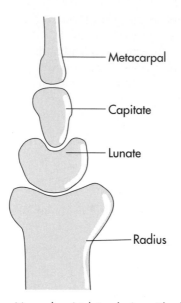

Fig. 68-2 Normal wrist lateral view. The long finger metacarpal, capitate lunate, and radius normally line up. If the lunate is dislocated, this alignment is disrupted.

Mechanism of Injury

Falling on an outstretched (dorsiflexed) hand results in navicular fractures.

Diagnostic Findings

1. Tenderness over the anatomic snuffbox and clinical suspicion. The scaphoid compression test may be more sensitive than snuffbox tenderness. Inward longitudinal pressure is applied along the axis of the thumb metacarpal. Pain in the wrist suggests scaphoid tenderness.
2. Decrease in grip strength.

X-Ray Films

A view of the wrist, including the navicular view, is indicated. The x-ray film may be normal, but if the patient has clinical snuffbox tenderness, it should be treated as a fracture.

Management

Nondisplaced fractures should have a long-arm cast, which includes the thumb, MCP joint, and the elbow. Immobilization is for 7 to 8 weeks unless no fracture was seen on the initial x-ray film, in which case the wrist should be reevaluated by x-ray examination in 7 to 10 days.

Even though nonunion and avascular necrosis of the navicular bone are rare in children, it is wise to have an orthopedist follow the child. If the fracture is displaced, an ED consultation should be obtained.

METACARPAL BONE FRACTURE

Mechanism of Injury

A direct blow to the hand produces the fracture.

Diagnostic Findings

1. Swelling and point tenderness
2. Deformity with displacement (need to assess the degree of rotation and angulation)
3. Types of fracture:
   a. *Boxer fracture:* fracture of the little-finger metacarpal head. Usually has good functional result with up to 35 to 40 degrees of volar angulation.
   b. *Bennett fracture:* fracture of the thumb metacarpal base into the joint. Unusual in children.

X-Ray Films

AP and lateral views of the hand are indicated.

Management

1. Immobilize for 3 to 4 weeks with splinting (often casting) from the midforearm to the distal phalanges. Splint the MCP joint at 45 to 90 degrees of flexion (to prevent MCP contracture) with the wrist in extension.
2. Once reduced and immobilized, recheck the fracture with x-ray examination to ensure that rotation and alignment have been corrected.
3. Bennett fractures, even if reduced, usually require internal fixation to hold reduction because of the opposing forces of the abductor pollicis longus and adductor pollicis.

In general, more deformity is tolerated in the ring and little fingers than in the thumb, index, or long-finger metacarpals.

PHALANGEAL FRACTURE

The phalanx is the most commonly fractured bone in children.

Mechanism of Injury

There is a direct blow to the tip of the finger, such as being caught in a car door.

Diagnostic Findings

1. Swelling and point tenderness of the phalanx.
2. Deformity with displacement. On flexion, the fingernails normally point toward the scaphoid tubercle. If they do not, there may be a rotational injury.

X-Ray Film
AP and lateral views are indicated. A true lateral view of the individual digits must be obtained, using the fingernail as a landmark.

Management

1. With the middle or distal phalanx, immobilize the fracture of the involved digit and the neighboring one in a finger splint. If involved, the long and ring fingers should always be splinted together because their lumbricales are mutually dependent.
2. If the proximal phalanx is fractured, use a dorsal splint that incorporates the wrist at 30 degrees of extension, the MCP joint flexed at 30 to 50 degrees, and the interphalangeal (IP) joint flexed at 10 to 15 degrees.
3. For open and intraarticular fractures, with or without displacement, that involve a large portion of the joint space, refer to a hand or orthopedic surgeon.
4. Rotational or angulation deformities are difficult to correct and require consulta-

tion. A fracture of the phalangeal neck is a transverse fracture through the neck of either the proximal or middle phalanx. Maintaining reduction is difficult, and loss of reduction may be functionally significant.
5. Epiphyseal fractures usually occur in the proximal phalangeal base of the little fingers—usually Salter type II. They require reduction and splinting to a neighboring phalanx, with flexion at the joint. Complete separation of the plate requires open reduction.

FINGER DISLOCATION

Ligaments and capsular structures in children are stronger than an epiphyseal plate. Trauma that might dislocate a finger in an adult may instead produce a fracture in a child. Dislocations are rare.

Mechanism of Injury

There is a blow to the tip of the finger.

Diagnostic Findings

1. Obvious deformity and tenderness at the joint
2. Swelling and inability to flex the finger
3. Complex dislocation if the MCP joint involved
   a. Phalanx displaced on metacarpal—not at 90 degrees, as in a simple dislocation, but more parallel, with slight displacement and less angulation
   b. Dimpling of palmar skin

X-Ray Films
These should be done before attempting reduction because there may be an underlying fracture. Dislocated bones are usually at 90 degrees to each other.

A complex fracture has widened joint space and parallel position. The sesamoid bone may be in the joint space, which often signifies the need for surgery.

Management

1. Refer to an orthopedist.
2. Reduce by hyperextension of the joint while pushing the distal bone over into position from above. Do not pull. Immobilize for 1 to 2 weeks.
3. After reduction, check for ligamentous instability and immobilize with splinting for 1 to 2 weeks.

BOUTONIÈRRE DEFORMITY

This is a rupture of the central slip of the extensor tendon at the PIP joint, with volar subluxation of the lateral bands.

Mechanism of Injury

A direct blow or laceration produces the deformity.

Diagnostic Findings

1. Tenderness and swelling over the dorsal PIP joint may make diagnosis clinically difficult.
2. The distal IP joint is held in extension while the proximal IP joint is held in flexion.
X-Ray Film
Fracture should be excluded.

Management

If fracture is not present, splint in extension and arrange for follow-up with a hand surgeon. Patients seen days after injury without treatment will probably need operative repair.

MALLET FINGER

This is a fracture of the base of the distal phalanx with disruption of the extensor tendons at the DIP joint. It is common in adolescents and may be a Salter type III epiphyseal injury. Younger children typically have a Salter type I or II injury.

Mechanism of Injury

There is blunt trauma, such as a blow to the tip of the finger from a softball or football striking the finger ("jammed finger").

Diagnostic Findings

1. The patient is unable to extend the distal phalanx because of terminal slip rupture, laceration of the terminal slip, or an avulsion fracture.
2. Tenderness and swelling of the DIP joint.
3. The finger is held with the distal phalanx flexed.
X-Ray Films
AP and lateral views of the digit are indicated. These views may show a chip fracture of the distal phalanx at the DIP joint.

Management

1. Fracture less than 25% of the joint surface (without subluxation) is splinted in hyperextension and the patient referred. The finger may be splinted on either the dorsal or volar surface, but the tape must be changed daily while the fingers are held in extension. Use foam and aluminum splints.
2. With fracture greater than 25% of the joint surface or a subluxed joint, operative reduction and fixation are required.
3. In older adolescents, injury may occur without fracture and the finger may be splinted with the DIP joints in hyperextension. Strict immobilization for 6 weeks is necessary.

GAMEKEEPER THUMB (SKIER THUMB)

This is injury to the ulnar collateral ligament of the thumb.

Mechanism of Injury

There is hyperextension of the MCP joint of the thumb (a common ski-pole injury with a fall on an outstretched hand while clasping the pole).

Diagnostic Findings

1. Swelling and tenderness over the ulnar aspect of the MCP joint of the thumb with increased pain on radial deviation of the MCP joint
2. Laxity of the joint with stressing

X-Ray Films

AP and lateral views are indicated to exclude an avulsion fracture of the proximal phalanx.

Management

1. Apply a thumb spica splint with the thumb in extension; splint remains for 6 weeks. Arrange for follow-up with a hand surgeon.
2. With stress instability greater than 30% to 45%, initial surgical repair is needed.

LACERATION

See Chapter 65: Soft Tissue Injuries.

Diagnostic Findings

1. Evaluate the wound to determine the depth of injury and involvement of underlying tissues, including vessels, nerves, muscles, tendons, ligaments, bones, and joints.
2. Sensation and motor function must be specifically tested, focusing on the three major nerves (radial, median, and ulnar), as well as sensation distal to the injury. Two-point discrimination is particularly useful. Each tendon must be evaluated. Consider the stance of fingers when the tendon was lacerated (p. 534).

Management

1. Use direct pressure and elevation to obtain hemostasis. Never use a clamp, hemostat, or deep suture. If extensive bleeding is associated with a finger laceration, an excellent field tourniquet can be achieved by cleansing the patient's finger and then slipping the hand into a sterile glove, snipping the end of the glove on the involved finger, and then rolling back the finger of the glove to provide exposure and tourniquet. These are also available commercially. Careful scrubbing is then done.
2. After sensory examination, infiltrate with lidocaine (Xylocaine) without epinephrine to facilitate cleansing and laceration repair. Epinephrine-containing medications should *not* be used. Slow infiltration and buffered lidocaine reduce pain (see Appendix to Chapter 65).
3. Partial tendon tears may or may not cause functional deficits, and these, as well as complete lacerations, require referral. Partial tendon lacerations may be associated with pain with use of the tendon, decreased tone (often with altered stance), weakness, or evidence of laceration of the tendon sheath.

   Extensor tendon repairs have an excellent prognosis, whereas flexor injuries, even with meticulous surgical technique, have a poorer prognosis.
4. Repair lacerations using either 4-0 or 5-0 nylon (e.g., Prolene, Ethilon, Surgilon) suture material on a P3 needle. Never use deep sutures.

   Do not suture if more than 8 hours since injury. Arrange for delayed closure at 48 to 72 hours if indicated.
5. Children require extensive dressing and splints to maintain position and thereby minimize further injury and facilitate repair.

In children with extensive injuries, particularly when there is associated tendon damage, the best position for splinting is the "hooded cobra." The wrist is in neutral position (long axis of forearm roughly lines up with long axis of thumb), the MCP joints are flexed to about 60 to 70 degrees, the IP joints are flexed 10 to 20 degrees, and the thumb is widely abducted. The first layer of dressing, when required, is a non-adherent material. The second layer maintains the position of the hand and is a noncircumferential, noncompressible material (e.g., fluffs or sponges), mostly occupying the palm and the dorsum of the hand, wrist, and forearm. The final layer should have decreasing tension and compression from the distal end, proximally. A plaster splint of 10 to 15 layers (or fiberglass) may be incorporated into the volar (palmar) side of the dressing.

FINGERTIP INJURIES

Crush injuries are common in children and may be associated with tuft fracture.

Mechanism of Injury

There is a blow to the distal phalanx between two firm objects.

Diagnostic Findings

1. Discoloration, swelling, local tenderness
2. Often associated with subungual hematoma
3. Possibility of associated nail bed injury
X-Ray Films
Views should be taken to exclude underlying fracture.

Management

1. *Subungual hematoma:* Drain with electric cautery or red-hot paper clip. Exclude fractures.
2. If there is a laceration, cleanse it thoroughly and use sutures sparingly, with only loose approximation of the skin.
3. If the nail bed is injured, with partial avulsion, or if it is lacerated, the nail should be left on to act as a splint and to protect the nail bed. If it is avulsed at the base and there is a transverse fracture of the distal phalanx, there is usually a laceration of

the nail bed. Under these circumstances the nail should be removed and the nail bed repaired to prevent distortion. Use 5-0 fine absorbable sutures (Vicryl, Dexon).
4. Distal tuft injuries usually heal without treatment other than good wound cleansing, dressing, and splinting.

AMPUTATION OF FINGERTIPS

This is common in children.

Management

1. If the subcutaneous tissue is intact, initial cleaning and debridement with a bulky dressing are adequate. It will heal well by secondary intention.
2. If there is partial laceration of the fingertip, it should be loosely approximated. Children heal remarkably well, and little is lost if the tissue becomes necrotic and demarcates and subsequently must be removed.
3. X-ray examination is necessary to ensure that there is no bony involvement. Consult a hand surgeon.
4. Amputation at or distal to the distal half of the fingernail may be treated with careful cleansing and debridement and covered with ointment and gauze and immobilized in a nonoperative fashion. Antibiotics are indicated if significant contamination is present. Such conservative treatment also may be useful in very distal (distal to insertion of extensor and flexor tendons of distal phalanx) amputations. Obtain consultation.
5. For the completely amputated digit, treatment depends on the availability of microsurgery. Wrap the amputated part in sterile gauze that has been soaked in lactated Ringer's solution, place and seal in a plastic bag, and then place in ice water. This prevents immersion and water logging. Rapid transport is essential.

WRINGER OR DEGLOVING INJURY
Mechanism of Injury

The involved limb is caught in roller, producing a crushing friction burn. A shearing force component is added if the individual attempts to pull away. This may also be seen when an extremity is run over by a car.

Diagnostic Findings

1. There is swelling of the involved soft tissue area.
2. Fractures are uncommon and depend on the type of force applied. Dislocations may occur.
3. Degloving and crushing injuries may coexist and result in deep soft tissue damage.

Complications
1. There is extensive hematoma and compartmental swelling with neurovascular compromise.
2. Skin slough is common if there is loss of vascular supply or a compartment syndrome.

Management

1. Control swelling by applying sterile occlusive dressing after cleansing the extremity.
2. Elevate the extremity, and hospitalize for observation for 24 hours.
   - In rare circumstances, with mild injury and assurance of good follow-up, the patient may be discharged with re-examinations every 12 hours. In such cases, splint the arm.
3. Fasciotomy of the forearm or carpal tunnel decompression may be needed because of neurovascular compromise.
4. Skin graft may be needed.

AMPUTATION OF THE HAND OR PARTS
Management

1. Examine hand completely. Preserve any viable tissue.

2. Clean the hand, wrap in sterile gauze, soak in lactated Ringer's solution, place in a plastic bag, and then put on ice.
3. X-ray hand to determine integrity.
4. Immediately refer to center capable of re-implantation.

RING ON A SWOLLEN FINGER
Management

Several alternatives exist:
1. Place a piece of string under the ring and from the distal end of the finger wrap it in close loops. Exert a slow pull on the proximal end, gently pulling the ring distally as the string unwinds.
2. Alternate at 5-minute intervals between soaking the finger in cold water and elevating the fingers. This is repeated for 30 minutes and oil (mineral or cooking) applied while the hand is elevated. With a steady motion, the ring is pushed off.
3. Cut the ring with a ring cutter.

SUBUNGUAL SPLINTER
Management

A splinter under the nail can be removed by gently shaving over the distal end of the splinter until the splinter can be exposed. A single-edge razor or scalpel can be used.

INFECTIONS
Felon

Mechanism of Injury
Improper trimming of nails or puncture wound to the volar aspect of the distal phalanx causes felons.

Diagnostic Findings
Swelling, erythema, and tenderness of the volar aspect of the distal phalanx are present.

Management
1. Drainage. Incision can be made at the site of maximum tenderness or laterally, tak-

ing care to avoid the neurovascular bundle. A Penrose drain promotes drainage. Incision and drainage should be carried out before the wound becomes fluctuant because intercompartmental pressure will produce ischemic necrosis.

2. Elevation, soaks.

Paronychia

Mechanism of Injury
Hangnail or any bacterial inoculum causes irritation leading to infection.

Diagnostic Findings
There is swelling, erythema, and tenderness alongside the nail, which may extend under the nail.

Management
1. Digital block is essential. Do *not* use epinephrine-containing anesthetics.
2. If relatively acute, lift the cuticle up around the entire nail to relieve pus and insert cotton wick to promote drainage. Continue treatment with soaks.
3. If chronic, excise medial or lateral edge of nail to permit drainage. Make a longitudinal cut in the outer portion of the nail and then grasp the free edge with a hemostat and remove the nail. Cover with Vaseline gauze.
4. Antibiotics may be used.

Acute Suppurative Tenosynovitis

Mechanism of Injury
Extension of local infection can involve the synovium.

Diagnostic Findings
1. Erythema and tenderness along the tendon sheath, often with maximal pain over metacarpal head.
2. Finger held in flexed position. Passive extension of DIP joint causes severe pain.

Management
1. Hospitalize.
2. Immobilize entire length of tendon.

3. Consider incision and drainage by an orthopedist.
4. Give high-dose antibiotics: nafcillin (or equivalent), 100 mg/kg/24 hr q4hr IV, in absence of penicillin allergy.

Palmar (Thenar and Midpalmar) Space Infection

Mechanism of Injury
Extension of a localized puncture wound, laceration, or an animal bite leads to infection.

Diagnostic Findings
Swelling, tenderness, and erythema are present.

Management
1. Hospitalize.
2. Arrange for incision and drainage by hand surgeon.
3. Administer antibiotics: nafcillin (or equivalent), 100 mg/kg/24 hr q4hr IV, in the absence of a penicillin allergy, unless Gram stain or culture indicates other choices.
4. Injection injuries from a paint gun usually need decompression by a hand surgeon.

Herpetic Whitlow

Etiology
Herpes simplex I virus is usually acquired from oral lesions.

Diagnostic Findings
1. In contrast to bacterial paronychia, the lesions are more blistered, the exudate is serous, and the pain is described as burning. The lesions may be subungual and difficult to see.
2. Gram stain of the exudate may show giant cells but no bacteria. If recurrent, viral cultures are useful.
3. Complications:
   a. Superimposed bacterial infection
   b. Recurrence and long, indolent course

Management

1. Splint the involved digit.
2. Oral analgesics may be useful.
3. In general, surgery is avoided because it spreads the infection. However, if the lesions are subungual, incision and drainage with decompression may increase the patient's comfort.
4. Topical acyclovir (Zovirax) 5% ointment may shorten the course and diminish recurrences.

REFERENCES

Bhende MS, Dandrea LA, Davis HW: Hand injuries in children presenting to a pediatric emergency department, *Ann Emerg Med* 22:1519, 1993.

Brook I: Aerobic and anaerobic microbiology of paronychia, *Ann Emerg Med* 19:994, 1990.

Seaberg DC, Angelos WJ, Paris PM: Treatment of subungual hematomas with nail trephination: a prospective study, *Am J Emerg Med* 9:209, 1991.

Stein A, Lemos M, Stein S: Clinical evaluation of flexor tendon function in the small finger, *Ann Emerg Med* 19:991, 1990.

69 LOWER EXTREMITY INJURY

SANDY MOON

PELVIC FRACTURE

The injury is usually incurred while the patient is a pedestrian or a passenger in an automobile collision. There are often major associated injuries, and the mortality rate is high.

Mechanism of Injury

Fracture results from blunt trauma to the pelvic area.

Diagnostic Findings

1. Local tenderness. Excessive movement or crepitus on pelvic rocking or pressure on the symphysis.
2. Because the pelvis is a bony ring, fractures of one part are usually associated with fractures elsewhere in the ring, particularly if the fracture is displaced. The ischiopubic ring follows this ring concept independently.
3. Blood loss. May be significant, with up to 2500 ml of hemorrhage common in adults. Massive retroperitoneal hematoma can occur with shock and vascular collapse.
4. Injuries to the bladder or urethra (see Chapter 64).
   a. If there is blood at the meatus or inability to void with a distended bladder, obtain a retrograde urethrogram before passing a catheter.
   b. If the urethra is intact, perform a cystogram followed by an intravenous pyelogram (IVP).
   c. Hematuria is present in 50% to 60% of cases, but only 10% will have significant injuries.
5. Rectal and vaginal examination. Direct vaginal and perineal injuries may occur, or the examination may demonstrate communication with an open fracture.
6. High association with head trauma.
7. Infrequent injuries to the obturator, femoral, or sciatic nerves.

X-Ray Films

These consist of anteroposterior (AP) and frog-leg projections. Multiple ossification sites are present and must not be confused with a fracture.

Management

1. Manage life-threatening injuries first (see Chapter 56).
2. Initiate intravenous (IV) fluids with normal saline or lactated Ringer's (LR) solution and, shortly thereafter, blood, if indicated. Massive hemorrhage is less common in pediatric pelvic fractures but ultimately determines mortality rate.
3. Involve general surgery, orthopedic, and urology consultants as needed.
4. Pneumatic antishock trousers, military antishock trousers (MAST), may be helpful in both the initial immobilization of the patient and subsequent therapy. Pediatric MAST suits are available.
5. If profuse bleeding is present, angiography may be required to localize the site.

6. Pelvic fractures with a gravid uterus present a major risk of fetal injury and death. Obstetrics consultation is necessary. Fetal distress must be assessed by monitoring scalp pH and heart tones. If evidence of distress is present, an emergency cesarean section may need to be considered. The mother and child must be cared for at an appropriate institution.

APOPHYSEAL INJURIES OF THE PELVIS

Normal pelvic apophyses, along the inferior aspect of the ischium and superior aspect of the iliac wing, can mimic nondisplaced avulsion fractures. These apophyses stay open until approximately 21 years of age. Sudden movement involving abduction or adduction of the thigh, as in sprinting, can cause injury to one or more of these apophyses.

HIP FRACTURE

This is rare in children.

Mechanism of Injury

A fall onto the hip region with transmission of a large energy force causes the injury.

Diagnostic Findings

1. Externally rotated and shortened.
2. Localized swelling and tenderness, with pain on movement of leg.
3. There is a large potential for loss of blood.
4. Children who have severe falls should have hips checked for range of motion and pain.

Management

1. Immobilization
2. Orthopedic consultation in the emergency department (ED)

HIP DISLOCATION: POSTERIOR

Posterior hip dislocation is rare in children, and there is usually an associated fracture. Anterior and obturator dislocations are less common.

Mechanism of Injury

Longitudinal forces applied to the knee with the hip and knee in 90-degree flexion and slight abduction (knee hits dashboard in car) produce a posterior dislocation.

Diagnostic Findings

1. Leg is shortened, internally rotated, and slightly adducted.
2. Associated fractures, especially posterior wall of acetabulum, and sciatic nerve injury (10%).

Complication

Avascular necrosis of the femoral head may follow, particularly if reduction is delayed.

X-Ray Films

AP and lateral views of the hip are indicated. A computed tomography (CT) scan of articular surfaces is excellent for spatial resolution.

Management

1. Reduction without delay, preferably by an orthopedist, using spinal or general anesthesia. If transfer of the patient is necessary, with a long transit time, reduce the dislocation to prevent aseptic necrosis. Traction in the line of deformity should be followed by gentle flexion of the hip to 90 degrees and then internal-to-external rotation.
2. Bed rest and long-term follow-up observation are essential.

HIP DISLOCATION: CONGENITAL

This should be diagnosed in infancy, when prognosis for recovery is excellent. An older child in whom the diagnosis has been delayed may limp or be unable to walk and should be referred to an orthopedist for care.

TOXIC SYNOVITIS OF THE HIP

This occurs in 1- to 7-year-old children, with a peak at 2 years of age. It often follows respiratory infection.

Diagnostic Findings

1. Inability to bear full weight. Child may limp and complain of knee pain (see Chapter 40).
2. Minimal (or no) pain on abduction and external rotation, with variably limited range of motion.
3. Complete blood count (CBC) is usually normal; erythrocyte sedimentation rate (ESR) is normal or slightly elevated.
   X-Ray Films
   These are usually normal or show small effusion.

Management

1. Self-limited. Symptomatic treatment with ibuprofen (10 mg/kg/dose q6hr PO) or naprosyn (7.5 mg/kg/dose q12hr PO), and follow-up observation.
2. Must be certain to exclude septic arthritis clinically or by arthrocentesis or incision and drainage if necessary. If any question, admit and evaluate.

LEGG-CALVÉ-PERTHES DISEASE (AVASCULAR NECROSIS OF THE FEMORAL HEAD)

This is a common cause of limp in 4- to 10-year-old children.

Diagnostic Findings

1. Limited hip movement, particularly internal rotation and abduction. Limp is common (see Chapter 40).

2. Tenderness over anterior capsule.
   X-Ray Films
   There is widened joint space between the ossified head and acetabulum, progressing to collapse of the head, increased neck width, and head demineralization. Radionuclide bone scintigraphy can evaluate for avascular necrosis of the bone.

Management

1. Bracing and protection of the hip
2. Orthopedic monitoring

EPIPHYSEAL SEPARATION OF THE HEAD OF THE FEMUR (SLIPPED CAPITAL FEMORAL EPIPHYSIS)

This is usually seen in obese or rapidly growing adolescent males (12 to 15 years) and may be bilateral.

Mechanism of Injury

1. Upward blow transmitted through the shaft of the femur.
2. The patient may have no history of trauma.

Diagnostic Findings

1. The leg may be shortened, externally rotated, and adducted. The patient may stand on toes with heel off the ground on one side to compensate for the discrepancy in leg length. Pain is felt with movement. Limitation of internal rotation and abduction.
2. Impaired weight bearing. Limp is present (see Chapter 40).
3. Pain on palpation. Pain may be referred to the knee, groin, or hip.
   X-Ray Films
   AP and frog-leg views are indicated. Widening and irregularity of the epiphyseal plate are noted. If displaced, it usually is downward and posterior.

Management

1. Often requires surgical reduction and immobilization for 12 weeks.
2. Follow-up observation is important to watch for avascular necrosis of the femoral head.

FEMORAL SHAFT FRACTURE
Mechanism of Injury

A direct blow to the thigh (bumper injury) produces the fracture.

Diagnostic Findings

1. Swelling, deformity, tenderness, and pain on movement.
2. Impaired weight bearing.
3. Possible significant blood loss, although rarely requires a transfusion.
4. Possible neurovascular compromise.
5. Rare fat embolus, especially with associated injuries of the hip, knee, or pelvis.
6. Epiphyseal-metaphyseal fractures may be the result of child abuse. Spiral fractures, especially in the prewalking child are concerns for child abuse.

X-Ray Films

AP and lateral views to cover entire femur, including hip, are indicated.

Management

1. Immediate reduction of the fracture with Hare or Thomas traction splinting
2. Orthopedic consultation for long-term therapy, using traction, external fixation, or internal rod, depending on the age of the child

THIGH MUSCLE INJURY/MYOSITIS OSSIFICANS
Mechanism of Injury

1. Most commonly direct blow/tear to muscle

2. More common with repetitive trauma
3. Common in quadriceps

Diagnostic Findings

1. Firm mass in muscle after acute hematoma phase
2. Progressive contracture of muscle
3. May see decreased passive knee flexion with quadriceps involvement

X-Ray Films

Early fluctuant calcification in soft tissues later becoming mature, woven bone superficial to the periosteum.

Management

1. Avoid reinjury and limit activity until pain free, nontender with normal motion with crutch ambulation.
2. Obtain orthopedic consultation for long-term therapy.

COLLATERAL LIGAMENT INJURY TO KNEE

The medial collateral ligament is most commonly affected.

Mechanism of Injury

A twisting injury or blow to the outer aspect of the knee causes ligamentous injury. A varus stress commonly involves the lateral collateral ligament, whereas valgus stress often injures the medial collateral ligament.

Diagnostic Findings

1. Pain on flexion and palpation.
2. Knee effusion.
3. Pain and instability with varus and valgus stress testing. With the knee extended, stress is applied to one side of the knee joint while applying counterpressure against the opposite side.

Valgus stressing, a lateral to medial force on the lateral aspect of the knee, is used to detect medial collateral ligament stability. Varus stressing, a medial to lateral force on the medial aspect of the knee, checks for lateral collateral ligament integrity.

The degree of ligamentous laxity varies, especially in children. Use the opposite knee for comparison.

X-Ray Films

AP and lateral views of the knee are indicated. Arthroscopy and MRI scan may be needed.

Management

1. Immobilize with knee immobilizer.
2. Avoid weight bearing.
3. Refer to orthopedist.

MENISCUS INJURY TO KNEE

The medial meniscus is most commonly affected. Meniscus injury is uncommon in children but does occur in adolescents.

Mechanism of Injury

This occurs with squatting or twisting injury. While the knee is weight bearing and slightly flexed, a twisting motion is applied. Internal rotation injures the medial meniscus, whereas external rotation damages the lateral meniscus.

Diagnostic Findings

1. Pain on flexion of joint. Knee may lock in flexion or prevent full extension.
2. Knee effusion, with tenderness over the involved meniscus.
3. McMurray maneuver. In a supine patient, hold the foot under the arch with one hand and cup the knee with the other. Flex the knee. The knee is then extended with the leg in internal or external rotation. A clicking or rattling on extension in internal rotation indicates a tear of the lateral meniscus and, on external rotation, involvement of the medial meniscus.

X-Ray Films

AP and lateral views of the knee are indicated. There may be a need for arthroscopy and MRI scan.

Management

1. Orthopedic consultation for immobilization, arthroscopy, and possible removal of the meniscus.
2. Definitive care is needed within 1 to 2 days.

CRUCIATE LIGAMENT INJURY TO KNEE

The anterior cruciate ligament is most commonly affected, with injury usually occurring in children older than 8 years of age.

Mechanism of Injury

Forcible hyperextension or abduction and external rotation of the leg damages the ligament, often associated with acceleration or deceleration.

Diagnostic Findings

1. Patient may feel or hear a pop of the knee if the anterior cruciate ligament is ruptured.
2. Effusion.
3. AP drawer sign. With the patient supine, hip 45 degrees, knee flexed 90 degrees, and foot resting on the table in external rotation: pushing or pulling produces sliding motion, indicative of ligamentous injury. If there is increased anterior mobility, anterior cruciate ligament instability is present; if there is increased posterior mobility, posterior cruciate ligament damage has occurred.
4. Lachman's test is the most sensitive: anterior drawer sign with the knee in 15 to 20 degrees flexion and then anterior stability test.

X-Ray Films

AP and lateral views of the knee are indicated. Small avulsion fragment of tibial spine should be excluded. Patient may need arthroscopy and MRI scan.

Management

1. Immobilization and orthopedic referral for evaluation for surgical repair
2. With associated tibial spine fracture, hospitalization and orthopedic consultation

PATELLAR DISLOCATION

This is most common in adolescent females.

Mechanism of Injury

1. Internal rotation of the leg or a direct blow to the outer aspect of the knee
2. Rare occurrence with forcible contraction of the quadriceps muscle

Diagnostic Findings

1. Displaced patella palpated lateral to normal position.
2. Effusion and tenderness over medial collateral ligament and along articular surface of patella.
3. Subluxation of patella usually reduced spontaneously. Sense of knee "giving out" or buckling.
4. Pain reproduced by pushing the patella laterally with the knee flexed at 30 degrees and the foot supported (patellar apprehension).
5. Possibility of associated fracture of medial border of patella or osteochondral fracture of the lateral condyle.

X-Ray Films

AP and lateral views of the knee and tangential (sunrise) view of the patella are indicated.

Management

1. Reduction by extending the knee and flexing the hip (relaxing quadriceps). Apply slight medial pressure to the patella. Often happens spontaneously.
2. Immobilize the knee in extension for 6 weeks, and have patient avoid weight bearing.
3. If recurrent, surgically reimplant the patellar tendon.

PATELLAR FRACTURE
Mechanism of Injury

Blunt force over the anterior aspect of the knee can fracture the patella.

Diagnostic Findings

1. Effusion and tenderness. Fracture may be palpable.
2. Extension of the knee is limited if the fracture is transverse with complete transection of the extensor tendon. The patient may also lose extensor function as a result of rupture of patellar or quadriceps tendons or fracture of the tibial tubercle.
3. If the fracture was caused by pressure applied through the femur, such as the knee hitting a dashboard, posterior dislocation of the hip must also be excluded.

X-Ray Films

AP and lateral views of the knee and tangential (sunrise) view of the patella are indicated.

Management

1. Immobilization of the knee in extension and referral
2. Possibility of hospitalization and surgery with complete fracture

DISTAL FEMUR OR TIBIAL PLATEAU FRACTURE
Mechanism of Injury

A direct blow or indirect valgus or varus stress is the cause of injury.

Diagnostic Findings

A knee effusion is commonly present.

X-Ray Films

AP and lateral views are indicated. The patient may need stress films after consultation with an orthopedist.

Management

Temporary immobilization and referral to an orthopedist are required.

KNEE DISLOCATION

This is usually associated with a fracture and is rare in childhood.

Mechanism of Injury

Severe trauma disrupting all ligaments permits the dislocation.

Diagnostic Findings

An obvious deformity of the knee is present.

Complications

Neurovascular compromise is common. With absence of peripheral pulse, immediate reduction (without x-ray studies) is required.

X-Ray Films

AP and lateral views are required before and after reduction if neurovascular status is intact before reduction.

Management

1. Immediate orthopedic referral and reduction, usually by internal fixation
2. Possible immediate vascular consultation

OSGOOD-SCHLATTER DISEASE

This is usually seen in active children 11 to 15 years of age during rapid growth period. Boys are more often affected.

Mechanism of Injury

Constant pulling of the patellar tendon on its insertion causes this partial separation of the tibial tubercle. Predisposing factors include patellar malposition and extensor mechanism malalignment.

Diagnostic Findings

1. Localized swelling, pain, and tenderness over the tibial tuberosity
2. Possibility of a partial avulsion of the tubercle

X-Ray Films

AP and lateral knee views are required. Tibial tuberosity is normally irregular in adolescents.

Management

1. Restrict activity in mild cases; immobilize the knee in extension for 2 to 4 weeks for all others.
2. With avulsed fracture, there is a possibility of nonunion or avascular necrosis, requiring surgery at later date.
3. Best followed by an orthopedist.

CHONDROMALACIA PATELLAE

This is softening of the patella.

Mechanism of Injury

A fall on a flexed knee or chronic, strenuous exercise such as jogging causes the damage.

Diagnostic Findings

1. Pain after exercise, with a sensation of the knee grating or giving out
2. Pain when sitting for long periods with the knee flexed or when walking up or down stairs
3. Pain and crepitus with palpation of the patella as it moves over its articular surface

X-Ray Film of Patella

The film is normal.

Management

Restriction of activity with strengthening of the quadriceps muscles is indicated. Antiinflammatory agents such as ibuprofen may be useful.

BURSITIS

Inflammation of any of various bursae around the knee, evidenced by swelling or pain.

Mechanisms of Injury

1. Usually overuse
2. May be secondary to direct blow with bleeding into bursa

Diagnostic Findings

Localized swelling and tenderness in prepatellar region (for prepatellar bursitis), in distal patellar tendon region (for deep infrapatellar bursitis), in proximal medial tibia (for pes anserinus bursitis), or over medial joint line (for tibial collateral ligament bursitis).

X-Ray Films
The film is normal.

Management

1. Varies by location
2. Includes ice, nonsteroidal antiinflammatory drugs (NSAIDs), compression, and restricted activity
3. Referral to orthopedist for possible aspiration or steroid injection

TIBIAL OR FIBULA FRACTURE (BOOT-TOP FRACTURE)

Mechanism of Injury

A direct blow or indirect stress to the bone produces the fracture.

Diagnostic Findings

1. Tenderness, swelling, deformity, and impaired weight bearing.
2. Spiral and oblique fractures usually are located at the junction of the middle and distal thirds, the weakest region of the tibia. Tibial shaft fractures associated with a fibular reciprocal fracture are considered eccentric if the fibular site is subcapital or malleolar in location. Children rarely have an eccentric fibular fracture, which may reflect the greater flexibility of the ligamentous structures anchoring the proximal and distal fibula in children.

Complications
1. Open fractures.
2. Distal neurovascular injuries are common (e.g., compartment syndrome). If the proximal third of the tibia is fractured, there may be injury at the bifurcation of the anterior and posterior tibial arteries.

X-Ray Films
AP and lateral views are indicated. The patient may not have a fracture seen on radiograph, but epiphyseal separation may have occurred. Toward the end of adolescence, the medial aspect of the distal tibial epiphysis closes first.

Management

1. Isolated fibular fractures are managed with a short-leg walking cast. Undisplaced tibial fractures can be immobilized in a long-leg posterior splint, with the patient non–weight bearing and followed as an outpatient for 4 to 6 weeks. Early orthopedic consultation.
2. Displaced closed tibial fractures require hospitalization for observation of circulatory status. Orthopedic consultation in ED.
3. Open fractures require immediate consultation for surgical cleansing and stabilization.

REFERENCE

Ciaralla L, et al: Femoral fractures: are children at risk for significant blood loss? *Pediatr Emerg Care* 12:343, 1996.

70 ANKLE AND FOOT INJURIES

SANDY MOON

ANKLE SPRAIN

Ankle sprain is a ligamentous injury. The talus articulates primarily with the tibia. The medial and lateral malleoli provide horizontal stability. On the medial side of the ankle, the deltoid ligament binds the medial malleolus to the talus and calcaneus. On the lateral side, stability is achieved by three ligaments (anterior talofibular, posterior talofibular, and calcaneofibular ligaments).

Mechanism of Injury

Twisting of the foot produces ankle sprains. Inversion (supination) and eversion (pronation) are more frequent than plantar and dorsiflexion injuries. Inversion is the most common.

Diagnostic Findings

Local swelling, discoloration, and tenderness with impaired weight bearing are present.
1. Tenderness anterior and inferior to the lateral malleolus (attachment of talofibular and calcaneofibular ligaments) is common with inversion injuries.
2. Eversion injuries damage the deltoid ligament that is important for ankle stability. Separation greater than 5 mm between the medial malleolus and talus is evidence of deltoid ligament injury. Deltoid ligaments, which almost never tear without associated fracture, have accompanying local tenderness.
   X-Ray
   Anteroposterior (AP), lateral, and mortise views are indicated. With severe sprain, after routine films rule out fractures; the ankle should be stressed to demonstrate stability of the ankle mortise.

Management

1. First-degree (mild sprain): ice and elevation; non–weight bearing for 3 to 4 days; once swelling is resolved, passive exercises; once patient starts walking, support with ankle wrap or stirrup splint. Early mobilization and weight bearing are acceptable in first-degree spraining.
2. Second-degree (partial tear): immobilization in plaster splint, cast or stirrup splint for 3 to 4 weeks. Adolescents: non–weight bearing; preadolescents: limited activity and placed in short walking cast.
3. Third-degree (complete tear): often requires surgical repair. Refer to consultant.

ANKLE FRACTURE

Lateral malleolus is the most common type of ankle fracture.

Mechanism of Injury

Usually an inversion or eversion injury is the cause.

Diagnostic Findings

1. Swelling, ecchymosis, and tenderness over the malleolus with impaired weight bearing.

2. Pain when the foot is directed toward the tibial surface.
3. Inversion injury produces oblique fracture of the medial malleolus and either horizontal fracture of the lateral malleolus or a tear of the lateral ligament. Eversion injury causes opposite damage.

X-Ray Films

1. AP and lateral ankle views.
2. Mortise if question of instability.
3. Yield on x-ray film is greatest in the presence of localized bone pain.
4. In adults, the predictability of an abnormality is greatest when there is pain near the malleolus, and either an inability to bear weight or bone tenderness at the posterior tip or edge of a malleoli. This may be applicable to children.

Management

1. Lateral malleolus: immobilization for 4 weeks and non–weight bearing.
2. Medial malleolus: immobilization and referral. Size of fragment determines therapy.

ANKLE FRACTURE-DISLOCATION

Mechanism of Injury

Severe force applied to the area of the tibiotalar interface causes the fracture-dislocation.

Diagnostic Findings

Obvious deformity and swelling are present.

X-Ray Films

1. AP, lateral, and mortise ankle views
2. Displaced talus (posterior and lateral to the tibia)
3. Prereduction and postreduction films

Management

1. Rapid reduction to reduce swelling and neurovascular compromise

2. Open reduction and internal fixation usually required for associated fractures

CALCANEAL FRACTURE

This is associated with a spinal compression injury and with fractures of the hip and knee in as many as 50% of cases.

Mechanism of Injury

A fall from a height on extended legs can produce a fracture of the calcaneus.

Diagnostic Findings

1. Local swelling, tenderness, impaired weight bearing, ecchymosis on the posterior sole of the foot.
2. Frequent associated injuries, especially vertebral.
3. Puncture wounds are discussed in Chapter 65.

X-Ray Films

AP, lateral, and calcaneal views are indicated. Bohler angle is flattened. Angle described by anterior and posterior halves of the superior cortex of the bone. Spinal films may be indicated.

Management

Compression dressing, immobilization, and orthopedic consultation are necessary.

SEVER'S DISEASE (CALCANEAL APOPHYSITIS)

This is a common entity in the 9- to 11-year-old youngster during rapid growth.

Mechanism of Injury

Mechanical stress and excessive tension on growing calcaneal apophysis.

Diagnostic Findings

1. Calcaneal apophysis is very tender to palpation, especially to transverse compression.
2. Achilles-plantar fascia complex may be tight.

X-Ray Films

Typically not helpful because calcaneal apophysis is often fragmented and dense in normal children.

Management

1. Rest the heel.
2. In very symptomatic patients, prescribe a short leg walking cast for 10 to 14 days.
3. Refer to an orthopedist.

METATARSAL FRACTURE
Mechanism of Injury

The base of the fifth metatarsal is fractured as a result of inversion, with avulsion of the insertion of the peroneus brevis tendon. Fractures of the metatarsal midshaft are usually crush injuries.

Diagnostic Findings

1. Local swelling with impaired weight bearing.
2. March fractures: hairline stress fractures at the base of the metatarsal, often after hiking, jogging, or jumping. Pain is usually over the second, third, or fourth metatarsals. X-ray film finding may be initially negative.

X-Ray Films

AP, lateral, and oblique views are indicated.

Management

1. Immobilization in a posterior short-leg splint or short-leg walker cast for 5 to 6 weeks.
2. March fractures of the fifth metatarsal:

hard-soled shoes or, with significant pain, a short-leg walking cast.
3. For displaced fracture, possible surgery. Refer to consultant.

PHALANGEAL FRACTURES
Mechanism of Injury

"Stubbing" on an immovable object produces the fracture.

Diagnostic Findings

Local swelling and tenderness are present over the involved phalanx. Subungual injuries are discussed in Chapter 68.

X-Ray Films

AP and lateral views of the toe are indicated.

Management

The injury is managed by splinting the toe to the adjacent one for 2 to 3 weeks using tape.

DISLOCATIONS OF BONES OF FOOT

These are uncommon but may occur at the phalangeal, metatarsophalangeal, talonavicular, subtalar, and tarsometatarsal joints.

Mechanism of Injury

A twisting movement with associated force applied to the foot causes this type of injury.

Diagnostic Findings

Obvious deformity, tenderness, and decreased motion are characteristic.

X-Ray Films

AP, lateral, and oblique views are indicated.

Management

1. Phalangeal and metatarsophalangeal dislocations can usually be reduced by manual

manipulation. After infiltration with local anesthetic, a compression splint is useful for several days before mobilization.

2. Other dislocations require either closed reduction with the patient under general anesthesia or open reduction, and the patient should be referred.

REFERENCES

Annis AH, Stiell IG, Stewart DG, et al: Cost effectiveness analysis of the Ottawa ankle rules, *Ann Emerg Med* 26:422, 1995.

Chande VT: Decision rules for roentgenography of children with acute ankle injuries, *Arch Pediatr Adolesc Med* 149: 255, 1995.

Esposito PW: Pelvis, hip and thigh injuries. In Mellon MB, Walsh WM, Shelton GL, et al, editors: *The team physician's handbook*, St Louis, 1990, Mosby.

Griffin LY: Common sports injuries of the foot and ankle seen in children and adolescents, *Orthop Clin North Am* 25:83, 1994.

XI

DIAGNOSTIC CATEGORIES

71 CARDIOVASCULAR DISORDERS

BACTERIAL ENDOCARDITIS
Reginald L. Washington

ALERT: In high-risk children, blood cultures are diagnostic in children with a new murmur; treatment for children with predisposing factors should be initiated. Primary prevention is essential during procedures in patients at increased risk.

Bacterial endocarditis is a life-threatening microbial infection of the endocardial surface of the heart, most commonly involving a heart valve. It is rare in children less than 2 years old.

Approximately 90% of children who have endocarditis have underlying structural heart disease, either congenitally or acquired (i.e., acute rheumatic fever) or as a result of acute rheumatic fever. Patients at greatest risk include those with cardiac abnormalities associated with jet formation and vortex shedding. Lesions include systemic-pulmonary arterial communications (tetralogy of Fallot and other cyanotic heart disease); ventricular septal defect; mitral stenosis and regurgitation; aortic stenosis; aortic insufficiency; bicuspid aortic valve; coarctation of the aorta; and pulmonary stenosis. High-velocity blood ejected into a chamber or vessel causes endocardial or intimal erosion and vegetations. Postoperative patients with artificial valves or conduits are at the highest continuous risk for endocarditis and represent an increasingly large percentage of patients with infectious endocarditis.

Bacteremia and infective carditis are associated with many predisposing events:

1. Dental cleaning, irrigation, or extractions, particularly with gingival bleeding
2. Tonsillectomy
3. Bronchoscopy
4. Cystoscopy or urethral catheterization
5. Sigmoidoscopy
6. Intravenous drug abuse
7. Manipulation of a suppurative focus

ETIOLOGY
Bacterial Infection

1. *Streptococcus viridans* accounts for 17% to 77% of cases and is increasingly associated with postsurgical and catheterization-related cases.
2. *Staphylococcus aureus* is causative in 5% to 40% of cases.
3. Other: *Streptococcus faecalis, Streptococcus pneumoniae, Haemophilus influenzae,* enterococci, gram-negative organisms. Rarely fungi are involved.

DIAGNOSTIC FINDINGS

1. Fever is the most consistent finding and is present in 87% of cases. It is often prolonged without other systemic manifestations.
2. A heart murmur is commonly present (90% of cases). Chest pain may be noted but is rare.
3. Anorexia, malaise, weight loss, chills, weakness, and arthralgias are reported.
4. Splenomegaly is present in 65% of patients; arthritis is also noted.
5. Peripheral manifestations: petechiae or purpura (vasculitis), Osler nodes (small, tender, intradermal nodules in the pads

of the fingers and toes), Janeway lesions (painless erythematous hemorrhagic maculae on the palms or soles), and linear splinter hemorrhages under the nails are uncommon in children.

6. Neurologic manifestations, including confusion, seizures, stroke, or severe headache.

7. A careful dental examination should be performed on all patients with endocarditis.

Complications

1. Congestive heart failure (CHF) most commonly occurs with involvement of the aortic or mitral valves. Pericardial effusion is noted in 21% of patients.

2. Neurologic complications occur in 34% of patients, including mycotic, embolic, and cerebral abscesses. *S. aureus* endocarditis presents the greatest risk.

3. Diffuse glomerulonephritis and renal failure.

4. Progressive cardiac destruction, including mycotic aneurysm, pericarditis, rupture of the sinus of Valsalva, obstructive heart disease, acquired ventricular-septal defect, and conduction defects.

Ancillary Data

1. A complete blood count (CBC) demonstrates a leukocytosis and mild hemolytic anemia. The erythrocyte sedimentation rate (ESR) is elevated in 71% to 90% of cases. Urinalysis shows microscopic hematuria. An electrocardiogram (ECG) may show prolonged PR interval or bundle branch block. Chest x-ray film may be abnormal.

2. Echocardiogram will demonstrate vegetative lesions in only 66% of patients but is useful in diagnosis and monitoring of treatment.

3. Blood cultures are 68% to 98% positive when three separate cultures are ob-

tained. This is crucial to the diagnosis and requires meticulous care to avoid contaminants.

MANAGEMENT

Initial stabilization of the cardiac and respiratory status must be achieved immediately, with oxygen and therapy for CHF (see Chapter 16).

Antibiotics

1. Antibiotics must be compatible with organisms suspected or proved, and they may require alteration once sensitivity data are available.

2. Antibiotic levels must achieve at least a 1:8 serum-bactericidal level at all times. Antibiotic levels (peak and trough) and potential toxicity must be constantly assessed.

3. Treatment course is 6 to 8 weeks. *S. viridans* infections usually require 6 weeks, whereas 8 weeks is the usual course for *S. aureus,* gram-negative organisms, or unusual pathogens or if the cause is unknown.

4. Therapy with a penicillin-type antibiotic and an aminoglycoside is recommended for their synergistic effect.

5. If the patient is allergic to penicillin, cephalothin (Keflin), 100 mg/kg/24 hr q4hr IV, or vancomycin, 40 mg/kg/24 hr q6hr IV, may be substituted for penicillin or nafcillin if indicated by sensitivity data.

Surgical Intervention

This is indicated if there is increasing CHF, if the infection is uncontrolled by antibiotics, or if recurrent septic emboli or extensive cardiac destruction is present. If a conduit or prosthesis is present, surgical removal and replacement may be required for adequate sterilization and control if medical management is not effective.

Etiologic agent	Drug	Dose
Unknown	Nafcillin (or equivalent) and	150 mg/kg/24 hr q4hr IV
	gentamicin	5.0-7.5 mg/kg/24 hr q8hr IV
S. viridans	Penicillin G and	300,000 units/kg/24 hr q4hr IV (maximum: 20 million units/24 hr IV)
	gentamicin	5.0-7.5 mg/kg/24 hr q8hr IV
S. aureus	Nafcillin (or equivalent) and	150 mg/kg/24 hr q4hr IV
	gentamicin	5.0-7.5 mg/kg/24 hr q8hr IV

Prevention

Prophylaxis of high-risk patients is mandatory in preventing bacterial endocarditis. Approximately 90% of children who have endocarditis have underlying heart disease, either congenitally or secondary to acute rheumatic fever (p. 566). Conditions at greatest risk include the following:

1. Prosthetic cardiac valves (including biosynthetic and homograft valves). These patients are at the highest continuous risk for endocarditis and represent an increasingly large percentage of patients.
2. Most congenital cardiac malformations (but not uncomplicated secundum atrial septal defect).
3. Surgically constructed systemic-pulmonary shunts.
4. Rheumatic and other acquired valvular dysfunction.
5. Idiopathic hypertrophic subaortic stenosis.
6. Previous history of bacterial endocarditis.
7. Mitral valve prolapse with mitral insufficiency or thickened leaflets (low risk).

At lower risk are patients with dilated secundum atrial septal defects, secundum atrial septum defects repaired without a patch over 6 months earlier, patent ductus ligation repaired at least 6 months earlier, and postoperative coronary artery bypass surgery.

Bacteremia and infective endocarditis are associated with many predisposing events:

1. All dental procedures likely to induce gingival bleeding (not including simple adjustment of an orthodontic appliance or shedding of deciduous teeth).
2. Tonsillectomy or adenoidectomy.
3. Surgical procedures or biopsy involving the respiratory mucosa.
4. Bronchoscopy, especially with rigid bronchoscopy.
5. Incision and drainage of infected tissue.
6. Genitourinary and gastrointestinal procedures, including cystoscopy, urethral catheterization, prostatic, urinary tract, gallbladder, or colonic surgery, esophageal dilation, colonoscopy, endoscopy with biopsy, or proctosigmoidoscopy. In addition, if infection is suspected or if the patient is at very high risk, prophylaxis is indicated for uterine dilation and curettage, cesarean section, therapeutic abortion, and sterilization. Many clinicians recommend that intrauterine devices should not be used in patients with a risk of endocarditis.

Specific regimens reflect the nature of the procedure, the relative risk of the patient, and the desired route of administration.

1. Antibiotic regimen for *dental and upper respiratory tract procedures.*
   a. Standard *oral regimens*
      (1) Amoxicillin, 2.0 gm PO 1 hour before procedure. See number 3.
      (2) For amoxicillin/penicillin-allergic patients: Clindamycin, 600 mg PO 1 hour before. See number 3.

b. Alternative regimens
  (1) For patients unable to take oral medications:
    (a) Ampicillin, 2.0 gm IV (or IM) 30 minutes before procedure. See number 3.
    (b) For ampicillin/amoxicillin/penicillin-allergic patients unable to take oral medications: Clindamycin, 600 mg IV 30 minutes before procedure. See number 3.
2. For genitourinary and gastrointestinal procedures:
  a. Standard regimen
    (1) Ampicillin, 2.0 gm IV (or IM), plus gentamicin, 1.5 mg/kg IV (or IM) (not to exceed 80 mg) 30 minutes before procedure, followed by amoxicillin, 1.0 gm PO 6 hours after the initial dose. Alternatively, ampicillin, 1 gm IV or IM 6 hours after the initial dose. See number 3.
    (2) For amoxicillin/ampicillin/penicillin-allergic patients:
      Vancomycin, 1.0 gm IV administered over 1 hour plus gentamicin, 1.5 mg/kg IV (or IM) (not to exceed 80 mg) 1 hour before the procedure. Complete injection/infusion within 30 minutes of starting the procedure. See number 3.
  b. Alternative oral regimen for low-risk patients
    (1) Amoxicillin, 2.0 gm PO 1 hour before procedure. See number 3.
3. Initial pediatric doses

Amoxicillin	50 mg/kg
Ampicillin	50 mg/kg
Clindamycin	20 mg/kg
Gentamicin	1.5 mg/kg
Vancomycin	20 mg/kg

Pediatric dose should not exceed total adult dose.

4. Oral regimens are more convenient, but parenteral regimens are more likely to be effective. Parenteral administration is recommended for patients with prosthetic heart valves, those who have had endocarditis previously, and those on rheumatic fever prophylaxis. A single dose of parenteral antibiotic may be adequate because of the short duration of most bacteremias. However, one or two follow-up doses may be given at 8- to 12-hour intervals in those patients judged to be high risk.
5. Patients undergoing cardiac surgery should have maximal prophylaxis beginning before surgery and continuing for no more than 1 day postoperatively. Nafcillin (or equivalent) or a first-generation cephalosporin is recommended. Vancomycin is a good alternative.
6. Patients with indwelling transvenous cardiac pacemakers should receive prophylaxis during all procedures, as should renal dialysis patients with indwelling arterial-venous shunts and individuals with ventriculoatrial shunts for hydrocephalus.

DISPOSITION

All patients with bacterial endocarditis require hospitalization in an intensive care unit (ICU) for monitoring, immediate laboratory evaluation, and initiation of antibiotics. Mortality rate, especially with conduits or prosthetic valves, is as high as 50%.

REFERENCES

American Heart Association: Prevention of bacterial endocarditis: recommendations by the American Heart Association, *JAMA* 277:1794, 1997.

Friedman R, Starke J: Infectious endocarditis. In Garson A, Bricker J, McNamara D, editors: *Science and practice of pediatric cardiology*, Philadelphia, 1990, Lea & Febiger.

Kaplan EL: Bacterial endocarditis prophylaxis, *Pediatr Ann* 21:249, 1992.

Parras F, Bouza E, Romero J, et al: Infectious endocarditis in children, *Pediatr Cardiol* 11:77, 1990.

Saiman L, Prince A, Gersony WM: Pediatric infective endocarditis in the modern era, *J Pediatr* 122:847, 1993.

MYOCARDITIS
Reginald L. Washington

ALERT: Cardiac dysfunction after an infectious illness requires rapid evaluation.

Myocarditis is an inflammatory lesion characterized by cellular infiltrate of the myocardium, usually predominantly mononuclear. Because of decreased myocardial contractility, CHF often results. Viral agents are most frequently the cause.

ETIOLOGY

1. Rheumatic fever (p. 566)
2. Infection
   a. Viral
      (1) Enterovirus; coxsackievirus A and B, echovirus, and poliomyelitis
      (2) Influenza A and B
      (3) Other: mumps, variola, vaccinia, varicella-zoster, rubella, hepatitis
   b. Bacterial: diphtheria, β-hemolytic streptococci, meningococci, staphylococci, salmonellae, tuberculosis
   c. *Mycoplasma pneumoniae*
   d. Fungal
   e. Congenital syphilis
   f. Parasitic diseases: toxoplasmosis, trichinosis, Chagas disease
3. Drugs: antibiotics, indomethacin
4. Other: collagen vascular disease, substance abuse

DIAGNOSTIC FINDINGS

The onset is usually gradual and preceded by an upper respiratory infection (URI) or a "flu-like" syndrome. The early symptoms may mimic a severe URI, and only after cardiac decompensation will the diagnosis become obvious. In rare cases, the myocarditis is isolated without preceding illness. The onset may be acute.

Cardiac examination may reveal tachycardia with a gallop rhythm, atypical systolic murmur, weak or distant heart sounds, and hepatomegaly. Evidence of CHF with pulmonary edema may be present with tachypnea, wheezing, rales, and respiratory distress. Infants may develop nonspecific findings of poor feeding and irritability.

There are associated signs and symptoms of the etiologic agent or condition.

Complications

1. Congestive cardiomyopathy and CHF
2. Constrictive pericarditis
3. Hemopericardium
4. Cardiac arrest and death

Ancillary Data

1. Chest x-ray film: cardiomegaly. Pericardial effusion may be present.
2. ECG.
   a. Tachycardia
   b. Decreased QRS-complex voltages
   c. Nonspecific elevation of ST segment and flattening or inversion of T waves
3. Arterial blood gas (ABG), with cardiac decompensation.
4. Echocardiogram: reveals dilated cardiac chambers with decreased function. Pericardial effusion may be present.
5. Other studies as indicated by etiologic considerations.

DIFFERENTIAL DIAGNOSIS

1. Infection: pericarditis (p. 564)
2. Autoimmune: acute rheumatic fever (p. 566)
3. Vascular: congenital heart disease

4. Other: endocardial fibroelastosis, glycogen storage disease

MANAGEMENT

1. Stabilize the cardiac and respiratory status in symptomatic patients.
2. Give oxygen at 3-6 L/min to all symptomatic patients. Assess airway patency and initiate intervention if necessary. Monitor ABG if indicated.
3. Improve cardiac contractility while reducing work loads in patients with CHF (see Chapter 16).
   a. Digoxin may be helpful but must be used with extreme caution because the inflamed myocardium is sensitive, and signs of toxicity appear with low dosages (see Table 16-2). In acute situations, pressor agents (see Table 5-2) may be required.
   b. Vasodilators such as nitroprusside may be used if cardiac function is not improved by digoxin and the preload is adequate.
   c. β-Blocking agents should not be used.
   d. Diuretic therapy: furosemide (Lasix), 1 mg/kg/dose q6-12hr prn IV (see Table 16-3).
   e. Dysrhythmia and conduction disturbances are common and require treatment (see Chapter 6).
4. Give antibiotics for defined bacterial causes.

DISPOSITION

The patient should be admitted to the hospital and monitored closely until the cardiovascular status has stabilized. The clinical course may be erratic. A cardiologist should be involved in initial care and follow-up observation.

REFERENCES

Greenwood RD, Nadas AS, Fyler DC: The clinical course of primary myocardial disease in infants and children, *Am Heart J* 92:549, 1976.

Martin AB, et al: Acute myocarditis: rapid diagnosis by PCR in children, *Circulation* 90:330, 1994.

Press S, Lipkind R: Acute myocarditis in infants, *Clin Pediatr* 29:73, 1990.

PERICARDITIS
Reginald L. Washington

ALERT: The possibility of cardiac tamponade must be ruled out.

There is a broad spectrum of inflammatory diseases that involve the pericardium and the pericardial space. Fluid accumulation may rapidly cause cardiac decompensation. Viral and autoimmune causes are most common, although pericarditis is often considered idiopathic.

ETIOLOGY

1. Infection
   a. Viral: coxsackievirus, influenza
   b. Bacterial: *S. aureus, S. pneumoniae,* β-hemolytic streptococci, *H. influenzae, Escherichia coli, Pseudomonas,* and meningococci
   c. Other: fungal, tuberculosis, parasitic
2. Autoimmune: acute rheumatic fever, polyarteritis nodosa, systemic lupus erythematosus
3. Metabolic: uremia
4. Postpericardiotomy syndrome

DIAGNOSTIC FINDINGS

A pericardial friction rub is often associated with sharp, stabbing pain, located in the midchest with radiation to the shoulder and neck. The rub is best heard at any point between the apex and left sternal border. It is intensified with deep inspiration and decreased by sitting up and leaning forward. It is differentiated from pleural friction rubs when the patient holds his or her breath.

If a pericardial effusion is present, the heart may appear big to percussion, and auscultation reveals distant, muffled heart sounds. Friction rub may be present. The presence of pulsus paradoxus (decrease in amplitude of blood pressure on inspiration—significant if above 15 mm Hg) indicates at least a moderate accumulation of pericardial fluid. This may be indicative of a cardiac tamponade, particularly if there is distension of the jugular veins, tachycardia, enlargement of the liver, peripheral edema, and, in rare cases, hypotension. Urgent intervention is required.

1. Dyspnea and fever may be present.
2. Associated signs and symptoms of the causative entity may be present.

Complication

Cardiac decompensation, often from cardiac tamponade, is a common complication.

Ancillary Data

1. Chest x-ray film: varies with the amount of pericardial fluid. As accumulation increases, the cardiopericardial silhouette enlarges, and the contours become obscured, often in the shape of a water bottle. Fluoroscopy demonstrates the absence of pulsations of the cardiac borders.
2. ECG.
   a. ST-T wave elevation with inverted T waves
   b. Decreased QRS-complex and T wave voltages
3. Echocardiogram: pericardial effusion is diagnostic.
4. Complete blood count (CBC), erythrocyte sedimentation rate (ESR), and cultures as indicated by potential etiologic agents.

MANAGEMENT

Cardiac function must be rapidly assessed and decompression of the pericardium achieved if necessary. If there is a large volume of pericardial fluid, a pericardiocentesis should be performed for diagnostic and therapeutic objectives (see Appendix A-5).

1. Fluid should be sent for cell count, glucose, protein, lactate dehydrogenase (LDH), Gram stain, and culture.
2. Rapid infusion of fluids may be necessary if the removal of pericardial fluid results in hypotension.
3. Resection of the pericardium through a surgical incision is often required after needle aspiration.

Treatment of the underlying disorder should be initiated:

1. Give antibiotics as appropriate for bacterial, fungal, tuberculosis, or parasitic disease. If a bacterial cause is likely and initial Gram stain is nondiagnostic, initiate nafcillin (or equivalent), 150 mg/kg/24 hr q4hr IV, and cefuroxime, 100-150 mg/kg/24 hr q8hr IV (or equivalent), pending culture results. A surgical pericardial window may be required.
2. Dialysis, if uremia is the cause.

Antiinflammatory agents are useful for autoimmune or idiopathic causes. They improve long-term resolution but are not helpful in the immediate situation if evidence of cardiac decompensation is present. Alternative regimens include the following:

1. Aspirin
   a. Load with 100 mg/kg/24 hr q4hr PO for 1 to 2 days and then reduce to 60 mg/kg/24 hr q6hr PO for 4 to 6 weeks.
   b. Ideal drug level: 15-25 mg/dl.
2. Indomethacin, 1.5-2.5 mg/kg/24 hr q6-8hr PO (maximum: 100 mg/24 hr), may be used instead of aspirin in older patients.
3. If no resolution with aspirin or indomethacin, initiate prednisone, 1-2 mg/kg/24 hr q6hr PO, for 5 to 7 days, and slowly taper. This should only be done in consultation with a cardiologist.

DISPOSITION

The patient should be hospitalized for observation. If any evidence of cardiac decompensation is present, intensive care and evaluation for potential pericardiocentesis are necessary.

In rare early cases without evidence of cardiac decompensation, outpatient status with close follow-up may be tried after cardiology consultation.

REFERENCE

Benzing G III, Kaplan S: Purulent pericarditis, *Am J Dis Child* 106:289, 1963.

Acute Rheumatic Fever

Acute rheumatic fever is a delayed, nonsuppurative, autoimmune disease occurring as a sequela of group A streptococcal infections. Skin infections do not generally place a child at risk. It peaks in 6- to 15-year-old children and is more common in inner cities and black populations. The average annual incidence is declining. However, there has continued to be a recent resurgence in many areas of the United States.

DIAGNOSTIC FINDINGS

The Jones criteria are the basis for making the diagnosis during the initial attack, which is based on two major manifestations *or* one major and two minor manifestations. Their presence indicates a high probability of acute rheumatic fever, if supported by evidence of a preceding group A streptococcal infection documented by increasing streptococcal antibody levels or a positive throat culture.

Major Manifestations

1. Carditis. Usually associated with a murmur of valvulitis. New murmur, tachycardia disproportionate to fever, and in rare cases, pericarditis and CHF. Mitral and aortic valve are most commonly involved. Some clinicians believe the diagnosis can be made in the presence of active carditis, even if it is the only a manifestation of the initial attack.

2. Polyarthritis. Most common but benign major manifestation. Two or more joints are involved, most commonly the ankles, knees, wrists, or elbows. Usually swelling, heat, redness, severe pain, tenderness to touch, and limitation of motion. Lasts about 4 weeks in untreated patients. Dramatic response to salicylates.

3. Sydenham chorea. Marked emotional lability with involuntary motor movements. Usually self-limited but may last several months.

4. Erythema marginatum. Rapidly spreading, ringed eruption, forming serpiginous or wavy lines primarily over the trunk and extremities. Transient and migratory. The rash is not pruritic or indurated and blanches with pressure.

5. Subcutaneous nodules. Variably sized, hard, painless nodes that are rare and seen most frequently in patients with carditis. Commonly found overlying joints, scalp, and spine. Also seen in rheumatoid arthritis and erythema nodosum.

Minor Manifestations

1. Clinical findings
   a. Arthralgia with pain in one or more joints without objective evidence of inflammation. Should not be used as additional criteria if arthritis is present.
   b. Fever (temperature >39° C) present early.
2. Laboratory findings
   a. Elevated acute-phase reactants (ESR or C-reactive protein) are usually noted in patients who have polyarthritis or acute carditis. They are often normal in patients who have chorea alone.
   b. Prolonged PR interval occurs frequently but does not constitute adequate criteria for carditis.
   c. Supportive evidence of group A streptococcal infection. The antistreptolysin (ASO) titer is the most widely

used streptococcal antibody test. Elevated or rising ASO titers provide reliable evidence of a recent group A streptococcal infection. A single titer is considered to be modestly elevated if it is at least 240 Todd units in adults and 320 Todd units in children. A positive culture result is suggestive.

The diagnosis of rheumatic fever can be made without strict adherence to the criteria in three circumstances: chorea, indolent carditis, and recurrent attacks of rheumatic fever.

Complications

1. Cardiac
   a. Dysrhythmias (see Chapter 6)
   b. Mitral or aortic valvular disease
   c. Pericarditis (p. 564)
   d. CHF (see Chapter 16)
2. Rheumatic lung disease: pleurisy or pneumonia
3. Renal disease: glomerulonephritis or interstitial nephritis
4. Recurrence

Ancillary Data

1. CBC, ESR, and C-reactive protein
2. Streptozyme measuring antistreptolysin (ASO), antihyaluronidase (AH), antistreptokinase (ASK), antideoxyribonuclease (ADNase), and antinicotinamide-adenine dinucleotidase (ANA-Dase)
3. Throat culture
4. ECG and chest x-ray film

DIFFERENTIAL DIAGNOSIS

See Chapters 16 and 27.

MANAGEMENT

1. Initial management must focus on cardiac stabilization, if necessary (see Chapter 16).
   a. Digoxin is the drug of choice (see Table 16-2).
   b. Furosemide (Lasix), 1 mg/kg/dose IV, may be useful (see Table 16-3).
2. Acute-phase reactions should be monitored throughout the course of disease as an indication of resolution.
3. Antibiotics should be given to all patients:
   a. Penicillin V, 25,000-50,000 units/kg/24 hr q6hr PO for 10 days; or
   b. Benzathine penicillin G alone (or with procaine) in the dosages specified below.

Weight (lb)	Benzathine penicillin G (units) (Bicillin)
<30	300,000
31-60	600,000
61-90	900,000
>90	1,200,000

4. Antiinflammatory agents:
   a. Aspirin for fever and joint pain
      (1) Initially give 100 mg/kg/24 hr q4-6hr PO for a maximum of 5000 mg/24 hr.
      (2) Maintain levels at 20 to 25 mg/dl.
      (3) After 1 week, decrease to 50 mg/kg/24 hr q6hr PO for an additional 4 to 6 weeks of therapy.
   b. Steroids with evidence of carditis or CHF
      (1) Begin prednisone 2 mg/kg/24 hr q12-24hr PO.
      (2) After 1 week, decrease to 1 mg/kg/24 hr for 1 week, and begin aspirin at 50 mg/kg/24 hr.
      (3) Taper prednisone over the next 2 weeks.
5. For chorea: Haloperidol, 0.01-0.03 mg/kg/24 hr q6hr PO (adult dose: 2-5 mg/24 hr q8hr PO), may be useful.
6. Bed rest.
7. Prevention: prophylactic antibiotics, using either oral penicillin VK (250,000 to 400,000 units q12hr PO) or every 3 weeks, benzathine penicillin (1.2 million units IM) injections.

Prophylactic antibiotics are given indefinitely to those with cardiac involvement and those with chorea initially. Those without cardiac involvement should receive antibiotics for at least 5 years. For penicillin-allergic patients, erythromycin (250 mg PO BID) or sulfadiazine (≤27 kg: 0.5 gm/day; >27 kg: 1.0 gm/day) may be used.

The duration of prophylaxis for persons who have had acute rheumatic fever (ARF) is as follows: Rheumatic fever without carditis: 5 years or until 21 years old, whichever is longer. Rheumatic fever with carditis but no residual heart disease: 10 years or well into adulthood, whichever is longer. Rheumatic fever with carditis and residual heart disease: at least 10 years since last episode and at least until 40 years of age, sometimes lifelong.

DISPOSITION

1. Admit patients to the hospital for stabilization and initiation of treatment.
2. On discharge, emphasize the importance of prophylactic antibiotics, as well as the increased risk of endocarditis if abnormal valves are present.

REFERENCES

American Heart Association: Guidelines for the diagnosis of rheumatic fever, *JAMA* 268:2069, 1992.

Dajani A, Taubenk, Ferrier F, et al: Treatment of adult streptococcal pharyngitis and prevention of rheumatic fever, *Pediatrics* 96:758, 1995.

DiSciascio G, Taranta A: Rheumatic fever in children, *Am Heart J* 99:635, 1980.

Hosier DM, Craenen JM, Teske DW, et al: Resurgence of acute rheumatic fever, *Am J Dis Child* 141:730, 1987.

Kaplan EL: Acute rheumatic fever, *Pediatr Clin North Am* 25:817, 1978.

Kaplan EC, Berrios K, Speth J, et al: Pharmacokinetics of benzathine penicillin Cr. Serum levels during the 28 days after intramuscular injection of 1,200,000 units, *J Pediatr* 115:146, 1989.

Lue HC, Wu MH, Wong JK, et al: Three versus four week administration of benzathine penicillin G: effects on incidence of streptococcal infections and recurrences of rheumatic fever, *Pediatrics* 975:984, 1996.

Majed HA, Shaltout A, Yousof AM: Recurrences of acute rheumatic fever: a prospective study of 79 episodes, *Am J Dis Child* 138:341, 1984.

DEEP VEIN THROMBOSIS

Although uncommon in children and adolescents, deep vein thrombosis does occur in the presence of one of a number of predisposing factors.

ETIOLOGY
Predisposing Factors

1. Trauma: injury to the endothelium
   a. Leg injury
   b. Pelvic injury
2. Vascular: stasis or reduction in venous return
   a. Extended bed rest or immobilization
   b. Cyanotic heart disease or CHF
3. Endocrine: hypercoagulability
   a. Pregnancy
   b. Birth control pills
4. Osteomyelitis

DIAGNOSTIC FINDINGS

The clinical diagnosis of deep vein thrombosis is unreliable, but several findings should be sought:

1. Leg warmth, tenderness, or swelling.
2. Homans' sign (unreliable) with the knee extended, dorsiflex the foot. Pain or soreness in the calf or increased muscular resistance to dorsiflexion is considered positive.
3. Pulmonary embolism in the absence of other sources.

Complications

Pulmonary Embolism

Clinically, pulmonary embolism (PE) is accompanied by dyspnea (58% to 81% of patients), pleuritic pain (72% to 84%), hemoptysis (30%), cough (50%), and anxiety. Physical examination reveals tachypnea, tachycardia, rales, and increased secondary heart sound (pulmonary component). Of these patients, 32% to 58% have evidence of deep vein thrombosis.

There may be few symptoms. The classic triad (hemoptysis, pleuritic chest pain, and dyspnea) is seen in only 28% of patients.

Helpful laboratory tests include the following:
1. ABG may demonstrate hypoxia, although 10% to 20% of patients with severe PE have normal ABG findings.
2. ECG may demonstrate nonspecific ST-T changes (SIQ3T3, RV1, S1, S2, S3).
3. Chest x-ray film result may be normal or show elevated hemidiaphragm, infiltrate, effusion, and segmental or subsegmental atelectasis.
4. Ventilation-perfusion scan is diagnostic.
5. Definitive diagnosis may require pulmonary arteriography.

Ancillary Data

1. CBC, platelet count, prothrombin time (PT), and partial thromboplastin time (PTT).
2. Venogram (usually only indicated in patients with uncertain diagnosis) to define the location, extent, and age of the thrombus. Doppler ultrasonography and plethysmography are useful techniques that may provide definitive or confirmatory diagnostic information.

DIFFERENTIAL DIAGNOSIS

1. Infection: cellulitis (p. 573)
2. Trauma
   a. A sudden onset of leg tenderness, redness, swelling, and a palpable venous cord with superficial thrombophlebitis. Pulmonary embolism can occur if the thrombus is in the proximal saphenous vein.
   b. Muscle contusion.
   c. Compartment syndrome.
   d. Torn medial head of the gastrocnemius muscle. History of acute onset of pain while exercising, usually while up on toes (basketball, tennis, or skiing).

MANAGEMENT

1. Elevate the leg.
2. Apply heat packs to the leg.
3. Bed rest.
4. Anticoagulation (an important part of therapy):
   a. Heparin is given as a continuous intravenous infusion.
      (1) Initial dose is 50 units/kg IV.
      (2) Continuous drip is 10-15 units/kg/hr IV.
      (3) Goal is to maintain PTT at two times control.
      (4) Heparin therapy should be given for 7 to 10 days, the last four concurrent with the administration of warfarin (Coumadin).
      (5) Antidote: protamine sulfate (1 mg IV for each 100 units of heparin given concurrently; 0.5 mg IV for each 100 units of heparin given in preceding 30 minutes, and so on); maximum: 50 mg/dose.
         NOTE: No heparin effect is present in normal patients 4 hours after cessation of therapy.
   b. Oral warfarin (Coumadin) should be initiated 4 to 5 days after beginning anticoagulation with heparin.
      (1) Dosage is 0.1 mg/kg/24 hr PO (adult: 2-10 mg/24 hr PO).
      (2) Dosage should be titrated to maintain PT at two times control.
      (3) Duration of effect is 4 to 5 days.
      (4) Therapy should be continued for 4 to 6 weeks.
      (5) Antidote: vitamin K (infants: 1-2 mg/dose IV; children and adults: 5-10 mg/dose). Fresh-frozen plasma may be given for a more immediate effect.

c. Contraindications to anticoagulation therapy are as follows:
   (1) Active bleeding or blood dyscrasia
   (2) Cerebrovascular hemorrhage
   (3) Pregnancy
   (4) Poor compliance
   d. Drug interactions with warfarin include antibiotics, barbiturates, thyroid medications, prostaglandin inhibitors (aspirin), alcohol.
5. Fibrinolytics. Their use should be initiated only after consultation with the admitting physician and consulting hematologist.

DISPOSITION

All patients should be hospitalized if the diagnosis is proved or suspected, the latter group until diagnostic studies have excluded the diagnosis.

REFERENCES

Bernstein B, Coupey S, Schonberg SK: Pulmonary embolism in adolescents, *Am J Dis Child* 140:667, 1986.
David M, Andrew M: Venous thromboembolic complications in children, *J Pediatr* 123:337, 1993.
Hirsh J: Heparin, *N Engl J Med* 324:1565, 1991.

72 DERMATOLOGIC DISORDERS

ACNE

Acne vulgaris occurs in as many as 85% of children, with the onset between 8 and 10 years of age in 40%. Neonates may develop a self-limited form of acne in the first 4 to 6 weeks of life in response to maternal androgens. This form requires no treatment.

Acne results from outlet obstruction of the follicular canal with accumulation of sebum and keratinous debris. Sebaceous follicles are primarily located on the face, upper chest, and back. Acne is a multifactorial process involving anaerobic pathogens such as *Propionibacterium acnes*.

DIAGNOSTIC FINDINGS

Obstruction of the follicle leads to a wide, patulous opening filled with stratum corncum cells known as opcn comedones or "blackheads," which are commonly seen early in adolescent acne. Obstruction beneath the opening of the neck of the sebaceous follicle produces cystic lesions known as closed comedones or "whiteheads," which can progress to inflammatory acne with papules, pustules, cysts, and also draining sinus tracts that result in permanent scarring.

MANAGEMENT
Mild to Moderate Acne

Topical keratolytic agents are usually adequate in 80% to 85% of adolescents. These agents inhibit bacterial growth and have a comedolytic and sebostatic effect. The two most commonly used are benzoyl peroxide gel in 5% concentration and retinoic acid 0.05% cream. Either agent may be used once a day, or if there is significant inflammation, retinoic acid cream may be applied to acne-bearing skin in the evening and the benzoyl peroxide gel may be applied in the morning. If necessary, the frequency may be increased to twice a day.

Moderate to Severe Acne

In the presence of marked disease with tremendous inflammation, oral antibiotics should be initiated. Tetracycline, 0.5-1.0 gm/24 hr PO, is given for 2 to 3 months until lesions are suppressed. This should not be done in children less than 9 years old or if any potential of adolescent pregnancy exists.

Severe Cystic Acne

Severe cystic disease may additionally need oral retinoids; 13-cis-retinoic acid (isotretinoin [Accutane]) may be started at an initial dose of 40 mg once or twice daily PO. It should not be used in women of childbearing age and requires careful monitoring.

DISPOSITION

All patients may be followed on a regular basis to ensure compliance with the treatment regimen and to monitor progress. The management is directed at control and not eradication, with a response expected in 4 to 8 weeks.

See Chapter 42: Rash.

Atopic Dermatitis (Eczema)

Atopic dermatitis is both an acute and a chronic dermatologic problem, often associated with asthma or allergic rhinitis. There is often a family history of allergic disorders.

DIAGNOSTIC FINDINGS

The severity of the disease varies tremendously. Exacerbations are associated with erythema and edema, as well as crusting and weeping. Lesions are often intensely red at the center, gradually tapering out at the periphery and fading into normal skin. Patients have thickened, lichenified skin areas. Some have symmetrically distributed coin-shaped patches of dermatitis, primarily in the extremities. This is called nummular eczema.

Intense itching is often present, causing excoriation and secondary bacterial infection. In the absence of acute dermatitis, children with eczema often have dry skin with a fine, gritty feel.

Most children have their initial episode in the first few months of life, with the condition resolving by 2 years of age. Recurrences occur between 5 and 8 years and again at puberty.

The pattern varies with the age of the child.

1. Infants typically have fine, scaly erythematous patches on the extensor surface and face, which are generally symmetric in location but not severity.
2. Children primarily have symmetric involvement of the flexor surfaces. The lesions may be papules with plaques.
3. Adolescents have dry, scaly lesions over the hands, feet, and genitalia.

Complications

1. Secondary bacterial infection from *Staphylococcus aureus*
2. Secondary infection from herpes simplex virus (eczema herpeticum)

Ancillary Data

Cultures of the infected sites are useful.

DIFFERENTIAL DIAGNOSIS

Eczema must be differentiated from superficial infections and inflammatory processes caused by the following:

1. Seborrheic dermatitis (p. 585)
2. Contact dermatitis (p. 577)
3. Tinea corporis (p. 577)

Other unusual conditions that may be considered in children include psoriasis (thick, reddened, well-defined plaques with silvery scales on the exterior surface of the arms, legs, and pressure areas), Wiskott-Aldrich syndrome (eczema, thrombocytopenia, purpura, and immunodeficiency), and acrodermatitis enteropathica (zinc deficiency).

MANAGEMENT
Acute Exacerbation

Mild Disease

1. If there is no significant weeping or crusting, hydration is required. This is best achieved by bathing the child in water with an emollient (e.g., Alpha Keri oil) and then applying Eucerin to the involved areas without drying off the youngster. Do not use soap because it is drying. Cetaphil may be a soap substitute.
2. If there are well-circumscribed areas with marked erythema, hydrocortisone cream (1% four times a day) is useful for short periods and should be applied before the Eucerin.

Moderate to Severe Disease

1. For significant weeping and crusting, hydration is essential. The parent should use the following schedule for 2 to 3 days.
   a. During the day, apply wet compresses (gauze or soft dish towels) that are damp but not soaking with warm water. Keep them wet and remove them every 5 minutes, reapplying damp ones for a total of 15 minutes of treatment. Repeat three to five times/day.
   b. At night, bathe the child. Have the child wear cotton pajamas that are wet (not soaked) with warm water. Then

put on a pair of dry pajamas over the wet ones. If severe, apply wet dressings over topical steroids at night for 5 to 7 nights.

c. Do not use soap.

2. Topical steroids are usually necessary. They should be applied after the wet-compress treatment, before putting on the child's pajamas.

   a. Fluorinated steroids are particularly effective but should not be used on the face or intertriginous areas:

      (1) Fluocinolone acetonide cream, 0.01% (Synalar)

      (2) Triamcinolone cream, 0.01% (Kenalog)

   b. Hydrocortisone cream (1%) may be used on facial areas.

3. Antipruritic (antihistamines) agents are useful to reduce scratching and may produce some sedation:

   a. Diphenhydramine (Benadryl), 5 mg/kg/24 hr q6hr prn PO (over the counter); or

   b. Hydroxyzine (Atarax, Vistaril), 2 mg/kg/24 hr q6hr prn PO.

4. Antibiotics are often indicated if evidence of secondary bacterial infection is present.

   a. Dicloxacillin, 50 mg/kg/24 hr q6hr PO for 10 days; or

   b. Cephalexin (Keflex) or cephradine (Velosef), 25-50 mg/kg/24 hr q6hr PO for 10 days.

   c. Mupirocin 2% (Bactroban) may be a topical alternative for treatment of small areas of group A streptococcal infection.

Ongoing Management

This is crucial to minimizing acute problems.

1. Hydration should be maximized with daily baths and with application of Eucerin to the wet skin without drying off the child. If the problem is mild, lubricating creams such as Nivea may be easier to use. This is particularly important in dry areas or those that are recurrent problems. Some recommend placing bath oils, such as Alpha Keri, in the water.

2. Use of soap should be discouraged because it is a drying agent. Cetaphil lotion cleanser may be used as a soap substitute.

3. Occlusive ointments such as Vaseline should not be used.

4. Fingernails should be kept short to minimize scratching.

DISPOSITION

Most children can be sent home with appropriate management as described earlier. Hospitalization is indicated with severe disease, particularly if evidence of bacterial infection, eczema herpeticum, or poor compliance exists, or if the child fails to respond to home management.

Parental Education

1. Maintain skin hydration and reduce scratching. Patience and persistence are required.

2. Avoid skin-sensitizing agents that cause contact dermatitis: wool, soaps, chlorine, detergents, etc.

3. Call your physician if the following occur:

   a. There is increasing redness, crusting, pustules, large blisters, or evidence of fever or toxicity.

   b. No response is seen in 2 to 3 days.

4. Follow-up observation is essential. Keep appointments.

CELLULITIS AND PERIORBITAL CELLULITIS

Cellulitis is an acute suppurative infection of the skin and the subcutaneous tissue.

ETIOLOGY

Cellulitis is caused by bacterial infection (Table 72-1). Streptococcal organisms are common because the incidence of *H. influenzae* has

TABLE 72-1 Cellulitis: Etiologic Characteristics and Treatment

Etiology	Special clinical characteristics	Antibiotics
Streptococcus pneumoniae	Facial	Penicillin G, 25,000-50,000 units/ kg/24 hr q4hr IV; **if PO:** penicillin V, 25,000 units (40 mg)/kg/24 hr q6hr PO
Staphylococcus aureus	Often preexisting break in skin	Nafcillin, 100-150 mg/kg/24 hr q4hr IV; **if PO:** dicloxacillin, 50 mg/kg/24 hr q6hr PO (*or* cephalo- sporin: cephradine/cephalexin, 25-50 mg/kg/24 hr q6hr PO)
Group A streptococci	Often preexisting break in skin; rapidly spreading erythema, indu- ration, pain, lymphadenitis	Penicillin G, as above
Haemophilus influenzae	Facial; periorbital; purplish swelling; <9 yr	Cefotaxime, 50-150 mg/kg/24 hr q6-8hr, *or* ceftriaxone, 50-75 mg/kg/24 hr q12hr IV, *or* cep- furoxime, 50-100 mg/kg/24 hr q6-8hr IV
Anaerobes (*Clostridium perfringens*)	Possibly preexisting injury with necrotic tissue; dirty, foul- smelling, seropurulent discharge	Penicillin G, as above

decreased as a result of widespread immu- nizations.

DIAGNOSTIC FINDINGS

The lesions are generally erythematous, with swelling, tenderness, and edema. The edges are indefinite.

1. Common sites of involvement are the face and periorbital region, neck, and extremities.
2. Often, a preexisting break exists in the skin caused by animal or insect bites, lac- erations, abrasions, or chickenpox.
3. The violaceous (purplish) swelling associ- ated with facial cellulitis can be caused by most pathogens, not only *H. influenzae.*
4. *Lymphangitis* appears as red lines spread- ing rapidly from the focus of infec- tion in the direction of regional lymph nodes. It is most common with group A streptococci.

5. *Erysipelas* presents as a small deeply erythematous area of the skin; borders are irregular and raised. An elevated advancing edge is painful to touch. Area is indurated and lymphangitis may be present. Group A streptococcus is usually causative.

Often concomitant fever, malaise, and re- gional lymphadenopathy are present. Periorbital cellulitis is often accompanied by otitis media and systemic bacterial infection at other sites. Sinusitis, especially ethmoiditis, may be a pre- disposing condition.

Complications

1. Bacteremia with secondary focus.
2. Infection of underlying joint or bone. Sub- cutaneous air implies myonecrosis sec- ondary to clostridial infection.
3. Deeper involvement of the orbit (Table 72-2).

TABLE 72-2   Periorbital Cellulitis: Differentiating Clinical Features

| | Clinical feature | | | |
Condition	Lid erythema with swelling	Ophthalmoplegia	Proptosis	Acuity
Periorbital cellulitis	Common	Absent	Absent	Absent
Orbital cellulitis	Common	Common	Common	Variable
Subperiosteal abscess	Absent	Absent	Lateral	Absent
Orbital abscess	Common	Common	Common	Common
Cavernous sinus thrombosis*	Common	Common	Common	Common

Modified from Barkin RM, Todd JK, Amer J: *Pediatrics* 62:390, 1978.
*Plus papilledema, meningismus, prostration, and cranial nerve involvement.

Ancillary Data

Although empiric treatment is usually appropriate, when widespread cellulitis involves the face or periorbital region or in cases of systemic toxicity, additional data are useful:

1. Blood culture results in the toxic child. Positive results are common with facial cellulitis, whereas they usually are negative in patients with extremity cellulitis.
2. White blood cells (WBC) elevated with a shift to the left.
3. Needle aspiration of the edge of the lesion with a 23- to 25-gauge (face) or 18-gauge (extremity) needle, after thorough povidone-iodine preparation of the insertion site may be considered in very toxic children or those who are not responding rapidly to appropriate antibiotic management. The needle is inserted at an angle while maintaining negative pressure with a 10-ml syringe. If no material is obtained, 0.5 ml of nonbacteriostatic saline solution is injected and the material withdrawn. Aspirate is sent for Gram stain and culture. Aspiration of periorbital cellulitis should be done only if the edge extends beyond the orbit.
4. Urine counterimmune electrophoresis (CIE) may be a useful diagnostic adjunct, if Gram stain and culture are negative.
5. CT scan of the orbit may be necessary to determine the extent of the infection, thereby differentiating periorbital or preseptal cellulitis from deep orbital cellulitis. Evaluation of the sinuses may be useful in excluding an accompanying sinus infection.

DIFFERENTIAL DIAGNOSIS
Infection

1. Erysipelas is an infection with acute lymphangitis of the skin that must be differentiated from less invasive group A streptococcal infections. There is erythema with marked induration. The margins are raised and clearly demarcated. Fever, vomiting, and irritability may be present.
2. Osteomyelitis or septic arthritis is difficult to differentiate from simple cellulitis. Bone scans and aspirates are useful.
3. Lymphadenitis or abscess (particularly cervical) may have an overlying cellulitis. With appropriate treatment, the cellulitis will resolve rapidly, leaving a clearly defined lymph node. Abscesses should demonstrate fluctuance.
4. Periorbital or preseptal cellulitis must be distinguished from other infections of the orbit (see Table 72-2). Spread to deeper structures is rare. Although the computed

tomography (CT) scan gives a definite answer about the extent of involvement, the physical examination should delineate the structures involved.

Allergy

Insect bites may cause a tense, warm, erythematous area. The history of insect exposure, presence of an entry point, and partial response to antihistamines is helpful in differentiation.

Trauma

After known or unknown trauma, contusions or hematomas may develop. In addition, environmental stresses such as hypothermia (frostbite), sunburn, or chemical burns may produce tissue injury.

MANAGEMENT

Antibiotics are the major form of treatment. The choice of antibiotics must reflect the likely etiologic agents, the toxicity of the patient, and the involved site, as well as information from Gram stain and culture of the needle aspirate. A total course of 10 days is required, often with a combination of parenteral and oral medications.

1. Patients with only a localized cellulitis (not involving the face and with no evidence of systemic toxicity) can usually be treated as outpatients on an empirical basis:
   a. Dicloxacillin, 50 mg/kg/24 hr q6hr PO; or cefazolin (Ancef) or cephradine (Velosef), 25-50 mg/kg/24 hr q6hr PO for 10 days
   b. With lymphangitis consistent with a group A streptococcal infection, penicillin alone: penicillin V, 25,000 units (40 mg)/kg/24 hr q6hr PO for 10 days
2. Patients with systemic toxicity or facial involvement require parenteral therapy. If the organism is unknown, the following guidelines are used.

a. For patients less than 9 years of age with toxicity or with large areas of involvement or facial location:
   (1) Cefotaxime, 50-150 mg/kg/24 hr q6-8hr IV, or ceftriaxone, 50-75 mg/kg/24 hr q12hr IV, or cefuroxime, 50-100 mg/kg/24 hr q6hr IV.
   (2) If there is a break in the skin, thereby increasing the likelihood of *S. aureus*, nafcillin (as above) should be used in addition to one of the cephalosporins suggested above, the latter to cover *H. influenzae*.
b. For patients older than 9 years of age: nafcillin, as above.
c. Erysipelas usually requires penicillin G (50-100,000 units/kg/24 hr q4hr IV) initially in addition to above therapy. Resolution of fever occurs in 24 hours.
d. After resolution of the cellulitis and defervescence: change to oral medications for a total course of 10 days. These agents may include amoxicillin, Augmentin, cephalosporin, dicloxacillin, or trimethoprim-sulfamethoxazole, depending on presentation, isolates, and sensitivity.

DISPOSITION

Patients with only localized cellulitis and no involvement of the face or systemic toxicity may be followed closely as outpatients. Nontoxic patients with periorbital cellulitis may be discharged after IM ceftriaxone, 150 mg/kg/dose, with reevaluation for improvement in 6 to 12 hours; others require hospitalization.

Parental Education

1. See that the child takes all medications and keeps appointments for follow-up observation.
2. Call your physician if the following occur:
   a. Fever increases.

b. The area of cellulitis increases or becomes fluctuant.

c. Underlying joint or bone remains tender or painful once cellulitis has resolved.

REFERENCES

Powell KR: Orbital and periorbital cellulitis, *Pediatr Rev* 16:163, 1995.

Powell KR, Kaplan SB, Hall CB, et al: Periorbital cellulitis, *Am J Dis Child* 142:853, 1988.

Schwartz GR, Wright SW: Changing bacteriology with periorbital cellulitis, *Ann Emerg Med* 28:617, 1996.

CONTACT DERMATITIS

Contact irritant dermatitis results from contact with an exogenous substance. It may be caused primarily by an irritant, such as an alkali or a detergent, or by prolonged contact of the skin with urine and feces as in diaper dermatitis (p. 578). It is usually mild in nature.

Allergic contact dermatitis is lymphocyte-mediated and caused by a variety of substances, including plants (poison ivy or poison oak), topical medications, shoes, nickel, and cosmetics.

DIAGNOSTIC FINDINGS

1. The distribution and patterning of the lesions, as well as the history of contact, are diagnostic. The lesions often are limited to exposed contact surfaces, and they may be sharply delineated or have bizarre symmetric distribution.

2. The dermatitis is initially erythematous with edema but may progress to vesicle formation, weeping, and crusting.

MANAGEMENT

The offending allergen or irritant, if identifiable, should be removed.

Severe, Generalized, Allergic Contact Dermatitis

A short course of systemic steroids is indicated if extensive involvement exists over the body, face, or genitalia, especially if edema is significant. Exacerbation may occur if therapy is not prolonged enough.

1. Prednisone is given 1-2 mg/kg/24 hr q6-24hr PO for 1 week and then tapered over the next 2 weeks for a total therapeutic period of 3 weeks.

2. Therapy may be initiated parenterally: dexamethasone (Decadron), 0.25 mg/kg/dose IV or IM.

Moderate Allergic Contact Dermatitis

Topical steroids and compresses are adequate as described for atopic dermatitis (p. 572).

Mild Allergic or Irritant Contact Dermatitis

1. Topical steroids are usually adequate.

2. Hydration of the involved area may be useful and, after baths, application of Eucerin or Nivea. Others prefer applying compresses of tepid water, saline, or Burow's solution to weeping areas to dry up the involved region.

DISPOSITION

1. Patients may be discharged but followed until resolution occurs.

2. Patch testing may be useful in defining potential allergens that should be avoided.

DERMATOPHYTOSIS

See Table 72-3.

ANCILLARY DATA

1. Wood's light. In dark room, shine Wood's light. Obtain fluorescence.

2. KOH prep. Place specimen taken from

TABLE 72-3   Dermatophytoses: Clinical Characteristics

	Location	Diagnostic findings	Differential diagnosis	Management
Tinea capitis	Scalp, hair	Initially, noninflammatory—bald, scaly patch; 2-8 wk; inflammatory phase—edematous nodule with pustule (kerion)	Alopecia areata (scalp within normal limits); trichotillomania; pyoderma	Griseofulvin
Tinea corporis	Nonhairy parts of body	Dry, scaly, annular lesion with clear center	Pityriasis rosea, atopic dermatitis	Topical
Tinea pedis	Feet	Vesicle, erosion of fourth and fifth toes, extending to other toe and arch of foot; adolescent	Atopic or contact dermatitis	Topical
Tinea fachei	Face	Erythematous, scaly lesion; butterfly distribution	Systemic lupus erythematosus	Topical
Tinea cruris	Groin	Sharply demarcated erythematous, scaly lesion; scrotum not involved; adolescent		Topical
Tinea unguium	Nails	Nail is thickened, friable; subungual debris; nail discoloration; adolescents	Psoriasis	Griseofulvin and topical; possibly surgery (if poor response)

just inside the advancing border of the infection on slide. Add 1 to 2 drops of 10% to 20% KOH; place cover glass on slide and heat gently (do not boil); do microscopic examination. Ideally, the hyphae are seen branching.

3. Culture. Sabouraud agar or dermatophyte test medium (DTM). Latter turns red if dermatophyte is present. Incubate up to 4 weeks.

MANAGEMENT (see Table 72-3)

1. Topical. Apply cream or solution two to three times/day for at least 1 week after eruption has cleared. May take 2 to 4 weeks.
   a. Tolnaftate (Tinactin)
   b. Clotrimazole (Lotrimin) (over-the-counter)
   c. Miconazole (MicaTin)
   d. Haloprogin (Halotex)

2. Tinea capitis and unguium. Oral griseofulvin (microsize: 10 mg/kg/24 hr; or ultramicrosize: 5-10 mg/kg/24 hr) given PO for 6 weeks (hair) or 3 months (nails). Ultramicrosize is better absorbed. Culture before starting griseofulvin therapy. Supplement griseofulvin with twice weekly shampooing with selenium sulfide suspension.

   Selenium sulfide, 1% to 2.5%, may be adjunctive therapy for tinea capitis.

3. Kerion. Requires prednisone, 1-2 mg/kg/24 hr for 1 month, usually in consultation with a dermatologist.

DIAPER DERMATITIS AND CANDIDIASIS

Diaper dermatitis is a result of prolonged contact with urine or feces, leading to chemical irritation and associated dampness and maceration. Candidiasis secondary to *Candida albicans* is usually associated with prolonged dermatitis in the diaper region; 80% of diaper dermatitides that last more than 4 days are colonized with *Candida,* even before the classic rash appears.

DIAGNOSTIC FINDINGS

Diaper dermatitis has a clinical presentation of diffuse erythema with vesiculation and isolated erosions in the diaper area. Satellite papules on an erythematous base caused by *C. albicans* usually develop when the dermatitis has been present for more than 3 days (also called *Monilia*). This may be associated with white plaques on an erythematous base on the buccal mucosa, which is known as *thrush*.

DIFFERENTIAL DIAGNOSIS

Other entities that must be distinguished include contact dermatitis (p. 577), atopic dermatitis (p. 572), and bullous impetigo (p. 581).

MANAGEMENT

1. Remove the irritant.
   a. Change diapers frequently.
   b. Leave the baby without a diaper as much as possible. Naps are a particularly good time. Overnight, use triple diapers and rubber pad.
   c. Fasten diapers loosely.
      (1) If cloth diapers are used, double rinse them. Alkalinity may be reduced by adding dilute vinegar (1 cup in washer tub of water or 1 oz in 1 gallon). Do not use plastic pants.
      (2) If disposable diapers are used, punch a few holes in the plastic liner. Newer superabsorbent diapers may reduce dermatitis.
   d. Keep the skin clean, washing gently with warm water. Superfatted or nonirritating soaps (Neutrogena, Basis, Lowila) may be used sparingly. Cetaphil lotion cleanser may also be used.

2. If any evidence of satellite lesions associated with candidiasis is present, initiate application of nystatin cream to the involved area during diaper changes. Continue for 2 to 3 days after resolution of the diaper dermatitis.
   a. With marked erythema mix hydrocortisone cream (1%) with the nystatin and apply to the diaper area until the erythema has decreased. Other alternatives to nystatin include miconazole and clotrimazole. Do not use fluorinated steroid preparations.
   b. Treat oral white plaques (thrush) with nystatin oral suspension: 1 ml in each side of the mouth QID for 2 to 3 days after clearing.
      An alternative is fluconazole (load of 6 mg/kg/dose followed by 3 mg/kg/dose once a day orally).

Complication

A complication is secondary bacterial infection.

DISPOSITION

Patients may be sent home.

Parental Education

1. Initiate more frequent diaper changes and avoid skin-sensitizing agents.
2. Expose the diaper area to air when possible and avoid airtight occlusion caused by such things as rubber pants.
3. Do not use cornstarch or ointments in the diaper area.
4. Call your physician if the following occur:
   a. Satellite lesions develop in the diaper area.
   b. White plaques develop in the mouth.
   c. Evidence of bacterial infection, including crusting, pustules, or large blisters is present.
   d. No resolution occurs in 1 week.

REFERENCE

Janniger CK, Thomas I: Diaper dermatitis: an approach to prevention employing effective diaper care, *Cutis* 52: 153, 1993.

Eczema (see p. 572)

Erythema Multiforme

Erythema multiforme is a self-limited, hypersensitivity reaction with a broad spectrum of presentations, including toxic epidermal necrolysis and Stevens-Johnson syndrome.

ETIOLOGY: PRECIPITANTS

1. Infections
   a. Viral: herpes simplex, Epstein-Barr (EB) virus—infectious mononucleosis, enterovirus
   b. Other: group A streptococci, *Mycoplasma pneumoniae*
2. Intoxications: sulfonamides, penicillin, barbiturates, phenytoin

DIAGNOSTIC FINDINGS

Classically, erythema multiforme is a monomorphous eruption.

1. Initially it presents as symmetric, concentric, and erythematous lesions, primarily on the dorsal surfaces of the hand and extensor surfaces of the extremities. The palms and soles are often involved while the trunk is spared. The lesions become papular with an intense erythematous periphery and cyanotic center appearing as target or iris lesions. They may become bullous.
2. There may be a prodrome of fever, headache, sore throat, cough, rhinorrhea, and lymphadenopathy.
3. The skin lesions evolve over 3 to 5 days with resolution over 2 to 4 weeks. They may recur.

Toxic Epidermal Necrolysis (Lyell Disease)

1. Drug induced, it represents a severe form of erythema multiforme with cleavage of the skin below the epidermis and dermal layer resulting in full-thickness necrosis of the epidermis.
2. Rarely, the lesions progress to produce severe confluent erythema and bullae with subsequent shedding of the epidermis, predominantly over the extremities, face, and neck.
3. Patients have a positive Nikolsky sign at the site of the lesions, whereby minor rubbing results in desquamation of underlying skin.
4. Extensive loss of superficial epidermis may occur, with subsequent fluid losses and complications paralleling those of a second-degree burn.
5. Patients are usually toxic, with high fever, malaise, and anorexia.

Stevens-Johnson Syndrome

1. A variant of erythema multiforme, the cutaneous lesions extensively involve the mucosal membranes and affect at least two sites (conjunctivae or mucosa of mouth, genitalia, or nose).
2. Blisters form and subsequently unroof with formation of extensive hemorrhagic crusts on the mucosal surface.
3. Patients are usually toxic and have difficulty with fluid intake.
4. A prodrome 1 to 14 days before the onset of mucocutaneous lesions is noted, including malaise, nausea, vomiting, sore throat, cough, myalgia, and arthralgia.

Complications

1. Dehydration from surface losses or poor fluid intake
2. Secondary bacterial infections
3. Chronic dry eye or mild chronic symblepharon

Ancillary Data

1. Throat culture to rule out group A streptococci
2. Data related to fluid status if dehydration is present (see Chapter 7)
3. Other tests related to defining precipitants

DIFFERENTIAL DIAGNOSIS

1. Differential consideration of toxic epidermal necrosis: staphylococcal scalded-skin syndrome or Ritter's syndrome in newborn (pp. 586 and 712). Patients are sick with fever.
2. Differential consideration of Stevens-Johnson syndrome: Kawasaki syndrome (mucocutaneous lymph node syndrome) (p. 710).

MANAGEMENT

1. Supportive care is essential: fluid management, antipruritics, and analgesics.
2. For toxic epidermal necrolysis, see Chapter 46 on burns for discussion of management of fluids, etc. (steroids have no value in therapy).
3. For Stevens-Johnson syndrome careful attention to fluid management, oral hygiene, and eye care is important.
   a. If fluid intake is a problem, discomfort may be decreased by having patient gargle with a solution containing equal parts of Kaopectate, diphenhydramine (Benadryl), and 2% viscous lidocaine (Xylocaine). The dose of the 2% viscous lidocaine (Xylocaine) should not exceed 15 ml q3hr or 120 ml in 24 hours in the adult (proportionately less in child). The patient should not eat or drink for 1 hour after application because of the danger of aspiration. Antacids such as Maalox or Mylanta are equally effective.
   b. Mouth washes with half-strength peroxide, if tolerated, are useful.
   c. If there is extensive involvement of the eye, consult an ophthalmologist.

If possible the precipitant should be identified. There is *no* clear role for steroids.

DISPOSITION

Patients with uncomplicated illness may be followed as outpatients, with instructions to watch for more extensive involvement.

Patients with toxic epidermal necrolysis should be hospitalized for fluid and skin management unless there is very minimal involvement and follow-up observation is excellent. Dermatologic consultation should be obtained.

The ability to maintain hydration and the extent of involvement dictate the disposition of patients with Stevens-Johnson syndrome.

REFERENCES

Assier H: Erythema multiforme with mucous membrane involvement and Stevens-Johnson syndrome are clinically different disorders with distinct causes, *Arch Dermatol* 131:539, 1995.

Prendiville JS, Hebert AA, Greenwald MJ, et al: Management of Stevens-Johnson syndrome and toxic epidermal necrolysis in children, *J Pediatr* 115:881, 1989.

IMPETIGO

ETIOLOGY: INFECTION

Impetigo is a bacterial infection caused by group A streptococci or *S. aureus* (bullous impetigo).

DIAGNOSTIC FINDINGS

An erythematous area evolves into numerous thin-walled vesicles, often overlying areas of abrasion or trauma. The vesicles are quickly unroofed, leaving a superficial ulcer that becomes covered with a thick, honey-colored crust. These spread centrifugally and may coalesce into larger lesions.

Less commonly, the vesicles may become

Weight (lb)	Benzathine penicillin G (units)	Bicillin C-R (units) (900,000 benzathine : 300,000 procaine)
<30	300,000	300,000 : 100,000
31-60	600,000	600,000 : 200,000
61-90	900,000	900,000 : 300,000
>90	1,200,000	NA

bullae that coalesce. When ruptured, they leave a discrete round lesion. This is *bullous impetigo*, usually caused by *S. aureus.*

Lesions most commonly occur on the face and extremities or in areas of trauma.

Complications

1. Acute glomerulonephritis secondary to nephrogenic strains of streptococci
2. Ecthyma: streptococcal infection with extension through all layers of the epidermis, resulting in a firm, dark crust with surrounding erythema and edema

Ancillary Data

Very rarely, a culture of the lesion is indicated if there is doubt about the diagnosis.

MANAGEMENT

Local skin care may be helpful. Soaking with water combined with some abrasion is useful in removing the crusts.

Antibiotics are indicated for all patients.

1. For lesions that consist primarily of erythema and crusts (the most likely causative organism is group A streptococci):
   a. Penicillin V, 25,000-50,000 units/kg/24 hr q6hr PO for 10 days; or
   b. Benzathine penicillin G (Bicillin C-R), usually given 900,000:300,000 IM as a single injection according to the schedule listed above.
2. For bullous impetigo (resulting from *S. aureus* infection): dicloxacillin, 50 mg/kg/24 hr q6hr PO for 10 days.

3. Alternative antibiotics:
   a. Erythromycin, 30-50 mg/kg/24 hr q6hr PO for 10 days; or
   b. Cephalexin (Keflex) or cephradine (Velosef), 25-50 mg/kg/24 hr q6hr PO for 10 days, which may be particularly useful because of the potential significance of *S. aureus* in poorly responsive infections; or
   c. Mupirocin 2% (Bactroban) ointment is a topical treatment equal to oral medication.

DISPOSITION

All uncomplicated patients may be sent home.

Parental Education

1. Have your child take all medication.
2. Remove the crust with soaking and minimal abrasion.
3. Minimize sharing of towels, sheets, etc.
4. Bring any other children with similar lesions in for treatment.

Patients are not infectious 24 hours after initiating treatment.

REFERENCES

Demidovich CW, Wittler RR, Ruff ME, et al: Impetigo: current etiology and comparison of penicillin, erythromycin and cephalexin therapy, *Am J Dis Child* 144: 1313, 1990.

Dogan R, Bar-David Y: Comparison of amoxicillin and clavulanic acid (Augmentin) for the treatment of nonbullous impetigo, *Am J Dis Child* 143:916, 1989.

Mertz PM, Marshall DA, Eaglstein WH, et al: Topical mupirocin treatment of impetigo is equal to oral erythromycin, *Arch Dermatol* 125:1069, 1989.

Rice RD, Duggan AK, DeAngelis C: Cost-effectiveness of erythromycin versus mupirocin for the treatment of impetigo in children, *Pediatrics* 89:210, 1992.

Lice (Pediculosis)

Lice or crabs primarily affect the head or pubic areas and are transmitted by person-to-person spread. They cannot live beyond 3 days without human contact.

DIAGNOSTIC FINDINGS

Excoriated papules or pustules are noted in the scalp or perineum. The louse is often seen in the hair or on hats or underwear. Gelatinous nits are often noted as tightly adherent white specks on the shaft of the hair.

Intense nocturnal pruritus may be present.

Complications

Complications consist of secondary bacterial infection such as impetigo (discussed previously).

MANAGEMENT

Several pediculicides are commonly available:

1. RID (purified pyrethrins): Apply about 1 oz undiluted to infested area until entirely wet and allow to remain for 10 minutes. Wash thoroughly. A second treatment is usually needed in 7 to 10 days. Available over-the-counter.
2. NIX (permethrin 1%) creme rinse. After washing hair, saturate with creme rinse, allow to remain for 10 minutes, then rinse. Single application usually adequate, although some recommend a second treatment a week later. Available over-the-counter. The hair should be combed with a nit comb.
3. Lindane (Kwell): Apply about 1 oz (adult) or Kwell shampoo to either the scalp or pubic region and work into a lather, frequently adding small amounts of water. Scrub the hair well for 4 minutes and rinse thoroughly. Removal must be thorough because of the potential for contact dermatitis or central nervous system (CNS) toxicity. One treatment is usually adequate but some prefer to repeat in 10 days. For an adult, 1 to 2 oz is enough; prescribe smaller amounts for children. Do not give extra medication or use in pregnant women.
4. Other preparations are available as well. Some suggest applying olive oil or petrolatum to the hair to kill the nits in conjunction with the above medications.

If the nits are present in the eyelashes or eyebrows, apply petrolatum (Vaseline) carefully to the area overnight once. Do not have the parents mechanically remove them, because this tends to produce eye trauma.

Although the nits are dead in the hair, they may stay tightly adherent. Remove by washing the hair with warm vinegar for about 30 minutes to loosen the nits and then mechanically remove them with a fine-toothed comb.

Treat symptomatic contacts; for example, treat all nonpregnant sexual contacts.

All the child's bed linens and clothes that have recently been worn should be machine washed and dried using the hot cycle of dryer for at least 20 minutes. Hats and other headgear that are difficult to wash should be put away, in a sealed plastic bag for 10 to 14 days. Children may return to school after one treatment.

Antihistamines may be necessary for pruritus, which may continue for several weeks: diphenhydramine (Benadryl), 5 mg/kg/24 hr q6hr PO, or hydroxyzine (Atarax, Vistaril), 2 mg/kg/24 hr q6hr PO.

Pinworms

Enterobius vermicularis are ½-inch, white, threadlike worms that infect the perianal region.

DIAGNOSTIC FINDINGS

1. Children complain of perianal itching. In rare cases, with persistent irritation, an associated vulvovaginitis may be present.
2. Worms may be seen by parents.

Ancillary Data

A piece of transparent adhesive tape or special kit is gently touched to the perianal region. The sticky side is applied to a glass slide for examination for ova by light microscopy. The highest yield is at night.

DIFFERENTIAL DIAGNOSIS

Pinworms should be distinguished from irritation, fissures, or contact dermatitis in the perianal region.

MANAGEMENT

1. One of two drugs should be used:
   a. Mebendazole (Vermox) for children older than 2 years; 100-mg chewable tablet PO once (repeat in 1 week); or
   b. Pyrantel (Antiminth), 11 mg (0.2 ml)/kg/dose (maximum: 1 gm) PO once (repeat in 1 week).
2. Family members or contacts with perianal irritation or itching should be similarly examined and treated. Asymptomatic contact need not be treated.

Parental Education

Children are usually infected by other children, many of whom carry pinworms but are asymptomatic. Good personal hygiene, with particular attention to hand washing, may reduce the chance of infection.

PITYRIASIS ROSEA

Pityriasis rosea affects children and adolescents and is of unknown cause.

DIAGNOSTIC FINDINGS

1. Initially, a round, scaly, erythematous patch (2 to 4 cm) with central clearing develops, usually on the trunk. This herald patch precedes the generalized eruption by an average of 10 days and may be confused with tinea corporis.
2. Multiple erythematous macules develop and progress to small, rose-colored papules, primarily over the trunk. The individual lesions are oval shaped, 1 to 2 cm in size, and follow the wrinkle or cleavage lines of the skin. This creates a "Christmas tree" distribution on the back.
3. In black children, distribution varies, being primarily on the proximal extremities, inguinal and axillary areas, and the neck.
4. Patients may initially have pruritus but later become asymptomatic.
5. The rash may last for several months, marked by resolution and recurrences.

MANAGEMENT

1. Reassurance is of primary importance. Contact irritants should be avoided.
2. Antihistamines may be useful if itching is severe:
   a. Diphenhydramine (Benadryl), 5 mg/kg/24 hr q6hr PO; or
   b. Hydroxyzine (Atarax, Vistaril), 2 mg/kg/24 hr q6hr PO.
3. Ultraviolet light (either natural or sunlamp) may hasten the resolution.

SCABIES

Scabies is caused by the mite *Sarcoptes scabiei* and requires close person-to-person contact for transmission. The female mite cannot live beyond 2 to 3 days without human contact.

DIAGNOSTIC FINDINGS

1. Lesions appear as erythematous papules associated with S-shaped linear burrows.

a. They are primarily located on the dorsum of the hand, interdigital web spaces, elbows (extensor surface), wrists, anterior axillary fold, abdomen, and genitalia. The head and neck are rarely involved.

b. There is intense nocturnal pruritus, which may continue for up to 1 week after successful treatment.

2. Infants often have an associated acute dermatitis with excoriations and crusting. In addition to the normal distribution, they also have involvement of the head, neck, palms, and soles.

Complications

Impetigo (p. 581) is a secondary bacterial infection.

Ancillary Data

Microscopic examination for mites, eggs, or feces may be done by placing a drop of mineral oil at the advancing end of a burrow and unroofing the burrow with a scalpel. The specimen is then placed on a microscope slide, a cover glass applied, and the material examined by light microscopy.

MANAGEMENT

Two scabicides are primarily used, although Lindane is preferred.

1. Lindane (Kwell lotion) is applied to dry skin in a thin layer from the neck down. The lotion is left on for 8 hours and the patient is then bathed thoroughly to remove residual lotion. Removal must be complete because of the potential of contact dermatitis and CNS toxicity. It should not be used in pregnant women or children less than 1 year old. One treatment is usually adequate, although a retreatment is sometimes necessary 1 week later, particularly in infants and children with many lesions.

In adults, 1 to 2 oz is usually adequate, with proportionately smaller volumes in children.

2. Crotamiton 10% (Eurax cream) is applied from the neck down, with particular attention to folds and creases, and repeated in 24 hours. After 48 hours the child should be thoroughly bathed.

3. Permethrin topical cream (Elimite) has low toxicity and is effective; 1 to 2 oz is applied to the entire body and left on for 12 hours before being rinsed off. A second treatment in 7 to 10 days is suggested but is not always needed.

All members of the household and sexual contacts should be treated. (Lindane should not be used in pregnant women.) All the child's bed linens and clothes that have recently been worn should be machine washed. Blankets and other items that are difficult to clean should be put away for 4 days. After one treatment, children can return to school.

Antihistamines may be necessary for prolonged pruritus: diphenhydramine (Benadryl), 5 mg/kg/24 hr q6hr PO, or hydroxyzine (Atarax, Vistaril), 2 mg/kg/24 hr q6hr PO. Itching may continue for 1 week after treatment.

REFERENCE
Rasmussen JE: Scabies, *Pediatr Rev* 15:110, 1994.

Seborrheic Dermatitis

Seborrheic dermatitis is caused by the overproduction of sebum in areas rich with sebaceous glands, including the scalp, face, midchest, and perineum. It is commonly seen during the first few months of life and in adolescents at puberty.

DIAGNOSTIC FINDINGS

1. The involved areas are minimally erythematous, dry, and scaly with a greasy sensation. Lesions have more intense color and periphery, with clearing at cen-

ter. Edges are sharply demarcated. Weeping and edema are not present.

2. Newborns particularly have problems with the scalp and may develop "cradle cap."

MANAGEMENT

1. In infants the scalp may be treated by washing with minimal abrasion (washcloth or soft brush) in an effort to remove the scales. Do not use oils.
2. In children and adolescents, shampoos such as Sebulex or those containing selenium sulfide, combined with abrasion, may be helpful.
3. Hydrocortisone cream (1%) is used in markedly involved areas, except for the scalp.
4. Resolution usually occurs within 1 week. Recurrences may be noted.

STAPHYLOCOCCAL SCALDED SKIN SYNDROME

ETIOLOGY
Infection

S. aureus, phage group II, produces an exotoxin (exfolitin) in the patient. The bacteria typically colonize in the patient without overt infection.

DIAGNOSTIC FINDINGS

1. Staphylococcal scalded-skin syndrome may be generalized in the newborn (Ritter's disease) and the child. Patients may be febrile and irritable.
2. An erythematous eruption develops primarily on the face (perioral and periorbital), the flexor area of the neck, and the axilla and groin, with accompanying tenderness of the skin, progressing to a tender scarlatiniform rash over 1 to 2 days.
   a. Edema of the face develops, with crusting around the eyes and mouth and sparing of mucous membranes.
   b. Patients have a positive Nikolsky's sign,

whereby the epidermis separates with only minor trauma.
3. If the erythema does not progress but desquamates, the patient merely has a scarlatiniform rash.
4. Some patients develop only a localized involvement with the evolution of large bullae with clear or purulent fluid. This is bullous impetigo (p. 581).

Complications

1. Dehydration from fluid losses
2. Systemic infection with *S. aureus*
3. Toxic shock syndrome (p. 721)

Ancillary Data

Bacterial culture of involved areas may be done.

DIFFERENTIAL DIAGNOSIS

1. Erythema multiforme, toxic epidermal necrolysis (p. 580)
2. Group A streptococcal infection: impetigo or scarlatiniform rash (p. 581)

MANAGEMENT

1. Patients require support with fluids and analgesia.
2. Local treatment with warm compresses may be helpful. However, if the loss of epidermis is extensive, the protocol for management of burns should be implemented (see Chapter 46).
3. Antibiotics should be initiated for all patients:
   a. Dicloxacillin, 50 mg/kg/24 hr q6hr PO for 10 days
   b. Parenteral antibiotics (nafcillin or equivalent) for toxic patients

DISPOSITION

Most patients should be hospitalized for local skin care, monitoring of fluids, and antibiotics.

Sunburn

Sunburn results from overexposure to ultraviolet (UV) light. Phototoxic agents that sensitize skin to sun include sulfonamides, tetracycline, hydantoin, barbiturates, chlorpromazine, chlorothiazide, coal tar derivatives, perfumes, celery, and parsnips.

DIAGNOSTIC FINDINGS

1. The exposed skin is erythematous and tender in the first few hours. With significant burns, it will become erythematous and edematous over the next 6 to 12 hours and ultimately blister by 24 hours.
2. Patients may have concomitant chills, headache, and malaise (see Chapter 50).
3. Photosensitizing agents should be considered, including sulfonamides, diphenhydramine, phenothiazines, and tetracyclines.

MANAGEMENT

1. Cool baths or wet compresses are helpful in relieving the pain and burning; repeat three to four times per day for 10 minutes each. Bland emollients (Eucerin, Nutraderm, Lubriderm) may be helpful.
2. Aspirin or indomethacin (1-3 mg/kg/24 hr q6-8hr PO in children over 14 years) is useful in the management of severe sunburn if begun within 12 hours.
3. Steroids have no proven role.

DISPOSITION

Patients may be sent home.

Parental Education

1. Avoid overexposures in the future, particularly if the child is taking a photosensitizing agent.
2. Use sunscreens with a skin-protective factor (SPF) of at least 15 before exposure in the future. Reapply after swimming or active sweating.
3. Push fluids to maintain hydration.

REFERENCE

Hebert AA: Photoprotection in children, *Adv Dermatol* 8:309, 1993.

Urticaria

ETIOLOGY

1. Allergy
   a. Drugs: penicillin, salicylates, narcotics
   b. Foods: nuts, shellfish, eggs
   c. Inhalants
   d. Insect bites (p. 306)
2. Infections
   a. Viral: hepatitis, EB virus (infectious mononucleosis)
   b. Parasites
3. Trauma: mechanical, thermal (cold and heat), sun or solar
4. Autoimmune: systemic lupus erythematosus, inflammatory bowel disease
5. Neoplasms

DIAGNOSTIC FINDINGS

1. Eruption is a rapidly evolving, erythematous, raised wheal with marked edema. The edema is well circumscribed and tense. The lesions are markedly pruritic.
2. Subcutaneous extension of the edema, known as angioedema, occurs in as many as 50% of children with acute urticaria.
3. If associated with anaphylaxis, there may be respiratory or circulatory compromise (see Chapter 12).

Ancillary Data

No tests are indicated initially except to define the cause.

TABLE 72-4 Categories of Warts and Appropriate Management

Common	Filiform	Flat	Plantar	Venereal
DIAGNOSTIC FINDINGS				
Solitary papule, irregular scaly surface; found anywhere	Projection from skin on narrow stalk; lip, nose, or eyelids	Flat-topped, skin-colored papule; face or extremity	Smooth papule level with skin surface on weight-bearing surfaces	Multiple confluent papules, irregular surface; genital mucosa or adjacent skin (condylomata acuminata)
MANAGEMENT				
Cryotherapy, salicylic acid paint (periungual: cantharidin, salicylic acid paint)	Surgery	Retinoic acid, salicylic acid paint	Salicylic acid plaster, salicylic acid paint	Podophyllin, cryotherapy

MANAGEMENT

1. Avoid etiologic conditions.
2. Ensure that there is no associated respiratory compromise. If present, begin therapy immediately as outlined in Chapter 12.
3. Antihistamines and epinephrine are the hallmarks of therapy:
   a. Diphenhydramine (Benadryl), 5 mg/kg/24 hr q6hr PO, IM, or IV; or
   b. Hydroxyzine (Atarax, Vistaril), 2 mg/kg/24 hr q6hr PO (causes less associated fatigue).
   c. With poor response, addition of pseudoephedrine (Sudafed), 4-5 mg/kg/24 hr q6hr PO.
   d. An alternative for recurrent or persistent allergic urticaria are histamine (H_2) blockers such as cimetidine (Tagamet), 20-30 mg/kg/24 hr q4-6hr PO (adult: 300 mg q6hr PO).
   e. Epinephrine (1:1000), 0.01 ml/kg/dose (maximum: 0.35 ml/dose) SC q20min prn, up to three doses if rapid clearing of rash is desired.
4. Refer for a more complete evaluation of patients with recurrent or persistent urticaria beyond 4 to 6 weeks.

REFERENCES

Mahwood T, Janniger CK: Childhood urticaria, *Cutis* 52:78, 1993.

Moscati RN, Moore GP: Comparison of cimetidine and diphenhydramine in the treatment of acute urticaria, *Ann Emerg Med* 19:12, 1990.

WARTS AND MOLLUSCUM CONTAGIOSUM

Warts are viral-induced, intraepidermal tumors caused by human papovavirus. They are often asymptomatic, although those on pressure-bearing surfaces may be painful. Spontaneous resolution occurs in 9 to 24 months. Warts may be categorized by their appearance and location (Table 72-4).

MANAGEMENT TECHNIQUES
(Listed in Table 72-4)

1. Cryotherapy. Cotton swab is dipped in liquid nitrogen, applied to the center of the wart until it is white, and maintained for 20 to 30 seconds.
2. Salicylic acid paint. Salicylic acid in concentration above 10% is applied to wart twice a day for 2 to 4 weeks. On thick surfaces salicylic acid, 16.7%, and lactic acid, 16.7%, in flexible collodion are used. A weaker concentration (10%) is used on flat warts.
3. Salicylic acid plaster. Cotton plaster with salicylic acid (40%) is cut to size of wart and taped to skin; it remains for 3 to 5 days and is then replaced. Wart is treated for 2 to 3 weeks.
4. Retinoic acid (0.1% cream) is applied once or twice a day, with resolution in 2 to 4 weeks.
5. Cantharidin is applied directly to periungual warts, and the warts are then covered with tape for 24 hours.
6. Podophyllin (25%) is applied to venereal warts and washed off thoroughly in 4 hours. May need to be repeated in 1 week. Because it is neurotoxic, it must not be used on an extensive area or at home.

Molluscum contagiosum is a white or whitish-yellow papule with central umbilication caused by a poxvirus. Grouped genital lesions are common, often surrounded by an area of dermatitis. Wright stain of the contents of the papule reveals epidermal cytoplasmic viral inclusions.

Sharp dermal curettage is the treatment of choice if removal is desired. This may leave a small scar. Spontaneous resolution occurs in 2 to 3 years.

REFERENCES

Rosekrans JA: Dermatologic disorders. In Barkin RM, editor: *Pediatric emergency medicine: concepts and clinical practice*, ed 2, St Louis, 1997, Mosby.

Weston WL, Lane AT, Morelli JC: *Color textbook of pediatric dermatology*, ed 2, St Louis, 1996, Mosby.

73 Ear, Nose, and Throat Disorders

DENTOALVEOLAR INFECTIONS

Toothaches and associated dentoalveolar infections usually are caused by untreated dental caries, although they may be related to failing dental restorations.

DIAGNOSTIC FINDINGS

1. Patients usually complain of local or generalized dental or facial pain, often exacerbated by heat, cold, sweets, air, and chewing pressure.
2. The affected tooth usually has an obvious defect, such as dental caries or broken or lost restoration.
3. Facial swelling is commonly noted. Dentoalveolar swelling or fistula also may be present.

Complications
1. Facial cellulitis (p. 573)
2. Bacteremia
3. Loss of tooth

Ancillary Data

Dental x-ray film, if available, is helpful.

DIFFERENTIAL DIAGNOSIS

1. Dentoalveolar or periodontal abscess.
2. Newly erupting tooth.
3. Traumatic dental injury.
4. Broken dental restoration.
5. Foreign object embedded in tissue.
6. *Dental stains* may be mistaken for caries in a tooth. Normal teeth have some color variation. Stains also may be caused by external agents that can be removed with cleaning; such stains (green, orange, or black) result from poor hygiene or from excessive use of certain foods or beverages, smoking, or liquid medications (iron). Intrinsic conditions that lead to dental staining include problems in the neonatal period (biliary atresia, hepatitis, erythroblastosis, or maternal tetracycline ingestion), trauma, excessive fluoride, or previous tetracycline ingestion between 3 months and 8 years of age.

MANAGEMENT
Toothache without Infection

1. Evaluation of legitimate need for analgesics, which children rarely require
2. Dental referral within 24 hours

Toothache with Localized Infection

1. Initiation of antibiotics: penicillin V, 25,000-50,000 units (15-30 mg)/kg/24 hr q6hr PO for 7 to 10 days
2. Consideration of analgesics
3. Dental referral within 24 hours

Dental Infection with Cellulitis

1. Hospitalize.
2. Initiate antibiotics.
   a. Give nafcillin (or equivalent), 150 mg/kg/24 hr q4hr IV.
   b. Switch to dicloxacillin once parenteral therapy is no longer indicated at a

dosage of 50 mg/kg/24 hr q6hr PO for a total course of 10 days.

3. Consult with dentist to evaluate need for incision and drainage, extraction of tooth, or open drainage. Dentist will attempt to relieve pain, treat infection, and provide appropriate follow-up as necessary for extraction or root canal treatment, restoration, or dental prosthesis.

REFERENCES

Josell SD, Abrams RE: Common oral and dental emergencies and problems, *Pediatr Clin North Am* 29:705, 1982.

Kureishi A, Chow AW: The tender tooth: dentoalveolar, pericoronal and periodontal infections, *Infect Dis Clin North Am* 2:163, 1988.

Epistaxis (Nosebleed)

Nasal bleeding normally originates in the anterior portion of the nasal septum (Kiesselbach area), which accounts for 90% of cases.

ETIOLOGY

1. Trauma: nose picking, foreign body, repeated hard blowing with associated upper respiratory infection, nasal fracture.
2. Allergic rhinitis or polyp.
3. Bleeding dyscrasia, aspirin ingestion, anticoagulants, leukemia.
4. Vascular: telangiectasia, hemangioma. Hypertension is an unusual association.

DIAGNOSTIC FINDINGS

Active bleeding from one or both nostrils is present. Examination of the nose reveals an inflamed area at Kiesselbach plexus. Predisposing causes should be defined.

Complication

Although epistaxis is usually self-limited, extensive bleeding may cause anemia or shock.

Ancillary Data

Rarely are any laboratory data indicated unless there are suggestions of systemic disease. A bleeding screen (complete blood count [CBC], platelet count, prothrombin time [PT], partial thromboplastin time [PTT], and bleeding time) for recurrent epistaxis is indicated if there is a history of significant bleeding with lacerations, circumcision, etc., spontaneous bleeding at other sites, or a positive family history (see Chapter 29).

MANAGEMENT

1. Apply constant pressure over the anterior nares for a minimum of 10 minutes. Preceding this, the patient should blow the nose to remove clots. Optimally, have the patient remain sitting with head forward to avoid draining blood posteriorly into the airway or esophagus.
2. If pressure is unsuccessful, place a piece of cotton soaked in 0.25% phenylephrine (Neo-Synephrine), or epinephrine (1:1000) and 1% cocaine in the nose, and then apply pressure for 10 minutes.
3. If anterior bleeding continues or the problem is recurrent, cauterize the bleeding site with application of a silver nitrate stick for 3 seconds. Do not cauterize children with bleeding problems.
4. Apply petrolatum (Vaseline) daily for 4 to 5 days to decrease friability of the anterior nasal mucosa.

If posterior bleeding is present, a posterior pack (and Foley catheter) may be inserted by an otolaryngologist.

DISPOSITION

Patients can usually be discharged. If a posterior pack is inserted, the patient must be admitted. Admission should be seriously considered if bilateral anterior packs are used. Appropriate allergy management, if indicated, should be instituted. Hematologic or otolaryngologic consultation is rarely indicated.

Parental Education

1. Increase home humidity. Minimize nose trauma and picking.
2. Apply Vaseline daily to anterior nares for 4 to 5 days.
3. If bleeding recurs, apply pressure for a full 10 minutes, compressing the soft and bony parts of the nose, pressing downward toward the cheeks with thumb and forefinger.
4. Call your physician if there are unexplained bruises, if large amounts of blood are lost, or if bleeding cannot be controlled by pressure.

REFERENCES

John DG, Alison AI, Scott DJA, et al: Who should treat epistaxis? *J Laryngol Otol* 101:139, 1987.
Padgam N: Epistaxis: anatomical and clinical correlates, *J Laryngol Otol* 104:308, 1990.

FOREIGN BODIES IN THE NOSE AND EAR

Foreign bodies found in the nose or ear commonly include inanimate objects (e.g., toys, earrings), vegetable materials, and insects. The nose is a common site in children less than 3 years; the ear is a common site in those less than 8 years.

DIAGNOSTIC FINDINGS

1. A patient with *nasal* foreign bodies has nasal obstruction or unilateral foul-smelling discharge. The object often may be visualized.
2. A patient with a foreign body in the *ear* often has pain or discharge from the external ear canal. Often, there is a history either of inserting an object into the ear or of a buzzing sound associated with an insect. The object may be visualized.

MANAGEMENT

Cooperation is essential through immobilization, sedation, or anesthesia. Good visualization, an excellent light source, and proper equipment are necessary. Button batteries should be promptly removed.

Nasal Foreign Bodies

Have the child blow the nose vigorously, then try suction. If unsuccessful, proceed with other techniques.

1. Vasoconstriction. Use topical epinephrine (1%) applied with a cotton-tipped swab, sprayed phenylephrine (0.25%), or cocaine (1%) before instrumentation individually or in combination.
2. Use forceps if the object can be grasped. Suction and hook or loop may be useful for larger objects.

If these maneuvers are unsuccessful and there is room, a lubricated No. 8 Foley catheter may be passed beyond the object and inflated with 2 to 3 ml water (with the patient in reverse Trendelenburg position). Then the Foley catheter is withdrawn.

Ear Foreign Bodies

Several techniques are useful in attempting to remove objects.

1. If an insect, kill it before removal by inserting alcohol.
2. Irrigate. Direct the stream of water beyond the object to flush it out. Do not use with vegetable matter (the material may swell) or if the tympanic membrane is perforated.

   NOTE: A useful irrigation technique is to cut off the needle of a large butterfly (18-gauge) catheter, leaving the pliable section of tubing. The ear is then easily irrigated with water and the fluid aspirated from the canal. A pulsating water device also may be used.
3. Mechanical removal: Use forceps for small objects, hooks, or loops.

DISPOSITION

If the foreign body cannot be removed, patients should be referred to an otolaryngologist for ambulatory management.

REFERENCES

Baker MD: Foreign bodies of the ears and nose in childhood, *Pediatr Emerg Care* 3:67, 1987.

Brownstein DR, Hodge D III: Foreign bodies of the eye, ear and nose, *Pediatr Emerg Care* 4:215, 1988.

Kavanagh KT, Litovitz T: Miniature battery foreign bodies in auditory and nasal bodies, *JAMA* 255:1470, 1986.

ACUTE NECROTIZING GINGIVITIS

This is an acute, contagious oral infection of adolescents and young adults involving the gingival tissues.

ETIOLOGY: INFECTION

It is caused by spirochete *Borrelia vincentii.*

DIAGNOSTIC FINDINGS

1. History of recent emotional or physical stress (rarely epidemic). Fatigue may be a factor.
2. The classic triad is intense, unremitting pain; punched-out interdental papillae covered with a white pseudomembrane; and foul odor from the mouth.
3. Rarely associated with regional lymphadenopathy, malaise, and fever.

Complications

Without treatment there is bone loss and loosening of teeth.

DIFFERENTIAL DIAGNOSIS

1. Infection: acute viral and bacterial infections
2. Leukemic gingivitis

MANAGEMENT

1. Give penicillin V, 25,000-50,000 units (15-30 mg)/kg/24 hr q6hr PO for 10 days.
2. Refer to dentist and follow-up with observation for tissue debridement. Surgery may be necessary.

CERVICAL LYMPHADENOPATHY

The cervical lymph nodes course along the carotid sheath and drain the head and neck. The superior node group has afferents from the tongue, tonsils, nose, teeth, and the back of the head and neck. It becomes inflamed with potential suppuration from infections in these areas.

ETIOLOGY: INFECTION

1. Bacterial: group A streptococci, *S. aureus,* typical and atypical mycobacteria
2. Viral: infectious mononucleosis, enterovirus, rubella
3. Other: cat-scratch fever (see p. 304), toxoplasmosis, histoplasmosis, tuberculosis, mucocutaneous lymph node syndrome (Kawasaki syndrome)
    NOTE: Lymphadenopathy may be an early finding of human immunodeficiency virus (HIV)–positive patients.

DIAGNOSTIC FINDINGS

1. History should be obtained for rapidity of progression, recent travel, exposure to tuberculosis, contact with cats, and concurrent systemic signs and symptoms.
2. Pyogenic lesions have a unilateral, visible, firm, tender, discrete swelling early in the disease, which may progress to generalized swelling, erythema, and tenderness that becomes fluctuant. Patients usually are febrile and become increasingly toxic with extension of the process. There may be pain on neck movement.
3. Nonpyogenic organisms have a more insidious course. Tuberculosis, histo-

plasmosis, or toxoplasmosis should be considered if mass is associated with a child more than 10 years of age; persistent, unexplained fever or weight loss; fixation of mass with overlying skin, skin ulceration, supraclavicular location, no local tenderness, or increasing size 3 cm or more in diameter.

4. Cat-scratch fever (see p. 304) is caused by a small, pleomorphic gram-negative bacterium. Regional lymphadenopathy of an extremity occurs about 14 days (range: 3 to 50 days) after the scratch.

5. Palpable head and neck nodes are detected in 45% of normal children and 34% of neonates. Younger children most commonly have nodes in the occipital and postauricular areas, whereas older children have them predominantly in the cervical and submandibular regions.

Complications

Suppuration and spontaneous drainage of the lymph node occurs.

1. Exteriorly, this is a problem for cosmetic reasons.
2. Nodes caused by atypical mycobacteria may chronically drain.
3. Interior drainage may involve multiple neck structures, with significant morbidity.

Ancillary Data

1. White blood cells (WBC) with differential (shift to left).
2. Throat culture for group A streptococci.
3. Monospot and Streptozyme.
4. Intermediate-strength purified protein derivative (PPD) test (usually <10 mm with atypical disease but may be negative).
5. Aspiration of the node with an 18-gauge needle if there is no resolution of signs and symptoms in 48 hours. Biopsy may also be considered, particularly if nonpyogenic organism is suggested.

a. Care should be exercised if atypical mycobacteria are considered because of the potential for chronic drainage.
b. Culture for bacteria and mycobacteria should be done, as well as Gram and acid-fast stains.
c. If a formal surgical incision and drainage (I and D) is performed, similar cultures should be obtained.

6. Computed tomography (CT) scan of the neck may be indicated in toxic patients and those with large nodes that are not rapidly responsive to therapy. Ultrasonography is useful in defining the nature of a neck mass.

DIFFERENTIAL DIAGNOSIS

Considerations must include those entities that cause *stiff neck* (p. 730).

1. Infection: parotitis (most commonly mumps). This infection obliterates the angle of the jaw, is associated with parotid tenderness, and is often bilateral.
2. Neoplasm: lymphoma, leukemia, metastatic carcinoma.
3. Congenital: bronchial cleft or thyroglossal duct cyst.
4. Hemangioma or cystic hygroma.

MANAGEMENT

Management of cervical lymphadenopathy must proceed in an orderly fashion, and other etiologies should be considered if the patient's initial response is slow. Total resolution may occur over many weeks.

1. Initiate antibiotics for at least 10 days after appropriate cultures are obtained.
a. Cephalexin (Keflex) or cephradine (Velosef) or equivalent, 25-50 mg/kg/24 hr q6hr PO; or
b. Erythromycin, 30-50 mg/kg/24 hr q6hr PO; or
c. Dicloxacillin, 50 mg/kg/24 hr q6hr PO.
d. Some prefer a more limited coverage

initially: penicillin V, 80,000 units (50 mg)/kg/24 hr q6hr PO, given for 48 hours if the node is not fluctuant initially. This is a relatively high dosage.

e. If clinical improvement is noted, the therapy is continued.

f. If the patient is toxic or the lymph node is fluctuant, large, or markedly tender, initiate parenteral antibiotics (nafcillin [or equivalent], 150 mg/kg/24 hr q4hr IV). I and D may be required, depending on the child's toxicity, comfort, and the node's size, warmth, fluctuance, and localization. This is often done in the operating room.

g. If the lymphadenopathy is slow to resolve on routine antibiotics, clindamycin, 10-25 mg/kg/24 hr q6hr PO (or 15-40 mg/kg/24 hr q6-8hr IV), may be initiated to ensure gram-positive and anaerobic coverage.

h. Consider other antibiotics if the Gram stain or culture of the node aspirate reveals less common organisms, such as *H. influenzae.*

2. Treatment of atypical mycobacterial infections is controversial. Excision provides the best cure rate. Some clinicians treat with rifampin after surgery. Infectious disease consultation is indicated.

DISPOSITION

1. Patients may be followed at home unless there is significant toxicity, marked fluctuance, tenderness or erythema of the lymph node, or I and D is required. Close follow-up observation is essential.

2. Surgical consultation is necessary for patients with fluctuant or unresponsive nodes.

Parental Education

Lymphadenopathy may require several months for complete resolution. For children followed at home, the parent should understand the following:

1. Treatment requires very high-dose antibiotics. The child should take all doses.

2. Your physician should be called if the following occur:

   a. Swelling increases or becomes more red, tender, or fluctuant.

   b. Systemic toxicity develops.

REFERENCES

English CK, Wear DT, Margileth AM, et al: Cat-scratch disease, *JAMA* 259:1347, 1988.

Wright JE: Cervical lymphadenitis in childhood: which antibiotic agent? *Med J Aust* 150:150, 1989.

ACUTE MASTOIDITIS

The middle ear communicates with the mastoid air cells, leading to concurrent infections if acute otitis media (AOM) is improperly treated.

ETIOLOGY

Acute mastoiditis is caused by bacterial infection identical to those organisms causing AOM, most commonly *S. pneumoniae, H. influenzae,* group A streptococci, *S. epidermidis,* and a number of anaerobes. *H. influenzae* is less common in children older than 8 years of age.

DIAGNOSTIC FINDINGS

AOM is followed by pain, edema, and tenderness over the mastoid area. Postauricular swelling, resulting from a subperiosteal abscess, may cause severe pain and displace the pinna forward, making the ear prominent.

Complications

1. Infection: meningitis and intracranial abscess

2. Paralysis of facial nerve

3. Sensorineural hearing loss

Ancillary Data

1. Mastoid x-ray film shows clouding of the septa of the mastoid bone (48%). Bony destruction and resorption of air cells eventually occur (12%). CT scan may provide definitive anatomic data.
2. Tympanocentesis, culture, and Gram stain of aspirated material may be useful.

DIFFERENTIAL DIAGNOSIS

Acute mastoiditis should be differentiated from other infections. Postauricular lymphadenitis is difficult to differentiate.

1. Postauricular tenderness and erythema overlie a distinct node and do not diffusely involve the mastoid.
2. There is often an associated external otitis media.

MANAGEMENT

1. Initiate antibiotics pending culture and sensitivity results.
   a. For children 8 years or older:
      (1) Cefotaxime, 50-150 mg/kg/24 hr q6-8hr IV, or cefuroxime, 100 mg/kg/24 hr q6-8hr IV, or ceftriaxone, 50-75 mg/kg/24 q12hr IV
   b. For children older than 8 years:
      (1) Ampicillin, 100-200 mg/kg/24 hr q4hr IV
      NOTE: Once the illness begins to resolve, oral antibiotics may be continued for a total course of 4 weeks of treatment.
   c. Many use clindamycin, 15-40 mg/kg/24 hr q6-8hr IV, and ultimately, 10-25 mg/kg/24 hr q6hr PO to ensure gram-positive and anaerobic coverage, the route reflecting response and toxicity. This is particularly important in patients with poorly responsive or chronic disease.
2. Analgesia may be given, including codeine, 0.5 mg/kg/dose q4-6hr PO, or meperidine (Demerol), 1 mg/kg/dose q3-4hr IM, as indicated.
3. If the patient's condition worsens or a subperiosteal abscess develops, a postauricular I and D with a mastoidectomy should be performed by an otolaryngologist.

DISPOSITION

Hospitalization and consultation with an otolaryngologist usually are required.

REFERENCES

Ogle JW, Lauer BA: Acute mastoiditis: diagnosis and complications, *Am J Dis Child* 140:1178, 1986.

Scott TA, Jackler RK: Acute mastoiditis in infancy: a sequela of unrecognized acute otitis media, *Otolaryngol Head Neck Surg* 101:683, 1989.

ACUTE OTITIS MEDIA

ALERT: Extreme irritability or lethargy may imply concurrent meningitis or other systemic infection.

Acute otitis media (AOM) is a suppurative effusion of the middle ear accounting for one third of office visits of children who are ill.

ETIOLOGY: INFECTION

Infection often follows evidence of eustachian tube dysfunction caused by either obstruction or abnormal patency. Pathogens include the following:

1. Bacteria (Table 73-1). No bacteria are isolated in up to 30% of patients studied, whereas *S. pneumoniae*, *H. influenzae*, and *Moraxella catarrhalis* are the most common pathogens identified.
2. Viral: parainfluenza, respiratory syncytial virus, rhinovirus, influenza, adenovirus, and enterovirus.
3. *Mycoplasma pneumoniae*: associated with bullous myringitis, as are other pathogens.
4. Other: tuberculosis.

TABLE 73-1   Acute Otitis Media: Common Pathogens and Treatment

Age group/ condition	Common pathogens	Antibiotics[a]	Daily dosage[b] (mg/kg/24 hr)	Frequency/ route	Minimum duration	Comments
<2 mo	S. pneumoniae, H. influenzae, group A streptococci, S. aureus, gram-negative enteric	Ampicillin; **and** gentamicin **or** cefotaxime	100-200 5.0-7.5 50-100	q4hr IV q8hr IV q8hr IV	3-7 days, then appropriate PO	Appropriate if signs of systemic illness; tympanocentesis may be indicated; hospitalize; if no signs, symptoms, or toxicity, use older child regimen
Infants, toddlers, and adolescents[f]	S. pneumoniae, H. influenzae, M. catarrhalis, group A streptococci	Amoxicillin; **or** erythromycin and sulfisoxazole[c]; **or** erythromycin and trimethoprim-sulfamethoxazole; **or** Augmentin[d]; **or** cefaclor; **or** cefixime[e]; **or** azithromycin; **or** clarithromycin	30-50 30-50 100-150 30-50 8.0 40 20-40 (amox) 20-40 8 10 mg (day 1) 5 mg (days 2-5) 15	q8hr PO q6hr PO q6hr PO q6hr PO q12hr PO q8hr PO q8hr PO q24hr PO q24hr PO q12hr PO	10-14 days 10-14 days 10-14 days 10-14 days 10-14 days 10-14 days 10-14 days 10-14 days 5 days 10 days	
Refractory		Sulfisoxazole; **or** trimethoprim-sulfamethoxazole; **or** amoxicillin	100-150 8.0 40 20	q6hr PO q12hr PO q8hr PO	14 days 14 days 14 days	Use after initial course; if no resolution, consider tympanocentesis
Recurrent		Sulfisoxazole, **or** trimethoprim-sulfamethoxazole	50-75 4.0 20	q12hr PO q24hr PO	2-4 mo 2-4 mo	Otolaryngologist and audiologist may be helpful

[a]Additional acceptable antibiotics are available but are either broader in spectrum or more costly.
[b]See Formulary (p. 858) for adult (maximum) doses.
[c]Available as a single combination (Pediazole).
[d]Amoxicillin-clavulanate.
[e]Other cephalosporins include cefpodoxime, cefprozil, and cefuroxime. Cefuroxime (30 mg/kg/24 hr) may be efficacious with 5 days therapy.
[f]There is increasing evidence that H. influenzae is an important pathogen in this age group; therefore broader spectrum antibiotics are also appropriate therapies.

Predisposing factors include associated upper respiratory infection, nasotracheal intubation, and Down syndrome. American Indians, Eskimos, and infants with straight eustachian tubes also are at higher risk.

DIAGNOSTIC FINDINGS

1. Lethargy, irritability and other behavioral changes, ear pain, fever, and accompanying respiratory symptoms. Drainage may be present if the tympanic membrane has ruptured. In the older child, hearing loss may occur.
2. Tympanic membrane (TM).
   a. Full visualization is essential, often necessitating the removal of cerumen and debris, using irrigation (provided no perforation is present) or a cerumen spoon. The presence of cerumen does not preclude the diagnosis of AOM.

   A useful irrigation technique is to cut the needle off a large butterfly catheter (18 gauge), leaving only the pliable tubing. The ear then can be easily irrigated with subsequent aspiration of the fluid from the canal. A pulsating water device also may be useful.
   b. TM has increased vascularity and erythema with obscured landmarks.
   c. Pneumatic otoscopy is a reliable means of determining whether an effusion is present. Decreased mobility accompanies AOM, often with bulging or retraction unless the TM is perforated.
   d. The optimal position of the child for the examination varies with the examiner and the child. Many prefer to have the child supine on the examining table, restrained by an adult or by specific pediatric restraints. In the partially cooperative child, the child may be seated in the parent's lap, face-to-face, and hugged tightly; the child's legs are wrapped around the parent's waist. One of the parent's arms embraces the child while the other holds the child's head.

Complications

1. Persistent AOM after an initial course of antibiotics occurs in 25% of patients. A second course of antibiotics is appropriate. If AOM persists after completion of a second or third course, referral to an otolaryngologist and tympanocentesis usually are indicated for diagnostic and therapeutic purposes. On the basis of culture results, an additional course of antibiotics is initiated and follow-up observation is arranged. Many prefer inserting tympanometry tubes after a third course with little response.
2. Recurrent AOM occurs when a child has had three episodes of AOM in 6 months or four in 12 months.
   a. It is particularly common in children who had their first episode of AOM before 1 year of age. In children who have six or more episodes of AOM before 6 years of age, 49% had their initial episode during the first year of life.
   b. Prophylactic antibiotics (especially following episodes of otitis media) or pressure-equalizing tubes are indicated.
3. Perforations occur when sufficient pressure in the middle ear develops, which may produce external otitis media (p. 601) or a transient conductive hearing loss. Local and systemic therapy is indicated.
4. Serous otitis media (SOM) occurs in 42% of children after an episode of AOM and usually resolves without intervention. Temporary hearing losses may occur, and such children should be referred for audiologic evaluation if the loss persists beyond 3 months.
5. Conductive hearing loss may be present with AOM and SOM. If persistent, intervention with pressure-equalizing tubes may be appropriate.

6. Mastoiditis, common before the antibiotic era, now is rare (p. 595).
7. Cholesteatoma, a saclike structure lined by keratinized, stratified, squamous epithelium with accumulation of desquamating epithelium or keratin in the middle ear, may be caused by recurrent AOM. It may result in erosion of the bone and progressive enlargement of the otic antrum.

Ancillary Data

1. Tympanocentesis is indicated in symptomatic patients less than 8 weeks of age, in immunocompromised children, and in those with persistent AOM beyond multiple treatment courses. It is useful in defining pathogens, and the material should be Gram stained and cultured. In rare cases, tympanocentesis may be used to relieve severe pain. Puncture of the bullae associated with tense bullous myringitis results in immediate relief.

   The tympanocentesis is performed by using a slightly bent 3 inch 18-gauge spinal needle attached to a 1-ml syringe. After visualization of the tympanic membrane using an otoscope, the lens is moved sideways to allow access and the needle inserted with aspiration into the inferior, posterior portion of the membrane. This procedure may also be done under a binocular scope by an otolaryngologist.
2. Tympanometry with an electrical acoustic impedance bridge measures compliance of the tympanic membrane and middle ear. It is useful in confirming findings on examination of children more than 7 months.
3. Audiologic evaluation is indicated in children with persistent or recurrent otitis media, especially if there has been an effusion for more than 3 months.
4. Nasopharyngeal and throat cultures are not helpful.

DIFFERENTIAL DIAGNOSIS

AOM should be differentiated from ear pain caused by the following:
1. Infection
   a. External otitis media (p. 601)
   b. Mastoiditis (p. 595)
   c. Dental abscess (p. 590)
   d. Peritonsillar abscess
   e. Sinusitis
   f. Lymphadenitis
   g. Parotitis
2. Trauma: foreign body perforating the tympanic membrane or, if still present, external otitis media; barotrauma; instrumentation
3. Serous otitis media or eustachian tube dysfunction
4. Impacted third molar
5. Temporomandibular joint dysfunction

Heavy (≥20 cigarettes/day) maternal smoking increases the risk of recurrent AOM in the first year of life.

MANAGEMENT

The patient must be evaluated to be certain that a more significant infection, such as meningitis, is not present.
1. Antibiotics are generally used for children with AOM. However, meta-analysis has suggested that symptoms may resolve spontaneously. The choice of antibiotics varies with the child's age, allergies, the seriousness of the infection, compliance, and etiologic agents (see Table 73-1).
   a. Children less than 2 months require broad-spectrum coverage, usually administered parenterally as an inpatient if there is any evidence of systemic illness.
   b. There is increasing evidence that *H. influenzae* is an important pathogen in children older than 9 years and therefore broader coverage may be indicated (e.g., amoxicillin) in that age group as well.

c. A single dose of ceftriaxone, 50 mg/kg/dose IV or IM, is efficacious and may be useful in selected children.

d. Children with bullous myringitis, which is frequently associated with *M. pneumoniae*, also require treatment for other organisms considered to be pathogens in the age group. If pain is severe, myringotomy may be indicated.

e. From 60% to 90% of patients improve within 72 hours of initiating therapy.

2. Decongestants and decongestant-antihistamine combinations given either systemically (antihistamines or vasoconstrictors) or nasally are not effective in altering the course.

3. Eardrops may be useful in the treatment of external otitis media resulting from perforation (polymyxin B [Lidosporin] or cortisporin suspension) or to relieve pain (glycerin [Auralgan] or mineral oil).

4. Antipyretics and analgesics such as acetaminophen or aspirin should be initiated.

5. Recurrent AOM is initially treated with prophylactic, low-dose antibiotics, including amoxicillin, 20 mg/kg/24 hr q12-24hr PO; or sulfisoxazole, 50-75 mg/kg/24 hr q12hr PO; or trimethoprim-sulfamethoxazole, 4/20 mg/kg/24 hr q24hr PO.

Tympanostomy tubes may be considered in children with bilateral effusions if prolonged prophylactic antibiotics are unsuccessful or there is a bilateral conductive hearing loss. Adenoidectomy may have an additional benefit if tubes do not decrease the incidence of recurrent AOM although this is controversial. Antihistamines and decongestants do not have proven efficacy.

The role of steroids is under investigation.

DISPOSITION

1. Children may be followed at home if no other serious systemic infection is present, with a follow-up appointment in 2 to 3 weeks.

2. Children less than 2 months of age and those with significant toxicity or immunodeficiencies should be hospitalized.

3. Patients with persistent (after two courses) or recurrent AOM should be followed by an otolaryngologist.

Parental Education

1. The entire course of antibiotics should be taken even if the child is better.

2. Antipyretics (acetaminophen or aspirin) may make the child feel better.

3. A return appointment in 2 to 3 weeks should be made to evaluate the response.

4. Call your physician if the following occur:

   a. There is no improvement in 36 hours or the fever continues beyond 72 hours. If the signs and symptoms continue, the antibiotic may have to be altered to ensure treatment of resistant *H. influenzae* (change to sulfisoxazole, trimethoprim with sulfamethoxazole, or third-generation cephalosporin).

   b. Child becomes increasingly irritable or lethargic.

   c. Child develops vomiting or diarrhea.

REFERENCES

American Academy of Pediatric Otitis Media Guideline Panel: Managing otitis media with effusion in young children, *Pediatrics* 94:766, 1994.

Bernard PAM, Stenstrom RJ, Feldman W, et al: Randomized controlled trial comparing long-term sulfonamide therapy to ventilation tubes for otitis media with effusion, *Pediatrics* 88:215, 1991.

Celin SE, Bluestone CD, Stephenson J, et al: Bacteriology of acute otitis media in adults, *JAMA* 266:2249, 1991.

Committee on Drugs, AAP: Guidelines for monitoring and management of pediatric patients during and after sedation for diagnostic and therapeutic procedures, *Pediatrics* 89:1110, 1992.

Del Mar C, Glasziou P, Hayem M: Are antibiotics indicated as initial treatment for children with acute otitis media? A meta-analysis, *BMJ* 314:1526, 1997.

Gates GA, Avery CA, Prihoda TJ: Effectiveness of adenoidectomy and tympanostomy tubes in the treatment of chronic otitis media with effusion, *N Engl J Med* 317:1444, 1987.

Giebink GS, Canafax DM, Kempthorne J: Antimicrobial treatment of acute otitis media, *J Pediatr* 119:495, 1991.

Green SM, Rothrock SE: Single dose of intramuscular ceftriaxone for acute otitis media in children, *Pediatrics* 91:23, 1993.

Isaacson E, Rosenfield RM: Care of the child with tympanotomy tubes: a guide for the pediatrician, *Pediatrics* 93:924, 1996.

Kramer II, Kramer AM: The phantom earache: temporomandibular joint dysfunction in children, *Am J Dis Child* 139:943, 1985.

Mandel EM, Casselbrant ML, Rockette HE, et al: Efficacy of 20 versus 10-day antimicrobial treatment for acute otitis media, *Pediatrics* 96:5, 1995.

Mandel EM, Rockette HE, Bluestone CD: Efficacy of amoxicillin with and without decongestant-antihistamine for otitis media with effusion in children: results of a double blind, randomized trial, *N Engl J Med* 316:432, 1987.

Paradise JL, Bluestone CD, Rogers KD, et al: Efficacy of adenoidectomy for recurrent otitis media in children previously treated with tympanostomy tube placement: results of parallel randomized and non-randomized trials, *JAMA* 263:2066, 1990.

Roberts DB: The etiology of bullous myringitis and the role of mycoplasma in ear disease: a review, *Pediatrics* 65:761, 1980.

External Otitis Media

External otitis media is an inflammatory reaction of the external ear canal.

ETIOLOGY

1. Infection
   a. Perforated tympanic membrane with drainage of pus
   b. Impetigo
   c. Herpes simplex
   d. Furunculosis associated with *S. aureus*
2. Dermatitis referred to as "swimmer's ear," causing irritation and damage
3. Foreign body

DIAGNOSTIC FINDINGS

1. Severe pain (particularly on movement of the tragus) and drainage are common.
2. Systemic signs are uncommon.
3. The external ear canal is swollen with drainage, erythema, and edema. The tympanic membrane is intact and mobile with normal color (unless caused by perforation).

Complications

Malignant external otitis media (caused by *Pseudomonas* organisms) is uncommon.

Ancillary Data

Culture of the discharge is not helpful because it often grows *Pseudomonas* or *S. aureus* organisms, not necessarily reflecting the true pathogens.

DIFFERENTIAL DIAGNOSIS

Ear pain from external otitis media should be differentiated from pain caused by infections such as the following:

1. AOM (p. 596)
2. Dental infection (p. 590)
3. Mastoiditis (p. 595)
4. Posterior auricular lymphadenopathy

MANAGEMENT

1. If no perforation is present, the ear may be irrigated with saline.
2. Eardrops (suspension if perforated) such as polymyxin B (Lidosporin or Cortisporin) should be initiated: 2 to 3 drops, four to six times a day inserted into the ear. If significant swelling is present, a cotton wick should be inserted after soaking in an otic-drop suspension until direct application is possible. Many ear solutions and suspensions contain neomycin, which may cause contact dermatitis in 1 of every 1000 patients. If burning is

noted and problematic, may use ophthalmologic drops, such as gentamicin or tobramycin as the eardrops.

3. Systemic antibiotics are not indicated unless the underlying condition requires such treatment.
4. Foreign bodies, if present, should be removed.

DISPOSITION

Children may be followed at home and reevaluated if there is no resolution in 4 to 5 days.

Acute Parotitis

ETIOLOGY: INFECTION

1. Viral (nonsuppurative)
   a. Mumps (the most common etiologic agent)
   b. Other: coxsackievirus and parainfluenza virus
2. Bacterial (suppurative)
   a. *S. aureus* and *S. pneumoniae*
   b. Obstruction from stricture, calculi, or foreign material (food) often present
3. Fungi: *Candida* organisms

DIAGNOSTIC FINDINGS

1. Nonsuppurative parotitis (e.g., mumps) is an insidious disease with slow onset of fever and earache accompanied by tenderness and enlargement of the parotid gland.
   a. The ear lobe is pushed upward and outward, and the angle of the mandible is obscured.
   b. The orifice of Stensen's duct is edematous and erythematous and exudes a clear fluid.
2. Suppurative parotitis is caused by an anatomic stricture.
   a. Systemic toxicity is present.
   b. The area of the parotid is painful and tender with overlying erythema.
   c. A purulent discharge is noted at Stensen's duct.

Complications

1. Mumps may have an associated encephalitis or orchitis.
2. Suppurative parotitis may follow an episode of nonsuppurative infection.

Ancillary Data

1. Serum amylase level is elevated in acute infectious parotitis and normal in recurrent parotitis.
2. Culture of the drainage from Stensen's duct may be helpful if the suppurative parotitis is unresponsive to antibiotics.
3. Sialogram is rarely helpful.

DIFFERENTIAL DIAGNOSIS

1. Infection: cervical lymphadenopathy (p. 593)
2. Recurrent parotitis: usually unilateral and may occur as many as 10 times before spontaneous resolution
3. Neoplasm
4. Hemangioma

MANAGEMENT

1. Nonsuppurative parotitis, most commonly mumps, resolves without therapy. Discomfort may be reduced by avoiding citrus fruits such as oranges and lemons.
2. Suppurative parotitis requires antibiotic therapy:
   a. For nontoxic children: dicloxacillin, 50 mg/kg/24 hr q6hr PO
   b. For systemically ill children: nafcillin (or equivalent), 100 mg/kg/24 hr q4hr IV
3. If suppurative parotitis is present, surgical consultation should be sought early. Often probing of Stensen's duct or early I and D

is desirable to avoid damage to the facial nerve and to facilitate resolution.

DISPOSITION

All patients may be followed at home unless they are toxic or have fluctuant parotitis, requiring parenteral therapy.

Parental Education

Mumps is contagious until the swelling has disappeared, usually 6 days into the illness.
1. Avoid citrus fruits because they stimulate the parotid gland with resultant pain.
2. Call your physician if the following occur:
   a. The swelling has not resolved in 7 days.
   b. Erythema, increasing tenderness, or pain develops over the parotid gland.

REFERENCE

Meyer C, Cotton RT: Salivary gland disease in children: a review, *Clin Pediatr* 26:314, 1986.

PERITONSILLAR ABSCESS

Tonsillar infections occasionally suppurate beyond the tonsillar capsule into surrounding tissues.

ETIOLOGY

Bacterial infection is caused in the following manners:
1. Most commonly by group A streptococci
2. Uncommonly by *H. influenzae, S. pneumoniae, S. aureus*
3. By normal mouth flora, including anaerobes (occasionally implicated)

DIAGNOSTIC FINDINGS

These infections have a rapid onset.
1. Toxicity accompanied by fever, severe sore throat, progressive trismus, drooling, alteration in speech ("hot potato voice"), and dysphagia are common.
2. Tonsil is unilaterally displaced medially with erythema and edema of the soft palate. Uvula deviates to the opposite side. The abscess may be fluctuant.

Complications

1. Extension beyond the tonsillar regions into the retropharyngeal or mediastinal spaces
2. Upper respiratory obstruction as a result of edema and swelling
3. Aspiration pneumonia secondary to spontaneous rupture

Ancillary Data

1. Aspirate culture and Gram stain
2. White blood cells (WBC) usually elevated with a shift to the left
3. Throat cultures for group A streptococcus

DIFFERENTIAL DIAGNOSIS

Peritonsillar abscess should be differentiated from infection caused by the following:
1. Severe pharyngotonsillitis from group A streptococci or infectious mononucleosis.
2. Parapharyngeal abscess with erythema and swelling of the lateral pharyngeal wall and brawny induration of the neck. Neck spasms and torticollis occur in children usually less than 5 years.
3. Peritonsillar cellulitis without definite abscess or displacement of the uvula. This can often be treated with high doses of penicillin and close follow-up observation.
4. Tetanus.
5. Dental infection.

MANAGEMENT

If there is any compromise of the airway, intervention should be an immediate priority.

1. Antibiotics should be initiated early in treatment: ampicillin, 100-200 mg/kg/24 hr q4hr IV.
   a. If resolution is slow: nafcillin (or equivalent), 100-150 mg/kg/24 hr q4hr IV, should be started. Another alternative is clindamycin, 15 to 40 mg q6-8hr IV.
   b. Antibiotics may be altered when results of culture and sensitivity are available.
2. Analgesia may be given: meperidine (Demerol), 1-2 mg/kg/dose q4-6hr IM.
3. I and D is required if the abscess is fluctuant, the child is toxic, or if there is no resolution after 48 hours of therapy.
   a. Needle aspiration may initially be both diagnostic and therapeutic.
   b. Definitive I and D should be carried out in the operating room.
4. Tonsillectomy is indicated on an elective basis 3 to 4 weeks after resolution of the inflammation unless improvement is slow, in which case it may be done on an emergent basis.

DISPOSITION

Patients should be admitted to the hospital for antibiotics and drainage. An otolaryngologist should be involved in the management.

REFERENCE

Hardingham M: Peritonsillar infections, *Otolaryngol Clin North Am* 20:273, 1987.

Pharyngotonsillitis (Sore Throat)

Acute pharyngitis is commonly associated with tonsillitis resulting from inflammation of the throat, with associated soreness, fever, and minimal nasal involvement.

ETIOLOGY: INFECTION

1. Bacterial
   a. Group A streptococci
   b. Less common pathogens, including *Neisseria gonorrhoeae*, *H. influenzae*, *Neisseria meningitidis*, other streptococci, and *Corynebacterium diphtheriae*
2. Viral
   a. Adenovirus: patient may have accompanying conjunctivitis.
   b. Enterovirus: *herpangina* with associated fever, sore throat, dysphagia, vomiting, and small vesicles on the soft palate, tonsil, or pharynx.
   c. Influenza, parainfluenza, Ebstein-Barr (EB) virus (infectious mononucleosis), and herpes simplex (less frequent); 15% of patients with infectious mononucleosis also have group A streptococcus.
3. *M. pneumoniae:* common in school-age children

DIAGNOSTIC FINDINGS (Table 73-2)

Clinically, patients have a range of symptoms, making it difficult to differentiate group A streptococci from viral infections.

1. Infants with streptococcal infections commonly have excoriated nares and are listless.
2. Viral etiology is generally more likely in children up to 6 years of age.
3. Children less than 3 years of age who do have group A streptococcus typically have chronic, mucopurulent rhinitis, low-grade fever, and cervical adenitis.
4. Streptococcal infections in school-age children produce complaints of sore throat, accompanied by headache, vomiting, and abdominal pain. The peak age is 5 to 12 years.
5. Adults with streptococcal infections have tonsillar findings similar to the school-age group but rarely have abdominal pain or a

TABLE 73-2   Pharyngotonsillitis: Diagnostic Signs and Symptoms

	Group A streptococci			
	Infant	**School-age**	**Adult**	**Viral**
ONSET	Gradual	Sudden	Sudden	Gradual
CHIEF COMPLAINT	Anorexia, rhinitis, listlessness	Sore throat	Sore throat	Sore throat, cough, hoarseness, rhinitis, conjunctivitis
DIAGNOSTIC FINDINGS				
Sore throat	+	+++	+++	+++
Tonsillar erythema	+	+++	+++	++
Tonsillar exudate	+	++	+++	+
Palatal petechiae	+	+++	+++	+
Adenitis	+++	+++	+++	++
Excoriated nares	+++	+	+	+
Conjunctivitis	+	+	+	+++
Cough	+	+	+	+++
Congestion	+	+	+	+++
Hoarseness	+	+	+	+++
Fever	Low grade	High	High	Rare or low grade
Abdominal pain	+	++	+	+
Headache	+	++	++	+
Vomiting	+	++	++	+
Scarlatiniform rash	+	+++	+++	+
Streptococcal contact	+++	+++	I I I	+
ANCILLARY DATA				
Positive streptococcal culture	+++	++	+++	+
Elevated white blood cell count	++	++	+++	+

history of contact. It is uncommon in adults except during epidemics.

6. A scarlatiniform rash is diagnostic of streptococcal infection (infants rarely have the eruption).
7. Against a child having a group A streptococcal infection is the presence of rhinorrhea, cough, or hoarseness, as well as the absence of fever, tonsillopharyngeal erythema/exudate, and cervical adenitis.
8. Exudative pharyngitis accompanies group A streptococci, EB virus (infectious mononucleosis, p. 714), *Corynebacterium diphtheriae*, and adenovirus infections. Exudative pharyngitis is commonly caused by a virus in children less than 3 years and frequently caused by group A streptococci in children above 6 years. In children less than 6 years, group A streptococcus accounts for 10% to 20% of cases. Soft-palate petechiae are found with group A streptococcal and EB virus infections; vesicles or ulcers on the posterior tonsillar pillars with en-

terovirus infection; and ulcers on the anterior palate with adenopathy in herpes infections.

Complications

1. Group A streptococci: acute rheumatic fever (ARF) (p. 566) and acute glomerulonephritis (p. 800). Half of children with these sequelae have no history of an antecedent pharyngitis. ARF may be prevented if therapy is started within 7 to 9 days of onset of symptoms.
2. Otitis media (p. 596).
3. Cervical lymphadenopathy (p. 593).
4. Recurrent streptococcal pharyngitis (histories rarely reliable). Culture documentation is important.
5. Chronic adenotonsillar hypertrophy may lead to upper airway obstruction.

Ancillary Data

Throat cultures are indicated for patients with sore throat with or without fever to help exclude group A streptococci as the etiology.

1. Cultures should normally be evaluated only for group A streptococci, optimally using selective media, anaerobic methodology, bacitracin "A" discs, or antigen testing techniques. Swabs are best obtained by rotating them over both tonsillar areas. Repeat swabbing twice. A single culture may miss a small number of positive patients identified by duplicate specimens.
2. Infants should have their noses rather than their throats cultured.
3. Positive cultures with low colony counts may be indicative of the carrier states. To investigate this possibility, a serum Streptozyme must be ordered. Low titers are consistent with the chronic carrier state.
4. Symptomatic family members should have cultures.
5. If suggestive, culture for *C. diphtheriae*.
6. Rapid simple diagnostic tools to identify

group A streptococci make immediate diagnosis possible, simplifying management. The BioStar optical immunoassay (OIA) and other specific and sensitive assays appear to be more sensitive and specific than a single throat culture, thereby omitting the need for concurrent cultures in patients with negative rapid streptococcal tests. If other tests are used with significant false negative rates, it is essential to confirm negative test results with a routine throat culture.

MANAGEMENT

Symptomatic relief may be obtained by gargling with warm water, sucking hard candy, and initiating aspirin or acetaminophen (40-50 mg/kg/24 hr q6hr PO).

If the infection is streptococcal, antibiotic therapy should be administered for a total of 10 days of continuous therapy (unless given IM):

1. Penicillin VK, 25-50 mg (40,000-80,000 units)/kg/24 hr q6hr PO; or
2. Benzathine penicillin G administered IM once (usually given as 900,000:300,000 Bicillin C-R, which is 75% benzathine, because it hurts less). Dosing should be calculated by the amount of benzathine required:

Weight (lb)	Benzathine penicillin G (units)	Bicillin C-R (units) (900,000 benzathine: 300,000 procaine)
<30	300,000	300,000:100,000
31-60	600,000	600,000:200,000
61-90	900,000	900,000:300,000
>90	1,200,000	NA

3. Alternative antibiotics.
   a. Erythromycin, 30-50 mg/kg/24 hr q8hr PO. Erythromycin estolate (30-50 mg/kg/24 hr q6-8hr PO) has less gastrointestinal symptoms. It has the additional benefit of treating other potential pharyngeal pathogens such as *Chlamydia* organisms.
   b. Clarithromycin (Biaxin), 15 mg/kg/24 hr q12hr PO for 10 days.

c. Azithromycin (Zithromax), 10 mg/kg/24 hr q24hr PO first day, then 5 mg/kg/24 hr q24hr PO on days 2 through 5.

Symptomatic improvement is noted after early therapy with antibiotics. Treatment also allows children to return to school or day-care sooner, thereby decreasing the associated family disruption. Patients may return to school (work or day-care) 24 hours after beginning medication. The risk of acute rheumatic fever and acute glomerulonephritis developing is not increased if antibiotics are started within 7 days of the onset of symptoms.

Preliminary studies have shown equivalent cure rates may be achieved by a dosage in children of penicillin VK, 250 mg q12hr PO, or erythromycin, 20 mg/kg/24 hr q12hr PO for 10 days. Another alternative is cefadroxil (Duricef), 30 mg/kg/24 hr q24hr PO for 10 days (expensive).

Indications for tonsillectomy for recurrent sore throats are controversial, and the procedure should be considered only in selected cases. Symptomatic chronic adenotonsillar hypertrophy may require removal of the tonsils and adenoids. A 30-day course of amoxicillin/clavulanate in a dose of 40 mg amoxicillin/kg/24 hr q8hr PO, may reduce the need for surgery.

Evidence would suggest that the child with *problematic* group A streptococcal carriage may be treated with benzathine penicillin G as outlined *and* rifampin, 10 mg/kg/dose q12hr for eight doses PO. Clindamycin, 20 mg/kg/24 hr (maximum: 450 mg/24 hr) q8hr PO, for 10 days may be substituted for rifampin. Another regimen is to combine penicillin V, 250-500 mg q8-12hr for 10 days, and rifampin, 20 mg/kg/24 hr q24hr, for the last 4 days of the penicillin course.

DISPOSITION

Patients may be followed at home.

Parental Education

1. Medication should be taken for the full 10 days (unless given IM).

2. Symptomatic treatment may be helpful.
   a. Gargle with warm salt water (1 tsp in 8 oz glass).
   b. Suck hard candy.
   c. Take aspirin or acetaminophen (10-15 mg/kg/dose q6hr prn PO).
3. Family members who are symptomatic with fever, sore throat, anorexia, or headache should have cultures.
4. Children may return to school in 24 hours.
5. Call your physician if the following occur:
   a. Severe pain, drooling, difficulty swallowing or breathing, or big, swollen lymph nodes develop.
   b. There is evidence of infection elsewhere.
   c. The fever lasts longer than 48 hours.

REFERENCES

Bass JW: A review of the rationale and advantages of various mixtures of benzathine penicillin CR, *Pediatrics* 97:3960, 1996.

Berkowitz CD, Anthony BF, Kaplan EL, et al: Cooperative study of latex agglutination to identify group A streptococcal antigen on throat swabs in patients with acute pharyngitis, *J Pediatr* 107:89, 1985.

Bisno AT: Acute pharyngitis: etiology and diagnosis, *Pediatrics* 97:S949, 1996.

Doctor A, Harper MB, Fleisher CR: Group A beta-hemolytic streptococcal bacteremia: historical overview, changing incidence and recent association with varicella, *Pediatrics* 96:428,1995.

Gerber MA, Spadaccini LJ, Wright LL: Twice-daily penicillin in the treatment of streptococcal pharyngitis, *Am J Dis Child* 139:1145, 1985.

Gerber MA, Randolph MF, DeMeo KK, et al: Lack of impact of early antibiotic therapy for streptococcal pharyngitis on recurrence rates, *J Pediatr* 117:853, 1990.

Green SM: Acute pharyngitis: the case for empiric antimicrobial therapy, *Ann Emerg Med* 25:404, 1995.

Hofer C, Binns HJ, Tanz RR: Strategies for managing streptococcal pharyngitis, *Arch Pediatr Adolesc Med* 151:824, 1997.

Paradise JL, Bluestone CD, Bachman RZ: Efficacy of tonsillectomy for recurrent throat infection in severely affected children: results of parallel randomized and nonrandomized clinical trials, *N Engl J Med* 310:674, 1984.

Pichichero ME: Group A streptococcal tonsillopharyngitis: cost-effective diagnosis and treatment, *Ann Emerg Med* 25:390, 1995.

Portier H, Chavenet PK, Waldner A, et al: Five versus 10 day treatment of streptococcal pharyngotonsillitis: a randomized controlled trial comparing cefpodoxime proxetil and phenoxymethylpenicillin, *Scand J Infect Dis* 26:591, 1994.

Putto A: Febrile exudate tonsillitis: viral or streptococcal, *Pediatrics* 80:6, 1987.

Randolph MF, Gerber MA, DeMeo KK, et al: Effect of antibiotic therapy on the clinical course of streptococcal pharyngitis, *J Pediatr* 106:870, 1985.

Selafani AP, Ginsburg J, Shah MK, et al: Treatment of symptomatic chronic adenotonsillar hypertrophy with amoxicillin/clavulanate potassium: short- and long-term results, *Pediatrics* 101:675, 1998.

Tanz RR, Poncher JR, Corydon KE, et al: Clindamycin treatment of chronic pharyngeal carriage of group A streptococcus, *J Pediatr* 119:123, 1991.

Tanz RR, Shulman ST, Berthel MJ, et al: Penicillin plus rifampin eradicates pharyngeal carriage of group A streptococci, *J Pediatr* 106:876, 1985.

Retropharyngeal Abscess

ALERT: Retropharyngeal abscess requires immediate intervention to prevent respiratory obstruction.

Otitis media and nasopharyngeal infections may lead to suppurative adenitis of the small lymph nodes between the buccopharyngeal and prevertebral fascia. If untreated, this can lead to abscess formation, particularly in children less than 5 years of age.

ETIOLOGY

Retropharyngeal abscess results from bacterial infection commonly caused by group A streptococci, *S. aureus*, *Haemophilus* species (71% β-lactamase producer), and anaerobes (*Bacteroides*, *Peptostreptococcus*, and *Fusobacterium* species). It occurs by direct spread from nasopharyngitis, otitis media, vertebral osteomyelitis, or from wound infection after a penetrating injury of the posterior pharynx or palate.

DIAGNOSTIC FINDINGS

1. Nasopharyngitis or otitis media usually precedes the development of fever, difficulty swallowing, drooling, and severe throat pain. Meningismus may result from irritation of the paravertebral ligaments. Some patients complain of pain in the back of the neck or shoulder, precipitated or aggravated by swallowing.
2. Labored respirations with gurgling and hyperextension of the head are evidence of potential respiratory obstruction.
3. A definite unilateral posterior pharyngeal wall mass is present, often becoming fluctuant.

Complications

1. Obstruction of the trachea, esophagus, or nasal passages
2. Aspiration pneumonia if abscess ruptures. Possible dissection of purulent material into mediastinum
3. Sudden death if abscess erodes into major blood vessel

Ancillary Data

1. Lateral neck x-ray film. Demonstrates increased soft tissue mass between the anterior wall of the cervical spine and the pharyngeal wall. In a child the retropharyngeal soft tissue should not be greater than 5 mm at the level of C3 or 40% of the anteroposterior (AP) diameter of the body at C4 at that level. A CT scan, ultrasound examination, or magnetic resonance imaging (MRI) study is more sensitive in characterizing soft tissue swelling and defining the anatomy.
2. WBC: Increased with shift to left.
3. Cultures and Gram stain of purulent material. Obtained from I and D.

DIFFERENTIAL DIAGNOSIS

1. Infection: croup or epiglottitis
2. Trauma: foreign body

MANAGEMENT

1. Stabilize airway, if necessary. Monitor.
2. Initiate antibiotics immediately: nafcillin (or equivalent), 100-150 mg/kg/24 hr q4hr IV. Clindamycin, 15-40 mg q6-8hr IV, may also be considered.
3. Give analgesia: meperidine (Demerol), 1-2 mg/kg/dose q4-6hr IM.
4. I and D is indicated immediately if obstruction is present or an evolving abscess becomes fluctuant.
   a. Normally done in the operating room.
   b. The head is positioned down and hyperextended to minimize aspiration.

DISPOSITION

All patients require hospitalization, antibiotics, and immediate otolaryngologic consultation.

REFERENCES

Asmar BI: Bacteriology of retropharyngeal abscess in children, *Pediatr Infect Dis* 9:595, 1990.

Brook I: Microbiology of retropharyngeal abscesses in children, *Am J Dis Child* 141:202, 1987.

Morrison JE, Pashley NRT: Retropharyngeal abscesses in children: a 10-year review, *Pediatr Emerg Care* 4:9, 1988.

RHINITIS (COMMON COLD)

Nasopharyngitis, or rhinitis, is common among children and represents what is usually a self-limited process. Nasal rhinitis may be allergic in origin as well as infectious.

ETIOLOGY: INFECTION

1. Viral: rhinovirus, respiratory syncytial virus (RSV), adenovirus, influenza, and parainfluenza
2. Bacterial: *C. diphtheriae*, *H. influenzae*, *S. pneumoniae*, *N. meningitidis*

DIAGNOSTIC FINDINGS

Patients have nasal congestion, sneezing, and, commonly, a clear watery discharge. Throat irritation and pharyngitis may be associated. There are minimal constitutional symptoms.

Associated clinical findings may include lymphadenopathy, otitis media, sinusitis, pneumonia, croup, and bronchiolitis. Allergic rhinitis is usually accompanied by pale, swollen, and boggy nasal mucosa.

Ancillary Data

Nasal cultures should not be done because there is no way to interpret them unless nares are excoriated (group A streptococci).

MANAGEMENT

Symptomatic therapy is indicated by removing the discharge and attempting to decrease congestion.

1. In younger children, use a bulb syringe. May also use Neo-Synephrine nosedrops (0.25% phenylephrine) q4hr.
2. In older children, use a bulb syringe or prescribe blowing and decongestants. Oxymetazoline (Afrin) nosedrops (0.025% to 0.05%) q8-12hr may be useful. Routine antibiotic treatment of purulent nasopharyngitis is not useful. Antihistamine-decongestant combinations have little impact on the common cold.
3. Allergic rhinitis may be treated with antihistamines. The first choice is the inexpensive alkylamines such as chlorpheniramine (0.35 mg/kg/24 hr q6hr PO). Another alternative is clemastine [Tavist]). Some use a nasal spray such as oxymetazoline or Nasalcrom.

Parental Education

1. Place 2 to 3 drops of water or fresh salt water (tsp of salt in a cup of water) in

each nostril with the child lying on the back.

2. If old enough, have the child blow the nose.

3. With a baby, use a rubber bulb syringe to remove the mucus.

4. Use a vaporizer in the child's room during napping and sleeping.

5. For children older than 18 months of age, use decongestants such as pseudo-ephedrine and chlorpheniramine (can be obtained over the counter without prescription).

6. Call your physician if the following occur:
   a. Child develops a fever and is less than 3 months of age.
   b. The fever lasts longer than 24 to 48 hours.
   c. Child has difficulty breathing, is wheezing, or has croup or any other evidence of infection, such as red eye or ear pain.
   d. The skin under the nose becomes crusty.

REFERENCES

Hutton N, Wilson MH, Mellits ED, et al: Effectiveness of antihistamine-decongestant combination for young children with the common cold: a randomized, controlled clinical trial, *J Pediatr* 118:125, 1991.

Todd JK, Todd N, Damato J, et al: Bacteriology and treatment of purulent nasopharyngitis: a double blind, placebo controlled evaluation, *Pediatr Infect Dis* 3:226, 1984.

ACUTE SINUSITIS

ALERT: Sinusitis may be associated with intracranial and extracranial infections.

Swelling of the nasal mucosa and obstruction of the meatus result in an acute inflammatory reaction within the sinuses.

ETIOLOGY

1. Infections
   a. Common bacterial. *H. influenzae* accounts for 19% to 32% of positive aerobic cultures; *S. pneumoniae,* 9% to 28%; group A streptococci, 17% to 27%; *S. aureus,* 6% to 21%; and *Moraxella catarrhalis.*
   b. Fungal infections in diabetic and immunocompromised patients.
   c. Up to 93% of patients with chronic sinusitis have anaerobes (*Bacteroides* species and *Fusobacterium* species).
      NOTE: Cultures are nondiagnostic in as many as a third of patients.
2. Impairment of normal nasal physiologic processes with poor ventilation and increased secretions secondary to adenoidal hypertrophy, polyps, cleft palate, or allergies
3. Trauma
4. Dental infections with contiguous spread

DIAGNOSTIC FINDINGS

1. Rhinorrhea is present in 78% of patients, 64% having a purulent discharge. Cough, often worse at night (50%), sinus pain or headache (12%), and temperatures over 38.5° C (101° F) (19%) are reported. Concurrent upper respiratory tract infections are common; signs and symptoms are insidious. Malodorous breath *(fetor oris)* may be noted.

2. Only 8% of patients have tenderness overlying the frontal, ethmoid, or maxillary sinuses, whereas 76% have unequal or poor transillumination. Transillumination is of limited value in children because of the variable development of sinuses before age 8 to 10 years. Sphenoid sinusitis is associated with occipital or retroorbital pain and is rare in children. Swelling may be present over involved sinus.

3. Chronic sinusitis may have variable findings. Malaise, fatigability, and anorexia may be noted.

Complications

These occur in 4.5% of patients:
1. Periorbital infections, particularly ethmoid (p. 573)
2. Osteomyelitis of the sinus wall, most commonly the frontal (this appears as Pott's puffy tumor, a midfrontal swelling)
3. Brain, subdural, or epidural abscesses
4. Meningitis

Ancillary Data

1. Radiologic examination has variable reliability in young children. Normal sinus film results are helpful. Abnormal sinus film findings are difficult to interpret, although after 6 years of age the interpretation can be more definitive. The ethmoid sinuses develop completely by 7 years, and the maxillary sinuses shortly thereafter, while the frontal and sphenoid sinuses develop after puberty.

   Sinusitis appears as clouding, mucosal thickening, or air fluid levels within the sinuses, the latter being most helpful in defining an acute infection. CT scan (coronal, noncontrast) is the standard of diagnosis and may obviate the need for plain radiographs.

   Radiographs are indicated if the child is seriously ill, has had recurrent episodes, or has chronic disease or suspected suppurative complications.
2. Antral puncture by an otolaryngologist is indicated if there is severe pain unresponsive to medical management; sinusitis in a seriously ill, toxic child; an unsatisfactory response; suppurative complications; or if the patient is an immunocompromised host. A Gram stain and an aerobic and anaerobic culture should be done on the aspirated material.

DIFFERENTIAL DIAGNOSIS

1. Allergy
2. Foreign body in the nose (p. 592)
3. Neoplasm or polyp
4. Functional organic causes of headache (see Chapter 36)

MANAGEMENT

The symptoms in bacterial sinusitis usually resolve in 48 to 72 hours. Up to 20% of patients have a persistent nasal discharge after a 2-week course of antibiotics:

1. Antibiotic treatment for a 2- to 3-week course:
   a. Amoxicillin, 50 mg/kg/24 hr q8hr PO; or
   b. Augmentin (amoxicillin with clavulanic acid), 20-40 mg/kg/24 hr q8hr PO; or
   c. Erythromycin, 30-50 mg/kg/24 hr q6hr PO, *and* sulfisoxazole (Gantrisin), 150 mg/kg/24 hr q6hr PO (available as a combination drug: Pediazole); *or*
   d. Erythromycin (as in c) and trimethoprim-sulfamethoxazole (8 mg/40 mg)/kg/24 hr q12hr PO.
   e. Cefuroxime (Ceftin), 8 mg q24hr PO.
      NOTE: Failure to respond justifies the addition of specific coverage for *S. aureus* (dicloxacillin, 50 mg/kg/24 hr q6hr PO) and anaerobic organisms.
2. Decongestants and antihistamines are commonly used. Afrin or Neo-Synephrine nosedrops may be used for 2 days. Topical nasal steroids can help if allergic component suspected.
3. Desensitization rarely may be helpful if allergies are a contributory factor.
4. Sphenoid sinusitis requires aggressive antibiotic therapy (often parenteral),

sometimes in conjunction with surgical drainage.

5. The antibiotic management of chronic sinusitis should use another antibiotic after the above standard regimen:
   a. Clindamycin, 25-40 mg q6-8hr IV or 20 mg/kg/24 hr q8hr PO; or
   b. Cefoxitin (Mefoxin), 80-160 mg/kg/24 hr IV

DISPOSITION

1. Patients usually may be discharged and instructed to take oral antibiotics at home for 2 to 3 weeks. If symptoms do not resolve, patients should be referred to an otolaryngologist for assessment and possible irrigation of the antrum.
2. Patients with sphenoid sinusitis usually are hospitalized for parenteral therapy.

Parental Education

The parent should call the physician if the following occur:

1. Symptoms worsen or the patient has a fever or toxicity.
2. Symptoms have not improved markedly in 1 week and disappeared in 2 to 3 weeks.

REFERENCES

Bluestone CD: Medical and surgical therapy of sinusitis, *Pediatr Infect Dis* 3:513, 1984.

Goldenhersh MJ, Rachelefsky GS: Sinusitis: early recognition, aggressive treatment, *Contemp Pediatr* 6:22, 1989.

Hnatuk LAF, Macdonald RE, Papsin BL: Isolated sphenoid sinusitis, *J Otolaryngol* 23:36, 1994.

Johnson DL, Markle BM, Wiedermann BL: Treatment of intracranial abscesses associated with sinusitis in children and adolescents, *J Pediatr* 113:15, 1988.

Kovatch AL, Wald ER, Ledesma-Medina J, et al: Maxillary sinus radiographs in children with nonrespiratory complaints, *Pediatrics* 73:306, 1984.

Lew D, Southwick FS, Montgomery WW, et al: Sphenoid sinusitis: a review of 30 cases, *N Engl J Med* 309:1149, 1983.

Tinkelman DG, Silk HJ: Clinical and bacteriologic features of chronic sinusitis in children, *Am J Dis Child* 143:938, 1989.

Wald ER: Chronic sinusitis in children, *J Pediatr* 127:339, 1995.

Weld ER: Sinusitis in children, *Pediatr Infect Dis J* 7:S150, 1988.

Williams JW, Simel DC: Does this patient have sinusitis? *JAMA* 270:1242, 1993.

ACUTE STOMATITIS

Acute stomatitis is generalized inflammation of the oral mucosa.

ETIOLOGY AND DIAGNOSTIC FINDINGS
Infection

1. Herpes simplex causes distinct multiple small ulcers of the oral mucosa and generalized inflammation. In rare cases, other viruses (coxsackievirus) may cause diffuse ulceration, primarily on the palate, that lasts 7 to 10 days.
2. Thrush is caused by *Candida albicans*. The white plaques are predominantly on the buccal mucosa and tongue with generalized erythema.

Aphthous Stomatitis or "Canker Sores"

These are erythematous, indurated papules that quickly erode to become painful circumscribed necrotic lesions of the mucosa that do not involve the lips. Their onset is often related to physical or emotional stress, and they resolve spontaneously in 1 to 2 weeks.

Complication

Dehydration may result if oral intake is impaired by painful ulcers.

DIFFERENTIAL DIAGNOSIS

1. Infection: necrotizing ulcerative gingivitis (Vincent angina) (p. 593)

2. Trauma
   a. Acid, alkali, or other caustic agents (p. 366)
   b. Mechanical or thermal injuries

MANAGEMENT

1. These entities are self-limited but occasionally cause discomfort and interfere with intake so that some intervention is appropriate. Approaches to local analgesia include the following:
   a. Antacid (Maalox or Mylanta) gargled or swallowed to coat the mucosa; *or*
   b. 1% to 2% viscous lidocaine (Xylocaine) gargled or applied directly prn; *or*
   c. Mixture (1 part each) of lidocaine (2% viscous Xylocaine), diphenhydramine (Benadryl), and kaolin-pectin (Kaopectate), gargled prn.

NOTE: The dosage of the 2% viscous lidocaine (Xylocaine) should not exceed 15 ml q3hr or 120 ml in 24 hours in the adult (proportionately less in children). The patient should not eat or drink for 1 hour after application because of the danger of aspiration.

2. Frequent mouthwashes and alterations of diet to bland foods may help.

3. Thrush may be treated with nystatin (100,000 units/ml), using 1 ml (dropper) in each side of mouth four times/day, and continued 3 to 4 days after resolution.

DISPOSITION

Patients should be followed at home unless the hydration status requires inpatient therapy.

74 ENDOCRINE DISORDERS

ADRENAL INSUFFICIENCY

ETIOLOGY

1. Congenital: enzymatic defects, hemorrhage (birth injury), and hypoplasia
2. Infection
   a. Waterhouse-Friderichsen syndrome (adrenal hemorrhage), *Neisseria meningitidis*, *Streptococcus pneumoniae*
   b. Tuberculosis, histoplasmosis
3. Autoimmune disease
4. Withdrawal of steroid therapy or unusual stress in patient taking pharmacologic dosage of glucocorticosteroids (e.g., surgery, infection)

DIAGNOSTIC FINDINGS

See Table 74-1.

DIFFERENTIAL DIAGNOSIS

1. Acute insufficiency: infection, poisoning, diabetic ketoacidosis, hemorrhage
2. Addison's disease: central nervous system (CNS) disease such as tumor or anorexia nervosa

MANAGEMENT

1. Initial management: Restore intravascular volume with normal saline (0.9% NS), initially 20 ml/kg and then at a rate reflecting vital signs. When appropriate, correct levels of electrolytes and glucose and achieve acid-base balance. Hypotension may require pressor agents.

2. Adrenal corticosteroid replacement therapy (Table 74-2):
   a. Acute crises
      (1) Hydrocortisone (Solu-Cortef), 2 mg/kg/dose q4-6hr IV; *and*
      (2) Cortisone, 1-5 mg/kg/24 hr q12-24hr PO, to allow tapering of intravenous medications. Intramuscular cortisone therapy often is recommended initially to facilitate the transition to oral therapy once stabilization has occurred.
   b. Addison disease
      (1) Glucocorticoid
         (a) Hydrocortisone, 0.5 mg/kg/24 hr (15-20 mg/m^2/24 hr) q6-8hr PO; *or*
         (b) Cortisone, 0.5-0.75 mg/kg/24 hr (20 mg/m^2/24 hr) q6-8hr PO; *or*
         (c) Prednisone, 0.1-0.15 mg/kg/24 hr (4-5 mg/m^2/24 hr) PO
      (2) Mineralocorticoids
         (a) Fludrocortisone (Florinef), 0.05-0.1 mg/24 hr PO; *or*
         (b) Desoxycorticosterone, 1-5mg/24-48 hr IM
3. Give antibiotics when indicated.
4. Give corticosteroids for patients with adrenal insufficiency who are undergoing surgery.
   a. Administer hydrocortisone (Solu-Cortef), 1-2 mg/kg IV (or equivalent), before surgery. In an emergency, administer as preanesthetic drug. If elective, administer in four doses over 48 hours.

TABLE 74-1   Adrenal Insufficiency

Clinical manifestation	Acute	Chronic (Addison's disease)
Nausea/vomiting	+++	+++
Abdominal pain	++	++
Hypothermia	+	±
Hypotension	+++	+++
Dehydration	++	±
Failure to thrive	−	+
Fatigue/weakness	+++	+++
Confusion, coma	+	−
Hyperpigmentation	−	++
Hypoglycemia	++	++
↓ Na$^+$/↑ K$^+$	+++	+++

b. During anesthesia, administer hydrocortisone, 25 to 100 mg IV.

c. After surgery, give hydrocortisone, 0.5-1.0 mg/kg/dose q6hr IV, for 3 days and then taper to presurgical levels (if any).

DISPOSITION

Patients with acute adrenal crisis should be admitted to an intensive care unit (ICU). In cases of chronic illness, disposition must be determined by clinical status and ease of follow-up, which is essential.

REFERENCE

Urban MD, Kogut MD: Adrenocortical insufficiency in the child, *Curr Ther Endocrinol Metab* 5:131, 1994.

DIABETIC KETOACIDOSIS

ALERT: Start treatment early with hydration. Insulin may be given once a glucose determination has been made. Always look for a precipitating cause.

Diabetes mellitus has certain unique features in the pediatric age group. Children are more subject to infection, emotional and environmental stresses, increased caloric requirements, and extremes of activity and dietary patterns. These place the child with diabetes at risk of development of ketoacidosis.

Diabetic ketoacidosis (DKA) requires attention when a patient is hyperglycemic (>300 mg/dl), ketonemic (serum ketones large at >1:2 dilution), or acidotic (pH <7.1 or HCO$_3$ <12 mEq/L) and is experiencing glycosuria and ketonuria.

ETIOLOGY: PRECIPITATING FACTORS

A number of conditions cause DKA in a patient with well-controlled diabetes:

1. Infection: virus, bacteria (group A streptococci or abscess is common).
2. Intrapsychic: emotional or environmental stresses at home or school. Adolescents often manipulate their surroundings by becoming ill.
3. Drugs and diet: alteration of normal insulin dosage (poor compliance), steroids, birth control pills. Major change in diet.
4. Trauma: major trauma or surgery.
5. Endocrine: pregnancy, puberty, Cushing syndrome, hyperthyroidism.

DIAGNOSTIC FINDINGS (Box 74-1)

DKA is marked by tachypnea with Kussmaul respiration (deep, rapid pattern), tachycardia, orthostatic blood pressure changes, acetone on the breath, vomiting, dehydration, and mental status changes, which may lead to obtundation and coma. Abdominal pain is a common finding, often mimicking an acute surgical condition, which resolves with treatment of the acidosis.

It is imperative to document the history of diabetes mellitus, standard insulin regimen, past management, duration of symptoms, estimated weight loss, and presence of precipitating factors.

Patients not previously diagnosed may give a history of excessive or poor food intake, weight

TABLE 74-2 Adrenal Corticosteroids

Drug	Availability	Dose*	Frequency	Glucocorticoid effect†	Mineralocorticoid effect†
GLUCOCORTICOIDS					
Cortisone	IM: 25, 50 mg/ml PO: 5, 25 mg	0.25 mg/kg/24 hr 0.5-0.75 mg/kg/24 hr	q12-24hr q6-8hr	100 mg	100 mg
Hydrocortisone (Solu-Cortef)	PO: 5, 10, 20 mg IV/IM: 100, 250, 500 mg	0.5 mg/kg/24 hr Asthma§: 4-5 mg/kg/dose	q8hr q6hr	80 mg	80 mg
Prednisone	PO: 1, 5, 10, 20 mg, 5 mg/5 ml	0.1-0.15 mg/kg/24 hr Asthma: 1-2 mg/kg/24 hr	q12hr q6hr	20 mg	Little effect
Methylprednisolone (Solu-Medrol)	IV: 40, 125, 500, 1000 mg	Asthma§: 1-2 mg/kg/dose	q6hr	16 mg	No effect
Dexamethasone (Decadron)	IV/IM: 4, 24 mg/ml	Croup: 0.60 mg/kg/dose Meningitis: 0.15 mg/kg/dose	q6hr q6hr (16 doses)	2 mg	No effect
MINERALOCORTICOIDS					
Fludrocortisone (Florinef)	PO: 0.1 mg	0.05-1 mg/24 hr	q24hr	5 mg	0.2 mg
Desoxycorticosterone (DOCA)	IM: 5 mg/ml (in oil)	1-5 mg/24-48 hr	q24-48hr	No effect	2 mg

With long-term therapy, dose requires adjustment. Attempt QOD dosing when using pharmacologic doses. Long-acting preparations for physiologic replacement are available with monthly (or longer) activity.
*Physiologic replacement unless otherwise indicated.
†Equivalent doses required for same clinical effect.
§Asthma, status asthmaticus.

Box 74-1

DIAGNOSTIC FINDINGS IN DIABETIC KETOACIDOSIS

EARLY

Due to hyperglycemia
  Polyuria, polydipsia, polyphagia, visual disturbance
Due to muscle breakdown and dehydration
  Weight loss, weakness

LATE

Due to ketonemia
  Anorexia, nausea, vomiting, fruity acetone breath
Due to hyperosmolality
  Altered mental status
Due to acidosis
  Abdominal pain, Kussmaul respiration
Due to hypokalemia
  Ileus, muscle cramps, dysrhythmia

loss, or dehydration in the face of large urinary output. A dehydrated child with a normal or large urine flow must be considered diabetic until proved otherwise.

b. Those whose diabetes is in poor control have polyuria, polydipsia, polyphagia, and weight loss. Recurrent episodes of DKA often are associated with psychosocial dysfunction.

Complications

1. Dehydration with metabolic acidosis (differential of metabolic acidosis: p. 359).
2. Cerebral edema is unpredictable in onset, usually occurring within 8 to 12 hours after initiation of treatment. Seizures may be noted. Abrupt changes in mental status, pupillary changes, and posturing progressing to coma are associated with a mortality rate of up to 90%.

3. Adult respiratory distress syndrome (p. 44).
4. Death of CNS or metabolic complications.

Hyperosmolar nonketotic coma with glucose level of 800 to 1200 mg/dl rarely occurs in children; it occurs more often in adults. Patients may not be acidotic, but they do have hyperglycemia, hyperosmolality, and dehydration. They also may be comatose, presumably because of a relative water deficiency. This has been reported in children less than 2 years and in children with preexisting neurologic damage.

Ancillary Data

1. Electrolytes may be abnormal with an anion gap (p. 79) and must be monitored every 2 to 4 hours during stabilization.
   a. Hyponatremia resulting from urinary losses. Sodium level may be artificially depressed by hyperglycemia and hyperlipidemia. An estimate of the true serum sodium level may be derived as follows:

Corrected serum Na^+ (mEq/L) =
  Measured serum Na^+ (mEq/L) +
  [(Plasma glucose [mg/dl] − 100) × 0.016]

   b. A total body potassium deficit (the serum level may be normal). Serum potassium increases 0.5 mEq/L for each 0.1 decrease in pH.
   c. Acidosis with a low bicarbonate level and pH, the degree of decrease reflecting the severity of disease.
   d. Blood urea nitrogen (BUN) level is usually elevated.
2. Glucose level is elevated above 300 mg/dl with glucosuria and must be monitored every 1 to 2 hours until stable. Screening by Dextrostix or Chemstrip may provide a bedside estimate. Serum osmolarity should be determined if the glucose level is above 1000 mg/dl. Home blood glucose monitoring facilitates glucose control long-term and during illness.

3. Serum ketones are large at a dilution of 1:2 or above with ketonuria. Ketone measurements reflect acetoacetate but not beta-hydroxybutyrate. Because the latter dissociates to acetoacetate with clinical improvement, ketonemia may persist despite clinical resolution and should be checked every 2 to 4 hours until clear.
4. Urinalysis reveals glucosuria and ketonuria. The normal renal glucose threshold is about 180 mg/dl, but variability does exist.
5. Arterial blood gas (ABG) demonstrates a respiratory alkalosis superimposed on a metabolic acidosis.
6. Amylase level may be elevated; white blood cell (WBC) count is variable.
7. Electrocardiogram (ECG) may be used to assess serum potassium levels rapidly.
8. Cultures of throat, blood, urine, and cervix are done as indicated.
9. Glycosylated hemoglobin gives an excellent measure of the degree of long-term control.

MANAGEMENT
Initial Management

Initial stabilization must include intravenous fluids, cardiac monitoring, and determination of serum electrolyte, glucose, acetone, and BUN levels and venous (or arterial) pH. A bedside Dextrostix or Chemstrip test may facilitate management. Laboratory data should be repeated every 1 to 2 hours during the initial treatment periods. Vital signs, fluids, insulin, and urinary output must be monitored and followed on a flow sheet.

Initial therapy should begin with aggressive hydration, infusing 0.9% NS solution at a rate of 20 ml/kg over 30 minutes, and repeated until achieving partial reconstitution of vascular space and stabilization of blood pressure, pulse, and respiration.

After the initial bolus, fluid and electrolyte therapy must reflect maintenance and deficit requirements. Patients typically have an isotonic

10% dehydration (see Chapter 7). Deficits are calculated and carefully replaced on the basis of serum concentration with 0.45% NS with potassium salts.
• If the corrected sodium is 140 mEq/L or less, replace half of the deficit over first 16 hours and restore total deficit over 36 hours.
• If the corrected sodium is 140 mEq/L or more, restore total deficit evenly over 48 hours.

The rates often need to be increased because of the obligate excessive urinary losses and hemodynamic considerations. If the patient is significantly acidotic with pH less than 7.0 or HCO_3^- less than 10 mEq/L, sodium bicarbonate can be given in conjunction with half-normal (0.45% NS) solution, although its benefits are unproven. The bicarbonate deficit should be only partially corrected. In patients requiring sodium bicarbonate therapy, administer 1-2 mEq/kg over 30 minutes while monitoring the response. Normally, the pH does not need to be actively corrected above 7.0 because correction of intravascular volume will facilitate the return to normal values and excessive administration of sodium bicarbonate may lead to alkalosis shift of oxyhemoglobin dissociation and paradoxical cerebrospinal fluid (CSF) acidosis. Evidence would indicate that correction of severe acidosis (<7.0) with administration of bicarbonate does not affect outcome.

If neurologic changes are noted, infusion should be slowed and other monitoring and measurements initiated. Potassium must be added to the infusion early (after initial flush) because of the total body deficit. Potassium acetate may be substituted for potassium chloride if the patient is highly acidotic. Some clinicians prefer KPO_4 because of a relatively common phosphorus depletion.

Serum K+ (mEq/L)	Potassium infusate (mEq/L)
<3	40-60*
3-4	30
4-5	20
5-6	10

*Many patients may not tolerate peripherally. Significant risk for dysrhythmia.

Glucose should be added to the intravenous (IV) fluid infusion when the glucose level is less than 250 mg/dl (without stopping the infusion of insulin). One unit of insulin causes intracellular movement of 2 to 4 gm of glucose.

Those with mild to moderate disease who respond rapidly to the initial fluid management can be given oral hydration if vomiting has ceased and vital signs are stable with normovolemia.

Patients with only mild diabetes and without significant acidosis may be managed by oral hydration if vomiting is not a problem. Patients with nonketotic hyperosmolar diabetic coma respond to hydration, replacement of electrolyte deficits, and reduction of serum glucose and hyperosmolarity. Fluid therapy is primary.

Although the mechanism of evolution of cerebral edema is unknown, several observations about its management should be considered. The expansion of the treatment plan to 48 hours and use of a repair fluid containing 125 mEq/L Na^+ early may be protective. The failure of the serum sodium concentration to rise as glucose concentration declines is a marker for excessive administration of free water. A total fluid dose greater than $4 L/m^2/day$ may correlate with increased risk. Further data are required.

Insulin

Insulin is the second major component of therapy. Infusion must be related to the state of hydration, fluid management, and laboratory data. Several routes of administration are available.

Many insulin preparations are available, including semisynthetic human insulins. Regular crystalline insulin has an onset of 30 minutes, peaks at 2 to 4 hours, and has a duration of 6 to 8 hours. U100 preparations are commonly used.

1. Continuous regular insulin IV infusion causes a smooth fall in glucose level, with lower incidence of hypoglycemia and hypokalemia and better ongoing control of therapy. Optimally, glucose level falls 50-100 mg/dl/hr.

- Method: 50 units of regular insulin is mixed in 250 ml of 0.9% NS (0.2 units/ml) and infused at a rate of 0.1-0.2 units/kg/hr. Run insulin solution through IV tubing before initiating therapy.

2. Intramuscular injection of regular insulin is an acceptable alternative, 0.1-0.2 units/kg/hr injected intramuscularly.

Insulin administration should not be stopped when the glucose level is less than 250 mg/dl. The hourly insulin dose is lowered and glucose (5% to 10%) is added to the fluid to maintain a serum glucose level around 200-250 mg/dl. Insulin infusion or intramuscular (IM) injections should be stopped and subcutaneous (SC) insulin begun when the patient has negative serum acetone at a dilution of 1:2.

If an infusion is used, administer SC insulin 30 minutes before stopping the IV infusion. SC insulin is initiated at the rate of 0.25-0.5 units/kg q4-6hr. It is based on the serum glucose acetone. Rapid glucose monitoring devices facilitate this process.

As mentioned, regular insulin has an onset of 30 to 60 minutes, peaks at 2 hours, and has a duration of 6 to 12 hours, requiring administration on a routine basis before meals. A newer synthesized insulin analog called lispro (Humalog) has an earlier onset (5 to 15 minutes) and shorter duration (≤4 hr) but has not been approved for children 12 years of age or younger.

Long-acting insulin should be initiated as soon as possible. This therapy should be coordinated with the primary care provider. The sum of the short-acting insulin administered in the previous 24-hour period gives an approximation of the following day's requirement. Typically, patients require 0.6-0.8 unit/kg/day divided so that two-thirds dose is administered in the morning and one-third in the evening. A common insulin mixture is two-thirds isophane insulin suspension (NPH) and one-third regular insulin to provide a smooth pattern. NPH has an onset of 2 hours, peaks at 8 to 10 hours, and has a duration of 16 to 20 hours.

NOTE: Patients with newly diagnosed diabetes have a low initial insulin requirement. At the time of initial diagnosis, insulin requirement is high (≥1 unit/kg/24 hr). This requirement falls rapidly ("honeymoon period") to as little as 0.1-0.3 units/kg/24 hr for the next few weeks to months.

Insulin pumps have been introduced with the potential for markedly improved control.

DISPOSITION

Patients with significant DKA require hospitalization unless prolonged observation with monitoring equipment, personnel, and expertise is available in the ambulatory setting. Patients with pH less than 7.0, and HCO_3 less than 10 mEq/L, or altered mental status should be hospitalized early in treatment. In addition, those with intercurrent infections often require admission. Those with their first episode usually should be hospitalized for control and education, although ambulatory education is often used after stabilization.

Insulin therapy on discharge should be coordinated with the primary care provider. All diabetic patients require close follow-up observation with frequent blood glucose level monitoring at home. This must be ensured before discharge.

REFERENCES

Bonadio WA: Pediatric diabetic ketoacidosis: pathophysiology and potential for outpatient management of selected children, *Pediatr Emerg Care* 8:287, 1992.
Duck SC, Wyatt DT: Factors associated with brain herniation in the treatment of diabetic ketoacidosis, *J Pediatr* 113:10, 1988.
Finberg L: Why do patients with diabetic ketoacidosis have cerebral swelling and why does treatment sometimes make it worse? *Arch Pediatr Adolesc Med* 150:785, 1996.
Green SM, Rothrock SG, Ho JD, et al: Failure of adjunctive bicarbonate to improve outcome in severe pediatric diabetic ketoacidosis, *Ann Emerg Med* 31:41, 1998.
Harris GD, Fiordalisi I, Harris WL, et al: Minimizing the risk of brain herniation during treatment of diabetic ketoacidemia: a retrospective and prospective study, *J Pediatr* 117:22, 1990.
Hillman K: Fluid resuscitation in diabetic emergencies: a reappraisal, *Intens Care Med* 13:4, 1987.
Krane EJ, Rockoff MA, Wallman JK, et al: Subclinical brain swelling in children during treatment of diabetic ketoacidosis, *N Engl J Med* 312:1147, 1985.
Morris LP, Murphy MB, Kitabchi AE: Bicarbonate therapy in severe diabetic ketoacidosis, *Ann Intern Med* 105:836, 1986.
Rosenbloom A: Intracerebral crisis during treatment of diabetic ketoacidosis, *Diabetes Care* 13:22, 1990.
Rosenbloom AL, Schatz DA: Diabetic ketoacidosis in childhood, *Pediatric Ann* 23:284, 1994.
Sperling MA: Diabetic ketoacidosis, *Pediatr Clin North Am* 31:591, 1984.
White K, Kolman ML, Wexler O, et al: Unstable diabetes and unstable families: a psychosocial evaluation of diabetic children with recurrent ketoacidosis, *Pediatrics* 73:749, 1984.

FAILURE TO THRIVE

ALERT: Although feeding problems are often causative, organic conditions must be excluded. Prolonged delay in diagnosis and active intervention may result in long-term neurologic delays.

Growth failure in children occurs when the rate of weight gain is below that anticipated for a peer age group. Although a single measurement below the third or fifth percentile is suggestive, a decrease in the velocity of growth is diagnostic.

The most common pattern occurs when the weight is reduced out of proportion to the height; head circumference is normal. This is usually due to inadequate intake or malabsorption. Children with a proportional reduction in weight and height and a normal or increased head circumference is associated with constitutional dwarfism and endocrinopathies. When the head is small and the weight and height similarly reduced, the cause is usually related to CNS disease or intrauterine growth retardation.

ETIOLOGY

1. Inadequate caloric intake is usually primary, accounting for more than one half of cases.
2. Psychosocial problems are present in nearly one half of children.
   a. Parent-child dysfunction
      (1) Perinatal and neonatal factors related to bonding and emotional support
      (2) Developmental delays
   b. Family dysfunction
      (1) Socioeconomic limitations
      (2) Child abuse or neglect
      (3) Family discord
3. Organic conditions:
   a. Congenital: anatomic or metabolic inborn errors
   b. Gastrointestinal
      (1) Malabsorption
      (2) Liver disease
      (3) Obstructive disease
      (4) Gastroesophageal reflux (GER)
      (5) Food allergies
   c. Cardiopulmonary
      (1) Congenital or acquired heart disease
      (2) Cystic fibrosis
      (3) Chronic lung disease
   d. Renal
      (1) Renal failure or infection
      (2) Renal tubular acidosis
   e. CNS
      (1) Congenital, perinatal, or acquired disease
   f. Endocrine/metabolic
      (1) Thyroid, pituitary, diabetes mellitus, adrenal, parathyroid
      (2) Inborn errors of metabolism
   g. Immunologic/infection
      (1) Acquired immunodeficiency syndrome; severe combined immunodeficiency
      (2) Chronic infections: TB, HIV, parasites
   h. Toxic: heavy metal (lead), etc.

DIAGNOSTIC FINDINGS

1. Feeding technique, efficacy, pattern, and problems must be clearly defined. Calorie count may be useful.
2. Growth charts including weight, height, and head circumference (see p. 839) to determine patterns of growth and relationship between these three parameters. Physical, environmental, and social changes should be temporally noted on the chart.
3. Perinatal history, developmental milestones, family history including growth patterns and inherited diseases, and psychosocial issues and family function may be suggestive.
4. Beyond specific evaluation of growth parameters, the physical examination should focus on excluding potential etiologies. Neglect or abuse should be excluded.

Complications

1. Neurologic delays accompanying inadequate intake
2. Malnutrition, dehydration, anemia

Ancillary Data

1. Screening studies, including urinalysis and urine culture, electrolytes and glucose, WBC, and ESR. Stool for pH, reducing substances, blood, fat, and infectious agents.
2. Radiologic evaluation for bone age.
3. Chest x-ray study if any indication of cardiac or pulmonary disease.
4. Selective studies to exclude organic causes.

DIFFERENTIAL DIAGNOSIS

The important consideration is whether the changing velocity pattern reflects potential organic or nonorganic problems or the normal growth pattern for the child.

Potential etiologies beyond feeding and family problems should be excluded as suggested by the presenting findings and the pattern of relationship between growth patterns.

MANAGEMENT

1. Assuming acute fluid problems are corrected, the initial screening studies are obtained. If these are normal, a trial of feeding is usually initiated, focusing on techniques when caloric intake is thought to be inadequate. Measurement of intake and output and adjustments to formula, solids, etc. to maximize calories should be initiated.

   Close follow-up is essential and support provided. Family support must be initiated.

   If this is unsuccessful, admission and inpatient feeding and observation may be required.
2. If no improvement is noted or initial examination suggests an organic etiology, other diagnostic considerations must be excluded and treated.

DISPOSTION

1. Outpatient management is usually appropriate while feeding techniques are adjusted. Close follow-up and support are essential.
2. Admission may be required if the child is unstable, markedly malnourished, compliance uncertain, suspected to be abused, or likely to have a significant organic etiology.
3. Referral is appropriate for all patients to ensure continuity.

REFERENCE

Maggioni A, Lifshitz F: Nutritional management of failure to thrive, *Pediatr Clin North Am* 42:791, 1995.

THYROID DISEASE

THYROIDITIS

Chronic lymphocytic thyroiditis (Hashimoto disease) is an autoimmune disease. It accounts for most nontoxic goiters, with a peak incidence between 8 and 15 years and a female predominance of 4:1.

Diagnostic Findings

Thyroid enlargement is noted in more than 85% of patients—the thyroid usually is firm and nontender and has a cobblestone sensation. Patients rarely are symptomatic.

Ancillary Data (Table 74-3)

Levels of thyroglobin and microsomal antibodies may be elevated. Findings of function studies are usually normal.

Differential Diagnosis

1. Simple colloid goiter.
2. Infection. Suppurative thyroiditis has an acute onset of fever, dysphagia, sore throat, and painful, tender swelling in the area of the thyroid. Commonly it results from mixed aerobic and anaerobic organisms, *S. aureus* rarely is cultured. Antibiotics (penicillin or dicloxacillin) or surgical drainage is required.

Management

Patients with documented hypothyroidism should be treated with replacement doses of sodium L-thyroxine (100 $\mu g/m^2/24$ hr). Patients with euthyroidism are usually treated because in

TABLE 74-3   Thyroid Function Tests: Common Disorders of Thyroid Function

Disorder	Serum thyroxine (T$_4$)	Triiodothyronine (T$_3$) resin uptake	Serum thyrotropin (TSH)	Comments
Chronic lymphocytic thyroiditis				Thyroid antibody increased
Euthyroid	WNL	WNL to ↑	WNL to ↑	
Hypothyroid	↓	WNL to ↓	↑	
Hyperthyroid	↑	↑	↓	
Hyperthyroid	↑*	↑	↓	
Hypothyroid				
Primary	↓	↓	↑	
Secondary	↓	↓	↓	Decreased response TRH
TBG				
↓ TBG	↓	↑	WNL	Free thyroxin index normal
↑ TBG (pregnancy, birth control pills)	↑	↓	WNL	Free thyroxin index normal

Modified from Fisher DA: *J Pediatr* 82:187, 1973.
*May be normal or low in triiodothyronine toxicosis. *TRH,* Thyroid-releasing hormone; *TBG,* thyroid-binding globulin.

some hypothyroidism develops. Such treatment ordinarily reduces the goiter size.

Disposition

All patients should be followed at home for at least 6 months. If treatment was not initiated, they should be reevaluated at 6-month intervals to assess thyroid function.

HYPERTHYROIDISM
Etiology

1. Autoimmune (Graves' disease). Often associated with other autoimmune diseases. In about 10% of patients with chronic lymphocytic thyroiditis, hyperthyroidism develops.
2. Hypothalamic or pituitary dysfunction. Rare.
3. Congenital. Present in children of mothers who have or have had Graves' disease.

May persist to 6 to 12 months and may have postneonatal onset.

Diagnostic Findings

Patients usually have a gradual onset of symptoms, with an enlarged thyroid gland and associated decreasing school performance, weight loss, tachycardia, eye prominence and exophthalmos, motor hyperactivity with tremor, and increased sweating. Atrial fibrillation can be present.

Thyroid storm is very rare in children. It is manifested by acute onset of hyperthermia, tachycardia, sweating, and nervousness. It occurs almost exclusively in patients with preexisting hyperthyroidism, secondary to a diffuse toxic goiter (Graves' disease).

Complications
Hyperthyroidism can cause an elevated metabolic rate, with delirium, coma, and potentially, death.

Ancillary Data

See Table 74-3.

Differential Diagnosis

Hyperthyroidism should be differentiated from a neoplasm such as pheochromocytoma.

Management

Several management options exist.

1. Most clinicians inhibit synthesis of thyroid hormone and initiate oral antithyroid medication (propylthiouracil [PTU], 5 mg/kg/24 hr up to 300 mg/24 hr) for 3 to 4 years unless remission occurs earlier. Lugol solution (5 drops q8hr PO) is usually begun 1 hour after PTU.
2. Surgery is indicated for patients whose compliance is poor, for those whose glands are three to four times their normal size, and for those with adenomas or carcinomas. Patients must be euthyroid before surgery. The use of radioactive iodides in children is controversial.
3. Propranolol, 10-20 mg/dose q6-8hr PO, is useful initially for patients in a hypermetabolic state. In patients with thyroid storm, immediate therapy with propranolol, 1-2 mg/dose IV, initially, followed by oral therapy, is indicated. Propranolol is contraindicated in patients with congestive heart failure. Fluid deficits, hyponatremia, and hyperthermia should be corrected.
4. Congenital hyperthyroidism may initially be treated with Lugol solution, 1 drop q8hr PO.

Disposition

Patients generally can be followed clinically and chemically at home, with frequent visits for at least 3 to 4 years. Patients with thyroid storm require hospitalization.

HYPOTHYROIDISM

Etiology

1. Congenital: aplasia, hypoplasia, errors of metabolism, autoimmune disease, maternal ingestion of drugs or goitrogens during pregnancy
2. Autoimmune: chronic lymphocytic thyroiditis (Hashimoto thyroiditis)
3. Intoxication: iodides, radiation
4. Hypothalamic or pituitary dysfunction
5. Trauma: neck injury or surgery
6. Infection: viral (rarely aerobic or anaerobic bacteria)
7. Neoplasm: primary (carcinoma) or secondary infiltration

Diagnostic Findings

Clinical presentation varies, depending on the patient's age and duration of illness. Although most patients with congenital hypothyroidism are asymptomatic, they may be lethargic and eat poorly. Less commonly, hypotonia, prolonged jaundice, umbilical hernia, wide fontanel, or delayed growth is noted. Most states require neonatal screening, and the diagnosis should be made early.

In later childhood, patients exhibit growth retardation, delays in dentition, edema, poor performance (school and play), hoarseness, delayed tendon reflexes with flabby muscles, and a dull, placid expression.

Complications

Myxedema coma (usually caused by autoimmune [Hashimoto] thyroiditis, ^{131}I therapy, or surgery), is extremely rare but may accompany coma, hypothermia, hypoglycemia, and respiratory failure. Therapy is initiated parenterally.

Ancillary Data

See Table 74-3.

Management

Hormone replacement is initiated after obtaining laboratory specimens to evaluate function.

Levothyroxine (Synthroid) is a stable, synthetic hormone that can be given once a day. Dosage should be adjusted to maintain the serum thyroxine (T_4) level between 10 and 12 µg/dl.

Age	Dosage (µg/kg/24 hr)	Average levothyroxine/24 hr
<6 mo	8-10	25-50 µg
6-12 mo	6-8	50-75 µg
1-5 yr	5-6	75-100 µg
6-12 yr	4-5	100-150 µg
>12 yr	2-3	100-200 µg

In older children, there is usually less urgency, and the child should be started on a low dosage (25 µg/24 hr) that is increased every 2 to 4 weeks until full replacement is achieved. Patients should be monitored closely.

Therapy for myxedema coma should be initiated parenterally. The adult dose is 200 to 500 µg levothyroxine IV, followed by 50 µg/24 hr IV.

Disposition

Patients without complications should have therapy initiated and be followed as outpatients with laboratory tests repeated in 2 weeks. Serum thyroxine and serum thyrotropin levels are the tests of choice. Because excessive therapy in the infant may cause craniosynostosis and brain dysfunction, infants should be monitored at 3-month intervals in the first year of life.

REFERENCES

Lafranchi S: Thyroiditis and acquired hypothyroidism, *Pediatr Ann* 21:29, 1992.
Zimmerman D, Gan-Gaisand M: Hyperthyroidism in children and adolescents, *Pediatr Clin North Am* 37:1273, 1990.

75 Eye Disorders

JAMES B. SPRAGUE

CHALAZION AND HORDEOLUM

A *chalazion* is an inflammatory granulomatous nodule of the meibomian gland on an otherwise normal eyelid. It results from retained secretions of a gland. Physical discomfort, as well as some disfigurement from the mass effect of the nodule, may be present.

Hot compresses are used initially to encourage drainage. The chalazion may be incised and curetted by an ophthalmologist. It also may respond to steroid injection.

A *hordeolum (stye)* is a painful, tender, erythematous infection of the hair follicle of the eyelashes, usually resulting from *Staphylococcus aureus*. A hordeolum usually points and drains and may occur in multiple sites. Very rarely is it complicated by periorbital cellulitis (p. 575).

Hot compresses are useful; if a stye does not drain spontaneously, incision and drainage may be done. Topical medications probably are not helpful, and recurrent multiple lesions may respond to systemic antistaphylococcal agents.

CONJUNCTIVITIS

Infectious conjunctivitis is the most common cause of "red eye" in children and is usually benign and self-limited in older children. Bacterial conjunctivitis typically produces purulent discharge with polyps in the smear. The cornea is not involved and vision is unaffected; there is little pain. Viral disease causes keratoconjunctivitis with corneal involvement. These patients have pain, photophobia, and mildly decreased vision. The discharge is classically mucoid with mononuclear cells on the smear. Chlamydial disease may cause symptoms similar to those of viral keratoconjunctivitis. Diagnostic findings are summarized in Table 75-1.

ETIOLOGY AND DIAGNOSTIC FINDINGS

1. Infection:
   a. Bacterial
      (1) *Haemophilus influenzae:* bilateral and purulent
      (2) *Streptococcus pneumoniae:* purulent
      (3) *Neisseria gonorrhoeae:* usually occurs in the first days of life; large amount of hyperacute mucopurulent discharge; also occurs in sexually active individuals
      (4) *S. aureus:* rare
      (5) *Pseudomonas* organisms secondary to contact lens
   b. Viral
      (1) Adenovirus: mucopurulent discharge; associated pharyngitis in some
      (2) Herpes simplex: Dendritic pattern with corneal ulcer and keratitis; unilateral; vesicle on eyelid may

TABLE 75-1   Infective Conjunctivitis: Diagnostic Findings and Management

Cause	Epidemiology	Diagnostic findings						Management*
		Vision	Pain	Photophobia	Discharge/ microscopic	Cornea	Conjunctiva	
BACTERIA (a,d) *S. pneumoniae H. influenzae*	Bilateral, history of exposure	WNL	None	None	Purulent; PMN on smear	WNL	Injected papillary	Topical antibiotics
VIRAL (d)								
Adenovirus (b) types 8, 19, 3, and 7	Incubation: 5-14 days; history of exposure; systemic symptoms; preauricular node	Often decreased	FBS	±	Mucoid; mononuclear on smear	Punctate keratopathy	Injected follicles	Topical antibiotics for secondary bacterial infection
Herpes (c)	Unilateral; often secondary	±	FBS	+	Mucoid; mononuclear on smear	Dendrite	Injected follicles	Refer to ophthalmologist
Varicella (chickenpox)	"Pox" may involve lid, rarely cornea	WNL	±	±	Mucoid; mononuclear on smear	±	Injected follicles	Follow
CHLAMYDIA	May be recurrent if inadequately treated	WNL	±	±	Inclusion bodies (Giemsa); fluorescent antibody	WNL	Injected follicles	Erythromycin for 2-3 wk

FBS, Foreign body sensation; *PMN,* polymorphonuclear neutrophil; *WNL,* within normal limits.

*Do not prescribe topical analgesics for *prn* use.

(a) "Bacterial" conjunctivitis unresponsive to topical antibiotics more often results from viral agents or iritis than from insensitivity to antibiotics.

(b) Adenoviral conjunctivitis also is known as epidemic keratoconjunctivitis. Children should be kept out of school/daycare until resolution.

(c) Herpes simplex can be difficult to diagnose. Because steroids dramatically worsen herpes keratitis, they should *not* be prescribed without clear indications.

(d) Prolonged treatment with neomycin-containing antibiotics can cause local sensitivity.

be present; herpes type I is more common, although type 2 can occur through spread from genital lesions

 (3) Varicella: vesicle on lid; conjunctivitis

 c. *Chlamydia trachomatis:* purulent discharge beginning at 5 to 15 days of life; possible associated pneumonia

2. Allergy:
 a. Watery discharge with chemosis and edema of the conjunctiva, pruritic
 b. Bulbar conjunctivitis
 c. Rhinorrhea
 d. Seasonal allergy

3. Chemical: may occur bilaterally in newborns after delivery if silver nitrate drops are not well irrigated; in older children it is secondary to cosmetics, drugs, eyedrops, or aerosols.

4. Ophthalmia neonatorum (Table 75-2).
 a. Babies with conjunctivitis should have cultures and a stat Gram stain obtained to exclude *N. gonorrhoeae.* If the baby has gonorrhea or Chlamydia, it must

be treated systemically and the mother and her sexual partner evaluated.

DIFFERENTIAL DIAGNOSIS
(see Tables 75-1 and 75-2)

In addition to the various distinguishing etiologic agents that cause infectious or allergic conjunctivitis, a number of other entities must be considered.

1. Trauma
 a. Foreign body usually associated with pain, photophobia; vision may be normal; fluorescein finding positive (p. 434)
 b. Corneal abrasion (p. 437)
 c. Traumatic iritis is accompanied by blurred vision with severe acute unilateral pain; photophobia; flush around limbus
 d. Traumatic hyphema (p. 438)

2. Congenital
 a. Nasolacrimal duct obstruction
 b. Congenital glaucoma causes visual impairment with conjunctival injection,

TABLE 75-2   Neonatal Ophthalmia: Diagnostic Findings

Etiology	Incubation period	Diagnostic findings	Management
CHEMICAL Silver nitrate	24 hr	Diffuse injection; culture: negative	Wait and watch
GONOCOCCAL *Neisseria gonorrhoeae*	24-72 hr	Hyperpurulent; history of infected birth canal or infected contact; smear: typical gonococcus	Systemic and topical antibiotics; hospitalize
CHLAMYDIA (inclusion conjunctivitis) *Chlamydia trachomatis*	7-10 days	Indolent, although often purulent; history of infected birth canal; may have had partial response to topical antibiotics; no follicles in infant; smear: cytoplasmic inclusion; culture: negative	Systemic erythromycin or sulfonamides; exclude systemic disease
OTHER BACTERIA	2-5 days	Purulent or hyperpurulent	Topical antibiotics

photophobia, and a small or midsize fixed pupil; rare

3. Systemic disease: ataxia-telangiectasia, Kawasaki syndrome, juvenile rheumatoid arthritis

MANAGEMENT

1. If present, remove foreign bodies (p. 438).
2. Treat allergic conjunctivitis, if significantly symptomatic, with systemic antihistamines: diphenhydramine (Benadryl), 5 mg/kg/24 hr q6hr PO for 3 to 5 days, or hydroxyzine (Vistaril, Atarax), 2 mg/kg/24 hr q6hr PO.
3. Infectious conjunctivitis:
   a. Treat Chlamydia disorders with oral erythromycin (30-50 mg/kg/24 hr q6-8hr PO) *or* sulfisoxazole (Gantrisin) (150 mg/kg/24 hr q6hr PO).
   b. Refer those with herpes conjunctivitis to an ophthalmologist. Topical antiviral agents such as 1% trifluridine drops or 5% vidarabine ointments may be used.
   c. Treat bacterial and viral conjunctivitis with ophthalmic ointment or solution for 2 days beyond clearing.
      (1) Sulfacetamide (10% to 15%) or sulfisoxazole (4%) solution (drops) q2-4hr in eye; *or*
      (2) Sulfacetamide (10%) or sulfisoxazole (4%) ointment q4-6hr in eye; *or*
      (3) Polymyxin B-bacitracin (Polysporin) ointment q4-6hr in eye.
      (4) Tobramycin and gentamicin preparations are preferred by some.
   d. Gonococcal ophthalmia requires hospitalization, consultation, and systemic antibiotics. Term infants may be treated with aqueous penicillin G, 50,000 units/kg/24 hr q8hr IV for 7 days. An alternative antibiotic is ceftriaxone, 125 mg IM.

   e. Management tips:
      (1) Always exclude herpes simplex (fluorescein stain may be helpful).
      (2) Exclude corneal foreign body.
      (3) Warn parents to handle towels and pillowcases of the infected child with care.
      (4) Consider adenovirus in children who do not respond in 3 to 4 days.
      (5) Consider *Chlamydia* with a history of recurrence.
      (6) Consider intraocular disease (iritis, glaucoma) with "deep" pain unrelieved with topical anesthetics and with decreased vision and photophobia.
      (7) Think of allergy if the main symptom is itching. Look for modest discharge and thickened conjunctiva at the limbus.
      (8) Chlamydial conjunctivitis can be diagnosed with direct monoclonal fluorescent antibody, enzyme-linked immunosorbent assay (ELISA), or nucleic acid probe.
      (9) Topical steroids are best prescribed by an ophthalmologist.
      (10) Topical anesthetics should never be prescribed for prn use.
      (11) Bacterial cultures are rarely useful in older children.

DISPOSITION
Parental Education

1. Before using topical medication, remove the yellow discharge and dried matter from the eye with a wet cotton ball and warm water.
2. Place 2 drops of eyedrops in each eye every 2 to 4 hours (or as often as possible) while your child is awake until the eye is improving, then decrease the frequency.
   a. For younger children, only an eye ointment will be provided; it may be used

four times/day, but blurs vision. It also may be used for bad infections at bedtime in conjunction with the drops.

b. Continue the medication until your child has awakened for two mornings without discharge.

3. Your child may infect other people. Use of separate towels and washcloths, as well as careful hand washing, prevents infection.

4. Call your physician if the following occur:

a. The infection has not responded in 72 hours.

b. The eyelids become red or swollen.

c. The eyeball becomes cloudy or sores develop on it.

d. Vision becomes blurred.

e. The eye becomes painful or develops photophobia.

REFERENCES

Beinfang DC, Kelly LD, Nicholson DH, et al: Ophthalmology, *N Engl J Med* 323:956, 1990.

Fisher MC: Conjunctivitis in children, *Pediatr Clin North Am* 34:1446, 1987.

Heggie AD, Jaffe AC, Stuart LA, et al: Topical sulfacetamide vs oral erythromycin for neonatal chlamydial conjunctivitis, *Am J Dis Child* 139:564, 1985.

Laga M, Namara W, Brunham RC: Single-dose therapy of gonococcal ophthalmic neonatorum with ceftriaxone, *N Engl J Med* 315:1382, 1986.

Levin AV: Eye emergencies: acute management in the pediatric ambulatory care setting, *Pediatr Emerg Care* 7:367, 1991.

Maller JS: Eye disorders. In Barkin RM, editor: *Pediatric emergency medicine: concepts and clinical practice*, ed 2, St Louis, 1997, Mosby.

Powell KR: Orbital and periorbital cellulitis, *Pediatr Rev* 16:163, 1995.

76 GASTROINTESTINAL DISORDERS

ACUTE INFECTIOUS DIARRHEA

ALERT: Rapid assessment of the patient's state of hydration, complications, and likely etiologic agents is imperative. Fluid resuscitation may be required.

Acute infectious diarrhea is accompanied by an increase in stool number or water content. Commonly, a host of viral and bacterial agents and parasites is associated with unique epidemiologic and clinical characteristics (see Chapter 32).

ETIOLOGY AND DIAGNOSTIC FINDINGS
Rotavirus

Rotavirus accounts for 39% of patients requiring hospitalization for diarrheal disease. Antibody indicating past infection is noted in up to 90% of 2-year-old children. It occurs commonly in the cooler months, usually affecting children 6 to 18 months of age. Vomiting is a prominent early symptom, often preceding the onset of diarrhea, which is loose, relatively frequent (>5 stools/day), and rarely associated with mucus or blood. Respiratory symptoms may accompany the gastrointestinal (GI) symptoms that last for 2 to 3 days.

A rotavirus vaccine has been studied extensively, but further studies are still under way.

Other Viral Agents

Astrovirus causes findings similar to those of rotavirus but has about one half the incidence. Children from infancy to 7 years are predominantly affected. A winter peak is noted. Transmission is from person to person, and contaminated water and shellfish have been reported vehicles. Asymptomatic shedding has been noted.

Adenovirus-induced diarrhea lasts longer than that caused by rotavirus, having an incubation period of 3 to 10 days and lasting 5 to 12 days. Patients have watery diarrhea with vomiting, fever, and dehydration.

Calicivirus (Norwalk-like, snow mountain-like) is also similar to rotavirus, commonly occurring in children 3 months to 6 years. In developing countries, children often develop the infection after first decade of life. The illness lasts about 4 days after a 1-2-hour to 4-day incubation period. Person-to-person and fecal-oral transmission occurs; drinking water, cold food, and shellfish have also been implicated.

Salmonella Organisms

Multiple animal reservoirs (cattle, poultry, shellfish, rodents, and turtles) facilitate transmission. This is more common in warm months.

1. Gastroenteritis is the most common clinical presentation.
    a. It primarily affects children less than 5 years of age.
    b. Symptoms of fever, vomiting, and diarrhea begin 24 to 48 hours after exposure, diminishing over 3 to 5 days. Older children may have abdominal pain, often confused with an acute appendicitis.
    c. The stool is commonly loose and slimy with a foul odor. The green diarrhea variably has mucus, rarely is bloody,

631

and usually has polymorphonuclear leukocytes.

d. The reservoirs are animals, contaminated food or water, and humans. Animals that have frequently been incriminated include poultry, pet turtles, and livestock. Foods such as chicken, eggs, unpasteurized milk, and cantaloupes have been linked to outbreaks.

2. The white blood cell (WBC) count is usually elevated with a variable shift to the left.

3. Septicemia may occur because of the potential of penetrating the lamina propria. Meningitis, osteomyelitis, septic arthritis, endocarditis, pneumonia, and urinary tract infections (UTIs) have been reported. Children less than 1 year of age and those who have sickle cell disease or other hemoglobinopathies or who are immunocompromised are at increased risk of bacteria and should generally have a blood culture as part of the evaluation.

4. *Salmonella typhi* causes severe, prolonged disease with gastroenteritis associated with fever, malaise, headache, and myalgias. Hepatosplenomegaly and rose spots (2-mm maculopapular lesions) may appear.

Prolonged shedding of Salmonella organisms in the stool is a common finding; stool results are positive for several months.

Shigella Organisms

1. These are commonly spread by person-to-person transmission, occurring most often in children less than 5 years of age. There is commonly (in >50%) diarrhea in other household members.

2. Patients have rapid onset of fever, crampy abdominal pain, and diarrhea. Stools are watery and usually contain mucus, blood, and polymorphonuclear leukocytes.

3. Febrile convulsions are common, with a peak between 6 months to 3 years, particularly in children with a family history of seizures or a high peak temperature (p. 747). Meningismus and respiratory symptoms may be present.

4. WBC count usually is less than 10,000/mm^3 with a marked shift to the left. Blood culture results are usually negative.

Campylobacter Organisms

1. These are transmitted by contaminated food and person-to-person contact. Incubation period is 2 to 7 days, with a peak in children less than 6 years during warm months. Transmission occurs person to person and pet to person.

2. Although the patient may be asymptomatic, the onset of illness can be marked by high fever, myalgia, headache, abdominal cramps, and vomiting. Diarrhea is profuse, watery, mucousy, and bloody. Leukocytes are common. Resolution occurs in 2 to 5 days.

Yersinia enterocolitica

1. *Yersinia enterocolitica* occurs in sporadic cases in toddlers and teenagers during the cooler months after exposure to contaminated food or water or by person-to-person transmission. Incubation is 3 to 4 days.

2. In younger children, acute diarrhea, with fever and abdominal pain, is common. Stools contain rare leukocytes and blood. Older children with mesenteric adenitis have fever and right lower quadrant (RLQ) pain.

Enterotoxigenic or Invasive *Escherichia coli*

1. *Escherichia coli* may cause disease by production of an enterotoxin or by tissue

invasion. Classification of the mechanism by serogroup of the organism is unreliable. *E. coli* serotype 0157.H7 is associated with hemolytic-uremic syndrome.
2. Diarrhea is particularly severe in infants and young children. It may produce symptoms similar to those caused by cholera (profuse, watery diarrhea) or *Shigella* organisms (fever and systemic symptoms). Mucus, blood, and polymorphonuclear (PMN) leukocytes are found in the stool.

Food Poisoning

1. Staphylococcal food poisoning results from a common-source food that is usually poorly refrigerated. Vomiting, marked prostration, and diarrhea occur within 12 to 16 hours of ingestion.
2. *Clostridium perfringens* may produce abdominal pain and diarrhea within 8 to 24 hours of ingestion of contaminated food. Fever, nausea, and vomiting are rare. Resolution occurs in 24 to 48 hours.
3. *Clostridium botulinum*, although it does not cause diarrhea, may produce clinical symptoms within 12 to 36 hours (range: 6 hours to 8 days) of ingestion of foods— usually home-preserved vegetables, fruit, or fish. Honey may cause infantile botulism in children less than 1 year of age. Patients have nausea, vomiting, diplopia, dysphagia, dysarthria, and dry mouth. Ptosis, mydriasis, nystagmus, and paresis of extraocular muscles may be noted (p. 707).

Parasites

1. *Giardia lamblia* is the most commonly identified intestinal parasite. It is usually asymptomatic but may cause nausea, flatulence, bloating, epigastric pain or cramps, and watery diarrhea. The patient rarely has right upper quadrant (RUQ) pain and tenderness.
2. *Cryptosporidium* is associated with malabsorption or secretory diarrhea that is usually self-limited. Spread is via contaminated water supply, human-human transmission, or from infected animals. Although no treatment is usually required, paromomycin may be effective. It is a serious illness in immunocompromised patients.
3. *Isospora belli* is usually due to contaminated food and water and may be treated with trimethoprim-sulfamethoxazole. As is cyclospora, both are usually self-limited in immunocompromised hosts.
4. Diarrheal diseases associated with parasites are usually chronic in nature and are associated with multisystem disease and weight loss.

Clostridium difficile

This is associated with pseudomembranous colitis and with many cases of antibiotic-related diarrhea in adults and children. The most common agents are amoxicillin, ampicillin, cephalosporins, and clindamycin. Less often associated are tetracycline, erythromycin, sulfonamides, and trimethoprim. Children may be asymptomatic or have chronic diarrhea, often with abdominal cramping. Stools are bloody with very rare leukocytes.

It is commonly cultured from the intestine of newborns without consistent clinical significance. *C. difficile* is an uncommon cause of enterocolitis in children in the first year of life.

Traveler's Diarrhea

Traveler's diarrhea is a nonspecific term used to define diarrhea that often occurs during travel in foreign countries and that is not associated with a known pathogen. *E. coli* that produces a heat-labile enterotoxin is probably causative. Symptomatically, patients have abdominal cramps, tenesmus, vomiting, nausea, chills, anorexia, and watery diarrhea.

Complications

1. Dehydration (see Chapter 7)
2. Postinfectious malabsorption
   NOTE: Children often experience a temporary lactose intolerance and develop watery diarrhea when challenged with lactose (dairy) products. Lactose-free soy formulas should be used for 2 to 4 weeks.
3. Hemolytic-uremic syndrome (p. 801)
4. Acute tubular necrosis (p. 809)
5. Systemic extension of infection (e.g., meningitis, septic arthritis)

Ancillary Data

Cultures of the Stool

Cultures are useful in determining the bacterial cause of the acute diarrhea but should be reserved for those patients in whom the results will have a therapeutic or epidemiologic impact. Rectal swabs handled expeditiously provide a good culture source if stool is unavailable. Cultures should be routinely done in children less than 1 year of age who are febrile or toxic on arrival with diarrhea and who have PMN leukocytes in their stool. Cultures are also important if multiple members of the same family are ill, if any member of the family is a food handler, if patients have recently traveled extensively, or if symptomatic children are immunosuppressed or have hemoglobinopathy.

Fecal Leukocytes (Methylene Blue Smear of Stool)

This is a reliable test to determine the etiologic agent because more than 90% of diarrhea resulting from *Salmonella* or *Shigella* organisms have PMN leukocytes in the stool. Fecal leukocytes also are often found in patients with *Campylobacter* organisms, *Y. enterocolitica*, invasive *E. coli*, and *Vibrio parahaemolyticus*. This is an excellent screen to define that group of patients at greatest risk of having a bacterial pathogen.

A small amount of mucus is placed on a clear glass slide and mixed with 2 drops of methylene blue. A coverglass is placed on the slide, and nuclear staining occurs over 2 minutes. Microscopic examination for PMN leukocytes is performed, and the finding is positive when there are 5 white blood cells/high-powered field (WBC/HPF) or more.

Rotavirus Test

This may be identified by electron microscopy, radioimmunoassay, or the easier enzyme-linked immunosorbent assay (ELISA) test, which is commercially available. Similar technology exists for adenovirus and cryptosporidiosis.

Blood Tests

These are important if a significant abnormality of intake or output is present and should include electrolytes, blood urea nitrogen (BUN), and a complete blood count (CBC) with differential. All patients with any degree of dehydration or a prolonged course should have these studies performed. When the ratio of band forms over total neutrophils (segmented plus bands) is more than 0.10, *Shigella*, *Salmonella*, or *Campylobacter* organisms should be suspected. The WBC is usually less than 10,000/mm^3, with a marked shift to the left in patients with *Shigella* infection. In *Salmonella* infection, WBC is increased, with a mild shift to the left. A high WBC count is also found in patients with *Campylobacter* and *Yersinia* infections.

Ova and Parasites

Cultures are important if *Giardia* or other parasites are suspected. With *Giardia* organisms, cysts are present in formed stools and trophozoites in watery stool or duodenal aspirates.

Blood Cultures

These are indicated for infants and young children with high fever and significant toxicity, as well as in immunocompromised patients.

DIFFERENTIAL DIAGNOSIS

See Chapter 32.

MANAGEMENT

The initial assessment of the patient must focus on the magnitude and type of dehydration. Rapid correction of deficits as outlined in Chapter 7 is imperative.

Antibiotics (Table 76-1)

Antibiotics must be restricted to specific etiologic agents, especially *Shigella* infection. In general they are not useful in most diarrheal illnesses. The ultimate choice should reflect culture and sensitivity results, the patient's clinical status, and epidemiologic considerations.

Antibiotic therapy in patients with proved or suspected *Salmonella* infection is controversial because it prolongs the carrier state; however, it should be initiated in toxic patients less than 6 months, in those with suspected bacteremia, and in children who are immunosuppressed or have a hemoglobinopathy.

Campylobacter disorders may resolve symptomatically more rapidly after treatment with erythromycin.

Ciprofloxacin (500 mg BID PO for 3 to 5 days) may be an alternative treatment in children older than 17 years for *Campylobacter*, *Shigella*, and *Salmonella*.

C. difficile pseudomembranous colitis rarely requires antibiotic therapy but often actually responds to cessation of previous antibiotics. If indicated by either significant or ongoing symptoms, vancomycin, 40 mg/kg/24 hr q6hr PO (adult maximum: 2 gm/24 hr); or metronidazole, 15-40 mg/kg/24 hr q8hr PO, for 10 days may be useful.

TABLE 76-1   Antibiotic Indications in Infectious Diarrhea

Etiologic agent	Drug of choice	Dose: mg/kg/ 24 hr (adult: gm/dose)	Route/frequency	Comments
Salmonella	Ampicillin **and** gentamicin*	200-400 (1 gm) 5-7.5 (80 mg)	IV q4-6hr IV q8hr	Only in toxic patient when bacteremia is a concern; prolongs carrier status
Shigella	Trimethoprim-sulfamethoxazole; **or**	8-10/40-50 (double strength)	PO q12hr	Preferred, depending on sensitivity; treat 5 days
	Ceftriaxone; **or**	50-100	IV/IM q12-24hr	Treat for 5 days
	Ampicillin	50-100 (0.5 gm)	PO q6-8hr	Do not use amoxicillin; may give parenterally for very toxic patients
Campylobacter	Erythromycin	30-50 (0.5 gm)	PO q6-8hr	Effectiveness unproved; reduces length of excretion
Yersinia entero- colitica	Trimethoprim-sulfamethoxazole	8-10/40-50	PO q12hr	With severe toxicity, may use tetracycline (>8 yr old) and aminoglycoside; controversial
Giardia	Furazolidone; **or** Metronidazole	6-8 (0.1 gm) 15 (0.25 gm)	PO q6hr PO q8hr	7-10 days; suspension available 5 days

*Controversial. Generally, antibiotics are indicated only for invasive disease or for those at risk of invasive disease. Other approaches include third-generation cephalosporin (ceftriaxone, cefotaxime); ampicillin and chloramphenicol; trimethoprim-sulfamethoxazole (IV). Drug must reflect local sensitivity patterns and treatment approaches.

Antidiarrheal Agents

Agents like kaolin and pectin suspensions have no defined value. Diphenoxylate and atropine (Lomotil) cause segmental contraction of the intestines, retarding movement of intestinal contents. It may have a detrimental effect on recovery from *Shigella* organisms. Special care is required because of the frequency of overdose in children. Loperamide (Imodium) may have a similar role by decreasing peristalsis. Initial oral dose of loperamide for the first day for a 13- to 20-kg child is 1 mg TID; for a 20- to 30-kg child, 2 mg BID; for a child more than 30 kg, 2 mg TID. After the first day, the child is given a 0.1 mg/kg/dose after each unformed stool up to the maximum daily dose noted above. Others use a dose of 0.4-0.8 mg/kg/24 hr q6-12hr PO in children greater than 2 years up to a maximum of 2 mg/dose.

Antispasmodics

Their role is controversial, and they are rarely indicated.

Bile Acids

In children with prolonged diarrhea, primarily of a secretory nature that does not respond to a clear liquid or NPO regimen, bile acids may contribute to GI irritation; stools are usually green. A short course of aluminum hydroxide (Amphojel), 2.5 to 5.0 ml (to 1 tsp) q6hr or with meals PO for 2 to 4 days, may be useful in recalcitrant diarrhea. Cholestyramine (Questran), available in 4-gm packages, also absorbs and combines with bile acids when 1 gm/24 hours is administered to infants less than 1 year (up to 4 gm/24 hours in older children). Both also bind bacterial enterotoxins and fatty acids.

Prostaglandin Inhibitors

Hormonally or prostaglandin-mediated secretory diarrhea may be treated pharmacologically if traditional dietary manipulations are ineffective. Aspirin, indomethacin, and non-steroidal antiinflammatory agents may be indicated empirically.

Traveler's Diarrhea Prophylaxis

Prevention through attention to strict sanitary guidelines is mandatory. If necessary, treatment should focus primarily on support, including fluid management and restricted diet. Recent guidelines recommend against routine prophylaxis because adverse reactions occur in 2% to 5% of patients. The decision to use prophylaxis must be individualized, reflecting the underlying health of the patient and the circumstances of the prospective travel. For mild diarrhea in adolescents and adults, antimotility agents such as diphenoxylate with atropine (Lomotil) may have a very limited role, supplementing fluid therapy. More severe diarrhea (>3 stools in 8 hours with nausea, vomiting, or fever) is treated with doxycycline (children >8 years) or trimethoprim-sulfamethoxazole. Reduction in diarrhea may also be achieved by bismuth subsalicylate, 2 tablets QID or 30 ml q30min for 3 hours. Loperamide, 4 mg (adult) initially, then a 2-mg capsule after each unformed stool for 2 days (maximum: 8 capsules/day) may also be effective.

Drugs normally are prescribed for the patient, who carries them along in the event of illness. They are not given prophylactically. Oral hydration must be simultaneously instituted.

DISPOSITION

All patients with serious toxicity, dehydration, abnormal electrolytes, or a history of significant noncompliance should be hospitalized for IV therapy. In addition, admission should be sought for patients with sickle cell disease, hemoglobinopathies, or compromised immune systems. Oral rehydration may be attempted in nontoxic children under close observation.

Once the deficit has been restored and abnormal losses reduced, clear liquids (Pedialyte, Ricelyte, or Lytren) should be initiated slowly. If an adequate response is noted, a soy formula can be tried with slow progression.

Patients with minimal or no dehydration may be followed at home with careful fluid management and close follow-up observation.

Parental Education

1. Give only clear liquids; give as much as the child wants. The following may be used during the first 24 hours:
   a. Rehydralyte, Ricelyte, or Lytren
   b. Defizzed, room-temperature soda for older children (>2 years) if diarrhea is only mild
   c. Gatorade
2. If your child is vomiting, give clear liquids *slowly.* In younger children, start with a teaspoonful and slowly increase the amount. If vomiting occurs, let the child rest for awhile and then try again. About 8 hours after vomiting has stopped, your child can gradually return to a normal diet.
3. After 24 hours, your child's diet may be advanced if the diarrhea has improved. If only formula is being taken, mix the formula with twice as much water to make up half-strength formula, which should be given over the next 24 hours. Applesauce, bananas, and strained carrots may be given if your child is eating solids. If this is tolerated, your child may be advanced to a regular diet over the next 2 to 3 days.
4. If your child has had a prolonged course of diarrhea, it may be helpful in the younger child to advance from clear liquids to a soy formula (Isomil, ProSobee, or Soyalac) for 1 to 2 weeks. Children older than 1 year with significant findings may do better with minimal cow's milk products (milk, cheese, ice cream, or butter) for several days.
5. Do not use boiled milk. Kool-Aid and soda are not ideal liquids, particularly for younger infants, because they contain few electrolytes.
6. Call the physician if the following occur:
   a. The diarrhea or vomiting is increasing in frequency or amount.

b. The diarrhea does not improve after 24 hours of clear liquids or resolve entirely after 3 to 4 days.
c. Vomiting continues for more than 24 hours.
d. The stool has blood or the vomited material contains blood or turns green.
e. Signs of dehydration develop, including decreased urination, less moisture in diapers, dry mouth, no tears, weight loss, lethargy, or irritability.

REFERENCES

Ashkenazi S, Dinari G, Zegulknov A, et al: Convulsions in childhood shigellosis, *Am J Dis Child* 141:208, 1983.
Barkin RM: Acute infectious diarrheal disease in children, *J Emerg Med* 3:1, 1985.
Cohen MB: Etiology and mechanisms of acute infectious diarrhea in infants in the United States, *J Pediatr* 118:534, 1991.
DeWitt TG, Humphrey KF, McCarthy P: Clinical predictors of acute bacterial diarrhea in young children, *Pediatrics* 76:551, 1985.
DuPont HL, Ericsson CD, Johnson DC, et al: Prevention of travelers' diarrhea by the tablet formulation of bismuth subsalicylate, *JAMA* 257:1347, 1987.
Herrmann JE, Taylor DN, Echeverria P, et al: Astroviruses as a cause of gastroenteritis in children, *N Engl J Med* 324:1757, 1991.
Kelly CP, Pothoulakis C, LaMont JT: *C. difficile* colitis, *N Engl J Med* 330:257, 1994.
Krajden M, Brown M, Petrasek A, et al: Clinical features of adenovirus enteritis: a review of 127 cases, *Pediatr Infect Dis J* 9:636, 1990.
Listernick R, Zieseri E, Davis AT: Outpatient oral rehydration in the United States, *Am J Dis Child* 140:211, 1986.
Pickering LK: Therapy of acute infectious diarrhea in children, *J Pediatr* 118:S119, 1991.
Varsana I, Eidlitz-Marcus T, Nussinovitch M, et al: Comparative efficacy of ceftriaxone and ampicillin for treatment of severe shigellosis in children, *J Pediatr* 118:627, 1991.

GASTROINTESTINAL FOREIGN BODIES

Although most foreign bodies inadvertently swallowed by the inquisitive child pass without incident, they may lodge at points of physiologic narrowing, including the cricopharyngeal muscle, the carina or aortic arch, Schatzki ring, or the cardioesophageal junction. They also may get stuck at the ligament of Treitz. Children rarely insert foreign bodies into the rectum.

DIAGNOSTIC FINDINGS

Most patients are asymptomatic, and the foreign body passes without difficulty. When the foreign body does lodge in the esophagus, the patient may be anxious and have difficulty swallowing.

Physical examination usually is unremarkable. It is important to be certain that there is no evidence of any airway foreign body.

X-ray films are indicated if there is any question of an airway foreign body or if the patient is symptomatic. Some recommend that an x-ray film be taken in asymptomatic patients at 24 hours to assure that the object has passed and thereby minimize the number of x-ray films obtained.

More recently, investigators have been studying the reliability of metal detectors in defining the location of a metallic foreign body.

1. Coins that are in the esophagus lie in the frontal plane (full circle can be seen) while those in the trachea lie sagittally and appear end-on in a posteroanterior (PA) chest film.
2. Objects commonly become lodged at the proximal thoracic inlet; the cricopharyngeus muscle, the aortic arch, or the carina.
3. A lateral chest view supplementing the AP view may be helpful if there is any question of localization.
4. If the foreign body is not found on the chest films, an abdominal film should be obtained. If it still cannot be located, a contrast study may be indicated.
5. For reference, a dime is 17 mm, a penny is 18 mm, a nickel is 20 mm, and a quarter is 23 mm in diameter.

DIFFERENTIAL DIAGNOSIS

Foreign bodies in the trachea are differentiated by history, physical examination, and x-ray film (p. 791).

MANAGEMENT

Historically, asymptomatic patients have been managed without intervention or diagnostic studies and with reassurance. Most foreign bodies, whether round, irregular, or sharp (e.g., pins) pass without difficulty. Evidence, however, has suggested that 17% of patients with coin ingestions were without symptoms. Therefore it is appropriate to consider chest radiographs, including the cervical esophagus, in patients ingesting coins if there is any question of symptoms, poor compliance, or if follow-up observation will be difficult.

All patients should be instructed to watch for fecal passage of the object and report any symptoms including pain, tenderness, obstruction, or signs of perforation immediately to permit further diagnostic and therapeutic steps.

1. Esophageal foreign bodies:
   a. If the object is sharp or has sharp projections and it is lodged, remove it by endoscopy. Endoscopy may be used for other types of objects as well. Obtain a film before attempting retrieval.
   b. Other foreign bodies (e.g., coins) that become lodged in the distal esophagus in the asymptomatic patient for less than 24 hours may be observed during the first 24 hours. If they do not subsequently move over the first 24 hours, they may be removed by endoscopy. Some institutions with radiologic assistance pass a Foley catheter beyond the foreign body, blowing up the balloon with a radiopaque substance and gently pulling out the material. The procedure should be done under fluoroscopic control, with an nasogastric (NG) tube having been passed initially to empty the stomach. Preparations should be made in the event that the patient aspirates the foreign body, a risk that is minimized by placing the patient in Trendelenburg position.

   If a single coin was ingested in the preceding 24 hours in a patient without prior esophageal disease or surgery and no respiratory distress, a single pass of a Hurst bougie dilator may be effectively passed through the mouth in an upright position.

Dilator size is as follows:

1-2 yr	28 Fr
2-3 yr	36 Fr
4-5 yr	36 Fr
>5 yr	40 Fr

2. Foreign bodies lodged in the stomach (usually distal antrum) usually can be watched for 2 to 3 weeks unless they have corrosive potential, such as button batteries (p. 368).

3. Foreign bodies lodged at the ligament of Treitz:

   a. Round objects may be watched for up to 1 week, awaiting passage, unless the patient has evidence of obstruction or perforation.

   b. Elongated objects such as pencils should be observed for 6 to 8 hours and, if no movement is noted, removed either by endoscopy or surgery.

4. Rectal foreign bodies:

   a. If large, they usually require general anesthesia to facilitate removal.

   b. Small objects can be removed through an anoscope. Preparation of the patient with oral (PO) or rectal (PR) mineral oil may be useful.

5. Button batteries lodged in the esophagus should be removed endoscopically. If they have passed beyond the pylorus, the patient may be observed in the asymptomatic patient. Batteries less than 15 mm in diameter in the stomach may also be observed; batteries more than 15 mm in diameter should be viewed on x-ray film again in 48 hours and if still in the stomach retrieved at that time (see Chapter 55).

6. Although without proved efficacy, some clinicians continue to believe that glucagon (0.03-0.1 mg/kg/dose IV; adult: 1 mg/dose) may have some value in the management of esophageal foreign bodies.

DISPOSITION

Asymptomatic patients may be discharged with close follow-up observation if the foreign body is lodged in an anatomic site not requiring urgent removal. Symptomatic patients and those requiring removal should be hospitalized.

REFERENCES

Bendig DW: Removal of blunt esophageal foreign bodies by flexible endoscopy without general anesthesia, *Am J Dis Child* 140:789, 1986.

Caravati EM, Bennett DL, McElwee NE: Pediatric coin ingestion, *Am J Dis Child* 143:549, 1989.

Hodge D, Tecklenburg F, Fleisher G: Coin ingestion: does every child need a radiograph? *Ann Emerg Med* 14:443, 1985.

O'Neill JA, Holcomb GW, Neblet WW: Management of tracheobronchial and esophageal foreign bodies in childhood, *J Pediatr Surg* 18:475, 1983.

Ros SP, Cetta F: Successful use of a metal detector in locating coins ingested by children, *J Pediatr* 120:753, 1992.

Sacchetti A, Carraccio C, Lichtenstine R: Hand-held metal detection identification of ingested foreign bodies, *Pediatr Emerg Care* 10:204, 1994.

Schunk JE, Harrison AM, Correl HM, et al: Fluoroscopic Foley catheter removal of esophageal foreign bodies in children: experience with episodes, *Pediatrics* 94:709, 1994.

Sheizh A: Button battery ingestions in children, *Pediatr Emerg Care* 9:224, 1993.

VIRAL HEPATITIS

Acute viral hepatitis commonly is classified as hepatitis A (predominantly fecal-oral transmission), hepatitis B (largely parenteral), and hepatitis C, D, and E (non-A/non-B [transfusion related]) on the basis of serologic and clinical data (Table 76-2).

What used to be called "non-A, non-B hepatitis" is caused by three specific viruses, hepatitis C, D, and E.

1. Hepatitis C is the most common form of non-A, non-B posttransfusion hepatitis. Perinatal and sexual transmission is uncommon. Vertical transmission occurs in high-risk mothers (intravenous [IV] drug abusers, sexually transmitted disease [STD], human immunodeficiency virus

TABLE 76-2 Hepatitis: Characteristics of Virus Types

	A	B	C	D	E
Virus type Antigen	RNA HAVAg	DNA HBsAg, HBcAg, HBeAg	RNA HCVAg	RNA HDVAg	RNA HEVAg
Serologic diagnosis	IgM anti-HAV (may persist 4 mo)	Anti-HBs Anti-HBc Anti-HBe	Anti-HCV	Anti-HDV (IgM, IgG)	Anti-HEV
Epidemiology Transmission	Fecal-oral, contaminated water/food, oral-anal sex	Parenteral blood products, sexual, perinatal, child to child in household	Parenteral, perinatal, and sexual	Coinfection or superinfection with HBV	Fecal-oral (see A)
Onset	Acute	Insidious	Insidious with relapse	Coinfection	Acute
Incubation period Chronicity	2-6 wk No	2-6 mo Infants: 90% Adults: 6%-10%	6-12 wk 50%-80%	2-8 wk 2%-70%	6 wk No
Symptoms	90%-95% children <5 yr asymptomatic; flulike symptoms early; jaundice may last 1-3 wk; may be fulminant	Asymptomatic to fulminant; insidious onset with prolonged jaundice	Acute or chronic; more mild than B; often anicteric	Acute or chronic	Icteric or anicteric hepatitis; usually self-limited
Management	Supportive Prevent spread (hygiene, IG)	Supportive	Supportive May be role for α-interferon with chronic hepatitis C	Supportive α-interferon may be beneficial	Supportive
Vaccine	Yes	Yes	No	No	No

[HIV]). It is characterized by an acute infection after an incubation period of 6 to 12 weeks. Disease is mild or subclinical. Chronic disease may occur, producing chronic active hepatitis in 35% to 50% of patients and cirrhosis in 20%.
2. Hepatitis D may cause epidemics in high-risk patients. Coinfection with hepatitis B may occur; 5% progress to chronic disease. Superinfection with hepatitis B may occur.
3. Hepatitis E is enterically transmitted and has an incubation period of 6 weeks. It occurs more commonly in males, most notably in those 15 to 39 years of age. The incubation is 6 weeks.

Patients may have variable types of hepatitis, including acute icteric, anicteric, acute fulminant, and subacute. Most infections are self-limited.

DIAGNOSTIC FINDINGS (see Table 76-2)

Epidemiologic and diagnostic findings vary.
1. Patients generally have a prodromal, pre-icteric phase with malaise and anorexia.
2. Jaundice develops, accompanied by scleral icterus (bilirubin >2.5 mg/dl) and pruritus.
3. The abdomen may be distended. Palpation of the right upper quadrant over the liver demonstrates the greatest tenderness. Splenomegaly is variably present.
4. Evidence of serum sickness is present with hepatitis B. Arthralgia, myalgia, erythematous or maculopapular rash, and fever are noted. Patients may develop myocarditis or pericarditis, with symptoms of pleuritic chest pain and friction rubs.

Complications

1. Fulminant hepatitis. A poor prognosis is seen with hepatitis B when associated with a prolonged prothrombin time (PT) (>4 over control), unresponsive to large doses of vitamin K, elevated bilirubin level (>20 mg/dl), leukocytosis (>12,500 WBC/mm^3), and hypoglycemia.
2. Chronic active hepatitis.
3. Hepatorenal syndrome with edema and ascites.
4. Hepatic encephalopathy marked by altered mental status, seizures, and coma. Tremor, asterixis, and hyperreflexia may be present.
5. Bleeding diathesis.

Ancillary Data

1. WBC count usually is normal.
2. Prothrombin time is prolonged. Other bleeding studies are normal.
3. Liver functions are elevated. Transaminase and bilirubin levels are elevated for weeks in hepatitis A and months in hepatitis B. Bilirubin level greater than 20 mg/dl is consistent with severe disease. Glutamyl transferase level greater than 300 units/L is consistent with biliary atresia or alpha$_1$-antitrypsin deficiency.
4. Urine is dark with urobilinogen and bilirubin.
5. Serologic studies are important in differentiating the type of hepatitis.
   a. Hepatitis A antibody (IgM) is diagnostic of an acute infection, whereas hepatitis B antibody (IgG) is evidence of previous infection.
   b. Serologic tests for hepatitis B are listed below.

Hepatitis B antigen/antibody	Interpretation
Surface antigen (HBsAg)	Carrier or acutely infected
Antibody to surface antigen (Anti-HBs)	Prior infection with HBV; immunity after vaccine
e Antigen (HBeAg)	Carrier with high risk of transmitting HBsAg
Antibody to e antigen (Anti-HBe)	HBsAg carrier with low risk of infectiousness
Antibody to core antigen (Anti-HBc)	Prior HBV infection (not immunization)
IgM antibody to core antigen (IgM Anti-HBc)	Acute or recent HBV infection

6. Detection of HCV-RNA is the best means of confirming hepatitis C.
7. Hepatitis D is detected by the presence of hepatitis D antigen. Chronic illness may be indicated by high titer levels found at 2 to 4 weeks.
8. Serologic evaluation may be diagnostic for hepatitis E virus antigen. Electron microscopy of infected stools may be useful.
9. If indicated, other studies should be done to exclude other causes of hepatitis.

DIFFERENTIAL DIAGNOSIS

1. Infection/inflammation
   a. Viral: infectious mononucleosis (Epstein-Barr [EB] virus), cytomegalovirus, herpes simplex
   b. Toxoplasmosis
   c. Cholangitis
2. Metabolic disorders
   a. Cholelithiasis
   b. Wilson's disease
   c. Gilbert's disease and Dubin-Johnson syndrome
3. Drugs
   a. Alcohol
   b. Analgesic: aspirin, acetaminophen
   c. Anesthetic: halothane
   d. Antibiotic: erythromycin estolate, sulfonamides, tetracycline, rifampin, carbenicillin
   e. Antituberculosis: isoniazid, rifampin
   f. Others: phenytoin, phenothiazine, morphine
4. Congenital disorder: biliary atresia (infants)

MANAGEMENT

Most patients need careful follow-up observation and monitoring to ensure that their liver functions are normalizing and that hydration is maintained.

Patients with impending liver failure require a host of supportive measures:
1. Respiratory and cardiovascular support
   a. Oxygen and active airway management if necessary
   b. Maintenance of intravascular volume
2. Central nervous system (CNS) support, if encephalopathy is present
   a. Decrease of protein intake
   b. NG tube with administration of neomycin, 50-100 mg/kg/24 hr q6hr, via the tube
   c. Treatment of cerebral edema
      (1) Fluid restriction: 75% of maintenance
      (2) Steroids: dexamethasone, 0.25 mg/kg/dose q6hr IV; controversial
      (3) Mannitol: 0.25-1.0 gm/kg/dose q6hr IV
      (4) Hyperventilation (if ventilatory support is necessary)
3. Other
   a. Give diuretics for fluid overload.
      (1) Furosemide (Lasix), 1-2 mg/kg/dose q2-6hr IV or PO
      (2) Spironolactone (Aldactone), 1-3 mg/kg/24 hr q6-8hr PO
   b. Maintain glucose at 100-150 mg/dl.
   c. Support nutrition.
   d. For bleeding, administer fresh-frozen plasma (10 ml/kg/dose q12-24hr IV) and vitamin K (infants: 1-2 mg/dose IV slowly; children and adults: 5-10 mg/dose IV).
   e. Treat infections and GI bleeding appropriately.
   f. Isolate patient.
      NOTE: Other modalities that have been attempted without proved benefit include exchange transfusions and dialysis.
4. Trials of alpha interferon have demonstrated normalized liver function in patients with chronic hepatitis C; 50% responders relapsed when therapy ceased. Alpha interferon may produce transient beneficial effects for hepatitis D.
5. Immunization against hepatitis B may be useful.

Preventive Measures

Hepatitis A

Hepatitis A vaccine is currently available for children 2 years of age or older. It is recommended for the following people:

1. Travelers to areas with intermediate to high rates of endemic hepatitis A
2. Children living in defined or circumscribed communities with high endemic or periodic outbreaks of HIV infection
3. Patients with chronic hepatitis

Those with *household contacts* should receive 0.02 ml/kg IM of immune serum globulin (IG) as soon after exposure as possible. IG is not indicated beyond 2 weeks after exposure. Administration of IG also should be considered in the following circumstances:

1. In day-care centers with children more than 2 years of age who are toilet trained, give IG to all children in the day-care room when there is a case in an employee or child of employee in contact with index case.
2. In day-care centers with children who are not toilet trained, give IG to all employees and children if there is a case in an employee or child or in the household contacts of two enrolled children.
3. If recognition of outbreak is delayed by 3 weeks or there are cases in three or more families, consider administering IG to all staff and children and household contacts of children 3 years of age or younger.
4. Give IG to those who have personal contact with individuals with hepatitis in an institutional setting.
5. Exposure in classrooms or other places in schools has not generally posed a significant risk of infection. Hospital personnel caring for patients with hepatitis A are not routinely treated. Emphasis should be on good hand-washing technique.
6. Preexposure prophylaxis for travelers to areas where hygiene is poor may be done by giving immediately before departure a dose of immune serum globulin, 0.02

ml/kg for children, for stays less than 3 months, 0.06 ml/kg for children for stays 3 months or longer, and 2 ml IM to adults traveling for less than 3 months, and 5 ml for longer stays.

Hepatitis B

Preexposure prophylaxis is available from a vaccine prepared from formalin-inactivated subunits derived from hepatitis B surface antigen (HBsAg) from plasma of carriers or genetically engineered recombinant HB vaccine. A three-dose series is recommended, administering the vaccine at days 1, 30, and 180 to high-risk individuals.

For children less than 10 years of age, give 10 µg plasma-derived HB vaccine (0.5 ml) or 5 µg (0.5 ml) of recombinant vaccine. Older children and adults get 20 µg (1 ml) or 10 µg (1 ml) of the respective vaccines. Immunosuppressed patients may receive twice the recommended dose of plasma-derived HB vaccine. Children in this group include those from families with hepatitis B virus infection or chronic carriers, those in institutions for the mentally retarded, and those receiving large amounts of blood and blood products.

Postexposure prophylaxis must reflect the type of exposure (blood or percutaneous needle stick or mucosal membrane) and HBsAg of the donor.

1. For those with exposure to blood known to be HBsAg positive: Exposure may be percutaneous, ocular, or through mucosal membrane. A single dose of hepatitis B immunoglobulin (HBIG) (0.06 ml/kg or 5.0 ml for adult) should be given as soon as possible after exposure and within 24 hours if possible. Hepatitis B vaccine 1 ml (20 µg) (children less than 10 years: 0.5 ml) should be given as an IM injection at a separate site as soon as possible but within 7 days of exposure, with second and third doses given at 1 month and 6 months after the first dose. If HB vaccine is refused, repeat HBIG in 1 month.

2. For those with exposure to blood of unknown HBsAg status:
    a. High-risk patient exposure (e.g., those with Down syndrome who are institutionalized, dialysis patients, drug abusers).
    b. Initiate hepatitis B vaccine three-dose regimen. Consider HBIG, 0.06 ml/kg (adult: 5.0 ml), as well.
    c. Low-risk patient exposures should be individualized. Vaccine should be considered. Therapy may be delayed if status can be determined within 7 days of exposure.

Sexual contacts of persons with acute hepatitis B infections are at increased risk of acquiring the disease. A single dose of HBIG (0.06 ml/kg or 5.0 ml in adult) should be given to susceptible individuals who have had sexual contact with an HBsAg-positive person if it can be given within 14 days of the last sexual contact. A second HBIG dose should be given in cases of heterosexual exposures if the index patient remains HBsAg positive 3 months after detection. Subsequent doses of hepatitis B vaccine should be given at 1 and 6 months.

Newborns of mothers who are HBsAg positive are at risk of hepatitis B virus transmission. HBIG (0.5 ml) IM should be administered within 12 hours of birth. In addition, HB vaccine (0.5 ml) should be given at the time of administration of HBIG and 1 month and 6 months later. HBsAg testing should be done at 6 months in consultation with appropriate experts. Infants born to mothers who have not been screened for HBsAg should receive vaccine and HBIG at birth and the vaccine schedule completed as provided in routine immunization.

Routine immunization of infants is now recommended against hepatitis B. Immunization is done during the first few days of life, and subsequently at 1 to 2 and 18 months of age. Routine immunization of older children is also feasible.

Hepatitis Non-A/Non-B

Management is the same as for hepatitis A, although some recommend IG, 0.06 ml/kg IM, after exposure to blood.

REFERENCES

American Academy of Pediatrics, Committee on Infectious Diseases: Prevention of hepatitis A infections: guidelines for use of hepatitis A vaccine and immune globulin, *Pediatrics* 98:1207, 1996.

Clemens RM, Safary A, Hepburn A, et al: Clinical experience with an inactivated hepatitis A vaccine, *J Infect Dis* 171:514, 1995.

Hadler SC, Erbon JJ, Matthews D, et al: Effect of immunoglobulin on hepatitis A in day-care centers, *JAMA* 249:48, 1983.

Lemon SM: Type A viral hepatitis: new developments in an old disease, *N Engl J Med* 313:1059, 1985.

Morton TA, Kelen GD: Hepatitis C, *Ann Emerg Med* 31:381, 1998.

Report of the committee on infectious diseases, Elk Grove, Ill, 1991, American Academy of Pediatrics.

PANCREATITIS

ETIOLOGY

1. Infection
    a. Viral: mumps, hepatitis, EB virus, coxsackievirus
    b. *Mycoplasma pneumoniae*
    c. Kawasaki syndrome
2. Trauma: blunt, penetrating, or surgical
3. Intoxication
    a. Diuretics: thiazides, furosemide
    b. Prednisone, oral contraceptive agents
    c. Antibiotics: rifampin, tetracycline, isoniazid
4. Congenital: biliary tract anomalies
5. Structural
    a. Biliary tract disease
    b. Cholelithiasis
6. Systemic illness
    a. Systemic lupus erythematosus
    b. Kawasaki syndrome
    c. Cystic fibrosis
    d. Diabetes mellitus

DIAGNOSTIC FINDINGS

1. Abdominal pain is the primary complaint, either of insidious or sudden onset. Upper quadrant or epigastric constant or intermittent pain is reported. It may radiate to

the back or neck. Relief is obtained in the knee-chest position.

2. Abdominal tenderness and distension are noted, with decreased bowel sounds and ascites. Cullens (bluish periumbilical discoloration) and Grey Turner (discoloration of the flank) signs are indicative of pancreatic necrosis and only occur late.

3. Low-grade fever, nausea, vomiting, and lethargy may be present.

Complications

1. Hypotension and shock secondary to third-space losses and intravascular volume depletion

2. Acute respiratory distress syndrome with left-sided pleural effusions and pneumonitis

3. Pancreatic pseudocyst or abscess, usually with delayed onset

4. Disseminated intravascular coagulation

Ancillary Data

1. Electrolyte levels are normal. Glucose level may be increased.

2. Hypocalcemia is a bad prognostic sign.

3. Elevation of amylase level peaks at 12 to 24 hours, which may return to normal in 48 to 72 hours. Lipase level rises early and normalizes less rapidly. A determination that is useful for patients whose serum amylase level is not diagnostic is clearance values calculated from spot urine and serum values:

$$\frac{C_{amylase}}{C_{creatine}} = \frac{Amylase\ (urine)}{Amylase\ (serum)} \times$$

$$\frac{Creatinine\ (serum)}{Creatinine\ (urine)} \times 100$$

This ratio is normally equal to 1% to 4%. A value greater than 6% indicates pancreatitis.

NOTE: Amylase level may be elevated in abdominal trauma and infection, not specifically causing pancreatitis.

4. Liver functions are elevated, particularly the bilirubin level.

5. X-ray films may demonstrate pleural effusions, atelectasis, pneumonitis, and an intestinal ileus or sentinel loop.

DIFFERENTIAL DIAGNOSIS

1. Infection.
   a. Peritonitis and other causes of surgical abdomen
   b. Pneumonia
2. Trauma. It is essential to differentiate pancreatitis from other abdominal organic involvement. Peritoneal lavage may be necessary. Consider child abuse.

MANAGEMENT

1. Stabilization is of primary importance, with initial attention to fluid therapy, usually requiring IV replacement of deficits (see Chapter 7). In cases of trauma, it is imperative to be certain that other organs are not involved. Glucose and calcium abnormalities may require intervention.

2. An NG tube attached to suction should be begun and the patient made NPO until pain has subsided for several days.

3. Analgesia may be used. Meperidine (Demerol), 1 mg/kg/dose q4-6hr IM or IV, is the drug of choice.

4. When the patient can tolerate food, a bland, low-fat diet should be used, often requiring pancreatic enzyme supplements. Until that time, IV alimentation is appropriate.

5. Once the patient is stabilized, antacids or cimetidine may be useful.

DISPOSITION

1. Patients require hospitalization for IV fluids, gastric suction, and monitoring.

2. Long-term follow-up observation is essential because of the delayed onset of pancreatic pseudocyst and abscess.

REFERENCES

Mader TJ, McHugh TP: Acute pancreatitis in children, *Pediatr Emerg Care* 8:157, 1992.

Weizman Z, Durle PR: Acute pancreatitis in childhood, *J Pediatr* 113:24, 1988.

REYE SYNDROME

ALERT: Vomiting and behavior changes after an acute illness require rapid evaluation and intervention.

Reye syndrome is an acute, noninflammatory encephalopathy with altered level of consciousness, cerebral edema without perivascular or meningeal inflammation, and fatty metamorphosis of the liver, probably secondary to mitochondrial dysfunction. It is a multisystem disease with a biphasic history marked by an infectious phase followed by an encephalopathic stage. There have been reports of the syndrome in children between 4 months and 14 years, with an average age of 7 years and a peak occurrence between 4 and 11 years. It often follows a viral infection: influenza B and chickenpox are particularly implicated. Salicylate ingestion may be a predisposing factor. The incidence of the disease has dramatically increased.

The term *Reye-like syndrome* has been used to describe a variety of pathologic conditions resulting from defects in urea and fatty acid metabolism, toxicologic injury, and impaired gluconeogenesis.

DIAGNOSTIC FINDINGS

1. A prodrome of respiratory or GI symptoms is consistently present for 2-3 days.
2. Vomiting develops and is followed in 24-48 hours by an encephalopathic phase with marked behavioral changes, including delirium and combativeness, disorientation, and hallucination. The deteriorating level of consciousness reflects increasing intracranial pressure. Obtundation and coma may follow, associated with seizures, hyperventilation, and hypothermia. Progressive stages have been outlined, based on the progression of findings in cephalocaudal progression of brainstem dysfunction:
   - **0.** Alert, wakeful
   - **I.** Lethargy, follows verbal comments, normal posture, purposeful response to pain, brisk pupillary light reflex, and normal oculocephalic reflex
   - **II.** Combative or stuporous, inappropriate verbalizing, normal posture, purposeful or nonpurposeful response to pain, sluggish pupillary reaction, and conjugate deviation on doll's eyes maneuver
   - **III.** Comatose, decorticate posture, decorticate response to pain, sluggish pupillary reaction, conjugate deviation on doll's eyes maneuver
   - **IV.** Comatose, decerebrate posture and decerebrate response to pain, sluggish pupillary reflexes, and inconsistent or absent oculocephalic reflex
   - **V.** Comatose, flaccid, no response to pain, no pupillary response, no oculocephalic reflex
3. Hepatomegaly and pancreatitis may be present.
4. In children less than 1 year of age, vomiting is mild and the predominant findings are apnea, hyperventilation, seizures, hepatomegaly, and hypoglycemia.

Complications

Children in stages IV or V and those progressing rapidly from stage I to III have a poor prognosis.
1. Acute respiratory failure
2. Cerebral edema with herniation, reflecting progression of increased intracranial pressure (ICP) (10%)
3. Cardiac dysrhythmia
4. Death (10%)

Ancillary Data

1. Plasma ammonia levels are usually greater than or equal to 1 times normal values

(normal: 40-80 µg/dl). Transiently present for 24 to 48 hours after the onset of mental status changes. A level above 300 µg/dl is associated with a poor prognosis.

2. Elevated serum transaminase levels (usually three times normal) and other liver function tests, osmolality, and amylase level. Normal or slightly elevated bilirubin level. Variable BUN and electrolyte levels. Decreased glucose level, particularly in children less than 4 years of age.

3. Decreased liver-dependent clotting factor (II, VII, IX, and X) levels, with prolonged prothrombin time and partial thromboplastin time. Fibrinogen level may be decreased. Normal platelets.

4. Arterial blood gas (ABG), lumbar puncture (assuming no evidence of increased ICP), blood cultures, and toxicology screen to exclude other potential causes and to monitor the patient.

5. Computed tomography (CT) scan to exclude intracranial lesions (e.g., abscess) if diagnosis is uncertain. Scan demonstrates cerebral edema.

6. Percutaneous liver biopsy may be useful in patients with an atypical presentation, including infants less than 1 year in recurrent episodes and familial cases, and in nonepidemic cases without an antecedent infection or vomiting.

DIFFERENTIAL DIAGNOSIS (see Chapter 15)

1. Infection
   a. Meningitis/encephalitis (p. 725)
   b. Sepsis
   c. Viral: chickenpox or hepatitis
2. Endocrine/metabolic disorders
   a. Hypoglycemia (see Chapter 38)
   b. Hypoxia
   c. Amino/organic-acid inborn errors of metabolism
3. Intoxication: salicylates, acetaminophen, ethanol, lead, camphor (see Table 54-2)
4. Trauma: head
5. Vascular: intracranial hemorrhage

MANAGEMENT

1. General supportive care is crucial in determining the ultimate outcome. Dehydration may be present but should not be fully corrected because of the concurrent cerebral edema. Serum glucose level should be kept between 125 and 175 mg/dl, with a serum osmolality less than 310 mOsm/kg water.

2. Stages I and II require frequent monitoring of vital and neurologic signs, IV infusion of D10W-D20W, and correction of fluid and electrolyte abnormalities.

3. Stages III-V require aggressive support and intervention:
   a. Supportive measures
      (1) Monitoring of venous and arterial pressures; NG tube; and urinary catheter for intake and output measurement
      (2) Respiratory support including intubation, mechanical ventilation, and hyperventilation, if indicated
      (3) IV infusion of D15W at two-thirds maintenance after cardiovascular stabilization to maintain urine output at 1 ml/kg/hr
      (4) Seizure control: phenytoin (Dilantin) loading of 10-20 mg/kg/dose, with maintenance at 5 mg/kg/24 hr q6hr IV; does not cause sedation; monitor level
      (5) Control of temperature
   b. Metabolic abnormalities. Maintenance of glucose between 125 and 175 mg/ dl, using glucose and insulin (1 unit/5 gm of glucose given) infusion.
   c. For coagulation abnormalities:
      (1) Fresh-frozen plasma, 10 ml/kg/ dose q12-24hr IV or prn
      (2) Vitamin K, 1-10 mg/dose IV slowly
      (3) Exchange transfusion rarely indicated
   d. Intracranial monitoring to measure efficacy of a number of therapeutic modalities. Maintain ICP 15 to 18 mm Hg or less and cerebral perfusion

pressure (CPP) greater than 50 mm Hg. Measures may be tried individually or concurrently, depending on patient response.

(1) Mannitol, 0.25-0.5 gm/kg/dose IV infusion over 20 minutes. May repeat q2hr as needed. Monitor osmolality of serum, keeping below 210 mOsm/kg water.

(2) Hyperventilation to maintain $Paco_2$ at 25 mm Hg.

(3) Furosemide (Lasix), 1-2 mg/kg/dose q4-6hr IV.

(4) Head elevation.

(5) Muscular paralysis: pancuronium (Pavulon), 0.05-0.1 mg/kg/dose q1-2hr prn IV. Patient must be intubated with respiratory support.

(6) Pentobarbital (Nembutal), 3-20 mg/kg, by IV slowly while monitoring blood pressure. Maintain level at 25-40 µg/dl by maintenance infusion of 1-2 mg/kg/hr. Barbiturate coma is maintained for 2 to 3 days while monitoring other parameters if alternative approaches have not been successful (see Chapter 57).

4. Treat complications.

DISPOSITION

All patients require admission to an intensive care unit (ICU) capable of intracranial monitoring. Appropriate consultation should be sought.

REFERENCES

Committee on Infectious Diseases (AAP): Aspirin and Reye's syndrome, *Pediatrics* 69:810, 1982.

Hurwitz ES, Barrett MJ, Bregman D, et al: Public health service study on Reye's syndrome and medications, *N Engl J Med* 313:849, 1985.

Orlowski JP, Gillis J, Killam HA: A catch in the Reye, *Pediatrics* 80:638, 1987.

Rogers MF, Schonberger LB, Hurwitz ES, et al: National Reye's syndrome surveillance, *Pediatrics* 75:260, 1985.

Conditions Requiring Surgery

APPENDICITIS

ALERT: Severe RLQ pain requires urgent surgical consultation.

Diagnostic Findings

Clinical symptoms and signs vary, depending on the degree of inflammation and whether perforation has occurred. The hydration status of the patient may also affect the clinical presentation; most patients are 5% to 10% dehydrated. Patients classically have a low-grade fever and loss of appetite. Symptoms progress to include pain followed by vomiting.

1. The crampy abdominal pain initially is periumbilical but gradually shifts to the RLQ over the ensuing 4 to 12 hours. Tenderness is maximal over the McBurney point, located 4 to 6 cm from the iliac crest, along the line drawn between the iliac crest and the umbilicus. The patient is most comfortable in the supine position with the legs flexed. With rupture of the appendix, there is initial pain relief but subsequent worsening as a result of peritonitis.

2. RLQ guarding and rebound are present. Bowel sounds may be diminished. With perforation, there is less localization and more generalized peritoneal signs are present.

3. Rectal examination may demonstrate tenderness, greatest on the right.

4. Psoas sign: With the patient in the left lateral decubitus position, pain is elicited by passive extension of the right thigh. This suggests abdominal or pelvic peritoneal inflammation.

5. Obturator sign: With the patient in the supine position, pain is produced by flexion and internal rotation of the right thigh. This suggests pelvic inflammation.

6. In children less than 2 years of age, the diagnosis is particularly difficult because

of the nonspecific nature of the clinical picture. The morbidity rate is high because about 90% of such patients are not diagnosed until perforation has occurred. About one third of these patients have been seen by a physician 24 to 48 hours before admission.

a. Vomiting, lethargy or irritability, crying spells, and feeding problems are noted.

b. Concurrent illness (URI, otitis media, or gastroenteritis) may confuse the diagnostic picture.

c. The abdomen is diffusely tender, with decreased or absent bowel sounds, guarding, and tenderness on rectal examination. Patients are febrile and urinary retention may occur.

d. Tachypnea with short respiratory excursions may result from diaphragmatic irritation by peritonitis.

7. Mantrel's score may have some value:

Migration of pain to RLQ	1
Anorexia or acetone in urine	1
Nausea/vomiting	1
Tenderness to RLQ	2
Rebound tenderness	1
Elevated temperature	1
Leukocytosis (WBC >10,000/mm³)	2
Shift to left of WBC (>75% neutrophils)	1

A score of 7 or higher is highly suspicious; 5 to 6 indicates the patient should be observed and followed closely; 4 or less has a low likelihood of appendicitis. Further study is still needed of this scoring system.

Complications

1. Peritonitis. Perforation is associated with delay in treatment and with younger children.
2. Intraabdominal or pelvic abscess.
3. Ileus or obstruction.
4. Pyelophlebitis.
5. Sepsis and shock.

Ancillary Data

1. WBC. Elevated above $15,000/mm^3$ in about 40% of patients, with 93% having a shift to the left (percentage of neutrophils: >50% for 1- to 5-year-old children, >65% for 5- to 10-year-old children, and >75% for 10 to 15-year-old children).

2. C-reactive protein (CRP) may be useful. An increase of 1 mg/dl or more on the second CRP after 4 to 12 hours of observation is reliable. A CRP of more than 6 mg/dl is suggestive.

3. Urinalysis. May demonstrate minimal pyuria secondary to ureteral irritation (must exclude UTI). It also will assist in assessment of hydration.

4. Chest x-ray film to exclude pneumonia, particularly lower lobe.

5. Abdominal x-ray film (three-way view includes supine and upright abdomen and anteroposterior [AP] chest).
   a. Abnormal gas pattern with decreased gas, air-fluid levels, or diffuse small-bowel dilation
   b. Free peritoneal air
   c. Thickening of abdominal wall
   d. Appendolith (about 10% of cases)
   e. Abscess in RLQ
   f. Scoliosis
   g. Obliteration of psoas muscle margin

6. Ultrasonography. Increasingly used to confirm the diagnosis of abscess by experienced clinicians. Studies have demonstrated it to be 89% to 94% specific and 85% to 94% sensitive. It is operator dependent.

7. CT scan is a useful adjunct and is equally specific to ultrasonography.

8. Barium enema may on occasion be useful as a diagnostic modality to demonstrate other pathologic conditions.

9. Laparoscopy. Indicated for patients with relative contraindications to surgery and an equivocal examination. Videoscopic surgery is widely used for definitive removal of the appendix.

TABLE 76-3   Right Lower Quadrant Pain: Diagnostic Considerations

	Infection/inflammation	Neoplasm	Congenital
Systemic	Influenza		
Skin	Herpes zoster Cellulitis		
Abdominal wall			Inguinal hernia
Pulmonary	Pneumonia		
Gastrointestinal tract	**Mesenteric adenitis** **Gastroenteritis** (*Salmonella,* *Shigella, Yersinia,* typhoid) **Appendicitis** Peritonitis Meckel's diverticulum Cholecystitis Duodenal ulcer Hepatitis	Hodgkin's disease Carcinoma	Intussusception Obstruction Meckel's diverticulum
Kidney/ureter	**Pyelonephritis** **Cystitis** Perinephritic abscess	Wilms' tumor	Hydronephrosis
Reproductive tract	**Pelvic inflammatory disease** **Salpingitis** Tuboovarian Pelvic abscess	Endometriosis	Testicular torsion
Spine	Osteomyelitis		

Differential Diagnosis (Table 76-3)

Children who are misdiagnosed as having appendicitis are more likely to have had pain of more than 2 days' duration and a temperature above 38.3° C and to appear lethargic and irritable. The accuracy of the diagnosis is increased by admitting and observing children who have equivocal findings on examination.

Management

1. Focus initial management on stabilization of the patient.
   a. IV hydration, initially with 20 ml/kg of D5W 0.9% normal saline (NS) solution or D5W lactated Ringer's (LR) solution over 1 hour if any deficit exists (see Chapter 7)
   b. NG tube; patient NPO
   c. Oxygen if the patient is in marked distress
   d. Lowering of temperature by cooling blanket or antipyretics
2. Involve surgical consultant early.
3. If any evidence of peritonitis or perforation exists, begin antibiotics:
   a. Ampicillin, 100-200 mg/kg/24 hr q4hr IV; *and*
   b. Clindamycin, 30-40 mg/kg/24 hr q6hr IV; *and*
   c. Gentamicin, 5.0-7.5 mg/kg/24 hr q8hr IV or IM. Cefoxitin (Mefoxin), 80-160 mg/kg/24 hr q4-6hr IV, is used by some surgeons.
4. Give analgesia, if necessary, but only after the diagnosis is certain and the decision to operate has been made: meperidine

Autoimmune	Trauma	Intrapsychic	Vascular	Endocrine/metabolic
	Black widow spider bite	Functional		Diabetic ketoacidosis
				Acute prophyria
	Contusion			
	Muscle rupture			
Regional enteritis	**Impacted feces**		Mesenteric infarct	
Ulcerative colitis				
				Renal calculi
				Mittelschmerz
				Dysmenorrhea
				Ovarian cyst
				Threatened abortion
				Ectopic pregnancy

(Demerol), 1-2 mg/kg/dose IM (maximum: 50-100 mg/dose)

5. Perform surgery.

Disposition

All patients require admission for surgical management.

Patients for whom the diagnosis is uncertain may often benefit from 12 to 24 hours of observation to allow the disease to progress and define itself.

REFERENCES

Balthazar EJ, Binbaum BA, Yer J, et al: Acute appendicitis: CT and ultrasound correlation in 100 patients, *Radiology* 190:31, 1994.

Bond GR, Tully SB, et al: Use of Mantrel's score in childhood appendicitis: a prospective study of 187 children with abdominal pain, *Ann Emerg Med* 19:1014, 1990.

Brender JD, Marcuse EK, Koepsell TD, et al: Childhood appendicitis: factors associated with perforation, *Pediatrics* 76:301, 1985.

Chen SC: C-reactive protein in the diagnosis of acute appendicitis, *Am J Emerg Med* 14:101, 1996.

Crady SK, Jones JS, Wyn T, et al: Clinical validity of ultrasound in children with suspected appendicitis, *Ann Emerg Med* 22:1125, 1993.

Dickson AP, MacKinley GA: Rectal examination and acute appendicitis, *Arch Dis Child* 60:666, 1985.

Garcia C, Rosenfeld NS, Markowitz RI, et al: Appendicitis in children: accuracy of barium enema, *Am J Dis Child* 141:1309, 1987.

Northrock SG, Skeach G, Rush JJ: Clinical features of misdiagnosed appendicitis in children, *Ann Emerg Med* 20:45, 1991.

Vignault F, Filiatrault D, Brandt ML, et al: Acute appendicitis in children: evaluation with ultrasound, *Pediatr Radiol* 176:501, 1990.

Zoltie N, Cust MP: Analgesia in the acute abdomen, *Ann R Coll Surg Engl* 68:209, 1986.

Hernia, Inguinal (SEE P. 662)

ALERT: Although repair of an inguinal hernia is done electively, incarceration requires urgent surgery.

Inguinal hernias in children represent 37% of all surgical procedures in the pediatric age group. The hernia results from the failure of the processus vaginalis to obliterate in males and the canal of Nuck to close in females. Right-sided (60%) hernias are more common than left-sided (30%) hernias; 10% are bilateral.

An increased incidence of inguinal hernias is associated with increases in peritoneal fluid volume (ventriculoperitoneal shunt, peritoneal dialysis, ascites), abdominal tumors, genitourinary abnormalities (exstrophy of bladder, hypospadias, epispadias), connective tissue disorders, mucopolysaccharides, cystic fibrosis, and intersex syndromes.

DIAGNOSTIC FINDINGS

Parents report a bulge or mass in the groin that enlarges with crying and Valsalva maneuver. A smooth, firm, sausage-shaped nontender or slightly tender mass can be seen and palpated in the groin. During reduction, there is a gurgling or "swoosh" sound.

The hernia is usually reduced before being seen. A "silk glove" sign may be noted by rubbing the index finger over the spermatic cord at the pubic tubercle. A slippery feel similar to that of two layers of silk rubbing together is noted.

The hernia may incarcerate or become strangulated, resulting in signs and symptoms of intestinal obstruction. Perforation may also occur.

DIFFERENTIAL DIAGNOSIS

1. Hydrocele is an outpocketing of the peritoneum and lack of complete obliteration of the processus vaginalis. The transillumination finding is positive. A communicating hydrocele changes in size and is associated with an inguinal hernia. Hydroceles usually resolve by 1 year of age (see p. 662).
2. Lymphadenopathy.
3. An undescended or high-riding testicle may retract spontaneously.
4. Urologic problems, including testicular torsion and epididymitis, may occur.

MANAGEMENT

If evidence of intestinal obstruction or perforation exists, immediate intervention is required in stabilization and preparation for surgery.

Hernias that are easily reduced should be scheduled for semielective surgery. Discharge and close follow-up observation can be arranged after careful instructions related to recognition of incarceration or strangulation and the need for immediate intervention are provided.

Incarcerated hernias that do not easily reduce spontaneously should have gentle, persistent pressure applied. If this does not work, place the patient in a Trendelenburg position with cold compresses over the inguinal area. Sedatives may also be used. Surgical consultation should be initiated for repair. Patients are usually admitted for observation and early surgery.

Strangulated hernias cannot be reduced and require immediate surgical intervention.

REFERENCE
Sparnon AL, Kiely EM, Spitz L: Incarcerated inguinal hernia in infants, *BMJ* 293:376, 1986.

Hirschsprung's Disease
James C. Mitchiner

ALERT: Intestinal obstruction in the newborn or infant requires a careful and expeditious evaluation.

Hirschsprung's disease or congenital megacolon results from congenital aganglionosis of the distal colon and rectum, leading to failure of effective peristalsis through the aganglionic segment. It is the most common cause of partial intestinal obstruction in early infancy and occasionally in childhood.

DIAGNOSTIC FINDINGS

Neonates may fail to pass meconium in the first 24 hours of life. They also may be constipated, often not until 2 to 3 weeks of age. Paradoxically, diarrhea caused by mucosal ulcerations in the proximal dilated segment may develop. Vomiting and failure to thrive may occur.

Bowel obstruction usually is present, with a distended, tympanitic abdomen, hyperactive or high-pitched bowel sounds, and a history of vomiting. Rectal examination reveals an absence of stool in the ampulla, often followed by evacuation of gas and liquid stool after the examiner's finger is withdrawn.

Complications

1. Acute necrotizing enterocolitis secondary to *Clostridium difficile* with cecal perforation, rectal bleeding, pneumoperitoneum, and pericolic abscess
2. Acute appendicitis
3. Malnutrition
4. Reversible urinary tract obstruction (hydronephrosis, hydroureter, and recurrent UTIs)
5. Septicemia, particularly in newborns

Ancillary Data

1. CBC and electrolytes as indicated by clinical condition.
2. Abdominal x-ray film. May show distended, gas-filled proximal segment. May be normal.
3. Barium enema. Shows a normal diameter in the aganglionic segment associated with a dilated proximal segment tapering at the rectosigmoid. Once the dilated segment is defined, it is not necessary to com-

plete the study and, in fact, it may be dangerous. A postevacuation film taken 12 to 48 hours later shows residual barium.
4. Rectal biopsy. Ideally performed in the stable patient whose diagnosis is uncertain; often follows an equivocal barium enema and is performed proximal to the anorectal junction, 2 to 3 cm above the rectal columns. Specimen must be of sufficient depth to include both the mucosal and muscular layers for proper diagnosis. General anesthesia is usually necessary. Acetylcholinesterase activity, which is high in Hirschsprung's disease, should be obtained from the biopsy material.
5. Manometry demonstrates paradoxic contraction of the internal anal sphincter.

DIFFERENTIAL DIAGNOSIS

1. Congenital disorders:
   a. Colonic or ileal atresia
   b. Hypoplastic left colon syndrome
2. Infection/inflammation: neonatal sepsis, megacolon, necrotizing enterocolitis, ulcerative colitis.
3. Endocrine disorders: hypothyroidism and adrenal insufficiency.
4. Trauma: anal fissure.
5. Intoxication: drug-induced hypomotility (anticholinergics, narcotics).
6. *Acquired constipation* usually occurs after 2 years of age, with associated incontinence, abdominal pain, and obstruction. Stools usually are large in caliber, with increased stool in the ampulla. Barium enema shows a diffuse megacolon.

   In contrast, Hirschsprung's disease may occur in the newborn period with symptoms of failure to thrive but only rarely with associated incontinence or abdominal pain. The stool is thin and ribbonlike, with decreased frequency and little stool in the ampulla. Barium enema demonstrates a localized constriction with proximal dilation.

MANAGEMENT

1. Initial hydration and gastric decompression with an NG tube to suction are essential in the management of acute obstruction.
   a. Fluids: D5W 0.9% NS solution at 20 ml/kg over the first hour, then deficit and maintenance replacement
   b. With evidence of obstruction: institution of NG decompression
   c. Surgical consultation
2. After stabilization, a barium enema is indicated if enterocolitis and perforation are not present and, if suggestive, a rectal biopsy performed by a pediatric surgeon or gastroenterologist.
3. In general, surgery is the definitive treatment if the biopsy shows no ganglion cells and high acetylcholinesterase (ACE) activity.
   a. The goal is to place normal ganglion-containing bowel within 1 cm of the anal opening.
   b. Acute surgical therapy decompresses the bowel obstruction by a loop colostomy. The stoma must contain normal bowel.
   c. After the colostomy, the bowel can be adequately cleansed and definitive procedure done electively at a later date.
   d. Staging is unnecessary in a relatively well child.

REFERENCES

Doig CM: Hirschsprung's disease and mimicking conditions, *Dig Dis* 12:106, 1994.

Foster P, Cowan P, Wrenn EL Jr: Twenty-five years of experience with Hirschsprung's disease, *J Pediatr Surg* 25:531, 1990.

Hendren WH, Lillehei CW: Pediatric surgery, *N Engl J Med* 319:86, 1988.

Sullivan PB: Hirschsprung's disease, *Arch Dis Child* 74:5, 1996.

Vinton NE: Gastrointestinal bleeding in infancy and childhood, *Gastroint Clin North Am* 23:93, 1994.

Worman S, Ganiats TG: Hirschsprung's disease: a cause of chronic constipation in children, *Am Fam Physician* 51:487, 1995.

INTUSSUSCEPTION

James C. Mitchiner

ALERT: Classic signs of abdominal pain, vomiting, and bloody stool with mucus are not always present. Altered mental status may be noted.

Intussusception occurs when the proximal bowel invaginates into the distal bowel, resulting in infarction and gangrene of the inner bowel. It commonly occurs in children less than 1 year of age and is usually of the ileocolic type.

A lead point is more commonly found in older children with conditions such as Meckel's diverticulum, polyp, duplication, lymphoma, lymphoid hyperplasia, foreign body, cystic fibrosis, Henoch-Schönlein purpura, or after surgery.

DIAGNOSTIC FINDINGS

1. Classically, patients have an acute onset of intermittent fits of sudden intense pain with screaming and flexion of the legs. The episodes occur in 5- to 20-minute intervals. Vomiting, often bilious, commonly occurs, accompanied by passage of blood and mucus ("currant jelly stool") via the rectum. This classic triad is present in less than half of patients. Not all patients have gross or occult blood.
2. The abdomen is often distended and swollen, with a palpable mass and absent cecum in the right iliac fossa. Peristaltic waves may be present. The rectal and bimanual examinations may reveal bloody stool and a palpable mass.
3. Altered mental status may occur, marked by lethargy, behavioral changes, irritability, somnolence, and listlessness. These changes may precede abdominal findings and must be viewed as an important finding in this condition.

Complications

1. Perforation of bowel with peritonitis
2. Shock and sepsis
3. Reintussusception

Ancillary Data

1. Abdominal x-ray film results are positive in 35% to 40% of patients.
   a. Decreased bowel gas and fecal material in the right colon
   b. An abdominal mass
   c. The apex of the intussusception outlined by gas
   d. Small-bowel distension and air-fluid levels secondary to mechanical obstruction
2. Barium enema is both diagnostic and therapeutic and is up to 75% successful at achieving reduction.
   a. The success of reduction may partially reflect the duration: 32% of enemas were therapeutic when present more than 24 hours, whereas the success rate was 74% when the intussusception had been present for a shorter duration. The more distal the intussusception, the lower the ability to reduce it radiographically.
   b. A nonlubricated catheter is inserted into the rectum. Under fluoroscopic observation the barium solution flows, filling by means of gravity. The intussusception is identified, and reduction is manifested by free filling of the small intestine proximal to the point of obstruction. The procedure should be performed only by an experienced radiologist after surgical consultation.
   c. Up to three attempts of 3 minutes each may be tried. Sedation of the patient may be helpful in successfully performing the procedure. The abdomen should not be palpated or compressed during the study. Hydrostatic studies

have also been successful in achieving reduction.
   d. Of patients with intussusception, 97% have no lead point. More than two thirds of those with an identifiable lesion were in children older than 2 years.
   e. Contraindications to performing a barium enema include necrotic, gangrenous bowel, abdominal free air, peritonitis or an unstable patient with shock, anemia, or acidosis.
3. Ultrasonography may be useful as a noninvasive screening technique to evaluate intussusception.
   a. Sensitivity is 100% and specificity is as high as 98%.
   b. The typical appearance is a "donut" structure, with a hyperechoic core surrounded by a hypoechoic rim of homogeneous thickness.
   c. Interpretation is highly operator dependent.

DIFFERENTIAL DIAGNOSIS (see Chapters 24 and 35)

1. Infection
   a. Acute gastroenteritis
   b. Appendicitis
2. Infantile colic
3. Intestinal obstruction or peritonitis (e.g., volvulus, postoperative complication, tumor)
4. Incarcerated hernia
5. Testicular torsion

MANAGEMENT

1. Once intussusception is suspected, patients should have an IV line established and rehydration initiated. A bolus of D5W 0.9% NS, at 20 ml/kg, over 45 to 60 minutes should be given and repeated if there is any evidence of a deficit.

2. Surgical consultation should be obtained.
3. An abdominal x-ray film series should be taken and, if indicated, a barium enema.
4. If the barium enema is successful at reducing the intussusception, the patient should be hospitalized for observation because of the risk of recurrence and for continuous IV therapy. Because a small risk of perforation of the necrotic bowel also exists, the child should be observed by serial physical examinations and monitoring of vital signs and WBC.
5. Surgery is indicated immediately if the barium enema is unsuccessful or contraindicated. If evidence of peritonitis or perforation is present, initiate antibiotics, including ampicillin, 100-200 mg/kg/24 hr q4-6hr IV, and clindamycin, 30-40 mg/kg/24 hr q6hr IV, and gentamicin, 5.0-7.5 mg/kg/24 hr q8hr IV, before surgery. Some surgeons use cefoxitin (Mefoxin), 80-160 mg/kg/24 hr q4-6hr IV. Adults and children more than 4 years of age commonly need surgery because of the high incidence of pathologic lead points.

REFERENCES

Bhisitku DM, Listernick R, Shkolnik A, et al: Clinical application of ultrasonography in the diagnosis of intussusception, *J Pediatr* 121:182, 1992.

Collins DL, Pinckney LE, Miller KE, et al: Hydrostatic reduction of ileocolic intussusception: a second attempt in the operating room with general anesthesia, *J Pediatr* 115:204, 1989.

Hickey RW, Sodhi SK, Johnson WR: Two children with lethargy and intussusception, *Ann Emerg Med* 19:390, 1990.

Little KJ, Danzyl DF: Intussusception associated with Henoch-Schönlein purpura, *J Emerg Med* 9:29, 1991.

Losek JD: Intussusception: don't miss the diagnosis, *Pediatr Emerg Care* 9:46, 1993.

Losek JD, Fiete RL: Intussusception and the diagnostic value of testing stool for occult blood, *Am J Emerg Med* 9:1, 1991.

McCabe JB, et al: Intussusception: a supplement to the mnemonic for coma, *Pediatr Emerg Care* 3:118, 1987.

Ong NT, Beasley DW: The leadpoint in intussusception, *J Pediatr Surg* 25:640, 1990.

Rachmel A, Rosenbach Y, Amir J, et al: Apathy as an early manifestation of intussusception, *Am J Dis Child* 137:701, 1983.

Stein M, Alton DJ, Daneman A: Pneumatic reduction of intussusception: 5-year experience, *Radiology* 183:681, 1992.

Stephenson CA, Seibert JJ, Strain JD, et al: Intussusception: clinical and radiographic factors influencing reducibility, *Pediatr Radiol* 20:57, 1989.

Vinton NE: Gastrointestinal bleeding in infancy and childhood, *Gastroenterol Clin North Am* 23:93, 1994.

Winslow BT, Westfall JM, Nicholas RA: Intussusception, *Am Fam Physician* 54:213, 1996.

MECKEL'S DIVERTICULUM

James C. Mitchiner

ALERT: Meckel's diverticulum must be considered in patients with rectal bleeding or RLQ pain.

Meckel's diverticulum is the most common congenital malformation of the GI tract, resulting from the persistence of the omphalomesenteric duct remnant. Symptomatic diverticula usually contain gastric mucosa and are proximal to the ileocecal valve. Most cases occur by 2 years of age, a third of which are symptomatic during infancy.

DIAGNOSTIC FINDINGS

1. Although many patients remain asymptomatic with a diverticulum, patients with diverticulitis have crampy, RLQ abdominal pain associated with nausea, vomiting, and anorexia. Symptoms are caused by narrowing of the diverticular mouth as a result of peptic strictures, fecal material, granulomas, foreign bodies, tumors, etc.
2. Perforation may be present, associated with abdominal guarding, decreased bowel sounds, and fever.
3. Obstruction produces distension with abdominal pain.

4. Lower GI hemorrhage may be present in 40% of patients with Meckel's diverticulum. Children have painless rectal bleeding, which may be episodic. The stool blood is usually bright red or dark but rarely tarry. Anemia may be present.

Complications

1. Small bowel obstruction, often from obstruction of the ileum, is the most common complication. Causes include intussusception of the diverticulum into the ileum and volvulus.
2. Massive GI bleeding.
3. Perforation of the diverticulum with peritonitis.
4. Diverticular hernia (Littre's hernia). The diverticulum may present as either a femoral or inguinal hernia.

Ancillary Data

1. WBC count is often elevated and the hematocrit (Hct) decreased if significant bleeding has occurred.
2. Stool has bright red or dark red blood.
3. Abdominal x-ray examinations are not diagnostic but may demonstrate free air if perforation has occurred or distension and air-fluid levels when obstruction is present.
4. Radionuclide scan, with sodium technetium pertechnetate to identify ectopic gastric mucosa, is diagnostic. False-positive x-ray findings are rare, whereas false-negative x-ray findings may occur in as many as 30% of cases. In children, it has a sensitivity of 85% and a specificity of 95%. Diagnostic accuracy may be improved with the addition of pentagastrin, which stimulates metabolism of the ectopic gastric mucosa, and cimetidine, which enhances retention of radionuclide in the mucoid cells.

DIFFERENTIAL DIAGNOSIS

1. Rectal bleeding, most commonly resulting from intestinal polyps, intussusception, volvulus, and anal fissures (see Chapter 35)
2. RLQ pain: appendicitis (p. 648)
3. Small bowel obstruction caused by intussusception or volvulus
4. Other causes of peritonitis

MANAGEMENT

1. Depending on the degree of rectal bleeding and obstruction, patients may require resuscitation and blood products. An NG tube should be inserted for gastric decompression.
2. A rapid evaluation of the patient, including a surgical consultation, is usually required.
   a. Laboratory studies (CBC, electrolytes, glucose, blood, type and crossmatch, and urinalysis) should be rapidly obtained.
   b. If the cause of the bleeding is uncertain, a rapid radiologic evaluation of the patient should be completed, including abdominal flat plate, sigmoidoscopy, technetium scan, and barium enema, depending on likely causes and the patient's clinical status.
3. If evidence of peritonitis or perforation is present, IV antibiotics should be initiated; with a combination of ampicillin, 100-200 mg/kg/24 hr q4-6hr IV; and clindamycin, 30-40 mg/kg/24 q6hr IV; and gentamicin, 5.0-7.5 mg/kg/24 hr q8hr IV. Some surgeons use cefoxitin (Mefoxin), 80-160 mg/kg/24 hr q-6hr IV.
4. Surgical laparotomy is the definitive diagnostic and therapeutic procedure. A wedge diverticulectomy, which includes excision of the diverticulum and a wedge of ileum, should be performed in most symptomatic cases.

DISPOSITION

1. All patients should be admitted for evaluation and treatment.
2. A surgical consultation is required.

REFERENCES

Brown CK, Olshaker JS: Meckel's diverticulum, *Am J Emerg Med* 6:157, 1988.

Kilpatrick ZM, Aseron CA: Isotope detection of Meckel's diverticulum causing acute rectal hemorrhage, *N Engl J Med* 287:653, 1972.

Mackey WC, Direen P: A fifty-year experience with Meckel's diverticulum, *Surg Gynecol Obstet* 156:56, 1983.

Rossi P, Gourtsoyiannis N, Bezzi M, et al: Meckel's diverticulum: imaging diagnosis, *AJR Am J Roentgenol* 144:567, 1996.

Rutherford RB, Akers DR: Meckel's diverticulum: a review of 148 pediatric patients, with special reference to the pattern of bleeding and to mesodiverticular vascular bands, *Surgery* 59:618, 1966.

Vinton NE: Gastrointestinal bleeding in infancy and childhood, *Gastroenterol Clin North Am* 23:93, 1994.

PYLORIC STENOSIS

Ronald D. Lindzon

ALERT: Pyloric stenosis should be suspected in neonates 3 to 6 weeks old with postprandial, nonbilious vomiting. Projectile vomiting is not always present.

Hypertrophic pyloric stenosis results from hypertrophy and hyperplasia of the circular antral and pyloric musculature, resulting in gastric outlet obstruction. Although it has been reported in infants from birth to 5 months, it most commonly occurs at 3 to 4 weeks of life. White males are more frequently affected, and there is a familial incidence.

DIAGNOSTIC FINDINGS

1. Gradual onset of vomiting between 3 and 4 weeks is common. This progresses to become forceful or projectile, nonbilious emesis. An associated esophagogastritis is present in 20% of children, producing blood-tinged vomitus. The child is hungry and easily refed. Constipation is common.
2. Visible peristaltic waves may be observed traveling from the left upper to the right upper quadrant. These are best visualized postprandially and before emesis.
3. A palpable pyloric "olive" or tumor is present below the liver edge and just lateral to the right rectus abdominis muscle. It is best felt after emesis or when an NG tube has been placed on low intermittent suction.
4. Dehydration with varying degrees of lethargy may be present. This is often a hypochloremic alkalosis.
5. Jaundice may be present (8%) as a result of glucuronyl transferase deficiency. It clears after surgery.

Complications

1. Dehydration with metabolic alkalosis and, in rare cases, shock
2. Esophagitis, gastritis, or gastric ulceration, with upper GI hemorrhage or perforation
3. Failure to thrive and secondary neurologic sequelae

Ancillary Data

1. Electrolyte, BUN, and glucose determinations to evaluate hydration and nutrition. Bilirubin evaluation if patient has jaundice. CBC to exclude infection.
2. X-ray film.
   a. Abdominal plain film demonstrates gastric dilation.
   b. Barium swallow is indicated if suspected diagnosis is unconfirmed by physical examination. It reveals "string" or "beak" sign (fine elongated pyloric canal) and delayed gastric emptying. Rarely is pyloric obstruction complete.
   c. Abdominal ultrasonography provides reliable confirmation on the basis of the anatomy of the pylorus.

DIFFERENTIAL DIAGNOSIS (see Chapter 44)

1. Infection/inflammation
   a. Gastroenteritis or sepsis
   b. Esophagitis or gastritis
2. Endocrine disorders: adrenal insufficiency (adrenogenital syndrome)
3. Congenital disorders: hiatal hernia, intestinal obstruction, atresia, malrotation
4. Chalasia or poor feeding technique

MANAGEMENT

1. Once the diagnosis is considered, patients should have an IV line inserted and fluid deficits corrected. Initially give D5W 0.9% NS at 20 ml/kg IV over 30 to 60 minutes, and then compute deficit and maintenance replacements. Aggressive management of the inevitable hypokalemia is essential in correcting the electrolyte imbalance and alkalosis.
2. An NG tube should be inserted and placed on intermittent low suction.
3. Surgical consultation should be obtained early in the evaluation. Some surgeons feel comfortable performing a pyloromyotomy in symptomatic patients with a palpable pyloric mass without further evaluation.
4. Surgery is indicated once the fluid and electrolyte status is stable.
   a. In rare cases, conservative medical management has been attempted, but it results in prolonged hospitalization and significant morbidity.
   b. Pyloromyotomy is performed and is associated with low morbidity and mortality.

DISPOSITION

All patients require hospitalization and surgery.

REFERENCE

Breaux CW, Georgeson KE, Royal SA, et al: Changing patterns in the diagnosis of hypertrophic pyloric stenosis, *Pediatrics* 81:213, 1988.

VOLVULUS

ALERT: Acute onset of abdominal pain and obstruction in the child older than 1 year of age requires evaluation for volvulus.

Volvulus is a closed-loop obstruction with massive distension resulting from the twisting of a section of intestine on its own axis. Although uncommon in children, the rare cases that are reported occur in the first few days of life and between 2 and 14 years of age.

The condition may result from congenital malrotation, the presence of a long and freely mobile mesentery, Meckel's diverticulum, or surgical adhesions. It may occur without malrotation. Sigmoid volvulus is most often seen, although gastric (along axis joining lesser and greater curvatures), midgut, and transverse colon volvulus have been reported.

DIAGNOSTIC FINDINGS

1. Sudden onset of crampy abdominal pain, often greater in the lower quadrants, is common. In rare cases, patients have progressive or intermittent pain over several days or weeks, associated with sporadic twisting. Pain increases with worsening distension.
2. Marked intestinal obstruction is present with sigmoid volvulus, the degree reflecting the competency of the ileocecal valve. Tenderness is present, but guarding and peritoneal signs appear only if complications of peritonitis develop.
3. The rectum is empty of stool. Bloody stool is uncommon.
4. Anorexia and vomiting commonly occur.

Complications
1. Perforation with peritonitis
2. Dehydration

Ancillary Data
1. CBC and electrolytes
2. X-ray films

a. Abdominal films show dilated, gas-filled loops with colonic distension. No gas is present in the rectum.

b. Barium enema (very carefully performed) demonstrates in sigmoid volvulus that the sigmoid colon has a circular pattern and that barium stops at the junction of the sigmoid and left colon.

DIFFERENTIAL DIAGNOSIS

1. Congenital disorders
   a. Intussusception (usually occurs in children <1 year of age)
   b. Hirschsprung's disease
2. Inflammatory disorders
   a. Colitis with megacolon
   b. Peritonitis
3. Uremia

MANAGEMENT

1. Initial stabilization should provide for oxygen, replacement of fluid deficits, and surgical consultation.

2. If peritonitis is present, if it develops, or if reduction is not achieved, immediate surgical repair is necessary. Triple antibiotics should be initiated: ampicillin, 100-200 mg/kg/24 hr q4hr IV; and clindamycin, 30-40 mg/kg/24 hr q6hr; and gentamicin, 5.0-7.5 mg/kg/24 hr q8hr IV or IM.

3. The necessity for surgical repair on a semielective basis of a sigmoid volvulus in a child whose volvulus has been hydrostatically reduced is controversial. Children, in contrast to adults, have a decreased risk of recurrence.

REFERENCES

Leonidas JC, Magio N, Soberman N, et al: Midget volvulus in infants: diagnosis with ultrasound, *Radiology* 179:491, 1991.

Seashore JH, Touloukian RJ: Midget volvulus: an ever-present threat, *Arch Pediatric Adolesc Med* 148:43, 1994.

77 GENITOURINARY DISEASES

EPIDIDYMITIS

ALERT: Testicular torsion must be excluded in patients with testicular pain.

ETIOLOGY: INFECTION

1. Infection
   a. Commonly caused by *Neisseria gonorrhoeae* and *Chlamydia trachomatis*
   b. Uncommon organisms, especially important in younger age group; coliform and *Pseudomonas* bacteria
   c. Virus
2. Trauma
3. Chemical: reflux of sterile urine into ejaculatory duct
4. Systemic disease: Kawasaki syndrome, Henoch-Schönlein purpura, sarcoid
5. Idiopathic

DIAGNOSTIC FINDINGS

1. Usually, there is a gradual onset of scrotal and groin pain with edema.
2. Initially, the epididymis is tender and swollen, with a soft, normal testicle. This evolves to diffuse tenderness and edema of the epididymis and testicle, often involving the scrotal wall as well.
3. The patient may have a history of trauma, lifting, or heavy exercise.
4. Dysuria, frequency of urination, and urethral discharge may be present.

Ancillary Data

1. White blood cells (WBC) may be elevated.
2. Urinalysis and urine culture.
3. Gram stain and culture of urethral discharge.
4. Children less than 2 years and older patients with reflux should be investigated urologically.

DIFFERENTIAL DIAGNOSIS

See p. 664.

MANAGEMENT

The most important part of the management is to be certain of the diagnosis. If there is any question that a testicular torsion exists, immediate urologic consultation should be obtained.

1. For epididymitis, institute scrotal support, bed rest, and analgesia.
2. Start antibiotics (dose for boys >45 kg or 100 lb)
   a. Give amoxicillin, 3 gm PO once, *and* probenecid, 1 gm PO once, or ceftriaxone, 250 mg IM once.
   b. Follow (for boys >8 years of age) with tetracycline, 500 mg q6hr PO, or doxycycline, 100 mg q12hr PO, for 10 days. Children less than 9 years should receive erythromycin, 50 mg/kg/24 hr q6hr PO.
   c. If a specific organism is identified, alter antibiotics as appropriate.

DISPOSITION

Patients may be sent home with supportive care and antibiotics.

REFERENCES

Likitnukul S, McCracken AH, Nelson JD, et al: Epididymitis in children and adolescents, *Am J Dis Child* 141:41, 1987.

Turek PJ, et al: Normal epididymal anatomy in boys, *J Urol* 151:726, 1994.

HERNIAS AND HYDROCELES

HERNIAS (see p. 652)

Hernias result from persistence of the processus vaginalis.

Diagnostic Findings

Patients usually have intermittent, localized swelling in the groin or labia, sometimes accompanied by irritability, pain, abdominal tenderness, or limp.

1. Incarcerated hernias occur when the intestine becomes trapped in the sac, usually before 3 years of age.
2. Strangulated bowel has a compromised blood supply, leading to necrosis. It is tender and swollen, and the overlying skin is usually edematous with a red or violaceous color. It is rare in pediatric patients for the hernia to strangulate. However, in female patients the ovary or uterus may incarcerate, preventing easy reduction.
3. Intestinal obstruction may occur.

Management

1. Uncomplicated hernias may be repaired electively.
2. Incarcerated hernias can usually be reduced manually, after sedation, with gentle, prolonged pressure and elevation of the foot of the bed. Such patients should be hospitalized for observation and then urgent repair 12 to 24 hours after edema has resolved.
3. Strangulated hernias require immediate surgical intervention.

HYDROCELES

Hydroceles occur with closure of the processus vaginalis at the abdominal end and fluid accumulation in the sac.

Diagnostic Findings

1. The testicle appears large, surrounded by a fluid-filled sac. This usually resolves by 6 months of age. The sac is transilluminated.
2. If the size of the sac (or amount of fluid) changes from day to day, it is considered to communicate and is associated with a hernia.
3. A varicocele may exist, feeling like a collection of "worms."

Management

1. Noncommunicating hydroceles resolve by 6 months of age.
2. Communicating hydroceles or those that are still present at 12 months of age require surgical intervention for repair of the associated hernia.
3. Hydroceles of adolescents should be explored because of the potential for underlying neoplasm.

REFERENCE

Skoog SJ, Roberts KP, Goldstein M, et al: The adolescent varicocele: what's new with an old problem in young patients? *Radiation* 100:112, 1997.

PENILE DISORDERS

See also Chapter 64.

PHIMOSIS

Phimosis is a narrowing of the foreskin with an inability to retract the prepuce over the glans because of poor hygiene or chronic infection. Normally, retraction is possible by 4 years of age. If obstruction to urinary flow occurs, early circumcision (or dorsal slit) may be necessary.

PARAPHIMOSIS

Paraphimosis occurs when the foreskin retracts and is caught proximal to the coronal sulcus with subsequent swelling and venous congestion, potentially causing compromise of the vascular supply to the glans. It usually occurs with manipulation, masturbation, intercourse, or irritation.

After sedation, an ice and water mixture (usually in a rubber glove) is placed over the foreskin and glans for 3 to 4 minutes. With gentle, continuous, circumferential pressure on the glans for 5 minutes, the foreskin usually slips over. If the foreskin does not slip easily, the shaft of the penis should be held between the thumb and fingers of one hand (after 5 to 10 minutes of squeezing to reduce swelling) and the glans pushed down into the prepuce with a slow, steady pressure with the free thumb. Alternatively, the shaft may be held in both hands with the thumb on the glans and the foreskin pulled forward over the glans in a slow, steady motion. A dorsal slit with later circumcision rarely is indicated.

In newborns with a plastibell circumcision, the ring may slip behind the glans onto the shaft of the penis and cannot be slipped forward. In such event, an attempt should be made to reduce the swelling with cold compresses and steady continuous circumferential pressure. The ring also can be cut off.

BALANITIS

Balanitis is a chronic irritation and inflammation of the foreskin and glans, usually a result of poor hygiene. The foreskin is red and swollen with a collection of smegma. There is often a concurrent diaper dermatitis.

Hot baths and local care are usually sufficient for treatment.

CIRCUMCISION COMPLICATIONS

Newborn male circumcision is a reflection of cultural, religious, and family beliefs. Some advocate circumcision because of data that penile cancer and urinary tract infections (UTIs) may be reduced in incidence, as well as other penile disorders discussed earlier.

Intraoperative complications include hemorrhage, localized and systemic infection, Fournier syndrome, necrotizing fasciitis, and meatal problems (stenosis or ulcers). Hemorrhage is rare and usually controlled with pressure or application of silver nitrate. The plastibell device may restrict venous return or be retained past 10 days, in which case it should be removed.

Other nonacute problems may cause skin excess/asymmetry/redundancy, concealed penis, skin bridges or chordae, and meatal abnormalities.

REFERENCE

Baskin LS, Canning DA, Snyder HM, et al: Treating complications of circumcision, *Pediatr Emerg Care* 12:62, 1996.

TESTICULAR TORSION

ALERT: Acute onset of testicular pain and tenderness requires immediate urologic consultation.

ETIOLOGY

1. Congenital. A freely mobile testis suspended on a long mesorchium ("bell clapper") is usually present bilaterally.
2. Trauma. Scrotal trauma or exercise may precede the torsion, but torsion can occur at rest or may awaken the patient from sleep.

DIAGNOSTIC FINDINGS

Intermittent or constant testicular pain, which is sudden and intense in onset, occurs. Rarely, it may be gradual in onset with progression of severity. The testicle is tender, high riding, and often horizontal. Scrotal edema is present. The contralateral testis often has a horizontal axis. Nausea and vomiting often accompany the testicular pain.

The peak incidence is in 3-year-old children, and it is uncommon after the age of 30 years.

Complications

Testicular necrosis will occur within 6 to 8 hours of torsion.

Ancillary Data

1. Doppler examination of the testicle demonstrates decreased pulsatile flow in the affected testicle. Normally, flow is equal in both testicles.
2. Technetium nuclear scan has decreased perfusion and is 90% sensitive and specific for testicular torsion but should not delay surgery inordinately. It is less accurate in children less than 10 years of age.

DIFFERENTIAL DIAGNOSIS

Diagnostic considerations must be rapidly excluded in evaluating the patient with testicular pain. Table 77-1 summarizes significant findings.

TABLE 77-1   Testicular Pain: Diagnostic Considerations

Condition	Diagnostic findings	Ancillary data
TESTICULAR TORSION	Sudden onset; may follow trauma or occur during sleep or vehicle ride; nausea, vomiting Physical examination: tender testicle with horizontal lie; abdominal or flank pain; palpable cord twist Peak incidence 13 years of age; uncommon in those over 30 years of age	Urine: normal Technetium scan: decreased activity Doppler examination: decreased flow
TRAUMA	Sudden onset with history of trauma Physical examination: pain and swelling of testicle; hematoma may be present; findings reflect injury	Urine: normal Technetium scan: variable Doppler examination: variable
EPIDIDYMITIS	Usually gradual onset; uncommon in boys before puberty; groin pain; may be associated with trauma, lifting, exercise; recent instrumentation Physical examination: tender epididymis present early with a soft normal testicle whereas later, diffuse tenderness of epididymis and testicle is noted; febrile; prostatic tenderness	Urine: pyuria, bacteriuria Technetium scan: increased activity Dopper examination: normal or increased flow
TUMOR	Gradual onset unless hemorrhage Physical examination: hard, irregular, and usually painless testicle	Urine: normal Technetium scan: normal Doppler examination: normal

For *acute scrotal swelling* a broader list of entities should be considered. *Painful* swelling with a tender testicle may be caused by testicular torsion, trauma with a hematocele, and epididymitis or orchitis. A nontender testicle and painful swelling may be secondary to an incarcerated hernia or torsion of the appendix testicle. In cases of *painless* swelling with an enlarged testicle, a testicular tumor or antenatal testicular torsion must be considered. If the testis is normal, underlying abnormality may include a hydrocele, an incarcerated hernia, Henoch-Schönlein purpura, or generalized edema, or the swelling may be idiopathic.

MANAGEMENT

1. Testicular torsion is a urologic emergency. If there is any question regarding the diagnosis, immediate consultation is required. Doppler and nuclear scans should be performed.
2. Surgical detorsion is indicated immediately. If this is unavailable, local detorsion by outward twisting (toward the outer thigh) may be cautiously attempted. Edema usually precludes local detorsion from being successful. This procedure may be monitored by Doppler examination, verifying return of blood flow.
3. Analgesia is useful after the diagnosis is certain and the decision made to operate.

DISPOSITION

All patients require immediate hospitalization for surgical detorsion and bilateral fixation. Necrosis usually results if torsion has existed for several hours when the cord is twisted three to four complete turns. Various degrees of atrophy have been reported after detorsion.

Salvage is 70% if the torsion has existed for 8 to 12 hours, whereas it is 80% to 90% if it has been present for less than 8 hours. For torsion greater than 12 hours, salvage is 20%.

REFERENCES

Herzog LW, Alvarez SR: The frequency of foreskin problems in uncircumcised children, *Am J Dis Child* 140:254, 1986.

May DC, Lesh P, Lewis S, et al: Evaluation of acute scrotum pain with testicular scanning, *Ann Emerg Med* 14:696, 1985.

Petrack MM, Hafeez W: Testicular torsion versus epididymitis: a diagnostic challenge, *Pediatr Emerg Care* 8:347, 1992.

Schul MW, Keating MA: The acute pediatric scrotum, *J Emerg Med* 12:565, 1993.

78 Gynecologic Disorders

Gynecologic Examination

The gynecologic examination of the prepubescent patient requires patience, sensitivity, and a modified approach to the examination. It is crucial to provide a careful explanation and to move slowly while constantly reassuring the patient and parents. This usually precludes the necessity for an examination under anesthesia. The most shy children are often those in the 11 to 13 years age group who are just experiencing puberty.

Younger girls are best examined in the presence of their mothers. Examination of the external genitalia by inspection and palpation can usually be accomplished while the child is on the mother's lap. If appropriate, having the child assist the examiner by separating the labia may be reassuring to the child. The examiner should simultaneously depress the perineum. Particular attention should be focused on observation for trauma, foreign bodies, lacerations, discharges, vesicles, ulcers, and adenopathy. Labial adhesions are common in young children, usually secondary to irritation or inflammation. They may spontaneously separate by 12 months, but this process may be facilitated by topical application of Premarin cream nightly for 2 weeks.

Next, the child should be placed in the knee-chest position with her buttocks held up in the air and apart by an assistant. The girl is asked to lie on her abdomen with bottom up and to let her stomach and back sag. Instrumentation is rarely necessary; the short vagina of the pre-pubertal girl allows enough visualization to rule out foreign bodies and other lesions. Samples of secretions, discharges, and seminal fluid for culture, cell cytology, or forensic examination may be obtained by using a moistened Q-tip or an eye dropper. A small vaginoscope or small nasal speculum should be used if direct visualization is necessary.

All discharges should be evaluated both for *Candida (Monilia)* and *Trichomonas* organisms, using a wet saline and KOH preparation. Trichomoniasis, bacterial vaginosis, and candidiasis samples can be collected with a cotton swab inserted into the vagina without needing a speculum. Gram stain and culture of all discharges on a minimum of Thayer-Martin or Transgrow medium also should be done.

Palpation may be required to establish abdominal tenderness and the position of the cervix and to exclude foreign bodies or other masses. A bimanual rectoabdominal or one-finger vaginal examination may be performed with the child on her back.

In the pubescent female, a careful examination should be done, with detailed explanations to maximize cooperation. The procedures should parallel those for the older female. A straightforward, noncondescending approach to the patient is crucial.

As a component of the examination, sexual maturity should be evaluated. Tanner stage I represents the prepubertal level; stage II, the early pubertal level; stages III and IV, intermediate levels of genital changes during puberty; stage V, adult level.

MENSTRUAL PROBLEMS

DYSMENORRHEA

Dysmenorrhea commonly has pain associated with menstruation, which is functional in more than 95% of patients. It may result from an increased secretion of prostaglandins causing contractility of the myometrium during a period of falling progesterone levels. Emotional problems or sexual maladjustment may rarely be contributory. Infrequently, endometriosis (rare in children), chronic pelvic inflammatory disease (PID), or anomalies of the müllerian ducts or genitourinary tract may be present as a cause of dysmenorrhea. There is a high correlation with dysmenorrhea in the mother. As many as 29% of girls 12 to 17 years have pain severe enough to interfere with normal activity; 14% of girls miss an average of 12 to 15 days of school per year because of cramps.

Diagnostic Findings

Crampy abdominal pain in the lower to middle abdomen with radiation to the back and thighs commonly is associated with the menses, often beginning 6 to 18 months after menarche. The discomfort normally commences within 1 to 4 hours of the menstruation, continues for up to 24 hours, and may vary in severity from month to month. In rare cases, the pain begins before bleeding and continues for several days. Nausea, vomiting, and diarrhea may be noted. Emotional problems should be suspected if the pain occurs at menarche or begins with anticipation of menses. Patients may be anxious and irritable with edema and weight gain or a sense of bloating. Patients also may be fatigued and depressed.

Premenstrual syndrome (PMS), a distinct luteal-phase disorder, starts 7 to 10 days before menses and includes symptoms of weight gain, fatigue, headache, pelvic pain, and emotional lability. It is uncommon in adolescents, usually occurring in the late twenties and thirties.

With functional dysmenorrhea physical examination is usually normal. A pelvic examination is indicated to exclude organic causes.

Management

1. Appropriately treat organic causes.
2. If functional, reassurance is of primary importance. Hot baths, heating pads, and relaxation may be used. Mild analgesics may be helpful. Aspirin is particularly useful because it is also a prostaglandin inhibitor and should be tried first, but it may produce increased bleeding.
3. If further intervention is appropriate, have the patient use a prostaglandin inhibitor on the first day of menses and take for 2 to 3 days as necessary for pain control. It may be more effective for some patients to begin medication a day before onset of menstruation. Several options exist:
   a. Naproxen (Naprosyn): 375 to 500 mg initially, followed by 250 to 375 mg q8-12hr PO (maximum: 1250 mg/24 hr).
   b. Ibuprofen (Motrin): 400 mg q6hr PO (maximum: 1200 mg/24 hr). Many find an initial dose of 800 mg to be useful. Available as over-the-counter medication (Nuprin or Advil 200 mg).
4. If discomfort continues to be significant, may initiate oral contraceptives for 3 to 6 months. If the patient is sexually active, oral contraceptives (if there are no contraindications) are particularly useful.

   Contraindications to the use of oral contraceptives include the following:
   a. Pregnancy
   b. History of thromboembolic disease
   c. History of cerebrovascular accident (CVA) or myocardial ischemia
   d. History of neoplasm
   e. Hepatic dysfunction
   f. Hypertension
5. Arrange follow-up every 2 to 3 months to provide reassurance and to monitor the clinical response.

PREMENSTRUAL EDEMA

Edema, bloating, and irritability may precede the onset of menstruation. Management includes mild salt restriction, and if the condition is severe, some clinicians suggest initiating diuretic therapy 3 to 4 days before the onset of menses and continuing for a total of 5 to 7 days. Hydrochlorothiazide (HydroDiuril), 25 mg/24 hr PO, is appropriate.

MITTELSCHMERZ

Mittelschmerz is thought to be caused by ovulatory bleeding into the peritoneal cavity. It is typically dull and aching, occurring midcycle and predominantly in one lower quadrant. It sometimes lasts 6 to 8 hours but may be severe and cramping, lasting for several days. Distinguishing it from pain caused by appendicitis, torsion or rupture of an ovarian cyst, ectopic pregnancy, and so forth, may be difficult.

1. Physical examination is usually normal.
2. Therapy includes reassurance, mild analgesia, and local application of heat.

DYSFUNCTIONAL UTERINE BLEEDING (HYPERMENORRHEA OR MENORRHAGIA)

Dysfunctional uterine bleeding is related to anovulatory cycles resulting in hyperplasia of the endometrium from continuous estrogenic stimulation. It often is associated with irregular menses and results when flow is frequent, heavy, and prolonged. It usually is painless. It may result from dietary changes, stress, diabetes mellitus, as well as from a number of endocrine conditions (hypothyroidism or hyperthyroidism, ovarian tumor, or adrenal insufficiency). Other causes of vaginal bleeding (see Chapter 43) must be excluded before treatment. Patients should have a hematocrit to assess the severity of bleeding, as well as routine and orthostatic vital signs.

Management

Management depends on the significance of the bleeding.

1. *Minimal bleeding* with little discomfort may be treated with reassurance and follow-up observation.
2. *Moderate bleeding* often requires pharmacologic intervention:
   a. Medroxyprogesterone (Provera), 10 mg/24 hr PO for 5 days.
      (1) This is the most common approach, and bleeding usually stops in 3 to 5 days.
      (2) If bleeding persists with subsequent menses, the patient takes 10 mg/24 hr for 5 days at the beginning of expected menstruation for three cycles, at which time normal cycles should resume.
   b. A combination of estrogen and synthetic progestin given in 21-day cycles separated by 7 days without therapy usually regulates the menstrual cycle. Active bleeding may be controlled by administration of up to four tablets at the time of the ED visit, followed by a tapering dose over the next few days down to one tablet per day during a 21-day cycle.
3. *Severe bleeding* requires hospitalization, treatment of anemia, and high-dose conjugated estrogens such as Premarin, 40 mg/dose q4hr IV for up to 24 hours (maximum: 6 doses), until bleeding stops. Circulatory resuscitation may be required.
   a. Once bleeding has stopped, a high estrogen-progestin oral preparation is begun: Ortho-Novum 5 mg or equivalent; 2 tablets are given initially, followed by 1 tablet QID PO and gradually tapered over 1 month. The patient is placed on a cycle of Ortho-Novum, 2 mg, or equivalent for 2 to 3 months.
   b. Gynecologic consultation is suggested.

Iron-deficiency anemia in menstruating adolescents often can be prevented by treating with supplemental iron and vitamin C (enhances oral iron absorption) and by monitoring response.

PELVIC INFLAMMATORY DISEASE
(VULVOVAGINITIS AND VAGINAL
DISCHARGE—P. 671)

Pelvic inflammatory disease (PID) encompasses a spectrum of illnesses that are seen with increasing frequency in adolescents. Asymptomatic or uncomplicated genital infections may involve only the urethra, vagina, or cervix, but they may become disseminated, resulting in generalized PID.

Although PID is normally considered a sexually transmitted disease and pelvic disease occurs almost exclusively in sexually active women, nonsexual transmission is possible, but rare, particularly in children. Factors contributing to sensitivity include foreign bodies such as an intrauterine device (IUD), instrumentation and other trauma, pregnancy, and menstruation. Most cases of gonococcal disease occur within 7 days of the onset of menses.

ETIOLOGY: INFECTION

1. *Neisseria gonorrhoeae*
2. Nongonococcal (often mixed) infection
   a. *Chlamydia trachomatis* (most common of nongonococcal etiologies)
   b. Anaerobes: *Bacteroides, Peptostreptococcus,* and *Peptococcus* organisms
   c. Aerobes: *Escherichia coli, Proteus* organisms, *Gardnerella vaginalis (Haemophilus vaginalis)*
   d. *Mycoplasma hominis* or *Ureaplasma urealyticum*

DIAGNOSTIC FINDINGS
Endometritis, Salpingitis, Parametritis, or Peritonitis

Complicated PID may be divided into acute, subacute, and chronic categories on the basis of the onset of symptoms, severity of findings, and number of previous episodes. In general, *N. gonorrhoeae* produces more severe symptoms and a more acute onset, and it usually is associated with the menstrual cycle, whereas *Chlamydia* infection is more commonly associated with an insidious course of pelvic pain. However, this differentiation is not reliable for the individual patient.

Acute PID

1. Patients usually have high fever. Vital signs reflect the severity of abdominal inflammation, including endometritis, salpingitis, parametritis, or peritonitis.
2. Abdominal pain is continuous, usually bilateral, and most severe in the lower quadrants. Only 10% of patients have unilateral pain, which should prompt consideration of ectopic pregnancy, appendicitis, cyst disease, or urinary origin. Peritonitis with rebound, guarding, and decreased bowel sounds may be present. Liver tenderness may result from perihepatitis (Fitz-Hugh and Curtis syndrome).
3. Cervical and adnexal tenderness is present and increases with movement. Uterine bleeding and vaginal discharge may be noted.
4. Clinical criteria to make the diagnosis of PID include the following:
   a. All three of the following:
      (1) Lower abdominal tenderness
      (2) Cervical motion tenderness
      (3) Adnexal tenderness
   b. Plus one or more of the following:
      (1) Oral temperature above 38.3° C
      (2) Leukocytosis more than 10,000 WBC/mm^3
      (3) Erythrocyte sedimentation rate (ESR) greater than 29 mm/hr
      (4) Laboratory documentation of cervical infection with *N. gonorrhea* or *T. vaginalis*
      (5) Inflammatory adnexal mass on pelvic examination or ultrasonography

Subacute PID

1. Patients often have low-grade fever and few systemic signs.
2. Moderate abdominal, cervical, and adnexal tenderness are present.

Chronic PID

Patients have recurrent episodes of abdominal pain, backaches, vaginal discharge, dysmenorrhea, and menorrhagia.

Complications

1. Infection/inflammation
   a. Peritonitis
   b. Tuboovarian abscess; 85% of adolescents have adnexal enlargement or tuboovarian abscess
   c. Endometriosis
   d. Salpingitis
   e. Perihepatitis
   f. Recurrent PID
2. Endocrine disorders
   a. Infertility. After first episode (10% to 12%), second episode (23% to 35%), and third episode (50% to 75%)
   b. Ectopic pregnancy (risk increased in subsequent pregnancies)
3. Chronic pelvic pain

Ancillary Data

1. White blood cells (WBC) count and ESR often are elevated. Hematocrit may be decreased with extensive bleeding. An elevated ESR (>15 mm/hr) is seen 75% of the time. WBC count is elevated in about 60% of patients.
2. Culdocentesis or laparoscopy is useful for patients with acute abdominal pain and potential pelvic pathologic conditions. Purulent cul-de-sac fluid may be present in either ruptured appendicitis or extensive PID. Unclotted blood suggests adnexal cyst rupture or ectopic pregnancy. A clear tap containing serous fluid occurs with PID, ruptured ovarian cyst, and other entities causing peritoneal reaction.
3. Bacterial culture and Gram stain.
   a. Gram stain of a cervical culture for *N. gonorrhoeae* can be useful. It is positive if gram-negative diplococci are present in or closely associated with polymorphonuclear (PMN) leukocytes; it is equivocal if only extracellular organisms or atypical intracellular gram-negative diplococci are present.

   Finding *N. gonorrhoeae* identifies a patient at high risk for PID, but the correlation with the infecting organism of an upper tract infection is not close enough to suffice as a basis for therapy.

   Gram stain of urethral discharge is reliable in males.
   b. Thayer-Martin (or Transgrow) culture and, if complicated, anaerobic cultures.
4. *Chlamydia* endocervical swab screening is reliable and easily available. Clear as much mucus as possible off the cervix before obtaining the specimen to prevent a false-negative result. Immunofluorescent staining and enzyme-linked immunosorbent assay tests are available.
5. Ultrasonography to define masses, adnexal enlargement, tuboovarian abscess, exclude ectopic pregnancy, or localize IUD, if indicated.
6. Pregnancy test, if indicated.
7. Serologic test for syphilis.

DIFFERENTIAL DIAGNOSIS

1. Infection/inflammation
   a. Urethritis
   b. Urinary tract infection (p. 815)
   c. Appendicitis, diverticulosis (p. 648)
   d. Peritonitis
   e. Gastroenteritis
   f. Mesenteric lymphadenitis
   g. Pancreatitis
   h. Inflammatory bowel disease
   i. Endometriosis
2. Endocrine disorders
   a. Ovarian cyst, torsion, tumor
   b. Ectopic pregnancy (p. 679)
   c. Spontaneous abortion
   d. Diabetic ketoacidosis

MANAGEMENT

Prescribed doses in the following section are for adolescents (>45 kg or 100 lb) and adults who are not pregnant.

Support includes parenteral fluids, analgesics, nasogastric (NG) tube (if ileus is present), and bed rest, as indicated.

1. Cefoxitin, 2 gm IV q6hr (or cefotetan 2 gm q12hr IV or equivalent); *plus* doxycycline, 100 mg q12hr IV or PO, for at least 48 hours after clinical improvement followed by doxycycline, 100 mg q12hr PO for a 10- to 14-day course. This regimen provides optimal coverage for *N. gonorrhoeae* and *C. trachomatis*.

2. Clindamycin, 900 mg (15-40 mg/kg/24 hr) IV q8hr; *plus* gentamicin load, 2 mg/kg/dose IV, followed by maintenance of 1.5 mg/kg/dose q8hr IV; *plus* doxycycline, 100 mg q12hr IV or PO, continued for at least 48 hours after clinical improvement; followed by doxycycline, 100 mg q12hr PO, for a 10- to 14-day course, or clindamycin, 600 mg q8hr PO for a 14-day course. This approach is preferred when a predominant facultative/anaerobic infection is probable (i.e., IUD-related). When pyogenic complications are suspected as a result of anaerobes or gram-negative findings, consider addition of clindamycin, 450 mg q6hr PO.

3. If doxycycline is not tolerated, an alternative is erythromycin, 40 mg/kg/24 hr q6hr PO.

4. When a patient does not require hospitalization and responds within 48 hours of initiation of treatment to outpatient therapy, an ambulatory regimen may be used. Cefoxitin, 2 gm IM (or equivalent), with probenecid, 1 gm PO; *plus* doxycycline, 100 mg q12hr PO for 10 to 14 days.

5. Reculture in 4 to 7 days and rescreen 4 to 6 weeks after completing treatment.

6. Children less than 45 kg should be treated with ceftriaxone, 100 mg/kg/24 hr q12hr IV or IM; *and* erythromycin, 40 mg/kg/24 hr q6hr IV.

Disposition

Hospitalization is indicated under the following circumstances:

1. Uncertain diagnosis, requiring further evaluation
2. Possibility of surgical emergencies such as appendicitis, ectopic pregnancy, or peritonitis
3. Moderate to severe disease with fever, nausea, vomiting, peritonitis, and leukocytosis
4. Suspicion of a pelvic mass or abscess
5. Pregnancy
6. Poor compliance or inability to take oral medications
7. Failure to respond to outpatient therapy
8. Recurrent episodes consistent with chronic PID
9. Any consideration of sexual abuse

Many clinicians recommend that all patients with PID, particularly younger women, be hospitalized to reduce complications, maximize long-term fertility, and emphasize the potential severity of the disease. Indwelling IUDs commonly are removed. A single episode of tubal infection results in tubal closure in 14% of women, and the rate of ectopic pregnancies is five times greater than in women without a pelvic infection.

VULVOVAGINITIS AND VAGINAL DISCHARGE (PELVIC INFLAMMATORY DISEASE—P. 669)

Vulvovaginitis and vaginal discharges are common problems of prepubertal and pubescent females, although the common causes vary with age.

A careful history should focus on the presence of accompanying pruritus and odor, and it should define the quality, duration, and volume of the discharge. Other illnesses (diabetes, infections) should be excluded, medications defined (e.g., contraceptives, deodorant sprays, douches, antibiotics), and menstrual history, sexual activity, previous infections, and symptoms in sexual partners clarified. Vaginal discharge associated with cervical motion or adnexal tenderness usually is associated with PID (p. 669).

PREPUBESCENT FEMALE
Nonspecific Causes

Poor hygiene or an allergic reaction usually are causative. Cultures show a variety of organisms, most of which are normal flora. Substances responsible for allergic responses in younger children include bubble bath and, in adolescents and adults, sanitary napkins, chemical douches, and deodorant and contraceptive sprays.

Diagnostic Findings
The discharge is thin and mucoid, and the introitus is painful, erythematous, and swollen. Patients may have a positive history of contact with an irritant. Dysuria may occur.

Management
1. Improved perineal hygiene with particular attention to ensure that the child wipes from front to back after bowel movements
2. Frequent changes of white cotton underpants
3. Avoidance of bubble baths and other irritating substances
4. Sitz baths: may be useful 2 to 4 times/day, washing the area with a very mild soap and allowing to air dry
5. For severe cases: 1% hydrocortisone cream for 2 to 3 days
6. If there is no resolution in 2 to 3 weeks: systemic ampicillin (or amoxicillin), 250 to 500 mg q6hr PO, for 10 days

Foreign Body

Articles commonly found in the vagina include paper products, vegetable matter, and in older patients, forgotten tampons. The discharge is blood tinged and foul smelling. Physical examination should reveal the foreign body. It often can be palpated on rectal examination.

Pinworms (p. 583)

Vulvovaginitis is secondary to irritation and itching of the perineum.

Physiologic Leukorrhea

A clear, sticky, nonirritating discharge may develop at the onset of puberty secondary to estrogen stimulation and irritation; it ceases once menarche occurs.

It is common for children in the first few days of life to have a thin vaginal discharge. This discharge may become bloody at 5 to 10 days because of withdrawal of maternal estrogens.

Infection

The infectious causes specified for the pubescent female may cause vulvovaginitis in the younger child and should be diagnosed and treated with weight-specific doses of drugs as outlined in the discussion of the postpubescent female.

Nonsexual transmission of sexually transmitted disease is uncommon in prepubescent females beyond the neonatal period. In general, sexual abuse should be considered, particularly in the presence of gonorrhea, *Chlamydia trachomatis*, *Trichomonas vaginalis*, and condyloma acuminatum.

Although uncommon, *Shigella* organisms can cause a chronic, purulent, blood-tinged discharge that is foul smelling. There may be no associated diarrhea. *E. coli* and group A streptococci also have been associated with vulvovaginitis.

POSTPUBESCENT FEMALES

Causes specified for the prepubescent female also occur after puberty, although the infectious agents discussed here are more common.

Gonorrhea/Chlamydia

Although *N. gonorrhoeae* may cause vaginitis in prepubescent girls, it is more often associated with cervicitis and salpingitis in the pubescent female (p. 671). *C. trachomatis* infection is common.

Diagnostic Findings

1. Patients have a vaginal (urethral in males) discharge that is yellow-green and purulent or mucopurulent. However, 60% to 80% of females (and 10% of males) are asymptomatic. Infection is most likely to occur in proximity to menses. Symptomatic patients have discharge, dysuria, frequency, variable cervical tenderness, and proctitis.

   a. Cervicitis in postpubertal females is marked by purulent discharge, dysuria, and dyspareunia. The cervix is hyperemic and tender on touch but not on movement.

   b. Urethritis occurs in boys and rarely, in girls. It is associated with purulent discharge and dysuria.

2. Complications:

   a. PID (p. 669).

   b. Disseminated gonorrhea, often associated with polyarthritis or polytenosynovitis. Endocarditis and meningitis are rare.

   c. Polyarthritis, most commonly the wrist, ankle, or knee (see Chapter 27).

   d. Monoarticular arthritis.

3. Ancillary data (p. 670):

   a. Swab or aspirate of discharge (and also of rectum and pharynx, when appropriate) is cultured on Thayer-Martin, Transgrow, or similar medium. Urethral or cervical discharge may reveal intracellular gram-negative diplococci on Gram stain. Rectal cultures should be done in females (and males if appropriate) because rectal culture result is positive in 5% of cases with negative cervical culture findings.

   b. Immunofluorescent staining of endocervical swab for *Chlamydia*.

   c. Syphilis serologic tests should be obtained (Venereal Disease Research Laboratory [VDRL] test or equivalent).

   d. Other studies that may be considered include pregnancy test, human immunodeficiency virus (HIV) antibody, hepatitis B screen, and urinalysis.

Management

Most clinicians believe that despite the isolated nature of an infection, concurrent treatment for *N. gonorrhoeae* and *C. trachomatis* is required.

1. Doses for uncomplicated vulvovaginitis, urethritis, epididymitis, proctitis, or pharyngitis in prepuberal children less than 45 kg or 100 lb.

   a. Ceftriaxone, 125 mg IM, or spectinomycin, 40 mg/kg (maximum: 2 gm) IM; **plus**

   b. Erythromycin, 40 mg/kg/24 hr (maximum: 2 gm/24 hr) q6hr PO for 7 days, *or* azithromycin, 20 mg/kg (maximum: 1 gm) PO.

2. Doses for uncomplicated endocervicitis, urethritis, epididymitis, proctitis, or pharyngitis in those older than 8 years of age and in nonpregnant adults weighing more than 45 kg or 100 lb.

   a. Ceftriaxone, 125 mg IM, *or* cefixime (Suprax), 400 PO, *or* ciprofloxacin, 500 mg PO; **plus**

   b. Doxycycline, 100 mg q12hr PO for 7 days, or azithromycin, 1 gm PO.

3. Disseminated gonococcal infections such as arthritis and dermatitis syndrome should be treated as follows:

   Ceftriaxone, 50 mg/kg/24 hr (maximum: 1 gm/24 hr) q24hr IV/IM for 7 days; **plus** doxycycline or azithromycin (children <8 years of age or pregnant women use erythromycin).

4. Conjunctivitis:

   Ceftriaxone 50 mg/kg (maximum: 1 gm) IM.

5. Pharyngeal gonococcal infections should be treated with ceftriaxone 125 mg IM. An alternative in adolescents and adults is ciprofloxacin.

6. Patients who are potentially incubating syphilis (seronegative, without clinical signs) may be cured by regimens that include ceftriaxone and a 7-day regimen of doxycycline or erythromycin.

7. Follow-up cultures from the infected site should be obtained 4 to 7 days after treatment. Positive culture findings often are caused by new exposures and require retreatment.

Disposition

Patients who have evidence of peritoneal signs or sepsis (arthritis, liver tenderness) should be hospitalized. Others may generally be followed at home. If outpatient management has failed or compliance is unlikely, close follow-up and frequent contacts may be required.

Candida albicans (Monilia)

This is an oval-budding fungus. Patients predisposed to this infection include diabetic individuals, those with recent antibiotic or oral contraceptive use, and those who are pregnant or use nylon undergarments.

Diagnostic Findings

1. The discharge is thick and white and resembles cottage cheese, often occurring 1 week before menses. There often is associated dysuria, intense pruritus, and dyspareunia. The vulva is red and edematous, with excoriations secondary to the intense itching.

2. A slide prepared by placing 1 drop of KOH (10%) on a small amount of discharge and covering with a coverglass will reveal branching filaments, yeastlike budding hyphae, or both.

Management

1. Sitz baths may provide symptomatic relief.

2. Topical treatment may include any of the following:
   a. Miconazole (Monistat): 1 applicator full before bed for 7 to 14 days. Also available as miconazole, 200-mg supposi-

tory (Monistat 3) that requires only 3 days of therapy.
   b. Clotrimazole (Gyne-Lotrimin), 100-mg vaginal tablet or 1% cream, before bed for 7 days.
   c. Nystatin cream or suppository (Mycostatin or Nilstat): two applications/day until symptoms are relieved; then before bed for a total of 10 days.
   d. Ketoconazole (Nizoral), 200 mg q12hr PO, for 5 days in adults. Longer treatment may be required.

3. Discontinue oral antibiotics or contraceptives, if possible.

Trichomonas vaginalis

Diagnostic Findings

1. Discharge is thin, frothy, malodorous, and yellow-green. Commonly, patients have itching, erythema, pain, and burning of the vulvovaginal area, with cystitis or urethritis. The cervix typically has red, punctate hemorrhages. In rare cases (10%), patients have abdominal pain.

2. A wet mount, with saline, of the cervical discharge will reveal motile, flagellated organisms, slightly larger than a leukocyte. Direct immunofluorescence with monoclonal antibodies may hold promise for rapid detection.

Management

1. Sitz bath or wet compresses for symptomatic relief

2. Metronidazole (Flagyl): 250 mg TID PO for 7 days or 2 gm as single dose PO. The sexual partner should be treated with metronidazole, 2 gm PO as a single dose.
   a. Younger children may receive 15 mg/kg/24 hr, divided into three doses for 10 days.
   b. Patients must not drink alcohol during the course of therapy. Do not give during pregnancy. Use clotrimazole, 100-mg vaginal tablet, before bed for 7 days.

Haemophilus vaginalis (Gram-Negative Pleomorphic Coccobacilli) (*Gardnerella vaginalis*)

Diagnostic Findings
1. Discharge is gray or clear, with a fishy smell. Gram stain shows multiple organisms and PMN leukocytes. Pruritus and burning may be present.
2. Microscopic examination will reveal epithelial cells coated with small refractile bacteria ("clue cells"). PMN leukocytes are common. Mixing the discharge with 10% KOH liberates a fishy, aminelike odor.

Management
Systemic treatment is most effective. Topical treatment can be used for symptomatic relief only.
1. Systemic:
   a. Metronidazole (Flagyl), 1 gm/24 hr q12hr PO for 7 to 10 days (children: 35 mg/kg/24 hr) or 2 gm PO as single dose (with second dose in 48 hours; *or*
   b. Clindamycin, 600 mg/24 hr q12hr PO for 7 days.
2. Topical:
   a. Metronidazole gel, 0.25%, 5 gm intravaginal BID in 5 days.
   b. Clindamycin cream, 2%, 5 gm intravaginal at bedtime for 7 days.
3. Treatment of the sexual partner does not influence relapse or recurrence rates.

Herpes Simplex, Type 2

Although both types 1 and 2 can cause infections of the vagina, vulva, and cervix, type 2 is the more common.

Diagnostic Findings
1. Grouped vesicles progress to ulcers in the perineal area, associated with bilateral tender inguinal nodes, pain, burning, and itching. Systemic illness may be present. Each episode of infection is usually self-limited but may last for a prolonged period with recurrence. It is particularly important to determine whether the patient is pregnant because of the fetal risk.
2. Wright or Giemsa stain of a vesicle has giant multinucleated cells and inclusion bodies.

Management
1. Sitz baths or wet compresses
2. Analgesics, if necessary
3. Acyclovir (Zovirax)
   a. *Oral* therapy shortens the symptomatic period by reducing the number of new lesions and duration of pain, dysuria, and constitutional symptoms while shortening the shedding of virus. This efficacy has been documented in primary herpes when treatment is initiated early (within 6 days of onset) in the *first episode.*
   • Dose: 200 mg q4hr while patient is awake (5 doses/day) PO for 10 days
     Treatment of the initial infection does not prevent recurrences.
     Treatment of *recurrent* episodes may shorten the healing time.
   • Dose: 200 mg five times per day for 5 days initiated within 2 days of onset
     Suppression of recurrences with long-term therapy has been useful in severe disease. The frequency of episodes decreases, but once the drug is discontinued, the frequency returns to the pretreatment level, with a first episode after medication that is often severe. Dose: 400 mg q12hr PO for up to 6 months.
   b. *Topical* 5% ointment is less effective in decreasing symptoms but may be used every 6 hours for 7 days.

REFERENCES
Abramowicz M: Treatment of sexually transmitted diseases, *Med Lett Drugs Ther* 32:5, 1990.
American Academy of Pediatrics: *Report of the Committee of Infectious Diseases*, ed 24, Elk Grove, Ill, 1997, American Academy of Pediatrics.
Corey L, Spear PG: Infections with herpes simplex viruses, *N Engl J Med* 314:686, 1986.
Emans SJ, Goldstein DP: *Pediatric and adolescent gynecology*, ed 3, Boston, 1990, Little, Brown.

Fleming DT, McQuillan GM, Johnson RE, et al: Herpes simplex virus type 2 in the United States, 1976 to 1994, *N Engl J Med* 337:1105, 1997.

Friedland LR, Kulick RM, Biro FM: Cost effectiveness decision analysis of intramuscular ceftriaxone versus cefixime in adolescents with gonococcal cervicitis, *Ann Emerg Med* 27:299, 1996.

Golden N, Cohen H, Gennari G, et al: The use of pelvic ultrasonography in the evaluation of adolescents with pelvic inflammatory disease, *Am J Dis Child* 141:1235, 1987.

Guinan ME: Oral acyclovir for treatment and suppression of genital herpes simplex virus infection, *JAMA* 255:1747, 1986.

Krieger JN, Tam MR, Stevens CE: Diagnosis of trichomoniasis, *JAMA* 259:1223, 1988.

Magid D, Douglas JM, Schwartz JS: Doxycycline compared with genital *Chlamydia trachomatous* infection: an incremental cost effective analysis, *Ann Intern Med* 124:389, 1996.

Martin DH, Mroczkowski TF, Dalu ZA, et al: A controlled trial of single dose azithromycin for the treatment of chlamydial urethritis and cervicitis, *N Engl J Med* 327: 921, 1992.

Sanders LL, Harrison HR, Washington AE: Treatment of sexually transmitted chlamydial infections, *JAMA* 255:1750, 1986.

Sirnick A, Melzer-Lange M: Gynecologic and obstetric disorders. In Barkin RM editor: *Pediatric emergency medicine: concepts and clinical practice*, ed 2, St Louis, 1997, Mosby.

COMPLICATIONS OF PREGNANCY

Benjamin Honigman

The diagnosis of pregnancy is made on the basis of clinical presentation, a host of urine or serum pregnancy tests, and ultrasonography. Pregnancy causes secondary amenorrhea. Women also have breast fullness and tenderness, darkening of the areola, enlargement of the nipples, and protrusion of Montgomery glands. Fatigue, lassitude, nausea, and vomiting are commonly present early in pregnancy. Urinary frequency may be reported. About 6 weeks after the last menses, early changes of softening of the uterine isthmus and violaceous coloration of the vulva, vagina, and cervix become evident. At about 8 weeks the uterus is enlarged with early changes of softening of the cervix (Hegar sign), and a bluish hue of the mucosa of the cervix and vagina (Chadwick sign) is present.

The physiology of pregnancy forms the basis for pregnancy testing. About 14 days before the next expected menstruation, ovulation is triggered by a surge of luteinizing hormone (LH). Nine days later (1 to 2 days after implantation), human chorionic gonadotropin (hCG) becomes detectable. The hCG maintains the corpus luteum of pregnancy, supporting the secretion of estrogen and progesterone.

The hCG is a sialoglycoprotein with alpha and beta subunits. The beta subunits are immunologically specific. Initially, hCG increases 1.9- to 2.0-fold every day for the first 30 days of pregnancy so by the expected day of menstruation, the hCG level is 50 mIU/ml. By 6 weeks' gestation (2 weeks after the first missed period), the level is 3000 mIU/ml, later peaking at 8 to 12 weeks with a level of 20,000-100,000 mIU/ml. During the third trimester, the level may decline.

A number of pregnancy tests are available to the clinician. Older bioassays have been replaced by immunoassays with varying sensitivities.

1. Enzyme-linked or solid-phase immunoassays of urine or serum are simple, can be performed within minutes, and are sensitive to an hCG level of 25-50 mIU/ml. They can detect pregnancy within 7 to 10 days of conception and are the preferred pregnancy tests for routine testing.

2. Home pregnancy urine tests routinely use hemagglutination inhibition (HAI) or latex agglutination inhibition (LAI) techniques. They can detect hCG at a sensitivity of 150-4000 mIU/ml (3 to 6 weeks' gestation). Errors occur from not using a concentrated first morning urine, excessive liquid intake, proteinuria, hematuria, and ingestion of psychotropic drugs.

3. Quantitative hCG levels can help in assessing fetal viability but not location. Because hCG levels double every 2 to 3 days in early pregnancy, serial quantitative measurements can be used to ensure normal embryonic growth. Ectopic and aborted

pregnancies are usually characterized by plateauing or declining levels, although 15% to 20% ectopic pregnancies may have normal increases in hCG. An abnormally high level may be associated with multiple gestations or molar pregnancies.

4. The hCG levels disappear completely 2 to 3 weeks after spontaneous or induced pregnancy loss.

5. Progesterone has also been used as a marker of early pregnancy; however, because of cost, lack of availability, and overlap of levels in normal and abnormal pregnancies they are rarely used in the emergency department. Levels 15 mg/ml or less are rarely associated with a viable fetus.

Location and viability of early pregnancy is best determined with ultrasonography. Transabdominal ultrasonography can demonstrate a "sac" at 6 weeks' gestational age (hCG levels approximately 3500 mIU/ml). A transvaginal ultrasound can detect a sac at 4 to 5 weeks (approximately 1500 mIU/ml).

Use of pregnancy testing and ultrasonography will help guide the clinician in decisions regarding viability and location of early pregnancy (Fig. 78-1).

The emergency physician most commonly is faced with one of a number of complications of pregnancy that must be considered in the differential diagnosis of presenting complaints.

All of these patients require monitoring of vital signs with orthostatic blood pressure readings and a hematocrit.

ABORTION

ALERT: Always consider ectopic pregnancy in pregnant patients having pain or bleeding.

Threatened Abortion

Diagnostic Findings

1. Vaginal bleeding during the first trimester of pregnancy; pain may be present.

2. Enlarged and nontender uterus, appropriate for dates. The cervix is closed.

3. *Inevitable abortion*: the os is open without tissue.

4. If the initial hCG is within normal range, there is a 79% chance of a favorable outcome.

Management

1. Reassurance: 30% to 40% of these patients carry pregnancy to term.

2. Bed rest with bathroom privileges at home. Any blood pooled in the vagina during rest will become apparent when the patient stands, giving the impression of profuse bleeding.

   NOTE: Patients with an open os will abort eventually and should be under continuing observation. An outpatient dilation and curettage (D & C) may be indicated in patients in whom the os is open (inevitable abortion).

Incomplete Abortion

Diagnostic Findings

1. First trimester bleeding accompanied by cramps and cervical dilation.

2. Enlarged, mildly tender uterus. The cervix admits a ring forceps beyond the internal os without resistance. Do not attempt to introduce forceps if the uterus is large enough to be felt by abdominal examination.

   Products of conception may be visible in the os.

Bleeding may be profuse.

Management

1. Remove any material from the cervical os. This should reduce bleeding.

2. Place oxytocin (Pitocin), 20 units in 1000 ml of D5W, and infuse over 1 to 2 hours.

3. Consult a gynecologist for an outpatient D & C.

4. With Rh incompatibility administer Rho (D antigen) immune globulin (RhoGAM).

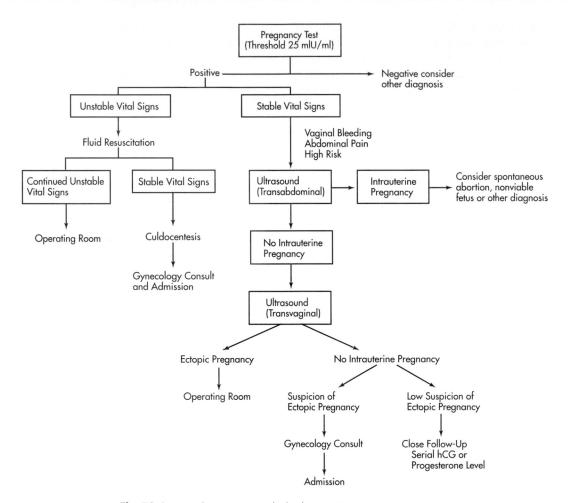

Fig. 78-1 Evaluation to exclude diagnostic ectopic pregnancy.

Normally, a hematocrit (Hct) and blood type determination should be obtained.

Complete Abortion

Diagnostic Findings
1. Complete expulsion of products of conception during the first trimester.
2. Small, firm, and nontender uterus. The cervix admits a ring forceps beyond the internal os. Products of conception are in the vagina or previously have been expelled.
3. Hct with complete blood count (CBC) and type and hold. Rh determination.

4. There is a 50% decrease in hCG every 12 to 48 hours; usually less than 5 mIU/ml after 3 to 7 days.

Management
1. Gynecologic consultation for D & C. (Some clinicians are now deferring this procedure.)
2. RhoGAM for Rh incompatibility.

Missed Abortion

Diagnostic Findings
1. Threatened or incomplete abortion is followed by decrease in bleeding to a

brownish discharge. The symptoms of pregnancy decrease.
2. Small uterus for gestational date and variably will admit ring forceps.
3. Hematocrit with CBC and type and hold. Rh determination.

Management
1. If 12 weeks or less: D & C
2. If more than 12 weeks: oxytocin drip (see earlier discussion) and hematologic monitoring for hypofibrinogenemia and disseminated intravascular coagulation (DIC)
3. With Rh incompatibility, administration of RhoGAM

ECTOPIC PREGNANCY

ALERT: Amenorrhea, abdominal pain, and vaginal bleeding accompanying symptoms of pregnancy must be rapidly investigated. The triad of abdominal pain, abnormal vaginal bleeding, and mass is present in 45% of patients.

Ectopic pregnancies (EPs) are normally (95%) tubal. Less than 3% are cornual, ovarian, or abdominal. Predisposing factors include PID, previous tubal surgery or EP, an IUD, or endometriosis. The incidence is greatest in women 35 to 44 years and lowest in 15 to 24 year-olds, although rates in this age group are increasing.

Diagnostic Findings

Ruptured Ectopic Pregnancy
Abdominal pain is invariably present. Sudden onset of pain associated with vaginal spotting in a pregnant female is very suggestive of a ruptured ectopic pregnancy. The pain may be described as sharp, dull, or aching, and it may be continuous or intermittent, reflecting episodes of intraperitoneal bleeding. Shoulder and back pain suggest peritonitis.
1. Rebound tenderness is present, and in rare cases, a bluish ecchymotic area around the umbilicus (Cullen sign) may develop if there has been a rupture.
2. The cervix is usually tender and the cul-de-sac full. Adnexal tenderness is present and, variably, a mass. The uterus is smaller than expected for gestational age.
3. Initial amenorrhea followed by vaginal bleeding can range from spotting to heavy flow; 15% to 30% of patients have a normal menstrual history; 15% rupture before a missed period, whereas 50% have abnormal bleeding before any pain.
4. Patients often experience vomiting and nausea (morning sickness), amenorrhea, and in rare cases, breast engorgement and other suggestions of pregnancy.
5. Patients often demonstrate hypotension, tachycardia, and dyspnea.

Unruptured Ectopic Pregnancy
Unruptured ectopic pregnancies are difficult to diagnose because abdominal pain may be the only symptom. A pelvic mass is present in only one half of patients. Thus women of childbearing age with abdominal pain should have a pregnancy test.

Complications
1. DIC (p. 683)
2. Fertility problems and recurrent ectopic pregnancies
3. Death from hemorrhagic shock

Ancillary Data
1. Hematocrit with CBC and type and cross-match
2. Pregnancy test. The test used should reflect the days since the last menses. Although ectopic pregnancy usually has a range of hCG of 150-800 mIU/ml, it may be as low as 10 mIU/ml. In selected cases, serial quantitative determinations may be useful.
3. Ultrasonography. A valuable diagnostic aid, it should be performed immediately in all patients at high risk for EP or those with continued pain. If the patient complains only of bleeding, careful follow-up and ultrasonography in 24 to 48 hours can

be done. Most adolescents should have early ultrasonography to ensure reliable follow-up and disposition. About one third of women with an EP with β-hCG values less than 1000 mIU were identified by transvaginal ultrasonography. One in 30,000 pregnancies involves simultaneous intrauterine and extrauterine pregnancies.

4. Culdocentesis. A useful diagnostic test that is indicated if there is a question of EP or infection or to differentiate abdominal from pelvic pathologic conditions before surgery for an acute abdomen. The aspirate results are categorized as follows:
   a. Normal tap: straw-colored fluid
   b. Dry tap: nondiagnostic, requiring a repeat tap or other diagnostic procedure (may occur with ectopic pregnancy before rupture)
   c. Positive diagnostic tap: bloody (nonclotting) aspirate with an Hct greater than 15%
5. Laparoscopy. Useful, particularly if available on an emergency basis, to make definitive diagnosis and initiate treatment.

Differential Diagnosis

In cases of pelvic pain with a positive pregnancy test, EP, intrauterine pregnancy, and spontaneous or threatened abortion must be considered.

Pelvic pain with a negative pregnancy test result may be caused by an EP (5% of symptomatic EPs have an hCG level <50 mIU/ml), Mittelschmerz, dysmenorrhagia, PID, appendicitis, neoplasm, adnexal torsion, endometriosis, fibroids, or adhesions, and ultimately pelvic congestion.

Management

1. For the unstable patient, intravenous (IV) fluids (crystalloid solution and blood),

military antishock trousers (MAST) suit (controversial), NG tube, and urinary catheterization for treatment and monitoring should be initiated.
2. Diagnostic evaluation should include ultrasonography, culdocentesis, or laparoscopy.
3. If diagnosis is confirmed, surgery is indicated to remove ectopic pregnancy and to ligate tube. Rarely, a tuboplasty is indicated for a single remaining tube in a nulliparous female. The hCG may be elevated for up to 24 days after surgery. In older patients with a large EP (hCG >5000 mIU/ml), methotrexate may have a role in chemically ablating the EP in consultation with a gynecologist.
4. For the stable patient with unconfirmed but suspected EP, hospitalization usually is indicated for further diagnostic evaluation.

ABRUPTIO PLACENTAE AND PLACENTA PREVIA

ALERT: Third trimester vaginal bleeding requires urgent evaluation.

Abruptio placentae is the premature separation of a normally implanted placenta, with peak incidence between 20 to 29 weeks and again at 38 weeks. It complicates 1% to 5% of minor abdominal blunt trauma in last trimester women experiencing such an injury.

Placenta previa occurs when the attachment of a placenta is located over or near the internal os. Its classification as total or partial is dynamic because of the changing location of the placenta with the progression of pregnancy.

Predisposing factors include abdominal trauma (abruptio placentae), hypertension, high parity, maternal age older than 35 years, and smoking.

Diagnostic Findings

Abruptio Placentae

Patients classically have vaginal bleeding and abdominal pain. The extent of pain reflects the degree of disruption of the myometrial fibers and intravasation of blood at the site of bleeding. Vaginal bleeding is variable and may be concealed. The uterus is uniformly tender but should be examined only when preparations have been made to perform a cesarean section using a double setup.

Hypotension is usually present. The decrease in blood pressure is often disproportionate to the amount of hemorrhage because of the concealed nature of the blood loss.

Placenta Previa

Vaginal bleeding is the prominent sign, varying from repeated episodes to profuse bleeding. The initial bleeding episode is classically minimal; the second episode may have profuse bleeding. The bleeding is painless. The cervix is boggy and easily admits a finger, but examination should be done only when preparations have been made to perform a cesarean section.

Hypotension is present, reflecting the amount of blood loss.

Complications
1. DIC (p. 683)
2. Acute tubular necrosis (p. 809)
3. Fetal death

Ancillary Data
1. Hematocrit is decreased. Type and cross-match should be sent to the laboratory.
2. Fibrinogen is decreased along with thrombocytopenia and coagulation abnormalities.
3. Ultrasonography will localize the placenta and is appropriate for the stable patient.

Differential Diagnosis

1. Trauma: laceration or other perineal injury
2. Endocrine disorders: complications of pregnancy including uterine rupture or marginal sinus bleeding, premature labor, or abortion

Management

1. Stabilization should include IV fluids and blood, NG tube, and urinary catheterization. DIC should be treated if present.
2. With a diagnosis of placenta previa, an attempt to stop labor should be made with a β-adrenergic agent such as terbutaline (0.25 mg).
3. Fetal heart tones and status should be monitored continuously.

The pelvic examination of the patient should be done only in the obstetric or operating suite, where double setup precautions are available and an immediate cesarean section can be performed. If the mother and fetus are stable, an ultrasound image may be useful in the initial assessment. The decision regarding vaginal delivery of the fetus is best done by the obstetric and pediatric consultants involved in the examination. Cesarean section usually is indicated if there is any evidence of fetal distress. Support personnel must be available to assist in the management of the unstable or potentially unstable patient.

REFERENCES

Abbot J, Emmans LS, Lowenstein SR: Ectopic pregnancy: ten common pitfalls in diagnosis, *Am J Emerg Med* 8:515, 1990.

American Academy of Pediatrics Committee on Adolescence: Adolescent pregnancy, *Pediatrics* 83:132, 1989.

Brown DL, Doubilet PM: Transvaginal sonography for diagnosing ectopic pregnancy, *J Ultrasound Med* 13:259, 1994.

Carson SA, Buster JE: Ectopic pregnancy, *N Engl J Med* 329:1174, 1993.

Dart RG, Kaplan B, Cox C: Transvaginal ultrasound in patients with low β-human chorionic gonadotropin values: how often is the study diagnostic? *Ann Emerg Med* 30:135, 1997.

Durham B, Lane B, Burbridge L, et al: Pelvic ultrasound performed by emergency physicians for the detection of ectopic pregnancy in complicated first-trimester pregnancy, *Ann Emerg Med* 29:338, 1997.

Gale CL, Stovall TG, Muran D: Tubal pregnancy in adolescence, *J Adolesc Health Care* 11:485, 1990.

Kaplan BC, Dart RO, Moskos M, et al: Ectopic pregnancy: prospective study with improved diagnostic accuracy, *Ann Emerg Med* 28:10, 1996.

Nederlof KP, Lawson HW, Saftlas AF, et al: Ectopic pregnancy surveillance, United States, 1970-1987, *MMWR* 39:9, 1990.

Olshaker JS: Emergency department pregnancy testing, *J Emerg Med* 14:59, 1996.

Stovall TO, Fing FW: Ectopic pregnancy, diagnostic and therapeutic algorithms minimizing surgical intervention, *J Reprod Med* 38:807, 1993.

79 HEMATOLOGIC DISORDERS

DISSEMINATED INTRAVASCULAR COAGULATION

Disseminated intravascular coagulation (DIC) is an acquired coagulopathy that may occur in a variety of clinical settings in which the clotting mechanism is triggered. This results in the deposition of thrombi within the microcirculation, consumption of coagulation factors (I, II, V, VIII) and platelets, and, ultimately, bleeding. The severity and clinical significance of DIC varies greatly between patients.

ETIOLOGY

The following are common triggers of DIC:
1. Infection
   a. Bacterial
      (1) Gram-negative sepsis
      (2) Meningococcemia (p. 713)
      (3) Gram-positive sepsis: *Streptococcus pneumoniae* and *Staphylococcus aureus*
   b. Viral
      (1) Herpes simplex
      (2) Measles
      (3) Chickenpox
      (4) Cytomegalovirus
      (5) Influenza
   c. Rocky Mountain spotted fever
2. Shock (see Chapter 5)
3. Respiratory distress syndrome and asphyxia
4. Trauma
   a. Burns (see Chapter 46)
   b. Multiple trauma (see Chapter 56)
   c. Snake bites (p. 311)
   d. Heat stroke (see Chapter 50)
   e. Head injury
5. Complications of pregnancy (p. 676)
6. Neoplasms
7. Necrotizing enterocolitis
8. Hemangioma
9. Intravascular hemolysis
   a. Incompatible blood transfusion
   b. Autoimmune hemolytic anemia

DIAGNOSTIC FINDINGS

The primary determinant of the clinical presentation is the triggering condition. In addition to the signs and symptoms related to that disease, a number of specific findings may be present with DIC.

1. Simultaneous evidence of diffuse bleeding and thrombosis, including petechiae, purpura, peripheral cyanosis, ischemic necrosis of the skin and subcutaneous tissues, hematuria, and melena
2. Prolonged bleeding from venipuncture and other sites of injury

Complications

1. Organ damage as a result of bleeding and infarction. May include gastrointestinal (GI) hemorrhage, hematuria, central nervous system (CNS) bleeding first appearing as mental status changes, apnea, seizures, and coma
2. Purpura fulminans: occurs as patchy hemorrhagic infarction of the skin and subcutaneous tissue
3. Complications of the precipitating event
4. Death from hemorrhage

Ancillary Data

1. Complete blood count (CBC) and peripheral blood smear.
   a. Evidence of hemolysis with fragmented red cells resulting from microangiopathy.
   b. Anemia may occur as a result of bleeding or hemolysis.
   c. Thrombocytopenia is usually present.
2. Coagulation studies. Typical findings include the following:
   a. Prolonged partial thromboplastin time (PTT) as a result of decreased consumable clotting factors (fibrinogen, II, V, VIII).
   b. Increased fibrin split (degradation) products.
   c. Increased fibrin monomer.
   d. Once the consumption of coagulation factors has ceased, values will normalize (fibrinogen and factor VIII in 24 to 48 hours; platelet count in 7 to 14 days).

DIFFERENTIAL DIAGNOSIS

1. Bleeding (see Chapter 29)
2. Precipitating conditions

MANAGEMENT

Initial attention must be directed toward stabilizing the patient and treating the underlying condition triggering DIC. If this precipitating event can be quickly reversed (e.g., shock, hypoxia, endotoxin release), further therapy is often unnecessary.

1. Administer fresh whole blood or packed red cells if there is significant hemorrhage.
2. Replacement of depleted coagulation factors is usually necessary with active or impending bleeding.
   a. Fresh-frozen plasma (FFP): fibrinogen (I) and other clotting factors (II, V, and VIII).
      (1) Usually deficient if hypoxia or acidosis is present
      (2) Administration of 10-15 ml/kg/dose IV repeated as indicated by follow-up coagulation studies
   b. Cryoprecipitate: fibrinogen (I) and factor VIII. Indicated only with no response to FFP. Does not correct deficiencies of other coagulation factors.
      (1) For infants: 1 bag cryoprecipitate/3 kg. For older children: 1 bag cryoprecipitate/5 kg.
      (2) Will usually raise fibrinogen to greater than 100 mg/100 ml, a level sufficient to promote hemostasis.
   c. Platelet concentrate: platelets plus aged plasma.
      (1) Usually deficient if triggered by infection
      (2) Administration of 1 platelet pack/5 to 6 kg or, for infants, 10 ml/kg should increase platelet count by 50,000 to $100,000/mm^3$
   d. Vitamin K (infants: 1-2 mg/dose IV slowly; children and adults: 5-10 mg/dose IV)
3. Heparin. Indicated in the presence of widespread thrombosis or active bleeding that cannot be controlled by replacement of clotting factors and platelets coupled with aggressive treatment of the triggering disorder. In this setting, the intent of heparin therapy is to block further consumption of clotting factors. It is not recommended until other therapies have failed. Heparin should be used early in the course of DIC associated with meningococcemia because of the frequent occurrence of fulminant thrombosis and tissue necrosis.
   • Heparin is administered preferentially by continuous IV infusion.
   a. Load with 50 units/kg IV.
   b. Give continuous drip of 10-15 units/kg/hr IV.

c. With purpura fulminans, give higher dosage if necessary: 20-25 units/kg/hr IV.

d. If bolus infusion is used, give four times the hourly dose q4hr IV.

- Replacement therapy with FFP and platelet concentrate should be continued after the initiation of heparin therapy to minimize bleeding risk.
- The efficacy of heparin therapy is monitored, measuring the fibrinogen level and, later, platelets and watching for increase and return to normal.

e. Unresponsive neonates. Exchange transfusion may occasionally be indicated for those who do not respond to normal medical management.

DISPOSITION

1. Most patients require admission to an intensive care unit (ICU) for treatment of the underlying disease as well as the DIC.

2. Critical care is required, with involvement of a hematologist and those with expertise in the management of the underlying pathologic condition.

REFERENCE

Feinstein DI: Diagnosis and management of disseminated intravascular coagulation: the role of heparin therapy, *Blood* 60:284, 1982.

HEMOPHILIA

Rochelle A. Yanofsky

ALERT: Minor pain often signifies deep muscle or joint bleeding requiring factor replacement. Any head trauma requires urgent intervention.

Hemophilia A (classical hemophilia) and hemophilia B (Christmas disease) are inherited as X-linked recessive conditions. However, as many as one third of cases are caused by recent genetic mutations, resulting in a negative family history of bleeding problems.

Hemophilia A and B are clinically indistinguishable. The diagnosis of both diseases is made on the basis of coagulation factor assays. Hemophilia A is characterized by a deficiency of factor VIII coagulant activity (with a normal level of von Willebrand factor); hemophilia B is characterized by a deficiency of factor IX. The normal range for factor VIII coagulant activity at all ages, and for factor IX activity after age 6 months, is 0.5-1.5 U/ml (or 50% to 150%).

Patients are classified as severe (factor VIII or IX coagulant level <0.01 U/ml [<1%]), moderate (factor VIII or IX coagulant level 0.01-0.05 U/ml [1% to 5%]), or mild (factor VIII or IX coagulant level low but >0.05 U/ml [>5%]). Patients with severe hemophilia bleed spontaneously; those with moderate hemophilia bleed with mild trauma; and those with mild hemophilia bleed with major trauma. Bleeding is usually deep-seated and delayed.

Type 2N von Willebrand disease may be confused with hemophilia A. The former disorder is autosomal recessive and is characterized by a shortened half-life of factor VIII coagulant activity caused by defective binding of that moiety to von Willebrand factor. Measures of factor VIII–von Willebrand factor binding are needed to establish the diagnosis; it cannot be distinguished from hemophilia A by standard coagulation factor assays.

The rare factor IX Leyden variant of hemophilia B is thought to be caused by a mutation at the androgen-sensitive promoter region of the gene. Patients with this variant of hemophilia B have severe hemophilia until age 15 years, after which their factor IX levels gradually increase, sometimes to levels as high as 0.50 U/ml (50%).

DIAGNOSTIC FINDINGS

Bleeding commonly occurs in muscles or joints, either spontaneously or as a result of minor trauma. A local tingling sensation and pain are often the first signs of bleeding. Hemophilia should be suspected in any male who bleeds excessively after trauma and in any male who has bled into joints or muscles. Common sites for bleeding include the following:

1. Musculoskeletal.
   a. Joints most commonly involved are the elbow, knee, and ankle. Joint tenderness, swelling, and limitation of range of motion may be present in the involved joint, but these are later findings. Septic arthritis may occur, but this is uncommon.
   b. Muscle bleeding in the forearm flexor group or the gastrocnemius muscle may cause a compartment syndrome.
   c. Signs of bleeding into the iliopsoas muscle may include lower quadrant abdominal pain and tenderness (may simulate appendicitis), pain in the groin or back, and limp. Compression of the femoral nerve may cause anterior thigh pain, as well as paresthesia, hypesthesia, weakness of the quadriceps muscle, and even permanent paralysis of the thigh flexors. The hip is held in flexion. Range of hip movement is full if the hip is kept flexed. The psoas sign is positive. Significant blood loss may occur.
2. Subcutaneous hematomas ("raised" bruises).
3. Intracranial. Bleeding may be subdural, subarachnoid, intraventricular, cerebellar, or cerebral. Without provocation, or after seemingly minor head trauma, patients may experience headache, vomiting, altered mental status, or seizures. With severe bleeding, signs of increased intracranial pressure may develop (see Chapter 57).
4. Spinal cord hematomas. May cause paralysis, weakness, back pain, and asymmetric neurologic findings.
5. Upper or lower GI bleeding. May be associated with hematemesis, melena, abdominal tenderness and distension, and shock. Intussusception is rare. Intraperitoneal or retroperitoneal hemorrhage may be present.
6. Retropharyngeal hematomas. May produce dyspnea, dysphagia, and potential GI or respiratory obstruction.
7. Mild hematuria is common.

Complications

1. DIC and thromboembolism have been reported with the repetitive use of large doses of low-purity factor IX (prothrombin complex) concentrates as well as with activated prothrombin complex concentrates, particularly with the concomitant use of antifibrinolytic agents (epsilon aminocaproic acid or tranexamic acid), or in the presence of liver dysfunction or other factors that would increase the risk of thrombosis.
2. Hepatitis, either hepatitis B or more commonly hepatitis C, may develop secondary to plasma-derived factor replacement therapy. All patients with hemophilia who are seronegative for hepatitis B should be immunized with recombinant hepatitis B vaccine. Hepatitis A and parvovirus may be transmitted in plasma-derived factor concentrates, despite the current viral attenuation processes used. In addition to the hepatitis B vaccine, it is probably worthwhile to administer the hepatitis A vaccine to patients that have tested negative for IgG antibodies to hepatitis A and who are likely to receive plasma-derived coagulation products.
3. Human immunodeficiency virus 1 (HIV-1). Plasma-derived factor VIII and factor IX concentrates in current use have been subjected to various methods of viral attenuation and appear to be safe in terms of transmission of HIV, HTLV, hepatitis B, and hepatitis C. Acquired immunodefi-

ciency syndrome (AIDS) has been documented in individuals with hemophilia who had previously received blood products contaminated with HIV-1. Evidence of immune dysfunction (AIDS-related complex, or ARC) is seen more commonly than full-blown AIDS in hemophiliacs who demonstrate HIV seropositivity. Hepatosplenomegaly, lymphadenopathy, lymphopenia, high levels of immunoglobulin G (IgG), thrombocytopenia, and Coombs' test positivity may be part of ARC.

4. Death may result from intracranial hemorrhage, underlining the necessity of rapid intervention in patients with head trauma (even minimal).

5. A cycle of repeated hemorrhages can occur into a "target" joint. The ensuing persistent inflammation and hyperemia can result in a chronic joint effusion (chronic synovitis), as well as progressive degeneration of joint bone and cartilage (hemophilic arthropathy). Primary or secondary prophylaxis with factor concentrate is sometimes used to minimize these problems.

6. Muscle wasting and contractures may develop as a result of bleeding into muscles or joints. A cyst may develop within muscle as a result of a previous intramuscular hematoma. A pseudotumor may develop as a result of an intraosseous or subperiosteal hematoma and may require surgical excision in addition to factor replacement therapy and local measures. Possible complications of pseudotumors include spontaneous rupture, fistula formation, nerve or vessel entrapment, and fracture of the adjacent bone.

7. A factor VIII (A) or factor IX (B) IgG inhibitor may develop (in about 20% to 33% of individuals with moderate or severe hemophilia A, and 1% to 4% of individuals with hemophilia B, usually during childhood), making the treatment of bleeding episodes more difficult. A bleeding episode that does not respond to factor replacement therapy should prompt investigations for an inhibitor.

Ancillary Data

1. CBC with hematocrit (Hct), if significant bleeding has occurred.

2. The CBC and differential, platelet count, PT, and thrombin time are normal, unless other diseases coexist. The bleeding time is usually normal but is not routinely done as part of the work-up for hemophilia. The PTT is prolonged. However, the degree of prolongation of the PTT varies, depending on the sensitivity of the reagent used and the severity of the deficiency. On occasion, the PTT may be normal in individuals with mild hemophilia. Assays for factors VIII and IX define the deficiency. These are useful in the initial evaluation (see Table 29-2).

    a. PTT is prolonged. Specific factor level is low.

    b. Factor replacement therapy for major bleeding episodes and perioperative management of hemostasis are guided by baseline coagulation factor assays.

    c. Urinalysis. Mild hematuria is common. Severe or persistent hematuria requires evaluation and factor replacement therapy.

3. Skeletal films are helpful when looking for degenerative joint changes or fractures; they are not used to assess acute hemarthroses. If symptoms of a retropharyngeal hematoma develop, a soft tissue lateral neck view will define the degree of swelling.

4. A computed tomography (CT) scan is indicated for anyone with head trauma and any neurologic symptoms, even if minimal. Evolving neurologic deficits require immediate factor replacement and often neurosurgical intervention.

5. Contrast studies of the genitourinary (GU)

and GI tracts are indicated for evaluation of serious bleeding from those sites.

6. Ultrasound examinations and CT scans are useful in defining the extent of a hematoma; they are particularly helpful for evaluating bleeding in retroperitoneal sites.

7. Aspiration of involved joints is indicated only if the cause is uncertain and infection is suspected. Hematologic consultation should be obtained before the procedure.

DIFFERENTIAL DIAGNOSIS

See Chapter 29.

MANAGEMENT

1. Stabilization of the patient requires intravenous (IV) fluids or blood for major hemorrhages. Airway management, if obstruction is present, must receive first priority.

2. Factor replacement should be initiated immediately as outlined in Tables 79-1 and 79-2 and Box 79-1. Do not waste factor concentrate. Use whole vials. Round dose up to the nearest vial.

   a. One unit (U) of factor VIII or IX equals the activity of factor contained in 1 ml of plasma.

   b. One unit of factor VIII/kg of body weight raises the patient's plasma level by approximately 0.02 U/ml (2%). The plasma half-disappearance time for factor VIII is about 12 hours.

   c. One unit of factor IX/kg of body weight raises the patient's plasma level by approximately 0.01 U/ml (1%). The yield is lower (0.008 U/ml or 0.8%) with high purity plasma-derived factor IX concentrates and may be even lower than this with recombinant factor IX concentrates. The plasma half-disappearance time for factor IX is about 24 hours.

   d. Available products for the treatment of bleeding episodes in hemophilia A include plasma-derived factor concentrates of intermediate, high, or very high purity, as well as recombinant factor VIII, concentrates (see Box 79-1). Cryoprecipitate is now used rarely in developed countries because of (among other things) the lack of viral inactivation processes for this product.

   Available alternatives for treatment of bleeding episodes in hemophilia B include plasma-derived factor IX concentrates of high and low purity, as well as recombinant factor IX concentrate (Box 79-2, p. 692).

   Plasma-derived factor concentrates are now subjected to various methods of viral attenuation. Lower purity plasma-derived factor concentrates may be immunosuppressive, particularly in individuals who are infected with HIV-1. Most children with hemophilia are treated with very high purity or recombinant factor concentrates to minimize this risk, as well as to reduce the risk of viral transmission. The more purified (and recombinant) products are considerably more expensive.

   e. Desmopressin acetate (DDAVP) will increase the factor VIII coagulant level to about two to three times the baseline value in patients with mild hemophilia A. However, considerable interpatient variation in response is seen. DDAVP may be given to patients with mild hemophilia A to treat mild bleeding episodes or to prepare them for minor surgery, as long as they have previously demonstrated an adequate rise in their factor VIII coagulant level after receiving DDAVP.

   DDAVP is usually given intravenously but can also be given subcutaneously or intranasally. The dosage of DDAVP for intravenous or

TABLE 79-1   Hemophilia A: Recommended Dosages of Factor VIII

Actual or potential site of bleeding	Initial dose* (factor VIII U/kg)	Subsequent doses* (factor VIII U/kg)	Comments
Joint or superficial muscles	25-50	25 q12-24hr prn	Several doses may be necessary. Rest, immobilization of involved muscles, or joint and physiotherapy may be needed. Calf/forearm bleeding is limb threatening (compartment syndrome). Use lower end of dose range for early/mild bleeding and higher doses for more severe/late bleeding.
Subcutaneous hematoma (enlarging)	20-25	Rarely needed	
Life-threatening situations†:			Significant blood loss may occur with retroperitoneal bleeding. Factor dosing is guided by factor assays. Evaluate for inhibitor before elective surgery. Perioperative and postoperative plans must be in place preoperatively.
Central nervous system hemorrhage	50	25 q12hr (or by continuous IV infusion as advised by local hemophilia center)	
Major trauma			
Tongue or neck bleeding with potential airway obstruction			
GI bleeding			
Retroperitoneal bleeding (including iliopsoas bleeding)			
Surgery: preoperative and postoperative care			
Hematuria (persistent or severe)	40-50	30-40 q24hr	Increase fluid intake. Rest. Prednisone (1-2 mg/kg/day) for 3-7 days may be useful. Look for cause. Antifibrinolytic agents are contraindicated.
Mouth bleeding or in preparation for dental work (tooth extraction or deep nerve block)	25-50	25 q12-24hr prn	Use of antifibrinolytic agent for 5-7 days will reduce the need for ongoing factor replacement.
Head trauma (no evidence of CNS bleeding)	50		Close follow-up observation.
Before spinal tap†	50		
Minor lacerations of skin: before suture placement and removal	25-50		
Before IM injections	15-25		Avoid IM injections if possible. If IM injection is required (e.g., immunization), give it with a small-bore (25-gauge) needle and apply firm pressure to the needle site for 10 minutes after the injection. Some comprehensive hemophilia centers do not routinely give factor replacement before an immunization.

*In individuals who have mild hemophilia A, DDAVP (desmopressin) is the treatment of choice rather than factor VIII concentrates for mild bleeding episodes.
†These cases should be treated in consultation with patient's comprehensive hemophilia center.

TABLE 79-2   Hemophilia B: Recommended Dosages of Factor IX

Actual or potential site of bleeding	Initial dose* (factor IX U/kg)	Subsequent doses* (factor IX U/kg)	Comments
Joint or superficial muscles	30-60	30-40 q24hr prn	Several doses may be necessary. Rest, immobilization of involved muscle or joint, and physiotherapy may be needed. Calf/forearm bleeding is limb threatening (compartment syndrome). Use lower end of dose range for early/mild bleeding and higher doses for more severe/late bleeding.
Subcutaneous hematoma (enlarging)	25-30	Rarely needed	
Life-threatening situations*: Central nervous system hemorrhage Major trauma Tongue or neck bleeding with potential airway obstruction GI bleeding Retroperitoneal bleeding (including iliop-soas bleeding) Surgery: preoperative and postoperative care	100	50 q24hr (or by continuous IV infusion as advised by local hemophilia center)	Significant blood loss may occur with retroperitoneal bleeding. Factor dosing is guided by factor assays. Evaluate for inhibitor before elective surgery. Perioperative and postoperative plans must be in place preoperatively.
Hematuria (persistent or severe)	80-100	40-50 q24hr	Increase fluid intake. Rest. Prednisone (1-2 mg/kg/day) for 3-7 days may be useful. Look for cause. Antifibrin-olytic agents are contraindicated.
Mouth bleeding or in preparation for dental work (tooth extraction or deep nerve block)	50	30-40 q24hr prn	Use of antifibrinolytic agent for 5-7 days will reduce the need for ongoing factor replacement but is relatively contraindicated when low purity or activated factor IX (prothrombin complex) concentrates are given.
Head trauma (no evidence of CNS bleeding) Before spinal tap*	100 100		Close follow-up observation.
Minor lacerations of skin: before suture placement and removal	40-80		
Before IM injections	25-40		Avoid IM injections if possible. If IM injection is required (i.e., immunization), give it with a small-bore (25-gauge) needle and apply firm pressure to the needle site for 10 minutes after the injection. Some comprehensive hemophilia centers do not routinely give factor replacement before an immunization.

*These cases should be treated in consultation with patient's comprehensive hemophilia center.

> **Box 79-1**
>
> **FACTOR TREATMENT PRODUCTS (AND MANUFACTURERS) FOR HEMOPHILIA A PATIENTS WITHOUT INHIBITORS OR WITH LOW-TITER/ LOW-RESPONDING INHIBITORS**
>
> a. Plasma-derived factor VIII, low purity:
>   Cryoprecipitate: Rarely need now in developed countries because of (among other things) lack of viral inactivation processes for this product.
> b. Intermediate purity plasma-derived factor VIII concentrates:
>   Humate P or Haemate P (Behringwerke/ Centeon)
>   Profilate-OSD (Alpha)
> c. High purity plasma-derived factor VIII concentrates:
>   Alphanate (Alpha)
>   Factor VIII HP (CRC-Bayer)
>   Koate-HP (Bayer)
> d. Very high (ultra) purity plasma-derived factor VIII concentrates:
>   Antihemophilic factor-M (American Red Cross)
>   Hemophil-M (Baxter/Hyland)
>   Monoclate-P (Centeon)
> e. Recombinant factor VIII concentrates (the concentrates listed are produced in cultured hamster cells, purified, and then stabilized with human serum albumin). Clinical trials are in progress evaluating a modified recombinant factor VIII concentrate that does not contain albumin:
>   Bioclate (Centeon)
>   Helixate (Centeon)
>   Kogenate (Bayer)
>   Recombinate (Baxter/Hyland)

subcutaneous use is 0.3 µg/kg/dose (or, 10 µg/m^2/dose, whichever is less) to a maximum of 20 µg/dose; for IV use, it is mixed with 50 ml of normal saline and infused over 20 to 30 minutes.

The dose of DDAVP nasal spray (Stimate) is 150 µg for individuals weighing less than 50 kg and 300 µg (i.e., 150 µg in each nostril) for individuals weighing less than 50 kg. The effect of intravenous DDAVP peaks 30 to 60 minutes after the drug is given; the effect of subcutaneous DDAVP peaks at 60 minutes; the effect of intranasal DDAVP peaks about 60 to 90 minutes after DDAVP is administered.

DDAVP can be given every 12 to 24 hours. Tachyphylaxis (diminishing effectiveness) may be noted when DDAVP is given more often than every 48 hours. DDAVP has a potent antidiuretic effect. In patients receiving IV fluids, care must be taken to avoid overhydration for 24 hours after the drug is given. Any IV fluids administered within 24 hours after DDAVP is given should contain the equivalent of normal saline (e.g., Ringer's lactate or D5W 0.9% NS).

f. A maxim in the management of bleeding episodes is "if in doubt, treat" with factor replacement therapy. Considerable controversy exists regarding the dosage of factor replacement therapy required to treat bleeding episodes. However, all agree that higher doses of factor replacement and longer duration of therapy are required to treat potentially life-threatening bleeding episodes and severe hemarthrosis.

Box 79-2

FACTOR TREATMENT PRODUCTS (AND MANUFACTURERS) FOR HEMOPHILIA B PATIENTS WITHOUT INHIBITORS OR WITH LOW-TITER/ LOW-RESPONDING INHIBITORS

a. Low purity plasma-derived factor IX (pro-thrombin complex) concentrates: (Contain significant amounts of activated factors II, VII, and X. May cause DIC or thrombosis if large amounts are given.)

    Bebulin VH (Immuno)
    Konyne 80 (Bayer)
    Profilinine SD (Alpha)
    Proplex T (Baxter/Hyland)

b. High purity plasma-derived factor IX concentrates: (Little or no thrombogenic potential. Virucidal methods for prevention of hepatitis C more rigorously tested than for purity factor IX concentrates.)

    Alphanine-SD (Alpha)
    Immunine (Immuno)
    Mononine (Centeon)

c. Recombinant factor IX concentrates:
    BeneFix (Genetics Institute Inc.): Contains no albumin. The rise in factor IX level may be lower than expected on the basis of the formula (described in the management section of the text) and should be measured to determine the yield in a given patient.

---

3. Postoperatively, or for management of serious bleeding episodes, the total daily dose of factor VIII (or IX) can be given by continuous IV infusion after an initial bolus dose. The continuous infusion method is superior to the intermittent bolus method in that the former achieves a constant therapeutic factor level and uses less factor concentrate than would be required by intermittent bolus dosing.

4. Secondary prophylaxis (with the infusion of factor VIII concentrate three times per week, or factor IX concentrate twice a week) is given to patients who are developing a "target" joint. Despite clinical improvement with secondary prophylaxis, many patients still have radiologic evidence of hemophilic arthropathy.

5. Studies performed in Europe show that primary prophylaxis (with factor VIII concentrate three times per week or factor IX concentrate twice a week, starting at age 1 to 3 years) is effective in preventing joint bleeding and joint damage. Studies are currently under way in North America evaluating primary prophylaxis.

6. Antifibrinolytic agents (epsilon aminocaproic acid and tranexamic acid) are available in IV, oral, and topical form and are useful adjuncts in the prevention or treatment of bleeding from the mouth, nose, or GI tract. The dosage of systemic epsilon aminocaproic acid (Amicar) is 50-100 mg/kg/dose (maximum: 6 gm/dose) q6-8hr IV or PO. The dosage of systemic tranexamic acid is 25 mg/kg/dose PO (maximum: 1.5 gm/dose) q6-8hr or 10 mg/kg/dose IV (maximum: 1 gm/dose) q8hr. Systemic antifibrinolytic therapy is usually administered for 5 to 7 days or until healing occurs. Antifibrinolytic drugs are contraindicated in the presence of hematuria and are not usually given in conjunction with the lower purity or activated prothrombin complex concentrates because of concern about the risk of thrombosis.

7. Prednisone, 1-2 mg/kg/24 hr, may be indicated for hematuria or for chronic synovitis resulting from recurrent hemarthroses.

8. Patients with moderate or severe hemophilia A or B may develop an inhibitor that is an IgG antibody to the transfused clot-

ting factor. The inhibitor may either be detected during routine screening or because of failure of bleeding episodes to resolve with appropriate factor replacement therapy. The inhibitor titer is measured in Bethesda units.

The treatment of bleeding episodes in patients with inhibitors is challenging and individualized. Treatment decisions are made on the basis of the severity of the bleeding, the inhibitor level, and the inhibitor response to transfused factor (i.e., a patient with hemophilia A who is a high responder has a marked rise in his inhibitor level about 5 days after factor VIII is given, whereas the level of inhibitor does not rise significantly in a "low-responding inhibitor" patient with hemophilia A after he is given factor VIII concentrate).

a. In hemophilia A or B patients who have a low inhibitor titer and are low responders, bleeding episodes are usually treated with higher doses of factor concentrate. More frequent dosing or continuous factor infusion may be required to achieve hemostatic factor levels.

In hemophilia A or B patients who have a high titer inhibitor or are high responders, bleeding episodes are treated with low purity or activated prothrombin complex concentrates, porcine factor VIII (for hemophilia A patients only), or recombinant factor VIIa (Box 79-3). Occasionally, the temporary removal of antibody by plasmapheresis can allow the short-term use of specific factor replacement for life-threatening or limb-threatening hemorrhage.

b. On a long-term basis, induction of immune tolerance may be attempted and is often successful. This involves the administration of large doses of factor VIII concentrate (or factor IX concentrate for hemophilia B patients), on a

---

Box 79-3

TREATMENT OPTIONS FOR HEMOPHILIA A OR B PATIENTS WITH HIGH-TITER OR HIGH-RESPONDING INHIBITORS

1. Prothrombin complex concentrates (see list of low purity factor IX complex concentrates listed in Box 79-2). Dose is 100 U/kg.
2. Activated prothrombin complex concentrates: Autoplex (Baxter/Hyland), FEIBA (Immuno). Dose is 50-75 U/kg. Risk of DIC or thrombosis.
3. Porcine factor VIII: Hyate C (Porton/Speywood). For hemophilia A patients only. Initial dose is 100-150 U/kg. May be used if the antibody to human factor VIII does not strongly react with porcine factor VIII. Propensity to cause anamnestic rise in antibody titer to both porcine and human factor VIII. May cause thrombocytopenia. Risk of transmission of porcine parvovirus with this product.
4. Recombinant factor VIIa: Novoseven or Niastase (Novo Nordisk). Not licensed yet. Limited availability on clinical study and on compassionate release basis.
5. Plasmapheresis.

---

daily or alternate-day basis, sometimes in conjunction with a short course of steroids, cyclophosphamide, or IV immunoglobulin. The factor VIII inhibitor level often falls with this therapy, although it may take several months for this to occur. Once the inhibitor has been eradicated, factor VIII replacement is administered every 2 to 3 days to prevent the reappearance of the inhibitor.

c. A hematologist should be consulted.

9. Other considerations include the following:
   a. Aspirin-containing medications are contraindicated.
   b. Intramuscular (IM) injections should

be avoided if possible. (See Tables 79-1 and 79-2 and Box 79-1 for factor replacement guidelines and suggested local measures for IM injections, including immunizations.)

c. Immobilization of affected areas and rest for 12 to 24 hours for acute muscle and joint bleeding. Analgesia is often required. Rehabilitation with physiotherapy may be required.

d. Hematology consultation for acute management and ongoing comprehensive care. The name and phone number of the director of the local comprehensive hemophilia center can be obtained during regular working hours by calling the National Hemophilia Society (for hemophilia centers in the United States) at 212-431-8541 or the Canadian Hemophilia Society at 800-668-2686.

e. Immediate surgical consultation for anterior compartment syndrome, intracranial bleeding, or spinal cord compression.

f. Methods for carrier detection and prenatal diagnosis are now available.

DISPOSITION

1. Most patients can be treated and discharged. Admission is required in the following circumstances:
   a. Head trauma, acute onset of headache, or spinal cord hematoma
   b. Retropharyngeal hematoma
   c. Muscle bleeding with impending or actual compartment syndrome
   d. GI bleeding
   e. Retroperitoneal or severe iliopsoas bleeding
   f. Poor patient compliance
2. Immediate consultation with a hematologist should be obtained under the following circumstances:
   a. Before any surgical or invasive procedure

b. Intracranial, retropharyngeal, or GI bleeding
   c. Bleeding in patients with inhibitors
3. Other consultants should be involved for specific indications.
4. All patients should be followed in a comprehensive hemophilia clinic.
5. Early treatment of joint and muscle bleeding, coupled with an aggressive physical therapy program, helps prevent prolonged disability. Home transfusion programs can expedite early intervention.

REFERENCES

Andrew M, Paes B, Johnston M: Development of the hemostatic system in the neonate and young infant, *Am J Pediatr Hematol Oncol* 12:95, 1990.

Cohen AJ, Kessler CM: Treatment of inherited coagulation disorders, *Am J Med* 99:675, 1995.

DiMichele D: Hemophilia 1996: new approach to an old disease, *Pediatr Clin North Am* 43:709, 1996.

Eyster ME, Gill FM, Blatt PM, et al: Central nervous system bleeding in hemophiliacs, *Blood* 51:1179, 1978.

Hoyer LW: Hemophilia A, *N Engl J Med* 330:38, 1994.

Morgan LM, Kissoon N, deVebber BL: Experience with the hemophiliac child in a pediatric emergency department, *J Emerg Med* 11:519, 1993.

National Hemophilia Foundation Medical and Scientific Advisory Council: Recommendations concerning HIV infection, hepatitis, and other transmissible agents in the treatment of hemophilia and related bleeding disorders (Medical Advisory #278), 1997.

Poon M-C, Israels SJ, Lillicrap DP, et al: Hemophilia and von Willebrand's disease: 1. Diagnosis, comprehensive care and assessment, *Can Med Assoc J* 153:19, 1995.

Poon M-C, Israels, SJ, Lillicrap DP, et al: Hemophilia and von Willebrand's disease: 2. Management, *Can Med Assoc J* 153:147, 1995.

Shopuick RI, Brettler DB: Hemostasis: a practical review of conservative and operative care, *Clin Orthop Rel Res* 328:34, 1996.

Silverman R, Kwiatkowski T, Bernstein S, et al: Safety of lumbar puncture in patients with hemophilia, *Ann Emerg Med* 22:1739, 1993

IDIOPATHIC THROMBOCYTOPENIC PURPURA

Idiopathic thrombocytopenic purpura (ITP) results from increased destruction of platelets on an autoimmune basis. It is associated with a spectrum of viral illnesses, including measles, rubella, mumps, chickenpox, infectious mononucleosis, and the common cold. Most cases of childhood ITP are self-limited; with 70% to 90% resolving within 6 months.

DIAGNOSTIC FINDINGS

1. An antecedent viral illness is reported in 50% of cases.
2. Symptomatic thrombocytopenia with abrupt onset of petechiae, purpura, and spontaneous bleeding of the skin and mucous membranes. Epistaxis and hemorrhage of the buccal mucosa are common. Bleeding usually responds to pressure.

Complications

1. Intracranial hemorrhage. Occurs in approximately 1% of patients, usually within the first 2 to 4 weeks. May be life threatening. Patients with headache or altered level of consciousness require emergency care.
2. GI bleeding.
3. Massive hematuria.
4. Chronic ITP. Thrombocytopenia of more than 6 month's duration. Most common in female children older than 10 years of age. Patients have a greater likelihood of associated autoimmune, collagen vascular, or malignant disease.

Ancillary Data

1. CBC, blood smear, and platelet count. Normal platelet count is 150,000-400,000 platelets/mm^3. In ITP patients, the platelet count is usually less than 100,000 platelets/mm^3 at the time of presentation. If the count falls to less than 20,000 platelets/mm^3, the patient is at risk of major hemorrhage.
2. Bone marrow puncture and analysis should be done early in the evaluation to confirm the diagnosis in patients with fewer than 50,000/mm^3 or when bone marrow disease is suspected. A normal or increased number of megakaryocytes is present in otherwise normal aspirate or biopsy. Some hematologists only recommend a bone marrow examination in patients with an atypical presentation.

DIFFERENTIAL DIAGNOSIS (PARTIAL)
Thrombocytopenia

1. Increased destruction of platelets
   a. Consumption
      (1) Microangiopathic state: hemolytic-uremic syndrome (HUS), DIC, local ischemic disease (necrotizing enterocolitis [NEC])
      (2) Prosthetic heart valves
      (3) Hyaline membrane disease (HMD)
   b. Autoimmune: systemic lupus erythematosus (SLE), Evans syndrome
2. Sequestration/maldistribution: splenomegaly or hypothermia
3. Decreased production of platelets
   a. Marrow infiltration: leukemia, lymphoma, storage disease, or solid tumor
   b. Marrow dysfunction
      (1) Congenital: Wiskott-Aldrich syndrome, etc.
      (2) Infection: viral
      (3) Drugs
         (a) Cytotoxic drugs
         (b) Anticonvulsants: phenytoin, carbamazepine, valproate
         (c) Antibiotics: sulfonamides, chloramphenicol, rifampin, trimethoprim with sulfamethoxazole

Platelet Dysfunction (Normal Count)

1. Congenital: von Willebrand syndrome
2. Drugs: aspirin, antihistamines, antibiotics (carbenicillin), nonsteroidal antiinflammatory agents
3. Uremia

Purpura and Petechiae without Thrombocytopenia or Platelet Dysfunction

These conditions include vasculitides such as Henoch-Schönlein purpura (HSP) and SLE and connective tissue disorders such as Ehlers-Danlos syndrome.

MANAGEMENT

Once the diagnosis is confirmed by bone marrow testing, expectant observation is indicated for several days, with close monitoring for developing CNS signs and symptoms. Because the antibodies responsible for ITP react with both patient and donor platelets, platelet transfusions are generally of little help in managing these patients. ITP is usually self-limited, with 80% of patients recovering spontaneously within 6 months.

Steroid Therapy

If the platelet count is less than 10,000 to 20,000/mm^3 or if there are extensive bleeding manifestations, most authorities recommend starting steroid therapy:

- Prednisone, 2 mg/kg/24 hr (maximum: 60 mg/24 hr) q8hr PO for 2 to 3 weeks; then taper at 5- to 7-day intervals.

Steroids lead to an increase in the platelet count by blocking reticuloendothelial consumption of antibody-coated platelets. They may also lessen the fragility of capillary membranes, causing a further decrease in bleeding.

The effects of steroid therapy are usually apparent by 48 to 72 hours, and more than 50% of children with ITP respond to steroids. However, the effect is transient and may only last as long as therapy is continued. If no initial response to steroids is noted or if the platelet count falls when they are discontinued, some suggest repeating a 4-week course after steroids have been discontinued for a month and the patient has been watched during that period. This should be done after consultation.

Emergent Intervention

If there is severe GI bleeding, epistaxis, hematuria, headache, or intracranial hemorrhage, emergent intervention is essential.

1. Red blood cell (RBC) transfusion for hypotension and anemia should be initiated.
2. Steroids are administered: hydrocortisone (Solu-Cortef), 4-5 mg/kg/dose q6hr IV, followed by prednisone, 2 mg/kg/24 hr PO q8hr. Others have suggested the use of methylprednisolone (Solu-Medrol), 30 mg/kg/24 hr PO for 7 days). Steroids may have an effect in 48 to 72 hours.
3. Hematuria may respond to pushing fluids.
4. Emergency splenectomy is usually necessary. Risk of infection is increased after surgery.
5. IV infusions of gamma globulin (1 gm/kg/dose IV over 4 to 8 hours up to three doses or 0.5 gm/kg/dose each day for 5 days) may be indicated in patients requiring a rapid rise in platelet count (surgery, trauma, or life-threatening mucosal or internal hemorrhages).
6. Platelet transfusions may be used with massive bleeding unresponsive to pressure. Adolescents and adults require 5 to 10 units, depending on size, age of platelet packs, and response. The half-life of transfused platelets is very short and usually fails to provide prolonged hemostasis.

Chronic ITP

This requires a sequential therapeutic plan:

1. Steroids: prednisone, as above.
2. If no improvement: splenectomy. The patient whose count does not improve with splenectomy should be evaluated for an accessory spleen by checking the blood smear for Howell-Jolly bodies and performing a spleen scan.
3. Immunosuppressive drugs such as vincristine and cyclophosphamide and IV immunoglobulins have been tried with some success.

DISPOSITION

1. Patients with platelet counts less than 50,000/mm^3 should be admitted for initial evaluation, monitoring, education, and treatment. A hematologist should be involved to perform a bone marrow examination and to assist in management. Asymptomatic patients with higher platelet counts may be monitored as outpatients after evaluation and monitored closely.
2. If no complications develop, the patient may be discharged after 3 days with close follow-up to ensure that thrombocytopenia resolves and no complications develop. Activity should be restricted and close follow-up evaluation ensured.

Parental Education

1. Watch for bleeding or any evidence of CNS abnormality.
2. Contact sports, as well as high-risk endeavors (e.g., skiing, diving), should be avoided.
3. Seat belts should be worn when the child travels in a car.
4. Young children (<4 years) can be fitted with padded helmets to decrease the risk of head trauma.
5. Aspirin and other drugs that inhibit platelet function should be avoided. The child should use a soft toothbrush and stool softener, and activity should be limited.

REFERENCES

Albayrak D, Islek I, Kalayei AG, et al: Acute immune thrombocytopenia: a comparison study of very high oral doses of methylprednisolone and intravenously administered immune globulin, *J Pediatr* 125:1004, 1994.

Bussel JB, Goldman A, Imbach P, et al: Treatment of acute idiopathic thrombocytopenia of childhood with intravenous infusions of gammaglobulin, *Pediatrics* 106:886, 1985.

Halperin DS, Doyle JJ: Is bone marrow examination justified in idiopathic thrombocytopenia purpura? *Am J Dis Child* 142:508, 1988.

Humbert JR, Sills R, editors: Controversies in treatment of idiopathic thrombocytopenic purpura in children, *Am J Pediatr Hematol Oncol* 6:147, 1984.

Stuart MJ, McKenna R: Diseases of coagulation: the platelet and vasculature. In Nathan DG, Oski FA, editors: *Hematology of infancy and childhood*, ed 3, Philadelphia, 1987, WB Saunders.

ONCOLOGIC PRESENTATIONS

Cancer is an important cause of death in children older than 1 year of age. Specific presentations may complicate the primary disease process. In as many as 7% of patients with cancer, the initial diagnosis was made in the emergency department (ED). Leukemia most commonly is manifested by pallor and weakness as well as hepatomegaly, petechiae, or ecchymoses, fever, tachycardia, or an abnormal white blood count. Children with CNS tumors were noted inconsistently to have headache, vomiting, fever, or balance problems. Children with non-CNS solid tumors had symptoms related to the location of the neoplasm.

FEVER AND NEUTROPENIA

Infection, inflammation, transfusion, medications, and tumor necrosis may cause fever in children with cancer. Children with neutropenia (<500/mm^3 polymorphonuclear leukocytes) and a fever require evaluation. Common bacterial pathogens include *S. pneumoniae*, *Streptococcus* species, *S. aureus*, *Klebsiella*, and *Enterococcus*. Fungal infections and *P. carinii* may also be noted.

After evaluation, expectant management is essential with a combination of antibiotics. Immunosuppressed patients in whom herpes simplex or varicella infection develops should receive acyclovir.

SUPERIOR VENA CAVA SYNDROME

Compression, infiltration, or thrombosis surrounding the superior vena cava may be causative, usually resulting from lymphoma or lung cancer. Patients have venous hypertension within the area drained by the superior vena cava. Periorbital, conjunctival, and facial swelling is present. Progression may lead to thoracic and neck vein distension, facial edema, tachypnea, plethora of the face, edema of the upper extremities, and cyanosis. Shortness of breath, cough, dyspnea, and chest pain may be reported.

Chest x-ray studies may reveal a mass, often associated with a pleural effusion. Irradiation and chemotherapy are therapeutic.

ACUTE TUMOR LYSIS SYNDROME

Lysis occurs 1 to 5 days after initiation of chemotherapy. Patients may experience renal failure, dysrhythmias, and neuromuscular symptoms. Uric acid, potassium, and calcium levels may be elevated. Allopurinol administration, hydration, and alkalinization of urine may be helpful.

HYPERVISCOSITY SYNDROME

Leukocytosis may develop, leading to sludging, decreased perfusion in the microcirculation, and vascular stasis. In acute myelogenous leukemia, hyperleukocytosis may occur with a white blood cell count greater than $200,000/mm^3$. Acute lymphocytic leukemia patients may tolerate up to $500,000/mm^3$.

Patients have retinopathy; neurologic findings include headache, dizziness, seizures, altered mental status, auditory disturbances, and hypotension, as well as respiratory, cardiac, and renal failure. Hydration may be helpful.

OTHER FINDINGS

Hyperuricemia may produce nephropathy, nephrolithiasis, and ultimately, renal failure. Treatment is administration of allopurinol, fluids, and alkalinization of urine. *Hypercalcemia* may be associated with tumors of the breast, ovary, lung, kidney, and thyroid. Ensuing com-

plications and *cardiac tamponade* may develop. *Neurologic* findings may be acute or chronic, usually as a result of direct involvement of the CNS.

REFERENCES

Bachman BT, Barkin RM, Brennan SA, et al: Hematologic and oncologic disorders. In Barkin RM, editor: *Pediatric emergency medicine: concepts and clinical practice*, ed 2, St Louis, 1997, Mosby.

Jaffe D, Fleisher G, Grosflam J: Detection of cancer in the pediatric emergency department, *Pediatr Emerg Care* 1:11, 1985.

Pizzo PA, Rubin M, Freifeld A, et al: The child with cancer and infection. I. Empiric therapy for fever and neutropenia and preventive strategies, *J Pediatr* 119:679, 1991.

Sickle Cell Disease

Thomas J. Smith

Roger H. Giller

Sickle cell anemia (SS disease) is an inherited disorder of hemoglobin synthesis, resulting from a single amino acid substitution (valine for glutamate) in the beta subunit of the hemoglobin molecule. Homozygotes for the sickle gene produce a predominance of sickle hemoglobin and develop symptomatic SS anemia. SS disease occurs in approximately 1 in 500 African Americans and occasionally may be seen in other racial groups from the Mediterranean region, the Middle East, and India. Sickle hemoglobin C (SC) disease and sickle-β-thalassemia are less common variants with similar but less severe clinical manifestations. Heterozygotes (AS) for the sickle gene produce both sickle (S) and normal adult (A) hemoglobin and remain asymptomatic carriers of the sickle trait except under conditions of severe hypoxia (including tourniquet surgery). These carriers are not anemic and do not demonstrate sickle cells in their blood smear. Newborn screening for sickle cell disease, when combined with extensive follow-up and education, significantly decreases patient mortality. Screening is now mandatory in 43 states. Identification of SS disease at birth enhances early recognition of sepsis and splenic sequestration, use of prophylactic penicillin and appropriate vaccines, and referrals to sickle cell centers.

DIAGNOSTIC FINDINGS (Table 79-3)

The clinical course of SS disease is a chronic illness punctuated by acute episodes ("crises") that threaten the life or comfort of the patient.

Anemia Crises

Sickling of erythrocytes results in chronic hemolytic anemia. Any process that further decreases the circulating red cell mass may produce a profound degree of anemia.

Aplastic Crisis
Impaired red cell production in the bone marrow may cause exacerbation of the chronic hemolytic anemia. Profound anemia may lead to high-output congestive heart failure. Hematocrit and reticulocyte counts are decreased relative to baseline values. Impaired erythropoiesis can be related to infection or folic acid deficiency. Recent evidence suggests that human parvovirus B19 infection is the predominant cause of aplastic crises in SS disease.

Hyperhemolytic Crisis
Acceleration of the already rapid rate of red cell destruction may occasionally cause worsening of the underlying anemia. Episodes may be related to concurrent G6PD deficiency or infection.

Splenic Sequestration Crisis
Young children with SS disease may suddenly pool a large portion of their peripheral blood volume in the spleen. This results in massive splenomegaly, severe anemia, and hypovolemic shock, evolving over a period of hours to days. It occurs most commonly between 4 months and 6 years of age, before autoinfarction of the spleen. It may be precipitated by infection.

Vasoocclusive Crises

Gelation of the abnormal hemoglobin within erythrocytes causes them to sickle, making them less deformable and leading to recurrent thromboses of the microvasculature. Local ischemia and tissue infarction result. Sickling is enhanced by dehydration, stasis, hypoxemia, acidosis, and hypertonicity. Bones, pulmonary parenchyma, abdominal viscera, and the CNS are the sites most often affected by the vasoocclusive process.

Musculoskeletal System
1. Bone pain, particularly of the extremities.
2. Dactylitis (hand-and-foot syndrome): symmetric, nonpitting edema of the hands and feet, accompanied by warmth and tenderness. Most common in children less than 4 years of age. Often, this may be the first manifestation of SS disease, alerting the clinician to evaluate the patient for this underlying disorder.
3. Aseptic necrosis of bone, particularly of the femoral or humeral head.
4. Leg ulcers.

Gastrointestinal Tract
1. Abdominal pain that is caused by a crisis is usually without peritoneal signs or decreased bowel sounds. In addition, the patient often has experienced this pain previously, and there has not been fever or an increase in the baseline white blood cell (WBC) count or band count.
2. Autosplenectomy by 5 years of age in those with SS disease.
3. Cholelithiasis caused by chronic hemolysis is increasingly prevalent after 10 years of age. Cholelithiasis may cause acute or insidious right upper quadrant pain and jaundice.
4. Hepatomegaly. A mild degree of enlargement is usually present, but it may progress because of one of the following:
   a. Acute hepatic sludging/right upper quadrant syndrome. Sickling may obstruct blood flow within the liver, leading to noncolicky right upper

TABLE 79-3 Sickle Cell Disease: Clinical Manifestations

Crisis	Category	Symptoms and signs	Evaluation	Management
Anemia	Aplastic	Fatigue, exercise intolerance, pallor, tachycardia, worsening anemia, low reticulocyte count	CBC, reticulocytes, bilirubin	Hospitalize, support intravascular volume, transfuse to replace RBC to slightly above baseline value
	Hyperhemolytic	As above, except high reticulocyte count, worsening icterus, increased bilirubin	As above	As above
	Splenic sequestration	Signs of anemia with splenomegaly (usually marked)	As above	As above; splenectomy may be necessary if recurrent problem
Vasoocclusive	Musculoskeletal	Pain, warmth, swelling, often in extremities (dactylitis)	CBC, reticulocytes (x-ray films of little help)	Pain control, hydrate
	Gastrointestinal	Pain, no peritoneal signs	CBC, reticulocytes, liver function tests; consider abdominal ultrasound for cholelithiasis	Pain control, hydrate
	Neurologic	Headache, focal neurologic findings, paralysis, seizures	CBC, reticulocytes, MRI of head without contrast	Hospitalize, hydrate, hematology consult, consider immediate RBC pheresis
	Priapism	Prolonged painful erection	CBC, reticulocytes	Pain control, hydrate, urology consultation; consider RBC transfusion or pheresis; avoid local heat or cold
Chest syndrome	Pulmonary	Chest pain, fever, tachypnea, hypoxia, focal pulmonary findings	CBC, reticulocytes, blood culture, pulse ox, ABG, CXR (V/Q scan of little help)	Hospitalize, hydrate, oxygen, antibiotics, hematology consult; may require RBC transfusion or pheresis if progressive
Infection	Fever	Fever with or without focal signs	CBC, reticulocytes, blood, and other appropriate cultures or x-ray films	Immediate antibiotics, may need hospitalization
	Pneumonia	See "Chest Syndrome"		See "Chest Syndrome"
	Osteomyelitis	Focal pain, warmth, swelling, fever; difficult to distinguish acutely from vasoocclusive crisis	CBC, reticulocytes, blood culture, plain film of site	Pain control, hydrate, consider aspiration; antibiotics only if diagnosis is clear

quadrant pain, progressive hepatomegaly, malaise, and jaundice.

b. Viral hepatitis usually secondary to prior blood transfusions.

c. Hepatic sequestration after infarction of the spleen.

Central Nervous System

Thrombotic or hemorrhagic strokes in those with SS disease occur in about 8% of patients. Patients may have severe headache, nuchal rigidity, focal neurologic findings, seizures, coma, or xanthochromic spinal fluid.

Priapism

Painful erections caused by obstruction of the venous drainage of the corpus cavernosum can be either "stuttering" (multiple short episodes) or prolonged (>24 hours).

Acute Chest Syndrome

Patients initially have chest pain, dyspnea, infiltrate, fever, leukocytosis, and rub or effusion. Pulmonary infarction often cannot be differentiated from pneumonia. Infarction usually occurs in children more than 12 years of age and may be associated with a painful crisis; infection is a more common trigger in younger children. The chest x-ray film is often clear initially with a positive ventilation-perfusion ($\dot{V}/\dot{Q}$) scan finding. Lower lobe involvement is common.

Infection

1. Functional asplenia leads to increased risk of serious bacterial infection. Sepsis, meningitis, pneumonia, and osteomyelitis occur with increased frequency and severity. Common causative organisms are listed in Table 79-4.

2. It is important to compare the WBC count to baseline WBC level. SS patients often have a high WBC level as a result of a hyperactive bone marrow.

3. The likelihood of bacterial infection is increased with more than 1000/mm^3 non-segmented neutrophils (bands) in the CBC.

4. Children with SC or sickle-β-thalassemia have a lower (but still high) risk of sepsis than do SS patients.

Other Diagnostic Findings

1. Impaired growth and delayed puberty are common.

2. Congestive heart failure (CHF) (see Chapter 16).

3. Psychosocial problems.

4. Retinopathy resulting from vasoocclusive phenomena. Marked by dilated and tortuous retinal vessels, microaneurysms, neovascularization, and retinal hemorrhage.

TABLE 79-4   Sickle Cell Disease: Infections

Infection	Common organisms	Initial antibiotic therapy*
Fever/presumed sepsis or meningitis	S. pneumoniae
H. influenzae	Cefotaxime, 150 mg/kg/24 hr (adult: 6 gm/24 hr) q6-8hr IV, or ceftriaxone, 100 mg/kg/24 hr (adult: 4 gm/24 hr) q12hr IV
Add vancomycin, 30-45 mg/kg/24 hr (adult: 2 gm/24 hr) q8-12hr IV for severe illness
Acute chest syndrome	S. pneumoniae
H. influenzae
M. pneumoniae	Cefotaxime or ceftriaxone as above; also, erythromycin, 40 mg/kg/24 hr q6hr PO; add vancomycin for severe illness
Osteomyelitis	Salmonella
S. aureus
S. pneumoniae	Cefotaxime or ceftriaxone as above and nafcillin, 100 mg/kg/24 hr q4hr IV, and gentamicin, 5-7.5 mg/kg/24 hr q8hr IV

*In critically ill children, more broad-spectrum antibiotics may be initiated. Therapy should be altered when culture and sensitivity data are available.

5. Premature births and spontaneous abortions are common during pregnancy.
6. Irreversible renal hyposthenuria is present in all patients by 5 years of age.
7. Hematuria may occur in both SS disease and sickle trait. Risk of urinary tract infections is increased.

Ancillary Data

1. CBC and reticulocyte count: abnormal. Baseline values for an individual patient are particularly important in the evaluation of acute problems (Table 79-5). Patients with sickle cell trait generally have no anemic or sickle cells on smear.
2. Hemoglobin electrophoresis confirms the diagnosis in coordination with the newborn metabolic screen. Early diagnosis allows initiation of preventative measures before the onset of signs or symptoms at 2 to 4 months. Solubility tests (e.g., Sickledex) are poor screening tests because they are insensitive during the newborn period. They do not distinguish between sickle cell disease and trait and fail to detect other hemoglobinopathies.
3. Unconjugated (indirect) bilirubin level is elevated (range: 1.5-4.0 mg/dl) because of chronic hemolysis. Other liver function test (LFT) results are normal unless there is supervening hepatobiliary disease (e.g., hepatitis, cholelithiasis, hepatic sludging).
4. Pulse oximetry and arterial blood gas (ABG). Helpful in the evaluation of pneumonia, pulmonary infarction, acute chest syndrome, CHF, and metabolic acidosis. Knowledge of baseline pulse oximetry is helpful.
5. Cultures: blood, urine, bone, cerebrospinal fluid (CSF) as indicated.
6. Urinalysis: hematuria common.
7. X-ray studies.
   a. Chest x-ray study: acute chest syndrome, infarction, infection, CHF. Film is especially indicated in febrile children as well as those with cough, chest pain, or physical findings suggesting chest findings.
   b. Abdominal x-ray or ultrasound study: cholelithiasis.
   c. Bone x-ray study: infarction, infection, aseptic necrosis. X-ray films usually cannot distinguish acute infarction from infection.
   d. Magnetic resonance imaging (MRI) scan: stroke.
8. Electrocardiogram (ECG): biventricular hypertrophy is common. Cor pulmonale may result from recurrent pulmonary infarcts.
9. Family studies. CBC with indices and reticulocyte count, blood smear, and hemoglobin electrophoresis on parents and siblings may help clarify the patient's diagnosis.

MANAGEMENT
Fluids

1. Maintain euvolemia. More fluids are only necessary if patient is hypotensive, dehydrated, or insensible losses are increased.

TABLE 79-5   Sickle Cell Disease: Hematologic Values

	Normal (AA) average	Sickle cell disease (SS) average (range)
Hematocrit (%)	36	22 (17-29)
Hemoglobin (gm/dl)	12	7.5 (5.5-9.5)
Reticulocytes (%)	1.5	12 (5-30)
WBC count (/mm³)	7500	20,000 (12,000-35,000)
Peripheral smear	Normal	Sickle cell present

Modified from Pearson HA, Diamond LK: In Smith CA, editor: *The critically ill child,* Philadelphia, 1985, WB Saunders.
NOTE: Patients with sickle cells trait have normal values and RBC morphology.

2. Administer 1 to 1¼ times maintenance fluids IV or PO during vasoocclusive crisis.
3. Monitor patient for dehydration, fluid overload, and high-output CHF. In splenic sequestration crisis, emergent fluid resuscitation with isotonic crystalloid, colloid, or blood is necessary to treat potential vascular collapse.

Blood Products

- Restore circulating RBC during aplastic or hyperhemolytic crises by administering packed RBC, 5-10 ml/kg over 3 to 4 hours.

If more rapid replacement of sickle erythrocytes is required (e.g., stroke, acute pulmonary syndrome, priapism), if CHF is present, or if there is concern about augmenting sickling because of increased blood viscosity after transfusion, partial exchange transfusion or red cell pheresis can be used.

- Reduction of cells containing sickle hemoglobin to 30% or more of the total circulating red cells effectively prevents further sickling. This can be accomplished by a chronic transfusion program with transfusions given every 3 to 4 weeks. Adequacy of transfusion therapy can be assessed by using the sodium metabisulfite sickling test or quantitative hemoglobin electrophoresis.

Oxygen

Hypoxia precipitates sickling and should be corrected when present, particularly in pulmonary disease, stroke, severe anemia, and CHF. Oxygen should be used to keep pulse oximetry at 92% or higher. Excessive oxygen may suppress reticulocyte count and exacerbate anemia.

Analgesia

1. Codeine, 4 mg/kg/24 hr q4-6hr PO.
2. Ketorolac (Toradol): above 2 years, 0.5-1 mg/kg/dose q6hr IV, 30 to 60 mg initially followed by 15 to 30 mg q6hr IV up to daily maximum of 150 mg. First parenteral nonsteroidal antiinflammatory agent.
3. Morphine, 0.1-0.2 mg/kg/dose q2-4hr IV. Maximum dose: 10 mg/dose. May need continuous infusion.
   NOTE: Prolonged use of meperidine (Demerol) should be prevented because of risk of seizures.
4. Hydromorphone (Dilaudid), 1-4 mg/dose q4-6hr PO (or IV). Not recommended for children less than 10 years of age.
5. Methylprednisolone, 15 mg/kg IV and repeated 24 hours later, decreased duration of pain but was associated with more rebound attacks. Not currently recommended.

A useful analgesic routine for inpatient management of severe pain may include the following. In most cases pain analgesia orders are not appropriate:

1. First 24 hours: morphine sulfate, 0.1-0.2 mg/kg/dose (maximum: 10 mg/dose) q2hr IV on a schedule. Monitoring is required. May supplement with ibuprofen or acetaminophen q4hr PO. Alternatively, ketorolac, 0.5-1.0 mg/kg/dose IV q6hr on schedule (maximum duration: 5 days) supplemented with morphine sulfate for breakthrough pain.
2. After 24 to 48 hours or when acute pain has diminished: taper parenteral dose by 20% daily but do not change interval. When one half of the starting parenteral dose is achieved, switch to oral analgesics every 4 hours and then slowly decrease interval to a prn basis.
3. Obviously, any regimen needs to be individualized.

Antibiotics

Antibiotics (see Table 79-4) should be given if any evidence of fever exists.

1. Cultures should be obtained before initiating treatment and should determine the ultimate choice of antibiotics.

2. A bacterial infection is more likely if there are more than 1000 bands/mm^3 but should be considered in all febrile patients.
3. The route of administration of antibiotics and the necessity of hospitalizing the patient are determined by the degree of toxicity and nature of systemic involvement. Prophylactic penicillin initiated by 4 months of age has been shown to reduce infection-related morbidity and mortality rates.
4. In chest syndrome and bone pain, it may be impossible to distinguish between infection and infarction. Chest syndrome should always be treated with appropriate antibiotics. With bone pain, it may be prudent to treat with hydration and analgesia and institute antibiotics only if symptoms persist 2 to 3 days.

Surgery

1. Cholecystectomy: symptomatic cholelithiasis
2. Splenectomy: recurrent splenic sequestration crises
3. Arthroplasty: aseptic necrosis of femoral or humeral head

Transfusion Therapy

Long-term transfusion therapy is 90% effective in preventing recurrent strokes after an episode of actual cerebrovascular accident (CVA). Therapy must be continued indefinitely. Chronic transfusions may also be required for recurrent chest syndrome or priapism.

DISPOSITION

1. Hospitalization is indicated for patients with splenic sequestration crisis, aplastic crisis with severe anemia, stroke, acute chest syndrome, suspected bacterial infection, severe or prolonged priapism, and severe vasoocclusive pain crisis in which parenteral analgesia or IV hydration is required. It is important not to prolong ambulatory management of such patients in the ED. Patients not responding in the first 2 hours with appropriate pain medication and hydration usually should be admitted.
2. Hydroxyurea. Hydroxyurea therapy significantly decreased the severity of anemia and frequency of vasoocclusive crisis in some children with SS disease. Nevertheless, it is a potent chemotherapeutic agent whose long-term toxicity is unknown and should be used by hematologists with expertise in chemotherapy.
3. Bone marrow transplant. Allogeneic bone marrow transplant from an HLA-identical sibling can change the hemoglobin electrophoresis pattern to that of the donor and eliminate sickle-related symptoms, without serious graft-versus-host disease. This is successful in 80% to 90% of children with SS who have undergone transplantation. The main problems are predicting the clinical severity of SS disease for any given child and finding a matched sibling donor.
4. Long-term follow-up is essential. Health maintenance considerations should include the following:
   a. Prophylactic penicillin. Consideration should be given to stopping this at age 5 although it is still under study.
   b. Pneumococcal, *H. influenzae*, meningococcal, and hepatitis B vaccines.
   c. Folic acid therapy (1 mg/day PO).
   d. Chronic transfusion therapy.
   e. Genetic counseling.
   f. Ophthalmologic examination for sickle retinopathy.
   g. Psychosocial counseling.
   h. Coordination of patient care and services through a comprehensive hemoglobinopathy program.

REFERENCES

Buchanan GR, Glader BE: Leukocyte counts in children with sickle cell disease, *Am J Dis Child* 132:398, 1978.

Charache S, Lubin B, Reid CD: Management and therapy of sickle cell disease, US Department of Health and Human Services, NIH Publication No. 91-2117, 1991.

DiMichele D: Hemophilia 1996: a new approach to an old disease, *Pediatr Clin North Am* 43:709, 1996.

Falletta JM, Woods GM, Verter JI, et al: Discontinuing penicillin prophylaxis in children with sickle cell anemia, *J Pediatr* 127:685, 1995.

Galloway SJ, Harwood-Nuss AL: Sickle cell anemia: a review, *J Emerg Med* 6:213, 1988.

Gaston MH, Verter JJ, Woods G, et al: Prophylaxis with oral penicillin in children with sickle cell anemia, *N Engl J Med* 314:1593, 1986.

Griffin TC, McIntire D, Buchanan GR: High dose intravenous methylprednisolone therapy for pain in children and adolescents with sickle cell disease, *N Engl J Med* 330:733, 1994.

Mills ML: Life-threatening complications of sickle cell disease in children, *JAMA* 254:1487, 1985.

Pollack CV, Sanders DY, Severance HW: Emergency department analgesia without narcotics for adults with acute sickle cell pain crisis: case reports and review of crisis management, *J Emerg Med* 9:445, 1991.

Poncz M, Kane E, Gill FM: Acute chest syndrome in sickle cell disease: etiology and clinical correlates, *J Pediatr* 107:861, 1985.

Scott J, Hillary CA, Brown ER, et al: Hydroxyurea therapy in children severely affected with sickle cell disease, *J Pediatr* 128:820, 1996.

Vermulen C, Counu F: Bone marrow transplantation for sickle cell disease: the European experience, *Am J Pediatr Hematol Oncol* 16:18, 1994.

Vichinsky E, Hurst D, Eaules A, et al: Newborn screening for sickle cell disease: effect on mortality, *Pediatrics* 81:749, 1998.

80 INFECTIOUS DISORDERS

ACQUIRED IMMUNODEFICIENCY SYNDROME

Children contract acquired immunodeficiency syndrome (AIDS) from their mothers during the perinatal period or through contaminated blood or blood products. The former accounts for 90% of new cases in the United States. Sexual activity is a rare mode of transmission in children but is obviously a major concern in adolescents and adults.

Human T lymphotropic virus type III (HTLV-III), called human immunodeficiency virus (HIV), is etiologic. It is tropic for T-helper (CD4) lymphocytes and macrophages, causing cell dysfunction, immune deficiencies, and death. Human retrovirus, of which HIV is one, uses enzyme reverse transcriptase to copy deoxyribonucleic acid (DNA) from the viral ribonucleic acid (RNA). The DNA is incorporated into human cellular DNA, where it can remain latent for months or years.

DIAGNOSTIC FINDINGS

Maternal HIV infections may be suspected if there is clinical evidence of infection or immunodeficiency. Intravenous drug abuse, sexual promiscuity, or residence in an area of high HIV prevalence also increases the risk. Perinatal transmission occurs in 25% to 40% of offspring of infected women. Breast milk has been implicated in the transmission of HIV infection. Infants may be small for gestational age or fail to thrive; problems develop by 3 to 6 months of age.

Older children have hepatosplenomegaly, lymphadenopathy, salivary gland enlargement, recurrent or persistent infections, and high immunoglobulin G (IgG) levels associated with AIDS-related complex (ARC), which ultimately progresses to AIDS. Chronic interstitial pneumonia *(Pneumocystis carinii)* may develop as well as other opportunistic infections. Otitis media, sinus infections, hepatitis, hepatosplenomegaly, failure to thrive, nephropathy, cardiomyopathy, malignancy, immune thrombocytopenia purpura, and chronic diarrhea are noted. Neurologic deficits may include developmental delay, generalized weakness with pyramidal signs, loss of milestones, and chronic or progressive encephalopathy with ataxia and seizures.

Common opportunistic infections in children include the following:

1. *P. carinii* pneumonitis
2. *Candida* esophagitis
3. Disseminated cytomegalovirus
4. Cryptosporidiosis
5. *Mycobacterium avium-intracellulare*
6. Chronic herpes simplex virus
7. *Cryptococcus*
8. Toxoplasmosis

Ancillary Data

1. Screening studies include HIV antibody testing by enzyme-linked immunosorbent assay (ELISA). If the result is positive, it should be repeated, and if the second test result is positive, the results should be confirmed by Western blot assay to

minimize false-positive results. If possible, obtain DNA PCR and P24 antigen tests. If the study findings are initially negative after a specific exposure, repeat screening may be warranted in 1 month. Informed consent to obtain these studies is sometimes appropriate.

2. Immune evaluation.
   a. Complete blood count (CBC) and differential
   b. T cell: delayed hypersensitivity skin test, complete T-cell subset, and mitogen and antibody stimulated lymphocyte blastogenesis
   c. B cell: quantitative immunoglobulins, preimmunization and postimmunization antibody levels, and B-cell enumeration
3. Other evaluations may include liver and renal function, chest x-ray examination, and lumbar puncture, usually in consultation with a center commonly caring for patients with AIDS.
   a. Patients with fever should generally have a CBC and differential, blood culture, chest x-ray examination, and other studies done to exclude specific infections. A more extensive evaluation is indicated for recurrent or unexplained fever.

MANAGEMENT

No definitive treatment exists. Supportive care is essential and parallels that for immunocompromised individuals, as outlined in Chapter 79. Referral for ongoing care is essential to ensure appropriate evaluation, continuity, and access to evolving protocols.

1. Opportunistic infections must be recognized and treated aggressively.
2. Zidovudine (ZVT) and Didanosine (DDI) are antiretroviral agents approved for use in HIV-infected children. ZVT administered during HIV infection pregnancies may reduce vertical transmission. Newer regimens, perhaps combined with cesarean section, may be prophylactic.
3. Provide psychologic support.
4. Use universal precautions.
5. The national AIDS hot line may be useful (800-342-AIDS).

REFERENCES

American Academy of Pediatrics Task Force on Pediatric AIDS: Guidelines for human immunodeficiency virus (HIV) infection in children and their foster families, *Pediatrics* 89:681, 1992.

Centers for Disease Control and Prevention: Guidelines: revised guidelines for prophylaxis against *Pneumocystis carinii* pneumonia for children infected with or permanently exposed to human immunodeficiency virus, *MMWR* 44(RR-4), 1995.

Falloon J, Eddy J, Wiener L, et al: Human immunodeficiency virus infection in children, *J Pediatr* 114:1, 1989.

Husson RN, Comeau AM, Hoff R: Diagnosis of human immunodeficiency virus infection in infants and children, *Pediatrics* 86:1, 1990.

Johnson JP, Nair P, Hines SE, et al: Natural history and serologic diagnosis of infants born to human immunodeficiency virus infected women, *Am J Dis Child* 143:1147, 1989.

Krasinski K: Antiretroviral therapy in children, *Acta Paediatr* 400(suppl 1):63, 1994.

Luzuriaga K, Bryan Y, Krogstad P, et al: Combination treatment with Zidovudine, Didanosine, and Nevirapine in infants with HIV type I infection, *N Engl J Med* 336:1343, 1997.

Moore RD, Hidalgo J, Dugland BW, et al: Zidovudine and the natural history of acquired immunodeficiency syndrome, *N Engl J Med* 324:1412, 1991.

Nicholas SW: Management of HIV positive children with fever, *J Pediatr* 119:521, 1991.

Rogers M, Caldwell M, Qwinn M, et al: Epidemiology of pediatric human immunodeficiency virus infection in the United States, *Acta Paediatr* 400(suppl 1):5, 1995.

BOTULISM

Botulism results from the ingestion of preformed toxins (e.g., canned vegetables), ingestion of spores in infant botulism (honey), or spore contamination of open wounds. *Clostridium botulinum* produces a neurotoxin that blocks the presynaptic release of acetylcholine. The incubation period of foodborne infection is

12 to 36 hours (range: 6 hours to 8 days), whereas it is 4 to 14 days with wound infections. Infant botulism has an incubation period of 3 to 30 days.

DIAGNOSTIC FINDINGS

1. A symmetric descending paralysis is noted, with weakness and equal deep tendon reflexes (DTRs).
   a. Pupils are fixed and dilated with oculomotor paralysis, blurred vision, diplopia, ptosis, and photophobia.
   b. Slurred speech, dysphagia, and sore throat are reported.
   c. Nausea, vomiting, vertigo, dry mouth, constipation, and urinary retention occur.
   d. Dyspnea and rales are commonly noted. In rare cases, secondary bacterial infection and total respiratory failure occur as a result of paralysis.
2. The sensorium and sensory examinations are normal.
3. If a wound is present, it may suppurate with gas formation.

Ancillary Data

1. *C. botulinum* toxin assay, if available
2. Lumbar puncture (LP) may have increased protein
3. Chest x-ray film and arterial blood gas (ABG) as indicated

DIFFERENTIAL DIAGNOSIS

Botulism should be distinguished from intoxication (see Chapter 54) caused by heavy metals or organophosphates (p. 385).

MANAGEMENT

1. Initially, focus on airway management, as well as other aspects of cholinergic blockage. Place a nasogastric (NG) tube and urinary catheter. All patients require intensive monitoring. In one study of 57 children with infant botulism, 77% were intubated and required mechanical ventilation.
2. Irrigate and debride all wounds.
3. Administer trivalent ABE antitoxin, available from the Centers for Disease Control and Prevention (days: 404-639-3670; nights: 404-639-2888) or a state health department.
4. Give antitoxin to individuals exposed to the source by ingestion.
5. Botulism may be prevented by boiling all foods adequately (more than 10 minutes). Children less than 1 year of age should not eat honey.

REFERENCES

Burmingham M, Walter F, Mecham C, et al: Wound botulism, *Ann Emerg Med* 24:1184, 1994.

Long SS, Gajewski JL, Brown LW, et al: Clinical laboratory and environmental features of infant botulism in Southeastern Pennsylvania, *Pediatrics* 75:935, 1985.

Shriener MS, Field E, Ruddy R: Infant botulism: a review of 12 years experience at the Children's Hospital of Philadelphia, *Pediatrics* 87:159, 1991.

DIPHTHERIA

Corynebacterium diphtheriae, a club-shaped, gram-positive, pleomorphic bacillus, produces an exotoxin that accounts for much of the systemic disease and its complications. The incubation period is 2 to 5 days.

DIAGNOSTIC FINDINGS

Four distinct clinical presentations have been described:

1. Pharyngeal-tonsillar: sore throat, fever, vomiting, difficulty swallowing, and malaise associated with a gray, closely

adherent pseudomembrane. It may progress to respiratory obstruction.

2. Laryngeal: less common. Initially occurs with hoarseness, loss of voice, and may extend into the pharynx.

3. Nasal: serosanguineous nasal discharge that may persist for weeks.

4. Cutaneous: sharply demarcated ulcer with membranous base. Common in the tropics.

Complications

These are primarily the result of the effects of exotoxin on organs beyond the respiratory tract.

1. Cardiac: myocarditis, endocarditis (p. 559), dysrhythmias (atrioventricular [AV] block, left bundle branch block) (see Chapter 6)

2. Respiratory obstruction and failure

3. Palatal and oculomotor palsy and peripheral polyneuritis (see Chapter 41)

4. Death, usually from respiratory or cardiac complications

Ancillary Data

1. Cultures (Loeffler medium and tellurite agar) and Gram stain

2. CBC (variable, platelets decreased)

3. Cardiac enzymes, electrocardiogram (ECG), and ABG as needed

DIFFERENTIAL DIAGNOSIS

See p. 604.

MANAGEMENT

1. Initially, focus on stabilization of the airway and treatment of cardiac dysfunction.

2. Give a Td booster to exposed, immunized, asymptomatic contacts. Give erythromycin (as below) to asymptomatic, unimmunized individuals for 7 days and begin immunization schedule as outlined in Appendix B-7.

3. Corticosteroids have no proven beneficial role in preventing ECG changes or neuritis.

Antitoxin

1. Sensitivity may be determined by diluting 0.5 ml serum in 10 ml saline or D5W. Give this slowly. Observe for 30 minutes and if no reactions, serum diluted 1:20 may be given at a rate of 1 ml/min.

2. If the membrane is pharyngeal or laryngeal and of less than 48 hours' duration, give 20,000 to 40,000 units of antitoxin; nasopharyngeal lesions, 40,000 to 60,000 units; and extensive disease of 3 days or more, 80,000 to 100,000 units.

3. With cutaneous disease, some recommend 20,000 to 40,000 units of antitoxin to prevent progression to toxic sequelae.

4. CDC may be a source of antitoxin (404-639-3670/2888).

Antibiotics

• Aqueous penicillin G, 100,000-150,000 U/kg/24 hr q4-6hr IV, for 7 to 10 days or procaine penicillin G, 25,000-50,000 U/kg/24 hr q12hr IM, for 14 days. Parenteral erythromycin is an alternative.

Once parenteral therapy is no longer required, a 10-day course of oral penicillin (or, with allergic patient, erythromycin) is begun:

1. Penicillin V, 25,000-50,000 units (15-30 mg)/kg/24 hr q6hr PO; or

2. Erythromycin, 30-50 mg/kg/24 hr q6hr PO.

Asymptomatic previously immunized close contacts should receive a booster immunization if they have not received a booster dose of diphtheria toxoid within 5 years.

Asymptomatic unimmunized (or unknown) close contacts should receive prophylaxis (erythromycin, 40-50 mg/kg/24 hr for 7 days, or benzathine penicillin G, 600,000-1,200,000 units IM).

All close contacts should be cultured.

DISPOSITION

Patients should be hospitalized for close observation and respiratory isolation. Carriers require antibiotics and immunization.

Parental Education

Active immunization should be encouraged.

REFERENCES

Report of the Committee on Infectious Disease, Elk Grove, Ill, 1997, American Academy of Pediatrics.

Thisyakorn USA, Wongvarich J, Kumpeng V: Failure of corticosteroid therapy to prevent diphtheritic myocarditis or neuritis, *Pediatr Infect Dis* 3:126, 1984.

KAWASAKI SYNDROME

Kawasaki syndrome is a multisystem disease affecting young children often less than 5 years of age and primarily in the late winter and early spring. Boys outnumber girls in incidence. It is also known as *mucocutaneous lymph node syndrome* (MCLS). Although it is self-limited, the major involvement of the coronary arteries results in significant morbidity. The cause is unproved but is thought to be related to lymphotropic retrovirus. There has been a reported association with house dust, mites, and rug shampoo.

DIAGNOSTIC FINDINGS

The syndrome is triphasic in clinical presentation. An *acute* febrile episode lasts for 7 to 10 days with the appearance of the six major diagnostic criteria. The *subacute* stage lasts 10 to 14 days up to 25 days from the onset with associated anorexia, desquamation, and cardiovascular complications and the highest risk of death. *Convalescence* lasts 6 to 8 weeks, and there may be a continuing period of high risk of death.

Six major criteria have been established in diagnosing the syndrome, at least five of which are required for confirmation of the diagnosis.

1. Fever greater than 38.5° C (usually 38.5° to 40° C) for at least 5 days. The fever begins abruptly and may last as long as 23 days (average: 11 days).
2. Discrete bilateral, nonexudative conjunctival injection, usually within 2 days of the onset of fever and sometimes lasting 1 to 2 weeks. Engorged vessels originate at the canthus and course toward the limbus.
3. Mouth changes appear 1 to 3 days after onset and may last 1 to 2 weeks.
   a. Erythema, fissuring, and crusting of the lips
   b. Diffuse, oropharyngeal erythema
   c. Strawberry tongue
4. Peripheral changes begin after 3 to 5 days and last 1 to 2 weeks.
   a. Induration of the hands and feet. May be edematous.
   b. Erythema of the palms and soles.
   c. Desquamation of the tips of fingers and toes 2 to 3 weeks after onset of illness.
   d. Transverse nail grooves are common during convalescence.
5. Erythematous, polymorphous rash concurrent with the fever and spreading from the extremities to the trunk. May be pruritic. The rash usually disappears in less than 1 week, but during the second week of illness, the patient may get desquamation at the junction of the nails and the tips of fingers and toes.
6. Enlarged lymph nodes, usually cervical and more than 1.5 cm. This is the last consistent major finding.
7. Other findings may include the following:
   a. Cardiovascular: coronary artery disease (see complications); ECG abnormalities
   b. Gastrointestinal: diarrhea, vomiting, abdominal pain, hydrops of the gall-

bladder, obstructive jaundice, perineal rash, pancreatitis
c. Blood: leukocytosis, increased erythrocyte sedimentation rate (ESR)
d. Genitourinary: urethritis, proteinuria, pyuria
e. Respiratory: pneumonia, cough
f. Joint: arthritis
g. Neurologic: meningismus, cerebrospinal fluid (CSF) pleocytosis, irritability, photophobia, uveitis, iritis

Complications

Coronary artery disease caused by arteritis, aneurysm, or thrombosis occurs in as many as 20% of patients, with onset as long as 45 days after the first fever. Half of these abnormalities resolve. Children less than 1 year and older than 5 years of age at onset of the disease are at greatest risk. The condition may be asymptomatic but accounts for the mortality rate of 1% to 2%. The risk is greatest during the subacute and convalescent periods; 70% of all deaths occur 15 to 45 days after the onset of fever. The severity of coronary artery involvement during the initial stages influences the regression of these lesions.

Congestive heart failure (CHF) is frequently observed, accompanied by carditis with complications such as dysrhythmias, pericarditis, mitral insufficiency, myocardial ischemia, or myocardial infarction. These increase the likelihood of coronary lesions.

Ancillary Data

1. CBC is usually elevated to more than 20,000/mm^3 with a predominance of neutrophils. Hematocrit (Hct) may be reduced.
2. Platelets are significantly increased, often as high as 1 million/mm^3.
3. ESR is elevated with a mean of 55 mm/hr. Serial monitoring may be useful.
4. Sterile pyuria and proteinuria may be present.

5. Elevated serum alanine aminotransferase level.
6. ECG is not diagnostic. Echocardiography or arteriography is often needed to define the extent of coronary artery disease and should routinely be considered initially and at 7 to 12 days into the illness.
7. The most common coronary artery involvement is simple dilation. Echocardiography may have a sensitivity and specificity of more than 95% in identifying abnormalities of the proximal coronary artery. Distal coronary artery abnormalities are rare in the absence of proximal involvement.
8. Gallium citrate ^{67}Ga scanning may be useful in demonstrating myocardial inflammation.
9. LP is indicated if meningismus is present.

DIFFERENTIAL DIAGNOSIS

Differentiating Kawasaki syndrome (Table 80-1) from other entities is particularly important for both acute care and for determination of the need for close, long-term follow-up observation.

The patient with Kawasaki syndrome is unlikely to have discrete intraoral lesions, exudative conjunctivitis, exudative pharyngitis, or generalized adenopathy.

1. Infection (see Table 80-1)
   a. Scarlatiniform rash: group A streptococci and *S. aureus*
   b. Measles
   c. Leptospirosis and rickettsial disease
   d. Staphylococcal scalded skin syndrome (p. 586) and toxic shock syndrome (p. 721)
2. Autoimmune: juvenile rheumatoid arthritis (JRA) and systemic lupus erythematosus (SLE)
3. Intoxication: acrodynia (mercury)
4. Erythema multiforme and Stevens-Johnson syndrome (p. 580)
5. Drug reaction: sulfonamides

TABLE 80-1   Kawasaki Syndrome: Diagnostic Considerations

Condition	Etiology	Diagnostic findings
Scarlatiniform rash (p. 289)	Group A streptococcus S. aureus	Diffuse erythroderma, prominent flexion creases; fingertip desquamation; pharyngitis; strawberry tongue
Scalded skin syndrome (Ritter syndrome in newborn) (p. 586)	S. aureus	Painful erythroderma with bullae and positive Nikolsky sign; toxic; may have fluid loss
Toxic epidermal necrolysis (erythema multiforme/ Stevens-Johnson) (Lyell syndrome) (p. 580)	Drug reaction	Confluent erythema with bullae desquamation prominent over extremities, face, and neck; positive Nikolsky sign; usually toxic with fever
Kawasaki syndrome (muco-cutaneous syndrome [MCLS]) (p. 710)	Unknown	Polymorphous erythroderma; desquamation of tips of fingers and toes; fever; conjunctival injection; red fissured lips; lymphadenopathy
Toxic shock syndrome (p. 721)	S. aureus	Diffuse erythroderma; desquamation, especially of palms and soles; fever; shock; multisystem involvement
Leptospirosis	Leptospira	Erythematous, macular, papular, petechial or purpuric rash; fever, conjunctivitis, pharyngitis, lymphadenopathy; multisystem (renal, liver, central nervous system) involvement

MANAGEMENT

1. Supportive care is essential, focusing on fluids, antipyretics, and treatment of CHF, if present (see Chapter 16).
2. Aspirin therapy is antiinflammatory, inhibits platelet function, and may reduce the tendency toward thrombosis and associated coronary artery disease. Initiate 100 mg/kg/24 hr q6hr PO through day 14 and then maintain on at least 3-5 mg/kg/24 hr q12-24hr PO for 6 to 8 weeks, when the platelet count and ESR should have returned to normal. Because of the impaired aspirin absorption, higher dosages may be required and it is imperative to monitor the serum level and maintain it at 20-25 mg/dl initially.
3. Steroids and antibiotics are not indicated. Steroids may actually increase the incidence of aneurysms.
4. High-dose intravenous immune gamma globulin (IVIG) combined with aspirin may decrease the frequency of coronary artery disease if given within 10 days of onset of the disease. An effective regimen is to administer 2 gm/kg as a single dose over 10 to 12 hours.

   Retreatment with IVIG may be necessary in 10% of children who have persistent (>48 to 72 hours) or recrudescent fever.
5. A cardiologist should be involved in the management to ensure immediate assessment and long-term follow-up observation.

DISPOSITION

1. All patients should be hospitalized early in their course for initial stabilization, in

addition to ensuring an adequate and rapid assessment to exclude other diagnostic possibilities.

2. Patients require follow-up for several years after the illness, with particular attention to coronary artery disease; 50% of aneurysms occur within 1 to 2 years. Many recommend special echocardiograms and delayed catheterization.

REFERENCES

Akagi T, Rose V, Benson LN, et al: Outcome of coronary artery aneurysms after Kawasaki disease, *J Pediatr* 121:689, 1992.

American Heart Association Committee on Rheumatic Fever, Endocarditis, Kawasaki Disease: Diagnostic guidelines for Kawasaki disease, *Am J Dis Child* 144:1210, 1990.

Barron KS, Murphy DJ, Silverman ED: Treatment of Kawasaki syndrome: a comparison of intravenously administered immune globulin, *J Pediatr* 117:638, 1990.

Burons JC, Mason WH, Glode MP, et al: Clinical and epidemiologic characteristics of patients referred for evaluation of possible Kawasaki disease, *J Pediatr* 118: 680, 1991.

Dajan A, Taubert K, Takahashi M, et al: Guideline for long-term management of patients with Kawasaki disease, *Circulation* 89:916, 1994.

Fujita Y, Nakamura Y, Sakata K, et al: Kawasaki disease in families, *Pediatrics* 84:666, 1989.

Ichida F, Fatica NS, O'Laughlin JE, et al: Epidemiologic aspects of Kawasaki disease in a Manhattan hospital, *Pediatrics* 84:235, 1989.

Koren G, Lavi S, Rose V, et al: Kawasaki disease: a review of risk factors for coronary aneurysm, *J Pediatr* 108:388, 1986.

Nakamura Y, Fujita Y, Nagai M, et al: Cardiac sequelae of Kawasaki disease in Japan: statistical analysis, *Pediatrics* 88:1144, 1991.

Newburger JW, Takahashi M, Beiser AS: A single intravenous infusion of gamma globulin as compared with four infusions in the treatment of acute Kawasaki syndrome, *N Engl J Med* 324:1633, 1991.

Rowley AH, Shulman SJ: Current therapy for acute Kawasaki syndrome, *J Pediatr* 118:987, 1992.

Shere NH, Spielberg SP, Grant DM, et al: Differences in metabolism of sulfonamides predisposing to idiosyncratic toxicity, *Ann Intern Med* 105:179, 1986.

Yahagawa H, Kawasaki T, Shigomatsu I: Nationwide survey on Kawasaki disease in Japan, *Pediatrics* 90:58, 1987.

MENINGOCOCCEMIA

Neisseria meningitidis is a gram-negative diplococcus responsible for a spectrum of clinical infections. Meningococcemia is life threatening and presents a diagnostic dilemma. In rare cases, *H. influenzae* can produce a comparable clinical picture.

DIAGNOSTIC FINDINGS

1. The onset varies, ranging from insidious to fulminant.
2. Patients have fever, malaise, headache, weakness, lethargy, vomiting, and arthralgia, as well as signs and symptoms of complicating conditions.
3. Two patterns of skin eruptions are noted:
   a. Pink maculopapular and generalized petechial rash, including palms and soles
   b. Purpuric and ecchymotic (often in a centrifugal distribution) associated with a very high mortality
4. Prognostically, unfavorable factors include the following:
   a. Presence of petechiae for less than 12 hours before hospitalization
   b. Shock
   c. Absence of meningitis (<20 WBC/mm^3 in CSF)
   d. White blood cells (WBC) normal or low (<10,000/mm^3)
   e. ESR normal or low (<10 mm/hr)
5. Survival is usually determined in the first 12 hours after treatment has begun.

Complications

1. Meningitis or meningoencephalitis (see Chapter 81)
2. Pericarditis (p. 564)
3. Cervicitis
4. Disseminated intravascular coagulation (DIC) (p. 683), Waterhouse-Friderichsen syndrome

5. Hypotension (see Chapter 5), cardiac collapse, and death

Ancillary Data

1. WBC, platelet count, and bleeding screens
2. Cultures of blood, spinal fluid, nasopharynx, and other involved organs
3. Skin scraping of the purpuric lesion may have positive culture. ·

DIFFERENTIAL DIAGNOSIS (see Table 42-2)

One study of children with fever and petechiae demonstrated that 20% had bacterial infections. Of these, 50% were caused by *N. meningitidis,* 30% by *H. influenzae* and the remainder by a variety of agents.

MANAGEMENT

Patients require immediate resuscitation (fluids, ventilation and airway support, and pressor agents, if necessary), supportive care, and treatment of complications.

Antibiotics

• Penicillin, 250,000 U/kg/24 hr q4hr IV (maximum: 20 million U/24 hr), for 7 to 10 days. Chloramphenicol for allergic patients; cefotaxime or ceftriaxone may also be considered.

Treatment of Contacts

Contacts are those who have slept or eaten in the same household as the index case or hospital personnel with intimate respiratory contact such as would occur with mouth-to-mouth resuscitation. Contacts should be clinically monitored.

Rifampin

1. Children: 10 mg/kg q12hr PO for 2 days
   • To administer to children, a liquid formulation can be prepared. Mixing the powder in vehicles such as applesauce can result in irregular absorption.
2. Adult: 600 mg q12hr PO for 2 days

DISPOSITION

1. All patients with systemic disease require admission to an intensive care unit (ICU) with provision for respiratory isolation.
2. Contacts require treatment and should notify the primary physician if fever, headache, stiff neck, or malaise develops. A vaccine is available for administration to high-risk groups; epidemic control may also be an indication.

REFERENCES

Berg S, Trollfors B, Alestig K, et al: Incidence, serogroups, and case-fatality of invasive meningococcal infections in a Swedish region 1975-1989, *Scand J Infect Dis* 24:333, 1992.

Harlens P, Garland J, Brook M, et al: Trends in mortality in children hospitalized with meningococcal infections, 1957 to 1987, *Pediatr Infect Dis* 8:8, 1989.

Olivareis R, Bouyer J, Hubert B: Risk factors for death in meningococcal disease, *Pathol Biol* 41:164, 1993.

Mononucleosis, Infectious

An acute viral illness caused by Epstein-Barr (EB) virus, infectious mononucleosis most frequently occurs in adolescents and young adults.

DIAGNOSTIC FINDINGS

1. Although the severity varies, most patients have a prodrome of 3 to 5 days with malaise, anorexia, nausea, and vomiting.
2. Patients rapidly develop high fevers, pharyngitis, lymphadenopathy, particularly cervical, and splenomegaly. Lymph nodes are usually symmetric, firm, discrete and mildly to moderately tender.
3. The symptoms may persist for weeks, particularly those associated with prodrome.

4. Young children may have fever, diarrhea, pharyngitis, otitis media, pneumonia, lymphadenopathy, hepatomegaly, and splenomegaly.
5. An erythematous, maculopapular rash may develop, commonly with the use of ampicillin. It is most prominent on the trunk and proximal extremities.

Complications

Complications are more commonly noted in adolescents than young adults.
1. Upper airway obstruction from marked tonsillar hypertrophy.
2. Splenic rupture, often preceded by abdominal pain secondary to splenomegaly. Risk is greatest between 14 and 28 days of illness.
3. Hepatitis (p. 639).
4. Autoimmune hemolytic anemia, leukopenia, and thrombocytopenia.
5. Encephalitis or Landry-Guillain-Barré syndrome (see Chapter 41). Oculomotor paralysis.
6. Pericarditis (p. 564).
7. Glomerulonephritis.
8. Orchitis.

Ancillary Data

1. WBC. Elevated, with a marked predominance of lymphocytes, 50% to 90% of which are atypical.
2. Thrombocytopenia.
3. Monospot test. Heterophil rarely indicated. Both results usually negative in children less than 5 years (EB virus titer may be needed). In adolescents and adults, positive test result is found during the second week of illness.

   Serologic diagnosis can be done by measurement of antibody to viral capsid antigen (VCA), which rises above 1:160 during acute infection.

4. Throat culture for identifying group A streptococci, which may be concurrently present; 15% to 18% of patients have group A streptococci.
5. Liver function tests with right upper quadrant (RUQ) tenderness.
6. ECG and ABG rarely indicated.

DIFFERENTIAL DIAGNOSIS

1. Infection
   a. Pharyngitis: group A streptococci, diphtheria, or viral
   b. Toxoplasmosis
   c. Infectious hepatitis
   d. Meningoencephalitis, viral
2. Neoplasm: leukemia or lymphoma

MANAGEMENT

1. Support and symptomatic care are required.
   a. Establishment of an airway, if obstructed
   b. Bed rest, fluids, and antipyretics
2. Steroids may be indicated for patients with complications of severe disease (e.g., severe hemolytic anemia, airway obstruction from tonsillar hypertrophy, thrombocytopenia): Solu-Cortef, 4-5 mg/kg/dose q6hr IV, or prednisone, 1-2 mg/kg/24 hr q6hr PO for 7 days and then tapering over 2 weeks.

DISPOSITION

Patients with significant symptoms and complications require hospitalization. Others may be sent home if hydration, observation, and support are adequate.

REFERENCE
Sumaya CV, Ench Y: Epstein-Barr virus infectious mononucleosis in children: clinical and general laboratory findings, *Pediatrics* 75:1003, 1985.

Pertussis (Whooping Cough)

Pertussis (whooping cough) is caused by *Bordetella pertussis* and occurs in all age groups, although its greatest morbidity rate is in children less than 1 year of age. It peaks in late summer and early fall. The incubation period is 7 to 10 days.

DIAGNOSTIC FINDINGS

Three stages categorize the progression of pertussis in children.

1. Catarrhal: minor respiratory complaints of fever, rhinorrhea, and conjunctivitis lasting up to 2 weeks.
2. Paroxysmal: severe cough associated with hypoxia, unremitting paroxysms, and vomiting. As many as 40 episodes/day may occur and go on for 2 to 4 weeks. In rare cases, it is associated with apnea.
3. Convalescent: residual cough.

The infant often has only a paroxysmal cough and rhinorrhea. Stages are indistinct. Adults often have only rhinorrhea, sore throat, and persistent cough.

Pertussis should be suspected in children less than 18 months with persistent respiratory illness and vomiting in poorly immunized children.

Partially immunized children will have less severe disease.

Complications

1. Pneumonia caused by secondary infection
2. Crepitus from subcutaneous or mediastinal emphysema
3. Pneumothorax
4. Seizures and encephalitis
5. Hypoxia
6. Apnea

Ancillary Data

1. WBC: markedly increased with a tremendous shift to the right (lymphocytosis)

2. Chest x-ray study: peribronchial thickening, infiltrates, and "shaggy" heart border
3. Culture: nasopharyngeal or cough plate on a Bordet-Gengou medium
4. Fluorescent antibody (FA) stain of nasopharyngeal swab (a rapid diagnostic technique)

DIFFERENTIAL DIAGNOSIS

Pertussis should be differentiated from other causes of pneumonia (p. 794).

MANAGEMENT

1. Of primary importance is pulmonary support, which may include oxygen, postural drainage, and rarely, intubation with sedation. Patients with severe paroxysms should be monitored to ensure that hypoxia and bradycardia are treated.
2. Antibiotics decrease the contagiousness of the patient: erythromycin, 30-50 mg/kg/24 hr (adult: 250 mg/dose) q6hr PO (if possible), for 7 to 14 days. It may also decrease the symptomatic course if given early in the catarrhal phase. Additional antibiotics should be given if there is evidence of superinfection.
3. Patients should be isolated. Those exposed may be treated with erythromycin, as above, for 10 days.
4. Pertussis immune globulin is not effective.
5. Corticosteroids and albuterol may reduce paroxysms of coughing. Further studies are required (p. 769).

DISPOSITION

1. Patients less than 1 year of age or those with any complication should be hospitalized for careful monitoring and pulmonary support.
2. Older children in the catarrhal phase or those experiencing only minor paroxysms may be discharged.

Parental Education

1. Importance of active immunization in disease prevention (see Appendix B-7).
2. Prophylaxis and isolation of household and other close contacts of pertussis cases should be considered.
   a. All household or other close contacts less than 1 year of age (regardless of DTP immunization status) should receive 14 days of oral erythromycin (40 mg/kg/24 hr q6hr PO)
   b. All household or other close contacts 1 to 7 years of age who have had less than 4 diphtheria tetanus pertussis (DTP) doses or whose last DTP was more than 3 years ago should receive 14 days of oral erythromycin, and many recommend a DTP immunization.
   c. Asymptomatic household or other close contacts need not be excluded from school if they are taking antibiotics or have up-to-date DTP immunization (four DTPs, the last within 3 years).
   d. Persons who have a positive laboratory test result for pertussis should be excluded from school or work until they have taken antibiotics for 14 days, although 7 days may be adequate.
   e. Adults and children with early symptoms who are household contacts should be excluded from school or work until they have completed 5 days of antibiotics.
   f. All household contacts 7 years or older should receive antibiotics if the last DTP was given 3 years ago or longer.
3. If the patient has been discharged, the parent should call their physician immediately if the following occur:
   a. Breathing difficulty recurs or worsens.
   b. Skin or lips turn blue.
   c. Restlessness or sleeplessness develops.
   d. Fluid intake decreases.
   e. Medicines are not tolerated.

REFERENCES

Cherry JD, Brunell PA, Golden GS, et al: Report of the task force on pertussis and pertussis immunization, *Pediatrics* 81:939, 1988.

Halperin SA, Bartoluss R, Langley JM, et al: Seven days of erythromycin estolate is as effective as fourteen days for the treatment of *Bordetella pertussis* infection, *Pediatrics* 100:65, 1997.

RABIES

Although rare, rabies in humans is a fatal viral disease resulting from skin or mucous membrane contact with an infected animal. The incubation is 10 days to several months after the initial exposure, the length reflecting the site and severity of the wound. The primary goal must be prevention.

DIAGNOSTIC FINDINGS

Initially, hypoesthesia or paresthesia is noted at the site of injury. Progression of symptoms, including hydrophobia, apprehension, and hyperexcitability associated with a clear sensorium, is rapid. Seizures, delirium, and lethargy are noted in the period before death in 5 to 7 days. Cardiovascular, respiratory, and central nervous system (CNS) instability may be noted in the interim.

Ancillary Data

Rabies virus may be isolated from the saliva or brain of infected individuals. Examination of the biting animal's brain by fluorescent antibody or Negri body identification, confirmed by viral isolation, provides additional verification.

MANAGEMENT

Although the mortality rate is extremely high, there have been several cases of survival with intense, supportive care.

Prevention of Rabies

Risk Factors

1. Bites and wounds inflicted by animals must be individually considered with regard to the risk of rabies. Skunks, foxes, coyotes, raccoons, wild dogs and cats, and bats are most commonly infected. Rodents (mice, rats, squirrels, chipmunks), rabbits, and hares are not normally considered to be risks.

2. The circumstances of the biting incident must be considered. Unprovoked attacks are more likely to indicate that the animal was rabid than are provoked attacks.

3. The type of exposure is a factor. Rabies is transmitted by the introduction of virus into open cuts or wounds in skin or via mucous membranes:

   a. Bite: any penetration of the skin by teeth

   b. Nonbite: scratches, abrasions, open wounds, or mucous membrane contaminated with saliva

4. Epizootic conditions of rabies in the area should be considered.

Management of the Biting Animal

1. Healthy domestic dogs and cats should be confined and observed for 10 days. If any suggestive signs develop, the animal should be killed and the head removed and shipped under refrigeration to the designated health department, provided there is risk of rabies in that area. Stray and wild dogs and cats should be killed and examined.

2. Wild animals that have bitten or scratched a person should be killed and the brain examined.

Local Treatment of Wound

1. Immediate and thorough washing and debridement are appropriate.

2. Tetanus prophylaxis should be given, if indicated.

Immunization (Table 80-2)

Antirabies immunization after exposure should include both passively administered antibody and vaccine, unless the patient has been immunized before exposure.

1. Read instructions for administration carefully on inserts of products. If immune globulin or vaccine is unavailable, call the CDC (404-639-3670 during working hours or 404-639-2888 on nights, weekends, and holidays).

2. Human rabies immune globulin (HRIG) is supplied in 2- and 10-ml (150 IU/ml) vials. It should be administered at a dose of 20 IU/kg. If anatomically feasible, approximately half the dose is used to infiltrate the wound and the remainder is given IM.

3. Human diploid cell rabies vaccine (HDCV) (Imovax Rabies) is administered IM in five 1-ml doses; the first dose is administered at the time of exposure, followed by the remaining doses at 3, 7, 14, and 28 days. Rabies vaccine absorbed (RVA) is another option.

4. Preexposure HDCV (Imovax Rabies) may be administered to at-risk individuals. In adults, give 1 ml IM in 3 doses at 0, 7, and 28 days with a booster every 2 years. May also give 0.1 ml intradermally using above schedule. If the antibody titer is 1:5 or above, may omit booster and monitor. RVA may also be used.

REFERENCE

Bernard KW, Mallonee J, Wright JC, et al: Preexposure immunization with intradermal human diploid cell rabies vaccine, *JAMA* 253:1059, 1987.

TETANUS

Tetanus results from puncture or other wounds with the introduction of *Clostridium tetani*, which produces a neurotoxin. Severe skeletal muscle hypertonicity occurs. The incubation period ranges from 3 days to 3 weeks (average: 8 days). Generally, the shorter the incubation period, the more severe the clinical presentation.

TABLE 80-2   Rabies Postexposure Prophylaxis Guide

Species of animal	Condition of animal at time of attack	Treatment of exposed human*
DOMESTIC		
Dog and cat	Healthy and available for 10 days of observation	None†
	Rapid or suspected rabid; unknown	HRIG and HDCV; consult public health officer†
WILD		
Skunk, bat, fox, coyote, raccoon, bobcat, and other carnivores	Regard as rabid unless proved negative by laboratory test or geographic area is known to be free of rabies‡	HRIG and HDCV
OTHER		
Livestock, rodents, rabbits, hares	Consider individually. Squirrel, hamsters, guinea pigs, gerbils, chipmunks, rats, mice, rabbits, and hares are almost never considered to be rabid.	

Adapted from American Academy of Pediatrics: *Report of the committee on infectious diseases,* Elk Grove, Ill, 1997. These recommendations are only a guide. They should be applied in conjunction with information about the animal species involved, the circumstances of the exposure, the vaccination status of the animal, and the presence of rabies in the region.
*All bites and wounds should immediately be thoroughly cleansed with soap and water. If antirabies treatment is indicated, both HRIG and HDCV should be given as soon as possible, regardless of the interval from exposure.
†During the usual holding period of 10 days, begin treatment with HRIG and HDCV at the first sign of rabies in the animal. The symptomatic animal should be killed immediately and examined.
‡The animal should be killed and tested as soon as possible. Holding for observation is not recommended. Discontinue treatment if test findings are negative.
HRIG, Human rabies immune globulin; *HDCV,* human diploid cell rabies vaccine.

DIAGNOSTIC FINDINGS

1. A wound is present in 80% of patients.
2. The onset of symptoms is marked by increased tone of the skeletal muscles initially involving the jaw and neck. This becomes generalized over the next 24 to 48 hours with spasms increasing in frequency and intensity.
   a. Trismus: inability to open the mouth because of spasms of the masseter muscles
   b. Peculiar, sustained facial distortion: risus sardonicus
   c. Opisthotonic posturing from spasms of neck and back
   d. Boardlike abdomen
   e. Stiff and extended extremities
3. A low-grade fever, headache, tachycardia, and anxiety are often present. The sensorium is totally normal.
4. Tetanus neonatorum occurs in the first 3 to 10 days of life, marked by muscle rigidity, particularly of the jaw and neck, difficulty swallowing, and irritability.

Complications

1. Respiratory: laryngospasm, pneumonia, pulmonary edema, and respiratory failure
2. Compression or subluxation injuries of the vertebrae

Ancillary Data

1. WBC: variably increased
2. LP: normal

3. ABG: indicated if there is respiratory compromise
4. Vertebral x-ray films: for patients with pain and severe opisthotonic posturing

DIFFERENTIAL DIAGNOSIS

1. Trauma: head and neck
2. Infection: dental abscess, peritonsillar abscess
3. Intoxication: phenothiazines, strychnine
4. Endocrine/metabolic: hypocalcemia (tetany)
5. Intrapsychic: hysteria, conversion reaction

MANAGEMENT

At Time of Exposure

1. Tetanus and diphtheria (Td) toxoid and tetanus immune globulin (TIG) are indicated (see schedule in Table 80-3 and Appendix B-7). DT (pediatric) may be used for children less than 6 years of age.
2. Wound cleansing and debridement must be done.

Treatment of Acute Disease

1. The patient must have immediate evaluation and support of the airway with oxygen and active intervention, when indicated.

2. Muscle spasms and associated pain must be controlled with the following:
   a. Diazepam (Valium), 0.1-0.3 mg/kg/dose q4-8hr IV or 0.1-0.8 mg/kg/24 q6-8hr PO; or
   b. Minimizing external stimuli.
3. Tetanus immune globulin antitoxin should be administered: 3000 to 6000 units IM with a portion infiltrated around the wound.
4. An antibiotic should be given: penicillin G, 100,000 U/kg/24 hr q4hr IV for 10 to 14 days.

Prevention

Active immunization (see Appendix B-7) is recommended.

DISPOSITION

1. All patients with tetanus require admission to an ICU.
2. Those individuals with tetanus exposure may be discharged after appropriate immunologic therapy.

REFERENCES

Brand DA, Acampora D, Gottlieb LD, et al: Adequacy of antitetanus prophylaxis in six hospital emergency rooms, *N Engl J Med* 309:636, 1983.

TABLE 80-3   Schedule for Td Toxoid and TIG at Time of Exposure

History of tetanus immunizations	Clean, minor wounds		All other wounds*	
	Td	**TIG**	**Td**	**TIG**
Uncertain or less than 3 doses	Yes	No	Yes	Yes
3 or more doses‡	Not§	No	Not‖	No

Adapted from *Report of the committee on infectious diseases,* American Academy of Pediatrics: 1997.
*Including but not limited to, contaminated wounds, as well as puncture wounds, avulsions and wounds resulting from missiles, crushing, burns, and frostbite.
†If only 3 doses of fluid toxoid have been previously received, a fourth dose of absorbed toxoid should be given.
‡Single dose of 3000 to 6000 units IM.
§Unless >10 yr have elapsed since the last dose.
‖Unless >5 yr have elapsed since the last dose.
Td, Tetanus diphtheria; *TIG,* tetanus immune globulin.

Richardson J, Knight A: The management and prevention of tetanus, *J Emerg Med* 11:737, 1993.

TOXIC SHOCK SYNDROME

Toxic shock syndrome (TSS) primarily affects menstruating young women; however, nonmenstruating females, men, and premenarcheal girls have also had the syndrome, usually associated with a definable site of infection.

ETIOLOGY: INFECTION

1. Although the pathophysiology remains unclear, a toxic shock syndrome toxin-1 (TSST-1) elaborated by coagulase-positive *S. aureus* (phage group I) is absorbed through the vaginal mucosa, causing systemic signs and symptoms.
2. There is a temporal relationship between tampon use, menstruation, and the onset of the syndrome.

DIAGNOSTIC FINDINGS

The onset of the illness is often preceded by a prodromal illness lasting less than 12 hours and including high fever, profuse diarrhea, and vomiting. Patients typically seek medical care 12 to 18 hours after prodromal illness, usually because of dizziness or confusion.

Clinically, TSS must include the following:
1. Fever (>38.9° C)
2. Rash (diffuse, blanching macular, erythematous, nonpruritic); erythroderma
3. Desquamation 1 to 2 weeks after the onset of illness, particularly on the palms and soles
4. Hypotension (systolic blood pressure 90 mm Hg for adults or <5% by age for children or orthostatic changes), usually with hypovolemia
5. Involvement of three or more of the following organ systems:
   a. Gastrointestinal (vomiting or diarrhea, usually at the onset of illness)
   b. Muscular (severe myalgia)
   c. Mucous membrane (vaginal, oropharyngeal, or conjunctival hyperemia)
   d. Renal blood urea nitrogen (BUN) or creatinine level at least twice elevated or above 5 WBC/HPF with no urinary tract infection (UTI)
   e. Hepatic (bilirubin, serum glutamic oxaloacetic transaminase [SGOT], or serum glutamic pyruvic transaminase [SGPT] level at least twice normal)
   f. Hematologic (platelets ≤100,000/mm^3)
   g. CNS (disorientation or alteration in consciousness without focal signs)
6. Negative results on the following tests, if obtained: serologic tests for Rocky Mountain spotted fever, leptospirosis, or measles and cultures of blood, throat, and CSF.
   NOTE: Blood culture may grow *S. aureus* (variable).

Patients often have a 2-day prodrome, comprised of fever, vomiting, diarrhea, and myalgia. Sore throat is a prominent complaint.

Group A streptococcal sepsis is similar to toxic shock syndrome; it is mediated by a pyrogenic exotoxin A elaborated by the streptococcus. Clinically, in addition to the primary infection, patients over several days develop erythroderma, hypotension, DIC, renal dysfunction, hypoalbuminemia, hypocalcemia, and respiratory failure. The onset of illness is often preceded by pain at the site of the skin lesion; local necrosis may occur. Patients may also have fever, chills, myalgia, diarrhea, and subsequent desquamation.

Complications

1. Cardiovascular collapse and shock with myocardial failure.
2. Adult respiratory distress syndrome with pulmonary edema. More common in children less than 10 years.
3. Coagulopathy with DIC is usually mild.
4. Recurrence. Usually mild, not meeting all criteria.

Ancillary Data

1. Hematology: increased WBC with shift to left, thrombocytopenia, and variable coagulation studies.
2. Chemistry: electrolyte, BUN, creatinine, and calcium levels. May be abnormal. Liver function and bilirubin level elevation are common.
3. Urinalysis: proteinuria and pyuria.
4. Cultures: vaginal culture for *S. aureus.* Blood, throat, and CSF culture results vary. Group A streptococcus should be sought, as well.
5. Chest x-ray study and ABG with any respiratory distress.

DIFFERENTIAL DIAGNOSIS

See Table 80-1.

MANAGEMENT

General supportive care is essential because of the multisystem involvement of the disease and the progressive nature of organ involvement.

1. Fluids for hypotension and abnormal loss from vomiting and diarrhea. Often very large volumes of fluids are required, with two to five times normal maintenance fluids being necessary. Fluids should not be restricted or diuretics administered without being able to maintain an adequate filling pressure.
2. Pressor agents may be required for significant hypotension unresponsive to fluid therapy: dopamine, 5-15 µg/kg/min IV constant infusion, often in combination with other pressors after volume deficits have been replaced. Echocardiography and Swan-Ganz catheter monitoring are indicated if myocardial failure is noted.
3. Ventilatory support with positive end-expiratory pressure (PEEP), particularly if adult respiratory distress syndrome (ARDS) with pulmonary edema is present.
4. If incriminated, removal of tampon and irrigation of vagina. Aggressive drainage of sites of staphylococcal infection must be achieved. Abscesses and empyemas always require surgical drainage.
5. Antibiotics should be initiated, although their role is unclear. They decrease the incidence of recurrence but do not clearly alter the course of the illness. The patient is given:
    a. Nafcillin, 100-200 mg/kg/24 hr (adult: 1 gm/dose) q4hr IV (or equivalent β-lactamase–resistant penicillin), for at least 7 days; *or*
    b. Cephalosporin: cephalothin (Keflin), 75-150 mg/kg/24 hr (adult: 1 gm/dose) q4hr IV.
6. Corticosteroids reduce the severity of illness and duration of fever if initiated within 2 to 3 days of illness: methylprednisolone (SoluMedrol), 10-20 mg/kg/24 hr IV.
7. Calcium supplementation is usually required.
8. Renal dialysis may be required if renal failure develops.
9. Group A streptococcal sepsis, in addition to the support noted, requires penicillin, 100,000 U/kg/24 hr q4hr IV.

DISPOSITION

Hospitalization is required of all patients with definite TSS because of the progression of findings. An ICU is usually indicated.

On discharge, long-term monitoring for renal and neuromuscular sequelae is essential.

REFERENCES

Bergovac J, Marton E, Lisic M, et al: Group A beta-hemolytic streptococcal toxic shock–like syndrome, *Pediatr Infect Dis* J 9:369, 1990.

Garbe PL, Arko RJ, Reingold AL, et al: *Staphylococcus aureus* isolates from patients with nonmenstrual toxic shock syndrome: evidence for additional toxins, *JAMA* 253:2538, 1985.

Resnick S: Toxic shock syndrome recent developments in pathogenesis, *J Pediatr* 116:321, 1990.

Todd JK, Ressman M, Caston SA, et al: Corticosteroid therapy for patients with toxic-shock syndrome, *JAMA* 252:3399, 1984.

Wiesenthal AM, Todd JK: Toxic-shock syndrome in children aged 10 years or less, *Pediatrics* 74:112, 1984.

TUBERCULOSIS

The resurgence of tuberculosis caused by *Mycobacterium tuberculosis* has been well documented because of coinfection in patients with HIV as well as the decline in access to rapid diagnosis and treatment and increasing immigration from high-prevalence countries. It results from the inhalation of aerosol droplets produced by individuals with infectious pulmonary tuberculosis. Children rarely transmit the disease because of the insufficient inoculum in their respiratory tract.

DIAGNOSTIC FINDINGS

The period from exposure until positive tuberculin skin test finding is usually 2 to 10 weeks. Most infections resolve without disease. Manifestations occur in the first 6 to 11 months, presenting either pulmonary or extrapulmonary findings. Extrapulmonary disease may include miliary tuberculosis, meningitis, and lymphadenitis, as well as renal, bone, and joint involvement.

Most patients are identified by routine skin testing or chest x-ray films.

Ancillary Data

1. Tuberculin Mantoux skin test (5 units). A positive test result is 15 mm or greater induration in healthy patients and 5 mm or greater in a patient with HIV infection, documented exposure, or radiographic evidence of disease. Induration of 10 mm or more is positive in patients from high incidence or medically underserved areas, as well as those from long-term care facilities. Additional consideration should be given to IV drug users and those who have diabetes, immunosuppression from steroid or other therapy, and end-stage renal disease.

2. Cultures should be obtained for isolation and identification of antibiotic sensitivity patterns. Gastric aspirate is often helpful, especially in children under a year of age.

3. Chest x-ray films on all patients with positive results should be obtained.

MANAGEMENT

1. Patients with a positive skin test result should be started on preventive therapy with isoniazid (INH), 10 mg/kg/24 hr for 9 months.

2. Uncomplicated pulmonary disease is treated with a 6-month course of INH (see above), rifampin (10-15 mg/kg/24 hr), and pyrazinamide (20-30 mg/kg/24 hr) for the first 2 months followed by twice-weekly INH (20-40 mg/kg/dose) and rifampin (10-20 mg/kg/24 hr) for the remaining 4 months.

3. Tuberculous meningitis, miliary disease, or bone/joint infection requires prolonged therapy and consultation.

REFERENCES

Barnes PF, Bloch AB, Davidson PT, et al: Tuberculosis in patients with human immunodeficiency infection, *N Engl J Med* 324:1644, 1991.

Committee on Infectious Disease: *Report of the Committee*, Elk Grove, Ill, 1997, American Academy of Pediatrics.

Hoge CW, Schwartz KB, Talkington DF, et al: The changing epidemiology of invasive group A streptococcal infections and the emergence of streptococcal shock-like syndrome: a retrospective population-based study, *JAMA* 269:384, 1993.

Huebner R, Schein M, Bass J: The tuberculin test, *Adv Pediatr Infect Dis* 8:23, 1993.

Jacobs R, Eisenach K: Childhood tuberculosis, *Adv Pediatr Infect Dis* 8:23, 1993.

Snider JDE, Roper WL: The new tuberculosis, *N Engl J Med* 326:703, 1992.

Starke JR, Jacobs RF, Jereb J: Resurgence of tuberculosis in children, *J Pediatr* 120:839, 1992.

81 NEUROLOGIC DISORDERS

BREATH-HOLDING SPELLS

Breath-holding spells may result after prolonged crying, producing cyanosis and, ultimately, loss of consciousness. They most commonly begin after 6 months of age and may continue until 4 years.

DIAGNOSTIC FINDINGS

1. Vigorous crying is precipitated by a fall or injury or by anger. The child subsequently becomes cyanotic, unconscious, and limp. The episodes are self-limited, lasting less than 1 minute.
2. Some evidence of disturbance at home or in the maternal-child interaction may be evident. Youth of parents, maternal depression, or difficulty in setting limits can usually be detected.

Complications

Tonic-clonic seizures may be noted as a result of cerebral anoxia.

DIFFERENTIAL DIAGNOSIS

It is usually easy to differentiate breath-holding spells from a seizure. Patients with seizures lose consciousness and then become cyanotic; the reverse is true with breath-holding spells, which rarely occur at night. It is important to note that cerebral anoxia may cause brief seizures with breath-holding spells.

MANAGEMENT

1. Reassurance and calmness of the parents must be emphasized. The episodes are self-limited. Behavior patterns that initiate breath-holding spells and secondary gain from that behavior must be reduced.
2. Anticonvulsants are not indicated. The focus must be on behavior modification and family support.

Parental Education

1. Minimize the events or factors that trigger the spells.
2. Attempt to be firm and consistent in management of behavior problems.
3. Call the physician if the nature, duration, or frequency of the breath-holding spells changes.

REFERENCES

DiMario FJ: Breath-holding spells in childhood, *Am J Dis Child* 146:125, 1992.

DiMario FJ, Chee CM, Berman PH: Pallid breath-holding spells: evaluation of the autonomic nervous system, *Clin Pediatr* 9:17, 1990.

Gordon N: Breath-holding spells, *Dev Med Child Neurol* 29:805, 1987.

MENINGITIS

ALERT: Infections elsewhere do not exclude the presence of meningitis. The younger the child, the less specific the presenting signs and symptoms. Unstable patients with suspected meningitis may require empirical treatment (after blood studies including culture).

ETIOLOGY: INFECTION

1. Bacterial
   a. The child's age is the predominant determinant of the common bacterial causes:

Age group	Predominant organism
<2 mo	*Escherichia coli*, group B streptococci (*S. agalactiae*), *Listeria monocytogenes*, *Haemophilus influenzae*, *Neisseria meningitidis*, *Streptococcus pneumoniae*
2 mo-9 yr	*H. influenzae*, *N. meningitidis*, *S. pneumoniae*
>9 yr	*N. meningitidis*, *S. pneumoniae*

   The incidence of *H. influenzae* meningitis has dramatically declined since the introduction of routine immunization.
   b. Ventriculoperitoneal (VP) shunt: 25% of patients with VP shunts have infections associated with alterations in the shunt, usually caused by *Staphylococcus epidermidis* and, less commonly, *Staphylococcus aureus*.
2. Viral: most commonly enteroviral (Table 81-1)
3. Fungal and *Mycobacterium tuberculosis*: uncommon, but consider if endemic

DIAGNOSTIC FINDINGS: BACTERIAL MENINGITIS

1. In younger children the initial presentation is nonspecific, including fever, hypothermia, dehydration, bulging fontanelle, lethargy, irritability, anorexia, vomiting, seizures, respiratory distress, or cyanosis (Table 81-2). Children less than 12 months of age are commonly toxic in appearance with impaired mental status. The diagnosis may therefore be difficult to confirm clinically; a lumbar puncture (LP) remains as the definitive test.
2. Older patients may have symptoms listed in item 1, as well as the more classic findings of nuchal rigidity, Kernig sign (pain on extension of legs), Brudzinski sign (flexion of the neck produces flexion at knees and hips), and headaches. Meningeal signs are present in 87% of children more than 12 months of age. Otitis media is often present.
3. Historically, the progression of illness, associated symptoms, exposures, and underlying health problems are important.
4. Partially treated children with bacterial meningitis less commonly have a temperature above 38.3° C and altered mental status. Immunization to prevent *H. influenzae* disease may also alter the presentation of children who ultimately develop meningitis as a result of this organism.
5. The distinction between a simple febrile seizure and a seizure-complicating meningitis is difficult to make in younger children and often requires an LP (p. 727).
6. Patients with a ventriculoperitoneal or other shunt may have a somewhat different presentation associated with a low-grade ventriculitis that includes headache, nausea, minimal fever, and malaise.

   The shunting device consists of three components. The ventricular catheter is passed into the anterior horns of the lateral ventricles through a right occipital or frontal burr hole. The catheter is attached subcutaneously to a reservoir that may be percutaneously tapped to obtain ventricular fluid. This reservoir is attached to a distal catheter containing a pump and one-way valve to regulate pressure and flow in the system. This distal catheter commonly passes into the peritoneum.

TABLE 81-1   Viral Meningoencephalitis

Agent	Epidemiology	Clinical manifestations
ENTEROVIRUS	Epidemic, with summer and fall peak incidence; all ages affected, particularly <12 yr	Most common; usually mild; rash often present; rarely with focal findings or sequelae
MUMPS	Epidemic, occurring year-round with increase in spring; all ages affected, particularly 2- to 14-year-old children	Mild-to-moderate meningoencephalitis accompanied by parotitis (>50%); focal findings and sequelae rare
HERPES SIMPLEX	Year-round; most commonly affecting patients <1 yr and >15 yr	Severe and progressive encephalitis; 50%-75% having focal findings; severe motor and mental deficits occur in as many as 75% of survivors; high mortality rate; treatment: acyclovir
OTHER		
California equine	Occurs in rural areas with peak incidence in June-Oct; 5- to 9-year-old children most commonly affected	Mild meningoencephalitis with accompanying seizures (50%) and focal findings (15%-40%); long-term behavioral problems (15%-20%)
St. Louis equine	Peaks in July-Oct; adults primarily involved	Commonly asymptomatic in children
Western equine	July-Oct peak incidence; primarily (20%-30%) affects infants	Sudden high fever with focal or generalized seizures, rare focal findings and coma; sequelae occur in > 50% of children affected in first year of life

TABLE 81-2   Bacterial Meningitis: Presentation By Age

Diagnostic findings	<2-3 mo	2-3 mo-2 yr	>2 yr
Apnea/cyanosis	Common	Rare	Rare
Fever	Common	Common	Common
Hypothermia	Common	Rare	Rare
Altered mental status	Common	Common	Common
Headache	Rare	Rare	Common
Seizures	Early finding	Early finding	Late finding
Ataxia	Rare	Variable	Early finding
Jitteriness	Common	Common	Rare
Vomiting	Common	Common	Variable
Stiff neck	Rare	Late finding	Common
Bulging fontanelle	Common	Common	Closed

To assess shunt function, the reservoir is pumped; this is normally done easily with a rapid refill of the reservoir in less than 3 seconds. If it cannot be depressed, there is a distal block, whereas if it pumps but does not refill, it is blocked proximally at the ventricular end. Pumping poorly may indicate a relative dysfunction. Pressure may be assessed by percutaneous needle access of the reservoir: High pressure indicates distal obstruction, whereas low pressure suggests proximal obstruction or overdrained ventricles. One third of obstructed shunts are infected. Withdrawing fluid from the shunt for analysis or because of abnormal pumping is usually done in conjunction with a neurosurgeon. A computed tomography (CT) study and plain radiographs comparing the present status with previous findings may be helpful in the assessment.

7. Aseptic (viral, fungal, mycobacterial) meningoencephalitis usually has a less toxic and acute clinical presentation. Diagnosis of encephalitis is often made on the basis of clinical evaluation (see Table 81-1).

Complications of Bacterial Meningitis

1. Cerebral edema with potential for increased intracranial pressure and herniation.
2. Septic shock and disseminated intravascular coagulation, particularly with *N. meningitidis*.
3. Bacteremia with associated hematogenous involvement of joints (particularly the hip), pericardium, and myocardium.
4. Inappropriate antidiuretic hormone (ADH) with hyponatremia.
5. Subdural effusion and empyema. Of patients aged 1 to 18 months, 39% have subdural effusions. Associated risk factors are young age, rapid onset of illness, low peripheral white blood count (WBC), and

high cerebrospinal fluid (CSF) protein level. Patients with subdural effusions are more likely to have seizures initially, but on long-term follow-up, there is no greater incidence of seizures, hearing loss, neurologic deficits, or developmental delay. No specific therapy is usually needed.

6. Anemia, especially with *H. influenzae*.
7. Of those patients with meningococcal or pneumococcal meningitis, 90% are afebrile by the sixth day, in contrast to only 72% of those with *H. influenzae* as the etiologic agent. Conditions associated with persistent fever include untreated disease, subdural effusion, nosocomial infection, phlebitis, and drug fever.

   The widespread use of dexamethasone (Decadron) in patients with bacterial meningitis has altered this pattern, particularly in children with *H. influenzae* disease. These children may have a relatively low temperature early in the illness with an elevated temperature becoming evident once steroids are stopped on day 4.
8. Neurologic findings, both transient and persistent, may include deficits in cranial nerves (particularly VI), hearing, vision, and retardation, as well as later behavioral problems. A long-term follow-up evaluation of children with bacterial meningitis noted that 14% had persistent deficits (10% sensorineural hearing loss and 4% multiple neurologic problems) 1 year after the illness; 7% had one or more late seizures not associated with fever.
9. Children with viral aseptic meningitis often are not toxic and without meningeal signs.

Ancillary Data

Lumbar Puncture (see Appendix A-4)

1. CSF is the basis for evaluation of the patient with clinical signs of meningitis.

Analysis of the fluid is essential (Table 81-3). Meningitis may exist in the absence of a CSF pleocytosis.

2. Partial treatment with antibiotics before LP rarely alters the CSF enough to interfere with an appropriate interpretation. The blood culture, CSF Gram stain, and latex agglutination are useful in identifying the causative organisms in patients receiving antibiotics before the LP is performed.

3. Although conflicting evidence exists regarding the potential risk of seeding the meninges with bacteria when performing an LP in the bacteremic patient, this consideration should not delay obtaining CSF in patients who are clinically at risk of having meningitis. The occurrence of meningitis after bacteremia is related to the organism causing the bacteremia rather than whether the patient had an LP.

4. If it is difficult to distinguish bacterial from viral meningitis on the basis of the initial CSF test, a repeat LP in 6 to 8 hours while the patient is observed closely without antibiotics is considered to be helpful by some clinicians. The second LP may demonstrate a marked decrease in the percentage of polymor-

TABLE 81-3   Cerebrospinal Fluid Analysis

	Normal			Bacterial	Viral
	Preterm*	Term	>6 mo		
Cell count (WBC/mm^3)†					
Mean	9	8	0	>500	<500
Range	0-25	0-22	0-4		
Predominant cell type	Lymph	Lymph	Lymph	80% PMN leukocyte	PMN leukocyte initially, lymphocyte later
Glucose (mg/dl)					
Mean	50	52	>40	<40	>40
Range	24-63	34-119			
Protein (mg/dl)					
Mean	115	90	<40	>100	<100
Range	65-150	20-170			
CSF/blood glucose (%)					
Mean	74	81	50	<40	>40
Range	55-150	44-248	40-60		
Gram stain	Negative	Negative	Negative	Positive‡§	Negative
Bacterial culture	Negative	Negative	Negative	Positive‡§	Negative

Modified from Sarff LD, Platt LH, McCracken GH Jr: *J Pediatr* 88:473, 1976; Portnoy JM, Olson LC: *Pediatrics* 75:484, 1985; and Rodriguez AF, Kaplan SC, Mason ED: *J Pediatr* 116:971, 1990.

*Infants <1000 gm have a mean cell count of 4 ± 3 WBC/mm^3 (range 0-14 cells/mm^3). The mean protein level is 150 ± 56 mg/dl (range 95-370 mg/dl) and glucose of 61 ± 34 mg/dl (range 29-217 mg/dl). Infants 1001-1500 gm have a mean cell count of 6 ± 9 WBC/mm^3 (range 0-44 cells/mm^3). The mean protein level is 132 ± 43 mg/dl (range 5-227 mg/dl) and glucose of 59 ± 21 (range 31-109 mg/dl).

†Total WBC/mm^3 by age in the normal child can be further delineated as follows (mean ± 2 SD): <6 wk: 3.7 ± 6.8; 6 wk-3 mo: 2.9 ± 5.7; 3 mo-6 mo: 1.9 ± 4.0; 6-12 mo: 2.6 ± 4.9; >12 mo: 1.9 ± 5.4

‡If Gram stain finding is negative, a methylene blue stain may distinguish intracellular bacteria from nuclear material.

§Of partially treated patients 85% will have a positive Gram stain result and >95% have positive culture findings. Counterimmunoelectrophoresis (CIE) may be helpful if the culture result is negative.

phonuclear neutrophil (PMN) leukocytes and an increase in lymphocytes in untreated patients with viral meningitis.

5. An LP may appropriately be delayed if the patient is hemodynamically unstable, if there is evidence of increased intracranial pressure, if infection is present in the area to be traversed by the needle, or if the procedure cannot logistically be performed. Obtain a blood culture before starting antibiotics; antibiotic administration should not be delayed.

   LP should be performed only cautiously, if at all, in the patient with suspected papilledema or increased intracranial pressure or in patients who are uncooperative. Consultation and CT scan usually are indicated.

6. Repeat LP may be done at 36 to 48 hours and 10 days after initiating therapy if the clinical response has been slow or the therapy inadequate. Otherwise, repeat LPs are rarely required.

7. Bloody spinal taps create a diagnostic dilemma.

   a. Hemorrhage into the subarachnoid space caused by bleeding results in an equal number of red blood cells (RBCs) in the first and last samples of fluid. The fluid should be xanthochromic after centrifugation.

   b. Although the appraisal may be inexact and fraught with errors, the number of leukocytes in spinal fluid obtained after a traumatic tap may be estimated.

      (1) 1000 RBC/mm^3 contribute 1-2 WBC/mm^3.

      (2) Number of WBCs introduced/mm^3.

      $$\frac{(\text{Peripheral WBC}) \times (\text{RBC in CSF})}{\text{Peripheral RBC count}}$$

      (3) The result is then compared with the actual number of WBCs counted in the CSF.

      (4) 1000 RBC/mm^3 in the CSF raises the protein about 1.5 mg/dl.

8. Cultures for tuberculosis or fungi may be done, if indicated.

9. Determinations of CSF lactic acid and lactate dehydrogenase (LDH) have not proved to be of value in the interpretation of the fluid.

10. A ratio of immature to mature neutrophils greater than 0.12 is associated with, and more sensitive for, the presence of bacterial meningitis than total peripheral WBC count. However, it is not sensitive enough to diagnose or exclude meningitis without an LP.

11. Approximately 90% of children with ventriculoperitoneal shunts with CSF white count greater than 100 cells/mm^3 are infected. The leukocyte count in the malfunctioning shunt is 18 WBC/mm^3 in contrast to an average of 156 WBC/mm^3 in an infected shunt. The CSF glucose level is usually normal and the organisms are less pathogenic.

12. The infant's airway should never be compromised during LP. This is particularly important in small infants who are held tightly, which could potentially cause suffocation or impaired central venous return.

Blood Cultures

These may provide bacteriologic confirmation of the infecting organism and should always be obtained. A blood culture is positive in nearly 100% of patients with *H. influenzae* meningitis, if pretreated children are excluded.

Cultures of Infected Sites

Aspirates of purpuric lesions, joints, and abscesses or middle ear infections should be obtained.

Counterimmunoelectrophoresis

Rapid bacteriologic diagnosis may be possible using antisera against capsular antigen to *H. influenzae*, type B; *S. pneumoniae*; *N. meningitidis*; and group B streptococcus. This is useful in children who have previously received antibiotics. The limited sensitivity and specificity restrict the usefulness of bacterial antigen detection tests (BADT) as a routine test.

Other Studies

1. Blood glucose should be obtained before performing LP.
2. WBC and platelets. The peripheral WBC count may be noted to increase after the LP.
3. Electrolytes. Should initially be obtained every 1 to 2 days to monitor for inappropriate ADH
4. Polymerase chain reaction (PCR) may be useful in making an early diagnosis of herpes and enterovirus.

Chest X-Ray Film

A film should be taken if there are associated respiratory symptoms.

CT Scan

A scan is indicated if there are focal neurologic signs or seizures or if there is clinical evidence of an intracranial mass effect. It is also appropriate if the patient had preceding trauma.

Subdural Taps

These should be done if there is evidence of increasing head circumference, expanding and bulging anterior fontanel, or continuing fever with poor clinical response (see Appendix A-6).

DIFFERENTIAL DIAGNOSIS
(see Chapters 15, 34, and 39)

Differential considerations in the patient with a stiff neck include meningitis, adenitis, osteomyelitis, trauma with secondary fracture, hematoma or muscle injury, tumor, hysteria, torticollis, and oculogyric crisis from drugs such as phenothiazines (p. 387).

Infection

Because of the nonspecific signs and symptoms, particularly in younger children, it is often difficult, without an LP, to distinguish meningitis from a number of other infections, for instance:

1. Pneumonia
2. Acute gastroenteritis with dehydra-

tion, particularly if caused by *Shigella* organisms
3. Acute illness associated with a febrile seizure
4. Less commonly, brain abscess, subdural empyema, and acute obstruction of a VP shunt

Vascular Disorder

Subarachnoid bleeding or a cerebrovascular accident may develop acutely and be associated with a systemic infection.

Intoxication

The stress of an acute infection may lead some individuals to overdoses, purposeful or accidental. Infection changes the kinetics of drugs like theophylline.

Trauma

Head trauma producing a subdural or epidural hematoma may be difficult to distinguish, sometimes necessitating a CT scan before the LP. Heatstroke may cause fever, dehydration, meningism, and marked changes in mentation.

MANAGEMENT

1. Initial management must focus on stabilizing the patient. Intravenous access should be established after ensuring adequate airway and ventilation. Assessment of vital signs with concomitant evaluation for hypoxia, dehydration, increased intracranial pressure, acidosis, electrolyte abnormalities, and disseminated intravascular coagulation (DIC), when appropriate, must be rapidly done.
2. An LP should be performed and rapidly analyzed.

Bacterial Meningitis

This requires immediate intervention.

Antibiotics

Antibiotics should be initiated parenterally using the Gram stain, patient's age, underlying disease, immunologic status of the patient, and allergy history as guides to selection. They should be altered once culture and sensitivity data are available. *S. pneumoniae* resistant to penicillin is becoming a more important pathogen. Although *H. influenzae* is less common because of widespread immunization, the organism may be resistant to ampicillin, chloramphenicol, or both (Box 81-1).

Cerebral Edema

An uncommon complication, it may develop with focal neurologic signs or evidence of herniation.

1. If the patient is intubated, hyperventilate to maintain $Paco_2$ at about 25 mm Hg.
2. Give mannitol (20% solution), 0.5-1.0 gm/kg/dose q4-6hr.
3. Give diuretic: furosemide (Lasix), 1 mg/kg/dose q4-6hr IV.

NOTE: Most patients who have symptomatic increased intracranial pressure (ICP)

Box 81-1
BACTERIAL MENINGITIS: ANTIBIOTIC TREATMENT

<6 wk

Unknown cause*	Ampicillin, 100-200 mg/kg/24 hr q4-6hr IV, *and* cefotaxime (or equivalent), 100-150 mg/kg/24 hr q8-12hr IV; **or** ampicillin, as above, *and* gentamicin, 5-7.5 mg/kg/24 hr q8-12hr IV (or tobramycin, 4-6 mg/kg/24 hr q8-12hr IV); if *S. pneumoniae* suspected by Gram stain or antigen testing, add vancomycin (30 mg/kg/24 hr q12hr IV)
E. coli	Cefotaxime, as above; treat 21 days or longer
Group B streptococci (*S. agalactiae*)	Penicillin G, 150,000-250,000 units/kg/24 hr q4-6hr IV, and gentamicin, as above; treat 14 days or longer
L. monocytogenes	Ampicillin, as above; treat 14-21 days or longer

6 wk-18 yr

Unknown cause†	Cefotaxime, 200 mg/kg/24 hr q6-8hr IV (or ceftriaxone, 100 mg/kg/24 hr q12hr IV or equivalent)
H. influenzae	Cefotaxime, 200 mg/kg/24 hr q6-8hr IV (or ceftriaxone, 100 mg/kg/24 hr q12hr IV, or ceftizoxime 200 mg/kg/24 hr q8hr IV) or equivalent
S. pneumoniae	Vancomycin, 30-45 mg/kg/24 hr q6hr IV, and ceftriaxone, 100 mg/kg/24 hr q12hr IV, pending sensitivities for 10-14 days,
N. meningitidis	Penicillin G, 250,000 units/kg/24 hr q4hr IV; treat 7-10 days‡

Duration of therapy in uncomplicated cases in children <2 mo of age is generally 14-21 days or longer. Older children may generally be treated for 7-10 days, depending on the response to therapy and the pathogen. Patients with complicated cases require longer duration.
*In preterm, low-birth-weight infant <1 mo, vancomycin (30 mg/kg/24 hr q12hr IV) and ceftazidime (100-150 mg/kg/24 hr q8hr IV) may be used because of risk of *S. aureus* and gram-negative bacilli.
†If *S. pneumoniae* is suspected, vancomycin and cefotaxime/ceftriaxone should be inititated until pathogen is identified and sensitivities completed.
‡Adult: 10 million-20 million units/24 hr q4hr IV.

and who require aggressive treatment as above should have an intracranial monitor placed by a neurosurgeon. Prognosis is improved if the cerebral perfusion pressure (CPP = difference between ICP and blood pressure [BP]) is greater than 30 mm Hg.

Seizures

Seizures should be treated with diazepam (Valium), 0.2-0.3 mg/kg/dose q5-10min IV (maximum: 10 mg), or lorazepam (Ativan), 0.05-0.15 mg/kg/dose IV. Phenobarbital or phenytoin should be initiated for maintenance therapy (see Chapter 21). Prophylactic anticonvulsants are generally not indicated.

Physical Examination

A complete examination, including head circumference, should be performed daily. Particular attention should be given to secondary complications such as septic arthritis or subdural effusion in performing daily examinations.

Fluid Therapy

This should be conservative, reflecting hydration and vital signs. After stabilization, fluids should be continued at 80% to 100% of maintenance requirements. Serum sodium level should be monitored and if decreased, spot urine and serum sodium and potassium levels and osmolality should be measured. If hyponatremia as a result of inappropriate ADH secretion occurs, fluid should be further restricted.

Steroids

Administration of steroids during the treatment of bacterial meningitis in children older than 6 weeks of age may reduce the incidence of subsequent hearing loss. Although steroids are often routinely used in bacterial meningitis, the exact benefit is under continuing study and results are somewhat conflicting. Dosage is dexamethasone, 0.6 mg/kg/24 hr q6hr IV, for first 4 days or 16 doses of therapy. The optimum time for starting dexamethasone is either before or concomitant with the first dose of parenteral antibiotics.

Steroids produce a more rapid improvement in the opening CSF pressure and CPP. They decrease meningeal inflammation and concentration of cytokines. They may also reduce the temperature during the first few days of therapy.

Disposition

All patients require hospitalization. Those with high-risk features (<1 year of age or demonstrating shock, coma, seizures, petechiae for <12 hours, low CSF glucose level, or very high CSF protein level) should be monitored very closely, often in an intensive care unit (ICU).

If the patient is seen initially in a setting without facilities to perform an LP and has signs and symptoms highly suggestive of bacterial meningitis, blood cultures should be obtained and parenteral antibiotics (IV preferably) administered before transport.

Coma, shock, respiratory distress, a low CSF white cell count (<1000 WBC/mm^3) at the time of admission have a poor prognosis in patients with *S. pneumoniae* meningitis. Worse sequelae in those with bacterial meningitis are associated with duration of symptoms more than 48 hours, prehospital seizure activity, presence of peripheral vasoconstriction, CSF cell count less than 1000/mm^3, and an admission body temperature 38° C or less.

Twenty-five percent of school-aged meningitis survivors have sequelae.

Chemoprophylaxis is indicated in the following situations.

1. Individuals who have had intimate contact with a patient with meningitis caused by *N. meningitidis* should receive prophylaxis: rifampin, 10 mg/kg/dose q12hr PO for 4 doses (adult: 600 mg/dose q12hr PO for 4 doses; children <1 month, 5 mg/kg/dose q12hr PO for 4 doses).

2. Prophylaxis for exposure to other systemic disease—especially meningitis caused by *H. influenzae*—is controversial but guidelines have been developed. Prophylaxis is recommended for all members of a household with children less than 4 years who have systemic *H. influenzae* type B disease. Prophylaxis in day-care settings is indicated if they resemble households such

as those with children less than 2 years in which contact is 25 hr/wk or more. It is also used if two or more cases of invasive disease occurred in attendees within 60 days. Dosage of rifampin is 20 mg/kg/dose (maximum: 600 mg/dose) q24hr PO for 4 doses. Some recommend reducing the dosage to 10 mg/kg/dose for infants less than 1 month. Efficacy is uncertain.

Exposed children who have a febrile illness should receive prompt medical evaluation and treatment should be initiated, if indicated.

3. Rifampin can be administered to children by having a liquid preparation formulated. Do not give to patients with liver disease or pregnant females.
4. Parents should be warned of the increased risk of children less than 1 year of age for secondary cases of *H. influenzae* meningitis.
5. In epidemic *Neisseria* meningitis, immunization of potential contacts is indicated.

With good clinical response, patients may be discharged within 24 hours after completion of antibiotic therapy. They should be followed closely, with particular attention to potential neurologic deficits and hearing loss.

All children should have audiologic evaluation. Children less than 2 years should have routine immunization to *H. influenzae* because the disease does not provide long-term immunologic protection.

Viral Meningitis or Meningoencephalitis
(see Table 81-1)

This requires supportive therapy.
1. If there is any concern regarding the reliability of the diagnosis, a repeat LP should demonstrate a marked decrease in the percentage of PMN leukocytes in 6 to 8 hours after the first study in untreated patients.
2. Most patients with viral meningitis should be hospitalized initially to ensure adequate fluid intake and pain management and to allow monitoring for deterioration. If herpes is considered, acyclovir may be initiated. Complications require aggressive management. After an initial assessment and stabilization period, patients may be discharged with close follow-up observation.
3. Although a definite treatment is unavailable, patients should be monitored closely on a long-term basis because of associated neurologic and learning deficits that may develop in subsequent months. Poor outcomes appear to be associated with young age, impaired consciousness, and abnormal oculocephalic responses.

REFERENCES
American Academy of Pediatrics, Committee on Infectious Diseases: Therapy for children with invasive pneumococcal infection, *Pediatrics* 99:289, 1997.
Arditi M, Herold BC, Yogev R: Cefuroxime treatment failure and *Haemophilus influenzae* meningitis: case report and review of literature, *Pediatrics* 84:132, 1989.
Blisitkul DM, Hogan AE, Tanz RR: The role of bacterial antigen detection tests in the diagnosis of bacterial meningitis, *Pediatr Emerg Care* 10:67, 1994.
Coant PN, Kornberg AE, Duffy LC, et al: Blood culture results as determinants in the organisms identification of bacterial meningitis, *Pediatr Emerg Care* 8:200, 1992.
Geiman BJ, Smith AL: Dexamethasone and bacterial meningitis: a meta analysis of randomized controlled trials, *West J Med* 157:27, 1992.
Grimwood K, Anderson VA, Bond L, et al: Adverse outcomes of bacterial meningitis in school-age survivors, *Pediatrics* 95:646, 1995.
Hamson SA, Risser W: Repeat lumbar puncture in the differential diagnosis of meningitis, *Pediatr Infect Dis* 7:143, 1988.
Jafari HS, McCracken OH: Dexamethasone therapy in bacterial meningitis, *Pediatr Ann* 23:82, 1994.
Kaaresen P, Flaegstad T: Prognostic factors in childhood bacterial meningitis, *Acta Paediatr* 84:873, 1995.
Kennedy CR, Duffy SW, Smith R, et al: Clinical predictors of outcome in encephalitis, *Arch Dis Child* 62:1156, 1987.
Key CB, Rothrock SC, Falk JL: Cerebrospinal fluid shunt complications: an emergency medicine perspective, *Pediatr Emerg Care* 11:265, 1995.
Kornelisse RE: Prognosis of pneumococcal meningitis, *Clin Infect Dis* 21:1390, 1995.

Lebel MH, Freis BJ, Syroglannopoulos GA, et al: Dexamethasone therapy for bacterial meningitis, *N Engl J Med* 319:964, 1988.

Lembo RM, Rubin DH, Krowchuk DP, et al: Peripheral white blood cell counts and bacterial meningitis: implications regarding diagnostic efficacy in febrile children, *Pediatr Emerg Care* 7:4, 1991.

Pomeroy SL, Holmes SJ, Dodge PR, et al: Seizures and other neurologic sequelae of bacterial meningitis in children, *N Engl J Med* 323:1651, 1990.

Quagliarella VJ, Scheld WM: Treatment of bacterial meningitis, *N Engl J Med* 336: 708, 1997.

Rodewald LE, Woodin KA, Szilagyi PG, et al: Relevance of common tests of cerebrospinal fluid in screening for bacterial meningitis, *J Pediatr* 119:363, 1991.

Rodriquez AF, Kaplan SL, Mason EO: Cerebrospinal fluid values in the very low birth weight infant, *J Pediatr* 116:971, 1990.

Rorabaugh ML, Berlin LE, Heldrich F, et al: Aseptic meningitis in infants younger than two years of age: acute illness and neurologic complications, *Pediatrics* 92:206, 1993.

Rothrock SG, Green SM, Wren J, et al: Pediatric bacterial meningitis: is prior antibiotic therapy associated with an altered clinical presentation, *Ann Emerg Med* 21:146, 1992.

Rubenstein JS, Yogev R: What represents pleocytosis in blood-contaminated ("traumatic tap") cerebrospinal fluid in children? *J Pediatr* 107:249, 1985.

Schaad UB, Suter S, Gianella B, et al: A comparison of ceftriaxone and cefuroxime for the treatment of bacterial meningitis in children, *N Engl J Med* 322:141, 1989.

Schaad UB, Wedgewood-Krucke J, Tschaeppoelee H: Reversible ceftriaxone-associated biliary pseudolithiasis in children, *Lancet* 2:1411, 1988.

Schlesinger Y, Sawyer MH, Storch GA: Enteroviral meningitis in infancy, potential role for polymerase chain reaction in pain management, *Pediatrics* 94:157, 1994.

Schoendorf KC, Adams WO, Kiely JL, et al: National trends in *Haemophilus influenzae* meningitis mortality and hospitalization among children, 1980-1991, *Pediatrics* 93:663, 1994.

Shohat M, Goodman Z, Ragovin H, et al: The effect of lumbar puncture procedure on blood glucose level and leukocyte count in infants, *Clin Pediatr* 26:477, 1987.

Snedeker JB, Kaplan SL, Dodge P, et al: Subdural effusion and its relationship with neurologic sequelae of bacterial meningitis in infancy: a prospective study, *Pediatrics* 86:163, 1990.

Taylor HG, Mills EL, Ciampi A, et al: The sequelae of *Haemophilus influenzae* meningitis in school-age children, *N Engl J Med* 323:1657, 1990.

Unhanand M, Mustafa MM, McCracken GH, et al: Gram-negative enteric bacillary meningitis: a twenty-one-year experience, *J Pediatr* 122:15, 1993.

Wald ER, Kaplan SL, Mason EQ, et al: Dexamethasone therapy for children with bacterial meningitis, *Pediatrics* 95:21, 1995.

Walsh-Kelly C, Nelson DB, Smith DS, et al: Clinical patterns of bacterial versus aseptic meningitis in childhood, *Ann Emerg Med* 21:910, 1992.

MIGRAINE HEADACHE

Migraines are recurrent headaches with initial intracranial vasoconstriction followed by extracranial vasodilation, producing a throbbing pain that may occur in any age group. A positive family history commonly is present (50%). There is a 3:1 prevalence in women. The headache often is precipitated by stress and may first develop during puberty. It is episodic and has a variable frequency.

DIAGNOSTIC FINDINGS

1. The *classic* headaches are unilateral but may be bilateral with a throbbing or pulsatile quality.
   a. They commonly are preceded by an aura, which may be visual (stars, spots, or circles), sensory (hyperesthesia), or motor (weakness), and are accompanied by abdominal pain, nausea, vomiting, anorexia, vertigo, ataxia, and syncope.
   b. Headaches subsequently become recurrent.
   c. Onset may be associated with exertion, stress, or coughing.
2. *Common* migraines may be generalized, without an aura—more common in younger children.
   • Generalized malaise, dizziness, nausea, and vomiting are prominent.
3. Less commonly, specific migraine complexes may be present.
   a. *Ophthalmoplegic* migraines cause unilateral eye pain with limitation of extraocular movement involving cranial nerves III, IV, and VI.

b. *Basilar* migraines involve the basilar artery, producing headaches, vertigo, ataxia, cranial nerve palsy, blindness, syncope, acute confusion without neurologic findings, cyclic vomiting, recurrent abdominal pain, and paroxysmal disequilibrium. Progressive mental status deterioration may be noted.

c. *Hemiplegic* migraines primarily cause transient motor deficits.

4. Migraines are often relieved by rest.

Ancillary Data

1. Electroencephalogram (EEG) may show slowing but is not diagnostically or therapeutically useful.

2. Tests to exclude other causes of headaches or specific presenting neurologic findings. Diagnostic studies should normally be obtained in children less than 6 years, those with large head circumference, and those who exhibit new neurologic signs, fail to return to a normal state of health, experience increasing frequency or severity, or experience personality changes.

DIFFERENTIAL DIAGNOSIS

See Chapter 36.

MANAGEMENT

1. Initial management must attempt to relieve pain. Many patients respond to mild analgesia such as acetaminophen or acetaminophen with codeine. Relief usually is achieved with sleep. Oxygen may be helpful.

2. Nonpharmacologic therapy should focus on trigger factors. Reducing stress and exertion and avoiding certain foods and oral contraceptives reduce the incidence rate. Biofeedback, relaxation therapy, psychotherapy, and hypnotherapy may be useful.

3. Once the diagnosis is established, *abortive* treatment of the acute episode is best achieved when medication is initiated early in the course.

a. If mild analgesics (acetaminophen, ibuprofen, naproxen) provide inadequate relief, aspirin, phenacetin, and caffeine combinations (Fiorinal or Fenbutal) should be initiated.

- In children less than 5 years of age, ½ tablet; in those 5 to 12 years, 1 tablet, repeated 1 hour later if no relief is obtained. Older children receive 1 to 2 tablets.

b. In the postpubertal child with classic migraine, Midrin (isometheptene mucate, 65 mg, dichloralphenazone, 100 mg, and acetaminophen, 325 mg) given at the onset of pain with an additional tablet 1 hour later may be useful.

c. Sumatriptan (Imitrex) (adult: 6 mg SC or 100 mg PO; SC dose may be repeated in 1 hour if no response to initial SC dose). The onset of response is rapid with 70% recovering within 1 hr; 35% have a recurrence during the subsequent 24 hours. There is limited experience in children. Sumatriptan is also available as a nasal spray.

d. If the patient arrives with a severe attack that has been going on for some time, chlorpromazine (Thorazine), 12.5 mg q20min IM up to a total adult dose of 37.5 mg, is helpful. Ketorolac (Toradol) is a parenteral nonsteroidal antiinflammatory agent given in children older than 2 years at a dosage of 1 mg/kg/dose q6hr IM. Adults are initially normally given 30-60 mg/dose followed by 15-30 mg/dose q6hr. This latter agent is as effective as meperidine and hydroxyzine in some studies.

e. If relief from a severe migraine is not achieved, ergotamine preparations may be used in subsequent attacks.

Ergotamine (1 mg with 100 mg caffeine) tablets should be used at the onset of pain and repeated every 30 minutes up to 3 doses per headache in children less than 12 years and no more than 6 doses per headache, regardless of age. Suppositories are available if the patient is vomiting (one suppository per headache for children <12 years and no more than two suppositories per headache for older patients). Caffeine potentiates the ergotamine by increasing absorption, but it may prevent sleep.

f. Other agents that may need to be considered in resistant patients include dihydroergotamine (DHE) (adult: 1 mg IM initially and repeat in 1 hour up to total dose of 3 mg. May be given IV to a maximum dose of 2 mg), given with Phenergan or other antiemetic. DHE appears to be effective in adults but there is limited experience in children.

Metoclopramide (Reglan) in a dose of 10 mg IV has been found useful in adults. Results of pediatric studies are pending.

4. *Long-term prophylactic* management of disabling migraines in adolescents and adults may include one of a number of agents. Often control is achieved by using a variety of agents that are attempted on an empiric basis.

a. Propranolol, 2 mg/kg/24 hr q8hr PO. Side effects include bradycardia, nausea, fatigue, hypotension, hypoglycemia, and depression. It is contraindicated in patients with asthma, congestive heart failure, or depression. Metoprolol (2-6 mg/kg/24 hr for adults) is recommended as a β blocker in patients with asthma.

b. Phenytoin (Dilantin), 3-5 mg/kg/24 hr q12-24hr PO. Side effects include drowsiness, impaired learning, idiosyncratic hypersensitivity, and gingival hypertrophy.

c. Amitriptyline (Elavil), 0.2-0.5 mg/kg/dose given at night, especially to older children with depressive characteristics. Side effects include dry mouth, dizziness, fatigue, and urinary retention.

d. Cyproheptadine (Periactin), 0.2-0.4 mg/kg/24 hr q6-8hr PO (maximum: 32 mg/24 hr), is an antihistamine that may cause weight gain and sedation.

e. Calcium channel blockers may be effective as well. Verapamil, 4-10 mg/kg/24 hr (240-480 mg/24 hr) TID PO, may be used.

DISPOSITION

1. Most patients can be sent home with appropriate acute and chronic medications and close follow-up observation.
2. Hospitalization is indicated only for severe pain.

REFERENCES

Bell R, Montoya D, Shuaib A, et al: A comparative trial of three agents in the treatment of acute migraine headache, *Ann Emerg Med* 19:1079, 1990.

Cooper PJ, Bawden HN, Camfield PR, et al: Anxiety and life events in childhood migraine, *Pediatrics* 79:999, 1987.

Duarte C, Dunaway F, Turner L, et al: Ketorolac versus meperidine and hydroxyzine in the treatment of acute migraine headache: a randomized prospective double blind trial, *Ann Emerg Med* 21:1116, 1992.

Ellis GL, Delaney J, De Hart DA, et al: The efficacy of metoclopramide in the treatment of migraine headache, *Ann Emerg Med* 22:191, 1993.

Igarashi M, May WN, Golden GS: Pharmacologic treatment of childhood migraine, *J Pediatr* 120:653, 1992.

Larkin GL, Prescott JE: A randomized, double-blind comparative study of the efficacy of ketorolac tromethamine versus meperidine in the treatment of severe migraine, *Ann Emerg Med* 21:919, 1992.

Olesen J: Understanding the biologic basis of migraine, *N Engl J Med* 331:1713, 1994.

Subcutaneous sumatriptan international study group: Treatment of migraine attacks with sumatriptan, *N Engl J Med* 325:316, 1991.

Welch KMA: Drug therapy of migraine, *N Engl J Med* 329:1476, 1993.

PSEUDOTUMOR CEREBRI

Benign intracranial hypertension or pseudotumor cerebri occurs when there is increased ICP in the absence of a local, space-occupying lesion or there is acute brain swelling accompanying an identifiable infectious or inflammatory process.

ETIOLOGY

Although the pathogenesis is unknown, pseudotumor cerebri is associated with a host of clinical entities:

1. Infection: upper respiratory tract (URI) infection, acute otitis media (AOM), roseola infantum, sinusitis
2. Allergy
3. Deficiency: anemia, including iron deficiency, leukemia, vitamin A deficiency, or overdose
4. Endocrine/metabolic disorders: steroid medication, oral contraceptive pills, uremia, hyperthyroidism, hypothyroidism, Addison disease, or galactosemia
5. Trauma: minimal head trauma
6. Vascular disorder: congenital or acquired heart disease
7. Intoxication: tetracycline, steroids, oral contraceptives, vitamin A
8. Idiopathic disorder

DIAGNOSTIC FINDINGS

1. Younger children may have only a bulging fontanelle with some irritability or listlessness.
2. Older children have headache, nausea, vomiting, and dizziness. Eye examination may reveal papilledema, sixth nerve palsy, diplopia, blurred vision, and enlarged blind spot.
3. The level of consciousness is relatively normal, given the signs of ICP.

Ancillary Data

1. LP: normal with the exception of increased pressure
2. CT scan: may be indicated to exclude mass lesion

DIFFERENTIAL DIAGNOSIS

1. Infection
   a. Meningitis or encephalitis: LP for evaluation
   b. Brain abscess: CT scan and subsequent LP
   c. Optic neuritis: slit-lamp examination
2. Trauma (subdural effusion or hemorrhage): subdural tap or CT scan
3. Neoplasm. CT scan (may be diagnostic)

MANAGEMENT

Although pseudotumor cerebri is a benign entity with an excellent prognosis, it is a diagnosis of exclusion, and other entities such as meningitis in the febrile child must be considered. Once the diagnosis is confirmed, treatment of the underlying disease is appropriate.

Adjunctive therapy, implemented in conjunction with a neurologist, may include the following:

1. Acetazolamide (Diamox), 5 mg/kg/dose (maximum: 250-375 mg/dose) q24-48hr PO; or
2. Serial LP.

Uncontrolled, increased ICP and papilledema may result in visual loss. The patient should therefore be followed by an ophthalmologist with testing of visual fields if possible.

REFERENCES

Amacher AL, Spence JD: Spectrum of benign intracranial hypertension in children and adolescents, *Child Nerv Syst* 1:81, 1985.

Lessell S: Pediatric pseudo tumor cerebri (idiopathic intracranial hypertension), *Surv Ophthalmol* 37:155, 1992.

SEIZURES

ALERT: If ongoing seizures are occurring, refer to status epilepticus (see Chapter 21).

A seizure or convulsion is a paroxysmal disturbance in nerve cells resulting in abnormalities in motor, sensory, autonomic, or psychic function. (See febrile seizures, p. 747.)

TABLE 81-4   Seizures: Cause By Age of Onset*

FIRST DAY OF LIFE

Hypoxia	Hyperglycemia
Drugs	Hypoglycemia
Trauma	Pyridoxine deficiency
Infection	

DAY 2-3 OF LIFE

Infection	Developmental malformation
Drug withdrawal	Intracranial hemorrhage
Hypoglycemia	Inborn error of metabolism
Hypocalcemia	Hypo/hypernatremia

DAY >4-6 MO

Infection	Developmental malformation
Hypocalcemia	Drug withdrawal
Hyperphosphatemia	Inborn error of metabolism
Hyponatremia	

6 MO-3 YR

Febrile seizures	Trauma
Birth injury	Metabolic disorder
Infection	Cerebral degenerative disease
Toxin	

>3 YR

Idiopathic	Trauma
Infection	Cerebral degenerative disease

*Differential considerations must be individualized.

ETIOLOGY (Tables 81-4 and 81-5)

The most common causes of acute onset of seizures in children often caused by lowering the threshold are infection, trauma, poor compliance, intoxications, and idiopathic disorders. Epilepsy accounts for most chronic seizure disorders.

By age of onset, specific causes are most common (see Table 18-4).

Classification

1. *Partial seizures*
   a. *Partial simple seizure* (consciousness retained)
      May have motor (Jacksonian), somatosensory (metallic, headache), autonomic (flushing, sweating), or psychiatric (déjà vu) symptoms.
   b. *Partial complex seizure* (consciousness impaired)
      Simple partial onset progressing to impaired consciousness or impaired at onset of seizure. Previously called psychomotor seizures. An aura that includes automatisms, alteration of perception, and hallucinations may occur before alteration of consciousness progresses.
   c. Partial seizures that secondarily generalize
2. *Generalized seizures* (involves both sides of brain)
   a. Nonconvulsive
      (1) *Absence seizures.* Characterized by brief lapse in awareness, sometimes accompanied by minor motor manifestations (staring, rhythmic eye blinking, head dropping) without postictal period. Previously called petit mal.
      (2) Atypical absence.
   b. Convulsive
      (1) *Myoclonic seizures.* Brief contractions that occur unilaterally or bilaterally.

TABLE 81-5   Seizures: Diagnostic Considerations

Condition	Diagnostic findings	Comments
EPILEPSY	Variable seizure types as described in this chapter	Multiple causes, including idiopathic
INFECTION		
Febrile (p. 747)	Fever; grand mal seizure; variable focal seizure; self-limited; peak: 5 mo–5 yr; high association with *Shigella*; LP normal	Must distinguish from meningitis
Meningitis (p. 725)	Fever, stiff neck, headache, Kernig, Brudzinski; in young child, dehydration, bulging fontanel, lethargy, irritability, vomiting, cyanosis; LP diagnostic	May be viral or bacterial
Encephalitis (p. 733)	Headache, fever, vomiting, irritability, listlessness, stupor, variable focal neurologic signs; LP may be diagnostic or equivocal	Epidemiology important; usually viral
Intracranial abscess	Insidious onset; fever; variable focal neurologic findings; CT scan diagnostic	
S/P DTP immunization	History of immunization, fever; seizure within 48 hr	May have permanent sequelae
Misc: pertussis, rabies, tetanus, syphilis	Disease-specific signs and symptoms	
Subacute bacterial endocarditis (p. 559)	Fever; usually insidious; focal neurologic findings; splenomegaly; embolic phenomenon; variable heart disease; positive blood cultures	
TRAUMA (Chapter 57)		
Concussion	History of trauma, variable abnormal neurologic examination; focal or grand mal seizure within 24 hr; CT scan variably WNL	May be recurrent; close neurologic monitoring; may not require anti-convulsants
Acute Subdural	Variable focal neurologic signs; change in mental status; progression with increased intracranial pressure; positive CT scan	Immediate neurosurgical intervention
Epidural	Lucid period after trauma; eventual lapse into coma with herniation	Immediate neurosurgical intervention
CONGENITAL (Chapters 10 and 11)		
Birth asphyxia	History of perinatal injury; neurologic abnormality; premature; low Apgar	Infection, placental insufficiency, difficult birth
Neurocutaneous syndrome	Pathognomonic skin findings; variably abnormal neurologic examination, family history; CT scan may be useful	

Continued

TABLE 81-5   Seizures: Diagnostic Considerations—cont'd

Condition	Diagnostic findings	Comments
INTRAPSYCHIC		
Breath-holding (p. 724)	Precipitated by crying, anger, injury, cyanosis, followed by loss of consciousness, may be opisthotonic; seizures rare and self-limited	Peak: 6 mo-4 yr; cyanosis precedes loss of consciousness; in seizures consciousness is lost first; usually maternal-infant problems
Hyperventilation		
Hysteria		
ENDOCRINE/METABOLIC		
Hypoglycemia (Chapter 38)	Sweating, pallor, syncope, vasovagal reaction; newborn: irritability, apnea, cyanosis, listlessness, poor feeding	Definition varies with age; glucose level: newborn <2500 gm (<20 mg/dl), term newborn (<30 mg/dl), older infant and child (<40 mg/dl)
Hyponatremia (Chapter 8)	Listlessness, variable stupor; associated condition (e.g., dehydration, head trauma, inappropriate ADH, Addison, water intoxication); usually temp <36.5° C	
Hypernatremia (Chapter 8)	Listlessness or irritability; associated condition (dehydration)	Rarely causes seizures unless rapid rehydration
Hypocalcemia	Muscle cramps, pain, Chovstek, Trousseau, variable increased intracranial pressure, headache	Common in premature, parathyroid deficiency
Hypomagnesemia	Tetany, tremor, irritability	Difficult to determine true body deficit
Kernicterus (Chapter 11)	Jaundice, developmental delay	Rare at present
Inborn errors		
Phenylketonuria (PKU)	Neurologically abnormal; developmental delay; variable acidosis; need urine and blood screen	
Amino and organic acidemia		
Uremia (p. 809)	Signs and symptoms of renal failure	

INTOXICATION (Chapter 54)

Aspirin
Amphetamine
Anticholinergics (e.g., tricyclics, phenothiazine)
Theophylline
Carbon monoxide
PCP, cocaine
Propoxyphene
Lead
Drug withdrawal (e.g., alcohol, anticonvulsants)

Signs and symptoms of associated drug intoxication or withdrawal

See Chapters 54 and 55 for complete listing

DEGENERATIVE/DEFICIENCY

Pyridoxine deficiency or dependence

Mentally retarded, anemia, diarrhea

Responds well to pyridoxine (5-10 mg IV/IM), then 0.3-0.5 mg/24 hr

Tay-Sachs disease

Blind, spasms, floppy, cherry-red spot

Eastern European background

Juvenile Huntington chorea

Rigidity, dementia

Metachromatic leukodystrophy

Incoordination, upper and lower neurologic signs

Other CNS diseases

Variable

NEOPLASM

Often focal neurologic findings

Glioma, most common; supratentorial lesions more likely to cause seizure

VASCULAR (Chapter 18)

Dysrhythmia

Irregular pulse, sudden event, abnormal ECG (e.g., long QT, block)

Intracranial hematoma
Cerebral
Extradural
Subarachnoid

Acute onset headache, neurologic findings; variable increased intracranial pressure

Associated with AV malformation, bleeding disorder (e.g., hemophilia), heart disease, sickle cell, trauma

Hypertensive encephalopathy (Chapter 18)

High blood pressure; vomiting, hyperpyrexia, ataxia, coma; facial paralysis

May be secondary to stroke

Embolism

Focal neurologic findings

Predisposing factors: heart disease, peripheral embolism

Transient ischemic attack infarct

Variable neurologic finding, dependent on site; fever; broad deficits; altered sensation

Differentiate from Todd paralysis

(2) Clonic, tonic, tonic-clonic seizures. Tonic movements reflect sustained muscle contracting resulting in limb and trunk rigidity. Clonic movements are rhythmic jerking and flexor spasms of the extremities.

(3) *Atonic* seizures. Abrupt loss of muscle tone, causing the child to collapse or drop.

DIAGNOSTIC FINDINGS

Patients usually have a history of seizures, but if ongoing seizures are present, evaluation and management as described in Chapter 21 should be implemented.

1. The initial assessment must determine the characteristics of the seizure, defining its focality or generalized nature, frequency, associated sensory and autonomic function, and behavioral changes. Predisposing factors such as fever, intoxications, perinatal asphyxia, trauma, and preexisting abnormalities in growth and development require definition.

2. A complete neurologic examination is essential, differentiating long-standing from acute changes. Evidence of asymmetry of findings, increased intracranial pressure, or infection must be carefully assessed.

Ancillary Data

Evaluation must reflect the nature of the seizure and potential causes.

Chemistries

A glucose determination should be performed on all patients: initially, Dextrostix or Chemstrip screening; electrolyte, Ca^{++}, Mg^{++}, and PO_4^{--} levels as indicated.

Hematology

For febrile patients, a complete blood count (CBC) and urinalysis should be done.

Lumbar Puncture

An LP should be performed in febrile patients, if indicated (p. 727). Evaluation of the fluid must include Gram stain (and methylene blue stain), culture, cell count, and glucose and protein levels. Seizures can cause some elevation of cells but never more than 20 WBC/mm^3 or more than 9 neutrophils/mm^3.

Cultures

In addition to a CSF culture and Gram stain in the febrile child, cultures of blood and urine should be obtained. Other cultures should be done as indicated.

X-Ray Film

1. A CT scan has a very low yield in generalized seizures without focal findings in the pediatric age group and is usually not required. It may be useful in cases with preceding head trauma or abnormal neurologic status.

   The CT scan of a patient with an acute seizure is usually normal if none of the following are present: malignancy, neurocutaneous disorder, recent closed head injury, recent CSF shunt revision, less than 6 months old, seizure of more than 15 minutes' duration, or recent onset of focal neurologic deficit.

2. A skull roentgenogram is indicated with evidence of trauma preceding the seizure and when a CT scan is not readily available.

3. Magnetic resonance imaging (MRI) may be useful for recurrent or progressive findings.

Drug Levels

1. Evaluation for possibility of ingestion (see Chapter 54).

2. Anticonvulsant medication levels if the patient is receiving chronic therapy. Subtherapeutic levels are a very common cause of seizures.

Subdural Tap (see Appendix A-6)

This may be indicated in the young child who has associated trauma or infection, particularly if the fontanel is full and the child is deteriorating. If stable, a CT scan may be diagnostic. Usually done in consultation with a neurosurgeon.

Electroencephalogram

An EEG is indicated to assess electrical seizure activity. The greatest yield in finding epileptiform abnormalities as a seizure focus is immediately after the seizure and declines with time. Nonspecific background changes may persist for 1 to 6 weeks after any type of seizure, including febrile or hypoxic breath-holding.

DIFFERENTIAL DIAGNOSIS

See Tables 81-5 and Box 81-2.

MANAGEMENT

1. Initial treatment of the patient with ongoing seizure activity (see Chapter 21) must include oxygen, dextrose, and anticonvulsants.
2. In the absence of active seizure activity, focus efforts on rapidly determining pos-

sible etiologic conditions and instituting specific treatment.

   a. Metabolic derangements require specific therapy to correct the abnormality.

   b. Seizures after trauma require immediate neurosurgical consultation and CT scan if the patient remains neurologically impaired.

   c. Infectious etiologies require antibiotics and supportive care.

3. If no cause is determined, consider anticonvulsants after consultation with a neurologist. At present, some controversy exists regarding the advisability of treating the first tonic-clonic seizure; many clinicians prefer to wait, pending subsequent seizures when a more definite diagnosis of epilepsy can be made. If medication is begun, loading is required (Table 81-6 and Box 81-3). Monotherapy is effective in about half the patients. Of those children who are not controlled by the first anticonvulsant, 42% had complete remission when their regimen was switched to a second anticonvulsant.

   a. If the patient is taking medication, increase anticonvulsant dosages, if subtherapeutic.

   b. If poor compliance is the basis for the low levels, reload the patient (in full or part, depending on the level) and educate about the importance of taking medications. Close follow-up observation with monitoring of the levels is necessary.

   c. Anticonvulsants usually are continued for at least 2 years after the last seizures. They may be stopped at that time, provided the child has been doing well.

   d. Erythromycin may decrease the metabolism of phenytoin and carbamazepine, requiring a reduction in anticonvulsant dose.

   e. Generic carbamazepine and primidone may have different bioavailability.

Box 81-2

CLINICAL ENTITIES SIMULATING SEIZURES

INFANT

Jitteriness
Apnea
Micturitional shivering
Tremor
Dysrhythmia

CHILD

Breath-holding spell
Micturitional/cough syncope
Night tremor/terrors
Migraine
Tics
Dysrhythmia

ADOLESCENT

Vasomotor syncope
Micturitional/cough syncope
Hyperventilation
Pseudoseizures
Orthostatic hypotension
Hysteria

TABLE 81-6   Common Anticonvulsants

Drug/availability	Primary indication	Maintenance dosage (mg/kg/24 hr) PO frequency	Loading dose* (mg/kg)	Serum half-life (hr)	Serum therapeutic range (µg/ml)
Carbamazepine (Tegretol) Susp: 100 mg/5 ml Tab: 100 (chew), 200 mg	Generalized tonic-clonic, partial seizures	10-40 (adult: 800-1600 mg/24 hr) BID		11-22	4-14
Clonazepam (Klonopin) Tab: 0.5, 1, 2 mg	Absence seizures, secondary for complex partial and tonic seizures	0.05-0.2 (adult: 1.5-2.0 mg/24 hr) BID		24-36	0.10-0.80
Diazepam (Valium) Vial: 5 mg/ml	Status epilepticus	NA	0.2-0.3 IV (<1 mg/min) 0.5 PR		
Ethosuximide (Zarontin) Syr: 250 mg/5 ml Cap: 250 mg	Absence seizures	20-40 (adult: 750-1750 mg/24 hr) QD or BID		24-42	40-100
Felbamate (Felbatol) Susp: 600 mg/5 ml Tab: 400-600 mg	Partial seizures, generalized tonic-clonic	15-45 (adult: 1200-3600 mg/24 hr) TID or QID		14-20	30-80
Gabapentin (Neurontin) Cap: 100, 300, 400 mg	Adjunctive drug for partial seizures Secondary drug for generalized tonic-clonic (>12 yr)	15-30 (adult: 900-2400 mg/24hr) TID		4-8	Unknown
Lamotrigine (Lamictal) Tab: 25, 100, 150, 200 mg	Generalized seizures, partial seizures, refractory absence seizures	3-5 QD (14 days), then BID (adult: 100-500 mg/24 hr) (no concurrent valproic acid)		12-48 (mean: 25)	2-4

Drug (formulation)	Seizure type	Oral dose	Loading/IV dose	Half-life (hr)	Therapeutic level
Lorazepam (Ativan) Vial: 2, 4 mg/ml	Status epilepticus	NA	0.05-0.10 IV	16	
Phenobarbital Elixir: 15, 20 mg/5 ml; Tab: 15, 30, 60, 100 mg; Vial: 65, 130 mg	Generalized tonic-clonic, partial seizures	2-6 (adult: 100-300 mg/24 hr) BID or QHS	15-20 IV (<1 mg/kg/min) IM erratically absorbed	48-72	15-35 (may be higher)
Phenytoin (Dilantin) Susp: 30, 125/5 ml; Tabs (chew): 50 mg; Cap: 30, 100 mg; Amp: 50 mg/ml; Amp (fosphenytoin—Cerebyx): 50 mg/ml equivalent	Generalized tonic-clonic, partial seizures	5-10 (adult: 200-400/24 hr) BID	10-20 IV; or IM, use fosphenytoin	6-30	10-20
Primidone (Mysoline) Susp: 250 mg/5 ml; Tab: 50, 250 mg	Generalized tonic-clonic, partial seizures	10-25 (adult: 750-1250 mg/24 hr) TID or BID		6-12	6-12 (or phenobarbital level)
Valproic acid (Depakene)‡ Syr: 250 mg/5 ml; Cap: 250 mg; Vial: 100 mg/ml (Depacon)	Generalized tonic-clonic	15-60 (adult: 1000-3000 mg/24 hr) TID or BID	Adult: 500-1000 mg IV followed by 500 mg q12hr (<20 mg/min)†	6-18	50-100
Vigabatrin (Sabril)	Partial seizures	40-80 (adult: 1500-3000 mg/24 hr)		5-17	Unknown

*When no specific loading dose specified, oral administration after several doses will achieve therapeutic range.

†IV dose administered over 60 minutes (<20 mg/min) for less than 14 days. Limited pediatric experience.

‡May become carnitine deficient.

Box 81-3

SUGGESTED ANTICONVULSANTS ALTERNATIVES BY SEIZURE TYPE

Partial seizures: CBZ, FBM, GBP, PHT, PRM, VPA

Generalized seizures
  Absence: ETX, VPA
  Tonic-clonic: CBZ, FBM, PB, PHT, PRM, VPA
  Myoclonic: BZD, FBM, VPA
  Atonic: BZD, FMB, VPA

Anticonvulsants listed alphabetically.
See Table 81-6 for drug identification and dosage.
BZD, Benzodiazapines.

---

4. Newborns require slightly different management (see Chapter 11).
5. A Glasgow Coma Scale score (p. 414) of 3 to 8 appears to be somewhat predictive of posttraumatic seizure. Prophylactic phenytoin may be indicated in consultation with a neurosurgeon.

DISPOSITION

1. Patients with first seizures of unknown cause are often admitted to the hospital for evaluation and control, as well as a response to parental anxiety.
2. After a period of observation, patients with chronic seizure disorders who are taking subtherapeutic doses or who require alteration in the therapeutic regimen can be discharged once the drugs are changed and follow-up evaluations arranged.
3. Patients with febrile seizures do not require hospitalization if no underlying life-threatening infection is detected, as outlined below.
4. All patients with seizure disorders require close follow-up of clinical status and therapeutic response. Assessment of anti-convulsant levels is periodically indicated. Patients with complex recurrent seizures should routinely be referred to a neurologist.

Parental Education

1. Give all medications as prescribed.
2. If a seizure does occur, institute seizure precautions to prevent the child from self-injury. Maintain the airway.
3. Close follow-up observation is very important. Please keep all appointments.
4. Call your physician if the following occur:
   a. There is any change in the pattern or frequency of seizure.
   b. There are behavior changes or problems with medication.

REFERENCES

Abramowicz M, editor: Drugs for epilepsy, *Med Lett Drug Ther* 37:37, 1995.

Callagham N, Garrett A, Goggin T: Withdrawal of anticonvulsant drugs in patients free of seizures for two years, *N Engl J Med* 318:942, 1988.

Camfield PR, Camfield CS, Gordon K, et al: If a first antiepileptic drug fails to control a child's epilepsy, what are the chances of success with the next drug? *J Pediatr* 131:821, 1997.

Chamberlain J, Altieri M, Futterman C, et al: Seizures in children, *Pediatr Emerg Care* 13:92, 1997.

Dodson WE, Pellock JM: *Pediatric epilepsy: diagnosis and therapy,* New York, 1993.

Hirtz DG: Generalized tonic clonic and febrile seizures, *Pediatr Clin North Am* 36:365, 1989.

Laxer K: Guidelines for treating epilepsy in the age of felbamate, vigabatrin, lamotrigine, and gabapentin, *West J Med* 161:309, 1994.

Lewis RJ, Yee L, Inkelis SH, et al: Clinical predictors of post-traumatic seizures in children with head trauma, *Ann Emerg Med* 22:1114, 1993.

Rider LG, Thapa PB, Del Beccaro MA, et al: Cerebrospinal fluid analysis in children with seizures *Pediatr Emerg Care* 11:336, 1995.

Scheuer ML, Pedley TA: The evaluation and treatment of seizures, *N Engl J Med* 323:1468, 1990.

Shinnar S, Berg AT, Moshe SL, et al: Risk of seizure recurrence following a first unprovoked seizure, *Pediatrics* 85:1076, 1990.

Vining EPG: Pediatric seizures, *Emerg Med Clin North Am* 12:973, 1994.

Vining EPG, Freeman JM: Seizures which are not epilepsy, *Pediatr Ann* 14:711, 1985.

Warden CR, Brownstein DR, Del Beccaro MA: Predictors of abnormal findings of computed tomography of the head in pediatric patients presenting with seizures, *Ann Emerg Med* 29:518, 1997.

FEBRILE SEIZURES

ALERT: Meningitis must be considered as a potential cause in the febrile child who has seizures.

Febrile seizures are generalized seizures occurring in children with febrile illnesses that do not specifically involve the central nervous system (CNS). They occur in 2% to 5% of children between 5 months and 5 years of age, with the peak incidence between 8 and 20 months.

ETIOLOGY: INFECTION

1. Upper respiratory tract infections are commonly present, representing more than 70% of underlying infections. Pharyngitis, otitis media, and pneumonitis are most common.
2. Gastroenteritis, urinary tract infections, measles, and immunizations such as diphtheria tetanus pertussis (DTP) are less common.
3. Roseola (exanthema subitum) is associated with a high fever, often complicated by a seizure before the onset of the rash.
4. *Shigella* organisms produce high fevers and a neurotoxin. Seizures are common.
5. Meningitis occurs in about 2% of children with fevers and seizures.

DIAGNOSTIC FINDINGS

1. Typically, there is a preceding infectious illness and high fever (usually >39° C). Patients have signs and symptoms of the underlying systemic infection. Of obvious importance is excluding meningitis; such patients commonly have lethargy, fever, headache, vomiting, etc. (p. 725).
2. Seizures are generalized tonic-clonic episodes lasting less than 15 minutes. Complex seizures occur when the episode lasts more than 15 minutes, is focal, or is followed by transient or persistent neurologic abnormalities.
3. Behavior and state of alertness are altered.
   a. Children are postictal.
   b. The underlying illness produces irritability, lethargy, and other changes in mental status.
4. Aggressive antipyretic therapy early in the management facilitates evaluation.

Complications

These are usually self-limited, although they may be recurrent or complex, resulting in hypoxia and self-injury.

Ancillary Data

Lumbar Puncture

LP is a useful part of the evaluation of the patient, particularly for those with a first febrile seizure (see Appendix A-4). It should generally be done in the following children:

1. Less than 1 year of age
2. Less than 2 years of age with a temperature of 41.1° C or more
3. Those who, after aggressive antipyretic therapy, remain irritable, lethargic, or demonstrate other abnormal behavior
4. When there is any question of the reliability of the examination, the caretaker, or follow-up

Other factors worthy of consideration include a prior physician visit within 48 hours, generalized seizure in the emergency department (ED), and focal seizure.

Evaluation of fluid should include Gram stain, culture, cell count, protein, and glucose.

Blood Glucose

This should be done immediately, either by quantitative methods or by Dextrostix/Chemstrip.

CBC with Differential

This is usually unreliable because of the demargination resulting from catecholamine release.

Electrolytes and Blood Urea Nitrogen

These are indicated if there is a preceding problem with intake or output. Ca^{++}, PO_4^{--}, and Mg^{++} determinations are not indicated in previously normal children outside the neonatal period.

Other Studies

Skull roentgenograms or CT scan is obtained if there is associated trauma. An EEG usually is not obtained, because it has little or no prognostic value, although transient abnormalities may be noted.

DIFFERENTIAL DIAGNOSIS (see Table 81-5)

1. Infection.
   a. CNS infection, including those caused by bacterial, viral, fungal or mycobacterial agents. LP is required for differentiation.
   b. Postinfectious encephalitis.
   c. Brain abscess with fever, seizures, and variable spinal fluid.
   d. Immunization, particularly DTP.
2. Intoxication.
   a. Hydrocarbon ingestion with aspiration pneumonitis, fever, and seizures
   b. Salicylate overdose
3. Intrapsychic problem. Breath-holding spells may occur during intercurrent febrile illness.

MANAGEMENT (see Chapter 21)

1. Patients with acute seizures require intervention with oxygen, suction, and maneuvers to minimize self-injury. Rarely is active airway management required. Establish venous access for drug administration. By the time patients arrive, they rarely are having seizures. If they are, give dextrose, 0.5-1.0 gm/kg/dose (2-4 ml D25W/kg/dose) IV.

2. Administer anticonvulsants (see Table 81-6) if patients continue to seize actively after airway and breathing stabilization:
   a. Diazepam (Valium): 0.2-0.3 mg/kg/dose IV given over 2 to 3 minutes at a rate not to exceed 1 mg/min. May repeat every 5 to 10 minutes if seizures continue (maximum total dose: 10 mg). Used to stop seizures.
   b. Lorazepam (Ativan): 0.05-0.15 mg/kg/dose IV over 1 to 3 minutes. Repeat dose rarely beneficial (maximum total dose in adult: 5 mg).
   c. Phenobarbital: 15-20 mg/kg/dose IV (25-50 mg/min or <1 mg/kg/min IV) or IM (erratic absorption), given as loading dose is an alternative, followed by maintenance. May be used as maintenance drug (3-5 mg/kg/24 hr IV, PO), as well as in the management of the patient who is seizing acutely.
   d. Phenytoin (Dilantin): 10-20 mg/kg/dose IV infusion (concentration of ≤6.7 mg/ml in saline solution, not water; not to exceed 40 mg/min or 0.5 mg/kg/min). Maximum loading dose: 1250 mg total dose. Maintenance dose of 5 mg/kg/24 hr IV or PO. Fosphenytoin (Cerebyx) is a new preparation that may be administered more rapidly IV without complications. It may also be given IM.
   e. Erythromycin may decrease metabolism of phenytoin, requiring a reduction in the anticonvulsant dose.
3. Patients who are not having active seizures require rapid evaluation and antipyretic therapy. Focus questioning on potential infectious sources, history of seizures, neurologic deficits, developmental problems, family history, medications, precipitating events, and preceding illness.
   • Antipyretic therapy should include acetaminophen, 10-15 mg/kg/dose q4-6hr PO, and tepid water sponging. Ibuprofen, 10 mg/kg/dose q6hr PO, may also be useful. Aspirin may also be used if

neither chickenpox nor influenza-like illness is present.

4. Obtain laboratory data, including an LP, as appropriate.
5. Treat underlying infections as appropriate.
6. Long-term anticonvulsants reduce, but do not eliminate, recurrent febrile seizures. Consider phenobarbital (5 mg/kg/24 hr q12-24hr PO after a loading dose) for certain patients (see Table 81-6):
   a. Those with two or more of the following risk factors:
      (1) Abnormal neurologic or developmental history before the seizures
      (2) Complex seizure: more than 15 minutes in length or one that is focal or followed by transient or persistent neurologic abnormalities
      (3) Positive family history for afebrile seizures in first-degree relative
   b. Children less than 12 months of age at the time of their first seizure.
   c. Another factor associated with a recurrence is the child only having a brief interval (<1 hour) between the onset of fever and the initial seizure.

      NOTE: Anticonvulsants are continued for 2 years if the patient remains seizure free, although this must be individualized. Intermittent use is of no value.
      • Family anxiety and other social factors may modify the decision to initiate anticonvulsants.
      • Learning disorders and hyperactivity may be associated with phenobarbital use. Anticonvulsants should be initiated only for appropriate reasons. Most children do not require medications.

DISPOSITION

1. Patients with simple febrile seizures may be discharged after appropriate fever control has been achieved. Underlying infections require treatment.

2. Patients requiring phenobarbital therapy may similarly be discharged with close follow-up observation and neurologic consultation after a loading dose has been given and maintenance therapy has been initiated. It is given normally for 2 years when deemed appropriate with dosage adjustment to accommodate growth. Intermittent phenobarbital is of no value.
3. Approximately 40% of children with a simple febrile seizure will have a recurrence, half of which occur within 6 months of the first episode.
4. Recurrent febrile seizures are also related to a fever less than 1 hour (44%) as well as a lower temperature at the time of the seizure. For each degree of increase in temperature from 101° F (38.3° C), 102° F, 103° F, 104° F, and 105° F (40.6° C), the risk was 35%, 30%, 26%, 20%, and 13%, respectively, of having a seizure.

Parental Education

Parental counseling is essential to provide reassurance. It is essential to discuss a number of issues:

1. Benign nature of febrile seizures in healthy children. Reassuring points include the high incidence (2% to 5%), the only slightly increased incidence of epilepsy in those defined as high risk, the low frequency of recurrences, and the rare incidence of death or sequelae.
2. Home treatment, which must include first aid to protect the airway and minimize self-injury. Fever control must be reviewed.
3. The risks and benefits of anticonvulsant therapy. It may reduce recurrences, but it has adverse effects.
4. The parent should call the physician after the initial evaluation if the following occur:
   a. Fever continues more than 36 hours; behavioral changes develop; severe vomiting, headache, nonblanching

rash, or stiff neck develops; or another seizure occurs.

b. The child is taking medication and becomes lethargic, hyperactive, or irritable or has a rash from phenobarbital. Sedation early in the course of treatment is common.

REFERENCES

American Academy of Pediatrics: Practice parameters: the neurodiagnostic evaluation of the child with a first simple febrile seizure, *Pediatrics* 97:169, 1996.

Anderson AB, Desisto MJ, Marshall PC, et al: Duration of fever prior to onset of a simple febrile seizure: a predictor of significant illness and neurologic course, *Pediatr Emerg Care* 5:12, 1989.

Berg AT, Shinnar S, Darefsy AS, et al: Predictors of recurrent febrile seizures, *Arch Pediatr Adolesc Med* 151:371, 1997.

Berg AT, Shinnar S, Hauser WA: A prospective study of recurrent febrile seizures, *N Engl J Med* 327:1122, 1992.

Bettis DB, Ater SB: Febrile seizures: emergency department diagnosis and treatment, *J Emerg Med* 2:341, 1985.

82 ORTHOPEDIC DISORDERS

SEPTIC ARTHRITIS

ALERT: Immediate drainage and antibiotics are indicated if the joint is to be salvaged.

Septic arthritis is an infection of the synovial membrane and joint space, resulting from either hematogenous spread or direct inoculation.

Predisposing factors include systemic bacterial infections, gonorrhea, and impaired immunologic status.

ETIOLOGY: INFECTION

1. *Staphylococcus aureus*: represents 20% to 30% of isolates and is often preceded by trauma
2. *Haemophilus influenzae*
   a. Most common in children less than 5 years of age but found in older children
   b. Often associated with infections elsewhere (meningitis)
3. Streptococci: group A, B, anaerobic, *Streptococcus viridans*
4. *Streptococcus pneumoniae*
5. *Neisseria gonorrhoeae*: primarily knee, wrist, and hand
6. Uncommon
   a. Gram-negative enteric: neonates and immunosuppressed
   b. *Pseudomonas* organisms: neonates, immunosuppressed; those with puncture wounds

DIAGNOSTIC FINDINGS

1. Patients inconsistently have systemic illness with fever, anorexia, and listlessness.
2. Local findings include pain and tenosynovitis, particularly with gonorrhea. The joints are tender, with warmth, swelling, effusion, and limitation of movement (see Chapter 40). It is primarily a monoarticular disease, involving the large, weight-bearing joints of the knee, hip, shoulder, wrist, and elbow. The patient may have concurrent osteomyelitis.
3. In one series of *H. influenzae* septic arthritis, 35% had associated otitis media and 30% had meningitis.

Complications

These involve damage to growth plate and joint cartilage, leading to poor growth and a stiff or destroyed joint.

Ancillary Data

1. White blood cells (WBC): variable; erythrocyte sedimentation rate (ESR): usually elevated and normalizes with recovery.
2. Blood cultures: positive in 50% of cases of nongonococcal disease and 20% of gonococcal infections.
3. Cultures of the cervix, rectum, and pharynx if gonorrhea is suspected: positive in 80% of patients with gonococcal disease.

4. Arthrocentesis and analysis of the synovial fluid, including glucose, cell count and differential, Gram stain, and culture (Table 82-1 and Appendix A-2). Negative cultures in gonococcal arthritis may occur.
5. X-ray films: plain films of joint.
   a. Early changes include joint fluid with capsular distension. If difficult to interpret, comparison views may help.
   b. Bony demineralization and subsequent cartilaginous and bony destruction may develop; however, radiographs may be normal and therefore are not adequately sensitive to be used as a screen.
6. Nuclear scan.
   a. Indicated when joint tap is contraindicated (overlying infection, small joints, axial skeleton involved).
   b. Technetium scan (^{99m}Tc): positive result within 24 hours of symptoms and may remain positive. Three-phase study may be helpful in differentiating from osteomyelitis (see p. 753).
   c. Gallium scan (^{67}Ga): result positive within 24 to 48 hours of symptoms but reverts to normal with adequate treatment.

DIFFERENTIAL DIAGNOSIS

There is significant overlap in ESR, temperature, and WBC in children with septic arthritis and transient synovitis of the hip.

See Chapter 27.

MANAGEMENT

1. Initial management must exclude other conditions in the differential diagnosis. Delay in treatment of septic arthritis exposes the patient to permanent joint damage.
2. Once septic arthritis is considered, the joint should be aspirated and the fluid analyzed (see Table 82-1).
3. The joint should be immobilized and physical therapy initiated once recovery is partially achieved.

Antibiotics

Initial antibiotics are selected on the basis of the Gram stain of the fluid obtained from the arthrocentesis and on drug allergies. Once final cultures and sensitivity data are available, the antibiotics may be altered.

TABLE 82-1 Common Synovial Fluid Findings

Category	Etiology	Appearance	Leukocytes (cells/mm^3)	Percentage of neutrophils	Percentage of glucose $\left[\dfrac{\text{synovial}}{\text{blood}}\right]$	Mucin* clot
Normal		Clear	<100	25	>50	Good
Bacterial	Septic arthritis	Turbid, purulent	>50,000	>75	<50	Poor
Inflammatory	Juvenile rheumatoid arthritis Rheumatic fever Mycobacterial, viral, and fungal arthritis	Clear or turbid	500-75,000	50	>50	Poor
Traumatic		Clear or bloody	<5,000†	<50	>50	Good

*For mucin clot: add 4 ml of water to 1 ml of synovial fluid supernatant. Mix in 2 drops of 5% glacial acetic acid. If normal, a tight rope of mucin will form. If infection or inflammation is present, clot will flake and shred.
†May have red cells.

For known organisms

S. aureus	Nafcillin, 100-200 mg/kg/24 hr q4hr IV, or an equivalent semisynthetic penicillin
H. influenzae	Cefotaxime, 150 mg/kg/24 hr q6-8hr IV; or ceftriaxone, 75 mg/kg/24 hr q12hr IV; or ceftizoxime, 150 mg/kg/24 hr q8hr IV
S. pneumoniae	Penicillin G, 100,000 U/kg/24 hr q4hr IV
N. gonorrhoeae	Penicillin G, as above

For unknown organisms

All patients	Nafcillin
Neonates	Add gentamicin, 5.0-7.5 mg/kg/24 hr q8-12hr IV or IM
Infants (≤5 yr)	Add cefotaxime or ceftriaxone

1. Clinical trials have substantiated the value of third-generation cephalosporins in the treatment of joint infections.
2. Traditionally, parenteral antibiotics are continued for a minimum of 2 weeks (gonococci, streptococci, and *Haemophilus* organisms) to 3 weeks (staphylococci, gram-negative enterics, and *Pseudomonas* organisms). Some investigators have used oral medications after 1 week of parenteral drugs associated with resolution of signs and symptoms while carefully monitoring clinical response. Serum levels, which must have a bactericidal level of at least 1:8, may be monitored in patients who respond slowly or require antibiotics achieving moderate levels. May also be used to monitor compliance.

Joint Drainage

1. Needle aspiration of the joint is attempted initially to relieve pressure and decompress the joint, unless surgical drainage is more appropriate. This also allows specimens to be obtained for evaluation.
2. Surgical drainage is indicated in the following situations:
   a. The hip, elbow, ankle, or shoulder is involved.
   b. Thick, purulent material is obtained.
   c. Adhesions are present, or inadequate decompression is achieved after 2 to 3 days of repeated needle aspiration.
   d. Response to therapy is poor after 36 to 48 hours of antibiotics.
   e. Long delay in the initiation of treatment has occurred.

DISPOSITION

All patients require hospitalization. Immediate orthopedic consultation should be obtained. The outcome is better in patients who are hospitalized and treated within 5 days of onset of symptoms.

REFERENCES

Barton LL, Dunkle LM, Habib FH: Septic arthritis in children, *Am J Dis Child* 145:898, 1987.

Becarre MA, Champoux AN, Bocherst, et al: Septic arthritis versus transient synovirus of the hip: the value of screening laboratory tests, *Ann Emerg Med* 21:1418, 1992.

Goldenberg DL, Reed JJ: Bacterial arthritis, *N Engl J Med* 312:764, 1985.

Rothbart HA, Glode MP: *Haemophilus influenzae* type b septic arthritis in children: report of 23 cases, *Pediatrics* 75:254, 1985.

Volberg FM, Sumner TE, Abramson JS, et al: Unreliability of radiographic diagnosis of septic hip in children, *Pediatrics* 73:118, 1984.

OSTEOMYELITIS

ALERT: Acute onset of limp or local tenderness, warmth, or erythema requires a careful evaluation. A prolonged course of antibiotics is indicated.

Acute osteomyelitis is an infection of bone, occurring most commonly by hematogenous spread but also associated with direct inoculation, which is secondary to open fractures, penetrating wounds, or surgical procedures. The metaphysis of the long bones, particularly the femur and tibia, is most commonly involved.

Factors predisposing an individual to osteomyelitis include trauma, systemic bacterial disease, drug abuse, sickle cell disease, and impaired immunologic status.

ETIOLOGY: INFECTION

1. *S. aureus:* accounts for 60% to 90% of isolates
2. *H. influenzae:* most common in children less than 3 years
3. *Pseudomonas* organisms: common in drug abusers and with osteomyelitis caused by penetrating injury of the foot, usually through a rubber-soled shoe in older children
4. Other organisms associated with infection:
   a. Streptococcal species: group A and B (in neonates usually B)
   b. *Staphylococcus epidermidis*
   c. *Salmonella* organisms: usually in patients with sickle cell disease
   d. Gram-negative enterics: usually in newborns
   e. Mycobacteria
   f. Fungal: usually in immunocompromised patients

DIAGNOSTIC FINDINGS

1. The clinical findings are extremely variable and the physician should be suspicious of osteomyelitis. Most patients have a fever and occasionally report a predisposing factor. Systemic disease may be present.
2. Patients may have a limp (see Chapter 40) and limitation of movement or merely a history of favoring the extremity.
3. Locally, patients inconsistently have tenderness, warmth, erythema, and pain over the involved site.
4. Children less than 1 year of age have little systemic toxicity.

Complications

1. Septic arthritis (p. 751). More common in infants.
2. Growth disturbance of the limb if there is disruption of the epiphyseal growth plate.
3. Chronic osteomyelitis with persistent infection, often a result of inadequate treatment.

Ancillary Data

1. WBC: often elevated, although most patients have counts between 5000 and 15,000 cells/mm^3.
2. ESR and C-reactive protein (CRP): commonly elevated; provides a useful parameter to assess the adequacy of treatment because it normalizes with resolution of inflammation. The CRP normalizes earlier than the ESR and correlates with a good outcome.
3. Blood cultures: positive in more than 50% of patients.
4. X-ray film: plain film of extremity.
   a. Soft tissue findings develop 3 to 4 days after the onset of symptoms:
      (1) Swelling of deep soft tissues next to metaphysis with displacement of fat lines
      (2) Obliteration of lucent planes between muscles
      (3) Subcutaneous edema
   b. Bony changes are noted 7 to 10 days after symptomatic onset:
      (1) Periosteal elevation
      (2) Lytic lesions
      (3) Sclerosis with new bone formation
5. Nuclear bone scan: technetium (^{99m}Tc).
   a. Twenty-four-hour delayed films may increase specificity. Three phase scan may have (1) increased flow on radionuclide angiogram, (2) increased activity on blood pool images, and (3) focal increased bone activity on delayed images. Cellulitis will show increased blood pool activity but normal soft tissue activity on delayed images.
   b. Often becomes abnormal 1 to 2 days after onset of symptoms with increased uptake in area of inflammation.
   c. May be falsely negative in up to 25% of cases, particularly in newborns and children less than 1 year.
   d. Uptake locally increased in osteomyelitis, septic arthritis, cellulitis, trauma, and neoplastic disease.

6. Aspiration of involved bone (usually done by orthopedist): provides definitive identification and sensitivity of etiologic organism.
   • Gram stain of aspirate may provide initial etiologic information.
7. Serum bactericidal titers may be useful in monitoring therapeutic regimens. However, the high serum levels achieved with many oral antibiotics decrease the importance of this measure.

DIFFERENTIAL DIAGNOSIS

1. Infection
   a. Septic arthritis (p. 751)
   b. Cellulitis (p. 573)
2. Trauma
   a. Local soft tissue injury
   b. Fracture
3. Neoplasm: Ewing tumor

MANAGEMENT

1. The key to appropriate management is early identification of the patient with osteomyelitis.
2. Cultures should be obtained before initiating therapy.
3. Aspiration of the lesions by an orthopedist is indicated. If pus is obtained, many clinicians recommend drainage and curettage. Open drainage also is indicated if there is poor response in the first 36 to 48 hours after initiation of therapy.
4. Immobilization of the involved extremity may minimize pain in the initial treatment stages during evaluation and stabilization.

Antibiotics

1. Give nafcillin (or other semisynthetic penicillin: methicillin or oxacillin), 100-200 mg/kg/24 hr q4hr IV (assuming no allergy). Alternative regimens include cefazolin or cephalothin, 100 mg/kg/24 hr q4-6hr IV.

2. Administer additional antibiotics if an organism other than *S. aureus* is suspected.
   a. In a child less than 5 years consider adding cefuroxime, 150 mg/kg/24 hr q6-8hr IV, to cover for *H. influenzae.*
   b. If the patient has sickle cell disease or is a neonate, a *Salmonella* organism or gram-negative enteric may be etiologic.
      • Give ampicillin, 200 mg/kg/24 hr q4hr IV, **and** gentamicin, 5.0-7.5 mg/kg/24 hr q8-12hr IV or IM. Prolonged therapy is indicated.
   c. With a puncture wound of the foot through a rubber-soled shoe or if the patient is a drug abuser and routine management is not adequate, a *Pseudomonas* organism should be considered and treated with the following:
      (1) Surgical drainage, as needed
      (2) Carbenicillin, 400-600 mg/kg/24 hr q4hr IV, and gentamicin, as above; or ceftazidime (Fortaz), 100-150 mg/kg/24 hr q8hr IV
3. In the routine care of osteomyelitis caused by *S. aureus*, patients are normally treated parenterally for 5 to 7 days, assuming decreased local inflammation and normalization of the ESR.
4. After the initial parenteral course and resolution of signs and symptoms, patients may be switched to oral therapy for 3 to 6 weeks. Studies suggest that with a good therapeutic response, the total treatment period may be reduced to as short as 3 weeks. Studies are under way to determine whether the shorter period leads to higher rates of recurrence.
   a. Dicloxacillin, 75-100 mg/kg/24 hr q6hr PO
   b. If the patient is allergic to penicillin: cephalexin, 50-100 mg/kg/24 hr q6hr PO, **or** clindamycin, 15-25 mg/kg/24 hr q6hr PO
5. Antibiotics may be modified by the results of Gram stain, culture, and sensitivity data.

6. During the phase of oral therapy, patients are often hospitalized to ensure continuing compliance.
7. Throughout the treatment course, serum bactericidal levels or serum antibiotic levels, if monitored, should achieve a bactericidal titer of 1:8 or greater.

DISPOSITION

1. Hospitalize all patients for therapy.
2. Obtain an orthopedic consultation. Infectious disease consultants also may be useful in the evaluation and long-term management of the patient, particularly if an unusual organism is suspected or identified.

REFERENCES

Chisholm CD, Schlesser JF: Plantar puncture wounds: controversies and treatment recommendations, *Ann Emerg Med* 18:1352, 1989.

Faden H, Grossi M: Acute osteomyelitis in children, *Am J Dis Child* 145:65, 1991.

Jacobs NM: Pneumococcal osteomyelitis and arthritis in children, *Am J Dis Child* 145:70, 1991.

Mustafa MM, Saez-Llorens X, McCracken GH, et al: Acute hematogenous pelvic osteomyelitis in infant and children, *Pediatr Infect Dis J* 9:416, 1990.

Peltola H, Unkila-Kallio L, Kallio MLT, et al: Simplified treatment of acute staphylococcal osteomyelitis of childhood, *Pediatrics* 99:846, 1997.

Unkila-Kallio L: Serum C-reactive protein, erythrocyte sedimentation rate, and white blood cell count in acute hematogenous osteomyelitis of children, *Pediatrics* 93:59, 1994.

83 PSYCHIATRIC DISORDERS

MANAGEMENT PRINCIPLES

The psychiatric examination of children and their families requires, above all else, sensitivity and a belief in one's own intuition. Data in the psychiatric evaluation may be "hard"—for example, an admission by the patient that he or she is suicidal or homicidal—but they may also be "soft." At times the only clue to an adolescent's violent inclination may be an uneasiness or anxiety on the part of the evaluator. Such feelings in the examiner, termed *countertransference,* can be used with great acumen to diagnose a variety of psychiatric ailments. If used appropriately, such data complement the more objective data obtained in a history.

The evaluator also must be willing to ask probing and difficult questions. Objectivity in the history taking will maximize the chances of the patient responding honestly and candidly. The examiner who is in a hurry or does not want to hear about certain aspects of the patient's behavior subtly encourages patients not to discuss their depression, suicidal ideation, or sexual perversions, for example. The examiner who is calm and maintains an empathic stance with patients will be amazed at how many describe really pressing psychiatric problems. The humbling statistic that nearly 50% of all patients who commit suicide have seen a physician sometime in the previous months speaks to the patient's wish to talk about problems and to get help, and, sadly, to the physician's frequent lack of responsiveness.

The approach to the preadolescent patient is usually different from that toward the adolescent. Initially, it is often appropriate to see the child's parents first and to gather as much history from them as possible. Then the child can be seen, usually alone, unless he or she is too stressed at being separated from the parents. The evaluator should first ask about the child's understanding of the evaluation. Clarifying that no shots will be given and that confidentiality will be maintained (unless information about the child being in danger emerges) can help loosen up a child. Even a 3-year-old child can communicate. Toys and drawings (which may reveal unconscious problems) should be saved for last. Particular attention should be paid to how the child relates to the examiner (oblivious? clinging?), to the youngster's activity level, and to how he or she relates to the parents. The question "How do you get along with friends?" posed to parents and child is the best single screening question for major psychopathology. If the child is isolated or has major interactive problems, a significant psychopathologic condition can be expected. If not, the child usually is in reasonable shape.

In contrast the adolescent should always be seen first and alone. The typical adolescent bristles at the idea that the evaluator is the parents' agent and thus must understand that the examiner is there to help him or her. This can be achieved through honesty and *objectivity* (regardless of personal morals and values). Teenagers can usually see through any falseness in the evaluator, who should try to leave his or her own adolescence in the waiting room and avoid the use of adolescent language that is not natural and who should not encumber the patient with personal feelings about such issues as marijuana, sex, and high school. Particular attention should be paid to such concerns as emancipation from family,* peer pressure, and heterosexual and homosexual exposure. These are the issues that dominate adolescent development and that lie at the root of an adolescent's psychiatric problems.

CONVERSION REACTIONS

Classic conversion reactions are rare, but conversion components of true physical illness may exist and conversion reactions may occur concomitantly with other serious psychopathologic conditions. The *initial* approach to a patient with a possible conversion disorder should be *both* medical and psychiatric. Conversion reaction is not a diagnosis of exclusion. Conversely, even when no physical cause is found to explain the loss of functioning, medical care should not be dropped because a large percentage of cases are subsequently found to have an etiologic organic pathologic condition.

DIAGNOSTIC FINDINGS

1. Loss of physical functioning, suggesting a physical disorder.
2. Psychologic factors as part of the symptoms.
    NOTE: Many investigators think it is possible to have simultaneous true organic abnormality and a conversion component.
3. Symptoms that are *not* conscious or voluntary. The loss of functioning is usually in the voluntary nervous system, rarely autonomic.

4. Symptoms that defy anatomic explanation usually have some symbolic significance that may reduce anxiety; they may become manifest at time of stress.
5. Associated findings.
    a. "La belle indifference" is probably of no value in verifying the diagnosis.
    b. Some symbolism may be involved in the development of the symptom (e.g., paralyzed arm prevents patient from hitting wife). The patient may try to emulate a relative's symptoms.
    c. A history of developing somatic symptoms is often present.
    d. Previous central nervous system (CNS) abnormality or trauma increases the risk for conversion disorder.
    e. Secondary gain is often present (i.e., the sick role is gratifying to the patient).

DIFFERENTIAL DIAGNOSIS

Conversion reactions should be differentiated from true organic pathologic conditions. Psychiatric disorders that must be excluded include the following:

1. Hypochondriasis: an unrealistic interpretation of normal body signs
2. Malingering: a conscious attempt to get attention through *voluntarily* feigned symptoms
3. Munchausen syndrome: an unconscious attempt to gain attention through voluntarily feigned symptoms
4. Depression: may occur with somatic symptoms without other signs of depression

MANAGEMENT

1. Conversion symptoms are often transient and disappear on their own. They may require hospitalization until they partially resolve.
2. Psychotherapy is indicated in refractory cases.
3. The patient may retrench and worsen if an attempt is made (especially ini-

---

*For the adolescent runaway, two resources may be useful: Runaway Hotline (800-231-6946) and National Runaway Switchboard (800-621-4000).

tially) to prove that the symptoms are emotional.

4. Any other underlying psychopathologic condition (e.g., schizophrenia) should be treated.

5. The prognosis is good, especially with acute onset, short duration of symptom(s), adequate premorbid personality, and minimal secondary gain from symptom. It is crucial to focus on the reduction of stress.

ACUTE PSYCHOSES

These patients require immediate attention to their level of self-destructiveness and potential for violence. If any doubt exists, the patient should be legally and physically restrained (e.g., with hospital guards) until these questions can be answered. Although psychiatrists disagree about subtypes of psychoses in childhood, several categories have merged as distinct diagnostic entities, which should be familiar to anyone involved in caring for pediatric emergencies. A child with an acute psychosis often seems "off" or detached. Accurate diagnosis and disposition are paramount because such children, when they arrive at an emergency setting, often have come from isolated, suspicious families that rarely frequent hospitals.

INFANTILE AUTISM
Etiology

1. Unproven former theories of "refrigerator parents" and abnormal rearing are being discarded in favor of a more dynamic cause involving organic factors (in the child) triggering aberrant parenting.

2. The illness is probably evenly distributed socioeconomically.

Diagnostic Findings

1. Age of onset is usually less than 30 months.
2. Highly unusual responses to environment (need for sameness, stereotypes), with poor social relations.

3. Gross deficits in language development. Abnormal speech patterns (echolalia, pronoun reversals).

4. Absence of delusions or hallucinations.

5. Commonly associated findings:
   a. Congenital blindness
   b. Retardation (70% have an IQ <70)
   c. Grand mal seizures before adolescence

6. Pockets of normal or even precocious development (e.g., unusual memory or ability to calculate quickly).

7. Abnormal auditory-evoked responses.

Differential Diagnosis

1. Mental retardation. Usually with uniform lags in development in all spheres (e.g., motor, social, language). Mentally retarded children ordinarily demonstrate some social relatedness.

2. Diffuse CNS disease (cytomegalovirus, phenylketonuria, hepatic encephalopathy).

3. Deafness. Audiogram will help differentiate.

Management

1. Multifaceted management (behavioral, structured educational program, psychotherapy) is indicated. Hospitalization should always be considered.

2. Neuroleptics may help symptoms of agitation, anxiety, and destructiveness (e.g., thioridazine [Mellaril] starting dosage: 0.5-1 mg/kg/24 hr q8-12hr PO [adult: 25 mg q8-12hr PO]). Titrate response.

The prognosis is very guarded and is best for children with a high IQ and good language development.

SCHIZOPHRENIA
Etiology

There are multiple causative theories, ranging from abnormal family patterns to a faulty neurotransmitter mechanism (dopamine hypothesis). Schizophrenia has a strong familial predilection.

Diagnostic Findings

1. Usual onset in late adolescence but may occur in earlier childhood
2. Lengthy prodrome of at least 6 months, during which patients exhibit gradual withdrawal from previous relationships and functioning
3. Delusions
4. Hallucinations (usually auditory)
5. Abnormal content of speech (loosening of associations)
6. Altered affect, which often is *inappropriate* to the content of speech (e.g., laughing while describing the death of a relative) but not predominantly euphoric or depressed
7. Associated findings
   a. Catatonia with either excitement or motoric rigidity.
   b. Excitation can be life threatening. Poor impulse control or paranoia can make these patients very dangerous.

Differential Diagnosis

1. Other nonorganic psychoses (manic-depression, which shows predominant mood problem).
2. Organic psychoses. Patient usually shows faulty cognition, which can be demonstrated with tests of memory (remembering three unrelated objects at 3 minutes) and orientation (to person, place, and time; disorientation to time is the first of these to be affected). Causes are multiple but, in the pediatric population, most commonly are ingestions (e.g., hallucinogens).
3. Reactive psychoses (also called schizophreniform psychoses). More acute and short-lived.
4. Acute grief reaction.

Management

The patient should be hospitalized for self-protection.

Neuroleptics

Neuroleptics usually should be administered after 1 to 2 days of hospitalization to see how well the patient will respond to a safe environment, unless the patient is agitated, combative, or in need of seclusion.

- Thiothixene (Navane), 10-30 mg/24 hr PO, or thioridazine (Mellaril), 200-800 mg/24 hr PO, reflecting the patient's age, size, and response to therapy

Side effects are important and must be considered (p. 387):

1. Acute dystonias, especially with high-potency neuroleptics (e.g., haloperidol [Haldol]). Treat with an anticholinergic agent (e.g., benztropine [Cogentin], 1 to 2 mg PO or IM q12hr).
2. Parkinsonian side effects. Treat with an anticholinergic agent (Cogentin as in 1).
3. Akathisias (motor restlessness). Difficult to treat and often requires adjusting dosage of neuroleptic.
4. Anticholinergic signs and symptoms, especially with low-potency neuroleptics (e.g., chlorpromazine, thioridazine [Mellaril]).
5. Tardive dyskinesias. Incidence increases with duration of treatment. May be "unmasked" when dosage of neuroleptic is lowered. No effective treatment at this time.
6. Rash, cholestatic jaundice.

Other Considerations

1. Electroconvulsive therapy only if all else fails or if patient is in acute danger (e.g., agitated catatonia or acutely suicidal)
2. Family and individual psychotherapy
3. Discharge planning and follow-up: crucial in preventing relapse
4. Prognosis: guarded

ORGANIC PSYCHOSES
Diagnostic Findings

1. Evidence for an organic cause: ingestion (hallucinogens, cocaine, amphetamines, over-the-counter anticholinergics); systemic illness; endocrine disorder (adrenal, thyroid); renal, cardiac, or liver failure; sensory deprivation (intensive care unit [ICU] "psychosis")
2. Cognitive impairment (memory and disorientation)
3. Predominantly visual hallucinations (if any) versus auditory hallucinations in schizophrenia

Management

1. Treatment of underlying disorder
2. Occasionally, seclusion, restraint, or neuroleptics (neuroleptics have sedative and anticholinergic properties and may be contraindicated)

MANIC-DEPRESSIVE PSYCHOSIS
Diagnostic Findings

Manic-depressive psychosis is rare in childhood and principally involves the following:
1. Increased motor activity
2. Flight of ideas
3. Euphoric or dysphoric mood change
4. Associated findings: spending binges, decreased need for sleep, grandiosity, delusions, hallucinations, increased sexual activity

Differential Diagnosis

Adolescents who have taken stimulants or phencyclidine (PCP) or who have sustained brain damage may have some of these findings.

Management

Patients should be hospitalized and given some combination of neuroleptic and lithium treatment.

DEPRESSION
Diagnostic Findings

Children may demonstrate signs and symptoms of depression, requiring recognition and intervention. Typically, patients have a variable appetite and some weight loss because of poor intake, whereas others gain weight as a result of increased appetite. Insomnia or hypersomnia is common, with a loss of interest and pleasure in usual activities. Depressed individuals have thoughts of worthlessness and self-reproach and suicidal ideation.

Management

Of primary importance is recognizing the depressed state of the patient and making referral for both short-term evaluation and long-term therapy. The urgency of such counseling must reflect the severity of the depression and ensure that there is no immediate danger to the patient from self-injury.

PSYCHOPHYSIOLOGIC PRESENTATIONS

A psychophysiologic illness has three components. The patient must (1) have an underlying biologic or genetic disposition to get a disease, (2) have a characteristic personality style, and (3) be in a stressful situation. Peptic ulcer disease and thyrotoxicosis are examples of such illnesses. Various illnesses are considered psychosomatic in that psychologic factors are seen as contributing to the actual disease process, but personality profiles and biologic markers and processes have yet to be delineated. The symptoms often are used to avoid undesirable activities, such as school phobias. The following are perhaps the most common presentations:
1. Rumination: An infant regurgitates and may have low weight, and symptoms worsen during separation from the mother.
2. Cyclic vomiting: In response to a subtle stress, a child vomits for several days and then is well for days to weeks.

3. Abdominal pain: This may result from a variety of physical conditions but also may be caused by a psychophysiologic illness (peptic ulcer, ulcerative colitis) or, possibly, anorexia nervosa. When no cause is found, abdominal pain may be a conversion symptom.

4. Headache: This very common symptom is usually transient in anxiety states but may be disabling when it is secondary to repressed anger, sexual wishes, etc.

5. Anorexia nervosa: Nonorganic extreme weight loss in the preadolescent or adolescent female; initially associated with voluntary dieting and a preoccupation with food. The patient has amenorrhea, withdrawal, depression, and an intense interest in physical activity that may lead to bradycardia and hypotension.

Differential considerations include hypopituitarism, ovarian dysfunction, malabsorption, or malignancy.

Behavioral modification with positive reinforcement is the basis for management to create a weight gain. The patient must be allowed to gain autonomy, effectiveness, and self-esteem, often requiring hospitalization for both psychiatric and medical therapy initially.

School phobia or school refusal may be manifested by one or more of the preceding problems. It is most common with the initial entrance into school, with change of school, or at the beginning of the school year. Anxiety and separation anxiety may be present. After excluding organic disease, it is best treated with insistence that the child attend school, providing reassurance and encouraging peer relationships.

Suicide Attempts

The incidence of suicide and suicide attempts in childhood is increasing. Any seemingly innocent ingestion or accident should raise the question of a suicide attempt. Furthermore, any child who appears depressed should be asked about suicidal ideation because suicide occurs most often in depressed individuals. Studies of suicidal individuals reveal that the risk of attempting or reattempting suicide is usually limited to a short crisis period. Therefore safeguarding the patient with hospitalization or well-established supports is paramount in suicide management.

DIAGNOSTIC FINDINGS

Evaluation of the patient who has attempted or is threatening suicide should include the following:

1. Try to discover the precipitant. Usually a loss or reminder of a loss (anniversary reaction) is causative, but simply an argument with parents can trigger an attempt.

2. Assess risk factors.
   a. Girls attempt suicide more often than boys, but boys are more successful.
   b. A chronic illness in the patient increases the risk.
   c. A family history of suicide is often found.
   d. A personal history of previous suicide attempt is an ominous sign.
   e. An intoxicated patient is at greater risk. Substance abuse is a risk factor.
   f. Depression in the patient increases the risk.
   g. Estrangement from a loved one is also a risk factor.
   h. A personality with any of the following characteristics increases risk: hopeless, hostile, impulsive, perfectionism, poor social skills.

3. Carefully evaluate the present illness and suicidal behavior.
   a. How *lethal* was the method of suicide (gun or hanging versus ingestion of a few Valium)? Always ask about suicidal intent and plan.
   b. Was suicide attempted in complete isolation, or had the patient considered that he or she might be found before dying?

c. Does any suicide note or afterthought explain a motivation?

d. Is the patient depressed or schizophrenic or taking drugs?

e. Would he or she try again if discharged?

Common pitfalls in evaluation include the following:

1. No one asks the patient about suicidal ideation or plan. Plan: Ask the patient directly.

2. On recovering from an overdose, the patient disappears. Plan: Always have patients guarded or in a locked unit until their freedom would not jeopardize them.

3. The physician or staff treats the patient roughly or unempathically. Plan: Treat suicidal behavior medically, *not* judgmentally.

MANAGEMENT

1. Treat the medical or surgical sequelae of the suicide attempt.

2. Protect the patient with hospitalization or sheltered environment if necessary.

3. Always include a psychiatrist in management. Ideally, this is done at the initial encounter to maximize insight into the precipitating event and to initiate discussion.

4. Try to shore up family and other sources of emotional support.

5. Remove all sources of potential self-injury if the patient is to return home.

6. Treat the underlying psychiatric illness:

a. Depression—antidepressants, psychotherapy. Warning: Remember that the lethal-dose ratio of tricyclic antidepressants is very low; dispense with caution.

b. Schizophrenia—neuroleptics and hospitalization are usually needed.

c. Intoxication or ingestion—do serial suicide evaluations and mental status examinations until return to baseline. Reevaluation is done when the patient is sober.

7. At discharge, carefully evaluate your alliance with the patient (i.e., will he or she call you prn and before the next attempt?).

POSTTRAUMATIC STRESS DISORDER

Anxiety may be associated with a known external traumatic event. The significance of the event relates to the degree of exposure, appraisal of threat, and the personal impact. The two most likely stressors are a serious threat to the child's, family member's, or close friend's life and witnessing injury or death as a result of an accident or physical violence. Stressors resulting in posttraumatic stress disorder in children may include the following:

• Kidnapping and hostage situation
• Exposure to violence, including terrorism, gang violence, sniper attacks and war atrocities
• Sexual or physical abuse
• Severe accidental injury, including burns and hit-and-run accidents
• Life-threatening illnesses and life-endangering medical procedures
• Train, airplane, ship and auto accidents
• Major disasters

DIAGNOSTIC FINDINGS

Clinically, children actually respond to stress in a fashion parallel to that of adults. Several behavioral patterns may be noted in the months after a specific event. The phenomenon is often reexperienced through dreams, repetitive plan, or distress at traumatic reminders. Children may try to regulate their emotions or behavior by avoiding specific thoughts, feelings, or situations associated with the trauma. Interest in usual activities may be reduced. Isolation and memory disturbances are common. Patients may exhibit an increased state of arousal with sleep disturbances, irritability, and hypervigilance.

MANAGEMENT

The presence of this problem must first be recognized and the child supported and counseled. This is essential for all those involved in the initial stabilization and long-term management of the child. The focus must be on assisting in the recognition of traumatic reminders that elicit anxiety as well as helping children to anticipate and understand the nature of the initial event. Family functioning strongly influences the child's reaction and recovery. The goals must be to restore a sense of personal security, validate and explain responses, and anticipate reminders. The school can also play a useful role.

SUBSTANCE ABUSE

Substance abuse is a major problem in the adolescent population. It is a significant risk factor in suicide and other psychiatric disorders. Substance abuse may result from, exacerbate, or uncover an associated psychiatric disorder. It should be considered in any patient who has psychiatric complaints or symptoms and may require toxicologic screens as outlined in Chapter 54.

REFERENCES

American Psychiatric Association: *Diagnostic and statistical manual of the mental disorders,* Washington, DC, 1987, American Psychiatric Association.

Aylward GP: Understanding and treatment of childhood depression, *J Pediatr* 107:1, 1985.

Barnett TM: Psychiatric and behavioral disorders. In Barkin RM, editor: *Pediatric emergency medicine: concepts and clinical practice,* ed 2, St Louis, 1997, Mosby.

Frame DS, Kercher EE: Acute psychosis: Functional versus organic, *Emerg Med Clin North Am* 9:123, 1991.

Garfinkel BD, Carlson GA, Weller ED, editors: *Psychiatric disorders in children and adolescents,* Philadelphia, 1990, WB Saunders.

Jari S, White M, Rosenberg LA, et al: Munchausen syndrome by proxy, *Int Psych Med* 22:343, 1992.

Maisami M, Freeman JM: Conversion reactions in children as body language: a combined child psychiatry/neurology team approach to the management of functional neurologic disorders in children, *Pediatrics* 80:46, 1987.

Pynoos RS: Post-traumatic stress disorder in children and adolescents. In Garfunkul BD, Carlson GA, Waller, editors: *Psychiatric disorders in children and adolescents,* Philadelphia, 1990, WB Saunders.

Schecker N: Childhood conversion reactions in the emergency department: general and specific features, *Pediatr Emerg Care* 6:46, 1990.

Terr LC: Childhood traumas: an outline and overview, *Am J Psychiatry* 148:10, 1991.

84 Pulmonary Disorders

ASTHMA

ALERT: All wheezing is not caused by asthma. The patient with asthma in severe respiratory distress may not wheeze. Oximetry and assessment of ventilation are essential for all patients. All patients with distress, tachypnea, or hypoxemia should receive oxygen.

Bronchoconstriction results from intrinsic mechanisms related to autonomic dysfunction or extrinsic sensitizing agents. A number of factors precipitate airway reactivity leading to hypoxia (Fig. 84-1).

An increase in intracellular cyclic adenosine 3'-5' monophosphate (AMP) resulting from the promotion of its biosynthesis (β-adrenergic agents) or inhibition of its degradation (theophylline) produces bronchodilation. Activation of the beta-adrenergic receptors on airway smooth muscle leads to the activation of adenylate cyclase and to an increase in the intracellular concentration of cyclic AMP. This increase leads to the activation of protein kinase A, which inhibits the phosphorylation of myosin and lowers intracellular ionic calcium concentrations, resulting in relaxation of the smooth muscle of the airways.

An increase in cyclic guanosine monophosphate (GMP), produced by parasympathetic stimulation from cholinergic receptors, causes bronchoconstriction. Parasympathetic agents such as atropine antagonize action of acetyl choline, inhibiting the release of cyclic GMP. The decrease in vagal tone and relaxation promotes bronchodilation.

ETIOLOGY: PRECIPITATING/AGGRAVATING FACTORS

1. Infection: associated with viral origin in 19% to 42% of cases
2. Allergic/irritant
   a. Environmental: pollen, mold, animal dander
   b. Occupational chemicals/allergens: chlorine, ammonia
   c. Irritants: smoke, pollutants, gases, aerosols
   d. A family history of asthma or parental smoking contributes to airway responsiveness at an early age.
   e. Environmental changes: moving to new home, vacation, etc.
   f. Food and additives
3. Exercise
4. Intrapsychic: emotional stress, phobias
5. Intoxication: bronchoconstrictors (propranolol, beta blockers, aspirin, nonsteroidal antiinflammatory drugs)

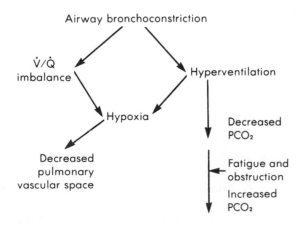

Fig. 84-1 Physiologic effect of bronchoconstriction.

DIAGNOSTIC FINDINGS

In managing the patient after initial stabilization of airway and breathing, it is essential to focus on the acute episode, as well as previous experiences and management of reactive airway disease. Medications (type, dose, and time of last dose), duration of acute symptoms, associated illness, history of aspiration, and exposure must be determined. In addition to specific issues related to pulmonary disease, it is important to estimate fluid intake and determine the pattern of response to previous episodes and medication.

History

1. Symptoms: cough, wheezing, chest tightness, sputum production, associated rhinitis, sinusitis, nasal polyposis, and atopic dermatitis. Pattern of symptoms in terms of seasonality, episodic versus continuous, onset, duration, frequency, and progression.
2. Precipitating and aggravating factors.
3. Pattern of disease related to age of onset and diagnosis, progression, previous evaluation, response to treatment, and ongoing management and evaluation. Prior hospitalizations and ventilatory support should be assessed.
4. Profile of typical exacerbation including prodromal signs and symptoms, temporal progression, management, and outcome.
5. Family history of allergy and asthma.
6. Medical history of patient focusing on other allergic manifestations, gastrointestinal disturbances, reactions to foods and drugs, croup, reflux, passive exposure to smoking, pneumonia, and early injury to lungs or airway associated with bronchopulmonary dysplasia (BPD), intubation, or congenital abnormalities.
7. Impact of disease on patient and family.
8. Living environment focusing on type of home and heating/cooling, humidifier, carpeting, pets, and exposure to smoke.

9. Assessment of family's and patient's perception of illness

Physical Examination

1. Labored respirations with retractions, nasal flaring, tachypnea, and tachycardia are present. Pulsus paradoxus may be present and, when combined with the degree of retractions, correlates with forced expiratory volume at 1 second (FEV_1). These are good indications of the severity of airway obstruction.
   a. Diffuse inspiratory and expiratory wheezing is noted with a prolonged expiratory phase. The patient with respiratory distress and without wheezing may not be moving enough air to generate air movement and may have a silent chest. This patient has severe disease.
   b. Rales and rhonchi may be present.
   c. Pulsus paradoxus may accompany severe asthma, pericardial tamponade, and pneumothorax. Its presence is determined by having the patient breathe quietly while the physician lowers the blood pressure cuff toward the systolic level. The pressure when the first sound is heard is noted. The pressure is further dropped until sounds can be heard throughout the respiratory cycle. A difference of 10 mm Hg or greater indicates the presence of pulsus paradoxus.
2. Patients may have cyanosis (usually confirmed by oximetry or arterial blood gases [ABGs]), diminished blood pressure, and fever as late findings.
3. Diaphoresis, agitation, somnolence, or confusion may result from hypoxia, hypercapnia, exhaustion, or drug intoxication, and the patient requires emergent intervention because of impending respiratory failure.
4. Status asthmaticus is present when a

patient has moderate to severe obstruction and fails to respond significantly to β-agonist agents administered in the initial treatment regimen.

5. Chronic cough may occasionally be the only presentation for ongoing mild reactive airway disease. The chest may sound clear, but wheezing can be induced by having the patient exercise. The condition requires a therapeutic trial of oral or inhaled bronchodilators.

Complications

1. Pneumothorax or pneumomediastinum.
2. Pneumonia.
3. Respiratory failure with Pao_2 less than 50 mm Hg and $Paco_2$ greater than 50 mm Hg at room air, sea level. These parameters may be useful, as will the pattern of progression of disease. Patients often have significant retractions, decreased or absent breath sounds, impaired mental status and agitation, decreased response to pain, and labored speech.
4. Dehydration.
5. Inappropriate antidiuretic hormone (ADH) secretion.
6. Theophylline overdose (p. 392).
7. Death resulting from respiratory failure with cardiac decompensation or dysrhythmias.

Ancillary Data

1. Oxygen saturation has important prognostic and therapeutic usefulness; oximetry may be more predictive of the need for admission than pulmonary function tests (PFTs). Furthermore, clinical assessment of hypoxemia does not correlate well with oximetry. Patients with a low initial oxygen saturation, even if they respond to nebulized albuterol, have been shown to be at high risk and require aggressive management and admission.

An increase in saturation in response to nebulization therapy in the emergency department (ED) does not necessarily mean a good outcome and may be transient. Furthermore, many children actually have a decreased oxygen saturation after nebulization therapy because of increased ventilation-perfusion mismatch caused by diffuse mucous plugging.

2. ABG measurements are recommended in children with relatively severe disease and those who have clinically impaired ventilation. Oximetry should not be viewed as a substitute for ABGs in severely ill children because it does not assess ventilation.
3. PFTs are useful in monitoring asthmatic patients and provide important prognostic information for an acute episode.
   a. The peak expiratory flow (PEF) rate and the FEV_1 have been proven useful in helping to assess the degree of airflow obstruction and severity. The technique, however, is not sufficient to make a diagnosis or fully evaluate physiologic impairment because it is effort dependent and measures only large-airway function. Furthermore, each patient must establish a "personal best" when he or she is well, with which measurements may be compared to assess the deterioration during an acute illness or to monitor chronic management (Table 84-1). It is particularly useful in following patients over time as an outpatient by using a peak flow meter. A PEF level of 50% to 80% of personal best signals caution, whereas a PEF level less than 50% suggests a medical alert. A level in the lower part of the 50% to 80% range should warrant greater concern.
   b. PFTs can measure a patient's response; the lack of improvement may reflect variable effort or worsening clinical condition.

TABLE 84-1   Predicted Average Peak Expiratory Flow (liters/minute) for Normal Children and Adolescents (Males and Females)

Height (inches)	Peak expiratory flow (L/min)	Height (inches)	Peak expiratory flow (L/min)
43	147	56	320
44	160	57	334
45	173	58	347
46	187	59	360
47	200	60	373
48	214	61	387
49	227	62	400
50	240	63	413
51	254	64	427
52	267	65	440
53	280	66	454
54	293	67	467
55	307		

From National Asthma Education Program: Guidelines for the diagnosis and management of asthma, Besthesda Md, 1991, National Institutes of Health, US Department of Health and Human Services, Publication 91-3042/3042A.

    c. Evaluation of patients with nonspecific symptoms of cough or shortness of breath on exertion may require PFTs to assess the contribution of broncho-constriction associated with "cough-variant asthma."

4. A variety of parameters are useful in estimating the severity of an acute exacerbation (Table 84-2).

5. A chest roentgenogram classically demonstrates hyperinflation and, in rare cases, an infiltrate. Children with increasing respiratory distress or who fail to respond as expected to conventional therapy should be studied to exclude an associated process that requires specific therapy or to eliminate other causes of wheezing. Any patient with signs suggestive of an air leak or foreign body aspiration should undergo x-ray studies. These are rarely indicated in children who respond well to initial therapy.

    The distinction between infiltrate and atelectasis may be difficult to make, both showing opacification on the roentgenogram.

	Infiltrate	Atelectasis
Diaphragm	Normal	Elevated
Mediastinal shift	None	Toward lesion
Air bronchogram	Common	Variable

6. Serum theophylline level is crucial in managing patients with an acute episode who were previously taking "therapeutic" doses of theophylline. Therapeutic levels are in the range of 10-20 µg/ml. Rapid assays of serum theophylline levels facilitate this process.

7. Complete blood count (CBC) may be useful in children who have been febrile. Optimally, it should be obtained before administration of β-adrenergic agents.

8. Electrolytes should periodically be monitored in the severely ill patient who is hospitalized to exclude inappropriate ADH secretion. Hypokalemia has been associated with prolonged use of albuterol.

DIFFERENTIAL DIAGNOSIS (see Chapter 20)

The differential considerations in the child with wheezing vary with the age of the child. In the *infant*, bronchiolitis, asthma, foreign body aspiration, gastroesophageal reflux, cystic fibrosis, cardiac disease, congenital and structural abnormalities (e.g., tracheoesophageal fistula, vascular ring), and upper airway congestion or obstruction must be excluded. *Older children* may have asthma, foreign body aspiration, pneumonia, or mediastinal tumors/lymph nodes. Cystic fibrosis and other chronic lung diseases also should be considered past infancy. Other diagnostic entities include the following:

1. Infection/inflammation:
   a. Pneumonia (p. 794)
   b. Bronchiolitis (p. 781)
   c. Aspiration
2. Trauma (see Chapter 62):
   a. Pneumothorax (may be spontaneous)
   b. Foreign body (p. 791)
3. Vascular disorder:
   a. Compression of trachea by vascular anomaly
   b. Pulmonary edema (see Chapter 19)
   c. Pulmonary embolism (p. 568)
   d. Congestive heart failure (CHF) (see Chapter 16)
4. Vocal cord dysfunction may mimic asthma. It is due to an adduction of the true and false vocal cords throughout the respiratory cycle and is often a response to stress or anxiety paralleling a conversion reaction.
5. Congenital disease:
   a. Cystic fibrosis
   b. Tracheoesophageal fistula or tracheal anomaly
6. Hyperventilation.
7. Intoxication: metabolic acidosis (may cause tachypnea) (p. 359), toxic inhalation.
8. Neoplasm: mediastinal or pulmonary.

MANAGEMENT (Fig. 84-2)

The patient is often the best indicator of both the severity of the attack and the most effective therapeutic regimen. If the history or physical examination suggests that asthma is not the most likely cause, an appropriate work-up (e.g., inspiratory and forced expiratory film, cardiac examination, fluoroscopy, bronchoscopy) should be initiated after stabilization of the patient's respiratory status. Emergency department and hospital management are outlined in Fig. 84-2.

1. When appropriate, stabilize airway, ventilation, and blood pressure, and correct acid-base abnormalities.
2. Administer humidified oxygen by nasal cannula or face mask at 3-6 L/min (30% to 40%) to all patients with significant wheezing.
3. Cardiac monitoring is important when administering adrenergic agents and theophylline, particularly in patients with moderate or severe disease (status asthmaticus).
4. Initiate oximetry early, preferably obtaining the first reading before oxygen is initiated.
5. Patients with severe asthma who are in respiratory failure, patients with persistent hypoxemia and hypercarbia on maximal therapy, and patients fatiguing or failing to respond to aggressive bronchodilation may require intubation. Fortunately, this is a rarely needed intervention.

Adrenergic Agents

Initially, a rapid-acting β-agonist bronchodilator is administered by inhalation. The choice of agent should reflect the clinician's experience, the child's age and level of cooperation, and the child's experience with therapeutic alternatives. In general, during the initial stabilization, agents may be given every 20 minutes or, with severe disease, continuously. Nebulized agents may be continued on an ongoing basis, the frequency reflecting the duration of effect, the clinical response, and severity of illness.

Nebulized inhalation administration is generally more effective than parenteral therapy and is the ideal route for administration of β-agonist agents. Albuterol and terbutaline are relatively pure β$_2$ agents, producing relatively

Text continued on p. 774

TABLE 84-2 Estimating Severity of Asthma Exacerbations*

	Mild	Moderate	Severe	Respiratory arrest imminent
SYMPTOMS				
Breathless	While walking	While talking (infant—softer, shorter cry; difficulty feeding)	While at rest (infant—stops feeding)	
Talks in	Can lie down Sentences	Prefers sitting Phrases	Sits upright Words	
Alertness	May be agitated	Usually agitated	Usually agitated	Drowsy or confused
SIGNS				
Respiratory rate	Increased	Increased	Often >30/min	
Use of accessory muscles; suprasternal retractions	Usually not	Commonly	Usually	Paradoxical thoracoabdominal movement
Wheeze	Moderate, often only end expiratory	Loud; throughout exhalation	Usually loud; throughout inhalation and exhalation	Absence of wheeze
Pulse/min	<100	100-120	>120	Bradycardia

Guide to rates of breathing in awake children:

Age	Normal rate
<2 mo	<60/min
2-12 mo	<50/min
1-5 yr	<40/min
6-8 yr	<30/min

Guide to normal pulse rates in children:

Age	Normal rate
2-12 mo	<160/min
1-2 yr	<120/min
2-8 yr	<110/min

Pulsus paradoxus	Absent <10 mm Hg	May be present 10-25 mm Hg	Often present >25 mm Hg (adult); 20-40 mm Hg (child)	Absence suggests respiratory muscle fatigue

FUNCTIONAL ASSESSMENT

PEF (% predicted or % personal best)	80%	Approximately 50%-80%	<50% predicted or personal best or response lasts <2 hr	
Pao_2 (on air)	Normal (test not usually necessary)	>60 mm Hg (test not usually necessary)	<60 mm Hg: possible cyanosis	
and/or				
Pco_2	<42 mm Hg (test not usually necessary)	<42 mm Hg (test not usually necessary)	≥42 mm Hg; possible respiratory failure	
Sao_2% (on air) at sea level	>95% (test not usually necessary)	91%-95%	<91%	

Hypercapnia (hypoventilation) develops more readily in young children than in adults and adolescents.

From the National Asthma Education and Prevention Program: *Guidelines for the diagnosis and management of asthma*, Bethesda, Md, 1997, National Institutes of Health, National Heart, Lung and Blood Institute, NIH Publication 97-4051A.
*Notes: The presence of several parameters, but not necessarily all, indicates the general classification of the exacerbation. Many of these parameters have not been systematically studied, so they serve only as general guides.

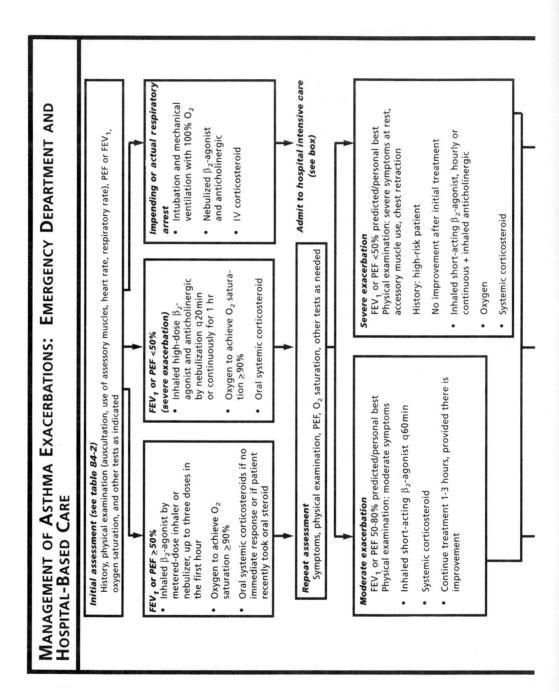

Management of Asthma Exacerbations: Emergency Department and Hospital-Based Care

Initial assessment (see table 84-2)
History, physical examination (auscultation, use of assessory muscles, heart rate, respiratory rate), PEF or FEV_1, oxygen saturation, and other tests as indicated

FEV_1 or PEF ≥50%
- Inhaled β_2-agonist by metered-dose inhaler or nebulizer, up to three doses in the first hour
- Oxygen to achieve O_2 saturation ≥90%
- Oral systemic corticosteroids if no immediate response or if patient recently took oral steroid

FEV_1 or PEF <50% (severe exacerbation)
- Inhaled high-dose β_2-agonist and anticholinergic by nebulization q20min or continuously for 1 hr
- Oxygen to achieve O_2 saturation ≥90%
- Oral systemic corticosteroid

Impending or actual respiratory arrest
- Intubation and mechanical ventilation with 100% O_2
- Nebulized β_2-agonist and anticholinergic
- IV corticosteroid

Repeat assessment
Symptoms, physical examination, PEF, O_2 saturation, other tests as needed

Moderate exacerbation
FEV_1 or PEF 50-80% predicted/personal best
Physical examination: moderate symptoms
- Inhaled short-acting β_2-agonist q60min
- Systemic corticosteroid
- Continue treatment 1-3 hours, provided there is improvement

Severe exacerbation
FEV_1 or PEF <50% predicted/personal best
Physical examination: severe symptoms at rest, accessory muscle use, chest retraction
History: high-risk patient
No improvement after initial treatment
- Inhaled short-acting β_2-agonist, hourly or continuous + inhaled anticholinergic
- Oxygen
- Systemic corticosteroid

Admit to hospital intensive care (see box)

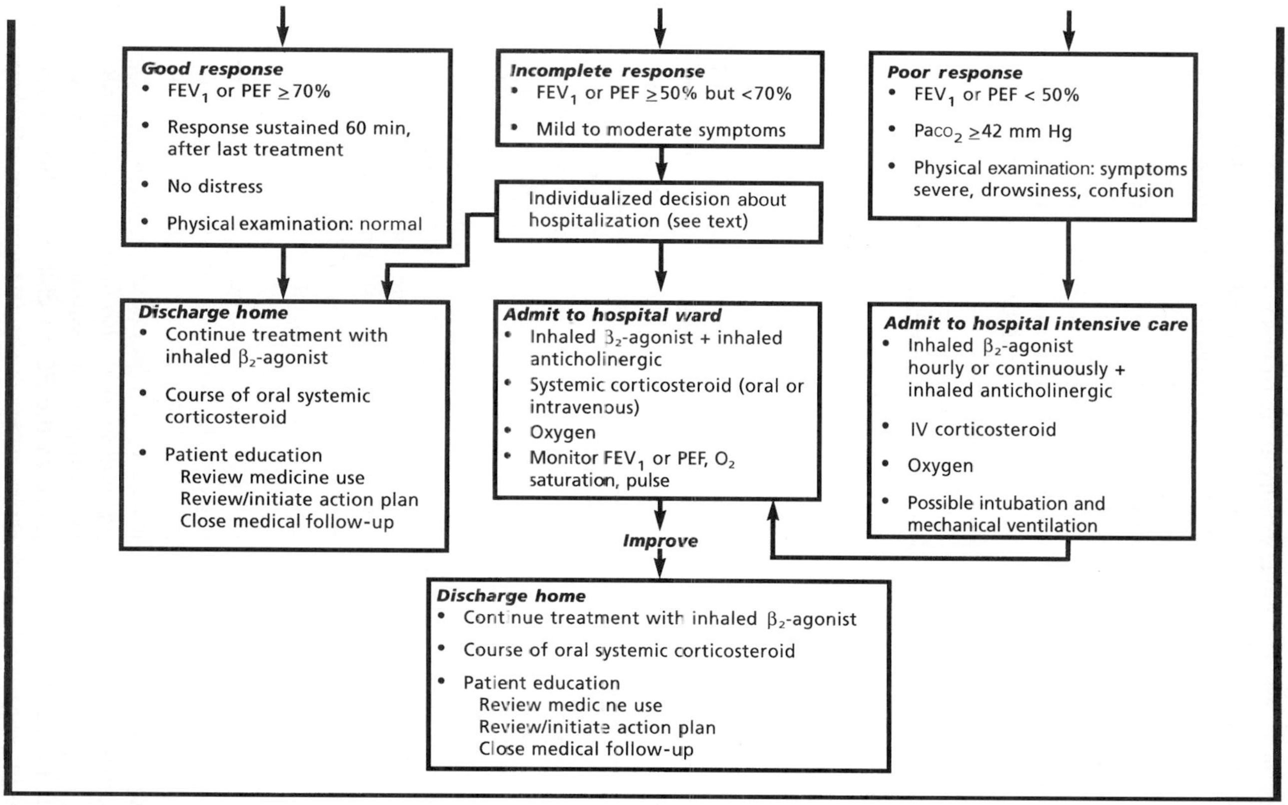
Good response
• FEV$_1$ or PEF ≥70%
• Response sustained 60 min, after last treatment
• No distress
• Physical examination: normal
Incomplete response
• FEV$_1$ or PEF ≥50% but <70%
• Mild to moderate symptoms
Individualized decision about hospitalization (see text)
Poor response
• FEV$_1$ or PEF < 50%
• Paco$_2$ ≥42 mm Hg
• Physical examination: symptoms severe, drowsiness, confusion
Discharge home
• Continue treatment with inhaled β$_2$-agonist
• Course of oral systemic corticosteroid
• Patient education
Review medicine use
Review/initiate action plan
Close medical follow-up
Admit to hospital ward
• Inhaled β$_2$-agonist + inhaled anticholinergic
• Systemic corticosteroid (oral or intravenous)
• Oxygen
• Monitor FEV$_1$ or PEF, O$_2$ saturation, pulse
Admit to hospital intensive care
• Inhaled β$_2$-agonist hourly or continuously + inhaled anticholinergic
• IV corticosteroid
• Oxygen
• Possible intubation and mechanical ventilation
Improve
Discharge home
• Continue treatment with inhaled β$_2$-agonist
• Course of oral systemic corticosteroid
• Patient education
Review medicine use
Review/initiate action plan
Close medical follow-up

Fig. 84-2 Management of asthma exacerbations: emergency department and hospital-based care.

(From National Asthma Education and Prevention Program: *Guidelines for the diagnosis and management of asthma*, Bethesda, Md, 1997, National Institute of Health, National Heart, Lung, and Blood Institute, NIH Publication 97-4051A.)

few cardiac side effects. The wide therapeutic indices of terbutaline and albuterol allow for safe administration of doses often exceeding traditional recommendations, with careful monitoring. During stabilization, most agents may be given two or three times as tolerated clinically to provide rapid bronchodilation. Often, a combination of a β agonist and ipratropium is most effective; in the severely ill child, the correct agents must be determined empirically or by prior experience in managing the specific child.

1. Albuterol (0.5% solution or 5 mg/ml) (Proventil, Ventolin): 0.03 ml (0.15 mg)/kg/dose up to a maximum of 1.0 ml (5.0 mg)/dose diluted in 2 ml of 0.9% NS administered q2-4hr by nebulization. Higher dosages up to 0.30 mg/kg have been shown to be safe and to result in greater pulmonary improvement. Treatments may be given more often as tolerated and clinically appropriate, especially in the early assessment and stabilization period. Continuous albuterol may be efficacious in the management of the seriously ill child. Peak of onset is 30 to 60 minutes, with a duration of 4 to 6 hours.

   Elevated CPK-MB enzyme levels have been noted with prolonged, continuous use, emphasizing the importance of ongoing cardiac monitoring.

2. Terbutaline (0.1% solution or 1 mg/ml for parenteral administration) (Brethine): 0.03 mg (0.03 ml)/kg/dose up to a maximum of 0.5 ml/dose in 2 ml 0.9% NS administered by nebulization q4hr or more often as tolerated, especially during early stabilization. Peak of onset is 30 minutes, with a duration of 3 to 4 hours. Use parenteral solution for nebulization.

Parenteral agents have limited usefulness because of the greater efficacy of inhaled agents, the associated side effects (headache and tachycardia), and the pain of injection. Parenteral administration may have a role in the uncooperative, severely ill patient or when inhalation therapy is logistically impractical (e.g., equipment, cooperation). Intravenous (IV) agents may ultimately have a role in the child who is in "extremis."

1. Epinephrine (Adrenalin) (1:1,000):0.01 (0.01 mg)/kg/dose to a maximum of 0.35 ml/dose given SC q20min up to a total of three administrations if tolerated and the heart rate less than 180/min. Peak onset is 15 to 30 minutes, with a duration up to 2 hours. Efficacy is less than inhaled agents. Significant α- and β-agonist side effects limit usefulness

   If this agent is used with a good response, some clinicians elect to administer SusPhrine (1:200), 0.005 ml/kg/dose (maximum: 0.15 ml/dose) SC, to achieve a longer duration of efficacy. The single vial ampule should be used to ensure consistency of dosage.

2. Terbutaline (0.1% solution) (Brethine): 0.01 ml/kg/dose to a maximum of 0.25 mg (0.25 ml)/dose SC q20min up to a total of three administrations if tolerated. Peak of onset is 30 minutes, and the duration is 3 to 4 hours. This is the best parenteral agent because of the reduced side effects, although the inhaled route is preferred. IV terbutaline may also be an effective alternative route once it is investigated.

3. Albuterol is available outside of the United States as an IV preparation with an initial loading dose of 1 µg/kg/min for 10 minutes followed by a continuous infusion of 0.2 µg/kg/min. The dose can be increased by 0.1 µg/kg q15min on the basis of the patient's response. The adult dose is 200 µg over 10 minutes IV followed by a continuous infusion of 3-12 µg/min. Studies also suggest that a single IV infusion of Salbumatol (15 µg/kg) given in the ED to children who do not respond to initial nebulization therapy may produce a rapid response. Similarly terbutaline is available elsewhere. Further data are required before these agents are readily accessible.

Status asthmaticus exists when the initial response to 2 to 3 doses of β-adrenergic agents is poor. Hypoxia, acidosis, and hypotension must be rapidly corrected and other causes of wheezing considered. The lack of improvement is often caused by airway obstruction from a prolonged inflammatory process, suggesting that steroid therapy may be useful in such patients.

Oral agents are useful in mild disease or as ongoing, chronic treatment. Albuterol (2 mg/5 ml) (Proventil) is an excellent option at a dosage of 0.1-0.15 mg/kg/dose q6-8hr PO up to a maximum of 4 mg/dose. It is also available in 2- and 4-mg tablets. Peak of onset is 1 to 2 hours, and duration is 4 to 6 hours.

Alternative agents include fenoterol (0.5% solution): less than 2 years, 0.1 ml/dose; 2 to 9 years, 0.2 ml/dose; greater than 9 years, 0.3 ml/dose. Procaterol, pirbuterol, and bitolterol have been studied, but there is only limited pediatric experience.

Metered-dose inhalers (MDIs) are available for many agents, including albuterol, terbutaline, steroids, and ipratropium. Such devices may routinely be used in children 6 years and older and with a spacer device in those older than 3 years. A spacer and mask device is available for children and has been found to be equally effective to the nebulizer when used appropriately, even in acutely ill children.

The optimal deposition of drug particles in the lower respiratory tract is achieved by using an oxygen/air flow of 6-7 L/min, diluted in a volume of 3.5 to 4.5 ml.

Anticholinergic Agents

1. Ipratropium (Atrovent): derivative of atropine with less cardiac effect; administered as an inhaled agent. Ipratropium (Atrovent) is available for nebulization in a 0.02% solution. The 500-µg unit dose is diluted in 2.2 ml for a total volume of 2.5 ml. Pediatric dosage is generally considered to be 250 µg/dose QID (one-half the adult dose). It is also available for MDI administration. The adult MDI dose is two inhalations (36 µg) QID. Safety and dosage studies in children show the agents to be beneficial in combination with a β agonist with less side effects than atropine. Peak of onset is 1 to 2 hours, and duration is 3 to 4 hours.

   NOTE: Ipratropium may not have an additive effect in patients with bronchiolitis.

2. Atropine: 0.02 mg/kg/dose up to a maximum of 2 mg/dose in 2 ml of 0.9% NS administered by nebulization q4-6hr or as tolerated.

Steroids

1. All patients with moderate or severe asthma (status asthmaticus) should receive a minimum of 3 to 4 days of steroid therapy. Administer methylprednisolone (SoluMedrol), 1-2 mg/kg/dose q6hr IV. This therapy shortens the length of hypoxia and hospitalization.

2. In children who are minimally to moderately ill and who have a good response to β-agonist agents, steroids may be initiated to facilitate recovery, often given orally or by MDI. Patients who respond only partially or who respond initially and then return for additional therapy may also benefit from steroids.

   In children with recurrent asthma, the severity of the attack may be reduced if steroids are administered in combination with albuterol at the first signs of upper respiratory tract infection and before any sign of wheezing. This is often initiated by parents who have been given specific guidelines. Begin prednisone or prednisolone, 1-2 mg/kg/24 hr q6-12hr PO, for 3 to 7 days. A liquid concentrated steroid preparation is prednisolone (Prelone), 15 mg/5 ml, although some prefer crushed prednisone tablets mixed with applesauce, yogurt, etc.

3. Patients who have taken steroids within 12 months (including those taking steroids administered by inhalation) or who

have a history of respiratory failure associated with asthma should have steroids initiated early for an acute exacerbation.

If more than four bursts have been given in 1 year, a brief course of glucocorticoids should be initiated for stress such as surgery.

4. Patients with severe asthma, particularly those with severe exacerbations, may benefit from long-term steroid therapy. Systemic steroids (prednisone, 1-2 mg/kg/24 hr q6-12hr PO) commonly are used initially for chronic therapy. Many patients requiring 20 mg or less of prednisone per day may be converted to inhalation administration with maintenance of good respiratory function and reduction of adverse reactions. Beclomethasone (Vanceril, Beclovent) is provided in an MDI delivering 42 µg/puff. Children 6 to 12 years receive 1 to 2 puffs q6-8hr (maximum: 10 puffs/24 hr), whereas older children and adults take 2 puffs q6-8hr (maximum: 20 puffs/24 hr).

Second-generation inhaled steroids (triamcinolone [Azmacort] and flunisolide [Aerobid]) have fairly short half–lives, whereas third-generation agents (fluticasone [Florent]) are usually effective in once-a-day or twice-a-day doses. The maintenance dose is 400 to 500 µg/day. A spacer or rinsing the mouth after inhalation reduces side effects such as oral thrush. The risk of systemic side effects with long-term use is undefined, including growth delay, cataracts, adrenal suppression, and immunosuppression.

Cromolyn

Cromolyn (Intal) bullets (each 20 mg): Adult dosage is 20 mg/dose; infant and neonatal dosage is 10 to 20 mg/dose. It may be given three to four times per day and has been used more commonly during acute management, although its efficacy in this role has not been documented. It is often used in conjunction with β-agonist agents, in those with exercise- or cold-induced problems and in conjunction with other elements of chronic therapy to reduce wheezing after an acute exacerbation.

Theophylline

Theophylline is rarely started after initial therapy with β-agonist agents and stabilization of the patient and then only after other approaches have been unsuccessful in achieving control. It has not been shown to benefit patients in hospital settings more than administering nebulized albuterol and steroids.

Parenteral, oral, and rectal preparations are available. All require appropriate loading before starting the patient on maintenance therapy.

If the patient is taking theophylline at the time of the encounter, it is imperative that the amount and time of the last dose and the duration of therapy be determined to decide whether a loading dose is necessary. A theophylline level is usually required in acutely ill patients.

1. If the patient is taking a subtherapeutic dose, half the loading dose may be given pending determination of the theophylline level.
2. Therapeutic theophylline is 10-20 µg/ml. 1 mg/kg of theophylline raises the theophylline concentration by about 2 µg/ml.
3. The dosage of theophylline must be adjusted to reflect changes in clearance. Alter the dosage as indicated for the following conditions:

Increase dose (clearance increased)	Decrease dose (clearance decreased)
Drugs: phenobarbital, phenytoin (Dilantin), rifampin, carbamazepine, marijuana	Illness: viral infections, fever, CHF, abnormal liver or renal function
Drugs: cimetidine, erythromycin, oral contraceptives	Other: infants <3 mo; pregnancy, especially third trimester
Diet: high protein, low carbohydrate, charcoal- broiled meat	
Smokers	
Other: hyperthyroidism, cystic fibrosis	

4. Dosage determination is made on the basis of lean body weight and must reflect serum theophylline levels. Aminophylline is about 85% theophylline.

5. The half-life of IV theophylline in children is approximately 2.5 hours; in adults it is 4.6 hours.

Parenteral Therapy

This is indicated for severe obstructive disease unresponsive to adrenergic agents. A loading dose is normally given over 20 minutes followed by an IV infusion of maintenance theophylline. The maintenance infusion may be mixed with aminophylline, 100 mg in 100 ml 0.9% NS (1 mg/ml of aminophylline or 0.85 mg/ml of theophylline).

The following doses of aminophylline (theophylline) are for patients not previously receiving theophylline products:

Age group	Loading dose* (mg/kg)	Maintenance dose* (mg/kg/hr)
1-6 mo	6-7 (5-6)	0.5 (0.4)†
6-12 mo	6-7 (5-6)	1.0 (0.85)†
1-9 yr	6-7 (5-6)	1.5 (1.2)
10-16 yr	6-7 (5-6)	1.2 (1.0)

*Aminophylline dose (theophylline dose).
†See more specific guidelines that follow.

In converting from maintenance IV infusion to sustained-release preparations, generally give the first dose of oral medication 1 to 2 hours before discontinuing the infusion. An approximation of the daily oral dose may be made by calculating the total infusion dose given over 24 hours.

Maintenance dosing of theophylline in infants *less than 1 year of age* requires careful monitoring of theophylline levels because of the variability in pharmacokinetics. Suggested guidelines are as follows:

1. Preterm infants up to 40 weeks postconception (postconception age = gestational age at birth + postnatal age): 1 mg/kg q12hr

2. Term infants either at birth or infants 40 weeks postconception:
   a. Up to 4 weeks postnatal: 1-2 mg/kg q12hr
   b. 4 to 8 weeks: 1-2 mg/kg q8hr
   c. Beyond 8 weeks: 1-3 mg/kg q6hr

Children less than 1 year of age and those with moderate to severe or recurrent disease should have levels measured within 6 to 12 hours of loading and then periodically. Tests done on fingerstick samples in 15 minutes make theophylline levels more readily available in the office or ED.

Oral Therapy

The oral approach may be used in children with chronic and recurrent disease on an ongoing basis. Routine use is unusual and should be viewed as an adjunct rather than primary treatment.

The loading dosage of theophylline is 6-7 mg/kg/dose as a single dose followed in 6 hours with a maintenance dosage of 4-5 mg/kg/dose q6hr PO. The dosage in children less than 1 year of age should be reduced. Short-acting formulations are particularly useful in children who only need sporadic theophylline for short periods because of brief flare-ups.

In the stable patient with a good response to initial β-adrenergic therapy, however, many clinicians prefer to begin sustained-release preparations after an initial loading with a short-acting theophylline. The daily dosage of sustained-release drugs should reflect the age of the child and measured theophylline levels. This approach may improve compliance.

Long-Term Oral Therapy

Long-term therapy with an oral theophylline preparation must reflect the therapeutic response and side effects. Other agents are generally considered to be the primary approach to management. Once a patient is stabilized after an acute episode, an oral dosage of 16 mg/kg/24 hr of theophylline is usually adequate but may be adjusted to the following daily *maximums:*

<1 yr:	maximum of 8 mg + 0.3 × age (wk)
1-9 yr:	maximum of 22-24 mg/kg/24 hr
9-12 yr:	maximum of 20 mg/kg/24 hr
12-16 yr:	maximum of 18 mg/kg/24 hr
>16 yr:	maximum of 12.5 mg/kg/24 hr (maximum: 600-800 mg/24 hr)

These dosages may be administered using short-term or long-term preparations. When approaching maximum recommended doses, levels must be measured.

The serum concentration should be maintained at 10-20 μg/ml and is the best measure of the appropriate dosage. On occasion, patients will do well with lower levels, whereas some require more than 20 μg/ml. Serious toxicity usually is not generally noted at less than a level of 30-40 μg/ml (p. 392).

Other Considerations: Theophylline

1. Combination drugs (often with ephedrine) have no advantage and are not recommended. Avoid preparations containing alcohol.

2. Solutions for rectal administration are available but may have a less consistent absorption pattern. Suppositories are very unreliable and are not recommended. Rectal solutions may be useful on a short-term basis for patients who are vomiting from an intercurrent illness if oral administration is precluded. Oral and rectal dosages are identical.

3. Theophylline toxicity results in tachycardia, dysrhythmias, irritability, and seizures, as well as nausea, vomiting, and abdominal pain (p. 392). Attention and achievement problems are usually associated with preexisting problems. It is imperative to ascertain that gastrointestinal symptoms are not evidence of toxicity.

Other Agents

1. $MgSO_4$ has been studied in the management of status asthmatic with some success. At a dosage of 25 mg/kg/dose over 20 minutes (adult: 2 gm/dose) in 100 ml of 0.9% NS, it has been found to be effective in patients older than 6 years of age who are unresponsive to adrenergic and anticholinergic agents.

2. Sedation has certainly been necessary as appropriate but only if ventilation is en-

sured. Ketamine is particularly useful because it is also a bronchodilator and has been administered in relatively low dosages (to reduce incidence of dysphonic reactions) with a loading dose of 0.1 mg/kg followed by an infusion of 0.5 mg/kg/hr.

3. Leukotriene-receptor antagonists have been noted to have a beneficial effect, serving as a complement to other agents for long-term management. Accolate (20-mg tablets) and zileuton [Zyflo] (20-mg tablets) are currently available for adult with extensive studies currently being undertaken in children. Montebukast (Sinqulair) has been approved for children 6 to 14 years of age in a dose of 5 mg/day taken in the evening.

DISPOSITION

1. Patients with moderate or severe asthma in status asthmaticus require immediate hospitalization and continuation of therapy initiated in the ED. Although parameters indicating admission are not well defined, risk factors include the following:

   a. Presence of symptoms for more than 24 hours.

   b. Marked retractions, hypoxia, or hypercapnia.

   c. Respiratory obstructions (PEF rate ≤10% of expected).

   d. Poor response to initial β-agonist agent (PEF rate ≤40% of expected). Failure to respond to initial ED management requires admission.

   e. History of hospitalization or respiratory failure.

   f. Multiple drug therapy; chronic or intermittent steroid use.

   g. Concurrent infection.

   h. Progressive fatigue.

   i. Multiple visits for episode.

2. A low oxygen saturation on admission to the ED (≤90% to 93% at sea level) has been

associated with a consistent need for hospitalization.

3. The patient who has mild disease and clears may be discharged with adequate oral therapy after appropriate loading before discharge. A more aggressive and perhaps more effective approach is to use home nebulizer machines in younger children and MDIs in older ones, with albuterol as the drug of choice. Steroids may be used in some children. Frequent telephone calls and visits are necessary.

4. Good follow-up (including monitoring of clinical response and frequency of exacerbations) is essential for all patients with asthma. Often psychiatric intervention is required because of the emotional component of asthma in many children.

Parental Education

1. Give all doses of medication.
2. Push clear liquids. Warm fluids are particularly helpful.
3. Try to keep your child calm.
4. Try to identify substances that precipitate attacks, and avoid them. Passive smoking may exacerbate wheezing.
5. Many patients develop reactive airway disease in response to an infection. Such children should take bronchodilator therapy (asthma medicine) at the first sign of a cough or respiratory infection if they do not take the medication every day.
   - Initiate inhalation treatments at the first sign of respiratory infection, with albuterol administered by nebulizer or MDI.
   - In children with recurrent problems, some clinicians may begin steroids at home.
6. Call your physician immediately if the following occur:
   a. Breathing difficulty recurs or worsens, color changes, restlessness develops, or fluid intake decreases, or if the child has difficulty speaking because of respiratory distress.
   b. Nausea, vomiting, or irritability develops because of the theophylline medicine or child is unable to take medication.
   c. Cough or wheezing persist or fever or chest pain develops.

REFERENCES

Abulhosn RS, Morray BH, Llewellyn C, et al: Passive smoke exposure impairs recovery after hospitalization, *Arch Pediatr Adolesc Med* 151:135, 1997.

Alario AJ, Lewander WJ, Dennhey P, et al: The relationship between oxygen saturation and clinical assessment of acutely wheezing infants and children, *Pediatr Emerg Care* 11:331, 1995.

Amirav I, Newhouse MT: Metered-dose inhaler accessory devices in acute asthma, *Arch Pediatr Adolesc Med* 151:876, 1997.

Barnett PU, Caputo GL, Baskin M, et al: Intravenous versus oral corticosteroids in the management of acute asthma in children, *Ann Emerg Med* 29:212, 1997.

Benton G, Thomas RC, Nickerson RG, et al: Experience with metered dose inhaler with a spacer in the pediatric emergency department, *Am J Dis Child* 143:678, 1989.

Browne GJ, Penna AS, Phung X, et al: Randomized trial of intravenous salbumatol in early management of acute severe asthma in children, *Lancet* 349:301, 1997.

Brunette MG, Lands L, Thibodeau LP: Childhood asthma: prevention of attacks with short-term corticosteroid treatment of upper respiratory tract infection, *Pediatrics* 81:624, 1988.

Chou KJ, Cunningham SJ, Cram EF: Metered dose inhaler with spacers versus nebulizers for pediatric asthma, *Arch Pediatr Adolesc Med* 149:201, 1991.

Christopher KO, Wood RP, Eckert RC, et al: Vocal-cord dysfunction presenting as asthma, *N Engl J Med* 308:1566, 1983.

Ciarallo L, Sauer AH, Shannon MJ: Intravenous magnesium therapy for moderate to severe pediatric asthma: results of a randomized placebo controlled study, *J Pediatr* 129:809, 1996.

Craig VC, Bigos D, Brill RJ: Efficacy and safety of continuous albuterol nebulization in children with severe status asthmaticus, *Pediatr Emerg Care* 12:1, 1996.

Cram EF, Weirs KB, Fagan MJ: Pediatric asthma care in US emergency departments, *Arch Pediatr Adolesc Med* 149:893, 1995.

DiGiulio GA, Kercsmar CM, Krug SE, et al: Hospital treatment of asthma: lack of benefit from theophylline given in addition to nebulized albuterol and intravenously administered corticosteroids, *J Pediatr* 122:464, 1993.

Emond SD, Camargo CA, Nowak RM: 1997 national asthma education and prevention guidelines: a practical summary for emergency physicians, *Ann Emerg Med* 31: 579, 1998.

Fugisang F, Pedersen S, Borgstrom L: Dose-response relationships of intravenously administered terbutaline in children with asthma, *J Pediatr* 114:315, 1989.

Geelhoed GC, Landau LI, LeSouef PN: Predictive value of oxygen saturation in emergency evaluation of asthmatic children, *BMJ* 297:395, 1988.

Geelhoed GC, Landau LI, LeSouef PN: Evaluation of Sao$_2$ as a predictor of outcome in 280 children presenting with acute asthma, *Ann Emerg Med* 23:1236, 1994.

Granit CC, Duggan AK, DeAngelis C: Independent parental administration of prednisone in acute asthma: a double blind placebo controlled crossover study, *Pediatrics* 96:224, 1995.

Hickey RW, Gochman RF, Chande V, et al: Albuterol delivered via metered-dose inhaler with spacer for outpatient treatment of young children with wheezing, *Arch Pediatr Adolesc Med* 148:189, 1994.

Howton JC, Rose J, Duffy S, et al: Randomized double blind placebo-controlled trial of intravenous ketamine in acute asthma, *Ann Emerg Med* 27:170, 1996.

Jagoda A, Shepherd SM, Spevitz A, et al: Refractory asthma: Part I: epidemiology, pathophysiology pharmacology and intervention. Part II: airway interventions and management, *Ann Emerg Med* 29:262, 275, 1997.

Jones LA, Gonzalez ER, Venitz J, et al: Evaluation of the theophylline assays in the emergency department setting, *Ann Emerg Med* 21:777, 1992.

Karem E, Levison H, Schuh S, et al: Efficacy of albuterol administered by nebulizer versus spacer device in children with acute asthma, *J Pediatr* 123:313, 1993.

Kudukis TM, Manthous CA, Schmidt GA, et al: Inhaled helium oxygen revisited: effect of inhaled helium oxygen during the treatment of status asthmaticus in children, *J Pediatr* 130:217, 1997.

Landwehr UP, Wood RP, Blager FB, et al: Vocal cord dysfunction mimicking exercise-induced bronchospasm in adolescents, *Pediatrics* 98:971, 1996.

Maneker AJ, Perack EM, Krug SE: Contribution of routine pulse oximetry to evaluation and management of patients with respiratory illness in a pediatric emergency department, *Ann Emerg Med* 25:36,1995.

Mower WR, Sachs C, Nicklin EL, et al: Pulse oximetry as a fifth pediatric vital sign, *Pediatrics* 99:681, 1997.

Pabon H, Monem G, al Kissoon N: Safety and efficacy of magnesium sulfate infusions in children with status asthmaticus, *Pediatr Emerg Care* 10:200, 1994.

Parks DP, Ahrens RC, Humphries T, et al: Chronic cough in childhood: approach to diagnosis and treatment, *J Pediatr* 115:S856, 1989.

Pearlman DS, Chervinsky P, LaForce C, et al: A comparison of salmeterol with albuterol in the treatment of mild-to-moderate asthma, *N Engl J Med* 327:1420, 1992.

Poirier MP, Pancioli AM, DiGuilio GA: Vocal cord dysfunction presenting as acute asthma in a pediatric patient, *Pediatr Emerg Care* 12:2 13, 1996.

Qureshi F, Zaritsky A, Lakkis H: Efficacy of nebulized ipratropium in severely asthmatic children, *Ann Emerg Med* 29:205, 1997.

Rappaport U, Coffman H, Guare R, et al: Effects of theophylline on behavior and learning in children with asthma, *Am J Dis Child* 143:368, 1989.

Rau II: Delivery of aerosolized drugs to neonatal and pediatric patients, *Respir Care* 36:514,1991.

Reijonen T, Korppi M, Kuikka U, et al: Antiinflammatory therapy reduces wheezing after bronchodilator, *Arch Pediatr Adolesc Med* 150:5 12, 1996.

Rosen LM, Yamamoto UG, Wiebe RS: Pulse oximetry to identify a high-risk group of children with wheezing, *Am J Emerg Med* 7:567,1989.

Schelleper A, Alcock D, Beaudry F, et al: Effect of therapeutic plasma concentration of theophylline on behavior, cognitive processing and affect in children with asthma, *J Pediatr* 118:449, 1991.

Schuh S, Parkin F, Rojan A, et al: High versus low dose frequently administered nebulized albuterol in children with severe acute asthma, *Pediatrics* 83:513, 1989.

Schuh S, Reider MJ, Canny G: Nebulized albuterol in acute childhood asthma: comparison of two doses, Pediatrics 86:509, 1990.

Schuh S, Johnson DW, Callahan S, et al: Efficacy of frequent nebulized ipratropium bromide added to frequent high-dose albuterol therapy in severe childhood asthma, *J Pediatr* 126:639,1995.

Wright AL, Holberg C, Martinez FD, et al: Relationship of parental smoking to wheezing and non-wheezing lower respiratory tract illnesses in infancy, *J Pediatr* 118:207, 1991.

Young S, LeSouef PN, Geelhoed GC, et al: The influence of family history of asthma and parental smoking on airway responsiveness in early infancy, *N Engl J Med* 324:1168, 1991.

Younger RE, Gerber PS, Herrod HG, et al: Intravenous methylprednisolone efficacy in status asthmaticus in childhood, *Pediatrics* 80:225, 1987.

BRONCHIOLITIS

ALERT: Patients with marked tachypnea, retractions, cyanosis, or decreased air exchange require immediate attention and hospitalization. Hydration status and oxygenation must be assessed.

Bronchiolitis is an acute lower respiratory infection producing inflammatory obstruction of the small airways and reactive airway disease. It commonly occurs in children less than 2 years of age, with the highest incidence in those less than 6 months. The relationship of bronchiolitis to asthma and later reactive airway disease is unclear at present. In contrast to asthma, which primarily has bronchoconstriction with secondary inflammation, bronchiolitis is primarily an inflammatory process with a bronchoconstrictive component that is variably present.

Children at greatest risk are preterm infants (<32 weeks' gestational age), those less than 6 months of age, and those with underlying cardiac, pulmonary, or immunologic problems. Older siblings or parental smoking increases the risk of bronchiolitis.

ETIOLOGY

Viral infection caused by respiratory syncytial virus (RSV) accounts for 90% of isolates. Parainfluenza, adenovirus, and influenza are less common.

DIAGNOSTIC FINDINGS

1. Most patients have a preceding respiratory tract infection followed by the onset of marked tachypnea (often >60/minutes) and diffuse wheezing.
   a. Most children appear well and are attentive, alert, and in no distress despite the tachypnea.
   b. Many have an accompanying otitis media, often bacterial, and viral pneumonia.

2. Patients with respiratory distress have marked retractions, nasal flaring, and cyanosis. With the progression of inflammation, air movement may decrease, with disappearance of audible wheezing. Vital signs may be altered.
3. Restless and apprehensive behavior may appear if hypoxia or fatigue is present.

Complications

1. Apnea is most commonly found in children less than 6 months of age who were born prematurely.
2. Dehydration may be exacerbated by the abnormal insensible losses from the rapid respiratory rate. Intake may be decreased because of the increased respiratory effort.
3. Bacterial pneumonia may result from secondary infection.
4. Pneumothorax may occur with severe obstructive disease.
5. Residual parenchymal and airway disease may result from any acute episode of bronchiolitis, causing long-term abnormalities in pulmonary function. The relationship to asthma and later pulmonary and allergic disorders is uncertain.
6. Atrial tachycardia.
7. Bronchiolitis fibrosa obliterans results from progressive fibrotic reaction, which obliterates the bronchioles.
8. Death in 1% to 2% of patients is secondary to respiratory failure.

Ancillary Data

1. ABG or oximetry is useful in assessing hypoxia and hypercapnia when the clinical examination is not conclusive. Continuous oximetry is often indicated, supplemented by an ABG if there is concern about ventilation or increasing fatigue.
2. Chest x-ray films demonstrate hyperinflation, often associated with a diffuse,

patchy infiltrate. These films are not required routinely. A pulmonary consolidation or atelectasis enhances a child's risk of requiring prolonged hospitalization.

3. Fluorescent antibody (FA) for RSV done on nasal washings is rapid and diagnostically important. A parallel test may be done for pertussis if that infection is a consideration.

DIFFERENTIAL DIAGNOSIS (see Chapter 20)

The most common considerations are asthma, pneumonia, and foreign bodies.

1. Asthma usually occurs in children older than 1 year of age (children with asthma generally experience more respiratory distress). Asthma is primarily caused by bronchoconstrictive disease, whereas bronchiolitis is primarily an inflammatory process.
2. Pneumonia may produce wheezing and asymmetric breath sounds. A chest x-ray film may be useful. Viral pneumonia often accompanies bronchiolitis.
3. Foreign bodies may be excluded by a negative history and normal inspiratory and expiratory films.
4. Other entities that should be excluded include CHF, cystic fibrosis, vascular ring, neoplasm, and toxic or smoke inhalation.

MANAGEMENT

1. The initial assessment should determine whether acute stabilization is required. Oxygen, airway intervention, and fluids may be initiated.
2. A trial of β agonists is worthwhile, particularly in the child with any degree of respiratory distress or tachypnea. Studies variably demonstrate clinical improvement after β agonists; mortality is not altered. One of a number of nebulized

agents may be used to determine efficacy in a specific child (p. 769):

a. Albuterol (0.5% solution) (Proventil, Ventolin): 0.03 ml (0.15 mg)/kg/dose diluted in 2 ml of 0.9% NS administered q2-4hr. Treatments may be given more often as tolerated and clinically appropriate, especially in the early assessment and stabilization. The concentration is 5 mg/ml.

b. Terbutaline (0.1% solution for parenteral administration) (Brethine): 0.03 mg (0.03 ml)/kg/dose 2 ml 0.9% NS administered q4hr or more often as tolerated, especially during early stabilization. Peak of onset is 30 minutes, and duration is 3 to 4 hours.

c. Oral albuterol (2 mg/5 ml) (Proventil) is another option in the mildly ill child at a dosage of 0.1-0.15 mg/kg/dose q6-8hr PO. Peak of onset is 1 to 2 hours, and duration is 4 to 6 hours.

d. The role of racemic epinephrine is under study and probably has a specific bronchodilator capacity.

e. Ipratropium (Atrovent) has no proven benefit.

3. The patient requires evaluation for signs of respiratory distress.

a. The patient who has a respiratory rate of more than 60/minutes or any evidence of hypoxia, hypercapnia, fatigue, or progression should be hospitalized for humidified oxygen therapy, fluids, and monitoring.

b. If respiratory failure is present or imminent (Pao_2 <50 mm Hg and $Paco_2$ >50 mm Hg), the patient should be in an intensive care unit (ICU) and active airway intervention initiated. Continuous positive airway pressure (CPAP) should be instituted if there is a rising respiratory rate or pulse, decreased responsiveness, decreasing Pao_2, or increasing Paco_2. Oxygen at 30% to 40% with 5 cm H_2O pressure may be used. Mechanical ventilation with intubation is necessary if CPAP fails or apneic spells are frequent.

4. Steroids have not been documented to be consistently beneficial in routine cases of bronchiolitis.

5. Aerosolized ribavirin may speed up improvement of illness in children with severe RSV lower respiratory tract disease, usually following documentation of the virus. Severe disease should be considered for such intervention if a prolonged (>3 days) hospitalization is anticipated or there is underlying cardiopulmonary abnormality. Special precautions are required for children who need mechanical ventilation.

6. Respiratory syncytial immunoglobulins (RSVIC or RespiGam) may reduce the risk of hospitalization when used prophylactically in high-risk children such as those with bronchopulmonary dysplasia or cardiopulmonary disease. It has been recommended in infants less than 2 years of age who have bronchopulmonary disease, infants who are receiving or have received oxygen within the last 6 months, infants less than 32 weeks' gestational age who are less than 6 months of age at the onset of RSV season, or those less than 27 weeks' gestational age who required ventilation, particularly when other risk factors are present. Risk factors may include multiple births, discharge from NICU during or right before RSV season, exposure to environmental pollutants, crowding, or sibling attending school. The dosage is 750 mg/kg/dose IV given monthly from October through May during the RSV season. A humanized monoclonal antibody against RSV is being studied and may offer greater flexibility.

DISPOSITION

The most serious risk factors are apnea, hypoxia on admission, radiopaque consolidation, atelectasis, congenital heart disease, prematurity, and immune suppression.

1. Patients should be hospitalized if there is any evidence of apnea, lethargy, or dehydration or if they have unreliable caretakers, live a long distance from a health care facility, or are premature.

   Factors associated with more severe illness include the following:
   a. "Ill" or "toxic" appearance
   b. Oxygen saturation less than 95% at sea level (the single best objective predictor)
   c. Gestational age less than 34 weeks
   d. Respiratory rate greater than 70 breaths/min
   e. Atelectasis indicated on chest x-ray study
   f. Less than 3 months old

2. Patients without respiratory distress, abnormal oximetry, or other modifying factors may be discharged with close follow-up observation.

Parental Education

1. Give all prescribed medications.
2. Push clear liquids. Do not worry about solids.
3. Humidified air may decrease congestion.
4. Call your physician if the following occur:
   a. Breathing effort/retractions increase.
   b. Cyanosis or apnea are noted.
   c. Fluid intake decreases.
   d. The child develops an increasing fever, toxicity, or fatigue.

REFERENCES

Andrade MA, Hoberman A, Glustein J, et al: Acute otitis media in children with bronchiolitis, *Pediatrics* 101: 617, 1998.

Donnerstein RL, Berg RA, Shebab Z, et al: Complex atrial tachycardia and respiratory syncytial virus infections in infants, *J Pediatr* 125:23, 1994.

Flores G, Horwitz RI: Efficacy of β₂-agonists in bronchiolitis: a reappraisal and meta-analysis, *Pediatrics* 100:233, 1997.

Gadomski AM, Lichenstein R, Horton L, et al: Efficacy of albuterol in the management of bronchiolitis, *Pediatrics* 93:907, 1994.

Hall CB, McBride JT: Vapors, viruses, and views: ribavirin and respiratory syncytial virus, *Am J Dis Child* 140:331, 1986.

Kellner JD, Ohlsson A, Gadomsici AM, et al: Efficacy of bronchodilator therapy in bronchiolitis: a metaanalysis, *Arch Pediatr Adolesc Med* 150:1166, 1996.

Klassen TP, Rowe PC, Sutcliffe T, et al: Randomized trial of salbutamol in acute bronchiolitis, *J Pediatr* 118:807, 1991.

Krilov LR, Lipson SM, Barone SR, et al: Evaluation of a rapid diagnostic test for respiratory syncytial virus (RSV): potential for bedside diagnosis, *Pediatrics* 3:903, 1994.

Leclair JM, Freeman J, Sullivan BF, et al: Prevention of nosocomial respiratory syncytial virus infections through compliance with glove and gown isolation precautions, *N Engl J Med* 317:329, 1987.

Navas L, Wang E, Carvalho VD, et al: Improved outcome of respiratory syncytial virus infection in a high-risk hospitalized population of Canadian children, *J Pediatr* 121:348, 1992.

Rodriquez WJ, Gruber WC, Welliver RC, et al: Respiratory syncytial virus (RSV) immune globulin intravenous therapy for RSV lower respiratory tract infection in infants and young children at high risk for severe RSV infections, *Pediatrics* 99:454, 1997.

Roosevelt G, Sheehan K, Grupp-Phelan J, et al: Dexamethasone in bronchiolitis: a randomised controlled trial, *Lancet* 348:292, 1996.

Sanchez I, DeKoster J, Powell RE, et al: Effect of racemic epinephrine and salbutamol on clinical score and pulmonary mechanics in infants with bronchiolitis, *J Pediatr* 122:145, 1993.

Schuh S, Canny G, Reisman JJ, et al: Nebulized albuterol in acute bronchiolitis, *J Pediatr* 117:633, 1990.

Schuh S, Johnson D, Callahan S, et al: Efficacy of frequent nebulized ipratropium bromide added to frequent high-dose albuterol in severe childhood asthma, *J Pediatr* 126:639, 1995.

Schweich PJ, Hurt TL, Walkley EI, et al: The use of nebulized albuterol in wheezing infants, *Pediatr Emerg Care* 8:184, 1992.

Wang EEL, Law BJ, Stephens D, et al: Pediatric investigator's collaborative network on infections in Canada: prospective study of risk factors and outcome in patients hospitalized with respiratory syncytial viral lower respiratory tract infection, *J Pediatr* 126:212, 1995.

CROUP AND EPIGLOTTITIS

ALERT: Ensure adequate airway. Differentiate croup from epiglottitis.

Epiglottitis requires that the patient be intubated. Always consider tracheitis, foreign body, and allergic croup in the differential diagnosis. A clinician skilled in airway management must accompany the patient until diagnosis and stabilization are complete.

Infections of the supraglottic area result in swelling of the laryngeal and epiglottic structures and may additionally involve the trachea as in croup (laryngotracheobronchitis).

ETIOLOGY

1. Infection:
   a. Croup is viral, and the agents include parainfluenza, RSV, and influenza.
   b. Epiglottitis is caused by *Haemophilus influenzae;* in rare cases, other bacteria may be causative. The incidence has decreased with the widespread use of *H. influenzae* vaccine. The condition is becoming increasingly prevalent in adults.
2. Allergy. Allergic croup is a rapid supraglottic swelling resulting from exposure to a precipitating or sensitizing agent.

DIAGNOSTIC FINDINGS (Table 84-3)

1. Respiratory failure may occur with both croup and epiglottitis; may have accompanying pulmonary edema.
2. Spasmodic or allergic croup has a rapid onset of croup syndrome after exposure to a precipitating factor and without a preceding viral respiratory infection as in infectious croup.
3. Other conditions resulting in upper airway obstruction and dyspnea must be considered in the history and physical examination.

TABLE 84-3   Comparison of Croup and Epiglottitis

	Croup	Epiglottitis
Age	6 mo-3 yr	Any age (peak: 2-5 yr)
Seasonal occurrence	Fall/winter	Any
Worst time of day	Night/early AM	Throughout day
Etiology	Viral	*H. influenzae*
Clinical signs/symptoms		
Onset	Insidious	Rapid
Preceding URI	Yes	Rare
Fever	<39.5° C	High
Toxic	No	Yes
Sore throat	Variable	Yes
Voice	Hoarse	Muffled
Drooling	None	Yes
Dysphagia	None	Yes
Cough	"Barking seal"	None
Preferred position	Variable	Prefers sitting
Stridor	Inspiratory/expiratory	Inspiratory
Epiglottis	WNL	"Cherry red"
Ancillary data		
WBC	WNL	High
Blood culture	Negative	Positive
ABG	Variable	Variable
X-ray, lateral neck (Fig. 84-4)	WNL	Enlarged epiglottis

4. Extraepiglottic foci commonly are associated with epiglottitis. Pneumonia, lymphadenitis, and otitis media are most common. Pulmonary edema occurs, not uncommonly, after relief of the obstruction.

DIFFERENTIAL DIAGNOSIS (see Chapter 20)

Stridor indicates that some degree of upper airway obstruction exists. Inspiratory stridor usually indicates a supraglottic lesion, whereas expiratory stridor usually emanates from a lower airway involvement. Common entities to consider include the following:

1. *Supraglottic* (extrathoracic)
   a. Viral infection.
   b. Bacterial infection: group A streptococcus, *Staphylococcus aureus*, anaerobes of the mouth *(Peptococcus,* *Bacteroides), Corynebacterium diphtheriae.* Retropharyngeal abscess (p. 608) and peritonsillar abscess (p. 603) must be considered.
   c. Epiglottitis: *H. influenzae.*
   d. Noninfectious: foreign body, trauma, caustic ingestion, neoplasm, angioneurotic edema.
   e. **Uvulitis** may be caused by a number of entities including *H. influenzae* and group A streptococcus. It may result from allergic exposures, angioneurotic edema, and caustic ingestions. Fever, dysphagia, and drooling are common.
2. *Infraglottic* or subglottic (laryngitis, laryngotracheitis, laryngotracheobronchitis)
   a. Viral: parainfluenza, influenza A and B, measles, adenovirus, RSV.
   b. *Mycoplasma pneumoniae.*

c. Of bacterial infections, which are usually secondary, the most important entity is **bacterial tracheitis.** This is secondary to superinfection of damaged trachea from an antecedent viral infection. It is commonly caused by *S. aureus, S. pneumoniae,* or *H. influenzae,* with accumulation of pus in the trachea causing a thick plug and ultimately leading to obstruction. It often is associated with pneumonia and appears clinically as a crouplike syndrome with toxicity and rapid progression. Active airway intervention often is required, combined with aggressive pulmonary drainage and toilet and appropriate antibiotics for potential pathogens.

MANAGEMENT (see Fig. 84-3)

1. The patient with upper airway obstruction from croup or epiglottitis requires urgent attention to do the following:
   a. Ensure adequate airway
   b. Differentiate croup from epiglottitis
   c. Provide ongoing management and airway stabilization
2. Respiratory failure caused by upper airway obstruction may occur. Airway intervention is indicated if hypoxia (Pao_2 <50 mm Hg with supplemental O_2) or hypercapnia ($Paco_2$ >50 mm Hg) is present, if the patient demonstrates evidence of fatigue, or if there is progressive anxiety or severe obstruction. Patients with epiglottitis (see following discussion) usually require intubation on a prophylactic basis. All patients requiring intubation should have the procedure performed with extreme care and maximal support, commonly under controlled conditions in the operating room with equipment and personnel mobilized (see Fig. 84-3). Often a smaller tube size is used to minimize the risk of subglottic stenosis. The tube should be well immobilized. There may be some consideration of bacterial tracheitis in children with severe disease before direct visualization and diagnosis, particularly in those with croup who require intubation.

3. After evaluation for respiratory failure, the epiglottis should be visualized to determine its configuration, size, and color. The epiglottis in the child is somewhat easier to see because it is at the level of C2-C3 rather than at the C5-C6 level as found in adults.
   a. If evidence of obstruction exists or if the clinical signs and symptoms are consistent with epiglottitis, visualization is optimally done in the operating room with clinicians experienced in surgical airway management (anesthesiologist, otolaryngologist, and surgeon) present. Patients should be preoxygenated and initially allowed to sit in their most comfortable position. Children are usually more comfortable sitting; a supine position may lead to acute obstruction. Minimize agitation. At the time of visualization, the patient care team must be prepared to intubate the child if obstruction occurs or epiglottitis is diagnosed (see Fig. 84-3).
   b. Some clinicians prefer to use a lateral neck x-ray film before visualization because of the potential risk of exacerbating the disease if the posterior pharynx is further inflamed. This technique may be useful if the child is not in severe respiratory distress and no evidence of obstruction exists, but direct controlled visualization is usually more desirable. *A clinician capable of intubating the patient must accompany the patient at all times.* Portable films should be considered. Classic findings of croup on lateral radiograph include ballooning of the hypopharynx with narrowing of the cervical trachea on inspiration and

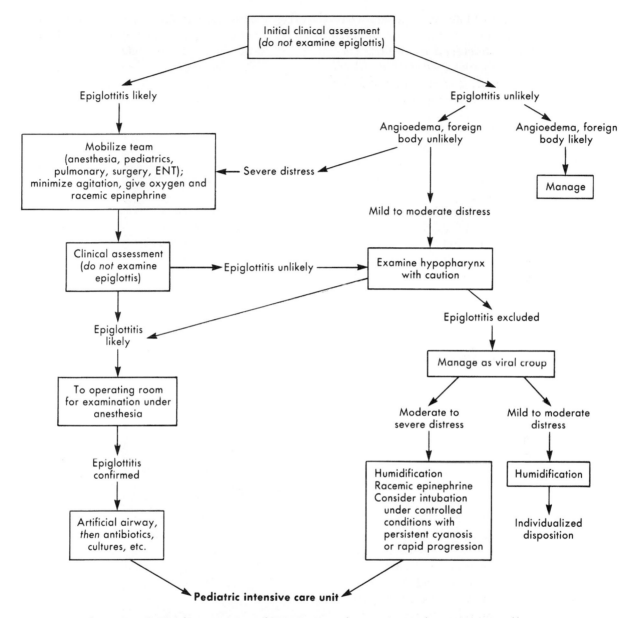

Fig. 84-3 Optimal assessment and management of upper airway obstruction caused by epiglottis or severe croup. Care must be individualized to reflect resources and logistic issues within a given institution.

ballooning of the cervical trachea on expiration (Fig. 84-4). The ratio of the aryepiglottic width to the body of the third cervical vertebrae is a useful parameter. When this ratio is 0.35 or more, it is 100% specific and 90% sensitive for epiglottis. Lateral neck radiographs in patients with epiglottitis may not be diagnostic in many patients. The rate of false-negative

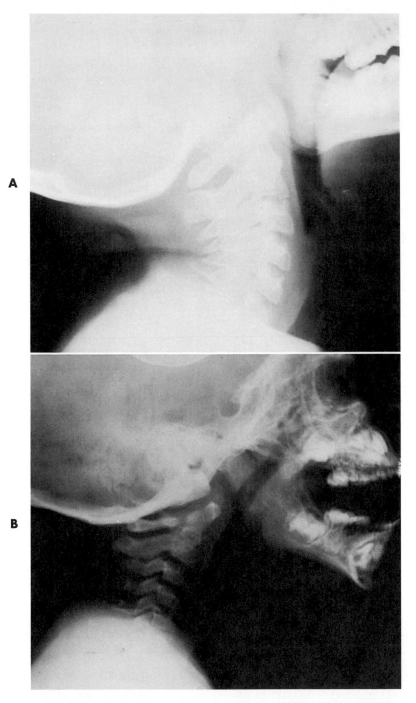

Fig. 84-4 Soft tissue lateral neck films. **A,** Normal. **B,** Markedly swollen epiglottis. Patients with epiglottitis have narrow valleculae and thick mass of tissue ("thumb" sign) extending from the valleculae to the arytenoids.

(Courtesy of S.Z. Barkin, Denver, Colo.)

results must be considered in approaching the evaluation of such patients radiographically.

Epiglottitis (see Fig. 84-3)

Immediate intervention is required. Initially, 100% oxygen should be given. The patient who is already obstructed may be ventilated by bag-mask positive pressure with a 100% oxygen bag. The patient should be intubated with an endotracheal or nasotracheal tube one to two sizes smaller than would normally be indicated. Topical 4% cocaine or topical epinephrine may be useful as may atropine (0.01-0.02 mg/kg IV), the latter decreasing the vagal response. After intubation, most patients are allowed to breath spontaneously with 4 to 6 mm Hg of CPAP and 40% Fio_2 (humidified). The CPAP helps stabilize the lungs after relief of the obstruction.

1. If time and clinical status permit, the optimal place to perform intubation (and visualize the epiglottis) is in the operating room with appropriate relaxation and with the assistance of an anesthesiologist and others experienced in airway management.

2. An otolaryngologist or surgeon should be available to assist if a surgical airway is required.

3. If personnel resources are limited, intubation, if necessary, can usually be achieved by a clinician skilled in pediatric airway management. The older child often can be intubated in the position of greatest comfort (usually sitting up and leaning forward). This means that in this circumstance clinicians have been successful in blindly intubating the child with the intubator behind the child (usually on stretcher with child). To be successful, this approach usually requires that the child (>6 years) be able to tolerate a 6-mm tube.

4. After intubation, patients are monitored in an intensive care unit. Blood cultures and other studies may be done and anti-biotics initiated. Patients usually remain intubated for 36 ± 14 (1 SD) hour.

5. Children should be reevaluated after 24 hours and then every 12 hours thereafter. The clinical course may be used to determine the timing of elective extubation and may include the following:
   a. Mild to moderate respiratory distress followed by improvement in edema and erythema of the epiglottis
   b. Moderate to severe respiratory distress followed by improvement in edema and erythema on two successive laryngoscopies
   c. Very severe respiratory distress followed by near-normal epiglottis and aryepiglottic folds

Intravenous Line

After airway stabilization, an IV line should be started if it has not already been initiated. Fluid status should be assessed and maintenance and deficit therapy (if any) initiated.

Antibiotics

Antibiotics should be given parenterally for at least 5 days (at which time they may be changed to oral therapy for a total course of 10 days):

- Cefotaxime, 50-150 mg/kg/24 hr q6-8hr IV, or ceftriaxone, 50-75 mg/kg/24 hr q12hr IV, or cefuroxime, 100 mg/kg/24 hr q6-8hr IV

Antibiotics may be altered to reflect sensitivity data from blood cultures obtained before beginning antibiotics.

Disposition

1. All patients require emergency admission to an ICU for airway management and monitoring. If transport is necessary, it should be arranged using an ambulance equipped for airway intervention, ventilatory support, and resuscitation. Trained personnel and an experienced physician should accompany the patient. *Transport without means to control the airway and ventilate the patient is inappropriate.* Ongoing involvement by an anesthesiologist, otolaryngologist, and critical care physician is helpful.

2. Patients may be extubated under controlled conditions after an average of 36 hours if clinical response indicates, and they usually may be discharged 4 to 6 days after admission.

Croup

If the epiglottis is normal and other entities within the differential are excluded, treatment for croup should be initiated.

Absence of Stridor at Rest

Humidified air is the mainstay of therapy and may be achieved by a variety of cool air vaporizers. Warm air humidifiers may be used, but they have the potential disadvantage of causing burns.

Parents should watch for changing breathing patterns. Stridor often worsens in the early morning hours.

1. Disposition. These patients may be sent home if parents can observe the child, administer fluids, and provide humidified air. Access to a phone and transportation in case the child deteriorates may serve to modify the disposition.
2. Parental education:
   a. Keep room humidified, preferably with a cool mist humidifier.
   b. Push clear liquids.
   c. Control fever to make the child more comfortable.
   d. Take your child who awakens with stridor outside for 5 minutes. If the stridor persists, take the child to the hospital.
   e. Call your physician immediately if the stridor worsens or if your child has more difficulty breathing, turns blue, begins drooling, becomes agitated or listless, has poor intake, or does not improve in 4 to 5 days.

Stridor at Rest

1. These patients should be observed for a long period or hospitalized. Humidified air remains the mainstay of therapy and may be achieved by vaporized rooms or mist tents. The latter has the disadvantage of decreasing patient visibility.
2. Racemic epinephrine (Vasonephrin) is useful for patients with stridor at rest and respiratory distress.
   a. Racemic epinephrine is administered by diluting the solution (2.25%) (<20 kg: 0.25 ml in 2.5 ml saline solution; 20 to 40 kg: 0.5 ml in 2.5 ml saline solution; >40 kg: 0.75 ml in 2.5 ml saline solution), which is administered by nebulizer with or without IPPB up to every 2 hours for increasing stridor at rest.
   b. The therapeutic effect lasts up to 4 hours, and the patient's clinical status often returns to the pretreatment level. However, this rebound may be avoided by initiating steroids at the time of administration of racemic epinephrine.
   c. Racemic epinephrine also has a bronchodilator effect.
3. Steroids may reduce the severity of disease, and they are indicated for patients requiring racemic epinephrine because of stridor at rest and respiratory distress. Many use it for less severe patients as well.
   a. Dexamethasone (Decadron), 0.6 mg/kg/dose IV, IM, or PO, is given for 1 to 4 doses q6-12hr.
   b. Early administration avoids rebound of racemic epinephrine.
4. Hydration must be maintained by oral or parenteral therapy. Antipyretics are often useful.
5. Oxygen without intubation rarely is indicated because hypoxia is usually an indication for airway intervention. Oxygen, when administered, should be given only in an ICU, where intensive monitoring and observation are possible. On occasion, intubation is required because of respiratory failure.

6. **Disposition.** Most patients with stridor at rest should be admitted for observation and therapy to a unit that provides close supervision and access to airway intervention, should it become necessary. Many patients with stridor at rest may resolve rapidly after treatment with racemic epinephrine and dexamethasone. If the patient is relatively asymptomatic 4 to 8 hours after the last nebulization treatment and there is good follow-up observation, early discharge may be contemplated on continuing dexamethasone with the assurance of careful monitoring.

Spasmodic or Allergic Croup

This is rapid in onset and usually treated very effectively with nebulized racemic epinephrine (0.25 to 0.50 ml [adult: 0.75 ml] diluted in 2.5 ml of saline). Patients respond dramatically but may require additional treatments in the ensuing 24 hours.

Patients with allergic croup should be hospitalized for observation, humidified air, and additional racemic epinephrine treatments.

REFERENCES

Aquino V, Terndrup TE: Uvulitis in three children: etiology and respiratory distress, *Pediatr Emerg Care* 8: 206, 1992.

Brilli RJ, Benzing G, Cotcamp OH: Epiglottitis in infants less than two years of age, *Pediatr Emerg Care* 5:16, 1989.

Cruz MN, Stewart G, Rosenberg N: Use of dexamethasone in the outpatient management of acute laryngotracheitis, *Pediatrics* 96: 220, 1995.

Donaldson JO, Maltby CC: Bacterial tracheitis in children, *J Otolaryngol* 18:101, 1989.

Fontanarosa DB, Polsky SS, Goldman GE: Acute epiglottitis, *J Emerg Med* 7:223, 1989.

Geelhoed GC: Sixteen years of croup in a Western Australia teaching hospital: effects of routine steroid treatment, *Ann Emerg Med* 28: 621, 1996.

Husby S, Agertoft L, Mortensen S, et al: Treatment of croup with nebulized steroids (budesonide), *Arch Dis Child* 68:353, 1993.

Johnson DW, Schuh S, Karen G, et al: Outpatient treatment of croup with nebulized dexamethasone, *Arch Pediatr Adolesc Med* 150:349, 1996.

Kairys SW, Olmstead EM, O'Connor GT: Steroid treatment of laryngotracheitis: a meta-analysis of the evidence from randomized trials, *Pediatrics* 83:683, 1989.

Kelley PB, Simon JE: Racemic epinephrine use in croup and disposition, *Am J Emerg Med* 10:181, 1992.

Kunkel NC, Baker MD: Use of racemic epinephrine, dexamethasone and mist in the outpatient management of croup, *Pediatr Emerg Care* 12:156, 1996.

Kuusela AU, Vesikari T: A randomized, double-blind placebo controlled trial of dexamethasone and racemic epinephrine in the treatment of croup, *Acta Paediatr Scand* 77:99, 1988.

Ledwith CA, Shea LH, Mauro RD: Safety and efficacy of nebulized racemic epinephrine in conjunction with oral dexamethasone and mist in the outpatient treatment of croup, *Ann Emerg Med* 25:331, 1992.

Liston SL, Gehrz RC, Siegel LG, et al: Bacterial tracheitis, *Am J Dis Child* 137:764, 1983.

Mauro RD, Poole SR, Lockhart CH: Differentiation of epiglottitis from laryngotracheitis in children with stridor, *Am J Dis Child* 142:679, 1988.

Rothrock SG, Pignatiello GA, Howard RM: Radiologic diagnosis of epiglottitis: objective criteria for all ages, *Ann Emerg Med* 19:978, 1990.

Rowe PC, Klassen TP: Corticosteroids for croup, *Arch Pediatr Adolesc Med* 150:344, 1991.

Skolnik NS: Treatment of croup: a critical review, *Am J Dis Child* 143:1045, 1989.

Super DM, Cartelli NA, Brooks LJ, et al: A prospective randomized double-blind study to evaluate the effect of dexamethasone in acute laryngotracheitis, *J Pediatr* 115:323, 1989.

Valdepena HG, Wald ER, Rose E, et al: Epiglottitis and *Haemophilus influenzae* immunization: the Pittsburgh experience, *Pediatrics* 96:424, 1995.

Waisman Y, Klein BL, Boenning DH, et al: Prospective randomized double-blind study comparing L-epinephrine and racemic epinephrine aerosols in the treatment of laryngotracheitis (croup), *Pediatrics* 89: 302, 1992.

FOREIGN BODY IN AIRWAY

ALERT: Laryngotracheal foreign bodies require immediate airway stabilization, by either removal of the material or surgical intervention. Foreign bodies may cause wheezing.

The clinical presentation of an airway foreign body will reflect the acuteness and location of the obstruction. Laryngotracheal foreign bodies typically produce an acute obstruction, whereas bronchial foreign bodies produce a more sub-acute course. Bronchial obstruction may result from a variety of mechanisms:

1. Check valve in which air is inhaled but not expelled leading to emphysema
2. Stop valve, which allows no inhaled air to pass, resulting in distal atelectasis
3. Ball valve in which the foreign body is dislodged during expiration but reimpacts on inspiration, resulting in atelectasis
4. Bypass valve producing a partial obstruction to inflow and outflow with decreased aeration on the affected side

Food and vegetable matter (nuts, seeds, grapes, raisins, hard candy, sausage-shaped meat such as hot dogs, or raw carrots) are most commonly aspirated by children. Objects are usually 32 mm or less; round objects are more likely to plug the airway completely. The highest risk period is from birth to 48 months; the peak age group is between 1 and 2 years (see Chapter 20).

DIAGNOSTIC FINDINGS

1. Although a history of aspiration is useful, the absence of a positive history does not exclude a foreign body.
2. Acute airway obstruction resulting from material in the laryngotracheal area causes acute, life-threatening respiratory distress. Cyanosis, apnea, stridor, wheezing, cough, and dysphonia may be present. Facial petechiae may appear as a result of increased intrathoracic pressure.
3. Subacute obstruction occurs with bronchial foreign bodies and, rarely, partial obstruction of the laryngotracheal segment. Clinically, patients develop air trapping, wheezing, cyanosis, a muffled voice, and cough. Atelectasis is commonly present. At least one component of the triad of wheezing, coughing, and decreased breath sounds is not present in 61% of patients.

Complications

1. Specific pulmonary complications may include atelectasis, pneumonia, erosion through the trachea and bronchus, and abscess.
2. Respiratory arrest occurs with any delay in clearing an acute obstruction. Attempts at removal of bronchial foreign bodies may produce total obstruction.
3. Dysrhythmias and other complications of hypoxia may develop, including a full cardiac arrest.
4. Pulmonary edema occasionally results from obstruction and increased intrathoracic pressure.

Ancillary Data

Relief of the obstruction should not be delayed awaiting results of ancillary data. Immediate intervention may be necessary. However, if obstruction is only partial, a number of ancillary diagnostic tests may be useful in defining the location of the foreign body and in considering other diagnostic entities.

1. ABG to determine hypoxia and ventilatory status.
2. Chest x-ray films, inspiratory and expiratory, to determine whether a bronchial foreign body is likely to be present. It is often important to distinguish a foreign body in the trachea from one in the esophagus. Foreign bodies lie in the plane of least resistance. Flat foreign bodies like coins in the esophagus lie in the frontal plane, appearing as a full circle on the posteroanterior (PA) view, whereas those in the trachea rest in the sagittal plane and will appear end-on in the PA chest x-ray film and flat on a lateral view.

   Radiopacity is a relative quality rather than an absolute property. Tracheobronchial tree findings may indicate obstruction (66%), atelectasis (13%), radiopaque foreign body (11%), and pneumonia (5%). Five percent were normal.

3. Soft tissue lateral neck.
4. Laryngoscopy. May be both diagnostic and therapeutic. Magill forceps or Kelly clamps can remove the foreign body under direct visualization of the laryngotracheal area.
5. Fluoroscopy may be useful. Tracheal foreign bodies may have a paradoxic movement.
6. Bronchoscopy is the definitive therapy but is also useful as a diagnostic tool. The procedure is rapidly and safely performed with fiber-optic equipment used by an experienced physician.

DIFFERENTIAL DIAGNOSIS (see Chapter 20)
MANAGEMENT

1. The initial stabilization of the patient with a foreign body involves attention to the airway while managing shock, respiratory or cardiac arrest, and the complications of hypoxia the patient has experienced. Concurrent with immediate resuscitation, other considerations in the differential diagnosis must be considered.
2. Efforts should be initiated on the first contact to relieve airway obstruction according to the guidelines of the American Heart Association. Attempts at clearing the airway followed by back blows and manual thrusts should be considered as an essential part of prehospital care and will, ultimately, determine the patient's prognosis.
3. If the child is acutely obstructed and obviously in respiratory distress, immediate intervention is required.
   a. If the infant is less than 12 months of age, the rapid increase in pressure resulting from five back blows may expel or loosen a foreign body because many of these lodge high in the trachea or throat. If the material is not expelled by the patient, five manual chest thrusts should be done immedi-

ately to provide a more sustained increase in pressure and airflow. Repeat as indicated.
   b. In older children, five manual abdominal (Heimlich) thrusts constitute the primary technique. Repeat as indicated. The chest wall compliance of older children reduces the efficacy of chest thrusts, and therefore that technique cannot be recommended.
   c. Blind probing of the airway to dislodge a foreign body is discouraged. The airway may be opened by the jaw thrust maneuver. If a foreign body is seen, it can be removed with the fingers or available instruments (Magill forceps or Kelly clamps).
   d. The above recommendations are made on the basis of the best available information, which suggests that a combination of maneuvers may be more effective than any single method, especially in the infant. These methods are under constant reevaluation.
4. If the above procedures are not rapidly successful, an attempt may be made to remove the foreign body with laryngoscopy and a Magill forceps or Kelly clamp.
5. Bronchoscopy is the definitive therapy and must be performed rapidly in all patients with unrelieved respiratory obstruction or in those with a bronchial foreign body present for more than 24 hours.
6. If these procedures are not available or immediately successful at relieving the obstruction, surgical intervention by cricothyroidotomy may be appropriate.
7. Postural drainage in an ICU, in combination with inhaled bronchodilators, is useful in removing nonvegetable matter foreign bodies that have been present in the tracheobronchial tract for less than 24 hours and that are not associated with respiratory distress. Bronchoscopy may, of course, be used instead.

DISPOSITION

1. Patients who have experienced significant hypoxia or any other complications of an upper airway foreign body should be hospitalized for monitoring if definitive therapy has been rendered either before arrival at the hospital or in the ED.
2. Patients with ongoing obstruction need emergent airway stabilization and critical care facilities.
3. The patient who has experienced a very transient episode of obstruction or choking and is free of distress or signs and symptoms referable to the incident may be followed closely as an ambulatory patient.

Parental Education

Small, hard foods such as nuts, seeds, raisins, hard candy, sausage-shaped meat, and raw carrots should not be given to small children unless cut into very small pieces. Parents should be taught the techniques of back blow and manual chest thrust for infants and abdominal thrust for older children.

REFERENCES

American Heart Association: Guidelines for cardiopulmonary resuscitation (CPR) and emergency cardiac care (ECC), *JAMA* 268:2171, 1992.

Blazer S, Naveh Y, Friedman A: Foreign body in the airway, *Am J Dis Child* 134:68, 1980.

Harris CS, Baker SP, Smith GA, et al: Childhood asphyxia by food: anatomical survey and overview, *JAMA* 251:2231, 1984.

Imaizuma H, Kaneko M, Nara S, et al: Definitive diagnosis and location of peanuts in the airway using magnetic resonance imaging techniques, *Ann Emerg Med* 23: 1379, 1994.

Kosloske AM: Bronchoscopic extraction of aspirated foreign bodies in children, *Am J Dis Child* 136:924, 1982.

Puhakka H, Svedstrom E, Kero P, et al: Tracheobronchial foreign body, *Am J Dis Child* 143:543, 1989.

Svedstrom E, Puhakka H, Kero P: How accurate is chest radiography in the diagnosis of tracheobronchial foreign body in children, *Pediatr Radiol* 19:520, 1989.

Schlass MD, Pham-Dang H, Rosales JK: Foreign bodies in the tracheo-bronchial tree: a retrospective study of 217 cases, *J Otolaryngol* 12:212, 1983.

PNEUMONIA

Pneumonia is an acute infection of the lung parenchyma presenting as an interstitial process involving either the alveolar walls or the alveoli.

ETIOLOGY AND DIAGNOSTIC FINDINGS: INFECTION (Table 84-4)

1. Respiratory findings (see Table 84-4) and tachypnea are often associated with pneumonia. The risk of pneumonia increases with age-specific respiratory rates:

<6 mo old	>59/min
6-11 mo old	>52/min
1-2 yr old	>42/min

2. Bacterial infection (Table 84-5).
   a. Common organisms: *Streptococcus pneumoniae, Haemophilus influenzae*, group A streptococci, and *Staphylococcus aureus*
   b. Unusual organisms
      (1) Pertussis: catarrhal stage followed by staccato, paroxysmal cough (p. 716).
      (2) *Pseudomonas aeruginosa*: usually in debilitated or immunocompromised patients, especially those with cystic fibrosis. May involve pulmonary tract, ear, sinus, or meninges.
      (3) *Klebsiella pneumoniae*: usually in infants, alcoholics, or those who are immunocompromised. Explosive pulmonary symptoms with gastroenteritis and neurologic findings. Chest roentgenogram shows bulging fissures.
      (4) Anaerobes such as *Peptostreptococcus* organisms, often as secondary infection or abscess.
3. Viral infections: RSV and parainfluenza predominant in children less than 2 years; influenza A and B in older children; other agents: adenovirus, measles, and chickenpox.

TABLE 84-4   Differentiating Features of Pneumonia

	Bacterial	Viral	Mycoplasma
Age	Any	<5 yr	5-15 yr
Season	Any	Epidemic	Any
Onset	Rapid	Gradual	Gradual
Toxicity	Severe	Mild/moderate	Mild
Fever	High	Moderate	Low
Chills	Common	Rare	Rare
Tachypnea	Moderate/severe	Mild/moderate	Mild/moderate
Cough	Productive, variable	Dry, variable	Dry, prominent
Myalgia/headache	None	Common	Headache, pharyngitis
Auscultation	↓ breath sounds, rales, rhonchi	Rare wheezes, rare rales	Very rare rales
Pleural effusion	Common	Very rare	Rare
Segmental consolidation	Common	Rare	Variable
Chest x-ray	Lobar consolidation	Interstitial, delayed resolution	Interstitial (more than physical examination would indicate)
White blood cells (cells/mm^3)	>10,000	Normal	Normal
Diagnostic procedures	Positive blood culture result; rarely, lung tap or thoracentesis	Viral culture, serologic evaluation	Cold agglutinin, complement fixation
Primary antibiotics	See Table 84-6	None	Erythromycin

TABLE 84-5   Bacterial Pneumonias: Diagnostic Findings

	Streptococcus pneumoniae	*Haemophilus influenzae*	Group A streptococci	*Staphyloccus aureus*
Age	≤4 yr	≤8 yr	>10 yr	<1 yr
Onset	Rapid	Gradual	Gradual	Rapid
Diagnostic features	Infant: poor feeding, cough, irritable. Child: fever, cough, toxic, abdominal pain	Fever, cough, toxic, otitis media (variable)	Fever, tachypnea, chill, pleuritic pain, hemoptysis	High fever, respiratory distress, nausea, vomiting
Complications	Bacteremia, Empyema, Effusion	Bacteremia, Meningitis, Empyema, Lung abscess, Bronchiectasis	Empyema (serosanguineous)	Pneumatocele, Empyema, Pneumothorax, Pyopneumothorax
Chest x-ray film	Lobar consolidation, Patchy bronchopneumonia	Unilateral lobar consolidation	Infiltrate	Segmental, lobar infiltrate

4. *Mycoplasma pneumoniae*: frequent in children older than 5 years.
5. *Chlamydia trachomatis.*
   a. Tachypnea, staccato cough, conjunctivitis, rarely toxic; fairly common in the second to sixth weeks of life
   b. Chest x-ray film: hyperexpansion; CBC; eosinophilia
6. *Mycobacterium tuberculosis.*
   a. History of exposure; fever, anorexia, cough.
   b. Chest x-ray film with hilar adenopathy and apical findings; sputum and gastric aspirates may be helpful. Purified protein derivative (PPD) skin test on patient and family should be done.
7. *Parasitic infection: Pneumocystis carinii.*
   a. Fever, tachypnea, cough, dyspnea, cyanosis; occurs in immunosuppressed or malnourished patients
   b. Chest x-ray film: diffuse interstitial pneumonitis; ABG; hypoxia, usually greater than would be indicated by chest x-ray study; lung aspirate or biopsy with methenamine-silver nitrate stain
8. Fungal infection.
   a. Coccidioidomycosis
      (1) Fever, pleuritis, productive cough with weight loss, anorexia, myalgias, headache, and rash
      (2) Chest x-ray study: pneumonia (interstitial), effusions, granuloma, cavitation
      (3) Skin test and complement-fixation test
   b. Histoplasmosis
      (1) Pulmonary cavitation, hemoptysis, variable hepatosplenomegaly, variable weight loss, lymphadenopathy
      (2) Chest x-ray film: pulmonary calcification; CBC; anemia
9. Rickettsial infection: Q fever.
   a. Fever, chest pain, headache, sore throat, chills, and respiratory symptoms; self-limited disease of 3 weeks
   b. Complement fixation

Ancillary Data

Laboratory studies must be individualized for the specific patient and the presenting clinical complex.

1. Chest roentgenogram: PA and lateral. In the absence of respiratory signs in children less than 8 weeks of age, abnormalities are unusual. Children with the following factors did not have pneumonia: illness in summer months, absence of cough, dyspnea, respiratory distress (grunting, flaring, retracting), respiratory rate less than 60 breaths/min, absence of rales, decreased breath sounds, presence of normal color, or white blood cell (WBC) count less than 19,000 cells/mm^3.
   a. Inspiratory and expiratory views may be useful in excluding a foreign body, if in doubt.
   b. Lateral decubitus can define an effusion.
2. CBC with differential.
3. ABG. For all patients with cyanosis, apnea, dyspnea, or respiratory distress. Oximetry may be useful if child has good ventilation.
4. Blood cultures. Positive result in 10% to 20% of all patients with bacterial pneumonias; 2.1% of ED patients with pneumonia have positive culture. Blood cultures should be obtained on patients requiring hospitalization (e.g., toxic, respiratory distress)
5. Counterimmunoelectrophoresis (CIE) may be useful in hospitalized patients with negative cultures.
6. Cold agglutinins. Positive correlation with titer of at least 1:64 to *Mycoplasma pneumoniae*. Place 4 drops of whole blood in small purple top tube (EDTA) placed on ice bath for at least 30 seconds. Then the tube is rolled on its side and observed for coarse flocculation.

Pulmonary Cultures

Invasive procedures are indicated for patients with severe toxicity and life-threatening infection, for those failing to respond to appropriate antibiotic therapy, and for those who are immunosuppressed.

Nasopharyngeal (NP) or throat cultures are of no value except for pertussis (NP swab) and viral cultures.

1. Sputum. Usually difficult to obtain in children and contaminated with mouth flora. Reliable only with productive cough and if single organism is recovered.
2. Tracheal suctioning by direct laryngoscopy. Fairly reliable but patient may have upper airway contamination.
3. Transtracheal aspiration. Difficult to do in children and usually should be avoided. Absolute contraindication is a bleeding diathesis or an uncooperative, young child.
4. Bronchoscopy with direct aspiration and brush border biopsy. Excellent approach yielding direct visualization with aspiration of good culture material. Requires equipment and experience, which are rarely available emergently.
5. Direct needle aspiration of the lung (useful in critically ill and immunocompromised children).
   a. Unless the infiltrate is in the upper lobes, the patient is placed in a sitting position and is told to take a deep breath and hold in expiration if old enough to cooperate. A needle (18- to 20-gauge, 1 to 1½ in) is inserted rapidly under negative pressure, along the top of the rib, with an attached syringe containing nonbacteriostatic saline solution. Patient requires hospitalization for observation after the procedure.
   b. Aspirate is excellent specimen for Gram stain and culture.
   c. Contraindications include hyperexpansion with air trapping, pneumothorax, bleeding diathesis, pulmonary hypertension, uncontrolled coughing or seizures, poor cooperation, and lack of facility to observe the patient after the procedure.

Thoracentesis (see Appendix A-8)

This is indicated for the removal of pleural fluid for either diagnostic or therapeutic purposes.

1. Patient is maintained in an upright position, and the site for thoracentesis is defined by x-ray film and physical examination.
2. Needle (18- to 20-gauge) with a 20-ml syringe is attached to a three-way stopcock. Using negative pressure, it is passed along the top of the ribs and fluid is withdrawn. The amount removed should reflect the degree of respiratory distress and that required for diagnosis. Patient must be hospitalized for observation after procedure.

Evaluation of the fluid should include Gram stain and culture, cell count and differential, protein, lactate dehydrogenase (LDH), and glucose.

DIFFERENTIAL DIAGNOSIS (see Chapter 20)

1. Allergy: asthma (p. 765)
2. Trauma
   a. Foreign body (p. 791)
   b. Drowning (see Chapter 47)
3. Atelectasis
4. Vascular disease
   a. CHF and pulmonary edema (see Chapters 16 and 19)
   b. Pulmonary embolism (p. 568)
5. Intoxication: hydrocarbon (p. 379)
6. Recurrent aspiration (gastroesophageal reflux, vascular ring, pharyngeal incoordination, H type tracheoesophageal fistula)
7. Congenital absence of lung, hemangioma, etc.
8. Neoplasm: primary or metastatic

MANAGEMENT

1. Most patients with pneumonia have only mild disease and require no immediate stabilization or airway support. However,

if respiratory distress is present, stabilization of the airway is of the highest priority.

   a. Initiate oxygen, optimally with humidification, if respiratory distress is present.

   b. Intubation may be indicated if respiratory failure (Pao_2 <50 mm Hg and $Paco_2$ >50 mm Hg) is present.

   c. ABG is indicated for moderately ill patient.

   d. Suctioning and postural drainage are useful adjunctive measures.

2. Initiate antibiotics with all cases of pneumonia in which bacteria or mycoplasmas are the suspected pathogens (Table 84-6).

   a. If appropriate, obtain cultures (blood and rarely lung tap) before initiating medication.

   b. Viral infections do not require antibiotics, although if the patient is toxic or having respiratory distress, antibiotics are indicated until culture results are available.

   c. Most patients may be treated with oral medications as outpatients.

   d. The initial choice must reflect common causes for the patient's age, allergies, signs and symptoms, and known bacterial sensitivity patterns.

   e. Antibiotic failures commonly result from resistant organisms (particularly *H. influenzae*), viral infections, or poor compliance.

   f. Organisms, such as tuberculosis and *Pneumocystis carinii*, require alternative therapy.

3. Bronchodilators are indicated if wheezing or reactive airway disease is present (p. 769).

4. Special considerations must be recognized in the management of the newborn (see Chapter 11).

DISPOSITION

Hospitalization rarely is necessary but is indicated if any of the following exist:

TABLE 84-6   Antibiotic Therapy for Bacterial Pneumonia

Age-group	Major etiologies	Antibiotic therapy PO	Antibiotic therapy IV
<2 mo*	*E. coli* Group B streptococci *S. aureus* *C. trachomatis*	Rarely given	Ampicillin, 100-200 mg/kg/24 hr q6-12hr, **and** gentamicin, 5-7.5 mg/kg/24 hr q8-12hr
2 mo-8 yr	Virus *S. pneumoniae*† *H. influenzae* *S. aureus* (rare)	Amoxicillin, 30-50 mg/kg/24 hr q8hr, **or** Augmentin **or** cefaclor	Ampicillin, 200 mg/kg/24 hr q4hr, **or** ceftriaxone, 50 to 100 mg/kg/24 hr q12hr IV.‡ **If poor response, add** nafcillin (or equiv), 100 mg/kg/24 hr q4hr
≥9 yr	Virus *S. pneumoniae*† *Mycoplasma* *S. aureus* (rare) Group A streptococci (rare) *H. influenzae* (rare)	Erythromycin, 30-50 mg/kg/24 hr q6hr	Ampicillin, 200 mg/kg/24 hr q4hr, **or** ceftriaxone, 50-100 mg/kg/24 hr q12hr IV; if poor response, consider erythromycin (PO) or nafcillin

*If *C. trachomatis* is suspected, **add** erythromycin, 30-50 mg/kg/24 hr q6hr PO.
†If *S. pneumoniae* is suspected and child is toxic, initially add vancomycin, 40 mg/kg/24 hr q6hr IV.
‡Other alternatives include cefuroxime, 100 mg/kg/24 hr q6-8hr IV, or cefotaxime, 50-150 mg/kg/24 hr q6hr IV.

1. Significant toxicity with high fever, dyspnea, apnea, cyanosis, or fatigue.
2. Any evidence of potential respiratory failure or progression.
3. Age less than 2 to 3 months.
4. Immunocompromised host: underlying disease (e.g., leukemia), drugs (steroids or other immunosuppressive agents), or sickle cell disease.
5. Patients with cystic fibrosis or other chronic pulmonary disease should be hospitalized for acute deterioration and distress with the aim of controlling the infection and instituting aggressive pulmonary toilet.
6. Pleural effusion or after lung aspiration or thoracentesis.
7. Unreliable home environment or questionable compliance.

Most patients may be discharged with appropriate medications.

1. Close follow-up must be ensured to assess the patient's condition after 24 and 48 hours to determine that resolution has occurred.
2. A repeat chest x-ray film should be obtained 4 to 6 weeks after the initial diagnosis in patients who have segmental or lobar infiltrates.

Parental Education

1. Give medication for entire treatment course.
2. Call or bring your child to the primary care physician in 24 hours to assess the response to treatment.
3. Perform postural drainage, if suggested.
4. Call your physician if the following occur:
   a. Your child is having more difficulty breathing or develops a high fever, more rapid breathing, increased retractions, cyanosis, or apnea.
   b. Your child has trouble taking medications or fluids.
   c. Your child is not afebrile and much improved in 48 hours.

REFERENCES

Courtoy I, Lande AE, and Turner RB: Accuracy of radiographic differentiation of bacterial from nonbacterial pneumonia, *Pediatrics* 28:261, 1989.
Denny FW, Clyde WA: Acute lower respiratory tract infections in nonhospitalized children, *J Pediatr* 108.635, 1986.
Hickey RW, Bowman MJ, Smith GA: Utility of blood cultures in pediatric patients found to have pneumonia in the emergency department, *Ann Emerg Med* 27: 721, 1996.
Inselman LA: Tuberculosis in children: an unsettling forecast, *Contemp Pediatr* 7:10, 1990.
Losek JO, Kishaba RG, Berens RJ, et al: Indications for chest roentgenograms in the febrile young infant, *Pediatr Emerg Care* 5:149, 1989.
Taylor J, DelBeccaro M, Done S, et al: Establishing clinically relevant standards for tachypnea in febrile children younger than 2 years, *Arch Pediatr Adolesc Med* 149: 283, 1995.

85 RENAL DISORDERS

JOSEPH T. FLYNN

ACUTE GLOMERULONEPHRITIS

Although glomerulonephritis is a histopathologic diagnosis, the term *acute glomerulonephritis* is commonly used to define the clinical presentation of hematuria, edema, and hypertension. The disease most commonly occurs between ages 3 and 7 and rarely less than 2 years.

Commonly, acute glomerulonephritis occurs as a sequela of a group A β-hemolytic streptococcal infection of either the pharynx or skin. (Infections with other bacteria, Mycoplasma, and certain viruses may produce an identical clinical picture.) The pathogenesis is poorly understood but probably results from the deposition of circulating immune complexes in the kidney. Although the disease is self-limited with careful clinical management, strict attention must be given to the initial evaluation, differential diagnosis, and recognition of complications.

DIAGNOSTIC FINDINGS

1. Usually a preceding streptococcal infection or exposure 1 to 2 weeks (average: 10 days) occurs before the onset of glomerulonephritis. An interval less than 4 days is associated with an exacerbation of preexisting disease rather than an initial attack.
2. Patients commonly have hematuria (90%), fluid retention and edema (100%), hypertension (60% to 70%), and oliguria (80%). Fever, malaise, and abdominal pain are frequently reported.

Complications

1. Circulatory congestion is sometimes noted with dyspnea, cough, pallor, and pulmonary edema.
2. Hypertensive encephalopathy with confusion, headaches, somnolence, and seizures may develop.
3. Anuria and renal failure occur in 2% of patients.

Ancillary Data

1. Urinalysis:
   a. Hematuria may be microscopic or gross. Erythrocyte casts are present in up to 80% of affected children.
   b. Leukocyturia and hyaline and granular casts are common.
   c. Proteinuria is usually less than 2 gm/m^2/24 hr.
   d. Urinary concentrating ability is preserved.
2. Fractional excretion of sodium (p. 811) may be reduced.
3. Antistreptococcal antibodies are present. Antistreptolysin O (ASO) is the most commonly ordered but is less specific than anti-DNAse B. The "streptozyme" panel screens for five different antistreptococcal antibodies and will almost always be elevated.
4. Total serum complement and specifically C3 is depressed in 90% to 100% of patients during the first 2 weeks of

illness, returning to normal within 6 to 8 weeks. Persistently low levels suggest that a chronic renal disease may exist.

5. Immunoglobulin G levels are elevated, often associated with rheumatoid factor titers greater than 1:32.
6. Anemia is present, possibly because of dilution. Thrombocytopenia is reported, and fibrinogen, factor VIII, and plasma activity may be acutely elevated.
7. Blood urea nitrogen (BUN) is elevated disproportionately to the serum creatinine. Hyponatremia and hyperkalemia may be present, specifically related to the degree of oliguria.
8. Chest roentgenogram may show cardiomegaly and pulmonary congestion.

DIFFERENTIAL DIAGNOSIS (see Chapter 37)

The diagnosis of poststreptococcal acute glomerulonephritis is established by the acute onset of edema, hypertension, and gross or microscopic hematuria with erythrocyte casts and proteinuria. Evidence of an antecedent streptococcal infection, decreased complement, and spontaneous improvement in the renal disease and its complications exists. Other diagnoses should be considered when the clinical syndrome is aberrant, the renal failure is severe, the individual's age does not fall within the predicted range, or resolution is prolonged.

MANAGEMENT

The initial focus must be on management of complications and evaluation of the extent of renal injury.

Fluid Overload

1. Fluid and sodium are restricted to maintain normal intravascular volume.
2. Diuretics may be required.

Hypertension (see Chapter 18)

1. Although a wide variety of drugs may be useful, the following are consistently effective:
   a. Diazoxide, 1-3 mg/kg/dose q6hr IV (potent vasodilator)
   b. Furosemide (Lasix), 1-2 mg/kg/dose IV (diuretic)
   c. Labetalol, 0.4-1.0 mg/kg/dose q4-6hr IV
2. For prolonged therapy, the following are given:
   a. Propranolol, 1 mg/kg/dose q6-8hr PO
   b. Hydralazine, 1-3 mg/kg/24 hr q6hr PO
   c. Isradipine, 0.2-0.6 mg/kg/24 hr q6-8hr PO

DISPOSITION

1. All patients who have evidence of uncontrolled hypertension, congestive heart failure, or azotemia should be hospitalized. Children without any of these problems can be followed at home but must have adequate medical care available, including frequent blood pressure measurements.
2. A nephrologist should be involved in the child's care.

REFERENCES

Mezzano S, Oliavarria F, Ardiles L, Lopez MI: Incidence of circulating immune complexes in patients with poststreptococcal glomerulonephritis and in patients with streptococcal impetigo, *Clin Nephrol* 26:61, 1986.

Roy S, Stapleton FB: Changing perspectives in children hospitalized with poststreptococcal acute glomerulonephritis, *Pediatr Nephrol* 4:585, 1990.

Travis LB, Kalia A: Acute nephritic syndrome. In Postlewaite RJ, editor: *Clinical paediatric nephrology*, Oxford, 1994, Butterworth-Heinemann.

HEMOLYTIC-UREMIC SYNDROME

Hemolytic-uremic syndrome (HUS) consists of the classic triad of renal failure, microangiopathic hemolytic anemia, and thrombocytopenia. Typical HUS follows an episode of bloody diarrhea or respiratory infection. It is primarily a disease of young children, usually occurring before 5 years of age. Predisposing factors include exposure to contaminated meat or to other children with gastroenteritis in day-care centers. It is more common in the late summer and early fall. Atypical HUS occurs in children without the predisposing factors noted above and may have a familial pattern. It has also been reported after exposure to certain medications, including oral contraceptives and cyclosporine.

HUS results from localized intravascular coagulation and endothelial injury within the kidney. The prostacyclin/thromboxane (coagulation/anticoagulation) equilibrium is disturbed.

The vascular endothelial cell injury produces swelling and detachment from the basement membrane with accumulation of a fluffy material. Clinical evidence of thrombotic microangiopathy is usually limited to the kidneys, although it may occur in extrarenal organs, including the colon, brain, and pancreas.

ETIOLOGY: INFECTION

1. Bacteria: Verotoxin-producing *Escherichia coli* serotype 0157:H7 is the most common organism involved. In a case-controlled study, evidence of *E. coli* 0157:H7 infection was found in 72% of patients studied. Other bacteria that have been implicated in HUS include *Shigella*, *Salmonella*, and group A streptococci.
2. Virus: Coxsackievirus, influenza, and respiratory syncytial virus (RSV).
3. Many other unspecified infections may trigger the disorder.

DIAGNOSTIC FINDINGS

1. Patients with typical HUS have a history of gastroenteritis with vomiting, bloody diarrhea, and crampy abdominal pain up to 2 weeks before the onset of HUS. The absence of a gastrointestinal (GI) pro-

drome is associated with a poor prognosis. Some patients experience respiratory infections before the illness.

2. The spectrum of clinical disease is highly variable, ranging from mild elevation of BUN without anemia to severe, total anuria produced by acute nephropathy with marked anemia and thrombocytopenia. In patients with anuria more than 8 days or oliguria more than 15 days chronic disease often develops, although 45% of those with HUS have no anuria and a third have no oliguria.
3. Patients may have marked hypertension, pallor, petechiae and easy bruising, hepatosplenomegaly, and edema. Hypertension occurs in as many as 50% of patients.
4. Central nervous system (CNS) findings occur relatively often, including irritability and lethargy, in some cases progressing to coma, seizures, and hemiparesis.

Complications

1. Atypical HUS is marked by recurrences, often without prodrome; mortality rate of 30%.
2. Renal failure, rarely progressing to end-stage renal disease. However, some renal abnormality may be found in up to 30% to 50% of all patients with HUS on long-term follow-up.
3. Bowel perforation or necrosis. In a recent Seattle outbreak, patients with severe GI involvement had an increased mortality rate.
4. Severe CNS findings including drowsiness, personality changes, and hemiparesis, progressing to cerebral infarction, seizures, and coma. Seizures occur in 40% of cases, especially in patients with hyponatremia or severe azotemia.
5. High output cardiac failure from volume overload. Rare myocarditis.
6. Pancreatic involvement with development of insulin-dependent diabetes mellitus.

Ancillary Data

1. Assessment of renal function (p. 811)
   a. Electrolytes (elevated K^+ level and acidosis may be present), BUN, creatinine, calcium (often low), and phosphorus levels (usually elevated).
   b. Urinalysis demonstrating hematuria and proteinuria.
   c. In dehydration the BUN is often elevated and should decrease by 50% over the first 24 hours of appropriate rehydration. If fall in BUN does not occur, HUS should be considered.
2. Hematologic findings
   a. A low hemoglobin (Hgb) level is usually present with red blood cells (RBCs) demonstrating a microangiopathic hemolytic anemia, with burr cells and fragments on peripheral smear.
   b. The white blood cell (WBC) count usually is elevated. A polymorphonuclear leukocyte count greater than 15,000/mm^3 is associated with severe manifestations.
   c. Platelets are often decreased to less than 50,000/mm^3.
   d. Coagulation studies are normal. Minimal evidence for disseminated intravascular coagulation (DIC) with fibrin split products is rarely found.
3. Arterial blood gas (ABG) for evaluation of acidosis and potential hypoxia
4. Bacterial and viral cultures, when appropriate, including stool for *E. coli* serotyping

DIFFERENTIAL DIAGNOSIS

1. Inflammation and infection:
   a. Ulcerative colitis is accompanied by bloody diarrhea and anemia. The length of illness may provide information.
   b. Surgical abdomen as a result of infection, perforation, or necrosis may be difficult to distinguish.
   c. An acutely dehydrated patient with acute tubular necrosis may have some parallel characteristics.
2. Trauma may be associated with hematuria and anemia from an acute blood loss.
3. Other causes of acquired hemolytic anemia (p. 208).

MANAGEMENT

1. The initial management, after establishing the diagnosis, should involve careful monitoring, assessing, and treating the volume status of the patient. Many patients have volume overload associated with electrolyte abnormalities, hypertension, and high output failure.
2. Renal failure requires attention to fluids and, when appropriate, treatment of hypertension, volume overload, hyperkalemia, acidosis, hypocalcemia, hyperphosphatemia, and other metabolic abnormalities. Consultation should be obtained.

   If routine medical management is ineffective, peritoneal dialysis usually is done when there is hypervolemia with oliguria or anuria, more than 24 hours of anuria, unresponsive electrolyte abnormalities, and life-threatening hyperkalemia in a patient in whom more conservative management is contraindicated.
3. Hgb less than 5 to 6 gm/ml or an hematocrit (Hct) less than 15% requires intervention. If the Hct is less than 20% and falling rapidly, and if there are symptoms of anemia (e.g., gallop rhythm or high output failure) or hypoxia, transfusion should be considered. It is crucial to initially transfuse only a small amount of blood slowly (5 ml/kg over 4 hours) to minimize volume overload. Blood pressure occasionally rises dramatically concomitant with or after the transfusion. If the patient is hyperkalemic, a transfusion should not be given until dialysis is established. Blood should be as fresh as possible.

4. Platelets have a shortened survival time, and transfused platelets may contribute to platelet plugging in the renal microvasculature. Platelet counts less than 10,000/mm^3 are uncommon; thrombocytopenia rarely requires specific therapy.

   Platelet transfusions (3 to 4 units or <15 ml/kg) are indicated only in children with active bleeding with a count consistently less than 20,000/mm^3, or in those with counts less than 50,000/mm^3 who are about to undergo invasive procedures.

5. Seizures are controlled with diazepam (Valium), 0.2-0.3 mg/kg/dose IV, repeated in 10 minutes as required or lorazepam (Ativan), 0.05-0.15 mg/kg/dose IV. Phenobarbital or phenytoin should be initiated for maintenance therapy (see Chapter 21).

   Prophylactic loading with phenytoin (10-20 mg/kg/dose IV administered at a rate of 0.5 mg/kg/min) is considered in patients with neuromuscular irritability (e.g., muscular twitching). Drug levels must be monitored.

6. Azotemia should be monitored. If the vomiting and diarrhea have ceased, limitation of dietary protein intake may limit azotemia (adequate calories to enable anabolism should be provided in the form of carbohydrates and fat). The indications and route of dialysis are somewhat controversial, but dialysis is usually initiated at a BUN level of 100-150 mg/dl or in the presence of clinical signs, including hyperkalemia, encephalopathy, etc.

7. Multiple investigational therapies have been attempted, including heparin, antiplatelet agents (aspirin or dipyridamole), fibrinolytic agents (urokinase), fresh-frozen plasma and plasma exchange, prostacyclin infusions, intravenous immunoglobulin G (IgG) infusions, and vitamin E therapy and shown to have varying success. Plasma exchange may be helpful if severe neurologic involvement is present. Consultation should be sought to determine the relative efficacy of each modality in each case.

DISPOSITION

1. Patients normally should be hospitalized initially for evaluation and treatment. A nephrology consultation should be sought.

2. In rare cases, patients may be discharged home if there is no clinical evidence of disease (normal blood pressure [BP], CNS status, and volume) and only minimal laboratory abnormalities (mildly hemolytic smear and normal Hgb, Hct, platelet count, and BUN and creatinine levels). If the patient is discharged, it is imperative to follow the patient (including laboratory parameters) to ensure that of the disease does not progress.

3. Given that siblings may get the disease, it is important that other household members be monitored as outpatients.

4. Long-term follow-up observation (>10 years) is indicated because of the possibility of delayed onset of renal failure and hypertension.

REFERENCES

Brandt JR, Fouser LS, Watkins SL, et al: *E. coli* 0157:H7–associated hemolytic-uremic syndrome after ingestion of contaminated hamburgers, *J Pediatr* 125:519, 1994.

Fitzpatrick MM, Walters MDS, Trompeter RS, et al: Atypical (non-diarrhea-associated) hemolytic uremic syndrome in childhood, *J Pediatr* 122:532, 1993.

Gravitz A, Rosmini F, Capioli A, et al: Haemolytic-uraemic syndrome in childhood surveillance and case control studies in Italy, *Pediatr Nephrol* 8:705, 1994.

Hahn JS, Havens PC, Higgins JJ, et al: Neurologic complications of hemolytic uremic syndrome, J *Child Neurol* 4:108, 1989.

Kelles A, Van Dyck M, Proesman W: Childhood haemolytic uraemic syndrome: long-term outcome and prognostic features, *Eur J Pediatr* 153:38, 1994.

Lopez EL, Devoto S, Fayad A, et al: Association between severity of gastrointestinal prodrome and long-term prognosis in classic hemolytic uremic syndrome, *J Pediatr* 120:210, 1992.

Martin DL, MacDonald KL, White KE, et al: The epidemiology and clinical aspects of the hemolytic uremic syndrome in Minnesota, *N Engl J Med* 323:1161, 1990.

Rizzoni G, Claris-Appiani A, Edefonti A, et al: Plasma infusion for hemolytic-uremic syndrome in children: results of a multicenter controlled trial, *J Pediatr* 112:284, 1988.

Rowe PC, Orrbine E, Ogborn M, et al: Epidemic *E. coli* 0157:H7 gastroenteritis and hemolytic-uremic syndrome in a Canadian Inuit community: intestinal illness in family members as a risk factor, *J Pediatr* 124:21, 1994.

Schulman SL, Kaplan BS: Management of patients with hemolytic uremic syndrome demonstrating severe azotemia but not uremia, *Pediatr Nephrol* 10:671, 1996.

Siegler RL: Management of hemolytic-uremic syndrome, *J Pediatr* 112:1014, 1988.

Siegler RL, Milligan MK, Burningham TH, et al: Long-term outcome and prognostic indicators in the hemolytic uremic syndrome, *J Pediatr* 118:195, 1991.

HENOCH-SCHÖNLEIN PURPURA

Henoch-Schönlein purpura (HSP) is an acute vasculitis of unknown etiology but associated with group A streptococcal, *Mycoplasma*, and viral (e.g., variccla, Epstein-Barr [EB] virus) infections; drugs (penicillin, tetracycline, aspirin, sulfonamides, and erythromycin); and allergens (insect bites, chocolate, milk, and wheat). It most commonly occurs in the winter months. A male predominance has been noted.

Multisystem involvement occurs primarily in children 2 to 11 years of age with progression of renal disease occurring more commonly in older children and adults (children: 5%; adults: 13% to 14%). Children less than 3 months commonly have only skin manifestations without gastrointestinal or renal involvement.

DIAGNOSTIC FINDINGS

1. Skin lesions are pathognomonic, beginning on the gravity-dependent areas of the legs and buttocks and the extensor surfaces of the arms. They begin as erythematous, maculopapular lesions that blanch and progress to become petechial and purpuric, at which time they are often palpable. They may be discrete, confluent, clustered, or individual. The entire body may be involved, although the lower extremities usually demonstrate the greatest eruption. A rash is the presenting symptom in 50% of patients. It may recur in 40% of patients within 6 weeks, often without systemic signs.
2. Colicky abdominal pain with diarrhea, often bloody, is commonly present. About 60% to 85% of patients have melena or hematemesis. Intussusception or perforation must be considered.
3. Nephritis associated with hematuria, proteinuria, and other nephrosis may develop. Renal involvement may begin after other symptoms and requires ongoing follow-up observation. Microscopic hematuria is common and carries a benign long-term prognosis; a "nephritic-nephrotic" presentation carries poor long-term prognosis.
4. Migratory polyarthritis, often transient, is present with greatest tenderness of ankles, knees, and wrist.
5. Other findings include soft tissue edema (scalp, ear, face, and dorsum of hands and feet), testicular pain, and parotitis.

Complications

1. Intussusception and abdominal distension.
2. Severe renal involvement progressing to nephritis. Renal involvement is the ultimate determinant of outcome and long-term sequelae and increases with advancing age.
3. CNS presentations include mental status change, hemiparesis, seizures, and intracranial hemorrhage.

Ancillary Data

1. Complete blood count (CBC) is variably elevated with left shift. Anemia may be present. Bleeding screen and platelet count are normal; erythrocyte sedimentation rate (ESR) is elevated.
2. Urinalysis reflects the degree of renal involvement. Hematuria, proteinuria, leukocytosis, and cylindruria may be noted.

If urinalysis is abnormal, other assessments of renal function are indicated.

3. Throat cultures for group A streptococci.
4. Blood cultures if bacteremia is a diagnostic consideration (i.e., fever or elevated WBC count).
5. Serum complement is normal.
6. Barium enema may be indicated to exclude intussusception if there is acute abdominal pain without evidence of perforation.
7. Renal biopsy is done in patients with severe nephropathy by a nephrologist after the acute phase of the illness. Mesangial IgA deposition is classically seen.
8. Skin biopsy of the purpuric lesions also demonstrates IgA deposition.

DIFFERENTIAL DIAGNOSIS

1. Infections, particularly those associated with petechial and purpuric eruption (e.g., meningococcemia, Rocky Mountain spotted fever) (see Table 42-1)
2. Thrombocytopenic purpura (platelet count should differentiate)
3. Nonthrombocytopenic purpura: Ehlers-Danlos syndrome, scurvy, massive steroid therapy, vasculitis
4. Glomerulonephritis
5. Intraabdominal abnormality: intussusception, trauma, appendicitis

MANAGEMENT

1. Supportive care. If evidence of GI hemorrhage or hypovolemia exists, initiate fluids and stabilization.
   a. Management of renal disease if there is abnormal function
   b. Evaluation for intussusception in patient with severe abdominal pain (p. 654)
   c. Exclusion of septicemic process
2. With significant GI pain and symptoms (once an acute abdomen is excluded), steroids may be useful: prednisone, 1-2 mg/kg/24 hr q12hr PO for 1 week. Steroids may also play a beneficial role in soft tissue and joint swelling and in preventing the progression of renal manifestations.
3. If acute renal failure or nephrosis is present, consult a nephrologist. Specific attention must be given to the control of blood pressure and intake and output. Treatment of more severe renal disease is controversial.

DISPOSITION

The patient should be hospitalized for observation and treatment unless skin manifestations are the only problem and close outpatient follow-up observation is possible. A poor prognosis is associated with children less than 6 years and with the presence of nephrotic syndrome or crescent formation in the glomeruli.

REFERENCES

Mollica F, LiVolti S, Garozzo R, et al: Effectiveness of early prednisone treatment in preventing the development of nephropathy in anaphylactoid purpura, *Eur J Pediatr* 151:140, 1992.
Robson W, Leung A: Henoch-Schönlein purpura, *Adv Pediatr* 41:163, 1994.
Rostoker G, et al: High-dose immunoglobulin therapy for severe IgA nephropathy and Henoch-Schönlein purpura, *Ann Intern Med* 120:476, 1994.

NEPHROTIC SYNDROME

Proteinuria occurs as a result of increased glomerular permeability in nephrotic syndrome. Most commonly affecting children less than 6 years of age, it is marked by massive proteinuria, edema, hypoalbuminemia, and hyperlipidemia.

ETIOLOGY

1. Primary renal disorders
   a. NIL or minimal change disease
   b. Focal glomerulosclerosis

c. Membranoproliferative glomerulone-phritis

d. Membranous glomerulonephritis

2. Intoxication: heroin, mercury, probene-cid, silver

3. Allergic reactions

   a. Poison ivy or oak, pollens

   b. Bee sting

   c. Snake venom

4. Infection

   a. Bacterial

   b. Viral: hepatitis B, cytomegalovirus, EB virus (infectious mononucleosis)

   c. Protozoa: malaria, toxoplasmosis

5. Neoplasm: Hodgkin's disease, Wilms' tumor, etc.

6. Autoimmune disorders: systemic lupus erythematosus

7. Metabolic disorder: diabetes mellitus

8. Cardiac disorders: congenital heart disease and congestive heart failure, pericarditis

9. Vasculitis: Henoch-Schönlein purpura, Wegener's granulomatosis

DIAGNOSTIC FINDINGS

1. Patients often report an upper respiratory infection or flulike symptoms before the development of edema. Because infection often exacerbates nephrotic syndrome, the physician should always look for an infection in the initial diagnostic evaluation or with patients who become unresponsive to steroids.

2. BP may be decreased if intravascular volume is depleted, or it may be increased with renal disease. Hypertension may be exacerbated by steroid therapy.

3. Patients have generalized peripheral edema and may have ascites with hepatomegaly.

4. Respiratory and cardiovascular status will reflect the extent of edema. Pleural effusion, pericardial effusion, pulmonary edema, and congestive heart failure may be present.

Complications

1. Infection. Patients are at increased risk of peritonitis and, if immunosuppressed, are susceptible to systemic infection. Septicemia, cellulitis, peritonitis, and pneumonitis are commonly caused by *S. pneumoniae*. They also are caused by *E. coli*, *Pseudomonas*, and *H. influenzae*.

2. Renal failure related to intravascular volume depletion.

3. Thromboembolism. Patients are hypercoagulable.

4. Protein-calorie malnutrition related to urinary protein losses.

5. Long-term effects of hypercholesterolemia, especially in patients who fail to respond to steroids.

Ancillary Data

1. WBC count to evaluate for infection.

2. Electrolytes, BUN, creatinine, calcium, and phosphorus levels. BUN and creatinine levels are elevated in 25% of children with minimal change nephrotic syndrome. Factitious hyponatremia (related to hyperlipidemia) is common.

3. Triglyceride and cholesterol levels. Plasma cholesterol carriers (low-density lipoprotein [LDL] and very low-density lipoprotein) are increased. Elevated lipid levels result from increased synthesis, as well as a defect in catabolism of phospholipid.

4. Hypoalbuminemia.

5. Spot urine protein/creatinine ratio greater than 1.0. A 24-hour urine collection is usually not routinely necessary. The protein level in a 24-hour urine collection is more than 3.5 gm protein/1.73 m^2/24 hr.

6. Further tests to evaluate potential cause only necessary in older children (Fig. 85-1). Should include serum complement (C3), ASO titer or streptozyme, antinuclear antibody (ANA), hepatitis studies (B and C), human immunodeficiency virus (HIV) when applicable.

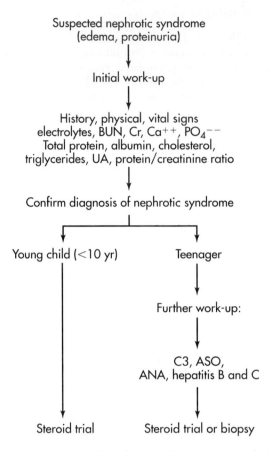

Fig. 85-1   Initial work-up and management of idiopathic childhood nephrotic syndrome.

7. Renal biopsy necessary only if poor prognostic signs are present:
   a. More than 10 years of age
   b. Decreased complement, positive ANA
   c. Failure to respond to steroids

DIFFERENTIAL DIAGNOSIS (see Chapter 37)

Diagnostic considerations in evaluating the patient with generalized edema include the following:
1. Renal: nephrotic syndrome, glomerulonephritis, renal failure
2. Cardiovascular: congestive heart failure, vasculitis, acute thrombosis
3. Endocrine/metabolic: hypothyroidism, starvation

4. Hematologic: hemolytic disease of the newborn
5. GI: cirrhosis, protein-losing enteritis, cystic fibrosis, lymphangitis
6. Iatrogenic: drugs (steroids, diuretics), water overload

MANAGEMENT (see Fig. 85-1)

1. After diagnosis and stabilization, the patient is begun on prednisone: 2 mg/kg (maximum: 80 mg/24 hr) divided BID PO for 4 to 6 weeks, then 1.5 mg/kg (maximum: 60 mg/dose) once every other morning PO for 4 to 6 weeks, then tapered. Of those patients who are going to respond, 73% do so within 14 days and 94% within 28 days. Other regimens have been suggested as well. Poor response to initial steroid therapy is generally predictive of a poor outcome.
   a. If remission (defined as clearing of proteinuria and return of serum albumin to normal) occurs and the patient relapses, begin prednisone again. Some children may be steroid dependent, relapsing as steroid dosage is tapered.
   b. After four relapses in less than 1 year or if the patient is steroid dependent, cytotoxic agents may then be considered. Either cyclophosphamide, 2 mg/kg/24 hr for 12 weeks, or chlorambucil, 0.2 mg/kg/24 hr for 12 weeks, is given in conjunction with prednisone, 1.0-1.5 mg/kg QOD. Consultation with a pediatric nephrologist should be obtained before cytotoxic agents are given.
   c. Patients who are steroid resistant (defined as failure to enter remission after more than 8 weeks of steroid therapy) are unlikely to have minimal change in disease and should be referred to a pediatric nephrologist for a renal biopsy. Drugs that may be useful in such patients include cyclosporine, "pulse" IV

SoluMedrol (with or without cytotoxic agents), and angiotensin-converting enzyme (ACE) inhibitors.

    d. Teenagers with nephrotic syndrome are less likely to be steroid sensitive than younger children, and early referral to a pediatric nephrologist should be considered.

2. Initiate sodium restriction (2-3 gm/day) to minimize edema formation. A high-protein diet, however, is not indicated and may increase urinary protein losses.

3. Give young children prophylactic low-dose amoxicillin (125 mg BID if <20 kg, 250 mg BID if >20 kg) when they are nephrotic because of the risk of infection with encapsulated organisms.

4. Avoid oral diuretics because of the increased risk of thrombosis.

DISPOSITION

1. Most children with uncomplicated nephrotic syndrome can be managed as outpatients.

2. Admit if complications are present:
    a. Renal insufficiency
    b. Severe, symptomatic hypertension
    c. Anasarca
    d. Thrombosis
    e. Peritonitis or other severe infection

3. Management of fluid overload (anasarca): Begin 25% albumin infusion, 2 gm/kg/day, over 24 hours; 6 to 8 hours after albumin infusion begun, give furosemide, 1 mg/kg/dose, q8-12hr. Observe carefully for complications of albumin infusion, including hypertension and pulmonary edema.

4. Provide IV antibiotics, heparinization, and antihypertensive therapy as indicated.

REFERENCES

Ehrich JHH, Brodehl J: Long versus standard prednisone therapy for initial treatment of idiopathic nephrotic syndrome in children, *Eur J Pediatr* 152:357, 1993.

Mendoza SA, Reznik VM, Griswold WR, et al: Treatment of steroid-resistant focal segmental glomerulosclerosis with pulse methylprednisolone and alkylating agents, *Pediatr Nephrol* 4:303, 1990.

Niaudet P, Habib R: Cyclosporine in the treatment of idiopathic nephrosis, *J Am Soc Nephrol* 5:1049, 1994.

Sakarcan A, Timmons C, Seikaly M: Reversible idiopathic acute renal failure in children with primary nephrotic syndrome, *J Pediatr* 125:723, 1994.

Schulman SL, Kaiser BA, Polinsky MS, et al: Predicting the response to cytotoxic therapy for childhood nephrotic syndrome: superiority of response to corticosteroid therapy over histopathologic patterns, *J Pediatr* 113:996, 1988.

Warshaw BL: Nephrotic syndrome in children, *Pediatr Ann* 23:495, 1994.

Wynn SR, Stickler GB, Burke EC: Long-term prognosis for children with nephrotic syndrome, *Clin Pediatr* 27:63, 1988.

ACUTE RENAL FAILURE

Acute renal failure occurs when there is a sudden impairment of the kidney's ability to regulate internal homeostasis. Once diagnosed, it is imperative that the cause be delineated rapidly to facilitate implementation of appropriate therapeutic steps. It may be prerenal (decreased perfusion of the kidney), intrarenal (damage to the kidney tissue itself), or postrenal (obstruction of the urinary tract).

ETIOLOGY

See Table 85-1.

DIAGNOSTIC FINDINGS (Table 85-2)

1. The history can provide some clue about the cause of renal failure.
    a. Prerenal patients have a history of decreased perfusion of the kidney. This may include dehydration from vomiting, diarrhea, diabetic ketoacidosis, decreased intravascular volume as a result of nephrotic syndrome, burns, or shock resulting from hemorrhage, sepsis, cardiac failure, or anaphylaxis.
    b. Intrarenal failure results from direct

TABLE 85-1   Common Causes of Acute Renal Failure

Prerenal (decreased perfusion of an intact nephron)*	Intrarenal (damage of the actual nephron)	Postrenal (downstream obstruction with initially intact nephron)*

Shock: hypovolemic
  Dehydration
  Hemorrhagic
  Diabetic ketoacidosis
  Burn
Shock: distributive
  Septic
  Anaphylactic
Shock: cardiogenic
Nephrotic syndrome with
  intravascular volume
  depletion from de-
  creased oncotic
  pressure
	Primary glomerular disease
	  Acute poststreptococcal nephritis
	  Membranoproliferative glomerulo-
	    nephritis
	  Rapidly progressive glomerulo-
	    nephritis
	Systemic disease
	  Henoch-Schönlein purpura
	  Hemolytic-uremic syndrome
	  Vasculitides
	  Bacterial endocarditis
	Systemic lupus erythematosus
	Nephrotoxins
	  Antibiotics (aminoglycoside,
	    methicillin)
	  Metals (gold, lead)
	  Antihypertensives (captopril)
	  Anticonvulsant (phenytoin)
	  Rhabdomyolysis (pigment damage
	    to nephron)
	  Radiocontrast materials
	  Nonsteroidal antiinflammatory drugs
	    (e.g., indomethacin, ibuprofen)
	  Organic solvent (carbon tetrachlo-
	    ride, methanol, toluene)
	Vascular
	  Renal vein thrombosis
	  Renal artery thrombosis or embolism
	Acute tubular necrosis (caused by
	    prolonged decreased perfusion)
		Posterior urethral valves
		Ureteropelvic junction (if bilateral)
		Stones (bilateral)
		Crystals
		  Sulfonamides
		  Uric acid
		Retroperitoneal fibrosis or tumor
		Trauma to collecting system
		Ureterocele
		Acquired urethral obstruction
		Abscess
		Constipation

*Prolonged obstruction or uncorrected hypoperfusion eventually leads to irreversible nephron damage.

intrinsic nephron damage occurring in glomerulonephritis (hematuria, proteinuria, edema, and hypertension), HUS (anemia, uremia, and thrombocytopenia), nephrotoxins, massive crush injuries, vascular catastrophes (renal thrombosis or embolic phenomena), overwhelming infection, or DIC.

  c. Postrenal failure results from obstruction, and is commonly seen in genitourinary (GU) malformations (posterior urethral valves, ureteropelvic junction obstruction), or in the presence of stone disease or abdominal masses. If of acute onset, this may be accompanied by abdominal and flank papain.

2. Physical examination can reflect the underlying renal and fluid abnormality:
  a. Hypovolemia (hypotension or orthostatic changes and tachycardia)
  b. Volume overload (increased blood pressure, edema, congestive heart failure)

TABLE 85-2   Differential Diagnosis of Acute Renal Failure

Prerenal	Intrarenal	Postrenal
Ultrasound: normal	Ultrasound: can have increased renal density or slight swelling	Ultrasonography: dilated bladder or kidney
Serum BUN-to-creatinine ratio >15:1		History and examination may be diagnostic
Urine Na^+ <15 mEq/L	Urine Na^+ >20 mEq/L	Indexes not helpful
Urine osmolality >500 mOsm/kg H_2O	Urine osmolality <350 mOsm/kg H_2O	
Urine-to-plasma creatinine ratio >40:1	Urine-to-plasma creatinine ratio <20:1 (often <5:1)	
Fractional excretion of Na^+ <1 (<2.5 in neonates)	Fractional excretion of Na^+ >2 (>2.5 in neonates)	

$$\text{Fractional excretion of } Na^+ = \frac{\text{Urine } Na^+ \text{ (mEq/L)}}{\text{Plasma } Na^+ \text{ (mEq/L)}} \times \frac{\text{Plasma creatinine (mg/dl)}}{\text{Urine creatinine (mg/dl)}}$$

Prerenal	Intrarenal	Postrenal
Urine sediment benign	Urine sediment "active" (casts, RBCs, WBCs, tubular cells)	Urine sediment benign

c. Obstruction (increased kidney size or large bladder)

d. Abdominal or flank mass

e. Signs of systemic infection or autoimmune disease

3. Patients may be oliguric (urine output <1 ml/kg/hr) or nonoliguric with a volume inappropriate to maintain hemostasis. Azotemia (increase in plasma concentration of nitrogenous waste products, i.e., BUN and creatinine) is present.

Complications

1. Fluid overload with associated congestive heart failure.

2. Hypertension from fluid overload or inappropriate renin production.

3. Azotemia with elevated potassium, BUN, and creatinine levels.

4. Dysrhythmias from hyperkalemia or hypocalcemia.

5. Hypocalcemia and high phosphorus level, leading to cardiac dysrhythmias, tetany, and altered mental status.

6. Acidosis from diminished H^+ secretion by kidney.

7. Hyperphosphatemia. High $Ca^{++} \times PO_4^{--}$ product (>70) can produce calcification in soft tissues and reciprocal hypocalcemia.

8. Altered level of consciousness, seizures, and coma from metabolic derangements (e.g., elevated BUN and potassium levels and decreased Ca^{++} levels), cerebral edema, and hypertension.

9. Bleeding resulting from platelet dysfunction associated with uremia. Anemia.

Ancillary Data

1. Electrolyte, Ca^{++}, PO_4^{--}, BUN, and creatinine levels, CBC, and platelets

2. Urinalysis with microscopic examination of urinary sediment

3. Urine sodium, creatinine, potassium, and osmolality

4. Renal ultrasonography, including Doppler assessment of arterial and venous flow

5. Chest x-ray film (helpful in assessing volume status)

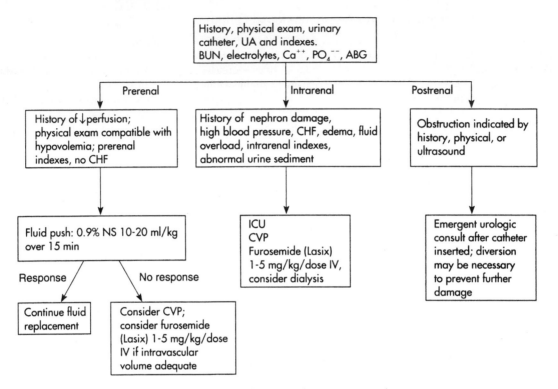

Fig. 85-2   Acute renal failure: initial assessment and treatment.

6. Electrocardiogram (ECG) and cardiac monitor

DIFFERENTIAL DIAGNOSIS

Combining data from history and physical examination, and serum, urine, and radiologic studies is the best method for differentiating among prerenal, intrarenal, and postrenal failure (see Table 85-2).

MANAGEMENT

Initial stabilization must focus on determining the cause and classification of the acute renal failure to permit appropriate therapeutic intervention. The initial approach is outlined in Fig. 85-2. Intake and urine output must be measured closely. A urinary catheter (6 months: 8 Fr; 1 to 2 years: 10 Fr; 5 years: 10 to 12 Fr; 8 to 10 years: 12 Fr) is usually necessary. Monitoring of central venous pressure (CVP) is helpful in following volume status.

Fluid Balance

Furosemide

Furosemide (Lasix) is a potent diuretic, and administration should be considered if the intravascular volume is adequate or overloaded according to CVP measurements.

1. Give 2-4 mg/kg/dose (high dosage to be used if creatinine is elevated).
2. If there is no response after two doses at maximum amount, do not continue because of potential nephrotoxicity and ototoxicity.
3. Do not give if evidence of obstruction is present.

4. A good response to diuretics is the formation of 6-10 ml/kg of urine over the subsequent 1 to 3 hours.

5. If patient responds to initial dose of furosemide, consider starting continuous infusion at 0.25-1.0 mg/kg/hr.

Administration of Fluids

If the patient remains oliguric or anuric, fluids should be administered to keep the patient intravascularly normal. Replace insensible (one third of maintenance fluid requirements) water losses with dextrose water, urine losses milliliter for milliliter with 0.45% NS, and other fluid losses (vomitus, diarrhea) milliliter for milliliter with Ringer's lactate or 0.45% NS. Composition of urine or other fluids being lost should be monitored and replacement fluid adjusted to maintain electrolyte balance.

Caloric requirements and protein intake must be considered. In general, protein intake should be limited to slow the rise of BUN, and adequate calories should be given in the form of carbohydrates and fat to enable anabolism.

Dopamine

A low-dose intravenous (IV) infusion of dopamine (1-5 µg/kg/min) increases renal blood flow and sodium excretion. It may be useful in ischemic renal injury.

Dialysis

Rapid referral for dialysis is mandatory for those patients with severe fluid overload or metabolic derangement who do not respond to the conservative measures listed above.

Hypertension (see Chapter 18)

Hypertension may be caused by fluid overload or high renin secretion. Any child having acute hypertension with a diastolic pressure greater than the 99th percentile for age should be treated parenterally because of the risk of seizures, encephalopathy, and other sequelae of hypertension. Only a mild reduction in pressure is needed in an acute situation, perhaps down to the 90th to 95th percentile blood pressure for age.

Parenteral Therapy

Parenteral therapy should be given sequentially, with observation for a response.

1. Furosemide (Lasix), 1 mg/kg/dose q6hr IV, facilitates action of vasodilators by volume contraction.

2. Diazoxide (Hyperstat), 1-3 mg/kg/dose by rapid infusion, may be repeated q30-60min. It is a vasodilator, and fluid infusion reverses severe hypotension.

3. Nitroprusside (Nipride) may be used instead of diazoxide: 0.5-10 µg/kg/min IV infusion (average: 3 µg/kg/min). A potent vasodilator, it requires constant monitoring. Nitroprusside provides the most exact method of controlling malignant hypertension because of its very short half-life. Buildup of thiocyanate (produced by breakdown of nitroprusside) limits the duration of time that nitroprusside can be used to 48 to 72 hours.

4. Hydralazine may be used if a slower acting, longer duration vasodilator is preferred in place of diazoxide or nitroprusside: 0.1-0.2 mg (rarely up to 0.5 mg)/kg/dose q4-6hr IV or IM. Use in combination with diazoxide to potentiate effect. Availability of hydralazine may be limited because it is being reformulated.

5. Another good option is labetalol, 0.4-1.0 mg/kg/dose, which may be repeated up to a total of 3.0 mg/kg over first hour of treatment. Labetalol can also be given by constant infusion at a dose of 0.25-3.0 mg/kg/hr.

6. Nicardipine is an IV calcium channel blocking agent that has been used in severe hypertension in both children and adults. It is given as a constant infusion at 1-3 µg/kg/min.

The choice of medication depends on urgency of treatment, knowledge of agents, and availability of monitoring equipment. Vasodilators may eventually cause compensatory tachycardia and may require the addition of a beta blocker such as propranolol (Inderal), 1 mg/kg/24 hr q6hr PO.

Hyperkalemia

Hyperkalemia causes membrane excitability with possible cardiac dysrhythmias. K^+ greater than 6.5 mEq/L can causes ECG changes consisting of peaked T waves and, eventually, widened QRS complex. Cardiac toxicity is enhanced by hypocalcemia, hyponatremia, or acidosis.

Potassium level greater than 7.0 mEq/L requires rapid intervention in the following sequence:

1. Calcium chloride 10%, 0.2-0.3 ml (20-30 mg)/kg/dose (maximum: 5 ml or 500 mg/dose), or calcium gluconate, 1.0 ml (100 mg)/kg/dose IV. Calcium chloride can cause bradycardia and should be given slowly over 5 to 10 minutes. It can also cause severe tissue necrosis if it extravasates so administration through a central line is preferred. Calcium gluconate can be given peripherally.
   a. It changes the cell-action potential, protecting the heart from dysrhythmias.
   b. It can be repeated up to four times or until serum calcium increases.
   c. Its effect lasts about 30 minutes.
2. $NaHCO_3$.
   a. Alkalosis helps exchange H^+ for K^+, thereby moving potassium intracellularly and normalizing membrane potential.
   b. $NaHCO_3$, 1-2 mEq/kg/dose IV push q2-4hr, or as required by pH is useful in emergent situations (as well as in combination with Kayexalate for asymptomatic hyperkalemia [K^+ <6.5 mEq/L]).
3. Glucose and insulin (to move K^+ intracellularly).
   a. Give glucose, 0.5-1.0 gm/kg, followed by 1 unit of insulin IV for every 4 gm of glucose infused; may repeat q10-30min.

b. Monitor Dextrostix/Chemstrip tests and glucose carefully. The effect lasts 1 to 3 hours.
4. Kayexalate (an ion exchange resin). Give 1 gm resin/kg/dose q4-6hr preferably mixed with 70% sorbitol PO (may use a nasogastric [NG] tube) or PR. For newborn give 1 gm/kg/dose with Kayexalate dissolved in 10% dextrose to make 25% solution.
   a. It is useful in combination with $NaHCO_3$ for K^+ less than 6.5 mEq/L.
   b. It may cause hypocalcemia and hypomagnesemia, gastric irritation, and diarrhea.
5. Albuterol by continuous nebulization may also be a helpful adjunctive measure. Like several of the measures listed, albuterol acts by shifting potassium intracellularly. Administration of Kayexalate or dialysis is still required for definitive treatment of hyperkalemia.

Metabolic Acidosis

Give $NaHCO_3$, 1-2 mEq/kg/dose q6hr IV push, as indicated by ABG, exercising care to avoid fluid overload. Alternatively, 75 mEq/L of $NaHCO_3$ can be added to IV fluids used for maintenance.

NOTE: If severe acidosis and fluid overload are present, rapid dialysis is mandatory.

Hyponatremia

Hyponatremia usually is a result of water overload. Water intake should be restricted to insensible plus extraordinary losses.

Hyperphosphatemia

Calcium carbonate, calcium acetate, or aluminum hydroxide should be given to bind dietary phosphorus. Aluminum is potentially toxic and should be used only for short-term therapy.

Rapid Dialysis (Peritoneal or Hemodialysis)

Indications are as follows:

1. Fluid overload refractory to medical management with congestive heart failure or hypertension
2. Severe hyperkalemia
3. Severe hyponatremia or hypernatremia
4. Unresponsive metabolic acidosis, particularly with fluid overload
5. BUN greater than 80 to 100 mg/dl, although not an absolute indication
6. Uremia producing alteration in consciousness or seizures

Technology has made dialysis possible for even the smallest infant. In the intensive care unit (ICU) setting, newer continuous renal replacement therapies (hemofiltration, hemodiafiltration) may be preferable because of the ability to give large volumes of parenteral nutrition and other fluids.

Other Considerations

Intravenous pyelograms and computed tomography (CT) scans with IV contrast should not be done in an individual with renal failure because of the risk of nephrotoxicity from the dye. Ultrasonography and renal scans are preferable for initial evaluation.

DISPOSITION

All patients require hospitalization and a nephrology consultation.

REFERENCES

Deal JE, Barratt TM, Dillon MJ: Management of hypertensive emergencies, *Arch Dis Child* 67:1089, 1992.
Feld L, Chachero S, Springate J: Fluid needs in acute renal failure, *Pediatr Clin North Am* 37:337, 1990.
Fildes RD, Springate JE, Field LE: Acute renal failure: management of suspected and established disease, *J Pediatr* 109:401, 567, 1986.
Foreman JW, Chan JCM: Chronic renal failure in infants and children, *J Pediatr* 113:793, 1988.
McClure RJ, Prasad VK, Brocklebank JT: Treatment of hyperkalemia using intravenous and nebulised salbutamol, *Arch Dis Child* 70:126, 1994.
Mehta RL: Therapeutic alternatives to renal replacement for critically ill patients in acute renal failure, *Semin Nephrol* 14:64, 1994.
Peter JR, Steinhardt GF: Acute urinary retention in children, *Pediatr Emerg Care* 9:205, 1993.
Sehic A, Chesney RW: Acute renal failure: diagnosis, *Pediatr Rev* 16:101, 1995.
Sehic A, Chesney RW: Acute renal failure: therapy, *Pediatr Rev* 16:137, 1995.
Thadhani R, Pascual M, Bonventre JV: Acute renal failure, *N Engl J Med* 334:1448, 1996.

URINARY TRACT INFECTION
Suzanne Z. Barkin

ALERT: Symptoms often are nonspecific. Appropriate cultures, treatment, and follow-up observation are required.

Urinary tract infections (UTIs) range from being asymptomatic to causing systemic disease associated with pyelonephritis. Long-term sequelae may include hypertension and chronic renal failure in some children with recurrent infections and vesicoureteral reflux.

ETIOLOGY: INFECTION

Bacteria causing most infections are normal rectal and perineal flora, including *E. coli*, *Klebsiella* organisms, enteric streptococci, and, rarely, *S. aureus* or *epidermidis*. Organisms gain entry into the GU tract by hematogenous spread in infants, whereas vesicoureteral reflux is the major risk factor in older children.

Uncommonly, viral, fungal, and mycobacterial agents are causative.

DIAGNOSTIC FINDINGS

Predisposing factors include poor perineal hygiene, the short urethra of females, infrequent voiding, and sexual activity. Circumcision may reduce the male's risk of a UTI developing.

Females have a higher incidence; the prevalence of UTIs in girls aged 2 months to 2 years is twice that of boys. Males with UTI have a high incidence of anatomic abnormality.

Symptoms in younger children are often nonspecific. The diagnosis in this age group is particularly important because it may indicate the presence of vesicoureteral reflux or another anatomic abnormality that may predispose the child to recurrent infections. In addition, the risk of renal scarring is greatest in children less than 1 year of age.

1. Neonates may have fever or hypothermia, poor feeding, failure to thrive, jaundice, sepsis, or cyanosis.
2. Infants may experience vomiting, diarrhea, fever, and poor feeding.
3. Older children have the more classic signs and symptoms of fever, abdominal pain, vomiting, enuresis, and urinary frequency, dysuria, and urgency.

Systemic toxicity accompanied by high temperatures, chills, and variably, costovertebral angle (CVA) pain often accompany upper urinary tract disease and pyelonephritis.

Historically, it is important to ascertain whether the patient has had previous episodes of infection. The physical examination should determine whether evidence of genitourinary malformations, hypertension, or poor growth exists.

The risk of recurrence is greatest in the first month after a UTI and increases with repeated infections.

Complications

1. Chronic renal failure resulting from recurrent pyelonephritis/reflux nephropathy.
   a. Incidence of scarring is greatest in children less than 1 year of age but can still be seen in older children.
   b. Scarring can be prevented by early detection and treatment of infection, and detection of vesicoureteral reflux.
2. Bacteremia.

3. Perinephric abscess.
4. Sepsis.
5. Urolithiasis is uncommon but may follow infection. Findings may include abdominal or flank pain, recurrent or persistent pyuria, and gross hematuria.

Ancillary Data

Urine Culture

Urine culture is the basis for making the diagnosis, and the quality of the specimen is an important determinant of the results. In asymptomatic or minimally ill patients, a clean-catch midstream specimen (CCMS) should be obtained after carefully cleansing the perineum and urethra. In patients who are toxic, specimens should be obtained by suprapubic aspiration (see Appendix A-7) or a straight catheterization, particularly in infants. In younger children the catheterization may be done by using a No. 5 Fr sterile feeding tube. The first 5 ml of urine is discarded and the remainder cultured. Bag urine is not satisfactory for adequate diagnosis.

1. The specimen must be cultured within 30 minutes or placed in a refrigerator. If not, the colony count may be elevated and is not reliable.
2. The interpretation of the culture varies with the method of collection (Table 85-3). Cultures that are uninterpretable

TABLE 85-3   Criteria for Diagnosis of UTI

Collection method	Probability of infection (based on colony forming units/ml*)		
	Unlikely	**Possible†**	**Likely**
Suprapubic	0		Any
Catheterization	$<10^3$	10^3-10^4	$\geq10^4$
CCMS‡	$<10^3$	10^4-10^5	$\geq10^5$

*Pure culture (single organims).
†If patient symptomatic or if dilute urine sample.
‡*CCMS*, Clean-catch midstream.

need to be repeated by a reliable method of specimen collection. Dilution (e.g., specimens that are not first morning void) or improper medium may lower the colony count. Other causes of low colony counts include recent antimicrobial therapy, fastidious organisms, bacteriostatic agents in urine, and complete obstruction of the ureter.

Urinalysis

Urinalysis is a useful diagnostic tool but not definitive. It may be normal in infants with UTI. Dilute urine specimens can be particularly misleading.

1. Pyuria (>5 WBC/HPF) is present in more than half of patients with UTI.
2. Causes of pyuria besides UTI include chemical (bubble bath) or physical (masturbation) irritation, other irritation, dehydration, renal tuberculosis, trauma, acute glomerulonephritis, respiratory infections, appendicitis, other abdominal and pelvic infections, gastroenteritis, and administration of oral polio vaccine.
3. The presence of leukocyte esterase correlates with the presence of pyuria, which is often but not always present with UTI.
4. A positive nitrite test implies that bacteria capable of fixing the nitrate normally found in urine have been present in the urine. A first morning urine is the optimal specimen.
5. Gram stain of urinary sediment is more reliable than dipstick methods of diagnosis and may be superior to the traditional urinalysis.

Radiologic Studies (Table 85-4)

These rarely are emergently indicated unless severe toxicity or evidence of obstruction is present. Those children who require radiologic evaluation after UTI include the following:

1. Infants less than 3 months of age
2. Males (increased association with anomaly)
3. Clinical signs and symptoms consistent with pyelonephritis
4. Clinical evidence of renal disease (e.g., high blood pressure or BUN or creatinine level)
5. After the second documented lower tract UTI in females, although some authorities recommend that these patients should be studied after the first infection

The optimal approach to evaluation remains controversial. Ultrasonography should be done in most settings (see Table 85-4) to evaluate renal size, evidence of hydronephrosis, and bladder abnormalities. However, the fluoroscopic voiding cystourethrogram (VCUG) is the most important screening test in children. The VCUG shows whether reflux is present and if so, its severity (graded I to V) while permitting visualization of the urethra, with its potentially correctable lesions. Many are substituting a nuclear cystogram for a fluoroscopic VCUG in females.

TABLE 85-4 Radiologic Evaluation of Children with Urinary Tract Infections

Age	Clinical setting	Imaging evaluation	
		Ultrasound	Voiding cystourethrogram
Infant <3 mo	Any infection	Within 2-3 days	Within 1-2 wk
Girls 3 mo-adolescence	Afebrile cystitis	As above	After second episode
	Febrile infection	As above	After first episode up to age 6 yr
Boys 3 mo-adolescence	Any infection	As above	Within 1-2 wk
Adolescent girls	Cystitis	After second or third episode within 12-18 mo	If ultrasonogram abnormal or if voiding dysfunction present

Adapted from Hellerstein S: *Pediatr Clin North Am* 42:1433, 1995.

In the acute setting, a normal renal ultrasonographic study does not exclude the diagnosis of pyelonephritis. The most sensitive test for demonstration of renal parenchymal involvement is the DMSA renal scan.

IVPs are performed less commonly because the nuclear DMSA scan is a more sensitive indicator of renal scarring. The optimal use of DMSA scans, however, is yet to be determined.

Blood Cultures

These are indicated in the febrile, toxic patient.

Blood Creatinine and Urea Nitrogen Levels

These should be obtained in patients with evidence of pyelonephritis, recurrent infections, or hypertension.

DIFFERENTIAL DIAGNOSIS

1. Trauma. Chemical (bubble bath) or physical (masturbation or perineal injury) irritation may cause discomfort.
2. Infection.
   a. Viral, mycobacterial, and fungal agents may cause similar symptoms with associated pyuria. Culture techniques need to be specific for these organisms.
   b. Vaginitis may cause irritation with comparable symptoms.
   c. Pinworms may cause perineal pain resulting from both inflammation and itching.
   d. Urethritis caused by *Neisseria gonorrhoeae* or *Chlamydia trachomatis* often is associated with a discharge. It may cause dysuria, suprapubic discomfort, and, in the male, prostatic or rectal tenderness.

MANAGEMENT

1. When UTI is suspected, an appropriate urine culture should be obtained. Suprapubic or catheterized specimens are indicated for moderately ill patients. A CCMS specimen for the minimally ill individual is appropriate and, if abnormal, should be repeated.
2. A urinalysis (UA) should be done. If normal, urine should be sent for culture. If pyuria or bacteriuria are found, the specimen should be sent for culture and the appropriate medication initiated. Urine sediment can also be Gram stained to assist in the diagnosis.
3. *A lower urinary tract infection (cystitis)* commonly has associated urinary symptoms of urgency, frequency, and dysuria. Appropriate management is to push fluids initially and to treat with antibiotics for a minimum of 10 days:
   a. Amoxicillin, 30-50 mg/kg/24 hr q8hr PO; or
   b. Trimethoprim (TMP) with sulfamethoxazole (SMZ), 8 mg TMP and 40 mg SMZ/kg/24 q12hr PO; or
   c. Cephalexin (Keflex), 25-100 mg/kg/24 hr q6hr PO; or
   d. Nitrofurantoin (Macrodantin), 5-7 mg/kg/24 hr q6hr PO.
      Final choice of antibiotics should reflect sensitivity and clinical response. Duration of therapy should be 7 to 10 days, except in adolescent girls with uncomplicated cystitis, in whom shorter regimens (1 to 3 days) may be adequate.
4. **Pyelonephritis** has associated systemic toxicity (temperature, chills, CVA tenderness) and requires broader coverage antibiotics. Until cultures and sensitivities are available (24 to 48 hours), a combination of one of the drugs noted above in No. 3 used in treating lower tract infection; **and** gentamicin or tobramycin, 5.0-7.5 mg/kg/24 hr q8-12hr IM or IV, should be given. For the patient with only moderate toxicity who is to be followed as an outpatient, administration of gentamicin, 2.0-2.5 mg/kg/dose (maximum: 80 mg/

dose), or ceftriaxone, 50 mg/kg/dose (maximum: 2.0 gm/dose) IM once, in combination with continuing oral therapy provides sufficient treatment pending isolation and determination of sensitivities in 24 to 48 hours. Cefixime (Suprax), 8 mg/kg/24 hr q12hr PO, is an excellent broad-spectrum antibiotic that may be useful in this setting. Those requiring hospitalization should be treated with standard parenteral daily doses.

5. If urinary dysuria, urgency, or frequency are predominant symptoms, temporary relief can be obtained with phenazopyridine (Pyridium), a urinary tract analgesic, at 12 mg/kg/24 hr orally in three doses q8hr up to 200 mg/dose for 1 to 3 days. Urine will turn orange.

6. Follow-up should be ensured in 48 hours to determine whether the patient is clinically improved and that the etiologic organism is sensitive to the medication. If there is any question, a repeat UA and urine culture should be obtained. Medication may need to be altered.

7. The patient should return in 14 days for a repeat UA and culture after a total course of antibiotics of 10 days. Close follow-up observation over the next year is appropriate because of the increased risk of recurrence. The greater the number of previous episodes, the more likely the infection will recur. In the first year the chance of recurrence is as high as 50%.

DISPOSITION

1. Patients who are toxic, pregnant, or compromised hosts; who are unable to maintain hydration or retain medications; or who have debilitating systemic disease should be hospitalized. In addition, those with previous renal disease associated with impaired function, foreign bodies (catheter), or stones should be hospitalized. Other criteria that should be considered include the likelihood of resistant organisms, failure on previous outpatient therapy, previous pyelonephritis within 30 days, and the reliability of the patient.

2. Most patients may be followed at home with appropriate antibiotic therapy. Compliance must be ensured and follow-up evaluation arranged in 1 to 2 days.

3. High-risk patients should be evaluated radiologically (see Table 85-4).
   a. If vesicoureteral reflux is present, the patient is typically maintained on prophylactic antibiotics (TMP/SMZ, 2 mg/kg/day of TMP given QHS) and a follow-up cystogram obtained in 12 to 18 months.
   b. Patients with recurrent UTI despite prophylaxis or with high-grade reflux should be referred to a pediatric urologist.

4. If signs of renal damage are present (elevated creatinine, proteinuria, or hypertension), refer to a pediatric nephrologist.

Parental Education

1. Give all of the medication. Call your physician if your child does not tolerate the medication.

2. A urine culture has been obtained. In 2 days you should contact your care provider to be sure that the child is taking the correct medicine and feeling better.

3. Two weeks after your initial visit, your care giver will want to see the child again for another culture. Periodic checks will be made over the next year.

4. To help prevent repeat infections, particularly in girls, try the following:
   a. Teach her to wipe correctly from front to back.
   b. Do *not* use bubble baths or let the soap float around in the bath.

    c. Treat constipation with mineral oil or a stool softener.

    d. Encourage frequent urination.

5. Call your physician if the following occur:

    a. Fever or pain with urination is not gone in 48 hours after beginning antibiotics.

    b. The child feels worse or does not tolerate the medication.

REFERENCES

Benador D, Benador N, Slosaan DO, et al: Cortical scintigraphy in the evaluation of renal parenchymal changes in children with pyelonephritis, *J Pediatr* 124:17, 1994.

Choi H, Snyder HM, Duckett JW: Urolithiasis in childhood: current management, *J Pediatr Surg* 22:158, 1987.

Dick PT, Feldman W: Routine diagnostic imaging for childhood urinary tract infection: a systematic overview, *J Pediatr* 128:15, 1996.

Durbin WA, Peter G: Management of urinary tract infections in infants and children, *Pediatr Infect Dis* 3:564, 1984.

Fine JS, Jacobson MS: Single-dose versus conventional therapy of urinary tract infections in female adolescents, *Pediatrics* 75:916, 1985.

Hellerstein S: Urinary tract infections, *Pediatr Clin North Am* 42:1433, 1995.

Hoberman A, Chao HP, Keller DM, et al: Prevalence of urinary tract infection in febrile infants, *J Pediatr* 123:17, 1993.

Lockhart GR, Lewander WJ, Cimini DM: Use of urinary gram stain for detection of urinary tract infection in infants, *Ann Emerg Med* 25:31, 1995.

Majad M, Rushton HG: Renal cortical scintigraphy in the diagnosis of acute pyelonephritis, *Semin Nucl Med* 22:98, 1992.

Lohr JA: The foreskin and urinary tract infections, *J Pediatr* 114:502, 1989.

Lohr JA, Donowitz LG, Dudley SM: Bacterial contamination rates in voided urine collection in girls, *J Pediatr* 114:91, 1989.

Naber KG: Cefixime in urinary tract infections (specific studies and literature in review), *Infection* 18(suppl 3):S132, 1990.

Pollack CV, Pollack ES, Andrew ME: Suprapubic bladder aspiration versus urethral catheterization in ill infants: success, efficiency and complication rates, *Ann Emerg Med* 23:224, 1994.

Stahl GE, Topf P, Fleisher GR, et al: Single dose treatment of uncomplicated urinary tract infections in children, *Ann Emerg Med* 13:705, 1984.

A PROCEDURES

Several procedures are unique to the pediatric patient. Others are done rarely and require some familiarity with the crucial landmarks. The descriptions included in this section are not meant to be inclusive but to serve as reminders of important aspects of techniques to those individuals who have had experience performing them in a supervised setting that included direct observation and instruction. This section is not intended to be a training manual for practitioners without previous experience in invasive procedures. Consent should be obtained when appropriate but should not delay lifesaving procedures in unstable patients.

Preparing a child for a procedure may facilitate the process and must be related to the child's age, developmental status, and ability to understand. Initially, determine what the parents know about the procedure and what they have told the child. Encourage the child to ask questions while presenting small amounts of information at a time. Describe the procedure in terms of what the child will feel, taste, see, or smell, while making the child as comfortable as possible. Appeal to older toddlers (2 to 4 years), who desire to please, by encouraging them to help, assist with the Band-Aid, or make choices when appropriate.

APPENDIX A-1: ARTERIAL PUNCTURES

Arterial punctures are used routinely to obtain heparinized blood for arterial blood gas (ABG) determinations. Most laboratories can make the determination with less than 1 ml of heparin-ized blood. A tuberculin syringe is filled with heparin that is then squirted out, allowing a small amount to remain in the hub. A 25-gauge needle is used in newborns and infants. The site is identified and prepared before puncture. After withdrawal of the needle, pressure should be applied to the site for at least 5 minutes.

1. The radial artery is the preferred site because of its stability and lack of an accompanying vein. It is entered tangentially (Fig A-1).
2. The posterior tibial artery, located between the medial malleolus and the Achilles tendon.
3. The femoral artery, which should be used only in life-threatening situations.

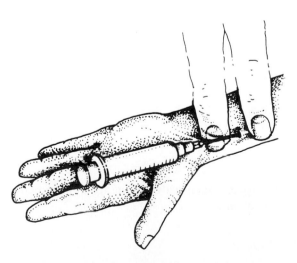

Fig. A-1   Localization of radial artery for puncture.

821

APPENDIX A-2: ARTHROCENTESIS

Arthrocentesis is essential in excluding infection in a joint that is acutely swollen or painful or that has limited range of motion.

SITE AND POSITION

Knee

The patient is placed on his or her back with the knee fully extended. The needle (18-gauge) is passed laterally or medially beneath the midpoint of the patella so that it enters the knee joint midway between the patella and the patellar grove of the femur.

Ankle

The ankle is approached either medially or laterally, reflecting the area of maximal swelling. For those with lateral swelling, the foot is placed in neutral position, and a 20- to 22-gauge needle is inserted horizontally 1 cm both medial and inferior to the tip of the lateral malleolus. Medial swelling also requires the foot to be in a neutral position, and the 20- to 22-gauge needle is directed horizontally just above and lateral to the medial malleolus, medial to the extensor hallucis longus tendon.

Elbow

Lateral aspiration is done by positioning the elbow joint at a 90-degree angle. The needle (20- to 22-gauge) is inserted perpendicularly, below the lateral epicondyle and above the olecranon process.

Hip

Arthrocentesis usually is done by an orthopedic consultant.

PROCEDURE

Aseptic technique is essential. The area should be shaved (if necessary) and the skin prepared with a povidone-iodine scrub, followed by cleansing with an alcohol scrub. The procedure is not routinely done in the presence of overlying cellulitis or a coagulation disorder.

Anesthetic agents (1% to 2% lidocaine) are infiltrated into the skin with a 23- to 25-gauge needle. A new bottle of anesthetic agent should be used to ensure sterility.

A large 18-gauge needle normally should be attached to a 5- to 10-ml syringe for aspiration of large joints (20- to 22-gauge for smaller joints). If large amounts of fluid are anticipated, the syringe may be connected to a stopcock and a larger syringe attached once free flow is established. Negative pressure usually is maintained.

COMPLICATIONS

Bleeding within the joint or in the subperiosteum may occur, as may infection. Strict aseptic technique must be maintained.

FLUID ANALYSIS (see Table 82-1)

Fluid obtained by arthrocentesis should always be analyzed completely. This analysis should include the following:

1. Cell count
2. Gram stain and culture, both aerobic and anaerobic
3. Protein and glucose
4. Examination for crystals (monosodium urate or calcium pyrophosphate dihydrate)
5. Mucin clot

APPENDIX A-3: VENOUS INFUSION

Obtaining venous access in the pediatric patient requires familiarity with potential sites and techniques, as well as expertise and patience. The choice of technique may require modification because of the nature of the injury or illness and the patient's condition, size, and fluid requirements.

PERIPHERAL VEIN PERCUTANEOUS PUNCTURE

Site

Peripherally, the preferred sites are the antecubital vein, veins on the dorsa of the hand and foot, and in the child less than 2 years of age, the scalp. The external jugular (p. 825) or femoral vein also may be used.

Position

1. The patient is immobilized to the extent necessary. For smaller children a papoose board may be useful.
2. Extremities require careful immobilization with tape (Fig. A-3, A). Hands may be better positioned if a small amount of cotton or gauze is placed under the wrist when using veins on the dorsum of the hand.

Preparation

1. Cleanse the area to be entered.
2. Shave the area if necessary (e.g., the head).

Tourniquet

1. Apply a tourniquet proximal to the point of venous access.
2. On the head a rubber band may serve as the tourniquet. Place a small amount of tape at one point on the rubber band to facilitate removal of the rubber band (Fig. A-3, B).

Needles and Cannulas

The choice is made on the basis of personal preference.

1. *Scalp vein needle.* May be used in all areas except for veins overlying joints. The inherent problem is the lack of true stability of the needle after it is inserted.
   a. Before inserting the needle, flush with saline solution, leaving the syringe attached until the skin is punctured. Once the skin is entered, remove the syringe to permit a flashback to appear on entering the vein.
   b. Insert the needle tangentially through the skin approximately 1 cm distal to the point of vein entry. Grasp the needle by the winged tabs. Advance

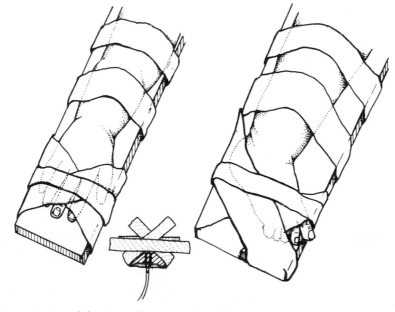

Fig. A-3   A, Immobilization of extremity for percutaneous venous puncture. Scalp vein needle taping.

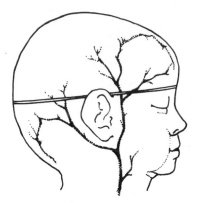

Fig. A-3   **B,** Location of scalp veins. Rubber band used for tourniquet.

the needle gently until the vein is entered and a flashback is visible. Unless the vein is large, do not thread the needle further.

c. Place a 1-cm wide tape over the needle at the point of entry to provide initial stabilization, and loop a second piece around the winged tabs.

d. Intermittently flush the needle to ensure patency and position.

e. Tape the needle carefully to minimize movement. Placement of a half medicine cup with the edges taped over the point of insertion and needle provides additional protection.

2. *Over-the-needle or through-the-needle catheter.* Inserted according to manufacturer's directions. Remember that once a flashback is noted in the over-the-needle catheter, the needle should be inserted 1 to 3 mm more to ensure that it is well into the vein before attempting to advance the catheter.

Intravenous Infusion

An intravenous (IV) infusion set should be attached after the patient is stabilized. In children less than 5 years of age, there should always be a volume-limiting device such as a Buretrol in line to prevent excessive fluid administration.

VENOUS CUTDOWN

Site

The greater saphenous vein is located anterior to the medial malleolus and medial to the anterior tibial tendon.

Position

The foot is immobilized with careful visualization of the malleolus.

Procedure

1. After cleansing, draping, and infiltrating locally with 1% lidocaine, apply a tourniquet.

2. Make a 1-cm transverse incision perpendicular to the vein, usually one fingerbreadth above and one fingerbreadth anterior to the medial malleolus.

3. Bluntly dissect down to the tibia in the direction parallel to the vein and identify the vein. Free the vein, and place two 3-0 Vicryl or silk sutures loosely around it.

   a. The distal suture is ligated to control venous return.

   b. The proximal suture is tied after the venous catheter has been placed. At this time it is left loose.

4. Some clinicians have recommended a more rapid approach. An incision from the posterior border of the malleolus is extended anteriorly to the "shin" or the anterior border of the tibia.

   A curved, closed hemostat pointing downward is scraped along the tibia from the anterior to the posterior aspect of the incision. All tissue is picked up and the hemostat is turned upward and opened. The saphenous vein is identified.

5. Another approach includes identification and isolation of the vein and subsequent cannulation using a guide-wire technique.

Catheterization

1. Select the appropriate size catheter. Using the proximal suture for traction, make a

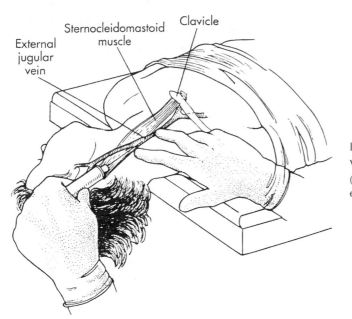

Sternocleidomastoid muscle
Clavicle
External jugular vein

Fig. A-3 **C,** Percutaneous external jugular vein puncture.

(From Barkin RM: *Pediatric emergency medicine,* ed 2, St Louis, 1997, Mosby.)

small flap incision in the anterior third of the vein with a No. 11 scalpel blade. The vein also can be cannulated by direct puncture, which does not require ligation.

2. Insert the catheter with traction from the proximal tie while elevating the vein flap. Remove the tourniquet and ensure that there is free flow.

3. Secure the catheter by tightening the proximal tie. Flush the vein with 1 to 2 ml of 1% lidocaine to overcome venous spasm, if necessary. Begin the IV infusion.

Closure

1. Close the wound with 4-0 Vicryl or Dexon sutures (some prefer silk or nylon), and further secure the catheter by extensive taping.

2. Cover with sterile dressing.

EXTERNAL JUGULAR VEIN
Site

The external jugular vein is easily accessible in children whose necks are not unduly short or obese. The vein courses from the angle of the mandible to the middle of the clavicle over the sternocleidomastoid muscle. The vein may be used for venipuncture, as well as for establishing peripheral or central venous access.

Position

The child is restrained in a supine position on a firm table. The head is rotated to the side away from the procedure and held off the edge of the table with the shoulders firmly touching the table (Fig. A-3, C).

Although the vein may be visible without additional measures, distension may be increased by placing the child in modified Trendelenburg position, by having the child cry, or by occluding the vein with a finger on the clavicle.

Catheterization

After the area is prepared and draped, the catheter is inserted.

1. If peripheral access is desired, the largest catheter that is easily inserted should be used.

2. If central access is desired, a guide-wire technique normally is used, as described on p. 829.
3. The IV infusion is attached, and the catheter secured.

INTRAOSSEOUS (IO) INFUSIONS

Bone marrow infusion provides a route to venous access when conventional routes are unavailable. The intramedullary vessels are supported by bone architecture and therefore accessible in children 6 years of age and younger because the tibial marrow is still actively producing red blood cells. The data would suggest that the greatest efficiency of the IO approach is in children 6 years of age or younger. This allows access into the sinusoids and ultimately the large medullary venous channels (Fig. A-3, D).

The technique is useful in life-threatening conditions requiring immediate venous access on a temporary basis for infusion of crystalloids and drugs. Besides fluids, numerous pharmacologic agents, including diazepam, inotropic agents, sodium bicarbonate, lidocaine, antibiotics, and insulin, have been administered without complications. The safety of infusion of hypertonic and strongly alkaline solutions has not been fully established on a long-term basis.

Bone marrow aspirate may be useful for laboratory studies such as blood culture and electrolytes.

Position

The patient is immobilized in the supine position. It is often useful to position a small sandbag under the leg, immediately behind the operative site. Restrain the leg.

Needle

Special intraosseous needles are available and are the optimal devices because of ease of use and the band that facilitates immobilization.

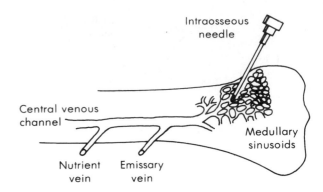

Fig. A-3   D, Venous drainage from marrow of long bone with intramedullary needle in place.

Other options are an 18- to 20-gauge spinal needle with stylet or a small 15- to 18-gauge bone marrow trephine needle.

Procedure (Fig. A-3, E)

1. Strict aseptic technique must be maintained.
2. Local infiltration with lidocaine is desirable but is often precluded by the emergent nature of the procedure and the depressed sensorium of the patient.
3. The needle is inserted perpendicular to the skin or at a 45- to 60-degree angle away from the epiphyseal plate. The proximal tibia or distal femur is preferred. If the tibia is used, a site two to three fingerbreadths below the tibial tuberosity is selected. A screwing motion is used to push the needle through the cortex.
4. The needle is in the marrow when there is a lack of resistance after the needle passes through the cortex and stands upright without support. Bone marrow is aspirated by the syringe, and the infusion flows smoothly.

Complications

The procedure is meant as a temporizing measure and should be replaced once stable access

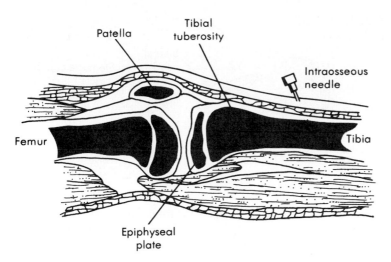

Fig. A-3   **E,** Intraosseous insertion of needle.

is achieved. Complications may include the following:

1. Osteomyelitis or abscess, usually from prolonged insertion.
2. Leakage around the needle, with compartment syndrome. If the needle comes out, it is difficult to insert in the same leg because of the leakage problem from a second puncture.
3. Potential injury to the bone marrow cavity.
4. Fat and bone marrow emboli.
5. Tibial fracture.
6. No impairment of bone growth has been observed.

CENTRAL VENOUS ACCESS

This involves the subclavian or internal jugular veins. The femoral vein also may be used and is preferred by many. Central venous access provides venous access, as well as measurement of central venous pressure.

Position

The patient is immobilized in Trendelenburg position (15 to 20 degrees) if condition permits, head turned away from site of puncture.

TABLE A-3, A   Approximate Conversion of French Size to Gauge to mm

French size	Gauge	mm
1	29	0.33
2	23/22	0.66
3	20/19	1.00
4	18/17	1.35
5	16/15	1.68
6	15/14	2

Site and Needle

The site is cleansed with povidone-iodine (Betadine), infiltrated with 1% lidocaine, and draped if time permits.

Needles, catheters, and guide wires are available as disposable kits from a variety of companies and are generally complete with catheters, guide wires, and needles. (Fig. A-3, A, and A-3, B and Table A-3, A).

Internal Jugular Vein

The vein runs posterior to the sternocleidomastoid muscle between its two heads and behind the anterior portion of the clavicular head as it courses to meet the subclavian vein just above the medial end of the clavicle.

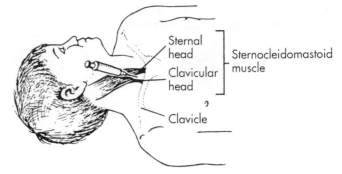

Fig. A-3 **F,** Percutaneous internal jugular vein insertion.

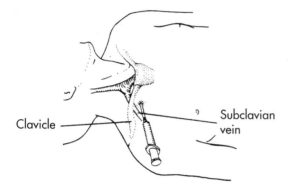

Fig. A-3 **G,** Subclavian vein puncture.

For the central or middle approach:

1. Landmarks are the triangle created by the sternal and clavicular heads of the sternocleidomastoid muscle and the clavicle at the base. The internal jugular vein is just behind the medial border of the clavicular head. The carotid artery is just medial to it.
2. The needle is inserted at the apex of the triangle at a 45-degree angle and aimed caudal and toward the ipsilateral nipple. The needle is inserted only 1 to 2 cm and blood should be free-flowing. If the vein is not entered, the needle is withdrawn and redirected slightly more laterally (Fig. A-3, F).
3. Once the vein is entered, the needle is left in place while the attached syringe is removed. The guide wire is then inserted through the needle.

4. The needle is then removed over the guide wire. A small cut is made at the point of skin entry and the catheter is inserted according to the manufacturer's directions.

Subclavian Vein

The vein crosses over the first rib and passes in front of the anterior scalene muscle and continues behind the medial third of the clavicle, where it unites with the internal jugular vein to form the innominate vein.

1. Estimate the length of the catheter needed by measuring from the site of insertion to the sternomanubrial angle.
2. Insert the needle infraclavicularly at the juncture of the middle and medial thirds of the clavicle parallel to the frontal plane. Direct it medially and slightly cephalad behind the clavicle toward the sternal notch.

    NOTE: It is often useful to place a finger in the suprasternal notch for reference (Fig. A-3, G).
3. Insert the needle with the bevel upward. Once the lumen of the vessel is entered, rotate it so that the bevel is directed caudally.
4. Attach the needle to a syringe and insert under negative pressure until a free flow of blood back into the syringe is achieved. The syringe is then removed and a thumb placed over the needle hub to prevent air embolization.
5. A supraclavicular approach is preferred by some clinicians. The site of insertion is

the angle and junction formed by the lateral border of the sternocleidomastoid muscle and the clavicle. The needle is inserted behind the sternocleidomastoid muscle and clavicle at an angle bisecting the angle formed by the landmarks and directed toward the contralateral nipple. The needle is advanced with the barrel of the syringe 5 to 10 degrees below the horizontal plane. The vein is entered 0.5 to 4.0 cm of depth. If unsuccessful, elevate the syringe 5 degrees above the horizontal plane.

Femoral Vein

The femoral vein may be cannulated by locating the femoral pulse and inserting a needle 2 cm distal to the inguinal ligament and 0.5 cm medial. The remainder of the approach using a guide wire is similar to other routes.

The Cannula

The *cannula* type determines the next step.

1. If the *catheter-through-the needle* technique is used, the catheter is slipped through the needle the appropriate distance and the needle is slid off the cannula once the cannula is in place. The catheter is never withdrawn through the needle because of the risk of shearing it.
2. If a *guide wire* is used, a wire guide is inserted through the needle and the needle is withdrawn. The dilator and overlying catheter are then fed over the wire and, once in place, the wire and dilator are removed.

Procedure

1. The IV infusion is attached with an inline manometer to measure central venous pressure (CVP).
2. The catheter is secured with suture through the skin and wrapped around the catheter. A sterile dressing is applied.
3. CVP is determined.

Cautions

1. A bright-red blood return indicates that an artery has been punctured. Remove the needle and apply pressure for a minimum of 10 minutes.
2. If unable to advance the catheter, remove the needle and catheter together. Never withdraw the cannula through the needle.
3. The right side usually is preferred, because the dome of the lung is lower on the right, it is a more direct path to the right atrium, and there is a smaller thoracic duct on the right.
   a. If there is pulmonary injury, such as a pneumothorax or major pulmonary contusion and a central line is to be placed for monitoring, place the central catheter on the side of the injury.
   b. If there is potential vascular injury to the subclavian, internal jugular, or innominate veins, place the catheter on the other side.
4. After insertion, a chest roentgenogram (anteroposterior [AP] or posteroanterior [PA] and lateral) should be obtained for defining placement, as well as excluding immediate complications.
   NOTE: Many believe that the external jugular is the safest approach, followed by the internal jugular technique.

Complications

These include pneumothorax, hemothorax, hydrothorax, air or catheter embolization, and brachial plexus injury. Preparations always should be made to treat them. Cervical hematomas are common, and although bleeding is usually trivial, it can produce occlusion of the airway. A common error, if a pneumothorax occurs, is to try to reverse it with too small an intrathoracic catheter. A thoracostomy should be performed with underwater drainage and, at times, additional suction.

UMBILICAL ARTERY AND VEIN

This is useful in the newborn (see Chapter 9).

APPENDIX A-4: LUMBAR PUNCTURE

Lumbar punctures (LPs) commonly are performed to exclude central nervous system (CNS) infection. It is important to exclude potential increased intracranial pressure on the basis of history and physical examination before performing the LP. If there is any question, a computed tomography (CT) scan should be obtained before the LP.

POSITION

The patient's position is crucial. The patient should be placed at the edge of a firm examination table and maintained in a position with the neck flexed and the knee drawn upward (fetal position). *The key to performing an LP is to properly position the child* (Fig. A-4).

1. The shoulders and back of the patient should be perpendicular to the table.
2. An alternative position for the small infant is to have the patient sitting, flexing the thighs up to the abdomen. This is recommended only if the holder and clinician are experienced with this approach.
3. In the preterm infant, the optimal position

is either the lateral recumbent one with the hips flexed and partial neck extension or the upright position. Full flexion of the neck may cause hypoventilation.

PROCEDURE

1. The patient's back is cleansed with a surgical solution—using povidone-iodine (Betadine)—and then draped. Steri-drapes are particularly useful, because they are adherent and do not obscure the landmarks.
2. Meticulous sterile technique is used.
3. Local anesthetic is used for children above 5 years of age who will cooperate more easily if the pain is minimized.

Site

The puncture is at the intersection of the line joining the superior portion of the iliac crest with the spine. This point is the spinous process of L4. The needle is optimally inserted at L3-L4 but may be inserted one space above or below.

Spinal Needle

This is a 22-gauge, 1-inch needle for children less than 5 years, increased to 3 inches long in older children and adults.

Fig. A-4   Position for lumbar puncture.

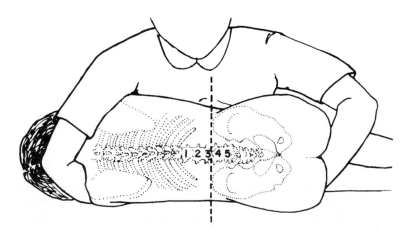

Insertion

The needle is inserted into the designated spot with the stylet in place.

1. The needle should be inserted perpendicular to the back and aimed toward the umbilicus.
2. In the younger child it is advisable to puncture the skin and allow the child to calm down and then to reassess the position before proceeding.
3. Younger children will not demonstrate the increasing resistance and "pop" noted in older children. It is advisable to frequently remove the stylet and examine the needle hub for fluid as the needle with stylet is advanced.

Manometry

This can be performed in cooperative children older than 5 years when it is important. A three-way stopcock and manometer are attached to the spinal needle and the pressure determined. Normal relaxed pressure is 5 to 15 cm of water.

Fluid Analysis (see Table 81-3)

Analysis of the cerebrospinal fluid (CSF) must be done expeditiously.

1. Tube No. 1: culture and Gram stain. If Gram stain result is negative: methylene blue. Cultures beyond routine bacterial ones should be specified.
2. Tube No. 2: protein and glucose. (Serum glucose level should be obtained before performing the LP.)
3. Tube No. 3: cell count. If bloody, it may be desirable to compare tube No. 1 and tube No. 3 cell count to determine whether the tap was traumatic.
4. A fourth tube may be collected for additional studies such as viral cultures.
5. The CSF pressure can be estimated (cm H_2O) by counting the number of drops in a specified counting period (seconds). Child must be relaxed and not crying.

Needle (gauge)	Length (in)	Counting period (sec)
22	1.5	21
22	3.5	39
20	3.5	12

6. Analysis is outlined in detail in Table 81-3, p. 728.

COMPLICATIONS

1. Cardiac respiratory arrest may result from the child being held too tightly, with subsequent respiratory arrest and impaired venous return. Children must be observed closely to prevent this problem.
2. Infection as a result of introduction of pathogens during the procedure may occur. Controversy exists as to the risk of performing an LP in the child with bacteremia. The risk is not substantiated, and this question should not serve to inhibit clinicians from doing necessary studies.
3. Herniation through the foramen magnum may occur because of antecedent increased intracranial pressure. If increased pressure is noted at the time of the procedures, only a small amount of fluid should be withdrawn and the needle quickly removed. The patient obviously requires immediate evaluation and treatment. Optimally an LP is avoided with such patients.
4. Headaches are more common in adults.
5. Intraspinal dermoids are avoided by using only needles with stylets.
6. Penetration of a nerve causes pain. In this case the needle is withdrawn and redirected.
7. Spinal cord hematoma occurs, particularly in patients with thrombocytopenia or coagulation defects.

Appendix A-5: Pericardiocentesis

Fluid collection in the pericardial sac, whether it results from effusion, infection, or hemorrhage, may be removed in the acute situation for both diagnostic and therapeutic reasons by pericardiocentesis. An ultrasonogram or echocardiogram may be an important diagnostic tool in the stable patient to establish the presence of an effusion. After this life-saving procedure, definitive surgical care is immediately indicated.

POSITION

The patient is supine, leaning backward at a 45-degree angle, supported by the bed or pillows (reverse Trendelenburg position).

SITE

The left subxiphoid is used, with the needle aimed cephalad and backward toward the tip of the left scapula (Fig. A-5). Some clinicians recommend aiming the needle toward the right scapula.

NEEDLE

An 18- or 20-gauge metal spinal needle (3 inch) is attached to a three-way stopcock and 20-ml syringe. One end of an alligator clip is attached to the needle's base and the other end to the V lead on an electrocardiogram (ECG). (Limb leads should be attached as usual.)

PROCEDURE

1. After preparing, cleansing, and draping the patient, the needle is inserted slowly under negative pressure through the puncture site, penetrating the diaphragm. As the pericardium is entered, there is a distinct "pop." A current of injury with ST-T wave changes will be noted if the epicardium is entered, and the needle should be withdrawn slightly.
2. Aspiration is performed. As little as 2 ml may be temporarily effective at relieving tamponade and improving cardiac output.
3. Vital signs should be monitored throughout the procedure.
4. Ultrasonography may facilitate this procedure.

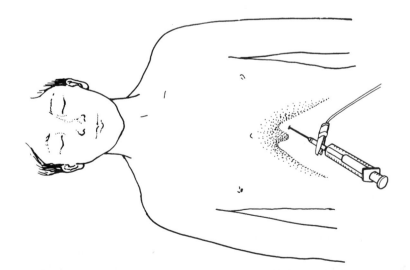

Fig. A-5   Position of needle for pericardiocentesis.

COMPLICATIONS

1. Pneumothorax.
2. Coronary artery injury or myocardial laceration.
3. Dysrhythmias.
4. Bleeding. In the stable patient, prothrombin time (PT), partial thromboplastin time (PTT), and platelet count may be obtained before the procedure.

APPENDIX A-6: SUBDURAL TAP

The subdural space is a noncommunicating space between the dura matter and the arachnoid membrane. Although a CT scan can delineate the presence of fluid in the subdural space, the tap is done to define the nature of the collection: hematoma, effusion, or empyema. This is commonly done in a conjunction with a neurosurgeon.

SITE

The *puncture site* is the lateral corner of the anterior fontanelle or further lateral along the suture. Optimally, this is at least 5 cm from the midline or 1 to 2 cm lateral to the edge of the anterior fontanelle, which is generally "open" until 12 months of age (Fig. A-6).

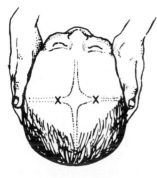

Fig. A-6   Puncture site for subdural tap.

POSITION

The patient is in the supine position with the head at the edge of an examining table. An assistant should immobilize the patient with the help of a papoose board.

NEEDLE

A *subdural needle* (short bevel) is used. If one is unavailable, a short spinal needle with a short bevel may be substituted. It is often advisable with this needle to place a hemostat on the needle at the point of entry to prevent excessive penetration.

PROCEDURE

1. The anterior two thirds of the scalp are shaved and surgically scrubbed with povidone-iodine solution (Betadine). Meticulous surgical technique is essential. The needle is inserted slowly at a right angle to the skin surface with total finger control. It is advanced slowly with the stylet in place until there is a sudden decrease in resistance, usually associated with a "pop," representing penetration of the dura.
2. The stylet is removed, and up to 15 to 20 ml of fluid is allowed to drain by gravity, avoiding aspiration. Normally, there are only a few drops in this space. Sometimes none is obtained.
3. In most cases, the procedure is repeated on the other side.
4. If excessive fluid is present or reaccumulates, repeat taps may be necessary over a period of time. A neurosurgeon should be consulted.

ANALYSIS OF THE FLUID

This should parallel the studies performed on specimens obtained by LP: culture, Gram stain, glucose, protein, and cell count (p. 728). A subdural effusion usually is associated with grossly xanthochromic or bloody fluid.

COMPLICATIONS

1. Infection resulting from introduction of pathogens during the procedure.
2. Bleeding from small vessels (lateral position of puncture site should be maintained to avoid superior sagittal sinus).
3. Removal of more than 20 ml/tap can produce CNS sequelae. If more than 20 ml is present, a neurosurgeon should be consulted.
4. Injury to the cerebral cortex if needle is inserted too deeply.

APPENDIX A-7: SUPRAPUBIC ASPIRATION

Suprapubic aspiration is a safe method to obtain urine from the newborn and infants less than 2 years of age because the distended bladder in this age group is primarily intraabdominal.

The infant's bladder must be full. Determining that the diaper has been dry for 45 minutes is good evidence of a full bladder. Dehydration reduces the success. Ultrasonographic confirmation of a full bladder may be helpful.

POSITION

The patient is restrained in the supine position.

SITE

The site is 2 cm (a fingerbreadth) above the symphysis.

PROCEDURE

1. Surgically cleanse the suprapubic area with povidone-iodine (Betadine).
2. Identify the pubic bone without contaminating the area of puncture.
3. Insert a 1-inch, 22-gauge needle attached to a 5-ml syringe at midline, angling the needle 10 to 20 degrees cephalad and advancing it through the skin under negative pressure at all times (Fig. A-7).

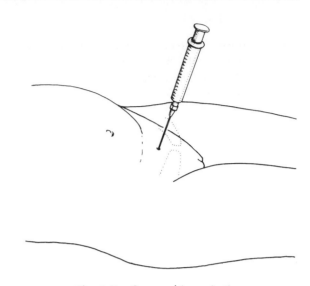

Fig. A-7   Suprapubic aspiration.

Entry into the bladder is indicated by return of urine. If no urine is obtained:

1. Angle the needle perpendicular to the frontal plane and try once more.
2. Avoid excessive probing or manipulation of the needle.
3. If no urine is obtained, try again in 15 minutes, or use a different technique, such as catheterization (an infant can be catheterized with a 3.5- or 5.0-Fr feeding tube).

COMPLICATIONS

These include gross hematuria (some hematuria usually will follow the procedure), anterior abdominal wall abscess, and bowel puncture. Peritonitis is uncommon.

APPENDIX A-8: THORACENTESIS

Thoracentesis is indicated to remove pleural fluid for diagnostic or therapeutic reasons or in the emergency treatment of a pneumothorax pending placement of a chest tube.

POSITION

For posterior or posterolateral approaches to fluid removal, the patient sits in a flexed position, leaning forward against a bed stand or chair back. A small infant may be held in the "burping" position.

1. If the patient is too ill to sit, the procedure may be performed with the patient lying on the involved side on a firm surface with a portion of the lateral chest wall extending over the edge of the bed. An alternative for gaining access to the lateral chest wall is for the patient to lie across two beds or examination tables with the involved side down.
2. If a pneumothorax is to be decompressed, the patient should be lying supine.

SITE

The site of puncture depends on the location of the pleural fluid. If a pneumothorax is being decompressed before placing chest tube (Fig. A-9), venting is done at the second or third intercostal space at the midclavicular line.

NEEDLE

An 18- or 19-gauge needle with a short bevel attached to a three-way stopcock and 10-ml syringe is used. If fluid is expected, plastic tubing is attached to the sidearm of the stopcock to facilitate removal of fluids.

Flexible cannulas over needle also are useful and may replace the needle. They decrease the risk of lung puncture and are particularly valuable for emergency intervention.

PROCEDURE

1. The patient is prepared and draped, and 1% lidocaine is infiltrated locally.
2. With sterile technique the needle or catheter over needle is inserted, passing over the superior edge of the rib under negative pressure, and advanced slowly. There is a sudden decrease in resistance once the pleural space is reached. A hemostat should be placed on the needle at the skin to prevent further penetration once the pleural space is entered.
3. Fluid is aspirated, the volume reflecting cardiopulmonary status and the therapeutic goals of the procedures.

ANALYSIS OF THE FLUID

This should include a culture, Gram stain, protein, glucose, lactose dehydrogenase (LDH), cell count, and a check for chyle (see below).

The distinction between transudate and exudate may be useful in differentiating the causes of pleural effusion. Transudates usually are associated with congestive heart failure, cirrhosis, nephrotic syndrome, acute glomerulonephritis, myxedema, and peritoneal dialysis. Exudates with proteins over 3 gm/dl occur with pulmonary infarction, neoplasms, infection (viral or bacterial such as *S. aureus*, *H. influenzae*, or streptococcus; tuberculosis; fungus; or para-

	Transudate	Exudate
Etiology	CHF, cirrhosis	Infection: bacterial, mycobacterial; infarction, neoplasm, pancreatitis
Protein	<3.0 gm/dl (PF/S <0.5)	>3.0 gm/dl (PF/S >0.5)
LDH	Low (<200 IU/L) (PF/S <0.6)	High (>200 IU/L) (PF/S >0.6)
Glucose	Same as blood	Variable (infection: low)
RBC	<10,000/mm^3	Variable (if >100,000/mm^3, consider infarction, trauma, neoplasm)
WBC	<1000/mm^3	>1000/mm^3 (infection)

PF, Pleural fluid; *S,* serum.

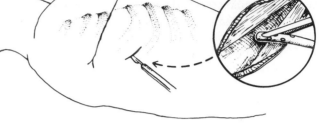

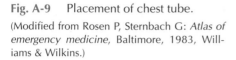

Fig. A-9   Placement of chest tube.
(Modified from Rosen P, Sternbach G: *Atlas of emergency medicine*, Baltimore, 1983, Williams & Wilkins.)

sites), collagen vascular disease, subphrenic abscess, trauma, and lymphatic abnormalities.

COMPLICATIONS

These include introduction of infection, pneumothorax, hemothorax, or pulmonary laceration. Hospitalize the patient to observe after the procedure.

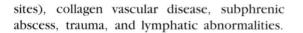

APPENDIX A-9: THORACOSTOMY

Chest tubes are used for the treatment of pneumothorax or hemothorax, often before making a definitive radiologic diagnosis (see Chapter 62). Management in newborns is discussed in Chapter 11.

INDICATIONS

1. Tension pneumothorax.
2. Traumatic moderate to large pneumothorax. A small (<10% simple) pneumothorax in a symptom-free patient (with no increase on repeat roentgenogram) may be observed in the hospital if general anesthesia or mechanical ventilation is not required for other injuries.
3. Any pneumothorax with respiratory symptoms.
4. Increasing pneumothorax after initial conservative therapy.
5. Pneumothorax in a patient who needs mechanical ventilation or general anesthesia.
6. Associated hemothorax.
7. Bilateral pneumothorax.

POSITION

The patient is supine with appropriate immobilization.

SITE

The site for insertion is at the fourth or fifth intercostal space in the midaxillary line.

TUBE SIZE

The tube should be the largest one that can be inserted. This is particularly important if a hemothorax is present.

1. The following are estimates of appropriate size:
   a. Newborn: 8 to 12 Fr
   b. Infant: 14 to 20 Fr
   c. Children: 20 to 28 Fr
   d. Adolescent: 28 to 42 Fr
2. The length of the tube should be approximated before insertion. All holes in the tube must be within the pleural cavity.
3. A Seldinger technique (tube-over-wire) may be an alternative to the traditional chest tube insertion.

PROCEDURE

1. The area is prepared, draped, and locally infiltrated with 1% lidocaine down to the rib and along the subcutaneous tissue to be tunneled.

2. The skin is incised with a scalpel parallel to the long axis of the rib. The incision should be adequate to permit manipulation of the tube (3 to 5 cm).

3. The area is bluntly dissected down to the rib with a clamp or scissors. If tunneling is desired, the dissection is continued across the intercostal space above the incision site and over the next rib. A clamp is then curved over the superior edge of the rib, dividing the intercostal muscles down to the parietal pleura, which is penetrated. The opening is enlarged by blunt dissection.

4. In older infants and children, a finger is inserted to ensure that there are no adhesions of the lung and that the tube will be inserted into the chest and not subdiaphragmatically.

5. The thoracostomy tube is grasped at the tip by a curved clamp and advanced through the tunnel and intercostal space into the chest. It is directed posteriorly and apically. The interspace is entered superior to the rib to avoid injuring the neurovascular bundle (Fig. A-9). All holes must be within the pleural cavity.

6. The tube is attached to an underwater seal. If there is a continuous air leak or an associated hemothorax, additional pleural suction may be needed up to 15 to 25 cm H_2O.

7. The tube is sutured in place and dressed with a sterile covering, often including a petrolatum-soaked gauze as an air seal.

8. A chest x-ray film should be obtained after the procedure.

COMPLICATIONS

1. Inserting the tube too low, causing penetration of the diaphragm and injury to the liver or spleen

2. Injury to the neurovascular bundle, causing persistent hemorrhage

3. Injury to the underlying lung

4. Air leak if the tube is not placed far enough to include all the holes in the pleural cavity, causing extensive subcutaneous emphysema and failure to reexpand the collapsed lung

5. Empyema

REFERENCES

Ahmed MY, Silver P, Wimroff L, et al: The needle-wire-dilator technique for insertion of chest tubes in pediatric patients, *Pediatr Emerg Care* 11:252, 1995.

Ellis RW, Strauss LC, Wiley JM, et al: A simple method of estimating cerebrospinal fluid pressure during lumbar puncture, *Pediatrics* 89:895, 1992.

Fiser BH: Intraosseous infusion, *N Engl J Med* 322:1579, 1990.

Fiser RT, Walker WM, Seibert JJ, et al: Tibia length following intraosseous infusion: a prospective radiographic analysis, *Pediatr Emerg Care* 13:186, 1997.

Glaeser PW, Hellmich JR, Szewczuga D, et al: Five-year experience in prehospital intraosseous infusions in children and adults, *Ann Emerg Med* 22:1119, 1993.

Orlowski JP, Julius CJ, Petras RE, et al: The safety of intraosseous infusion: risks of fat and bone marrow emboli to the lungs, *Ann Emerg Med* 18:1062, 1989.

Orlowski JP, Parembka DT, Gallagher JM, et al: The bone marrow as a source of laboratory studies, *Ann Emerg Med* 18:1348, 1989.

Orlowski JP, Parembka DT, Gallagher JM, et al: Companion study of intraosseous infusions of emergency drugs, *Am J Dis Child* 144:112, 1990.

Pollack CV, Pollack ES, Andrew ME: Suprapubic bladder aspiration vs. urethral catheterization in all infants: success, efficiency and complication rates, *Ann Emerg Med* 23:225, 1994.

Proter FL, Miller JP, Cole FS, et al: A controlled clinical trial of local anesthesia for lumbar puncture in newborns, *Pediatrics* 88:663, 1991.

Shockley LW, Butzier DJ: A modified well-guided technique for venous cutdown access, *Ann Emerg Med* 19:393, 1990.

B REFERENCE STANDARDS

APPENDIX B-1: GROWTH CURVES

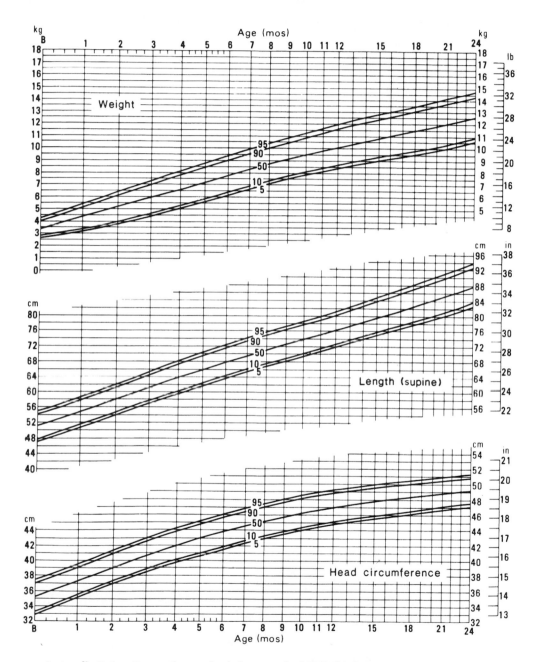

Appendix B-1 Percentile standards for growth: **BOYS (birth-24 mo).**

(Modified from National Center for Health Statistics [NCHS] growth charts, 1976.)

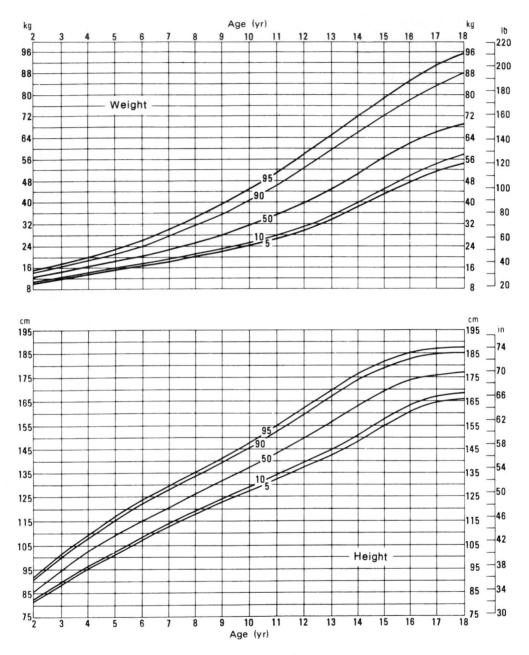

Percentile standards for growth: **BOYS (2-18 yr).**

(Modified from NCHS growth charts, 1976).

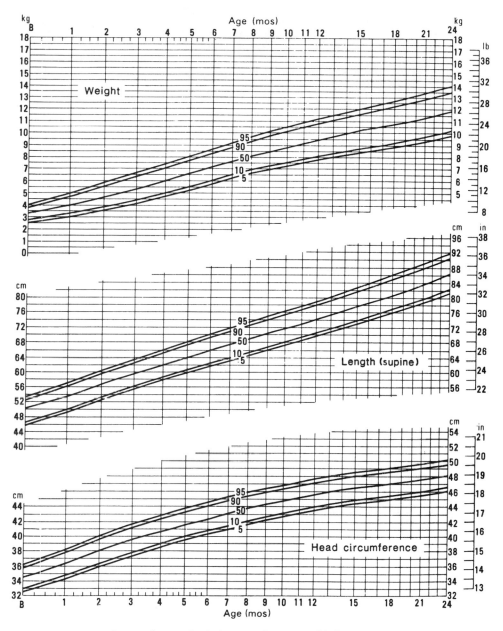

Percentile standards for growth: **GIRLS (birth-24 mo).**

(Modified from NCHS growth charts, 1976.)

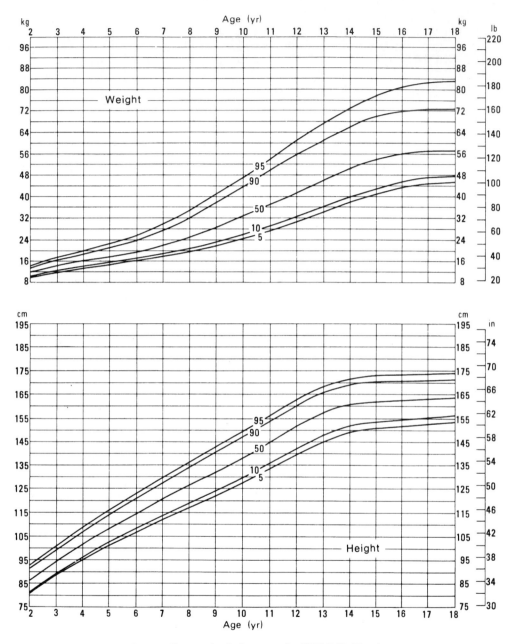

Percentile standards for growth: **GIRLS (2-18 yr).**

(Modified from NCHS growth charts, 1976.)

APPENDIX B-2: VITAL SIGNS AND ANCILLARY VENTILATORY SUPPORT

Age	Weight (kg)	Heart rate (average/min)	Respiratory rate	Blood pressure		ET tube		Suction catheter (Fr)	Chest tube (Fr)	Laryngoscopy blade
				Systolic	Diastolic*	ID† (mm)	Length (cm)			
Premature	1	145	>40			2.5	10	6	8-10	0 st
Newborn	1-2	135		42 ± 10	21 ± 8	3.0	11	6-8	10-12	1 st
Newborn	2-3	125		50 ± 10	28 ± 8	3.5	12	8		
1 mo	4	120	38 ± 10	60 ± 10	37 ± 8	3.5	13			
6 mo	7	130		80 ± 16	46 ± 16	3.5-4.0	14			
1 yr	10	125	39 ± 11	89 ± 29	60 ± 10	4.0-4.5	15	8-10	16-20	1 st
2-3 yr	12-14	115	28 ± 4	96 ± 30	66 ± 15	4.5	16	10	20-24	
4-5 yr	16-18	100	27 ± 6	99 ± 25	64 ± 25	5.0-5.5	17		20-28	2
6-8 yr	20-26	100	24 ± 6	See figures on pp. 844-845		5.5-6.0	18			
10-12 yr	32-42	75	21 ± 4			5.5-7.0	20	12	28-32	2-3
>14 yr	>50	70	20 ± 4			7.5-8.5	24		32-42	3

*Point of muffling (Nadas).

†Variability of 0.5 mm is common. Estimate: $\dfrac{16 + \text{age (yr)}}{4}$

95TH PERCENTILE OF SYSTOLIC AND DIASTOLIC BLOOD PRESSURE BY HEIGHT AND AGE, BOYS

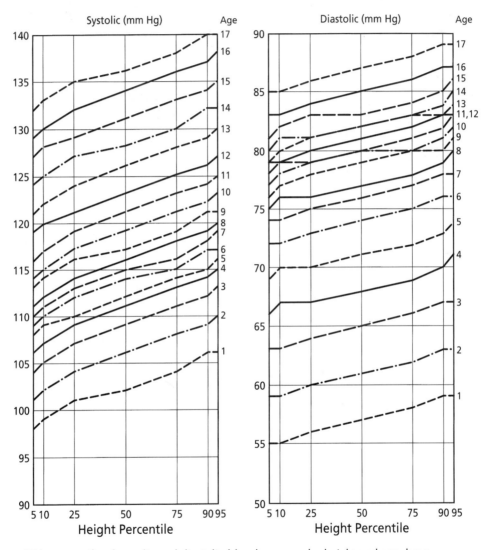

95th percentile of systolic and diastolic blood pressure by height and age, boys.

(From *Update on the Task Force Report (1997) on High Blood Pressure Control in Children and Adolescents: A working group report from the National High Blood Pressure Education Program.* National Institutes of Public Health, National Heart, Lung, and Blood Institute, NIH Publication No. 96-3790, 1996.)

95TH PERCENTILE OF SYSTOLIC AND DIASTOLIC BLOOD PRESSURE BY HEIGHT AND AGE, GIRLS

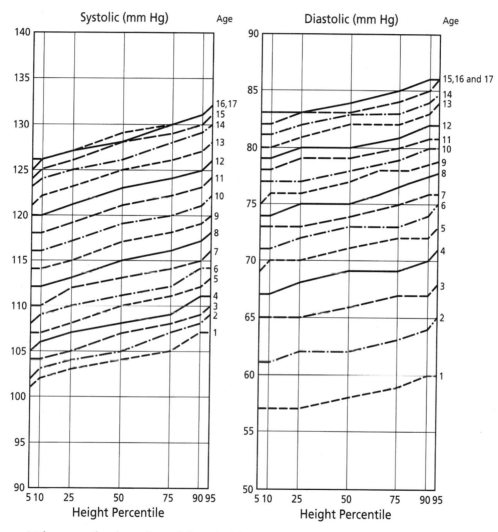

95th percentile of systolic and diastolic blood pressure by height and age, girls.

(From *Update on the Task Force Report (1997) on High Blood Pressure Control in Children and Adolescents: A working group report from the National High Blood Pressure Education Program.* National Institutes of Public Health, National Heart, Lung, and Blood Institute, NIH Publication No. 96-3790, 1996.)

Appendix B-3: Electrocardiographic Criteria

Age	Heart rate (/min)	QRS axis (degrees)	PR interval (sec)	QRS duration* (sec)
0-1 mo	100-180 (120)†	+75 to +180 (+120)	0.08-0.12 (0.10)	0.04-0.08 (0.06)
2-3 mo	110-180 (120)	+35 to +135 (+100)	0.08-0.12 (0.10)	0.04-0.08 (0.06)
4-12 mo	100-180 (150)	+30 to +135 (+60)	0.09-0.13 (0.12)	0.04-0.08 (0.06)
1-3 yr	100-180 (130)	0 to +110 (+60)	0.10-0.14 (0.12)	0.04-0.08 (0.06)
4-5 yr	60-150 (100)	0 to +110 (+60)	0.11-0.15 (0.13)	0.05-0.09 (0.07)
6-8 yr	60-130 (100)	−15 to +110 (+60)	0.12-0.16 (0.14)	0.05-0.09 (0.07)
9-11 yr	50-110 (80)	−15 to +110 (+60)	0.12-0.17 (0.14)	0.05-0.09 (0.07)
12-16 yr	50-100 (75)	−15 to +110 (+60)	0.12-0.17 (0.15)	0.05-0.09 (0.07)
>16 yr	50-90 (70)	−15 to +110 (+60)	0.12-0.20 (0.15)	0.05-0.10 (0.08)

QT interval‡

Rate/min	R-R interval (sec)	Q-T interal (sec)
40	1.5	0.38-0.50 (0.45)†
50	1.2	0.36-0.48 (0.43)
60	1.0	0.34-0.46 (0.41)
70	0.86	0.32-0.43 (0.37)
80	0.75	0.29-0.40 (0.35)
90	0.67	0.27-0.37 (0.33)
100	0.60	0.26-0.35 (0.30)
120	0.50	0.24-0.32 (0.28)
150	0.40	0.21-0.28 (0.25)
180	0.33	0.19-0.27 (0.23)
200	0.30	0.18-0.25 (0.22)

T-wave orientation

Age	V_1, V_2	aVF	I, V_5, V_6
0-5 days	Variable	Upright	Upright
6 days-2 yr	Inverted	Upright	Upright
3 yr-adolescent	Inverted	Upright	Upright
Adult	Upright	Upright	Upright

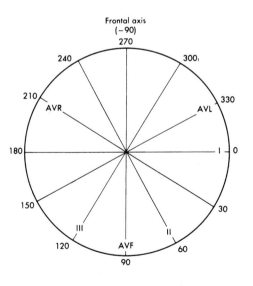

*If QRS duration is normal, add R + R′ and compare total (R + R′) with standards; R/S undefined because S can be equal to 0.

†Minimum-maximum (mean).

‡QT_c, $\dfrac{\text{measured Q-T interval (sec)}}{\sqrt{\text{R-R interval(sec)}}}$

QT_c should not exceed 0.45 in child <6 mo, 0.44 in children or 0.425 in adolescents/adults.

Adapted from Garson A, Jr, Gillette PC, McNamara DG: *A guide to cardiac dysrhythmias in children,* New York, 1980, Grune & Stratton, Inc; Guntheroth WGS: *Pediatric electrocardiography,* Philadelphia, 1965, WB Saunders.

Lead V₁			Lead V₆			
R-wave amplitude (mm)	S-wave amplitude (mm)	R/S ratio	R-wave amplitude (mm)	S-wave amplitude (mm)	R/S ratio	Age
4-25 (15)	0-20 (10)	0.5 to ∞ (1.5)	1-21 (6)	0-12 (4)	0.1 to ∞ (2)	0-1 mo
2-20 (11)	1-18 (7)	0.3 to 10.0 (1.5	3-20 (10)	0-6 (2)	1.5 to ∞ (4)	2-3 mo
3-20 (10)	1-16 (8)	0.3 to 4.0 (1.2)	4-20 (13)	0-4 (2)	2.0 to ∞ (6)	4-12 mo
1-18 (9)	1-27 (13)	0.5 to 1.5 (0.8)	3-24 (12)	0-4 (2)	3.0 to ∞ (20)	1-3 yr
1-18 (7)	1-30 (14)	0.1 to 1.5 (0.7)	4-24 (13)	0-4 (1)	2.0 to ∞ (20)	4-5 yr
1-18 (7)	1-30 (14)	0.1 to 1.5 (0.7)	4-24 (13)	0-4 (1)	2.0 to ∞ (20)	6-8 yr
1-16 (6)	1-26 (16)	0.1 to 1.0 (0.5)	4-24 (14)	0-4 (1)	4.0 to ∞ (20)	9-11 yr
1-16 (5)	1-23 (14)	0 to 1.0 (0.3)	4-22 (14)	0-5 (1)	2.0 to ∞ (9)	12-16 yr
1-14 (3)	1-23 (10)	0 to 1.0 (0.3)	4-21 (10)	0-6 (1)	2.0 to ∞ (9)	>16 yr

Chamber enlargement ("hypertrophy")

Right ventricular
1. RV1 >20 mm (>25 mm under 1 mo)
2. SV6 >6 mm (>12 mm under 1 mo)
3. Abnormal R/S ratio (V1 >2 after 6 mo)
4. Upright TV3R, RV1 after 5 days
5. QR pattern in V3R, V1

Left ventricular
1. RV6 >25 mm (>21 mm under 1 yr)
2. SV1 >30 mm (>20 mm under 1 yr)
3. RV6 + SV1 >60 mm (use V₅ if RV5 >RV6)
4. Abnormal R/S ratio
5. SV1 >2 × RV5

Combined
1. RVH and SV1 or RV6 exceed mean for age
2. LVH and RV1 or SV6 exceed mean for age

Right atrial
1. Peak P valve >3 mm (<6 mo), >2.5 mm (≥6 mo)

Left atrial
1. PII >0.09 sec
2. PV1 late negative deflection >0.04 sec and >1 mm

Maximal P-R interval (sec)						
Rate/min	<1 mo	1 mo-1 yr	1-3 yr	3-8 yr	8-12 yr	Adult
<60					0.18	0.21
60-80				0.17	0.17	0.21
80-100	0.12			0.16	0.16	0.20
100-120	0.12		0.16	0.16	0.15	0.19
120-140	0.11	0.14	0.14	0.15	0.15	0.18
140-160	0.11	0.13	0.14	0.14		0.17
>160	0.11	0.11				

APPENDIX B-4: NORMAL LABORATORY VALUES

DETERMINATION FOR

(S) = Serum
(B) = Whole blood
(P) = Plasma

ACID-BASE MEASUREMENTS (B)

pH: 7.38-7.42
Pao_2: 65-76 mm Hg
$Paco_2$: 36-38 mm Hg
Base excess: −2 to +2 mEq/L

ACID PHOSPHATASE (S, P)

Newborns: 7.4-19.4 IU/L
2-13 yr: 6.4-15.2 IU/L
Adult males: 0.5-11 IU/L
Adult females: 0.2-9.5 IU/L

ALANINE AMINOTRANSFERASE (SGPT) (S)

Newborns (1-3 days): 1-25 IU/L
Adult males: 7-46 IU/L
Adult females: 4-35 IU/L

ALKALINE PHOSPHATASE (S)

Age	IU/L
Newborns (1-3 days)	95-368
2-24 mo	115-460
2-7 yr	115-460
8-9 yr	115-345
10-11 yr	115-437
12-13 yr	92-403
14-15 yr	78-446
16-18 yr	35-331
Adults	39-137

AMMONIA (P)

Newborns: 9-150 μg/dl (53-88 μmol/L); higher in premature and jaundiced infants
Thereafter: 0-60 μg/dl (0-35 μmol/L) when blood is drawn correctly

---

*Values may vary with laboratory, technique, determination, underlying conditions, etc.

AMYLASE (S)

Neonates: undetectable
2-12 mo: levels increase to adult levels
Adults: 28-108 IU/L

ASPARTATE AMINOTRANSFERASE (SGOT) (S)

Newborns (1-3 days): 16-74 IU/L
Adult males: 8-46 IU/L
Adult females: 7-34 IU/L

BICARBONATE (P)

18-25 mEq/L

BILIRUBIN (S)

After 1 mo
  Conjugated: 0-0.3 mg/dl
  Unconjugated: 0.1-0.7 mg/dl

BLEEDING TIME

1-3 min

CALCIUM (S)

Premature infants: 3.5-4.5 mEq/L
Full-term infants: 4-5 mEq/L
Infants and thereafter: 4.4-5.3 mEq/L

CARBOXYHEMOGLOBIN (B)

<5% of total hemoglobin

CATION-ANION GAP (S, P)

5-15 mEq/L

CHLORIDE (S, P)

96-116 mmol/L

CHOLESTEROL (S, P)

Full-term newborns: 45-167 mg/dl
3 days-1 yr: 69-174 mg/dl
2-14 yr: 120-205 mg/dl
14-19 yr: 120-210 mg/dl
20-29 yr: 120-240 mg/dl
30-39 yr: 140-270 mg/dl
40-49 yr: 150-310 mg/dl
50-59 yr: 160-330 mg/dl

CHOLINESTERASE (S)

2.5-5 μmol/min/ml of serum (pseudocholinesterase)
2.3-4 μmol/min/ml of red cells

COMPLEMENT (S)

C3: 96-195 mg/dl
C4: 15-20 mg/dl

CREATININE (S, P)

Values in mg/dl

Age	Males	Females
Newborns (1-3 days)	0.2-1.0	0.2-1.0
1-3 yr	0.2-0.7	0.2-0.6
4-10 yr	0.2-0.9	0.2-0.8
11-17 yr	0.3-1.2	0.3-1.1
>18 yr	0.5-1.3	0.3-1.1

CREATININE CLEARANCE*

Newborns (1 day): 5-50 ml/min/1.73 m^2 (mean, 18 ml/min/1.73 m^2)
Newborns (6 days): 15-90 ml/min/1.73 m^2 (mean, 36 ml/min/1.73 m^2)
Infants (1 mo): 65 ml/min/1.73 m^2
Infants (2 to 12 mo): 85 ml/min/1.73 m^2
Adult males: 85-125 ml/min/1.73 m^2
Adult females: 75-115 ml/min/1.73 m^2

GLUCOSE (S, P) (SEE CHAPTER 38)

Premature infants: 20-80 mg/dl
Full-term infants: 30-100 mg/dl
Children and adults (fasting): 60-105 mg/dl

γ-GLUTAMYL TRANSPEPTIDASE (S)

0-1 mo: 12-27 IU/L
1-2 mo: 9-159 IU/L
2-4 mo: 7-98 IU/L
4-7 mo: 5-45 IU/L
7-15 mo: 3-30 IU/L
Adult males: 9-69 IU/L
Adult females: 3-33 IU/L

GLYCOHEMOGLOBIN (HEMOGLOBIN A_{IC}) (B)

Normal: 6.3%-8.2% of total hemoglobin
Well-controlled diabetic patients ordinarily have levels <10%

HEMATOCRIT (B) (SEE P. 209)

At birth: 44%-64%
14-90 days: 35%-49%
6 mo-1 yr: 30%-40%
4-10 yr: 31%-43%

HEMOGLOBIN ELECTROPHORESIS (B)

A_1 hemoglobin: 96%-98.5% of total hemoglobin
A_2 hemoglobin: 1.5%-4% of total hemoglobin

FETAL HEMOGLOBIN

At birth: 50%-85% of total hemoglobin
At 1 yr: <15% of total hemoglobin
1-2 yr: up to 5% of total hemoglobin
>2 yr: <2% of total hemoglobin

IMMUNOGLOBINS (S)

Age	IgG (mg/dl)	IgA (mg/dl)	IgM (mg/dl)
2 wk-3 mo	299-852	3-66	15-149
3-6 mo	142-988	4-90	18-118
6-12 mo	418-1142	14-95	43-223
1-6 yr	356-1381	13-209	37-239
6-12 yr	625-1598	29-384	50-278
>12 yr	660-1548	81-252	45-256

IRON (S, P)

Newborns: 20-157 μg/dl
6 wks-3 yr: 20-115 μg/dl
3-9 yr: 20-141 μg/dl
9-14 yr: 21-151 μg/dl
14-16 yr: 20-181 μg/dl
Adults: 44-196 μg/dl

IRON-BINDING CAPACITY (S, P)

Newborns: 59-175 μg/dl
Children and adults: 275-458 μg/dl

LACTATE DEHYDROGENASE (LDH) (S, P)

Newborns (1-3 days): 40-348 IU/L
1 mo-5 yr: 150-360 IU/L
5-12 yr: 130-300 IU/L
12-16 yr: 130-280 IU/L
Adult males: 70-178 IU/L
Adult females: 42-166 IU/L

LACTATE DEHYDROGENASE ISOENZYMES (S)

LDH_1 (heart): 24%-34%
LDH_2 (heart, red cells): 35%-45%
LDH_3 (muscle): 15%-25%
LDH_4 (liver [trace], muscle): 4%-10%
LDH_5 (liver, muscle): 1%-9%

MAGNESIUM (S, P)

Newborns: 1.5-2.3 mEq/L
Adults: 1.4-2 mEq/L

PARTIAL THROMBOPLASTIN TIME (PTT) (P)

Children: 42-54 seconds (varies with control)

PHOSPHORUS, INORGANIC (S, P)

Full-term infants:
  At birth: 5-7.8 mg/dl
  3 days: 5.8-9 mg/dl
  6-12 days: 4.9-8.9 mg/dl
1-10 yr: 3.6-6.2 mg/dl
Adults: 3.1-5.1 mg/dl

POTASSIUM (S, P)

Premature infants: 4.5-7.2 mEq/L
Full-term infants: 3.7-5.2 mEq/L
Children and adults: 3.5-5.8 mEq/L

PROTHROMBIN TIME (P)

Children: 11-15 seconds (varies with control)

SEDIMENTATION RATE (MICRO) (B)

<2 yr: 1-5 mm/h
>2 yr: 1-8 mm/h

SODIUM (S, P)

Children and adults: 135-148 mEq/L

UREA NITROGEN, BLOOD (BUN) (S, P)

<2 yr: 5-15 mg/dl
>2 yr: 10-20 mg/dl

PROTEIN (S)

Age	Total protein (gm/dl)	Albumin (gm/dl)	α_1 Globulin (gm/dl)	α_2 Globulin (gm/dl)	β Globulin (gm/dl)	Gamma globulin (gm/dl)
Birth	4.6-7.0	3.2-4.8	0.1-0.3	0.2-0.3	0.3-0.6	0.6-1.2
3 mo	4.5-6.5	3.2-4.8	0.1-0.3	0.3-0.7	0.3-0.7	0.2-0.7
>1 yr	5.4-8.0	3.7-5.7	0.1-0.3	0.4-1.1	0.4-1.0	0.2-1.3

*Creatinine clearance (ml/min/1.73 m^2) = $\dfrac{UV}{P} \times \dfrac{1.73}{SA}$

P, U, plasma or urinary concentration of creatinine (mg/dl); *V,* volume of urine divided by number of minutes in collection period (24 hr = 1440 min); *SA,* surface area (m^2).

APPENDIX B-5: CONVERSIONS, ESTIMATES, AND NOMOGRAMS

TEMPERATURE

To convert Celsius to Fahrenheit: ($\frac{9}{5}$ × temperature) + 32

To convert Fahrenheit to Celsius: (temperature − 32) × $\frac{5}{9}$

Celsius	Fahrenheit	Celsius	Fahrenheit
34.2	93.6	38.6	101.4
34.6	94.3	39.0	102.2
35.0	95.0	39.4	102.9
35.4	95.7	39.8	103.6
35.8	96.4	40.2	104.3
36.2	97.1	40.6	105.1
36.6	97.8	41.0	105.8
37.0	98.6	41.4	106.5
37.4	99.3	41.8	107.2
37.8	100.0	42.2	108.0
38.2	100.7	42.6	108.7

WEIGHT

To change pounds to grams: multiply by 454

To change kilograms to pounds: multiply by 2.2

If patient weighs ≥10 lb, the following are used, adding the intermediate value in pounds and ounces to determine the final conversion:

10 lb	4.53 kg	110 lb	49.89 kg
20 lb	9.07 kg	120 lb	54.43 kg
30 lb	13.60 kg	130 lb	58.96 kg
40 lb	18.14 kg	140 lb	63.50 kg
50 lb	22.68 kg	150 lb	68.04 kg
60 lb	27.21 kg	160 lb	72.57 kg
70 lb	31.75 kg	170 lb	77.11 kg
80 lb	36.28 kg	180 lb	81.64 kg
90 lb	40.82 kg	190 lb	86.18 kg
100 lb	45.36 kg	200 lb	90.72 kg

Growth Patterns

Birth weight (avg): 3.3 kg (7 lb 5 oz)

A newborn loses up to 10% of birth weight initially but should be up to birth weight again by 10 days.

An infant gains 30 gm (1 oz)/day for the first 1-2 mo

5 mo: birth weight should be doubled

12 mo: birth weight should be tripled

2 yr: birth weight should be quadrupled

Weight conversion table (pounds and ounces to grams)

Ounces	0 lb	1 lb	2 lb	3 lb	4 lb	5 lb	6 lb	7 lb	8 lb	9 lb
0		454	907	1361	1814	2268	2722	3175	3629	4082
1	28	482	936	1389	1843	2296	2750	3204	3657	4111
2	57	510	964	1418	1871	2325	2778	3232	3686	4139
3	85	539	992	1446	1899	2353	2807	3260	3714	4168
4	113	567	1020	1474	1928	2382	2835	3289	3742	4196
5	142	595	1049	1503	1956	2410	2863	3317	3771	4224
6	170	624	1077	1531	1984	2438	2892	3345	3799	4253
7	198	652	1106	1559	2013	2467	2920	3374	3827	4281
8	227	680	1134	1588	2041	2495	2948	3402	3855	4309
9	255	709	1162	1616	2070	2523	2977	3430	3884	4338
10	284	737	1191	1644	2098	2552	3005	3459	3912	4366
11	312	765	1219	1673	2126	2580	3034	3487	3940	4394
12	340	794	1247	1701	2155	2608	3062	3516	3969	4423
13	369	822	1276	1729	2183	2637	3090	3544	3997	4451
14	397	850	1304	1758	2211	2665	3119	3572	4026	4479
15	425	879	1332	1786	2240	2693	3147	3601	4054	4508

Estimates of Weight

4 to 8-year-old: $6 \times \text{Age} + 12 = \text{Weight (lb)}$
8 to 12-year-old: $7 \times \text{Age} + 5 = \text{Weight (lb)}$

LENGTH

To convert inches to centimeters: multiply by 2.54

To convert centimeters to inches: multiply by 0.394

Growth Patterns

Birth length (avg): 50 cm (20 in)
12 mo: birth length should be doubled

HEAD CIRCUMFERENCE
Growth Patterns

Birth head circumference (avg): 35 cm (14 in)
12 mo head circumference (avg): 47 cm (19 in)
Head circumference: grows 1 cm/mo during first 9 mo

BLOOD PRESSURE (ESTIMATE)

Systolic BP (mm Hg) = $2 \times \text{Age (yr)} + 80$
Diastolic BP (mm Hg) = $\frac{2}{3}$ systolic

OTHER CONVERSION FACTORS

To convert	To	Multiply by
1 mm Hg	psi	0.0193
1 cm H_2O	mm Hg	0.735
1 mm Hg	cm H_2O	1.259
1 cm	inch	0.3937
1 inch	cm	2.541
kg	pound	2.204
1 pound	kg	0.4536
1 Fr size	mm	0.33

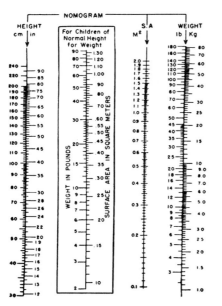

Nomogram for estimation of surface area. The surface area is indicated where a straight line that connects the height and weight levels intersects the surface area column; or the patient is roughly of average size, from the weight alone *(enclosed area)*.

(Modified from data of E Boyd by CD West.)

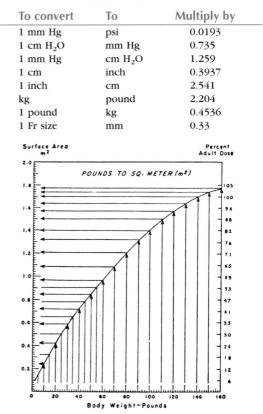

Relations among body weight in pounds, body surface area, and adult dosage. The surface area values correspond to those set forth by Crawford et al. (1950). Note that the 100% adult dose is for a patient weighing about 140 pounds and having a surface area of about 1.7 square meters.

(From Talbot NB, et al: *Metabolic homeostasis—a syllabus for those concerned with the care of patients,* Cambridge, 1959, Harvard University Press.)

From Vaughn VC, Behrman RE: *Nelson Textbook of Pediatrics,* ed 11, Philadelphia, 1967, WB Saunders.

APPENDIX B-6: DENVER DEVELOPMENTAL SCREENING TEST

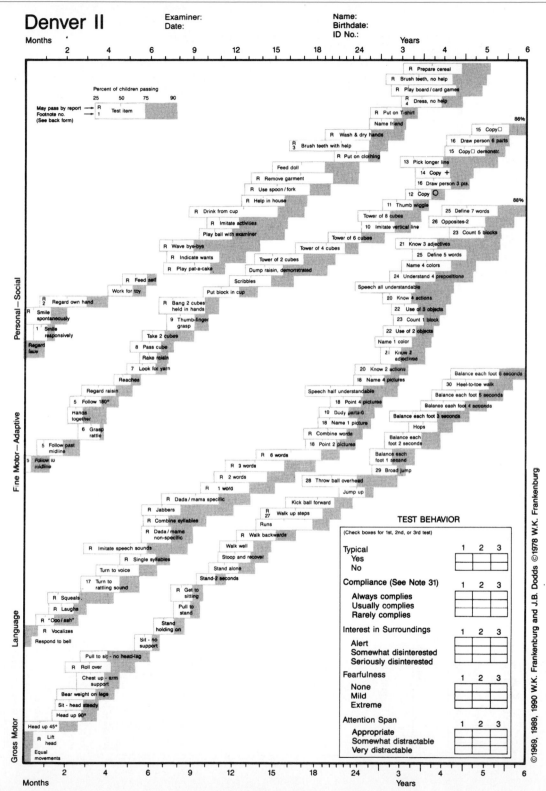

From Frankenburg WK, Dodds J, Archer P, et al: *Pediatrics* 89:91, 1992.

APPENDIX B-7: RECOMMENDED CHILDHOOD IMMUNIZATION SCHEDULE UNITED STATES 1998

Vaccines* are listed under the routinely recommended ages. [Bars] indicate range of acceptable ages for immunization. Catch-up immunization should be done during any visit when feasible. Shaded (ovals) indicate vaccines to be assessed and given if necessary during early adolescent visit.

Age ▶ / Vaccine ▼	Birth	1 mo	2 mo	4 mo	6 mo	12 mo	15 mo	18 mo	4-6 yr	11-12 yr	14-16 yr
Hepatitis B[†,‡]	Hep B-1	Hep B-2			Hep B-3					Hep B[‡]	
Diphtheria, tetanus, pertussis[§]			DTaP or DTP	DTaP or DTP	DTaP or DTP		DTaP or DTP[§]	DTaP or DTP[§]	DTaP or DTP	Td	
H. influenzae type b[‖]			Hib	Hib	Hib	Hib	Hib				
Polio[¶]			Polio[¶]	Polio		Polio	Polio	Polio	Polio		
Measles, mumps, rubella[**]						MMR	MMR		MMR[**]	MMR[**]	
Varicella[††]						Var[††]	Var[††]	Var[††]		Var[††]	

Approved by the Advisory Committee on Immunization Practices (ACIP), the American Academy of Pediatrics (AAP), and the American Academy of Family Physicians (AAFP).

*This schedule indicates the recommended age for routine administration of currently licensed childhood vaccines. Some combination vaccines are available and may be used whenever administration of all components of the vaccine is indicated. Providers should consult the manufacturers' package inserts for detailed recommendations.

† **Infants born to HBsAg-negative mothers** should receive 2.5 μg of Merck vaccine (Recombivax HB) or 10 μg of SmithKline Beecham (SB) vaccine (Engerix-B). The second dose should be administered at least 1 mo after the first dose. The third dose should be given at least 2 mo after the second, but not before 6 mo of age. **Infant born to HBsAg-positive mothers** should receive 0.5 ml hepatitis B immune globulin (HBIG) within 12 hrs of birth, and either 5 μg of Merck vaccine (Recombivax HB) or 10 μg of SB vaccine (Engerix-B) at a separate site. The second dose is recommended at 1-2 mo of age and the third dose at 6 mo of age. **Infants born to mothers whose HBsAg status is unknown** should receive either 5 μg of Merck vaccine (Recombivax HB) or 10 μg of SB vaccine (Engerix-B) within 12 hr of birth. The second dose of vaccine is recommended at 1 mo of age and the third dose at 6 mo of age. Blood should be drawn at the time of delivery to determine the mother's HBsAg status; if it is positive, the infant should receive HBIG as soon as possible (no later than 1 wk of age). The dosage and timing of subsequent vaccine doses should be based on the mother's HBsAg status.

‡Children and adolescents who have not been vaccinated against hepatitis B in infancy may begin the series during any visit. Those who have not previously received three doses of hepatitis B vaccine should initiate or complete the series during the 11- to 12-yr-old visit, and unvaccinated older adolescents should be vaccinated whenever possible. The second dose should be administered at least 1 mo after the first dose, and the third dose should be administered at least 4 mo after the first dose and at least 2 mo after the second dose.

§DTaP (diphtheria and tetanus toxoids and acellular pertussis vaccine) is the preferred vaccine for all doses in the vaccination series, including completion of the series in children who have received 1 or more doses of whole-cell DTP vaccine. Whole-cell DTP is an acceptable alternative to DTaP. The fourth dose (DTP or DTaP) may be administered as early as 12 mo of age, provided 6 mo have elapsed since the third dose, and if the child is considered unlikely to return at 15-18 mo. Td (tetanus and diphtheria toxoids) is recommended at 11-12 yr of age if at least 5 yr have elapsed since the last dose of DTP, DTaP, or DT. Subsequent routine Td boosters are recommended every 10 years.

‖Three *H. influenzae* type b (Hib) conjugate vaccines are licensed for infant use. If PRP-CMP (PedvaxHIB [Merck]) is administered at 2 and 4 mo of age, a dose at 6 mo is not required.

¶Two poliovirus vaccines are currently licensed in the United States: inactivated poliovirus vaccine (IPV) and oral poliovirus vaccine (OPV). The following schedules are all acceptable to the ACIP, the AAP, and the AAFP. Parents and providers may choose among these options:
1. Two doses of IPV followed by 2 doses of OPV.
2. Four doses of IPV.
3. Four doses of OPV.

The ACIP routinely recommends two doses of IPV at 2 and 4 mo of age followed by 2 doses of OPV at 12-18 mo and 4-6 yr of age. IPV is the only poliovirus vaccine recommended for immunocompromised persons and their household contacts.

**The second dose of MMR is routinely recommended at 4-6 yr of age but may be administered during any visit, provided at least 1 mo has elapsed since receipt of the first dose and that both doses are administered beginning at or after 12 mo of age. Those who have not previously received the second dose should complete the schedule no later than the 11- to 12-yr visit.

††Susceptible children may receive varicella vaccine (Var) at any visit after the first birthday, and those who lack a reliable history of chickenpox should be immunized during the 11- to 12-yr-old visit. Susceptible children 13 yr of age or older should receive two doses, at least 1 mo apart.

ADDITIONAL NOTES
Precautions and Contraindications

Minor illness or fever: Although immunizations are generally reserved for healthy patients, these are not contraindications. Deferring administration may lead to unimmunized children. However, if the fever or other manifestations suggest a moderate or serious illness, deferral is appropriate.

Immunocompromised children require special consideration, whether the condition is a congenital immunodeficiency, human immunodeficiency virus (HIV) infection, malignancy, or receipt of immunosuppressive therapy.

Egg Allergy

Children with egg allergy, even those with severe hypersensitivity, are at low risk of anaphylactic reactions to measles and mumps vaccine, singly or in combination; skin testing is not predictive of an allergic reaction. When vaccine is administered, it should be given as one injection and the child should be observed for 90 minutes with immediate availability of emergency equipment.

Influenza Vaccine (Inactivated)

Recommended in high-risk patients, including those with renal, metabolic, cardiac, or pulmonary disease, as well as immunocompromised hosts. The recommendations are reassessed *annually*, but in general, children 6 to 35 months of age receive 0.25 ml (split virus) twice given 4 weeks apart, those 3 to 12 years receive 0.5 ml (split virus) twice, and children more than 12 years should be given 0.5 ml (whole or split virus) once.

Pneumococcal Vaccine

Recommended for children older than 2 years of age who are at risk of severe pneumococcal infection. Indications are sickle cell disease; functional or anatomic asplenia; nephrotic syndrome or chronic renal failure; conditions associated with immunosuppression such as organ transplantation, drug therapy, or cytoreduction therapy; HIV infection, or cerebrospinal fluid (CSF) leaks.

Prematurity

The appropriate age for initiating most immunizations in the prematurely born infant is the usual recommended chronologic age. Vaccine doses should not be reduced for preterm infants. Studies are in progress.

Lapsed Immunizations

A lapse in the immunization schedule dose does not require reinstituting the entire series. If a dose of DTaP (or DTP), poliovirus vaccine, Hib or hepatitis B vaccine is missed, the next immunization should be given as if the usual interval had elapsed.

Adverse Reactions

Before administering a vaccine, previous adverse reactions should be sought. Unexpected events occurring soon after administration of any vaccine should be described in detail and reported to the Vaccine Adverse Events Reporting System (800-338-2382).

Informed Consent

Parents and patients should be informed about the benefits to be derived from vaccines in preventing disease in individuals and the risks of those vaccines. Questions should be encouraged to ensure that information is understood.

Health care providers should note in the patient's record the information that was provided. In addition, the date of administration of the vaccine, the manufacturer and lot of the vaccine, and the name of the provider should be recorded.

REFERENCES

American Academy of Pediatrics: *Report of the committee on infectious diseases,* ed 24, Elk Grove, Ill, 1997, The Academy.

Committee on Infectious Diseases, AAP: Poliomyelitis prevention recommendations for use of inactivated poliovirus vaccine and live oral poliovirus vaccine, *Pediatrics* 99:300, 1997.

Evans G: National childhood vaccine injury act: revision of the vaccine injury table, *Pediatrics* 98:1179, 1996.

Goldstein KP, Kviz FJ, Daum RS: Accuracy of immunization histories provided by adults accompanying preschool children to a pediatric emergency department, *JAMA* 270:2190, 1993.

Lindegren ML, Atkinson WL, Farizo KM, et al: Measles vaccination in pediatric emergency departments during a measles outbreak, *JAMA* 270:2185, 1993.

Robinson PE, Gausche M, Gerardi MJ, et al: Immunization of the pediatric patient in the emergency department, *Ann Emerg Med* 28:334, 1996.

Rodewald LE, Szilagyi PG, Humiston SG, et al: Effect of emergency department immunization rates and subsequent primary care visits, *Arch Pediatr Adolesc Med* 150:1271, 1996.

C FORMULARY

APPENDIX C-1: COMMON MEDICATIONS

Drugs	Dosages	Comments
Acetaminophen (Tylenol, Tempra) Drop: 80 mg/0.8 ml Elix: 160 mg/5 ml Tab: 80 (chew), 160 (junior), 325 mg Supp: 120, 325 mg	10-15 mg/kg/dose q4-6hr PO (adult: 10 gr/dose); (maximum: 3.6 gm/24 hr)	May give aspirin/ibuprofen for synergistic antipyretic effect; also see Codeine Tox: hepatic: overdose (Chapter 55)
Acetazolamide (Diamox) Tab: 125, 250 mg Cap (SR): 500 mg Vial: 500 mg/5 ml	Diuretic: 5 mg/kg/24 hr q6-24hr PO, IV (adult: 250-375 mg/24 hr) Epilepsy: 8-30 mg/kg/24 hr q6-8hr PO, IM, IV (maximum: 1 gm/24 hr)	Carbonic anhydrase inhibitor; IM painful; half-life: 4-10 hr; prophylaxis for high-altitude sickness; Table 16-3 Tox: hypokalemia, acidosis (long- term therapy), paresthesias
Acetylcysteine (Mucomyst) Soln: 10% (100 mg/ml) 20% (200 mg/ml)	Acetaminophen OD: load 140 mg/kg PO, then 70 mg/kg q4hr PO × 17 doses Nebulizer: 2-20 ml (10%) or 1-10 ml (20%) soln q2-6hr	Primary treatment for acetamino- phen overdose (Chapter 55); pulmonary mucolytic; IV preparation available (investi- gational) Tox: mucosal irritant, broncho- spasm
Acyclovir (Zovirax) Cap: 200 mg Vial: 500 mg/10 ml Ointment: 5%	Herpes genitalis: 200 mg q4hr (5 doses/24 hr) PO × 5-10 days Herpes neonatorum: 30 mg/kg/24 hr q8hr IV × 10 days Varicella: 80 mg/kg/24 hr q6hr PO × 5 days (maximum: 3200 mg/24 hr) q6hr PO × 5 days	IV therapy indicated in immuno- compromised patient; effective in newborn; modified dose for recurrent episode or suppres- sion; reduce with renal failure Tox: diaphoresis, hematuria, phlebitis (IV)
Adenosine (Adenocard) Vial: 3 mg/ml	0.1-0.2 mg/kg rapid (1-2 min) bolus; may repeat and double in 2 min if unsuccessful Adult: 6 mg IV as rapid (1-2 min) bolus; repeat 12 mg IV up to 2 times if no response in 2 min	No controlled studies in children but commonly used for parox- ysmal supraventricular tachy- cardia Tox: facial flushing, dyspnea, nausea, metallic taste

Many oral drugs may be given 3-4 times/day with more flexibility than implied by the specific intervals noted. Adult dose provided as guideline for maximum dose. *NB,* Newborns <7 days of age; *Pen,* penicillin; *SR,* sustained release; *Tox,* toxicity of drug.

Drugs	Dosages	Comments
Albumin 25% salt-poor albumin (25 gm/dl) 5% with 0.9% NS (5 gm/dl)	0.5-1 gm/kg/dose IV repeated prn	Salt-poor albumin has 0.6 mEq Na^+/gm; caution with hypervolemia, CHF
Albuterol (Proventil, Ventolin) Syr: 2 mg/5 ml Soln (inhalation): 0.5%: 5 mg/ml Tab: 2, 4 mg	Inhalation: 0.03 ml (0.15 mg)/kg/dose to maximum of 0.5-1.0 ml/dose diluted in 2 ml 0.9% NS; may repeat q20min × 3 or as needed Oral: 0.1-0.2 mg/kg/dose q6-8hr PO (maximum: 4 mg/dose)	β_2 Agonist with little cardiac effect; higher dosage more effective; available as MDI
Allopurinol (Zyloprim) Tab: 100, 300 mg	10 mg/kg/24 hr q6hr PO (<6 yr, 150 mg/24 hr; 6-10 yr: 300 mg/24 hr) (maximum: 600 mg/24 hr)	Titrate to serum uric acid level; reduce dosage with renal failure Tox: rash, hepatic, cataract
Aluminum hydroxide (Amphogel) Tab: 300, 600 mg Susp: 320 mg/5 ml **Maalox** (also magnesium hydroxide) Tab: 200/200, 400/400 mg Susp: 225/200 mg/5 ml	Peptic ulcer: 5-15 ml (adult: 15-45 ml) 1 and 3 hr after meals and before bed PO Prophylaxis GI bleeding Infant: 2-5 ml/dose q1-2hr PO Child: 5-15 ml/dose (adult: 30-60 ml) q1-2hr PO	Should be initiated early for prophylaxis; alternative includes cimetidine
Amantidine (Symmetrel) Syr: 50 mg/5 ml Cap: 100 mg	4.4-8.8 mg/kg/24 hr q12hr PO (>9 yr and adult: 100 mg q12hr PO or 200 mg q24hr PO)	Continue for at least 10 days and longer in unprotected high-risk patient with ongoing exposure to influenza A; only children >1 yr; effective if given early Tox: depression, CHF, psychosis, seizures
Amikacin (Amikin) Vial: 50, 250 mg/ml	15 mg/kg/24 hr q8hr IM, IV slowly over 30 min (maximum: 1.0 gm/ 24 hr) (NB: 15 mg/kg/24 hr q12hr)	Therapeutic peak level: <35 µg/ml: caution in renal failure (reduce dosage) Tox: renal, VIII nerve
Aminocaproic acid (Amicar) Syr: 250 mg/ml Tab: 500 mg Vial: 250 mg/ml	Load: 200 mg/kg PO (maximum: 6 gm); 100 mg/kg/dose q6hr PO (maximum: 24 gm/24 hr) × 5-7 days or until healing occurs Load: 100 mg/kg IV, then 33.3 mg/kg/hr IV up to 30 gm/24 hr	Useful for oral bleeding; also available for IV use; Chapter 79 Tox: thrombosis, rash, hypotension

Drugs	Dosages	Comments
Aminophylline		
	Load: 7.5 mg/kg PO; maintenance: 5 mg/kg/dose q6hr PO Load: 6 mg/kg IV slowly, maintenance: 0.8-1.2 mg/kg/hr IV Neonatal apnea load: 5 mg/kg; then 2-3 mg/kg q12hr PO	85% theophylline: therapeutic level: 10-20 µg/ml; neonatal apnea (Chapter 84) Tox: nausea, vomiting, irritability, seizures, dysrhythmias
Amiodarone (Cardarone) Tab: 200 mg	10 mg/kg/24 hr q12hr PO × 7-10 days, then reduce to 5 mg/kg/24 hr (maximum: 15 mg/kg/24 hr for 2-3 wk) (adult: load with 800-1600 mg/24 hr for 1-3 wk, then 600-800 mg/24 hr × 1 mo, then 200-400 mg/24 hr)	Little experience in children
Amoxicillin (Amoxil, Larotid) Susp: 125, 250 mg/5 ml Cap: 125, 250 mg	30-100 mg (average: 50 mg)/kg/24 hr q8hr PO (adult: 250-500 mg q8hr)	Do not use for *Shigella* Tox: similar to ampicillin but less diarrhea; see Penicillin G
Amoxicillin (AMX)-clavulanic acid (CLA) (Augmentin) Susp: 125 mg AMX/31.25 CLA/5 ml, 250 mg AMX/62.50 CLA/5 ml Tab: 250 mg AMX/125 CLA, 500 mg AMX/125 CLA Tab (chew): 125 mg AMX/31.25 CLA, 250 mg AMX/62.5 CLA	30-50 mg AMX/kg/24 hr q8hr PO (adult: 250-500 mg AMX q8hr PO)	Dosage is based on amount of amoxicillin; 2 tab 250 mg are not equivalent to 500 mg tab; β-lactamase inhibitor Tox: diarrhea, similar to amoxicillin
Amphotericin (Fungizone) Vial: 50 mg	0.6 mg/kg/24 hr IV over 1-4 hours; begin at 0.2 mg/kg/24 hr and increase dosage	May also be given intrathecal; only for severe fungal infection; initial test dose 0.1 mg/kg over 20-60 min Tox: fever, chills, bone marrow suppression
Ampicillin (Omnipen, Polycillin) Susp: 125, 250 mg/5 ml Cap: 250, 500 mg Vial: 250, 500, 1000 mg	50-100 mg/kg/24 hr q6hr PO (adult: 250-500 mg/dose PO); 100-400 mg/kg/24 hr q4-6hr IV (NB: 50-100 mg/kg/24 hr q12hr IV) (adult: 4-12 gm/24 hr IV)	Higher parenteral doses with severe infection: 3 mEq Na$^+$/gm Tox: rash (especially with infectious mononucleosis), diarrhea, superinfection; see Penicillin G

Many oral drugs may be given 3-4 times/day with more flexibility than implied by the specific intervals noted. Adult dose provided as guideline for maximum dose. *NB,* Newborns <7 days of age; *Pen,* penicillin; *SR,* sustained release; *Tox,* toxicity of drug.

Drugs	Dosages	Comments
Ampicillin (AMP)/Sulbactam (SUL) (Unasyn) Vial: 1.5, 3.0 gm	Adult: 1 gm AMP/0.5 gm SUL q6hr IV	Intraabdominal, gynecologic infections; semisynthetic β-lactamase inhibitor Little experience in children <12 yr
Aspirin (salicylate, ASA) Tab: 81 (chew), 325 mg Supp: 65, 130, 195, 325 mg	10-15 mg/kg/dose q4-6hr PO (adult: 10 gr or 650 mg/dose) Rheumatoid: 60-100 mg/kg/24 hr q4-6hr PO (maximum: 3.6 gm/24 hr PO)	Synergistic antipyretic effect with acetaminophen; avoid with chickenpox or influenza-like illness Therapeutic level: 15-30 mg/dl Tox: GI irritation, tinnitus, platelet dysfunction; overdose (Chapter 54)
Atenolol (Tenormin) Tab: 50, 100 mg	Hypertension: 1-2 mg/kg/dose q24hr PO (adult: 50 mg q24hr PO up to 100 mg q24hr PO)	Little experience in children; response seen in 1 wk; also available for IV use
Atropine Vial: 0.1, 0.4, 1 mg/ml	0.02 mg/kg/dose IV (minimum: 0.1 mg/dose) (adult: 0.6-1.0 mg/dose; maximum total dose 2 mg) q5min prn; may also be given ET	Infants require higher dose (0.03 mg/kg); organophosphate poisoning (0.05 mg/kg) (Chapter 54) Tox: dysrhythmias, anticholinergic
Azithromycin (Zithromax) Cap: 250 mg Pack: 1 gm	Otitis media: 10 mg/kg/24 hr q24hr PO followed by half dose on days 2-5 Pharyngitis: 12 mg/kg/24 hr q24hr PO × 5 days Uncomplicated genital chlamydia: 1 gm PO	Pharyngitis relapse high
Beclomethasone (Beclovent, Vanceril) MDI (inhalation: 42 µg/dose)	6-12 yr: 1-2 puffs QID >12 yr: 2 puffs QID	
Benztropine (Cogentin) Tab: 0.5, 1, 2 mg Vial: 1 mg/ml	>3 yr: 0.02-0.05 mg/kg/dose q12-24hr PO, IV Adult: 1-4 mg/dose IV	Pediatric dose not well established
Bethanechol (Urecholine) Tab: 5, 10, 25 mg Vial: 5 mg/ml	0.6 mg/kg/24 hr q8hr PO (adult: 10-30 mg QID PO) 0.15-0.2 mg/kg/24 hr SC (adult: 2.5-5 mg/24 hr)	

Drugs	Dosages	Comments
Bicarbonate, sodium (NaHCO$_3$) Vial: 8.4% (50 mEq/50 ml) 7.5% (44 mEq/50 ml) 4.2% (0.5 mEq/ml) for newborns	1 mEq/kg/dose q10min IV prn	Monitor ABG: dilute 1:1 with D5W or sterile water; incompatible with calcium, catecholamines Tox: alkalosis, hyperosmolality, hypernatremia
Bretylium (Bretylol) Vial: 50 mg/ml	5 mg/kg/dose IV followed prn by 10 mg/kg/dose q15min IV up to maximum total dose 30 mg/kg	Table 6-4; limited experience in children; use only after defibrillation and lidocaine unsuccessful Tox: nausea, vomiting, hypotension, bradycardia
Bumetanide (Bumex) Vial: 0.25 mg/ml Tab: 0.5, 1 mg	Begin with 0.015-0.1 mg/kg/dose q8-12hr IV up to a maximum of 0.3 mg/kg/dose or 10 mg/24 hr	Limited experience in children
Calcium chloride Vial: 10% (100 mg/ml-1.36 mEq Ca^{++}/ml)	20-30 mg/kg/dose IV (slow) (maximum: 500 mg/dose) q10min prn; 250 mg/kg 24 hr q6hr PO (mix 2% soln)	Monitor heart, avoid extravasation; caution in digitalized patient; incompatible with NaHCO$_3$ Tox: bradycardia, hypotension
Calcium gluconate Vial: 10% (100 mg/ml-0.45 mEq Ca^{++}/ml) Tab: 1 gm	100 mg/kg dose IV (slow) (maximum: 1 gm/dose) q10 min prn; 500 mg/kg/24 hr q6hr PO	See Calcium chloride
Captopril (Capoten) Tab: 12.5, 25, 50, 100 mg	1-6 mg/kg/24 hr q8hr PO (maximum: 450 mg/24 hr) (adult: initial 25 mg q8hr PO)	Table 18-2 Tox: renal, proteinuria, neutropenia, rash
Carbamazepine (Tegretol) Tab: 100 mg (chewable), 200 mg	10-40 mg/kg/24 hr q8-12hr PO (adult: 800-1600 mg/24 hr; begin 100-200 mg/dose q12hr PO with 100 mg/24 hr increments)	Therapeutic level: 4-14 µg/ml: Table 81-6 Tox: hepatic, nystagmus, nausea, aplastic anemia
Carbenicillin (Geopen, Geocillin) Vial: 1, 2, 5, 10 gm Tab: 382 mg	400-600 mg/kg/24 hr q4-6hr IV; 30-50 mg/kg/24 hr q6h PO (NB: 200 mg/kg/24 hr q12hr IV) (adult: 40 gm/24 hr IV; 2 gm/24 hr PO)	Used in combination therapy with aminoglycoside; 5.2-6.5 mEq Na$^+$/gm Tox: platelet dysfunction, rash; adjust dose with renal failure; see Penicillin G

Many oral drugs may be given 3-4 times/day with more flexibility than implied by the specific intervals noted. Adult dose provided as guideline for maximum dose. *NB,* Newborns <7 days of age; *Pen,* penicillin; *SR,* sustained release; *Tox,* toxicity of drug.

Drugs	Dosages	Comments
Cefaclor (Ceclor) Susp: 125, 250 mg/5 ml Cap: 250, 500 mg	20-40 mg/kg/24 hr q8hr PO (adult: 250-500 mg q8hr)	Active against ampicillin-resistant *H. influenzae*; second-generation cephalosporin Tox: renal, diarrhea, vaginitis; cross-reacts with penicillin
Cefadroxil (Duricef) Susp: 125, 250, 500 mg/5 ml Cap: 500 mg Tab: 1 gm	30 mg/kg/24 hr q12hr PO (maximum: 2 gm/24 hr)	Relatively long half-life; first-generation cephalosporin Tox: diarrhea, pruritus; cross-reacts with penicillin
Cefazolin (Ancef) Vial: 0.25, 0.5, 1 gm	25-100 mg/kg/24 hr q6-8hr IM, IV (NB: 40 mg/kg/24 hr q12hr) (adult: 2-12 gm/24 hr)	First-generation cephalosporin Tox: renal, hepatic, rash, phlebitis; cross-reacts with penicillin; adjust dosage with renal failure
Cefixime (Suprax) Syr: 100 mg/5 ml Tab: 200, 400 mg	8 mg/kg/24 hr q12-24hr PO (adult: 400 mg/24 hr)	Third-generation cephalosporin
Cefoperazone (Cefobid) Vial: 1, 2 gm	100-150 mg/kg/24 hr q8-12hr IV (maximum: 12 gm/24hr) Adult: 2-12 gm/24 hr q6-12hr IV slowly, IM	Third-generation cephalosporin; limited experience in children; half-life 2 hr Tox: diarrhea, hypersensitivity
Cefotaxime (Claforan) Vial: 1, 2 gm	50-150 mg/kg/24 hr q6-8hr IV, IM (neonatal meningitis: 100-150 mg/kg/24 hr q8-12hr) (adult: 1-2 gm q4-6hr up to maximum: 12 gm/24 hr)	Third-generation cephalosporin; excellent broad-spectrum coverage; meningitis, UTI, bacteremia, pneumonia, skin infection; half-life 1 hr Tox: hypersensitivity (cross-reacts with penicillin), phlebitis, pain (IM), diarrhea, colitis, renal, hepatic
Cefoxitin (Mefoxin) Vial: 1, 2 gm	80-160 mg/kg/24 hr q4-6hr IV (maximum: 12 gm/24 hr) PID: adult: 2 gm q6hr IV	Second-generation cephalosporin; good anaerobic coverage Tox: pain at site if IM injection, nausea, vomiting; adjust dosage with renal failure

Drugs	Dosages	Comments
Cefpodoxime (Vantin) Susp: 50, 100 mg/5 ml Tab: 100, 200 mg	10 mg/kg/24 hr q12hr PO (maximum: 800 mg/24 hr)	Second-generation cephalosporin
Cefprozil (Cefzil) Susp: 125, 250 mg/5 ml Tab: 250, 500 mg	15-30 mg/kg/24 hr q12hr PO (maximum: 1000 mg/24 hr)	Second-generation cephalosporin
Ceftazidime (Fortaz) Vial: 0.5, 1, 2 gm	100-150 mg/kg/24 hr q8hr IV (adult: 3-6 gm/24 hr)	Third-generation cephalosporin; limited CNS data Tox: diarrhea; cross-reacts with penicillin
Ceftizoxime (Cefizox) Vial: 1, 2 gm	150-200 mg/kg/24 hr q6-8hr IV (neonatal meningitis: 100-200 mg/kg/24 hr q8-12hr IV) (adult: 6-12 gm/24 hr)	Third-generation cephalosporin Tox: diarrhea; cross-reacts with penicillin
Ceftriaxone (Rocephin) Vial: 0.25, 0.5, 1, 2 gm	50-100 mg/kg/24 hr q12-24hr IV, IM (adult: 1-2 gm/dose q12-24hr IV, IM)	Third-generation cephalosporin; use in children >1 mo; less frequent administration; half-life 5-8 hr; reports of delayed CNS sterilization Tox: diarrhea, abnormal liver function, cholecystitis
Cefuroxime (Zinacef, Ceftin) Vial: 750, 1500 mg Tab: 125, 250, 500 mg	50-240 mg/kg/24 hr q6-8hr IV (adult: 4.5-9.0 gm/24 hr q6-8hr IV) 30 mg/kg/24 hr q12hr PO; >12 yr: 250-500 mg q12hr PO	Second-generation cephalosporin; oral formulation; higher dosage IV for meningitis but slower sterilization; useful for *H. influenzae* disease; do not use for neonatal meningitis, sepsis; oral form for nontoxic child with respiratory, skin, or urinary infections; 5 days oral treatment for otitis media
Cephalexin (Keflex) Susp: 125, 250 mg/5 ml Cap: 250, 500 mg	25-50 mg/kg/24 hr q6hr PO (adult: 250-500 mg/dose q6hr)	First-generation cephalosporin Tox: nausea, vomiting, renal, hepatic; cross-reacts with penicillin; adjust dosage with renal failure

Many oral drugs may be given 3-4 times/day with more flexibility than implied by the specific intervals noted. Adult dose provided as guideline for maximum dose. *NB,* Newborns <7 days of age; *Pen,* penicillin; *SR,* sustained release; *Tox,* toxicity of drug.

Drugs	Dosages	Comments
Cephalothin (Keflin) Vial: 1, 2, 4 gm	75-125 mg/kg/24 hr q4-6hr IM, IV (NB: 40 mg/kg/24 hr q12hr) (adult: 4-12 gm/24 hr)	First-generation cephalosporin Tox: renal, hepatic, phlebitis, neutropenia; cross-reacts with penicillin; adjust dosage with renal failure
Cephradine (Anspor, Velosef) Susp: 125, 250 mg/5 ml Cap: 250, 500 mg Vial: 0.25, 0.5, 1 gm	25-50 mg/kg/24 hr q6hr PO; 50-100 mg/kg/24 hr q6hr IM (deep), IV (maximum: 4 gm/24 hr)	First-generation cephalosporin Tox: renal, hepatic, nausea, vomiting, neutropenia, vaginitis, phlebitis, cross-reacts with penicillin; adjust dosage with renal failure
Charcoal, activated	1 gm/kg or 15-50 gm PO (adult: 50-100 gm/dose)	First dose may be mixed with 35%-70% sorbitol; may require NG tube for administration
Chloral hydrate (Noctec) Syr: 500 mg/5 ml (also 250 mg/5 ml) Cap: 250, 500 mg	Hypnotic: 50-100 mg/kg/24 hr q6-8hr PO (maximum: 1 gm/dose in children; 2 gm/dose in adults) Sedative: ½ hypnotic dose	Hypnotic dose often needed for sedation; do not use with renal, hepatic disease; two strengths of syrup
Chloramphenicol (Chloromycetin) Susp: 150 mg/5 ml Cap: 250 mg Vial: 1 gm (100 mg/ml)	50-100 mg/kg/24 hr q6hr IV (NB: 25 mg/kg/24 hr q12hr IV) (adult: maximum 2-4 gm/24 hr)	Tox: bone marrow suppression (reversible) and aplastic anemia; therapeutic level: 10-25 µg/ml
Chloroquine phosphate (Aralen) Tab: 500 mg (300 mg base)	10 mg base/kg/24 hr q24hr PO	Several forms available; see Appendix C-4
Chlorothiazide (Diuril) Susp: 250 mg/5 ml Tab: 250, 500 mg	10-20 mg/kg/24 hr q12hr PO (NB: 30 mg/kg/24 hr PO) (adult: 500-1000 mg q12-24hr PO)	Table 16-3 Tox: hyponatremia, hypokalemia, alkalosis; reduce dosage with renal failure
Chlorpheniramine (Chlor-Trimeton) Syr: 2 mg/5 ml Tab: 4 mg Tab/cap (SR): 8, 12 mg	0.35 mg/kg/24 hr q6hr PO (adult: 4 mg q4-6hr) Sustained release in children >12 yr: 16-24 mg/kg/24 hr q8-12hr PO	OTC antihistamine Tox: drowsiness, anticholinergic (Chapter 55), hypotension (IM)
Chlorpromazine (Thorazine) Syr: 10 mg/5 ml Tab: 10, 25, 50, 100 mg Cap (SR): 30, 75, 150 mg Supp: 25, 100 mg Vial: 25 mg/ml	0.5 mg/kg/dose q6-8hr PO, IM, IV prn (adult: 25-50 mg/dose) 1.0 mg/kg/dose q6-8hr PR prn (adult: 50-100 mg/dose PR)	Only children >6 mo old Tox: phenothiazine-extrapyramidal, anticholinergic (Chapter 55); often mixed with meperidine and promethazine (see Meperidine)

Drugs	Dosages	Comments
Cimetidine (Tagamet) Susp: 300 mg/5 ml Tab: 200, 300 mg Vial: 150 mg/ml	20-30 mg/kg/24 hr q6hr PO, IV (maximum: 2.4 gm/24 hr) (adult: 300 mg/dose q6hr PO)	Tox: diarrhea renal, neutropenia; reduce dosage with renal failure
Ciprofloxacin (Cipro) Tab: 250, 500, 750 mg	Adult: 250-750 mg q12hr PO	Should not be used in children <12 yr (probably causes arthropathy); reduce dosage if impaired renal function
Clarithromycin (Biaxin) Susp: 125, 250 mg/5 ml Tab: 250, 500 mg	15 mg/kg/24 hr q12hr PO Adult: 250-500 mg q12hr PO	Increases theophylline and car- bamazepine levels; do not refrigerate oral suspension
Clindamycin (Cleocin) Soln, topical: 1% Cap: 75, 150 mg Amp: 300, 600 mg	10-25 mg/kg/24 hr q6hr PO (adult: 600-1800 mg/24 hr PO) 15-40 mg/kg/24 hr q6-8hr IM, IV (NB: 15-20 mg/kg/24 hr q6-8hr IV) (maximum: 4.8 gm/24 hr IV)	Caution in renal, hepatic disease; topical solution useful for acne Tox: colitis, rash, diarrhea, phle- bitis; only for child >1 mo
Clonazepam (Klonopin) Tab: 0.5, 1, 2 mg	0.05-0.2 mg/kg/24 hr q8-12hr PO; start at 0.01 mg/kg/24 and add 0.25-0.5 mg/24 hr q3days until control (adult: 1.5-2.0 mg/24 hr) (maximum total dose: 20 mg/24 hr)	Therapeutic level: 0.013-0.072 μg/ml; caution in renal disease; titrate dosage slowly every third day; Table 81-6; previously Clonopin Tox: drowsiness, ataxia, personal- ity change
Clonidine (Catapres) Tab: 0.1, 0.2, 0.3 mg	0.005-0.01 mg/kg/24 hr q6hr PO (maximum: 0.9 mg/24 hr) (adult: 0.1 mg q12hr PO ini- tially; increase 0.1-0.2 mg/24 hr up to 2.4 mg/24 hr PO)	May be used acutely in hyperten- sion; widely used for ADHD (initial dose: 0.05 mg/24 hr) Tox: drowsiness, headache, dysrhythmia
Cloroquine phosphate (Aralen) Tab: 500 mg/300 mg base)	10 mg base/kg/24 hr q24hr PO	Several forms available; see Appendix C-4
Clotrimazole (Gyne-Lotrimin, Mycelex) Tab (vag): 100 mg Cream (vag): 1%	1 tablet or applicator-full vagi- nally nightly × 7-14 days	Tox: local irritation
Cloxacillin (Tegopen) Soln: 125 mg/5 ml Cap: 250, 500 mg	50-100 mg/kg/24 hr q6hr PO (maximum: 4 gm/24 hr)	Administer on empty stomach Tox: GI irritant, see Penicillin G

Many oral drugs may be given 3-4 times/day with more flexibility than implied by the specific intervals noted. Adult dose provided as guideline for maximum dose. *NB,* Newborns <7 days of age; *Pen,* penicillin; *SR,* sustained release; *Tox,* toxicity of drug.

Drugs	Dosages	Comments
Codeine Elix: 10 mg/5 ml (with antitussive) Tab: 15, 30, 60 mg Vial: 30, 60 mg/ml	Analgesic: 0.5-1.0 mg/kg/dose q4-6hr PO, IM (adult: 30-60 mg/dose) Antitussive: 1.0 mg/kg/24 hr q4-6hr PO (adult: 10-20 mg/dose)	Also available combined with acetaminophen 120 mg with 12 mg codeine/5 ml and tablets (acetaminophen 300 mg with 7.5 mg codeine [#1], 15 mg codeine [#2], or 30 mg codeine [#3]) Tox: dependence, CNS, and resp depression (Chapter 55)
Cortisone Tab: 5, 10, 25 mg Vial: 25, 50 mg/ml	Maintenance: 0.25 mg/kg/24 hr q12-24hr IM; 0.50-0.75 mg/kg/24 hr q6-8hr PO	Table 74-2
Cromolyn (Intal) Vial: 20 mg powder/soln	20 mg q6-8hr by nebulization	MDI may also be used to administer; for ongoing management of bronchospasm
Cyproheptadine (Periactin) Syr: 2 mg/5 ml Tab: 4 mg	0.25 mg/kg/24 hr q8-12hr PO (adult: 12-16 mg/24 hr)	
Dantrolene (Dantrium) Cap: 25 mg Vial: 20 mg	0.5 mg/kg/dose q12hr PO, then increase to 0.5 mg/kg/dose q6-8hr PO and increase up to maximum of 3 mg/kg/dose	Little information about use in children <5 yr; IV solution for surgical prophylaxis for malignant hyperthermia (1 mg/kg IV; repeat up to total dose of 10 mg/kg)
Deferoxamine (Desferal) Amp: 500 mg	If no shock: 90 mg/kg/dose q8hr IM (adult: 1-2 gm/dose × 1; maximum: 6 gm/24 hr) If shock: 15 mg/kg/hr IV	Urine turns rose colored if SI >TIBC in iron overdose; Chapter 55 Tox: urticaria, hypotension
Dexamethasone (Decadron) Vial: 4, 24 mg Elix: 0.5 mg/5 ml Tab: 1.5, 4, 6 mg	Croup: 0.25-0.6 mg/kg/dose q6hr IM, IV, PO Meningitis: 0.15 mg/kg/dose q6hr IV × 16 doses	Table 74-2
Dextrose D5W (0.5 gm/ml)	0.5-1.0 gm (2-4 ml D25W)/kg/dose IV	Dilute D50W 1:1 to prevent hypertonicity; draw glucose

Drugs	Dosages	Comments
Diazepam (Valium) Tab: 2, 5, 10 mg Vial: 5 mg/ml	Status epilepticus: 0.2-0.3 mg/kg/ dose IV (<1 mg/min) q2-5min prn (maximum total dose: child, 10 mg; adult, 30 mg) Sedation, muscle relaxation: 0.1-0.8 mg/kg/24 hr q6-8hr PO	If used for status epilepticus, must initiate additional drug; may be given as 0.5 mg/kg/dose PR; respiratory depression (Chapter 55); see flumazenil Tox: drowsiness, respiratory depression (increased with second drug)
Diazoxide (Hyperstat) Vial: 15 mg/ml	1-3 mg/kg/dose q4-24hr IV up to 150 mg/dose (fast); repeat in 30 min if no effect; may use inter- mittent smaller dose	Vasodilator: prompt (3-5 min) response (Table 18-2); also used to treat hyperinsulinemic hypoglycemia
Dicloxacillin (Dynapen) Susp: 62.5 mg/5 ml Cap: 125, 250, 500 mg	25-100 mg/kg/24 hr q6hr PO (adult: 125-500 mg/dose)	Do not use for NB; although optimally given on empty stomach, may have to use open capsule mixed with food Tox: GI irritant, see Penicillin G
Dicyclomine (Bentyl) Syr: 10 mg/5 ml Cap: 10, 20 mg	Children (>6 mo): 5-10 mg/dose q6-8hr PO; adult: 20-40 mg/dose q6-8hr PO	
Digoxin	See Tables 6-4 and 16-2	
Dimercaprol (BAL in oil) Amp: 100 mg/ml	Mild gold or arsenic poisoning: 2.5 mg/kg q6hr IM × 2 days, q8hr × 1 day, then q24hr × 10 days Severe arsenic or gold poisoning: 3 mg/kg q4hr × 2 days, q6hr × 1 day, then q12hr × 10 days Mercury poisoning: 5 mg/kg initially, then 2.5 mg/kg q12- 24hr × 10 days Lead encephalopathy: 4 mg/kg/ dose q4hr in combination with edetate calcium disodium × 2-7 days; if less severe, 3 mg/kg/ dose	

Many oral drugs may be given 3-4 times/day with more flexibility than implied by the specific intervals noted. Adult dose provided as guideline for maximum dose. *NB,* Newborns <7 days of age; *Pen,* penicillin; *SR,* sustained release; *Tox,* toxicity of drug.

Drugs	Dosages	Comments
Diphenhydramine (Benadryl) Elix: 12.5 mg/5 ml Cap: 25, 50 mg Vial: 10, 50 mg/ml	5 mg/kg/24 hr q6hr PO, IM, IV (maximum: 300 mg/24 hr) Anaphylaxis or phenothiazine overdose: 1-2 mg/kg/dose q6hr PO, IM, IV	Antihistamine: over the counter Tox: sedation, anticholinergic (Chapter 55); may inhibit breast milk
Diphenoxylate with atropine (Lomotil) Tab: 2.5 mg DPL/0.025 ATP Liq: 2.5 mg DPL/0.025 ATP/5 ml	0.3-0.4 mg DPL/kg/24 hr q6hr PO (adult: 2 tab QID PO)	Not recommended in children <2 yr; use liquid in children <13 yr; reduce dosage or dis- continue after control; prevent accidental ingestion
Dobutamine (Dobutrex) Vial: 250 mg	2-20 µg/kg/min IV infusion (maximum: 40 µg/kg/min IV) **Dilute:** 6 mg × weight (kg) in 100 ml D5W. Rate of infusion in µg/kg/min = ml/hr (1 ml/hr delivers 1 µg/kg/min); **or** 250 mg (1 vial) in 500 ml D5W = 500 µg/ml	Table 5-2
Docusate (Colace) Syr: 20 mg/5 ml Cap: 50, 100 mg	3-5 mg/kg/24 hr TID PO; (adult: 60-480 mg/24 hr)	
Dopamine (Intropin) Amp: 40 mg/ml Vial: 80 mg, 160 mg/ml	Low: 2-5 µg/kg/min IV drip Mod: 5-20 µg/kg/min IV drip High: >20 µg/kg/min IV drip **Dilute:** 6 mg × weight (kg) in 100 ml D5W. Rate of infusion in µg/kg/min = ml/hr (1 ml/hr delivers 1 µg/kg/min); **or** 200 mg (1 amp of 5 ml) in 500 ml D5W = 400 µg/ml	Table 5-2
Doxycycline (Vibramycin) Syr/susp: 25, 50 mg/5 ml Cap: 50, 100 mg Vial: 100, 200 mg	5 mg/kg/24 hr q12hr PO or IV slowly over 2-4 hr (adult: 100-200 mg/24 hr)	Do not use in children <9 yr of age Tox: GI irritant, hepatic, photo- sensitization, superinfection; adjust dosage with renal failure; BR
Droperidol (Inapsine) Vial: 2.5 mg/ml	0.1 mg/kg/dose IM, IV for anes- thetic premedication; 0.05 mg/kg/dose q4-6hr prn for nausea, vomiting (adult: 1.25-5 mg/dose IM, IV)	Monitor respirations; generally older children and adults

Drugs	Dosages	Comments
Edrophonium (Tensilon) Vial: 10 mg/ml	Test for myasthenia gravis: 0.2 mg/kg/dose and if no response in 1 min, give 1-mg increments up to maximum total dose of 5-10 mg IV (adult test dose: 2 mg) (NB: 1 mg single dose IV)	Have atropine available; may precipitate cholinergic crisis
Ephedrine Syr: 10, 20 mg/5 ml Tab/cap: 25, 50 mg	2-3 mg/kg/24 q4-6hr PO (adult: 25-50 mg q4-6hr PO)	Poor decongestant; potentiates side effects of theophylline without much therapeutic benefit (Chapter 84)
Epinephrine (Adrenalin) Vial (1:1000-1 mg/ml) (1:10,000-0.1 mg/ml) Sus-Phrine (1:200-5 mg/ml in oil)	Asthma: 0.01 ml (1:1000)/kg/dose (maximum: 0.35 ml/dose) q15-20min SC prn × 3; Sus-Phrine 0.005 ml/kg/dose (maximum: 0.15 ml) × 1 SC Asystole: 0.1 ml (1:10,000)/kg/dose (maximum: 5 ml/dose) IV initially; subsequent dose and initial ET dose is 0.1 mg/kg or 0.1 ml/kg of 1:1000 solution Shock: 0.05-1.0 µg/kg/min IV infusion **Dilute:** (for infusion in shock): 0.6 mg × weight (kg) in 100 ml D5W. Rate of infusion in 0.1 µg/kg/min = ml/hr (1 ml/hr delivers 0.1 µg/kg/min; **or** 1 mg in 500 ml D5W = 2 µ/ml	Inhalation (albuterol, terbutaline) therapy preferred for asthma; Sus-Phrine unreliable in dosing unless using single dose vial Use in shock only after isoproterenol and dopamine are ineffective; not effective with acidotic patient; Table 5-2 Tox: tachycardia, dysrhythmia, tremor, hypertension
Epinephrine, racemic (Vaponephrin) Soln: 2.25%	0.25-0.75 ml in 2.5 ml of sterile water or saline administered by nebulizer	Rebounds, always observe patient; often given with steroids; some bronchodilator effect
Erythromycin (Pediamycin, E.E.S., Erythrocin, E-Mycin, ERYC) Susp: 200, 400 mg/5 ml Tab: 200 (chew), 250, 400, 500 mg	20-50 mg/kg/24 hr q6hr PO (adult: 250-1000 mg/dose)	Also available as combination: erythromycin 200 mg + sulfisoxazole 600 mg/5 ml (Pediazole) Tox: GI irritant, rash
Ethambutol (Myambutol) Tab: 100, 400 mg	Initial TB treatment: 15 mg/kg q24hr PO Retreatment: 25 mg/kg q24hr PO	Multiple drug treatment indicated; monthly eye examination advised

Many oral drugs may be given 3-4 times/day with more flexibility than implied by the specific intervals noted. Adult dose provided as guideline for maximum dose. *NB,* Newborns <7 days of age; *Pen,* penicillin; *SR,* sustained release; *Tox,* toxicity of drug.

Drugs	Dosages	Comments
Ethanol		
100% (1 ml = 790 mg)	Methanol, ethylene glycol over-dose: 1 ml/kg over 15 min, then 0.15 ml (125 mg)/kg/hr IV	Maintain ethanol level at ≥100 mg/dl; Table 54-4
Ethosuximide (Zarontin)		
Syr: 250 mg/5 ml	20-40 mg/kg/24 hr q12-24hr PO; begin 250 mg q24hr (3-6 yr old) and increase 250 mg/24 hr at 4- to 7-day interval; maximum: 1.5 gm/24 hr	Therapeutic level: 40-100 μg/ml; Table 81-6
Cap: 250 mg		Tox: GI irritant, neutropenia, drowsiness, dizziness, head-ache
Factor VIII, IX		
	Tables 79-2 and 79-3	
Famciclovir (Famvir)		
Tab: 125, 250, 500 mg	Adult: 500 mg/dose q8hr × 7 days	Preferably begin within 12 hr of onset of rash; not studied in <18 yr olds
Famotidine (Pepcid)		
Tab: 20, 40 mg	1-2 mg/kg/24 hr q12-24hr IV, PO	
Susp: 40 mg/5 ml	Adult: 20-40 mg q24hr PO; 20 mg q12hr IV	
Vial: 10 mg/ml		
Fentanyl (Sublimaze)		
Amp: 50 μg/ml	1-5 μg/kg/dose IV slowly (adult: 50-100 μg/dose)	Narcotic; half-life: 20 min; monitor oxygenation and ventilation
Fexofenadine (Allegra)		
Cap: 60 mg	Adult: 60 mg q12hr PO	Antihistamine limited experience in children <12 yr
Fluconazole (Diflucan)		
Susp: 10, 40 mg/ml	*Oral candidiasis:* load, 6 mg/kg PO; then 3 mg/kg/24 hr PO	Usually treat 2-3 weeks
Tab: 50, 100, 200 mg		
Fludrocortisone (Florinef)		
Tab: 0.1 mg	0.05-0.1 mg/24 hr q24hr PO	
Flumazenil (Mazicon)		
Vial: 0.1 mg/ml	0.01 mg/kg initially, repeating 0.01 mg/kg q1min to a maximum total dose of 1 mg; adult: 0.2 mg IV initially; then 0.3 mg IV and then 0.5 mg if no response up to a cumulative dose of 3 mg	Management of suspected benzo-diazepine overdose
Folic acid		
Tab: 0.1, 0.4, 1 mg	0.2-1.0 mg/24 hr PO (adult: 1-3 mg/24 hr)	
Furazolidone (Furoxone)		
Liq: 50 mg/15 ml	*Giardia:* 6 mg/kg/24 hr q6hr PO (adult: 100 mg q6hr)	Do not use in children <1 mo; avoid alcohol; see Table 76-1
Tab: 100 mg		Tox: nausea, vomiting, rash

Drugs	Dosages	Comments
Furosemide (Lasix) Soln: 10 mg/ml Tab: 20, 40, 80 mg Amp: 10 mg/ml	1 mg/kg/dose q6-12hr IV initially (may repeat q2hr IV prn); 2 mg/kg/dose q2-12hr PO initially; may increase dosage by 1 mg/kg increments (maximum: 6 mg/kg/dose PO, IM, IV)	Rapid acting; Table 16-3 Tox: hypokalemia, hyponatremia, alkalosis, prerenal azotemia; ototoxicity
Gentamicin (Garamycin) Vial: 10, 40 mg/ml	5.0-7.5 mg/kg/24 hr q8hr IM, IV (maximum: 300 mg/24 hr) (NB: 5 mg/kg/24 hr q12hr) (adult: 3-5 mg/kg/24 hr q8hr)	Therapeutic peak level: 6-12 μg/ml; caution in renal failure (adjust dosage); slow IV infusion Tox: renal, VIII nerve
Glucagon Amp: 1 mg (1 unit)/ml	0.03-0.1 mg/kg/dose q20min SC, IM, IV prn (NB: 0.1-0.2 mg/kg/dose q4hr prn) (adult: 0.5-1.0 mg/dose)	Hypoglycemia: not adequate as only glucose support, especially in NB; treatment of propranolol (β-blocker) overdose
Glucose (see Dextrose)		
Griseofulvin Microsize (Grisactin, Grifulvin V) Susp: 125 mg/5 ml Tab/cap: 125, 250, 500 mg Ultramicrosize (Gris-PEG, Fulvicin P/G) Tab: 125, 250, 330 mg	Microsize: 10 mg/kg/24 hr q24hr PO (adult: 500-1000 mg q12-24hr PO) Ultramicrosize: 5 mg/kg/24 hr q24hr PO (adult: 250-500 mg/24 hr q12-24hr PO)	Give with meals; either formulation is adequate; treatment period of 4-6 wk Tox: renal, hepatic, neutropenia, rash, headache
Haloperidol (Haldol) Tab: 1, 2, 5, 10 mg Soln: 2 mg/ml Amp: 5 mg/ml, 100 mg/ml (decanoate)	Psychosis: 0.05-0.15 mg/kg/24 hr q8-12hr PO; begin at 0.5 mg/24 hr and increase Nonpsychotic behavior: 0.05-0.075 mg/kg/24 hr q8-12hr PO Adult: initial 0.5-2.0 mg/dose PO (maximum: 5 mg q8-12hr PO)	
Heparin (Liquaemin, Panheprin) Vial: 100, 1000, 5000, 10,000, 20,000, 40,000 units/ml	Load: 50-75 units/kg IV bolus Maint: 10-25 units/kg/hr IV infusion **or** 100 units/kg/dose q4hr IV Adult: load (5,000 units) with maint (20,000-30,000 unit over 24 hr IV continuous infusion **or** 5000-10,000 q4hr)	Titrate to maintain PTT at 2 times control; antidote: protamine Tox: bleeding, allergy rash, wheezing, anaphylaxis

Many oral drugs may be given 3-4 times/day with more flexibility than implied by the specific intervals noted. Adult dose provided as guideline for maximum dose. *NB,* Newborns <7 days of age; *Pen,* penicillin; *SR,* sustained release; *Tox,* toxicity of drug.

Drugs	Dosages	Comments
Hydralazine (Apresoline) Tab: 10, 25, 50, 100 mg Amp: 20 mg/ml	Crisis: 0.1-0.4 mg/kg/dose (1.7-3.5 mg/kg/24 hr) q4-6hr IM, IV prn (adult: 10-40 mg/dose) Maintenance: 0.75-3 mg/kg/24 hr q6-12hr PO (adult: 10-75 mg/dose q6hr PO)	Vasodilator, prompt (10-30 min response if IV) decrease BP; may also be given as 1.5 µg/kg/min IV infusion; limited availability in parenteral form (being reformulated); Table 18-2 Tox: tachycardia, angina, SLE-like syndrome; reduce dosage with renal failure
Hydrochlorothiazide (Esidrix, HydroDiuril) Tab: 25, 50, 100 mg	1-2 mg/kg/24 hr q12hr PO (NB: 2-3 mg/kg/24 hr PO) (adult: 25-100 mg q12-24hr)	Table 16-3 Tox: hyponatremia, hypokalemia, alkalosis; reduce dosage with renal failure
Hydrocortisone (Solu-Cortef) Susp: 10 mg/5 ml Tab: 5, 10, 20 mg Vial: 100, 250, 500, 1000 mg	Maintenance: 0.5 mg/kg/24 hr q8hr PO Asthma: 4-5 mg/kg/dose q6hr IV	Table 74-2
Hydroxyzine (Atarax, Vistaril) Syr/susp: 10, 25 mg/5 ml Tab (Atarax): 10, 25, 50 mg Cap (Vistaril): 25, 50, 100 mg Vial (Vistaril): 25, 50 mg/ml	2 mg/kg/24 hr q6hr PO (adult: 200-400 mg/24 hr q6hr PO) 0.5-1 mg/kg/dose q4-6hr IM prn (adult: 25-100 mg/dose q4-6hr IM prn)	Antihistamine, potentiates meperidine, barbiturates Tox: sedation, anticholinergic (Chapter 55); may inhibit breast milk
Ibuprofen (Motrin) Tab: 300, 400, 600, 800 mg Susp: 100 mg/5 ml Chewable: 50, 100 mg	40 mg/kg/24 hr q6-8hr PO (adult: 1.2 gm/24 hr)	Available over the counter as capsule (Nuprin, Advil 200 mg tab) (adult: 200-400 mg q4-6hr PO; maximum: 1.2 gm/24 hr) Tox: GI irritant, keratopathy, hematuria, retinopathy, rash
Imipenem (IMP)-**Cilastatin** (CIL) (Primaxin) Vial: 250 mg IMP/250 mg CIL, 500 mg IMP/500 mg CIL	60 IMP + 60 mg CIL/kg/24 hr q6hr IV (adult: 250-1000 mg IMP + 250-1000 mg-CIL/dose) (maximum: 50 mg/kg/24 hr **or** 4 gm/24 hr of each agent)	Limited experience in children but has been studied in those >3 mo Tox: phlebitis, diarrhea, renal
Imipramine (Tofranil) Tab: 10, 25, 50 mg	Enuresis: 25-75 mg at bedtime PO	
Immune serum globulin	Exposure to measles <1 yr of age (0.25 ml/kg IM) or immunocompromised (0.5 ml/kg IM); viral hepatitis type A contact within 14 days of exposure (0.02 ml/kg IM); and selected immunodeficiency disease; hepatitis B immune globulin (HBIG) is used with significant exposure to HBsAg-positive blood within 24 hr and 1 mo later (0.06 ml/kg/dose IM)	

Drugs	Dosages	Comments
Indomethacin (Indocin) Cap: 25, 50 mg	1-3 mg/kg/24 hr q6-8hr PO (maximum: 100-200 mg/24 hr)	Not approved in children <14 yr; may be used to close PDA (with CHF) in neonate; 0.1-0.2 mg/kg/dose q12hr up to maximum 0.6 mg/kg IV Tox: nausea, vomiting, headache, corneal opacity
Insulin	Table 74-3	
Iodoquinol	See Appendix C-4	
Ipecac, syrup of	6-12 mo: 10 ml/dose PO 12 mo: 15 ml/dose PO Adult: 30 ml/dose PO Give initial dose and may repeat × 1	Do not use in children <6 mo; push fluids; contraindicated in caustic ingestions and patients who are comatose or having seizures, Chapter 54
Ipratropium (Atrovent) MDI (18 µg/dose) Soln (0.02%): 500 µg in 2.5 ml	Adult: 2 inhalation (MDI) puffs QID; solution (500 µg/dose in 2.5 ml) by nebulization q6hr prn in adults; child: administer partial (half) adult dose	Efficacious as MDI or nebuliza- tion solution
Iron, elemental (Fe) (Fer-In-Sol, Feosol) Drop: 75 mg (15 mg Fe)/0.6 ml Syr: 90 mg (18 mg Fe)/5 ml Tab: 200 mg (40 mg Fe), 325 mg (65 mg Fe)	Therapeutic: 6 mg elemental Fe/kg/24 hr q8hr PO Prophylactic: 1-2 mg elemental Fe/kg/24 hr q8-24hr PO (maximum: 15 mg elemental Fe/24 hr)	Ferrous sulfate is 20% elemental iron (Fe) (Chapter 26) Tox: GI irritant (reduce by giving with food); overdose (Chapter 55)
Isoetharine (Bronkosol, Bronko- meter) Soln: 1% (10 mg/ml) Aerosol	Nebulizer: 0.25-0.5 ml diluted in 2.5 ml saline q4hr prn Aerosol: 1-2 puffs q2-4 hr prn	Administer by nebulizer; rarely used Tox: tachycardia, hypertension
Isoniazid (INH) Syr: 50 mg/5 ml Tab: 50, 100, 300 mg	10-20 mg/kg/24 hr q12-24hr PO (adult: 300 mg/24 hr)	Supplemental pyridoxine (10 mg/100 mg INH) needed in adolescents, adults Tox: peripheral neuropathy, hepatitis, seizure, acidosis

Many oral drugs may be given 3-4 times/day with more flexibility than implied by the specific intervals noted. Adult dose provided as guideline for maximum dose. *NB,* Newborns <7 days of age; *Pen,* penicillin; *SR,* sustained release; *Tox,* toxicity of drug.

Drugs	Dosages	Comments
Isoproterenol (Isuprel)		
Amp: 200 µg/ml	Shock: 0.05-1.5 µg/kg/min IV infusion; begin at 0.05 µg/kg/min and increase by 0.1 µg/kg/min increments (maximum: 1.5 µg/kg/min)	Table 5-2
Neb: 1:100, 200		Rarely used as bronchodilator
Aerosol		
	Nebulizer: 0.5 ml diluted in 2.5 ml saline q4hr prn	
	Aerosol: 1-2 puffs q2-4hr prn	
	Dilute: (for infusion in shock) 0.6 mg × weight (kg) in 100 ml D5W; rate of infusion in 0.1 µg/kg/min = ml/hr (1 ml/hr delivers 0.1 µg/kg/min); **or** 200 µg (1 ml) in 200 ml D5W = 1 µg/ml	
Ivermectin	See Appendix C-4	
Kanamycin (Kantrex)		
Vial: 37.5, 250, 333 mg/ml	15 mg/kg/24 hr q8hr IM, IV (maximum: 1 gm/24 hr) (NB: 15 mg/kg/24 hr q12hr)	Therapeutic peak level: 25-30 µg/ml; caution in renal failure (adjust dosage; infusion IV slowly
		Tox: renal, hearing
Ketamine		
Vial: 10, 50, 100 mg/dl	1 mg/kg/dose IV (maximum: 100 mg); 5 mg/kg/dose IM (maximum: 50 mg); 5-10 mg/kg PO (maximum: 50 mg)	Administer slowly; half-life 2½ hr, redistribution half-life 10-15 min; monitor
Ketorolac (Toradol)		
Syringe: 15, 30, 60 mg	1 mg/kg/dose q6hr IM (children >2 yr)	Limited experience in children <16 yr; do not give if patient hypovolemic
Tab: 10 mg	Adult: 30-60 mg IM initial, then 15-30 mg q6hr IM (maximum: 120 mg/24 hr); 10-20 mg q6hr PO	
Labetalol		
	0.4-1.0 mg/kg/dose IV slow push; repeat up to 3 mg/kg/hr IV (adult: 2 mg/min or 20 mg/dose; titrate 20-80 mg q10min; maximum: 300 mg)	Tox: hypotension; Table 18-2
Levothyroxine (Synthroid)		
Tab: 25, 50, 100, 200, 300 µg	Infancy: 7-9 µg/kg/24 hr PO; thereafter 100 µg/m²/24 hr PO (child: 3-5 µg/kg/24 hr PO)	Monitor T_4 and thyroid-stimulating hormone
Vial: 500 µg		

Drugs	Dosages	Comments
Lidocaine (Xylocaine) Vial (IV): 10, 20 mg/ml Vial (anesthetic): 10 mg (1%), 20 mg (2%),40 mg (4%)/ml	Load: 1 mg/kg/dose q5-10min IV prn to maximum of 5 mg/kg Maintenance: 20-50 µg/kg/min IV infusion Adult: load same; maintenance: 2-4 mg/min **Dilute** 150 mg × weight (kg) in 250 ml D5W; rate of infusion in µg/min = 10 × ml/hr	Antidysrhythmic; may be given ET (dilute 1:1); Table 6-4 Tox: seizures, drowsiness, euphoria, muscle twitching, dysrhythmias, and titrate dosage
Loperamide (Imodium) Cap: 2 mg Liq: 1 mg/5 ml	Children (>2 yr): 0.4-0.8 mg/kg/24 hr q6-12hr PO until diarrhea resolves (adult: 2 mg q8hr PO)	Limited efficacy; over the counter
Loracarbef (Lorabid) Cap: 200, 400 mg	Adult: 200-400 mg q12hr PO × 7 days	Urinary tract infection in children ≥13 yr
Lorazepam (Ativan) Vial: 2, 4 mg/ml	0.05-0.10 mg/kg/dose IV at rate 2 mg/min (adult: 2.5-10 mg/dose)	May consider repeating × 1 dose in 15-20 min if necessary
Magnesium hydroxide (see aluminum hyroxide) (Maalox)		
Magnesium sulfate Crystal: Epsom salt Vial: 100, 125, 250, 500 mg/ml	Catharsis: 250 mg/kg/dose PO (adult: 20-30 gm/dose PO) Hypomagnesemia: 25-50 mg/kg/dose q4-6hr × 3-4 doses IM or IV (adult: 1-4 gm/24 hr) Anticonvulsant: 20-100 mg/kg/dose q4-6hr IV (adult: 1 gm q6hr IV × 4)	Caution in renal failure; follow magnesium and calcium levels; Chapter 54 Tox: hypotension
Mannitol Vial: 20% (200 mg/ml) 25% (250 mg/ml)	Diuretic: 750 mg/kg/dose IV: do not repeat with persistent oliguria (adult: 300 mg/kg/dose) Cerebral edema: 0.25-0.5 gm/kg IV slowly over 10-15 min q3-4hr prn (maximum: 1 gm/kg/dose IV)	Maintain serum osmolality <320 mOsm/L; may be CNS rebound, intracranial monitor indicated Tox: hypovolemia, volume overload, hyperosmolality
Mebendazole (Vermox) Tab (chew): 100 mg	Pinworm: 100 mg PO, repeat in 1 wk Ascaris, hookworm: 100 mg q12hr PO × 3 days	Not studied in children <2 yr; see Appendix C-4 Tox: diarrhea

Many oral drugs may be given 3-4 times/day with more flexibility than implied by the specific intervals noted. Adult dose provided as guideline for maximum dose. *NB,* Newborns <7 days of age; *Pen,* penicillin; *SR,* sustained release; *Tox,* toxicity of drug.

Drugs	Dosages	Comments
Meperidine (Demerol) Syr: 50 mg/5 mg Tab: 50, 100 mg Vial: 25, 50, 100 mg/ml	1-2 mg/kg/dose q3-4hr PO, IM, IV prn (adult: 50-150 mg/dose) (maximum: 100 mg/dose in children)	75 mg meperidine = 10 mg morphine DPT, sedative cocktail (ratio 4:1:1) Meperidine (Demerol) 1-2 mg/kg/dose (maximum: 50 mg/dose) Promethazine (Phenergan) 0.25-0.5 mg/kg/dose (maximum: 12.5 mg/dose) Chlorpromazine (Thorazine) 0.25-0.5 mg/kg/dose (maximum: 12.5 mg/dose) Also potentiated by hydroxyzine Tox: CNS, respiratory depression, seizure, overdose (Chapter 55)
Metaraminol (Aramine) Vial: 10 mg/ml	0.01 mg/kg/dose IV prn **or** 1-4 µg/kg/min IV infusion	Tox: tachycardia, dysrhythmia, local tissue slough
Methicillin (Staphcillin) Vial: 1, 4, 6 gm	100-200 mg/kg/24 hr q4-6hr IM, IV (maximum: 12 gm/24 hr) (NB: 50-75 mg/kg/24 hr q8-12hr)	Equivalent to nafcillin, oxacillin Tox: interstitial nephritis (hematuria), bone marrow suppression; see Pencillin G
Methsuximide (Celontin) Cap: 150, 300 mg	Adult: 300 mg/24 hr q24hr PO × 1 wk; 300 mg/24 hr/wk increments q3wk prn (maximum: 1.2 gm/24 hr)	Petit mal seizures Tox: CNS symptoms, behavioral change, caution in liver, renal disease
Methyldopa (Aldomet) Tab: 125, 250, 500 mg Vial: 50 mg/ml Susp: 250 mg/5 ml	Crisis: 2.5-5 mg/kg/dose q6-8hr IV (maximum: 20-40 mg/kg/24 hr or 500 mg/dose IV) Chronic: 10 mg/kg/24 hr q6-12hr PO (maximum: 40 mg/kg/24 hr or total dose 2 gm/24 hr)	Table 18-2 Tox: somnolence, hemolytic disease, ulcerogenic; reduce dosage with renal failure
Methylene blue Vial: 1% (10 mg/ml)	1-2 mg/kg/dose IV q4hr prn	Use for methemoglobinemia
Methylphenidate (Ritalin) Tab: 5, 10, 20 mg	Initial dose (>6 yr): 5 mg in AM/PM PO; titrate; maximum: 60 mg/24 hr	Toxicity may be increased when combination therapy used
Methylprednisolone (Solu-Medrol) Vial: 40, 125, 500, 1000 mg	Asthma: 1-2 mg/kg/dose q6hr IV	Table 74-2; different preparation for intraarticular route

Drugs	Dosages	Comments
Metoclopramide (Reglan) Syr: 5 mg/5 ml Tab: 5, 10 mg Vial: 5 mg/ml	0.1 mg/kg/dose q6hr PO, IV Adult: 10-15 mg q6hr PO, IV	For gastroesophageal reflux, nausea, and vomiting; higher dosage (1 mg/kg/dose) may be used IV before chemotherapy to reduce vomiting
Metolazone (Zaroxolyn) Tab: 2.5, 5, 10 mg	0.2-0.4 mg/kg/24 hr q12-24hr PO Adult: 2.5-10 mg/24 hr PO	Little experience in children; useful when no response to other diuretics and decreased glomerular filtration rate; Table 16-3 Tox: azotemia, ↓ K^+, hypotension, lethargy, coma
Metronidazole (Flagyl) Tab: 250, 500 mg	*Haemophilus vaginalis (Gardnerella)* vaginitis: 500 mg q8hr PO × 7-10 days *Trichomonas vaginalis:* 15 mg/kg/24 hr q8hr PO × 7 days (adult: 250 mg q8h × 7 days) *Giardia lamblia:* 15 mg/kg/24 hr q8hr PO × 5 days (adult: 250 mg q8hr × 5 days) Amebiasis: 35-50 mg/kg/24 hr q8hr PO × 10 days (adult: 750 mg q8hr × 10 days)	IV form available for severe anaerobic infections Tox: nausea, diarrhea, neutropenia, urticaria, do not give to pregnant patient
Miconazole (Monistat) Vag cream (2%) Supp: 200 mg (Monistat 3)	*Candida (Monilia)* vaginitis: 1 applicator-full before bed × 7-14 days; supp: 200 mg before bed × 3 days	Systemic form available
Midazolam (Versed) Vial: 1.5 mg/ml	Conscious sedation: 0.05-0.10 mg/kg/dose (maximum: 5 mg) IV; 0.3-0.7 mg/kg PO; 0.4 mg/kg intranasal	Often used in combination with narcotic such as low-dose fentanyl, morphine, meperidine See Chapter 65.
Minoxidil (Loniten) Tab: 2.5, 10 mg	0.2-1.0 mg/kg/24 hr q24hr PO (adult: 10-40 mg q24hr PO) (maximum: 100 mg/24 hr)	Peripheral vasodilator; limited experience in children; increase dose gradually
Morphine Vial: 5, 8, 10, 15 mg/ml	0.1-0.2 mg/kg/dose (maximum: 10-15 mg/dose) q2-4hr IM, IV	Antidote: naloxone (Chapter 55) Tox: CNS, respiratory depression, hypotension

Many oral drugs may be given 3-4 times/day with more flexibility than implied by the specific intervals noted. Adult dose provided as guideline for maximum dose. *NB,* Newborns <7 days of age; *Pen,* penicillin; *SR,* sustained release; *Tox,* toxicity of drug.

Drugs	Dosages	Comments
Mupirocin 2% (Bactroban) Oint: 15 gm	Apply small amount TID	May substitute for systemic treatment of impetigo with small lesions
Nafcillin (Unipen) Vial: 0.5, 1, 2 gm	50-200 mg/kg/24 hr q4-6hr IM, IV (maximum: 12 gm/24 hr) (NB: 40 mg/kg/24 hr q12hr)	Equivalent to methicillin, oxacillin; IM painful; oral form available Tox: allergy, see Penicillin; low renal toxicity
Naloxone (Narcan) Amp: 0.4, 1.0 mg/ml	0.1 ml/kg/dose (minimum: 0.4 mg; maximum: 2.0 mg) IV	Narcotic antagonist; propoxyphene (Darvon) and pentazocine (Talwin) require very large doses to reverse; Chapter 55; may have role in septic shock
Naproxen (Naprosyn) Tab: 250, 375, 500 mg Susp: 125 mg/5 ml	2.5-5 mg/kg/dose q8hr PO (adult: 250-375 mg q8-12hr PO) (maximum: 15 mg/kg or 1250 mg for adult/24 hr) Dysmenorrhea: load 500 mg PO, then 250 mg q8-12hr PO	Nonsteroidal antiinflammatory Tox: GI irritant, vertigo, headache, platelet dysfunction; not approved for children <2 yr
Nifedipine (Procardia) Cap: 10, 20 mg	0.25-0.50 mg/kg q15-30min PO, sublingual, buccal (adult: 10-20 mg 1 dose)	Negative inotropic effect; contraindicated with intracranial hemorrhage
Nitrite, Amyl	Inhale pearl q60-120 sec	For cyanide poisoning, follow with sodium nitrite and sodium thiosulfate
Nitrite, Sodium (3%)	0.27 ml (8.7 mg)/kg (adult: 10 ml [300 mg]) IV slowly if Hgb 10 gm	For cyanide poisoning, precede with amyl nitrite and follow with sodium thiosulfate
Nitrofurantoin (Furadantin, Macrodantin) Susp: 25 mg/5 ml Tab: 50, 100 mg Cap: 25, 50, 100 mg	5-7 mg/kg/24 hr q6hr PO; chronic: 2.5-5 mg/kg/24 hr (adult: 50-100 mg/dose q6hr PO; chronic: 50-100 mg before bed PO)	Do not use for renal disease, G6PD deficiency, child <1 mo, pregnancy Tox: hypersensitivity
Nitroprusside (Nipride) Vial: 50 mg	0.5-10 µg (avg: 3 µg)/kg/min IV infusion **Dilute** 6 mg × weight (kg) in 100 ml D5W; rate of infusion in µg/kg/min = ml/hr **or** 50 mg (1 vial) in 100 ml of D5W = 500 µg/ml	Precise, rapid (1-2 min) BP control; requires constant monitoring; light sensitive; Tables 5-2 and 18-2 Tox: hypotension, cyanide poisoning (monitor thiocyanate level)

Drugs	Dosages	Comments
Norepinephrine (Levophed) Vial: 1 mg/ml	0.1-1.0 µg/kg/min IV infusion **Dilute:** 0.6 mg × weight (kg) in 100 ml D5W; rate of infusion in 0.1 µg/kg/in = ml/hr (1 ml/hr delivers 0.1 µg/kg/min); **or** 1 mg (1 ml) in 100 ml of D5W = 10 µg/ml	Table 5-2; titrate response
Norfloxacin (Noroxin) Tab: 400 mg	Adult: 400 mg q12hr PO	Quinolone antibiotic No pediatric recommendation because of risk of arthropathy
Nystatin (Mycostatin) Cream: 100,000 unit/gm Susp: 100,000 unit/ml Tab (vag): 100,000 unit	Thrush: 1 ml in each side of the mouth q4-6hr PO Diaper rash *(Candida):* apply cream with diaper changes (q2-6hr) Vaginitis: 1 tab in vagina before bed × 10 days	Continue oral and topical therapy for 2-3 days after clearing
Oxacillin (Prostaphin) Soln: 250 mg/5 ml Cap: 250, 500 mg Vial: 0.5, 1, 2, 4 gm	50-100 mg/kg/24 hr q6r PO (adult: 500-1000 mg q6hr PO); 50-200 mg/kg/24 hr q4-6hr IM, IV (maximum: 8 gm/24 hr) (NB: 25-50 mg/kg/24 hr q8-12hr IM, IV)	Equivalent to methicillin, nafcillin; oral form optimally given on empty stomach Tox: see Penicillin G
Pancuronium (Pavulon) Vial: 1, 2 mg/ml	Load: 0.04-0.1 mg/kg/dose IV (intubation: 0.06-0.1 mg/kg/dose IV) (NB: 0.02 mg/kg/dose IV) Maintenance: 0.01-0.02 mg/kg/dose q20-40min IV prn (NB: adjust on basis of loading dose)	Peak effect in 2-3 min; duration 40-60 min; must be able to support respirations
Paraldehyde (Paral) Soln: 1 gm/ml Amp: 1 gm/ml	Sedative: 0.15 ml (150 mg)/kg/dose PO, IM Anticonvulsant: 0.3 ml (300 mg)/kg/dose q4-6hr PR prn (maximum: 5 ml) (NB: 0.1-0.2 ml [100-200 mg]/kg/dose diluted in 0.9% NS q4-6hr PR prn; 0.15 ml/kg/dose q4-6hr IM, IV prn)	For PR, dissolve 1:2 in cottonseed, olive, or mineral oil; for IM, give deep; do not give if hepatic or pulmonary disease is present Tox: IV (pulmonary edema, CHF), IM (sterile abscess), PR (proctitis), respiratory depression

Many oral drugs may be given 3-4 times/day with more flexibility than implied by the specific intervals noted. Adult dose provided as guideline for maximum dose. *NB,* Newborns <7 days of age; *Pen,* penicillin; *SR,* sustained release; *Tox,* toxicity of drug.

Drugs	Dosages	Comments
Penicillin G (sodium or potassium salt) Susp: 125, 250 mg/5 ml Tab: 125, 250, 500 mg Vial: 1, 5, 20 million units	25-50 mg (40,000-80,000 units)/ kg/24 hr q6hr PO (adult: 300,000-1.2 million units/24 hr PO); 50,000-250,000 units/ kg/24 hr q4hr IM, IV (NB: 50,000-150,000 units/kg/24 hr q8-12hr IM, IV)	1 mg = 1600 units; salt content (1 million units contains 1.68 mEq Na^+ or K^+); PO erratically absorbed, give on empty stomach Tox: allergy (anaphylaxis, rash, urticaria), superinfection *(Candida)*, hemolytic anemia, interstitial nephritis; adjust dosage with renal failure

Penicillin G benzathine and Penicillin G procaine (Bicillin C-R 900/300)   900,000 units benz and 300,000 units proc/2 ml

	Benzathine pen G	*Benzathine/procaine pen G*
Weight (lb)	*(Bicillin L-A)*	*(Bicillin C-R 900/300)*
<30	300,000 units	300,000:100,000 units
31-60	600,000 units	600,000:200,000 units
61-90	900,000 units	900,000:300,000 units
>90	1,200,000 units	Not available

Drugs	Dosages	Comments
Penicillin V (Pen-Vee K, V-Cillin K) Susp: 125 mg (200,000 units), 250 mg (400,000 units) /5 ml Tab: 125, 250, 500 mg	25-50 mg (40,000-80,000 units)/ kg/24 hr q6hr PO (adult: 250-500 mg q6hr PO)	More resistant to destruction by gastric acid Tox: see Penicillin G
Pentamidine (Pentam) Vial: 300 mg	4 mg/kg/24 hr q24hr IM	May be given IV slowly
Pentobarbital (Nembutal) Elix: 20 mg/5 ml Cap: 30, 50, 100 mg Supp: 30, 60, 120, 200 mg Vial: 50 mg/ml	Sedation: 6 mg/kg/24 hr q8hr PO, PR, IM, IV (adult: 30 mg q6-8hr) Cerebral edema: load: 3-5 mg/kg slow IV; maintenance: 1-2 mg/kg/hr IV	Short-acting barbiturate; treatment of increased intracranial pressure must include monitor Pentobarbital to maintain intracranial pressure <15 mm Hg and barbiturate level 25-40 µg/ml; support respirations, monitor BP Tox: CNS excitement, respiratory depression, hypotension (Chapter 55)
Phenazopyridine (Pyridium) Tab: 100, 200 mg	6-12 yr of age: 100 mg q8hr PO (adult: 200 mg q8hr PO) × 1-3 days	Use until dysuria gone and diagnosis made; urine color orange/ red; avoid with G6PD deficiency Tox: hemolytic anemia, methemoglobinemia

Drugs	Dosages	Comments
Phenobarbital (Luminal) Elix: 20 mg/5 ml Tab: 8, 15, 30, 60, 90, 100 mg Vial: 65, 130 mg/ml	Seizures: load: 15-20 mg/kg PO, IM (erratic absorption), IV (<1 mg/kg/min); with status epilepticus and no response in 20-30 min, repeat 10 mg/kg IV (adult: 100 mg/dose IV q20min prn × 3) Maintenance: 2-6 mg/kg/24 hr q12-24hr PO (adult: 100-300 mg/24 hr PO) Sedation: 2-3 mg/kg/dose PO q8hr prn	May be used as first-line drug in status epilepticus (IV) or after seizures controlled by diazepam (Valium); Chapter 21 and 81 Therapeutic level: 15-35 µg/ml Tox: drowsiness, irritability, learning problems, CNS and respiratory depression with high dosages (Chapter 55) Reduce dosage with renal failure
Phentolamine (Regitine) Vial: 5 mg/ml	0.05-0.1 mg/kg/dose q1-4hr IV (adult: 2.5-5 mg/dose IV)	Specific for pheochromocytoma and MAO-induced hypertension; rapid onset; dose, especially PO, must be individualized; may be given as continuous infusion Tox: dysrhythmia, hypotension
Phenytoin (Dilantin, diphenylhydantoin) Susp: 30, 125 mg/5 ml Tab (chew): 50 mg Cap: 30, 100 mg Amp: 50 mg/ml Amp (fosphenytoin [Cerebyx]): 50 mg/ml equivalent	Seizures: load: 10-20 mg/kg PO, IV (<0.5 mg/kg/min unless using fosphenytoin); maintenance: 5-10 mg/kg/24 hr q12-24 hr PO (adult: 200-400 mg/24 hr PO) Dysrhythmia load: 5 mg/kg IV (<0.5 mg/kg/min) (adult: 100 mg/dose q5min prn up to 1 gm IV); maintenance: 6 mg/kg/24 hr q12hr PO (adult: 300 mg/24 hr PO)	Therapeutic level: 10-20 µg/ml: good for digoxin- and cyclic antidepressant–induced dysrhythmias; fosphenytoin has reduced toxicity and may be given IM; Chapters 21 and 81 Tox: nystagmus, ataxia, hypotension, gingival hyperplasia, SLE-like syndrome, hirsutism
Physostigmine (Antilirium) Vial: 1 mg/ml	Child: 0.02 mg/kg/dose up to 0.5 mg/dose IV (over 3 min) q10min prn (maximum total dose: 2 mg) Adult: 1-2 mg IV (over 3 min) q10min prn (maximum total dose: 4 mg in 30 min)	Anticholinesterase; use in life-threatening anticholinergic overdose (Chapter 55) Tox: neurologic, dysrhythmias

Many oral drugs may be given 3-4 times/day with more flexibility than implied by the specific intervals noted. Adult dose provided as guideline for maximum dose. *NB,* Newborns <7 days of age; *Pen,* penicillin; *SR,* sustained release; *Tox,* toxicity of drug.

Drugs	Dosages	Comments
Piperacillin (Pipracil) Vial: 2, 3, 4 gm	200-300 mg/kg/24 hr q4-6hr IV (maximum: 24 gm/24 hr) (NB: 100 mg/kg/dose q12hr IV)	Good *Pseudomonas* coverage Tox: neurologic, GI
Polystyrene sodium sulfonate (Kayexalate) Powder: 450 gm	1 gm/kg/dose q6hr PO or q2-6hr PR (adult: 15 gm PO or 30-60 gm PR q6hr)	1 level tsp = 3.5 gm; 4.1 mEq Na^+/gm: exchanges 1 mEq K^+ for 1 gm resin, which delivers 1 mEq Na^+ for each 1 mEq K^+ removed; mix 30%-70% sus- pension in D10W, 1% methyl- cellulose, or 10% sorbitol Tox: electrolyte problems, consti- pation
Pralidoxime (Protopam, 2-PAM) Vial: 1 gm	20-50 mg/kg/dose (maximum: 2 gm/dose) IV slow (<50 mg/min) q8hr prn × 3	Cholinesterase reactivator; use after atropine in organophos- phate overdose (Chapter 55); oral preparation for prophylaxis
Praziquantel (Biltricide)	See Appendix C-4	
Prazosin (Minipress) Cap: 1, 2, 5 mg	Initial: 5 µg/kg/dose PO; then up to 25 µg/kg/dose q6hr PO Adult: 1 mg q8-12hr PO; may increase slowly to 20 mg/24 hr	Limited experience in children
Prednisolone (Prelone) Soln: 15 mg/5 ml	Asthma: 1-2 mg/kg/24 hr q6hr PO	Liquid steroid preparation
Prednisone Tab: 5, 10, 20 mg Susp: 5 mg/5 ml	Maintenance: 0.1-0.15 mg/kg/24 hr q12hr PO Asthma: 1-2 mg/kg/24 hr q6hr PO	Table 74-2
Primidone (Mysoline) Susp: 250 mg/5 ml Tab: 50, 250 mg	10-25 mg/kg/24 hr q6-8hr PO; start at 125-250 mg, increase in 125-250 increments at 1-wk intervals (adult: initial 250 mg/24 hr PO; maintenance 750-1250 mg/24 hr q6hr PO)	Therapeutic level: 6-12 µg/ml (or phenobarbital 10-25 µg/ml); Table 81-6 Tox: sedation, nausea, vomiting, diplopia: reduce dosage with renal failure; see Phenobarbital
Probenecid (Benemid) Tab: 500 mg	Load: 25 mg/kg PO; mainte- nance: 40 mg/kg/24 hr q6hr PO (adult: 2 gm/24 hr); 25 mg/kg (adult: 1 gm) PO before ampicillin or penicillin treat- ment of *Neisseria gonorrhoeae*	Not recommended for children <2 yr Tox: GI irritant

Drugs	Dosages	Comments
Procainamide (Pronestyl) Tab/cap: 250, 375, 500 mg Vial: 100, 500 mg/ml	Load: 2-6 mg/kg/dose IV slow (<50 mg/min) (adult: 100 mg/dose IV slow q10min prn up to total load of 1 gm IV) Maint: 20-80 µg/kg/min IV (adult: 1-3 mg/min IV) or 15-50 mg/kg/24 hr q4-6hr PO (adult: 250-500 mg/dose PO)	IV must be given slowly at concentration <100 mg/ml; do not use with heart block; Table 6-4 Tox: GI irritant, SLE-like syndrome, dysrhythmias
Prochlorperazine (Compazine) Syr: 5 mg/5 ml Tab: 5, 10, 25 mg Supp: 2.5, 5, 25 mg Amp: 5 mg/ml	0.4 mg/kg/24 hr q6-8hr PO, PR (adult: 5-10 mg q6-8hr PO or 25 mg q12hr PR) 0.2 mg/kg/24 hr q6-8hr IM (adult: 5-20 mg/dose IM) (maximum: 40 mg/24 hr)	Only children >2 yr and >10 kg Tox: phenothiazine (extrapyramidal, anticholinergic) (Chapter 55)
Promethazine (Phenergan) Syr: 6.25, 25 mg/5 ml Tab: 12.5, 25, 50 mg Supp: 12.5, 25, 50 mg Amp: 25, 50 mg/ml	Nausea, vomiting: 0.25-0.5 mg/kg/dose q4-6hr PO, PR, IM prn (adult: 12.5-25 mg/dose) Sedation: 0.5-1 mg/kg/dose q6hr PO, PR, IM prn (adult: 25-50 mg/dose)	Often mixed with meperidine and chlorpromazine for DPT cocktail (see DPT cocktail—Meperidine) Tox: phenothiazine (sedation, extrapyramidal, anticholinergic) (Chapter 55)
Propantheline (Pro-Banthine)	1-2 mg/kg/24 hr q6hr PO (adult: 15-30 mg QID)	
Propranolol (Inderal) Tab: 10, 20, 40, 80 mg Vial: 1 mg/ml	Dysrhythmias: load: 0.01-0.1 mg/kg/dose (maximum: 1 mg/dose) IV over 10 min (adult: 1 mg/dose IV q5min up to total of 5 mg); maintenance: 0.5-1 mg/kg/24 hr q6hr PO (adult: 10-30 mg/dose q6-8hr PO) Hypertension: 0.5-1.0 mg/kg/24 hr q6-12hr PO (maximum: 320 mg/24 hr PO) Tetralogy spells: 0.1-0.2 mg/kg/dose IV repeated in 15 min prn Migraine prophylaxis: 10-60 mg q8hr PO Thyrotoxicosis: 10-20 mg q6-8hr PO	β-blocker; contraindicated in patient with asthma or CHF; Tables 6-4 and 18-2 Tox: dysrhythmias, hypoglycemia, hypotension, cardiac failure, bronchospasm, weakness; overdose treated with glucagon 0.1 mg/kg/dose IV 1-2 mg/kg/24 hr q6hr PO (adult: 15-30 mg QID)

Many oral drugs may be given 3-4 times/day with more flexibility than implied by the specific intervals noted. Adult dose provided as guideline for maximum dose. *NB,* Newborns <7 days of age; *Pen,* penicillin; *SR,* sustained release; *Tox,* toxicity of drug.

Drugs	Dosages	Comments
Propylthiouracil (PTU) Tab: 50 mg	Load: 5 mg/kg/24 hr q6-8hr PO (adult: 300 mg/24 hr); mainenance: $\frac{1}{3}$-$\frac{1}{2}$ of loading dose once patient is euthyroid (adult: 100-150 mg/24 hr)	Tox: blood dyscrasia, hepatic, dermatitis, urticaria, neuritis
Protamine Amp: 10 mg/ml	1 mg IV for each 100 units of heparin given concurrently; 0.5 mg IV for each 100 units of heparin given in previous 30 min, and so on; maximum: 50 mg/dose	Heparin antidote Tox: hypotension, bradycardia, flushing
Pseudoephedrine (Sudafed) Syr: 30 mg/5 ml Tab: 30, 60 mg	4-6 mg/kg/24 hr q4-6hr PO (adult: 60 mg q4-6hr PO)	Tox: irritability; use with caution in hypertensive patient
Pyrantel (Antiminth) Susp: 250 mg/5 ml	11 mg (~0.2 ml)/kg/dose PO once (maximum: 1 gm/dose); repeat in 1 wk	Do not use with preexisting liver disease, pregnancy Tox: nausea, vomiting, hepatic
Quinidine Tab: 100, 200, 300, 202 (SR), 300 (SR) mg Cap: 200, 300 mg	15-60 mg/kg/24 hr q6hr PO (adult: 300-400 mg q6hr PO)	Table 6-3 Tox: GI irritant dysrhythmias, hypotension, blood dyscrasia
Racemic epinephrine (Vaponefrin) Soln: 2.25%	<20 kg: 0.25 ml in 2.5 ml saline nebulizer; 20-40 kg: 0.5 ml; >40 kg: 0.75 ml	Rebound; observe child with croup following treatment; some bronchodilator effect
Ranitidine (Zantac) Tab: 150 mg Vial: 25 mg/ml	2-4 mg/kg/24 hr q12hr PO (adult: 150 mg q12hr PO; 50 mg q6-8hr IV; maximum: 400 mg/24 hr IV)	Limited experience in children; similar to cimetidine, fewer drug interactions
Reserpine (Serpasil) Elix: 0.25 mg/5 ml Tab: 0.1, 0.25, 0.5, 1 mg	0.02 mg/kg/dose q12hr PO (adult: 0.1-0.25 mg/24 hr)	Usually used in combination with another drug; rarely used; Table 18-2 Tox: severe depression, bradycardia, ulcerogenic

Drugs	Dosages	Comments
Ribavirin (Virazole) Vial: 6 gm/100 ml	20 mg/ml delivered as 190 µg/L in air for 12-18 hr/24 hr × 3 days	Use Viratek Small Particle Aerosol Generator; indicated in children at high risk of complications from RSV such as children with underlying heart or lung disease, AIDS, or severe disease
Rifampin (Rimactane, Rifadin) Cap: 150, 300 mg	10-20 mg/kg/24 hr q12-24hr PO (maximum: 600 mg/24 hr) Meningococcal prophylaxis: 10 mg/kg q12hr PO × 2 days (adult: 600 mg q12hr) *H. influenzae* prophylaxis: 20 mg/kg q24hr × 4 days (adult: 600 mg q24hr × 4)	Tox: hepatic, GI irritant, hemolytic anemia; turns urine red; lower dosage in children <1 mo
Rimantadine (Flumadine) Tab: 100 mg Syr: 50 mg/5 ml	5 mg/kg/24 hr q24hr PO (maximum: 150 mg/24 hr) Adult: 100 mg PO q12hr	Begin within 24-48 hr onset influenza A and continue for 48 hr after resolution
Secobarbital (Seconal) Cap: 30, 50, 100 mg Vial: 50 mg/ml	2-6 mg/kg/24 hr q8hr PO (adult: 60-120 mg/24 hr q8-12hr PO)	Short-acting barbiturate Tox: drowsiness, respiratory depression
Spectinomycin (Trobicin) Vial: 400 mg/ml	40 mg/kg/dose IM × 1 (adult: 2 gm IM × 1)	*N. gonorrhoeae* treatment; not good for syphilis Tox: dizziness, vertigo
Spironolactone (Aldactone) Tab: 25, 50, 100 mg	1-3 mg/kg/24 hr q8-12hr PO (adult: 25-100 mg/24 hr)	Useful adjunctive diuretic to maintain potassium; reduce dosage with renal failure; Table 16-3
Succinylcholine (Anectine) Amp: 20 mg/ml Vial: 0.5, 1 gm	1 mg/kg/dose IV (NB: 2 mg/kg/dose IV); maintenance: 0.3-0.6 mg/kg/dose q5-10min IV	Must be able to control airway; optimally premedicate with atropine
Sulfisoxazole (Gantrisin) Susp: 500 mg/5 ml Tab: 500 mg	Load: 75 mg/kg PO; maintenance: 120-150 mg/kg/24 hr q6hr PO (adult: 500-1000 mg q6hr PO) (maximum: 4-6 gm/24 hr)	Do not use in children <2 mo old: maintain good urine flow Tox: rash, Stevens-Johnson, neutropenia; reduce dosage with renal failure

Many oral drugs may be given 3-4 times/day with more flexibility than implied by the specific intervals noted. Adult dose provided as guideline for maximum dose. *NB,* Newborns <7 days of age; *Pen,* penicillin; *SR,* sustained release; *Tox,* toxicity of drug.

Drugs	Dosages	Comments

Sumatriptan (Imitrex)
   Syringe: 6 mg/0.5 ml
   Tab: 25, 50 mg
	Adult: initial dose 25 mg PO; may give up to 100 mg after 2 hr for maximum daily dose of 300 mg PO; 6 mg initial dose SC and may repeat ≤6 mg SC up to 12 mg/24 hr SC	Subsequent treatment should reflect initial doses; limited experience in children

Terbutaline (Brethine) Vial: 1 mg/ml	*Parenteral:* 0.01 ml (0.01 mg)/kg/dose (maximum: 0.25 ml/dose) q15-20min SC prn *Aerosol:* 0.03-0.05 mg (0.03-0.05 ml)/kg in 2.5 ml saline given q4hr (adult: 0.5-1.0 mg/dose)	β-Agonist for reactive airway disease; may have more prolonged effect than epinephrine; use parenteral solution for nebulization Tox: sympathomimetic

Tetracycline (Achromycin, Tetracyn)
   Syr: 125 mg/5 ml
   Tab/cap: 250, 500 mg
   Vial: 250, 500 mg (IM has lidocaine)
	25-50 mg/kg/24 hr q6hr PO (adult: 250-500 mg q6hr PO)
	15-25 mg/kg/24 hr q8-12hr IM (adult: 200-300 mg/24 hr q8-12hr IM)
	20-30 mg/kg/24 hr q8-12hr IV over 2 hr (adult: 250-500 mg/dose q8-12hr IV over 2 hr)
		Do not use in children <9 yr; parenteral (IM, IV) administration is rarely indicated
		Tox: GI irritant, hepatic, photosensitization, superinfection

Theophylline (Table 84-1)	Load: 6 mg/kg PO; maintenance: 4-5 mg/kg/dose q6hr PO Load: 5 mg/kg IV slowly: maintenance: 0.6-0.9 mg/kg/hr IV	Therapeutic level: 10-20 µg/ml; Chapter 84 for dosage details Tox: nausea, vomiting, irritability, seizures, dysrhythmias
Thiabendazole (Mintezol)	See Appendix C-4	
Thiopental (Pentothal) Vial: 0.5, 1 gm	Sedation: 2 mg/kg/dose IV; 2.5-5 mg/kg/dose PR (adult: 3-5 mg/kg/dose IV)	Respiratory monitoring imperative

Thioridazine (Mellaril)
   Susp: 25, 100 mg/5 ml
   Tab: 10, 15, 25, 50, 100 mg
	1-2.5 mg/kg/24 hr q8-12hr PO (adult: 75-300 mg/24 hr q8-12hr PO) (maximum: 800 mg/24 hr)	Do not use in children <2 yr; titrate dosage to response
		Tox: phenothiazine (Chapter 55)

Thiosulfate sodium (25%)	1.35 ml (325 mg)/kg (adult: 12.5 gm) IV slowly if Hgb 10 gm	
Ticarcillin (Ticar) Vial: 1, 3, 6 gm	200-300 mg/kg/24 hr q4-6hr IM, IV (maximum: 18-24 gm/24 hr) (NB: 150-225 mg/kg/24 hr q8-12hr)	Similar to carbenicillin; adjust dosage in renal failure; used in combination therapy

Drugs	Dosages	Comments
Tobramycin (Nebcin) Vial: 10, 40 mg/ml	3-7.5 mg/kg/24 hr q8hr IM, IV (maximum: 300 mg/24 hr) (NB: 4 mg/kg/24 hr q12hr)	Therapeutic peak level: 6-10 µg/ml: caution in renal failure (reduce dosage); slow IV infusion Tox: renal, VIII nerve
Trimethadione (Tridione) Soln: 200 mg/5 ml Cap: 300 mg Tab (chew): 150 mg	10-40 mg/kg/24 hr q12hr PO (adult: 900-2400 mg/24 hr q6-8hr PO)	Therapeutic peak level: 600-1000 µg/ml Tox: sedation, vision, headache
Trimethaphan (Arfonad) Vial: 50 mg/ml	50-150 µg/kg/min IV infusion (adult: 0.5-1 mg/min)	Constant monitoring required; tachyphylaxis; Table 18-2 Tox: ganglionic blocker (paralysis of pupils, bladder, bowels)
Trimethobenzamide (Tigan) Supp: 100, 200 mg Vial: 100 mg/ml	Adult: 200 mg/dose q6-8hr PR, IM	Limited experience in children; do not use in patients with acute onset vomiting
Trimethoprim (TMP)-sulfamethoxazole (SMX) (Bactrim, Septra) Susp: 40 mg TMP/200 mg SMX/5 ml Tab: 80 mg TMP/400 mg SMX: 160 mg TMP/800 mg SMX Amp: 80 mg TMP/400 mg SMX/5 ml	6-12 mg TMP/30-60 mg SMX/kg/24 hr q12hr PO (adult: 80-160 mg TMP/400-800 mg SMX q12hr PO) *Pneumocystis:* 15-20 mg TMP/75-100 mg SMX/kg/24 hr q6-8hr PO, IV *Severe UTI, Shigella:* 8-10 mg TMP/40-50 mg SMX/kg/24 hr q6-8hr PO, IV	Do not use in children <2 mo; rare indications for IV route; reduce dosage in renal failure Tox: bone marrow suppression, GI irritation
Valproic acid or valproate (Depakene) Syr: 250 mg/5 ml Cap: 250 mg Vial: 100 mg/ml (Depacon)	15-60 mg/kg/24 hr q8-24hr PO (adult: 1-3 gm/24 hr q8-24hr PO)	Therapeutic level: 50-100 µg/ml; Table 81-6; use in acute management of seizures is controversial; parenteral preparation available Tox: sedation, vomiting, rash, headache, hepatotoxic; increases phenobarbital level (20%) and decreases phenytoin level (50%-100%)

Many oral drugs may be given 3-4 times/day with more flexibility than implied by the specific intervals noted. Adult dose provided as guideline for maximum dose. *NB,* Newborns <7 days of age; *Pen,* penicillin; *SR,* sustained release; *Tox,* toxicity of drug.

Drugs	Dosages	Comments
Vancomycin (Vancocin) Vial: 500 mg Soln (oral): 1, 10 gm Pulvule: 125, 250 mg	30-40 mg/kg/24 hr q6hr IV (meningitis: up to 60 mg/kg/24 hr q6hr IV) (<500 mg/30 min) (maximum: 2 gm/24 hr) (NB: 30 mg/kg/24 hr q12hr IV) For *C. difficile* or pseudomembranous colitis: 40 mg/kg/24 hr q6hr PO	Reduce dosage if renal impairment; also available in oral preparation for staphylococcal enterocolitis and pseudomembranous colitis and *C. difficile* Tox: ototoxic, renal, rash, peripheral neuropathy
Vecuronium (Norcuron) 10 mg/ml	0.08-0.1 mg/kg/dose IV	Nondepolarizing muscle blockade; need to be able to control airway
Verapamil (Isoptin, Calan) Amp: 2.5 mg/ml	0.1-0.2 mg/kg/dose IV over 2 min repeated in 10-30 min prn (adult: 5 mg/dose IV)	Table 6-4; do not use if <1 yr old; largely replaced by adenosine Tox: bradycardia, hypotension
Vitamin K (Aquamephyton) Vial: 2, 10 mg/ml	NB, infant: 1-2 mg/dose IM, IV Child, adult: 5-10 mg/dose IM, IV	May give IV (<1 mg/min) but associated with hypotension and anaphylaxis
Warfarin (Coumadin) Tab: 2, 5, 7.5, 10 mg	0.1 mg/kg/24 hr q24hr PO Adult: 2-10 mg/24 hr q24hr PO after loading with 10-15 mg/24 hr PO × 2-3 days	Adjust dosage to maintain PT at 2 times normal (INR [International Normalized Ratio] between 2-3); antidote is vitamin K Tox: dermatitis

Appendix C-2: Simplified Schedule for Administration of Pediatric Resuscitation Drugs

Drug (availability)	Single dose	Route	Dose (ml) administered by weight									
			5 kg	10 kg	15 kg	20 kg	25 kg	30 kg	35 kg	40 kg	45 kg	50 kg
EPINEPHRINE (1:10,000)†												
(0.1 mg/ml)	0.01 mg/kg 0.1 ml/kg	IV	0.5	1	1.5	2	2.5	3	3.5	4	4.5	5
SODIUM BICARBONATE												
(1 mEq/ml)	1 mEq/kg 1 ml/kg	IV	5	10	15	20	25	30	35	40	45	50
ATROPINE												
(0.1 mg/ml)	0.02 mg/kg 0.2 ml/kg	IV, ET	1	2	3	4	5	6	7	8	9	10
CALCIUM CHLORIDE 10%												
(100 mg/ml)	20 mg/kg 0.2 ml/kg	IV	1	2	3	4	5	5	5	5	5	5
LIDOCAINE												
(20 mg/ml)*	1 mg/kg 0.05 ml/kg	IV, ET	0.25	0.5	0.75	1.0	1.25	1.5	1.75	2.0	2.25	2.5
FUROSEMIDE (Lasix)												
(10 mg/ml)	1 mg/kg 0.1 ml/kg	IV	0.5	1	1.5	2	2.5	3	3.5	4	4.5	5
DIAZEPAM (Valium)												
(5 mg/ml)	0.2 mg/kg 0.04 ml/kg	IV	0.2	0.4	0.6	0.8	1	1.2	1.4	1.6	1.8	2

Before using this schedule, it is essential to be certain that the concentration used is identical to that cited here. Clinical response and patient condition may modify this schedule (see Table 4-2). Drugs may often be administered intraosseous.
*Also available as 10 mg/ml.
†Second dose and ET dose is 0.1 mg/kg or 0.1 ml/kg of 1:1000 solution.

WEIGHT: 10 KG (22 lbs.)
ET SIZE: 4.0
LARYNGOSCOPE BLADE: 1-2
SUCTION CATHETER: 8 Fr
DEFIBRILLATION: 20 watt-sec
NG TUBE: 8 Fr
FOLEY: 8 Fr

AGE: 1 yr
PULSE: 125 beats/min
RESPIRATORY RATE: 39 ± 11 resp/min
BP: 96 ± 30 mm Hg

Emergency Medications

Drug (concentration)	Therapy dose range	Route*	Comments	Single dose	Dose administer
Epinephrine Syringe (1:10,000 = 0.1 mg/ml)	0.01 mg/kg (0.1 ml/kg) initial dose	IV	Maximum dose: 5 ml	0.1 mg	1 ml
Epinephrine (1:1,000 = 1 mg/ml)	0.1 mg/kg (0.1 ml/kg)	Second dose ET	Maximum dose: 5 ml	1 mg	1 ml
Bicarbonate, Sodium (1 mEq/ml)	1 mEq/kg (1 ml/kg)	IV	<1 yr dilute 1:1 with nonbacteriostatic H_2O	10 mEq	10 ml
Atropine (0.1 mg/ml)	0.02 mg/kg (0.2 ml/kg)	IV ET	Minimum dose: 0.1 mg; maximum dose: 2 mg; IV slowly	0.2 mg	2 ml
Calcium Cl 10% (100 mg/ml)	20 mg/kg (0.2 ml/kg)	IV	Maximum dose: 500 mg	200 mg	2 ml
Lidocaine 2% (20 mg/ml)	1 mg/kg (0.05 ml/kg)	IV ET	Maximum total dose: 5 mg/kg	10 mg	0.5 ml
Furosemide (Lasix) (10 mg/ml)	1 mg/kg (0.1 ml/kg)	IV	Maximum dose: 6 mg/kg	10 mg	1 ml
Diazepam (Valium) (5 mg/ml)	0.2 mg/kg (0.04 ml/kg)	IV ET	Maximum total dose: child 10 mg; adult 30 mg	2 mg	0.4 ml
Albuterol (soln: 5 mg/ml)	0.03 ml (0.15 mg)/kg/dose	NEB	May give as often as necessary; monitor	1.5 mg	0.3 ml in 2 ml saline
Naloxone (Narcan) (1 mg/ml)	0.1 mg/kg (0.1 ml/kg)	IV ET	If no response in 10 min may give up to 2 mg IV	1 mg	1 ml
Adenosine (3 mg/ml)	0.1 mg/kg (0.03 ml/kg) (rapid)	IV	May repeat in 2 min; maximum 12 mg initially	1 mg	0.33 ml
Dextrose 50% (0.5 gm/ml)	0.5 gm/kg (1 ml/kg)	IV	<1 yr dilute to D25W with nonbacteriostatic H_2O	5 gm	10 ml
Phenytoin (Dilantin) (50 mg/ml)	LOAD: (seizure) 15 mg/kg (0.3 ml/kg)	IV PO	NOT IM: IV give slowly in saline only; maximum dose: 1250 mg; DYSRHYTHMIA: 5 mg/kg/dose q5-20min prn × 2 IV	150 mg	3 ml
Phenobarbital (65 mg/ml)	LOAD: 15 mg/kg (0.23 ml/kg)	IV PO	Maximum dose: 300 mg; maintenance: 3-5 mg/kg/day	150 mg	2.3 ml

*Intravenous drugs may commonly be given intraosseous.

MIXING EMERGENCY DRUGS FOR CONTINUOUS INFUSION

Several alternative approaches to preparing medication for continuous infusion exist, and these are outlined on the following pages.

	Rule of 6s	Drug specific
Dopamine	6 × body wt (kg) equals mg of drug to be added to IV solution to make 100 ml D5W. Infusion of 1 ml/hr will deliver 1 μg/kg/min.	150 mg added to 250 ml D5W (600 μg/ml. Infusion of 1 ml/kg/hr delivers 10 μg/kg/min.
Dobutamine	Same as dopamine.	Same as dopamine.
Nitroprusside	Same as dopamine.	45 mg added to 250 ml D5W (180 μg/ml). Infusion of 1 ml/kg/hr delivers 3 μg/kg/min.
Isoproterenol	0.6 × body wt (kg) equals mg of drug to be added to IV solution to make 100 ml D5W. Infusion of 1 ml/hr will deliver 0.1 μg/kg/min.	1.5 mg added to 250 ml D5W (6 μg/ml). Infusion of 1 ml/kg/hr delivers 0.1 μg/kg/min.

Medication Drips for 10-kg child (p. 891)

Drug (concentration)	Therapy range	Conversion mixture	Add D5W	Add drug	Initial average dose (pump required)
Dopamine (40 mg/ml)	5-20 μg/kg/min IV drip	150 mg in 250 ml D5W = 600 μg/ml; 1 ml/kg/hr = 10 μg/kg/min	250 ml	3.75 ml	10 ml/hr
Dobutamine (25 mg/ml when mixed with 10 ml)	2-20 μg/kg/min IV drip	150 mg in 250 ml D5W = 600 μg/ml; ml/kg/hr = 10 μg/kg/min	250 ml	6ml	10 ml/hr
Nitroprusside (25 mg/ml)	0.5-10 (avg 3 μg) μg/kg/min IV drip	45 mg in 250 ml D5W = 180 μg/ml; 1 ml/kg/hr = 3 μg/kg/min	250 ml	1.8 ml	10 ml/hr
Isoproterenol (Isupel) (0.2 mg/ml)	0.05-1.5 μg/kg/min IV drip	1.5 mg in 250 ml D5W = 6 μg/ml; 1 ml/kg/hr = 0.1 μg/kg/min	250 ml	7.5 ml	10 ml/hr

APPENDIX C-3: PEDIATRIC EQUIPMENT GUIDELINES

The following supplies and equipment are modified from the recommendation by the American College of Emergency Physicians for pediatric patients in a general emergency department made in February 1995 (*Ann Emerg Med* 25: 307, 1995). Guidelines for prehospital equipment have also been developed (*Ann Emerg Med* 28: 699, 1998).

An emergency cart or other system to house all supplies, equipment, and drugs for a designated pediatric resuscitation area should be available.

NOTE: Numbers in parenthesis indicate the recommended number of items needed, if more than one.

Monitoring Devices

ECG monitor-defibrillator/cardioverter with pediatric and adult-sized paddles and hard copy recording capability; pediatric monitor patches
Otoscope/ophthalmoscope/stethoscope
Pulse oximeter with pediatric adapter
Sphygmomanometer
Doppler ultrasonographic blood pressure devices
Central venous pressure monitoring equipment
Rectal temperature probe
Hypothermia thermometer
Blood pressure cuffs (neonatal; infant; child; adult—arm, thigh)
End-tidal P_{CO_2} monitor and/or pediatric CO_2 detector
Blood gas kit

Vascular Access Supplies and Equipment

CVP kits, 3-8 Fr (4)
Catheter-over-needle devices, 16, 18, 20, 22, 24 (2 each)
Butterflies, 19, 21, 23, 25 (4 each)

Intraosseous needles, 16/18 gauge (4)
Umbilical vein catheters
Tourniquets (3), rubber bands
4×4 sponges
Povidone-iodine swabs (10)
Alcohol swabs
Tape, waterproof—½, 1, 2 in. (1 roll each)
Stopcocks (2)
T-connectors (3)
IV tubing, 30 inches (2)
Armboards (2 each size)
Tincture of benzoin
Povidone prep solution
Betadine ointment (2)
IV fluid/blood warmer
Infusion pumps, drip or volumetric, with microinfusion capability
IV administration sets and extension tubing
IV solutions
    Normal saline (0.9% NS)
    Ringer's lactate (LR)
    D10W
    D5W 0.2% NS

Respiratory Equipment and Supplies

Bag-valve-mask resuscitator, self-inflating (child and adult)
Suction devices
Laryngoscope handle with extra batteries and bulbs
Laryngoscope blades
    Curved: 2, 3
    Straight or Miller: 0, 1, 2, 3
Stylets for endotracheal tubes (infant and adult) (1 each)
Magill forceps
Endotracheal tubes
    Uncuffed sizes: 2.5, 3.0, 3.5, 4.0, 4.5, 5.0 (2 each)
    Cuffed sizes: 5.5, 6.0, 6.5, 7.0, 7.5, 8.0 (2 each)
Tracheostomy tubes
    Shiley tube sizes: 00, 0, 1, 2, 3, 4, 6
Oral airways
    Sizes: 0, 1, 2, 3, 4, 5

Nasopharyngeal airways
   Sizes: 12, 16, 20, 24, 28, 30 Fr
Clear oxygen masks (neonatal, infant, child, adult)
Nasal cannulae (child and adult) (2 each)
Oxygen cylinder, flow meter, tubing
Suction catheters
   Sizes: 6, 8, 10, 12, 14 Fr (2 each)
Yankauer suction tips (4)
NG tubes
   Sizes: 6, 8, 10, 12, 14, 16 Fr (2 each)
Tongue blades (5)
Lubricant (K-Y jelly) (4)

Medications

Activated charcoal
Adenosine
Albumin, 5%, 25%
Albuterol for inhalation
Antidotes immediately available:
   Cyanide kit
   Flumazenil
   Methylene blue
   Naloxone
Antipyretics
Atropine
Barbiturates
Benzodiazepines
Bicarbonate, sodium
β Blockers
Bretylium
Calcium chloride
Dextrose
Dexamethasone
Diphenhydramine
Dopamine
Epinephrine (1:1000 and 1:10,000)
Epinephrine, racemic (for inhalation)
Furosemide
Glucagon
Hydrocortisone
Insulin
Isoproterenol
Lidocaine
Magnesium sulfate
Mannitol

Methylprednisolone
Narcotics
Neuromuscular blocking agents
Succinylcholine
Pancuronium or vecuronium
Potassium chloride
Phenytoin
Procainamide
Verapamil

Specialized Pediatric Trays for the Following Procedures:

Tube thoracostomy and water seal drainage with chest tubes (8-40 Fr)
Thoracotomy tray
Cricothyrotomy including needle cricothyrotomy
Peritoneal lavage
Venous cutdown
Lumbar puncture
Umbilical vessel cannulation
Urinary catheterization: Foley catheters
   Sizes: 5-12 Fr (2 each)
Obstetric pack
Intracranial pressure monitoring*
Newborn kit

Fracture Management Devices

Femur splint (Hare traction)* (infant, child, and adult)
Spine board
Semirigid neck collars (child and adult)
Towel roll (or sandbag)
Extremity splints, various sizes

Miscellaneous Equipment

Infant scale
Heating source, overhead warmer preferred
CPR backboard
MAST trousers* (toddler, child, adult)
Infant formulas and oral rehydrating solutions

*Desirability depends on the clinical setting.

APPENDIX C-4: ANTIPARASITIC DRUGS

AMEBIASIS *(Entamoeba histolytica)*

Asymptomatic carrier — Iodoquinol (previously diiodohydroxyquin) 30-40 mg/kg/24 hr q8hr PO (adult: 650 mg/dose) × 20 days; **or** diloxanide furoate (Furamide) (CDC) 20 mg/kg/24 hr q8hr PO (adult: 500 mg/dose) × 10 days

Mild to moderate colitis — Metronidazole (Flagyl) 35-50 mg/kg/24 hr q8hr PO (adult: 750 mg/dose) × 10 days; **plus** iodoquinol, as above

Severe colitis — Metronidazole, as above × 10 days; **plus,** iodoquinol, as above

Extraintestinal — Metronidazole, as above × 10 days; **plus,** iodoquinol, as above

ASCARIASIS *(Ascaris lumbricoides)* — Mebendazole (Vermox) 100 mg q12hr PO × 3 days (children >2 yr); **or** pyrantel pamoate (Antiminth) 11 mg/kg/dose (maximum: 1 gm PO × 1 [one dose only])

BALANTIDIASIS *(Balantidium coli)* — Tetracycline 40 mg/kg/24 hr q6hr PO (children >8 yr only) (adult: 500 mg/dose) × 10 days; **or** iodoquinol 40 mg/kg/24 hr q8hr PO (adult: 650 mg/dose) × 20 days

CUTANEOUS LARVA MIGRANS or CREEPING ERUPTION (cutaneous hookworm) — Thiabendazole (Mintezol) 50 mg/kg/24 hr (maximum: 1.5 gm/dose) q12hr PO × 2-5 days; topical treatment also

CYSTICERCOSIS *(Taenia solium)* — Surgical excision most satisfactory; Praziquantel (Biltricide) 50 mg/kg/24 hr q8hr PO × 15 days (± steroids)

DIENTAMOEBIASIS *(Dientamoeba fragilis)* — Iodoquinol 40 mg/kg/24 hr q8hr PO (adult: 650 mg/dose) × 20 days

FILARIASIS ONCHOCERCIASIS *(Onchocerca volvulus)* — Ivermectin (Mectizan) (CDC) 150 µg/kg once and repeated every 3-12 mo

Other forms (LOA LOA, TROPICAL EOSINOPHILIA) *(Wuchereria bancrofti, Brugia malayi)* — Diethylcarbamazine (Hetrazan): *Day 1:* 1 mg PO (adult: 50 mg); *day 2:* 1 mg q8hr PO (adult: 50 mg/dose); *day 3:* 1-2 mg q8hr PO (adult: 100 mg/dose); *days 4-21:* 9 mg/kg/24 hr q8hr PO (adult: 9 mg/kg/24 hr q8hr PO)

FLUKES

Liver *(Opisthorchis viverrini)*
Lung *(Paragonimus westermani)*
Chinese liver *(Clonorchis sinensis)* — Praziquantel (Biltricide) 25 mg/kg/dose PO × 3 doses (doses to be taken in 1 day)

GIARDIASIS *(Giardia lamblia)* — Metronidazole (Flagyl) 15 mg/kg/24 hr (adult: 250 mg/dose) q8hr PO × 5 days; **or** Furazolidone (Furoxone) 6 mg/kg/24 hr (adult: 100 mg/dose) q6hr PO × 7-10 days; **or** tinidazole 50 mg/kg (maximum: 2 gm) PO once (adult: 2 gm PO once)

HOOKWORM
Necator americanus
Ancylostoma duodenale — Mebendazole (Vermox) 100 mg q12hr PO (children >2 yr) × 3 days; **or** pyrantel pamoate (Antiminth) 11 mg/kg/24 hr q24hr (maximum: 1 gm/24 hr) PO × 3 days

LEISHMANIASIS
Leishmania donovani (kala azar)
L. braziliensis (American mucocutaneous leishmaniasis)
L. mexicana, L. tropica — Stibogluconate sodium (Pentostam, Tricostam) (CDC) 20 mg/kg/24 hr (maximum: 800 mg/24 hr) q24hr IM, IV × 20-28 days; may need to repeat

Modified from Committee on Infectious Diseases: *Report of the Committee on Infectious Disease,* Elk Grove, Ill, 1997, American Academy of Pediatrics, 1997.

CDC: Available from the Centers for Disease Control Parasitic Drug Service, Atlanta; phone: (404) 639-3670. For emergencies on nights, weekends, and holidays: (404) 639-2888. Other resources include the information system for International Travelers at 404-639-1410 or 404-332-4555 and the National Center for Infectious Diseases (404-488-7760). Consult for recent recommendations.

MALARIA
  Prophylaxis
    For areas without chloroquine resistant *Plasmodium falciparum* — Chloroquine 5 mg base/kg (adult: 300 mg base) qwk PO, beginning 1 wk before potential exposure and continuing for 6 wk after last exposure; **plus** primaquine phosphate 0.3 mg base/kg (adult: 15 mg base) q24hr PO × 14 days after departure from endemic area
    For areas with chloroquine resistant *P. falciparum* — Mefloquine: 15-19 kg: ¼ tab; 20-30 kg: ½ tab; 31-45 kg: ¾ tab; >45 kg: 1 tab; adult: 250 mg PO qwk
  Treatment
    P. vivax, P. ovale — Chloroquine phosphate (Aralen, Nivaquine) 10 mg base/kg then 5 mg base/kg at 6 hr, 24 hr, and 48 hr after initial dose (adult: 600 mg base, then 300 mg base at 6 hr, 24 hr, and 48 hr)
    P. malariae — Chloroquine, as above
    P. falciparum (nonchloroquine-resistant) — Chloroquine, as above
    P. falciparum (chloroquine-resistant) — Quinine 30 mg/kg/24 hr (adult: 650 mg/dose) q8hr PO × 3-7 days; **plus** pyrimethamine-sulfaxodoxine <1 yr: ¼ tab; 1-3 yr: ½ tab; 4-8 yr: 1 tab; 9-14 yr: 2 tab; adult: 3 tab at once on last day of quinine; **plus** tetracycline 20 mg/kg/24 hr q6hr PO × 7 days if >8 yr **or** clindamycin 20-40 mg/kg/24 hr q8hr PO × 3-5 days

PINWORMS *(Enterobius vermicularis)* — Mebendazole (Vermox) 100 mg PO once (children >2 yr) (repeat in 1 wk) **or** pyrantel (Antiminth) 11 mg/kg/dose (maximum: 1 gm) PO once (repeat in 1 wk)

PNEUMOCYSTIS PNEUMONIA *(Pneumocystis carinii)* — Trimethoprim (TMP)-sulfamethoxazole (SMX) (Bactrim, Septra) 15 mg TMP, 75 mg SMX/kg/24 hr q6-8hr PO, IV × 14-21 days

SCHISTOSOMIASIS
  Schistosoma haematobium
  S. japonicum
  S. mansoni — Praziquantel (Biltricide) 40 mg/kg/24 hr PO × 2 doses in 1 day

TAPEWORMS
  Taenia saginata
  Taenia solium (see Cystercicosis)
  Diphyllobothrium latum — Praziquantel (Biltricide) 5-10 mg/kg PO once

TOXOPLASMOSIS *(Toxoplasma gondii)* — Pyrimethamine (Daraprim) 2 mg/kg/24 hr (adult: 25 mg/24 hr) q12hr PO × 3 days, then 1 mg/kg/24 hr q12hr PO × 4 wk (supplement with folinic acid 5-10 mg/24 hr): **plus** trisulfapyrimidines or sulfadiazine 100-200 mg/kg/24 hr (adult: 4-6 gm/24 hr) q6hr PO × 28 days

TRICHINOSIS *(Trichinella spiralis)* — Mebendazole (Vermox) 200-400 mg/dose (children >2 yr) q8hr PO × 5-10 days; steroids

TRYPANOSOMIASIS
  CHAGAS' DISEASE *(Trypanosoma cruzi)* — Nifurtimox (Lampit) (CDC) 1-10 yr: 15-20 mg/kg/24 hr q6hr PO × 90 days; 11-16 yr: 12.5-15 mg/kg/24 hr q6hr PO × 90 days; adult: 8-10 mg/kg/24 hr q6hr PO × 120 days

VISCERAL LARVA MIGRANS *(Toxocara canis)* — Diethylcarbamazine (Hetrazan) 6 mg/kg/24 hr q8hr PO × 7-10 days

WHIPWORM *(Trichuris trichiura)* — Mebendazole (Vermox) 100 mg q12hr PO × 3 days

*Associated with serious adverse reactions, including erythema multiforme, Stevens-Johnson, toxic epidermal necrolysis, and serum sickness. Discontinue if any mucocutaneous lesions develop.

INDEX

A

ABCs
  in advanced life support, 23-26
  in basic life support, 22-23, 22t
Abdomen
  examination of, in multiple trauma
    assessment, 407
  scaphoid, 95
  soft tissue injuries to, suture repair
    of, 502t
  surgical, vs. hemolytic-uremic syn-
    drome, 803
Abdominal disorders, chest pain
  from, 133, 134t
Abdominal pain
  acute, 197-199
    in abuse, 202t
    diagnostic considerations in, 198t
  with appendicitis, 648, 650t
  with dysmenorrhea, 667
  in ectopic pregnancy, 679
  Henoch-Schönlein purpura, 805
  initial nursing assessment of, 14t
  in pelvic inflammatory disease, 669
  as psychophysiologic presenta-
    tion, 762
  right lower quadrant, 648,
    650t-651t
  in sickle cell disease, 699
Abdominal thrusts, for foreign body
  airway obstruction, 793
Abdominal trauma, 476-486
  abdominal pain from, 198t
    in right lower quadrant, 651t
  blunt, 476
    management of, 481, 482
  chest pain from, 133t
  diagnostic findings in, 477-481
  from gunshot wounds, 477,
    485-486

Page numbers in *italics* indicate boxed
material and illustrations; *t* indicates
tables.

Abdominal trauma—cont'd
  management of, 481-486
    blunt trauma in, 481, 482
    general principles in, 481-482
    penetrating wounds in,
      485-486
    protocol for, *483*
    splenic injury in, 482, 484-485
  mechanisms of, 476-477
  from penetrating wounds,
    476-477, 481
    management of, 485-486
  from stab wounds, 477, 485
Abdominal wall defects, as postnatal
  emergency, 102-103
ABE antitoxin, 708
Abortion, 677-679
  complete, 678
  incomplete, 677-678
  missed, 678-679
  threatened, 677
  vaginal bleeding in, 291t
Abrasions
  corneal, 436, 437t
    irritability in, 274t
  foreign material in, 499-500
Abruptio placentae, 680-681
  vaginal bleeding in, 291t
Abscess
  vs. cellulitis, 575
  central nervous system, vomiting
    in, 295t
  cerebellar, ataxia in, 219t
  cerebral, headache in, 260t
  dental, headache in, 260t
  esophageal, respiratory distress
    in, 176t
  intracranial
    coma from, 137t
    seizures in, 739t
  orbital, 575t
  peritonsillar, 603-604
    dysphagia in, 237t
    respiratory distress in, 176t
  pulmonary, cough in, 228t

Abscess—cont'd
  retropharyngeal, 608-609
    central cyanosis in, 158t
    cough in, 228t
    dysphagia in, 237t
    respiratory distress in, 176t
    subperiosteal, 575t
    tuboovarian, 670
Absence seizures, 738
Abuse, 200-206
  in abdominal trauma assess-
    ment, 477
  diagnostic findings in, 200-203
  differential diagnosis of, 201t-202t
  history of, 200
  initial nursing assessment of, 14t
  management of, 203, *204*
  physical examination for, 201-202
  sexual, 205-206
Accelerated hypertension, 161, 163
  medications for, 165t
  syncope in, 191t
Acceleration-deceleration injuries,
  aortic injury from, 473-474
Acclimatization
  to heat, 330
  high-altitude, 327
Accolate, for asthma, 778
Accutane; *see* Isotretinoin
Acetaminophen
  antidote for, 356t
  dosage of, 858
  for febrile seizures, 748
  for fever, 241, 247, 248t
  poisoning/overdose of,
    363-364, *363*
  for sickle cell disease, 703
  for soft tissue injuries, 508t, 510
Acetazolamide
  for CHF with pulmonary edema,
    152t
  dosage of, 858
  for high-altitude sickness, 327, 329
  for metabolic alkalosis, 82
  for pseudotumor cerebri, 737

Antibiotics—cont'd
for urinary tract infections, 818
for volvulus, 660
Anticholinergics
antidote for, 356*t*
for asthma, 775
poisoning/overdose of, 369-371
seizures from, 741*t*
toxic syndrome from, 358
Anticoagulants; *see also* Heparin;
Warfarin
for deep vein thrombosis, 569-570
hematuria and proteinuria from,
265*t*
screening tests for, 222*t*
vaginal bleeding from, 292*t*
Anticonvulsants, 184-186
to reduce intracranial pressure, 420
for seizures, 744*t*-745*t*
febrile, 748, 749
guidelines for, 743
Antidepressants, cyclic
antidote for, 356*t*
poisoning/overdose of, 376-378
Antidiarrheal agents, 636
Antidiuretic hormone (ADH)
release of, 78-79
severe syndrome of inappropriate, 74
Antidotes, in poison management,
355, 356*t*-357*t*
Antidysrhythmic drugs, 61*t*-63*t*
Antiemetics, 299
Antifibrinolytic agents, for hemophilia, 692
Antihistamines
for allergic conjunctivitis, 629
for anaphylaxis, 126, 127
antidote for, 356*t*
for eczema, 573
for pityriasis rosea, 584
for pruritus
from lice, 583
from scabies, 585
for rhinitis, 609
for sinusitis, 611
for urticaria, 589
Antihypertensive drugs, 165*t*,
166*t*-169*t*, 169-170
Antiinflammatory agents
for acute rheumatic fever, 567
for pericarditis, 565
for soft tissue injuries, 510
Antilirium; *see* Physostigmine

Antimetabolites, acute diarrhea
from, 233*t*
Antiminth; *see* Pyrantel
Antipyretic therapy
for acute otitis media, 600
for febrile seizures, 748-749
for fever, 241
Antispasmodics, for acute infectious
diarrhea, 636
Antistreptolysin (ASO) titer, 566-567
Antithyroid medication, 624
Antitoxin
for botulism, 708
for diphtheria, 709
Antitussive medications, 230
Antivenin
for black widow spider bites, 308
for snake bites, 312, 313
Antral puncture, 611
Anxiety
acute diarrhea in, 234*t*
parental, irritability in, 273*t*
AOM; *see* Acute otitis media
Aortic aneurysm, dysphagia in, 238*t*
Aortic dissection, hypertension
from, medication for, 165*t*
Aortic injury, 473-474
Aortic stenosis, syncope in, 191*t*
AP drawer sign, 548
Apgar score, 86, 87*t*
Aphthous stomatitis, 612
Aplastic crisis, in sickle cell disease,
699, 700*t*
Apnea, 129-131
diagnostic considerations of,
130*t*-131*t*
as postnatal emergency, 117
posttraumatic, 416
of prematurity, 117
Apophyseal injuries of pelvis, 545
Apophysitis, calcaneal, 553-554
Apparent life-threatening event
(ALTE), 129, 187-188
Appendicitis, 648-651
acute abdominal pain from, 198*t*
acute diarrhea in, 233*t*
limp in, 278*t*
vomiting in, 295*t*
Apresoline; *see* Hydralazine
Apt test, 250
Aquamephyton; *see* Vitamin K
Aralen; *see* Chloroquine phosphate
Aramine; *see* Metaraminol
ARDS; *see* Adult respiratory distress
syndrome

Arfonad; *see* Trimethaphan
Arterial blood gases (ABG)
in asthma, 767
in bronchiolitis, 781
in pneumonia, 796
Arterial catheterization, umbilical,
90-91
nomogram for, *92*
Arterial punctures, procedure for, 821
Arteriogram, renal, for genitourinary
trauma, 490
Arteritis, temporal, headache in, 262*t*
Arthralgia, 214-217
Arthritis
juvenile rheumatoid
arthralgia and joint pain in, 215*t*
synovial fluid findings in, 752*t*
septic, 752-753
arthralgia and joint pain in, 214*t*
limp in, 277*t*
viral
arthralgia and joint pain in, 214*t*
limp in, 278*t*
Arthrocentesis, procedure for, 822
Arthroplasty, for sickle cell disease, 704
Arthropod/insect bites, 306-311
black widow spider, 308
brown recluse spider, 306-307
hymenoptera, 309
ticks, 309-311
ASA; *see* Aspirin
Ascariasis, medications for, 895
Ascaris lumbricoides, medications
for, 895
Ascites, vomiting in, 298*t*
Aspartate aminotransferase, normal
laboratory values for, 848
Asphyxia
hypoglycemia in, 269*t*
intrapartum, 94
Aspiration
cyanosis in, 158*t*
of foreign bodies, 792
meconium, 118-119
needle
of cellulitis, 575
of lung, for pneumonia, 797
suprapubic, procedure for,
834, *834*
transtracheal, pneumonia and, 797
Aspiration pneumonia, cough in,
228*t*

Sodium bicarbonate—cont'd
  for cyclic antidepressant poisoning/
    overdose, 378
  in diabetic ketoacidosis manage-
    ment, 618
  dosage of, 862
  for near-drowning, 322
  for postnatal hyperkalemia, 101
  in resuscitation, 31*t*
    for cardiopulmonary arrest, 30
    dosage of, 890, 891
    of newborns, 87*t*
Sodium nitrite
  for cyanide poisoning, 356*t*
  dosage of, 879
Sodium nitroprusside; *see also* Nitroprusside
  for congestive heart failure, 153
  for hypertensive emergencies,
    166*t*-167*t*
  for pulmonary edema, 174
  for shock, 49*t*
Sodium thiosulfate, for cyanide poisoning, 356*t*
Soft tissue, dental, assessment of, 442
Soft tissue injuries, 497-505
  diagnostic findings in, 497-498
  facial, management of, 428-430
  from fishhooks, 505
  management of, 498-505
    analgesia and sedation in,
     507-512
    antibiotics in, 504-505
    debridement in, 500
    hand/foot dressings and splints
     in, 504
    hemostasis in, 500
    hernia repair in, 504
    restraint, position, and draping
     in, 498-499
    wound closure in, 500,
     501*t*-503*t*, 504
    wound exploration, cleansing,
     and irrigation in, 499-500
  in multiple trauma assessment, 408
  parental education on, 505
  puncture wounds, 505
Solu-Cortef; *see* Hydrocortisone
Solu-Medrol; *see* Methylprednisolone
Sore throat, 604-607
  initial nursing assessment of, 15*t*
Spasmodic croup, 784
  management of, 791
  respiratory distress in, 177*t*

Spectinomycin
  dosage of, 886
  for gonococcal and chlamydial
    infections, 673
Sphenoid sinusitis, 610, 611-612
Spider bites, 306-308
Spinal cord hematoma
  in hemophilia, 686
  from lumbar puncture, 831
Spinal cord injury without radiographic abnormality
  (SCIWORA), 453-454
Spinal cord tumor, limp from,
  279*t*
Spinal needle, 830
Spinal shock, 454
Spinal taps, blood in, 729
Spine and spinal cord trauma,
  449-459
  diagnostic findings in, 450-457
    ancillary data in, 454-457
    cervical spine stability in, 453
    complications in, 454
    neurologic, 450, 451*t*, 453
    SCIWORA in, 453-454
    vital signs in, 450
  differential diagnosis of, 457
  disposition for, 458-459
  etiology of, 449-450
  management of, 457-458
  parental education on, 459
Spironolactone
  for CHF with pulmonary edema,
    152*t*
  dosage of, 886
  in hepatitis management, 642
  for hypertension, 165
Splenectomy, 484
  for idiopathic thrombocytopenic
    purpura, 696
  for sickle cell disease, 704
Splenic injury, 482, 484-485
Splenic sequestration crisis, in sickle
  cell disease, 699, 700*t*
Splinter, subungual, 541
Splints, 520-521
  of hand and foot soft tissue inju-
    ries, 504
  for hand and wrist lacerations,
    539, 540
Split tooth, 445
Sponging, for fever, 248
Spontaneous pneumothorax,
  at birth, 121

Sprains and strains, 521-522
  ankle, 552
  arthralgia and joint pain in, 214*t*
  initial nursing assessment of, 15*t*
  limp in, 277*t*
  management of, 519-520, 522
Sputum, pneumonia and, 797
SS disease; *see* Sickle cell disease
Stab wounds, abdominal, 477
  management of, 485
Staphcillin; *see* Methicillin
Staphylococcal food poisoning, 633
Staphylococcal scalded skin syndrome, 586
  vs. Kawasaki syndrome, 712*t*
Staphylococcus aureus
  acute otitis media from, 597*t*
  in animal bites, 303
  antibiotics for, 561*t*
  in bacterial endocarditis, 559
  bullous impetigo from, 581, 582
  cellulitis from, 574*t*
  meningitis from, 725
  osteomyelitis from, 754
    antibiotics for, 755
  pneumonia from, 794, 798*t*
    diagnostic findings in, 795*t*
  septic arthritis from, 751
    antibiotics for, 753
  in sickle cell disease, 701*t*
  staphylococcal scalded skin syn-
    drome from, 586
Staphylococcus epidermidis
  meningitis from, 725
  osteomyelitis from, 754
  in premature infants, 112
Status asthmaticus, 766-767, 775
Status epilepticus, 183-186
  medications for, 32*t*, 34*t*
STDs; *see* Sexually transmitted
  diseases
Stelazine; *see* Trifluoperazine
Stensen's duct, 602
Sternal fracture, 463-464
Steroids
  for acute rheumatic fever, 567
  for anaphylaxis, 127
  for asthma, 775-776
  for bacterial meningitis, 732
  for Bell's palsy, 284
  for contact dermatitis, 577
  for croup, 790
  in hepatitis management, 642
  for idiopathic thrombocytopenic
    purpura, 696